OPERATIVE TECHNIQUES IN SPORTS MEDICINE SURGERY

ALSO AVAILABLE IN THIS SERIES

OPERATIVE TECHNIQUES IN FOOT AND ANKLE SURGERY

Editor: Mark E. Easley
Editor-In-Chief Sam W. Wiesel

OPERATIVE TECHNIQUES IN ORTHOPAEDIC PEDIATRIC SURGERY

Editor: John M. Flynn
Editor-in-Chief Sam W. Wiesel

OPERATIVE TECHNIQUES IN ORTHOPAEDIC TRAUMA SURGERY

Editors: Paul Tornetta III
Gerald R. Williams
Matthew L. Ramsey
Thomas R. Hunt III
Editor-in-Chief Sam W. Wiesel

OPERATIVE TECHNIQUES IN SHOULDER AND ELBOW SURGERY

Editors: Gerald R. Williams & Matthew L. Ramsey
Editor-in-Chief Sam W. Wiesel

OPERATIVE TECHNIQUES IN ADULT RECONSTRUCTION SURGERY

Editors: Jarvad Parvizi & Richard H. Rothman
Editor-in-Chief Sam W. Wiesel

OPERATIVE TECHNIQUES IN HAND, WRIST, AND FOREARM SURGERY

Editors: Thomas R. Hunt III
Editor-in-Chief Sam W. Wiesel

OPERATIVE TECHNIQUES IN SPORTS MEDICINE SURGERY

Mark D. Miller, MD
EDITOR

S. Ward Casscells Professor of Orthopaedic Surgery
University of Virginia
Charlottesville, Virginia
Team Physician
James Madison University
Harrisonburg, Virginia

Sam W. Wiesel, MD
EDITOR-IN-CHIEF

Professor and Chair
Department of Orthopaedic Surgery
Georgetown University Medical School
Washington, DC

Wolters Kluwer | Lippincott Williams & Wilkins
Health
Philadelphia • Baltimore • New York • London
Buenos Aires • Hong Kong • Sydney • Tokyo

Acquisitions Editor: Robert A. Hurley
Developmental Editor: Grace Caputo, Dovetail Content Solutions
Product Manager: Dave Murphy
Marketing Manager: Lisa Lawrence
Manufacturing Manager: Ben Rivera
Design Manager: Doug Smock
Compositor: Maryland Composition/ASI
Copyright 2011

Two Commerce Square
2001 Market Street
Philadelphia, PA 19103

Printed in China

Library of Congress Cataloging-in-Publication Data

Operative techniques in sports medicine surgery / [edited by] Mark D. Miller ; Sam W. Wiesel, editor-in-chief.
p. ; cm.
Chapters derived from Operative techniques in orthopaedic surgery / editor-in-chief, Sam Wiesel. c2010.
Includes bibliographical references and index.
Summary: "Operative Techniques in Sports Medicine Surgery provides full-color, step-by-step explanations of all operative procedures in sports medicine. It contains the sports-related chapters from Sam W. Wiesel's Operative Techniques in Orthopaedic Surgery. Written by experts from leading institutions around the world, this superbly illustrated volume focuses on mastery of operative techniques and also provides a thorough understanding of how to select the best procedure, how to avoid complications, and what outcomes to expect. The user-friendly format is ideal for quick preoperative review of the steps of a procedure. Each procedure is broken down step by step, with full-color intraoperative photographs and drawings that demonstrate how to perform each technique. Extensive use of bulleted points and tables allows quick and easy reference. Each clinical problem is discussed in the same format: definition, anatomy, physical exams, pathogenesis, natural history, physical findings, imaging and diagnostic studies, differential diagnosis, non-operative management, surgical management, pearls and pitfalls, postoperative care, outcomes, and complications. To ensure that the material fully meets residents' needs, the text was reviewed by a Residency Advisory Board"—Provided by publisher.
ISBN 978-1-4511-0261-1
1. Sports injuries—Surgery. 2. Orthopedic surgery. I. Miller, Mark D. II. Wiesel, Sam W. III. Operative techniques in orthopaedic surgery.
[DNLM: 1. Athletic Injuries—surgery. 2. Orthopedic Procedures—methods. QT 261]
RD97.O64 2011
617.1'027—dc22

2010028466

---

10 9 8 7 6 5 4 3 2 1

Dedication

To my last child to leave the nest, Missy. I hope that all of our time together can be "quality time."

—Your loving father, MDM

CONTENTS

SECTION IV KNEE

SECTION V LEG

CONTRIBUTORS

Christopher R. Adams, MD
Orthopaedic Surgeon
Advanced Shoulder Orthopaedics
Jupiter, Florida

Julie E. Adams, MD
Assistant Professor of Orthopaedic Surgery
University of Minnesota
Minneapolis, Minnesota

Christina R. Allen, MD
Associate Clinical Professor of Orthopaedic Surgery
University of California
San Francisco, California

Michael J. Angel, MD
Orthopaedic Sports Medicine Fellow
Kerlan Jobe Orthopaedic Clinic
Los Angeles, California

Robert A. Arciero, MD
Professor of Orthopaedics
University of Connecticut Health Center
John Dempsey Hospital
Farmington, Connecticut

Steven A. Aviles, MD
Department of Orthopaedic Surgery
Iowa Orthopaedic Center
Mercy Hospital
Des Moines, Iowa

Frederick M. Azar, MD
Professor of Orthopaedic Surgery
University of Tennessee
Residency Program Director
Sports Medicine Fellowship Director
Campbell Clinic
Memphis, Tennessee

F. Alan Barber, MD
Fellowship Director
Plano Orthopedic Sports Medicine and Spine Center
Plano, Texas

Mark J. Billante, MD
Physician
Greater Austin Orthopaedics
Austin, Texas

Matthew T. Boes, MD
Raleigh Orthopaedic Clinic
Raleigh, North Carolina

Kevin F. Bonner, MD
Assistant Professor
Eastern Virginia Medical School
Jordan-Young Institute
Sentara Leigh Hospital
Virginia Beach, Virginia

Jesse C. Botker, MD
Orthopaedic Surgery Chief Resident
University of Minnesota
Minneapolis, Minnesota

Craig R. Bottoni, MD
Chief of Surgery
Assistant Chief Medical Officer
Aspetar Orthopaedic & Sports Medicine Hospital
Doha, Qatar

James P. Bradley, MD
Clinical Professor of Orthopaedic Surgery
University of Pittsburgh Medical Center
Pittsburgh, Pennsylvania

Anthony M. Buoncristiani, MD
Orthopaedic Surgeon
St. Luke's Wood River Medical Center
Ketchum, Idaho

Stephen S. Burkhart, MD
Director of Orthopaedic Education
The San Antonio Orthopaedic Group
The Orthopaedic Institute
San Antonio, Texas

Charles Bush-Joseph, MD, BA
Professor of Orthopaedic Surgery
Rush University Medical Center
Chicago, Illinois

J. W. Thomas Byrd, MD
Nashville Sports Medicine Foundation
Nashville, Tennessee

Eric W. Carson, MD
Associate Professor
Division of Sports Medicine
Department of Orthopaedic Surgery
University of Virginia
Charlottesville, Virginia

Mark S. Cohen, MD
Professor
Director, Hand and Elbow Section
Director, Orthopaedic Education
Department of Orthopaedic Surgery
Rush University Medical Center
Chicago, Illinois

Steven B. Cohen, MD
Assistant Professor of Orthopedic Surgery
Thomas Jefferson University
Rothman Institute Orthopaedics
Philadelphia, Pennsylvania

Brian Cole, MD, MBA
Professor
Section of Sports Medicine
Departments of Orthopaedic Surgery and Anatomy & Cell Biology
Section Head, Cartilage Restoration Center at Rush
Rush University Medical Center
Chicago, Illinois

Anne E. Colton, MD
Premier Orthopaedics
Broomall, Pennsylvania

John E. Conway, MD
Private Practice
Texas Health Harris Methodist Fort Worth Hospital
Fort Worth, Texas

David A. Coons, DO
Multicare Orthopedics and Sports Medicine
Tacoma, Washington

Andrew J. Cosgarea, MD
Professor, Orthopaedic Surgery
Director, Sports Medicine and Shoulder Surgery
Department of Orthopaedic Surgery
Johns Hopkins University
Lutherville, Maryland

Thomas M. DeBerardino, MD
Associate Professor of Orthopaedic Surgery
University of Connecticut Health Center
Farmington, Connecticut

David R. Diduch, MS, MD
Professor of Orthopaedic Surgery
Head Orthopaedic Team Physician
University of Virginia
Charlottesville, Virginia

Ivica Ducic, MD, PhD
Associate Professor
Chief, Peripheral Nerve Surgery
Department of Plastic Surgery
Georgetown University Hospital
Washington, District of Columbia

Jeffrey S. Earhart, MD
Resident
Department of Orthopaedic Surgery
Feinberg School of Medicine
Northwestern University
Chicago, Illinois

Gregory C. Fanelli, MD
Orthopaedic Surgery
Geisinger Sports Medicine
Danville, Pennsylvania

David L. Feingold, MD
Chief, Department of Orthopaedics
Olive View Medical Center
West Hills, California

Larry D. Field, MD
Clinical Instructor
Department of Orthopaedic Surgery
University of Mississippi School of Medicine
Director, Upper Extremity Service
Mississippi Sports Medicine and Orthopaedic Center
Jackson, Mississippi

Donald C. Fithian, MD
Director, San Diego Knee and Sports Medicine Fellowship
Kaiser Permanente, San Diego
El Cajon, California

Brett A. Freedman, MD
Orthopaedic Surgery
Walter Reed Army Medical Center
Washington, District of Columbia

Freddie H. Fu, MD, DSc, DPs (Hon)
Department of Orthopaedic Surgery
University of Pittsburgh Medical Center
Pittsburgh, Pennsylvania

John P. Fulkerson, MD
Clinical Professor of Orthopedic Surgery
University of Connecticut
Farmington, Connecticut

William E. Garrett, MD, PhD
Department of Orthopaedic Surgery
Duke University Medical Center
Durham, North Carolina

Jeffrey R. Giuliani, MD
Orthopaedic Surgery
Walter Reed Army Medical Center
Washington, District of Columbia

R. Timothy Greene, MD
Department of Orthopaedics
Orthopaedic and Neurosurgery Specialists
Greenwich, Connecticut

Christopher D. Harner, MD
Blue Cross of Western Pennsylvania Professor
Department of Orthopaedic Surgery
UPMC Center for Sports Medicine
Pittsburgh, Pennsylvania

Justin D. Harris, MD
Nebraska Orthopaedic and Sports Medicine
Lincoln, Nebraska

Laurence D. Higgins, MD
Department of Orthopaedic Surgery
Brigham and Women's Hospital
Boston, Massachusetts

MaCalus V. Hogan, MD
Resident Physician of Orthopaedic Surgery
Academic Orthopaedic Training Program
University of Virginia
Charlottesville, Virginia

Michael J. Huang, MD
Rocky Mountain Orthopaedic Associates, PC
Grand Junction, Colorado

Jeffrey M. Jacobson, MD
Resident
Department of Plastic Surgery
Georgetown University Hospital
Washington, District of Columbia

David R. Joestling, MD, FACS
Surgical Consults, PA
Edina, MN

Darren L. Johnson, MD
Professor and Chairman of Orthopaedic Surgery
University of Kentucky
Lexington, Kentucky

Sean M. Jones-Quaidoo, MD
Resident
Department of Orthopaedic Surgery
University of Virginia
Charlottesville, Virginia

Spero G. Karas, MD
Associate Professor of Orthopaedic Surgery
Emory University
Atlanta, Georgia

Jay D. Keener, MD
Assistant Professor
Department of Orthopaedic Surgery
Washington University
St. Louis, Missouri

Roland S. Kent, MD
Corresponding Member of USUHS Department of Surgery
Department of Orthopaedic Surgery
Navy Medical Center, Portsmouth
Uniformed Services University of Health Sciences
Portsmouth, Virginia

Sami O. Khan, MD
Resurgens
Snellville, Georgia

Christopher A. Kurtz, MD
Assistant Professor of Surgery
Uniformed Services University of the Health Sciences
Bethesda, Maryland
Chairman, Bone and Joint/Sports Medicine Institute
Naval Medical Center Portsmouth
Portsmouth, Virginia

Robert F. LaPrade, MD, PhD
Professor of Orthopaedic Surgery
University of Minnesota
Minneapolis, Minnesota

Christopher M. Larson, MD
Director of Education
Minnesota Sports Medicine Orthopaedic Sports Medicine Fellowship Program
Twin Cities Orthopaedics
Eden Prairie, Minnesota

Christian Lattermann, MD
Assistant Professor of Orthopaedic Surgery and Sports Medicine
Director of Center for Cartilage Repair and Restoration
University of Kentucky
Lexington, Kentucky

L. Scott Levin, MD, FACS
Chair of Orthopaedic Surgery
University of Pennsylvania School of Medicine
Philadelphia, Pennsylvania

Krishna Mallik, MD
Orthopaedic Surgery Sports Medicine and Arthroscopic Reconstruction
American Total Orthopedics
Scottsdale, Arizona

Elizabeth Matzkin, MD
Department of Orthopaedics
Tufts Medical Center
Boston, Massachusetts

Craig S. Mauro, MD
Chief Resident
Department of Orthopaedic Surgery
University of Pittsburgh Medical Center
Pittsburgh, Pennsylvania

Augustus D. Mazzocca, MD
Associate Professor
Department of Orthopaedics
University of Connecticut Health Center
John Dempsey Hospital
Farmington, Connecticut

David R. McAllister, MD
Professor of Orthopaedic Surgery and Chief of Sports
David Geffen School of Medicine at UCLA
University of California, Los Angeles
Los Angeles, California

Eric C. McCarty, MD
Chief of Sports Medicine & Shoulder Surgery
Associate Professor
Department of Orthopaedic Surgery
University of Colorado School of Medicine
Boulder, Colorado

Mark D. Miller, MD
S. Ward Casscells Professor
Department of Orthopaedic Surgery
University of Virginia
Charlottesville, Virginia
Team Physician
James Madison University
Harrisonburg, Virginia

Peter J. Millett, MD, MSc
Shoulder and Sports Medicine Specialist
Steadman-Hawkins Clinic
Vail, Colorado

Claude T. Moorman III, MD
Associate Professor of Surgery
Duke University
Durham, North Carolina

Craig D. Morgan, MD
Clinical Professor
Department of Orthopaedic Surgery
University of Pennsylvania School of Medicine
Morgan-Kalman Clinic
Wilmington, Delaware

Amir Mostofi, MD
Department of Orthopaedic Surgery
University of Connecticut Health Center
Farmington, Connecticut

Kevin P. Murphy, MD
Heekin Orthopaedic Specialists
Jacksonville, Florida

Brett D. Owens, MD
Assistant Professor of Orthopaedic Surgery
Keller Army Hospital
West Point, New York

Samuel S. Park, MD
Orthopaedic Surgery
Good Samaritan Hospital
Downers Grove, Illinois

Ralph W. Passarelli, MD
Clinical Instructor
Department of Orthopaedic Surgery
University of Pittsburgh Medical Center
Pittsburgh, Pennsylvania

Matthew T. Provencher, MD
Associate Professor of Surgery
Director, Orthopaedic Shoulder and Sports Surgery
Department of Orthopaedic Surgery
Naval Medical Center San Diego
San Diego, California

R. David Rabalais, MD
Clinical Assistant Professor of Medicine
Department of Orthopaedic Surgery
Louisiana State University Health Science Center
New Orleans, Louisiana

William G. Rodkey, DVM, Diplomate ACVS
Chief Scientific Officer
Steadman Hawkins Research Foundation
Vail, Colorado

Anthony A. Romeo, MD
Department of Orthopaedic Surgery
Rush University Medical Center
Chicago, Illinois

J. R. Rudzki, MD
Clinical Assistant Professor
Department of Orthopaedic Surgery
George Washington University School of Medicine
Washington, District of Columbia

John-Paul Rue, MD, CDR, MC, USN
Assistant Professor
Department of Surgery
Uniformed Services University of Health Sciences
Director of Sports Medicine
Department of Orthopaedic Surgery
National Naval Medical Center
Bethesda, Maryland

Marc Safran, MD
Professor of Orthopaedic Surgery
Stanford University
Stanford, California

Felix H. Savoie, III, MD
Lee C. Schlesinger Professor of Clinical Orthopaedics
Tulane University School of Medicine
New Orleans, Louisiana

John A. Scanelli III, MD
Resident
Department of Orthopaedic Surgery
University of Virginia
Charlottesville, Virginia

Robert C. Schenck, MD
Professor and Chairman
Department of Orthopaedics and Rehabilitation
University of New Mexico
Albuquerque, New Mexico

Jon K. Sekiya, MD
Associate Professor
MedSport—Department of Orthopaedic Surgery
University of Michigan
Ann Arbor, Michigan

Nicholas A. Sgaglione, MD
Associate Clinical Professor of Orthopaedic Surgery
North Shore Long Island Jewish Health System
Great Neck, New York

Benjamin S. Shaffer, MD
Washington Orthopaedics & Sports Medicine
Chevy Chase, Maryland

Ryan W. Simovitch, MD
Palm Beach Orthopaedic Institute
Palm Beach Gardens, Florida

Jeffrey T. Spang, MD
Assistant Professor of Orthopaedics
University of North Carolina
Chapel Hill, North Carolina

Matthew A. Stanich, MD
Resident
University of California, San Francisco
San Francisco, California

Erick S. Stark, MD
Tri-City Orthopedics
Oceanside, California

J. Richard Steadman, MD
Orthopaedic Surgeon and Principal
Steadman Hawkins Clinic
Vail, Colorado

Scott P. Steinmann, MD
Professor of Orthopedic Surgery
Mayo Clinic College of Medicine
Rochester, Minnesota

Rebecca M. Stone, MS, ATC
Minnesota Sports Medicine
Twin Cities Orthopedics
Eden Prairie, Minnesota

Robert T. Sullivan, BS, MD
Orthopedic Surgeon/Sports Medicine
United States Air Force Academy
USAF Academy, Colorado

Kenneth G. Swan, Jr., MD
Department of Orthopaedic Surgery
Robert Wood Johnson University Hospital
New Brunswick, New Jersey

Robert Z. Tashjian, MD
Department of Orthopaedics
University of Utah Orthopaedic Center
Salt Lake City, Utah

Richard J. Thomas, MD
OrthoGeorgia Orthopaedic Specialists
Macon, Georgia

Fotios P. Tjoumakaris, MD
Assistant Professor of Orthopaedic Surgery
University of Pennsylvania School of Medicine/Penn Sports Medicine
Philadelphia, Pennsylvania

Michael S. Todd, MC
Orthopaedic Surgery Service
William Beaumont Army Medical Center
El Paso, Texas

Daniel J. Tomaszewski, MD
Department of Orthopaedic Surgery
Geisinger Clinic
Danville, Pennsylvania

Bradley B. Veazey, MD
Assistant Professor
Department of Orthopaedic Surgery and Rehabilitation
Texas Tech University
Lubbock, Texas

Christian J. H. Veillette, MD, MSc, FRCSC
Assistant Professor
Division of Orthopaedic Surgery
University of Toronto
Toronto Western Hospital
University Health Network
Toronto, Ontario, Canada

Andrew J. Veitch, MD
Assistant Professor
Department of Orthopaedics and Rehabilitation
University of New Mexico
Albuquerque, New Mexico

Winston J. Warme, MD
Associate Professor of Orthopaedics and Sports Medicine
Chief of Shoulder and Elbow Surgery
University of Washington
Seattle, Washington

Jon J. P. Warner, MD
Professor of Orthopaedic Surgery
Chief of Harvard Shoulder Service
Partner's Health Care System
Massachusetts General Hospital
Brigham and Women's Hospital
Boston, Massachusetts

Daniel C. Wascher, MD
Professor
Department of Orthopaedics and Rehabilitation
University of New Mexico
Albuquerque, New Mexico

Carl H. Wierks, MD
Orthopaedic Chief Resident
Johns Hopkins Hospital
Baltimore, Maryland

Jocelyn R. Wittstein, MD
Resident
Department of Orthopaedic Surgery
Duke University Medical Center
Durham, North Carolina

Ken Yamaguchi, MD
Professor of Orthopaedic Surgery
Sam and Marilyn Fox Distinguished Professor of Orthopaedic Surgery
Chief of Shoulder and Elbow Service
Washington University School of Medicine
St. Louis, Missouri

PREFACE

When a surgeon contemplates performing a procedure, there are three major questions to consider: Why is the surgery being done? When in the course of a disease process should it be performed? And, finally, what are the technical steps involved? The purpose of this text is to describe in a detailed, step-by-step manner the "how to do it" of the vast majority of orthopaedic procedures. The "why" and "when" are covered in outline form at the beginning of each procedure. However, it is assumed that the surgeon understands the basics of "why" and "when," and has made the definitive decision to undertake a specific case. This text is designed to review and make clear the detailed steps of the anticipated operation.

Operative Techniques in Sports Medicine Surgery differs from other books because it is mainly visual. Each procedure is described in a systematic way that makes liberal use of focused, original artwork. It is hoped that the surgeon will be able to visualize each significant step of a procedure as it unfolds during a case.

Each chapter has been edited by a specialist who has specific expertise and experience in the discipline. It has taken a tremendous amount of work for each editor to enlist talented authors for each procedure and then review the final work. It has been very stimulating to work with all of these wonderful and talented people, and I am honored to have taken part in this rewarding experience.

Finally, I would like to thank everyone who has contributed to the development of this book. Specifically, Grace Caputo at Dovetail Content Solutions, and Dave Murphy and Eileen Wolfberg at Lippincott Williams & Wilkins, who have been very helpful and generous with their input. Special thanks, as well, goes to Bob Hurley at LWW, who has adeptly guided this textbook from original concept to publication.

SWW
January 1, 2010

ACKNOWLEDGMENTS

All book projects are a challenge and I certainly could not get as involved with them as I am without a lot of help. To my partners (especially David), my PAs (Jen and Jerry), the residents and fellows, and everyone I have had the pleasure to teach and learn alongside. Thank you!

—MDM

RESIDENCY ADVISORY BOARD

The editors and the publisher would like to thank the resident reviewers who participated in the reviews of the manuscript and page proofs. Their detailed review and analysis was invaluable in helping to make certain this text meets the needs of residents today and in the future.

Daniel Galat, MD
Dr. Galat is a graduate of Ohio State University College of Medicine and the Mayo Clinic Department of Orthopedic Surgery residency program.
He is currently serving at Tenwek Hospital in Kenya as an orthopedic surgeon.

Lawrence V. Gulotta, MD
Fellow in Sports Medicine/Shoulder Surgery
Hospital for Special Surgery
New York, New York

Dara Chafik, MD, PhD
Southwest Shoulder, Elbow and Hand Center PC
Tuscon, Arizona

GautamYagnik, MD
Attending Physician
Orthopaedic Surgery
DRMC Sports Medicine
Dubois, Pennsylvania

Gregg T. Nicandri, M.D.
Assistant Professor
Department of Orthopaedics (SMD)
University of Rochester
School of Medicine and Dentistry
Rochester, New York

Catherine M. Robertson, MD
Assistant Clinical Professor
UCSD Orthopaedic Surgery—Sports Medicine
San Diego, California

Jonathan Schoenecker, MD
Assistant Professor
Departments of Orthopaedics, Pharmacology and Pediatrics
Vanderbilt University
Nashville, Tennessee

Chapter 1 Shoulder Arthroscopy: The Basics

Elizabeth Matzkin and Craig R. Bottoni

DEFINITION

- The shoulder is a spheroidal multiaxial joint stabilized not only by its bony anatomy but also by the surrounding muscles and capsular structures.
- Arthroscopy is the process of visualization and examination of a joint using a fiberoptic instrument. All shoulder surgeons must be proficient in diagnostic arthroscopy of the shoulder.

ANATOMY

- The glenohumeral joint consists of the glenoid fossa of the scapula that articulates with the head of the humerus.
- The labrum is a "bumper" of fibrocartilaginous tissue around the rim of the glenoid that acts to deepen and enlarge the glenoid fossa and increase glenohumeral stability. The biceps tendon is anchored at the superior labrum and acts as a humeral head depressor and also aids in glenohumeral stability.
- The static stabilizers of the shoulder include the joint capsule and the glenohumeral ligaments—superior, middle, and inferior glenohumeral ligaments. These will be discussed in greater detail in subsequent chapters.
- The dynamic stabilizers of the shoulder are the rotator cuff muscles—supraspinatus, infraspinatus, subscapularis, and teres minor.
  - The scapular stabilizers—rhomboids, levator scapulae, trapezius, and serratus anterior—also contribute to dynamic stability of the shoulder.

PATHOGENESIS

- Shoulder injuries can occur secondary to trauma, microtrauma, or overuse injuries and can be activity- and age-dependent.
- Most patients under age 40 will have symptoms typical of overuse or instability, whereas patients over age 40 present more commonly with rotator cuff, impingement, inflammatory, or degenerative joint disease types of symptoms.

NATURAL HISTORY

- Shoulder injuries can be painful and lead to shoulder dysfunction.
- Recurrent shoulder instability decreases with age.[2]
- The frequency of rotator cuff tears increases with age.[1]
- If shoulder pathology is left unaddressed, pain, motion loss, degenerative changes, loss of function, and inability to participate in sports or work can occur.

PATIENT HISTORY AND PHYSICAL FINDINGS

- The most important part of the physical examination consists of taking an accurate history from the patient.
  - Was it a traumatic, nontraumatic, or overuse injury?
  - When and how did the injury occur?
  - Is the patient's complaint of pain, loss of motion, weakness, or inability to perform sports, activities of daily living, or work?
  - Is there pain at rest, only with activity, or while sleeping?
  - Are there any neurologic symptoms?
- Basic physical examination methods are summarized below. More specific examinations for different diagnoses will be described in other chapters in this section.
  - Observation of patient with shoulder pain from the front, back, and side
    - Identify any muscle atrophy and asymmetry of muscles, shoulder height, or scapular position.
  - Palpation of different parts of shoulder—sternoclavicular joint, acromioclavicular joint, greater tuberosity and rotator cuff, glenohumeral joint, biceps tendon, trapezium—to localize any areas of point tenderness, which may aid in differential diagnosis.
  - Passive and active range of motion—forward flexion, abduction, adduction, internal and external rotation
    - Loss of range of motion may indicate adhesive capsulitis, rotator cuff pathology (tendinitis or rotator cuff tear), or degenerative changes.
  - Resistive testing of deltoid, supraspinatus, infraspinatus, and subscapularis
    - Weakness of any muscles may indicate nerve injury, torn muscle or tendon, or weakness secondary to pain.
- Rotator cuff and scapular stabilizers: Look for atrophy, scapular winging, weakness with strength testing, and painful range of motion.
  - Provocative tests for rotator cuff tear include drop arm sign and liftoff or belly press for subscapularis.
  - Impingement tests include the Neer and Hawkins tests.
- Labrum: Catching, clicking, popping may indicate a labral tear; check for instability with provocative tests (load shift, apprehension test or crank test, relocation, O'Brien's).
- Multidirectional instability: Look for increased laxity inferiorly and in one other direction.
  - The sulcus sign demonstrates inferior laxity.
  - Check for the ability to voluntarily subluxate or dislocate the humeral head.
- Acromioclavicular joint: localized tenderness over the acromioclavicular joint and pain with cross-chest adduction and O'Brien's testing

IMAGING AND OTHER DIAGNOSTIC STUDIES

- Plain radiographs are used to assess different aspects of the shoulder joint.
  - Basic radiographs should consist of anteroposterior, axillary, and outlet views.
  - Special views may be obtained depending on shoulder pathology and will be discussed in subsequent chapters.

- Magnetic resonance imaging (MRI) and MRI arthrograms are also commonly obtained to aid in diagnosis because they are highly sensitive and specific in diagnosing many shoulder injuries.

DIFFERENTIAL DIAGNOSIS

- Impingement (internal or external)
- Rotator cuff tear
- Adhesive capsulitis
- Acromioclavicular joint injury or arthritis
- Labral tear
- Instability
- Biceps tendon pathology
- Degenerative arthritis
- Scapulothoracic dysfunction
- Cervical or neurologic
- Infection

NONOPERATIVE MANAGEMENT

- Nonoperative management for many different diagnoses may first consist of rest, nonsteroidal anti-inflammatories, physical therapy, and diagnostic and therapeutic injections.

SURGICAL MANAGEMENT

- A patient who has failed to respond to nonoperative management and continues to have symptoms consistent with his or her diagnosis is a candidate for shoulder arthroscopy.

Preoperative Planning

- Patient history and imaging studies are reviewed.
- The surgeon should have a good understanding of what pathology to expect at the time of arthroscopy to ensure that all appropriate equipment and instruments are available.
  - Patient positioning aids (arm holders, weights, beanbag, axillary roll)
  - Arthroscopic pumps or irrigation system
  - Video monitor, 30- and 70-degree arthroscopes
  - Arthroscopic cannulas
  - Shavers, burrs, suture anchors, arthroscopic instruments (probe, grasper, scissor, basket)
- An examination under anesthesia is performed to assess range of motion and stability.

Positioning

- Shoulder arthroscopy may be performed with the patient in either a beach-chair position or the lateral decubitus position (**FIG 1**).
- The beach-chair position requires a specially designed operating table attachment that ensures that the surgeon has adequate exposure to the patient's posterior shoulder and the patient's head is well supported.
  - The advantage of this position is that the shoulder can be freely manipulated throughout the procedure.
  - Commercially available arm holders can also be used to allow glenohumeral distraction and positioning without the need for an assistant.
- When using the lateral decubitus position (**FIG 1B**), the patient must be properly padded and the body supported with a beanbag, axillary roll, and pillows.

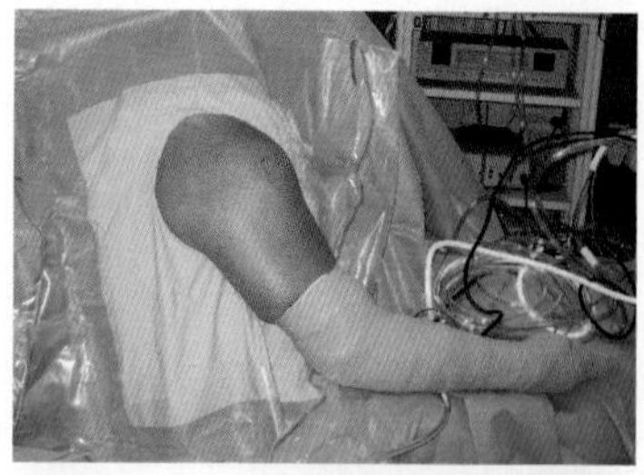

A

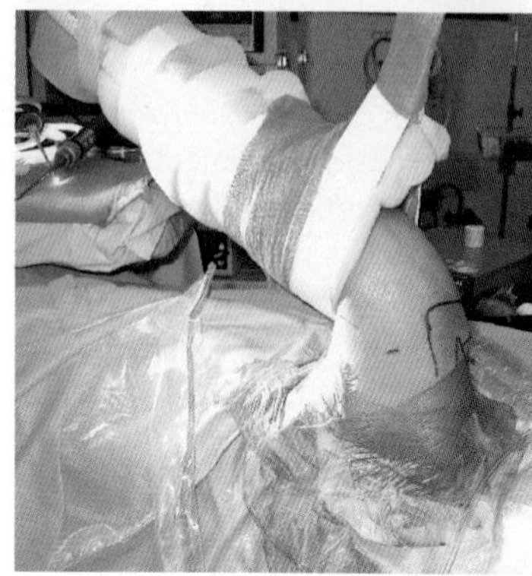

B

FIG 1 • **A.** Patient in beach-chair position with standard draping for right shoulder arthroscopy. **B.** Patient in right lateral decubitus position with shoulder distraction apparatus to abduct and distract the left upper extremity.

- The operative extremity is placed in a commercially available arm holder in approximately 70 degrees of abduction and 15 to 20 degrees of forward flexion, with 10 pounds of weight for traction. This allows for distraction of the glenohumeral joint and offers excellent visualization.

Approach

- The operating room should be set up to allow the surgeon easy access to the entire shoulder and permit optimal visualization of the video monitors and arthroscopic equipment.
  - The typical operating room setup is shown in **FIG 2**.
- The entire shoulder, arm, forearm, and hand and the exposed portion of the patient's hemithorax should be sterilely prepared after isolation with a clear U-drape. This will aid in keeping the patient dry in case fluid leaks under the surgical drapes.

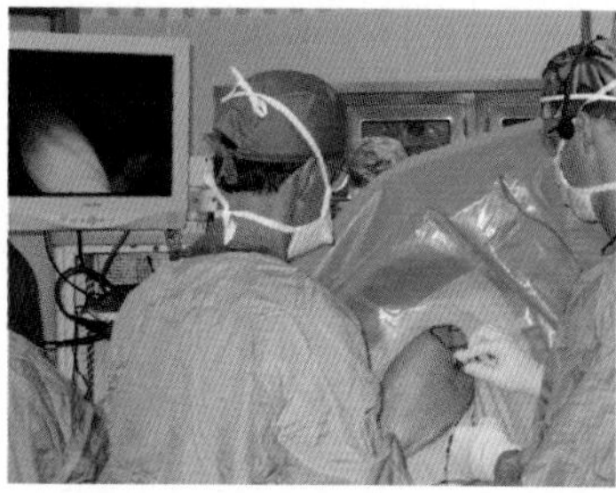

FIG 2 • Operating room setup to allow optimal visualization of monitor and arthroscopic equipment.

SETUP AND PORTAL PLACEMENT

- Once the patient is prepared and draped, the bony surface anatomy should be outlined with a surgical marking pen. This includes the clavicle, borders of the acromion (anteriorly, posteriorly, and laterally), the spine of the scapula, the acromioclavicular joint, and the coracoid (TECH FIG 1).

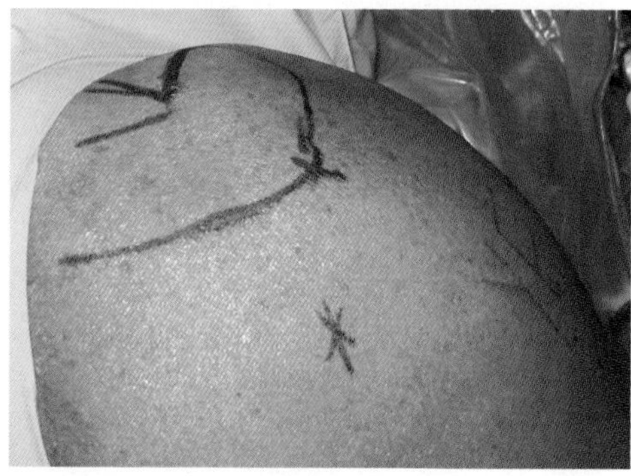

TECH FIG 1 • Right shoulder with preoperative markings identifying the acromion, clavicle, and expected portal sites.

- All expected portal sites should next be marked. For a basic diagnostic arthroscopy these should include a posterior, anterior, and if necessary lateral portal. Accessory portal locations required for specific procedures will be discussed in subsequent chapters.
  - Posterior portal: 2 to 3 cm inferior and 1 cm medial to the posterolateral border of the acromion. It is usually located in the "soft spot" of the posterior shoulder that can be palpated between the posterior rotator cuff muscles (infraspinatus and teres minor).
  - Anterior portal: This portal is marked just lateral to the tip of the coracoid process and inferior to the anterolateral acromial border. Care must be taken to ensure that all anterior portals are lateral to the coracoid to avoid damage to the neurovascular structures located medial to the coracoid.
  - Lateral portal: This portal is marked 3 to 5 cm lateral to the lateral margin of the acromial border. The location of this portal may change based on the intra-articular anatomy.
- Before starting the arthroscopic procedure, the surgeon ensures that all arthroscopic equipment (arthroscope, monitor, pump) is properly functioning.

INSERTION OF THE ARTHROSCOPE

- The posterior portal is created first.
  - A 5-mm skin incision is made using a number 11 scalpel.
  - All shoulder arthroscopy incisions should penetrate only the skin and no deeper to avoid injury to neurovascular structures and possible damage to articular surfaces.
- The arthroscope sheath and blunt obturator are then inserted into the glenohumeral joint (TECH FIG 2).
  - The trocar should be directed toward the coracoid. One hand can be used to stabilize the shoulder and the index finger used to palpate the coracoid tip.
  - The obturator should be directed just medial to the humeral head and into the space between the head and glenoid. There should be a "pop" once the capsule is penetrated and the cannula is within the glenohumeral joint.
  - Some surgeons prefer first to inject saline with a spinal needle into the glenohumeral joint. This expands the joint and allows a bigger target as well as, with fluid return, confirms that the arthroscope is in the proper place.
- The irrigation system and pump is turned on and the humeral head, glenoid, and biceps tendon are identified for quick orientation.
- A brief inspection of the glenohumeral joint can be performed to determine whether modification of the subsequent portals may be required.

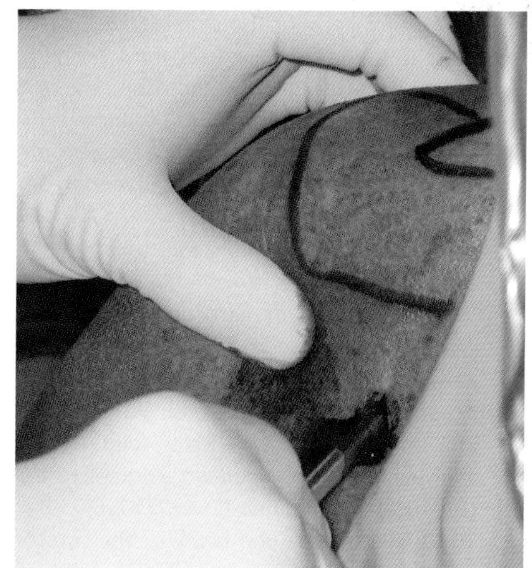

TECH FIG 2 • Arthroscope insertion. The trocar and arthroscopic cannula are directed toward the coracoid process. It enters the glenohumeral joint just lateral to the posterior glenoid labrum and approximately in the middle of the glenoid from superior to inferior. The surgeon's index finger is on the tip of the coracoid to help direct the trocar into the joint.

ESTABLISHING THE ANTERIOR PORTAL

- The anterior portal is next created. Depending on the intra-articular shoulder pathology to be addressed, a modified anterior portal may be needed; this is discussed in other chapters.
- For most standard arthroscopic procedures, the anterior portal may be created using either an inside-out or an outside-in technique.

Inside-Out Technique

- The arthroscope is placed within the rotator interval just inferior to the biceps tendon and held firmly against the anterior capsule. The camera is then removed while holding the cannula in position.
- A switching stick or Wissinger rod (a long metal rod that fits within the arthroscopic sheath) is inserted into the cannula and used to penetrate the anterior capsule and tent the skin.
- A small skin incision is made over the end of the switching stick.
- A cannula may then be passed over the switching stick and into the glenohumeral joint.

Outside-In Technique

- A spinal needle is inserted at the expected site of the anterior portal and into the joint (**TECH FIG 3**).
- Once the needle is visualized and its location deemed adequate, it is removed and a small skin incision is made at the site where the spinal needle was inserted.
- A cannula with its obturator is used to penetrate the anterior capsule into the glenohumeral joint under direct arthroscopic visualization.

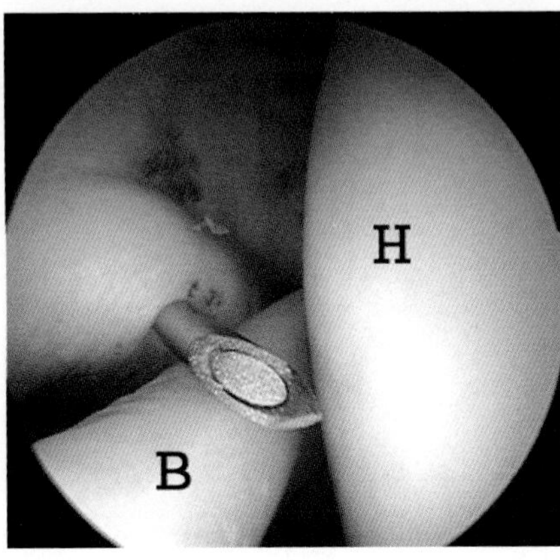

TECH FIG 3 • Spinal needle inserted in rotator interval to establish correct placement of anterior superior portal. The humeral head (*H*) and the long head of the biceps tendon (*B*) are clearly identified.

DIAGNOSTIC ARTHROSCOPY

Arthroscope in the Posterior Portal

- Diagnostic arthroscopy of the shoulder begins with the arthroscope in the posterior portal and a probe through the anterior portal. From this position, the following structures should be visualized and probed:
  - Articular surfaces of the humeral head and glenoid
    - The cartilage surface is evaluated, noting any chondral damage.
    - The glenoid cartilage may have a normal "thinned-out" appearance at its center.
    - Occasionally, the demarcation of the two ossific centers of the glenoid may be identified as a thin line on the chondral surface.
  - Subscapularis tendon and rotator interval
    - The integrity of the superior tendinous edge of the subscapularis and its attachment to the lesser tuberosity is evaluated (**TECH FIG 4A**).
    - The tissue quality and laxity of the rotator interval (the capsular tissue between the anterior edge of the supraspinatus and the superior edge of the subscapularis) is noted.
  - Superior and middle glenohumeral ligaments
    - The superior ligament is evaluated as it crosses between the subscapularis and biceps tendon and the middle ligament as it crosses the subscapularis tendon (**TECH FIG 4B**).
    - Variants may include a Buford complex (cord-like middle glenohumeral ligament) or even absence of the ligament altogether.
  - Superior labrum and biceps tendon
    - The biceps tendon is evaluated on both sides, using a probe to pull it into the joint to evaluate for hidden synovitis or fraying that exists as it leaves the joint and enters the bicipital groove (**TECH FIG 4C**).
  - Rotator cuff
    - The tendons of the rotator cuff are evaluated with the arthroscope looking superiorly. The rotator cuff tendon attachment to the humeral head should be smooth, without any fraying (**TECH FIG 4D**).
    - As the arthroscope is moved posteroinferiorly around the humeral head, the normal "bare spot" on the humeral head is easily identified by the lack of articular cartilage and the presence of nutrient foramen in the bone (**TECH FIG 4E**).
  - Inferior capsule and recess
    - The inferior capsular pouch and the capsular attachment to the humeral head are assessed (**TECH FIG 4F**).
    - Occasionally a humeral avulsion of the inferior glenohumeral ligament may occur here with or without a fragment of bone.

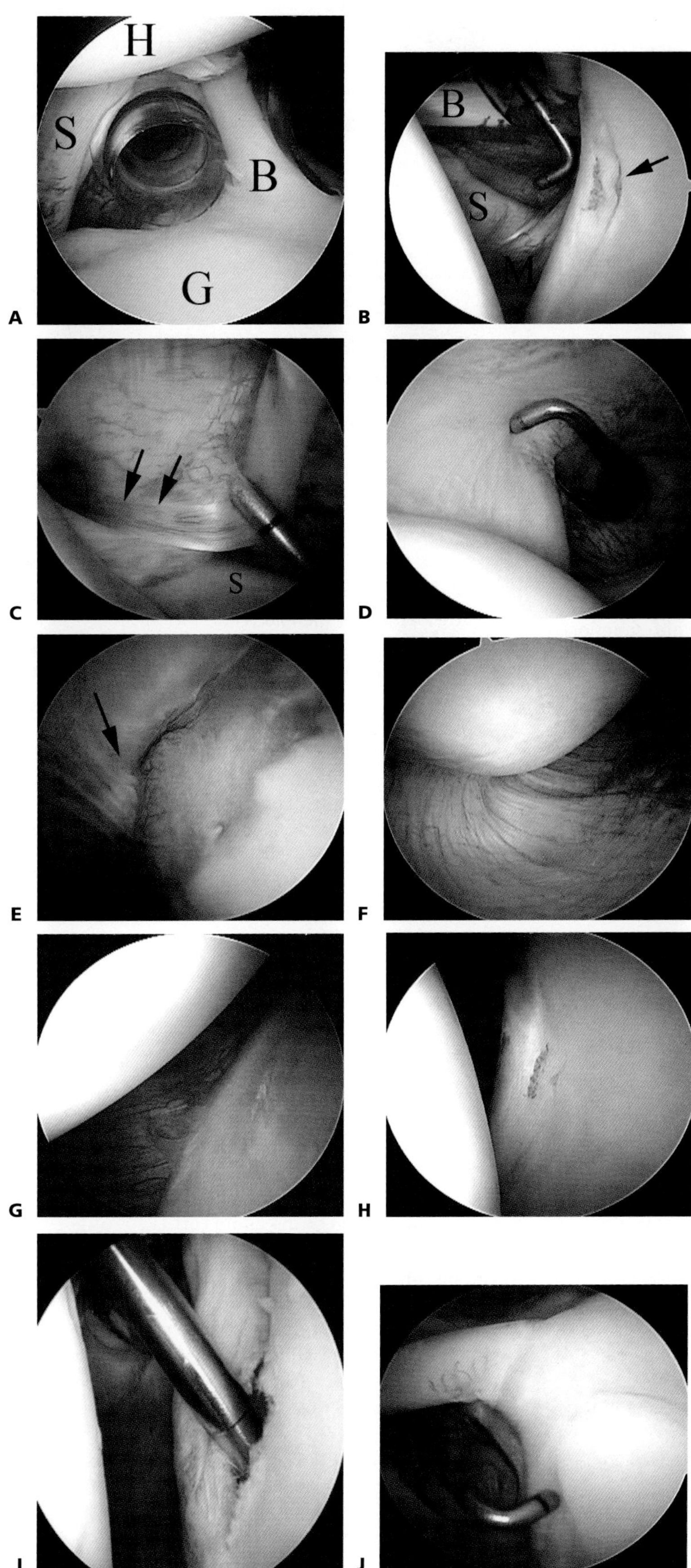

TECH FIG 4 • **A.** Left shoulder in lateral decubitus position with anterior superior and anterior inferior portals established. The biceps tendon (*B*) is between the two cannulas. The humeral head (*H*), glenoid (*G*), and superior edge of the subscapularis (*S*) are identified. **B.** Left shoulder in beach-chair position, with subscapularis (*S*), biceps tendon (*B*), and middle glenohumeral ligament (*M*) identified. The anterosuperior labrum is highly variable and in this case presents as a sublabral hole (*arrow*). **C.** The long head of the biceps can be pulled into the joint to inspect for synovitis (*arrows*), as shown in this shoulder. **D.** The anterior edge of the suprapinatus and the normal rotator cuff insertion are depicted in this image. **E.** As the arthroscope is swept posteriorly along the rotator cuff, the bare area of the humeral head is identified. This is a normal area devoid of articular cartilage. The transition between the posterior rotator cuff and the inferior capsule is identified (*arrow*). **F.** The inferior capsular pouch is seen attaching to the humerus. This is a common area to find loose bodies as they tend to fall to the most dependent aspect of the joint (in the beach-chair position). **G.** The inferior glenoid labrum can be visualized as the arthroscope is redirected superiorly from the axillary pouch. **H,I.** The anterior labral attachment is inspected. **H.** The labrum and capsular attachment are normal. **I.** There is a disruption in the attachment of the anteroinferior labrum (Bankart lesion). **J.** The superior labral attachment is probed.

- As the arthroscope is directed superiorly, the inferior labral attachment can be examined (**TECH FIG 4G**).
- Anterior band of the inferior glenohumeral ligament
  - This is the primary static stabilizer to anterior glenohumeral translation.
  - The anteroinferior labrum should be tightly attached to the glenoid (**TECH FIG 4H**). Detachment in this area is commonly referred to as a Bankart or Perthes lesion (**TECH FIG 4I**) and will be discussed in greater detail in Chapter SM-2.
  - Visualization of this ligament is facilitated when the ligaments and capsular tissues are loose and the arthroscope may easily pass into the anterior recess between the humeral head and glenoid. This is known as a "drive-through" sign and may represent multidirectional laxity.
- Biceps anchor
  - The superior labral attachment to the glenoid is probed to evaluate for a superior labral anterior to posterior (SLAP) lesion.[3]
  - Typically the superior labrum is well attached to the superior glenoid (**TECH FIG 4J**).
  - Normal variants such as a meniscoid superior labrum and variations of the biceps tendon (bifid tendon) are not uncommon. They must be differentiated from pathoanatomy that requires repair.

Arthroscope in the Anterior Portal

- The arthroscope is removed while keeping the sheath in the joint posteriorly. It is placed in the anterior cannula to allow evaluation of the posterior joint and to assess the rest of the joint from another viewpoint.

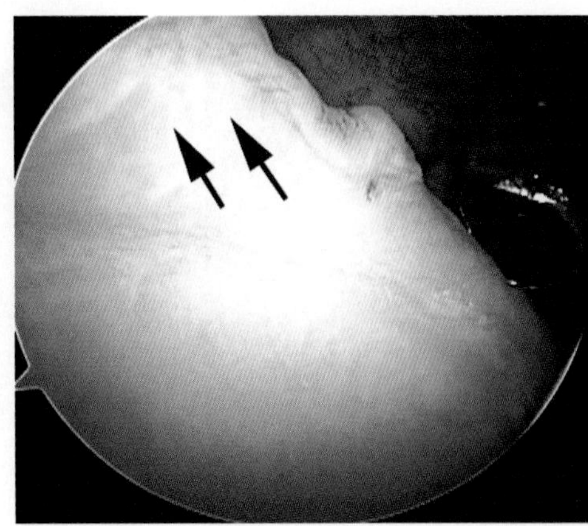

TECH FIG 5 • The arthroscope is now switched to the anterior portal to inspect the posterior labrum and capsule. The transition of the posterior labrum into the superior labrum and biceps attachment (*arrows*) is smooth.

  - The posterior labrum should be smooth and tightly attached to the glenoid (**TECH FIG 5**).
  - The scope is angled upward to assess posterior capsular attachment to the humeral head. If detached, this represents a reverse humeral avulsion of the glenohumeral ligament.
- Subscapularis and biceps tendon
  - The subscapularis recess and subscapularis attachment to the humeral head can be evaluated.
  - Loose bodies are occasionally found within the subscapularis recess.
  - Integrity and stability of the groove and the synovium of the biceps tendon are evaluated.

SUBACROMIAL ARTHROSCOPY (BURSCOSCOPY)

- Once the diagnostic glenohumeral arthroscopy is completed, the sheath and obturator are then directed into the subacromial space.
- This is done by placing the obturator tip just beneath the posterior acromion and then inserting it parallel to the acromion.
- If the arthroscope is inserted properly into the subacromial space anterior to the posterior bursal curtain, then the distended bursal space should allow for visualization of the subacromial structures.[3]
- At the surgeon's preference, a lateral portal may be created at this time.
- The inferior aspect of the acromion is evaluated and the coracoacromial ligament is identified.
  - The lateral and anterior aspects of the acromion are assessed.
  - The anterior acromial spur is evaluated if present.
- The arthoscope is oriented to look downward at the greater tuberosity and attachment of the rotator cuff.
  - A probe from the anterior or lateral portal is used to assess the rotator cuff integrity. The rotator cuff attachment should be smooth, without fraying or thinning of the tissue.
  - Internal and external rotation of the arm will allow for visualization of the entire cuff.
- The acromioclavicular joint is evaluated. The distal clavicle may be hidden behind thickened tissue. Further evaluation of this joint is discussed in Chapter SM-8.
- Once the subacromial space has been evaluated and all pathology has been addressed, the arthroscopic instruments and cannulas can be removed from the shoulder.
- The portals can be closed with a simple suture or subcuticular stitch.
- Wounds can be dressed and the shoulder placed in a sling for comfort or for rehabilitation purposes, depending on the procedure performed.

PEARLS AND PITFALLS

Indications	▪ The surgeon should have a clear understanding of patient history, physical examination, imaging studies, and pathology to be addressed.
Positioning	▪ Beach-chair or lateral decubitus position is used. The surgeon should ensure that the appropriate equipment is available in the operating room.
Portal placement	▪ The surgeon should have a full understanding of pertinent anatomy. Improper portal placement will make visualization and arthroscopic débridement and repair difficult.
Equipment	▪ The surgeon must make sure that all necessary equipment and instruments are available, including suture anchors for labral repair or rotator cuff procedures, multiple-size cannulas, sutures and passing instruments, shavers and burrs, and thermal or electrocautery.
Approach	▪ It is important to have a systematic, stepwise approach to diagnostic arthroscopy so that all structures are adequately visualized and no pathology is missed.

POSTOPERATIVE CARE

- The patient is placed in a sling for comfort. Allowable range of motion and exercises are tailored to the specific procedure performed and will be discussed in detail in the following chapters.
- Cryotherapy (a commercial ice unit) may be used.

OUTCOMES

- Shoulder arthroscopy is a safe and effective procedure. It allows for complete visualization of the glenohumeral joint and subacromial space and treatment of identified pathology.
- Outcome data for specific procedures performed are discussed in the following chapters.

COMPLICATIONS

- Failure to address all pathology with thorough diagnostic examination
- Infection
- Loss of motion or adhesive capsulitis

REFERENCES

1. Nove-Josserand L, Walch G, Adeleine P, et al. Effect of age on the natural history of the shoulder: a clinical and radiological study in the elderly. Rev Chir Orthop Reparatrice Appar Mot 2005;91:508–514.
2. Rowe CR. Acute and recurrent anterior dislocation of the shoulder. Orthop Clin North Am 1980;11:253–270.
3. Snyder S. Diagnostic arthroscopy. In: Snyder S, ed. Shoulder Arthroscopy, ed 2. Philadelphia: Lippincott Williams & Wilkins, 2003.

Chapter 2 Arthroscopic Treatment of Anterior Shoulder Instability

Robert A. Arciero, Augustus D. Mazzocca, and Jeffrey T. Spang

DEFINITION

- Glenohumeral stability depends on static and dynamic restraints to ensure stable yet unconstrained range of motion.
- Laxity is a physiologic term used to describe the passive translation of the humeral head on the glenoid.
- Instability is a pathologic state characterized by abnormal translation of the humeral head on or over the glenoid, leading to frank dislocation, functional impairments, or pain.
- The most common direction of glenohumeral instability is anteroinferior.
- Anterior instability may be traumatic (occurring with the arm in abduction and external rotation), acquired (subtle instability associated with repeated microtrauma), or atraumatic (multidirectional with underlying anatomic contributions).

ANATOMY

- The normal glenoid is broader inferiorly then superiorly (pear-shaped).
- The articulating surface of the humeral head is about three times the size of the corresponding glenoid cavity.[30]
- Static and dynamic stability must be provided by a complex interaction between the capsuloligamentous structures, the rotator cuff, the scapular stabilizers, and the biceps muscle.[6]
- The shallow bony glenoid is deepened by thicker articular cartilage on the periphery and the presence of the ringlike labrum.
- The fibrocartilaginous labrum increases the depth of the socket and prevents the head from rolling anteriorly over the glenoid. The superior labrum provides an attachment for the biceps, whereas the inferior labrum serves as an attachment for the glenohumeral ligaments.[7]
- The capsule and ligaments are intimately related and different geographic areas contribute to stability based on the anatomic position of the arm.
- The inferior glenohumeral ligament complex is the primary static restraint against instability from abduction angles of 45 to 90 degrees. The anterior band is the most important static restraint against anterior instability in the most common position of injury, the abducted and externally rotated arm (**FIG 1**).
- The superior and middle glenohumeral ligaments limit inferior translation and anteroposterior translation with the arm in adduction.
- The rotator cuff muscles and the long head of the biceps brachii provide critical dynamic stability by increasing joint compression.
- Less important contributors to joint stability include negative intra-articular joint pressure, articular version, and adhesion-cohesion forces.

PATHOGENESIS

- Trauma, especially athletic trauma, plays a significant role in recurrent anterior instability.
- Overhead athletes can present with more subtle instability.
  - Repetitive microtrauma contributes to the development of pathologic subluxation.
- Injury may result in subluxation and dislocation with spontaneous reduction or dislocation requiring reduction maneuvers.
- Traumatic anterior instability is most common in the young, athletic population.
  - In the 21- to 30-year-old age group the male/female incidence was reported as 9:1.[11]
- The Bankart lesion (detachment of the anterior inferior labrum and capsule) is considered the fundamental pathoanatomic lesion associated with anteroinferior instability. It may be present in about 90% of all traumatic glenohumeral dislocations (**FIG 2**).
- Recurrent dislocations lead to plastic deformation of the middle and inferior glenohumeral ligaments, contributing to laxity in the "sling" that is designed to restrict translation of the humeral head in abduction.
- Bone injuries to the humerus (such as the Hill-Sachs lesion) and the glenoid (bony Bankart or glenoid erosion) are known to contribute to increased glenohumeral translation, resulting in recurrent instability.
- Extensive soft tissue damage is rare but can include the humeral avulsion of the glenohumeral ligaments or a capsular tear.[24] In addition, the injured labral tissue may heal medially on the glenoid neck (the so-called anterior labroligamentous periosteal sleeve avulsion [ALPSA lesion]) leading to insufficiency of the inferior glenohumeral ligament and labral complex.[25]
- In the older patient with a traumatic dislocation, rotator cuff pathology must be ruled out. A thorough strength examination coupled with appropriate use of soft tissue imaging should alert the examiner to concomitant rotator cuff pathology.
  - Other soft tissue injuries (capsular tear and neurovascular injury) as well as glenoid and humeral head defects can occur in this age group.

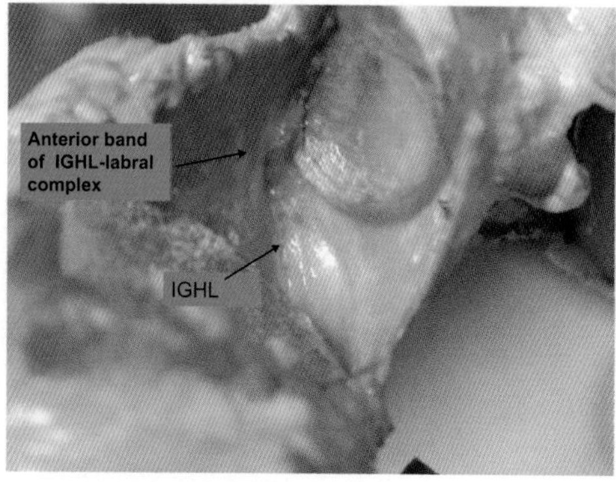

FIG 1 • Cadaveric image of the inferior glenoid humeral ligament and anteroinferior labral complex.

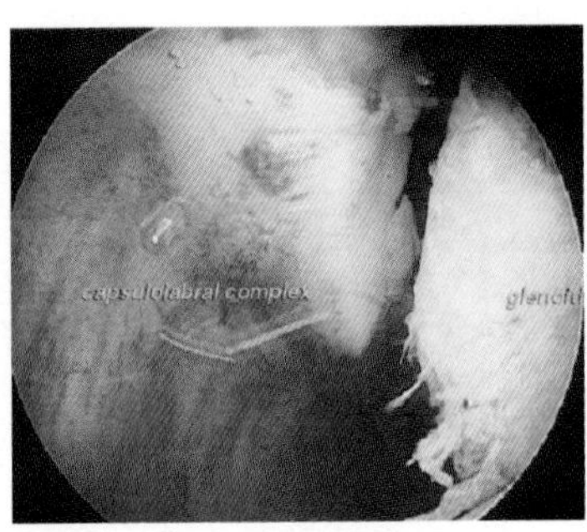

FIG 2 • Arthroscopic view of a Bankart lesion, left shoulder, sitting position, viewed from posteriorly.

NATURAL HISTORY

- Glenohumeral dislocation affects approximately 2% of the general population.[11]
- Few natural history studies exist with long-term follow-up.
  - A 10-year review of dislocation treated nonoperatively revealed a redislocation rate of about 66% for patients presenting under age 22.[12]
  - Other recent studies put the redislocation rate at 64% in those under 20.[34] The same author has recently reported a 25-year follow-up of patients under the age of 40 with an overall recurrence rate of 50%. Again patients under 20 years of age had recurrence rates of higher than 60%.[13] Another researcher examined a group of patients to determine if the need for surgery could be predicted after an initial dislocation. They reported a 55% recurrence rate but noted that younger patients, especially those involved in overhead or contact sports, were at increased risk.[29]
  - Older studies[23,27] report redislocation rates as high as 80% to 90% in patients under age 20.
- Older patients have much lower redislocation rates (14%).[28]
- Age is the most important predictor of recurrence rates after an initial dislocation. Activity level, especially collision or contact sports, may also increase recurrence rates but has not been definitively proven.
- Multiple authors have reported that early surgical reconstruction for primary dislocation decreases the risk of recurrence.[1,19,20,35] Further primary arthroscopic stabilization was observed to improve the quality of life, provide better outcome, and reduce recurrence rates.[26]

PATIENT HISTORY AND PHYSICAL FINDINGS

- The patient's age and activity level are critical to decision making. Prior surgical procedures should be reviewed in detail.
- There are five important questions in the history of instability:
  - Did the initial instability episode require a reduction?
  - What was the arm position for the first dislocation? The last dislocation?
  - What was the disability after the initial incident?
  - How many episodes of instability have occurred since the initial event? Were they dislocation or subluxation episodes?
  - What was the magnitude of the trauma associated with the initial event? Have subsequent events required similar force, or have they occurred with less provocation?
- The physical examination should begin with inspection from posterior to assess any muscular atrophy of the trapezius, supraspinatus, and infraspinatus and teres minor. Muscle atrophy may point out nerve injury.
- Generalized ligamentous laxity should be examined by testing a thumb hyperextension sign and elbow extension.
- Active and passive range of motion in all scapular planes should be recorded and compared with the contralateral shoulder.
- Strength testing should include all important shoulder musculature, with a focus on pain as limiting factor.
- The contralateral side is examined when doing the load and shift examination; positive findings indicate lax anterior stabilizers.
- It is critical to separate feelings of pain from instability relieved with Jobe relocation. A positive relocation maneuver may spotlight subtle instability.
- Axillary nerve function should be assessed by carefully testing motor function of the deltoid and examining sensory distribution.
- A positive posterior jerk test with pain and or crepitus illicited with posterior translation of the humeral head over the glenoid rim indicates posteroinferior capsular or labral pathology.
- When examining for the sulcus sign, the clinician should compare the result with the contralateral side. Failure of external rotation to eliminate the sulcus sign may indicate multidirectional instability or global laxity.
- Provocative maneuvers should be employed to evaluate shoulder stability.

IMAGING AND OTHER DIAGNOSTIC STUDIES

- Radiographs
  - Standard AP views of the arm with the arm in slight internal rotation: may show greater tuberosity fracture
  - AP views of the glenohumeral joint (**FIG 3A**)
  - West Point axillary view: may be used to assess bony avulsions of the inferior glenohumeral ligament, bony Bankart lesions, or anteroinferior glenoid deficiency[14]
  - Stryker notch view: may be used to examine and quantify a Hill-Sachs lesion
- Computed tomography
  - Bone defects are an important cause of failure for instability surgery.[2,32]
  - Three-dimensional reconstructions have been especially useful to quantify bone loss (**FIG 3B**).
  - Indications
    - Instability episodes while asleep
    - Instability episodes with minimal trauma after a primary instability episode that required manual reduction
    - Instability episodes at low degrees of humeral abduction
    - Failure of any prior instability procedure
    - Apprehension on examination at low degrees of humeral abduction
    - Remarkable laxity on load and shift test
    - Any bony lesion on radiographic evaluation
  - When bony deficiencies are identified, operative approaches must be adjusted accordingly. Careful consideration must be given to open instability procedures with bony augmentation in cases of bone involvement (Table 1).
- Magnetic resonance imaging
  - Contrast enhancement improves the ability to detect labral injury, rotator cuff tears, and articular cartilage lesions.

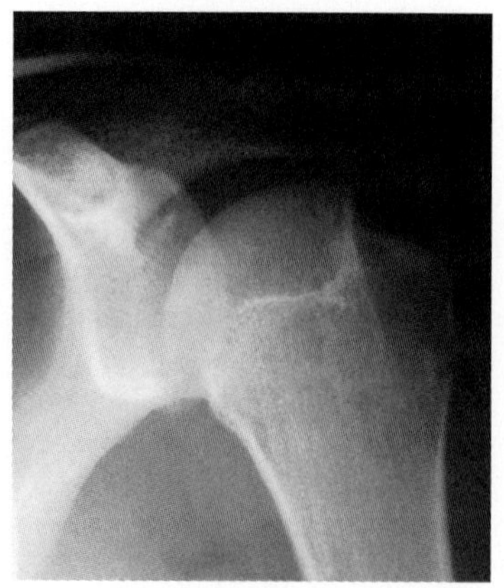
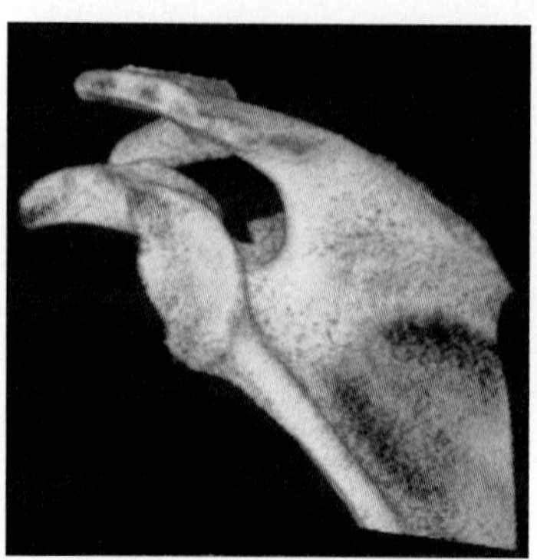
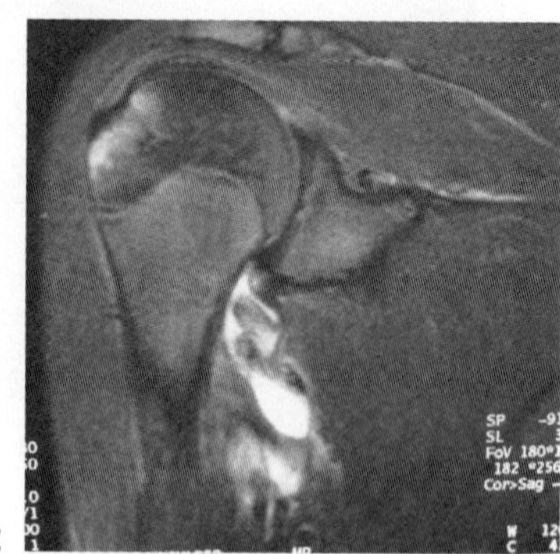

FIG 3 • **A.** AP radiograph showing defect in the humeral head. **B.** CT scan reconstruction showing erosion of the anteroinferior glenoid. **C.** MRI example of humeral avulsion of glenohumeral ligament lesion.

- It may identify humeral avulsion of the glenohumeral ligament lesions and capsular tears, allowing recognition of these infrequent but critical injuries (**FIG 3C**).

DIFFERENTIAL DIAGNOSIS

- Osseous lesions, including clavicle fractures, proximal humerus fractures, and scapular and glenoid fractures
- Soft tissue lesions, including deltoid contusions, acromioclavicular joint sprains, and rotator cuff injuries (more common in patients older than 40 years)
- Nerve lesions, including injuries to the axillary nerve, suprascapular nerve, and long thoracic nerve

NONOPERATIVE MANAGEMENT

- Nonoperative management has traditionally consisted of a period of immobilization followed by intensive physical therapy to improve proprioception and muscular balance around the shoulder girdle. A recent review noted that recommendations for positioning, length of immobilization, and outcomes are inconsistent at best.[3]
- Recent work by Itoi[14] suggested that immobilization in external rotation will reduce recurrence rates after magnetic resonance imaging demonstrates coaptation of the Bankart lesion with the arm in external rotation.[17] This same author reported a clinical series comparing immobilization in internal rotation versus external rotation after primary dislocation. Immobilization in external rotation reduced the risk of recurrence by 46%.[15]
- Failure of nonoperative management may be manifested in recurrent symptoms of instability (dislocations, subluxations, or pain) despite adequate nonoperative management and activity modification where appropriate.

Table 1 Arthroscopic Versus Open Treatment of Anterior Instability

Arthroscopic
Minimal to no bone defects—small, nonengaging Hill-Sachs, no glenoid bone loss
Unidirectional dislocators
Bankart or anterior labroligamentous periosteal sleeve avulsion (ALPSA lesion)
Proper surgeon experience

Open
Bone defects—large Hill-Sachs lesions (>25% articular surface), glenoid deficiencies >20%; "inverted pear" large "HAGL" (humeral avulsion of glenohumeral ligament); capsular deficiency or loss (thermal ablation)

Controversial patient populations
Patients with multidirectional instability or hyperlaxity
High-demand collision athletes

SURGICAL MANAGEMENT

- The guiding basis for the described arthroscopic technique is that restoration of the normal glenoid labrum anatomy and retensioning of the inferior glenohumeral ligament can be accomplished in a manner that mirrors the open method (**FIG 4**).

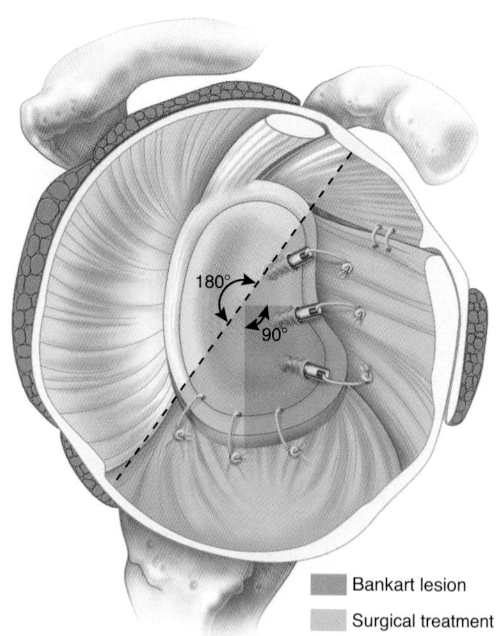

FIG 4 • Illustration of a surgical reconstruction with a 180-degree arthroscopic repair with three inferior plication sutures, three anchors repairing the labrum, and a rotator interval closure.

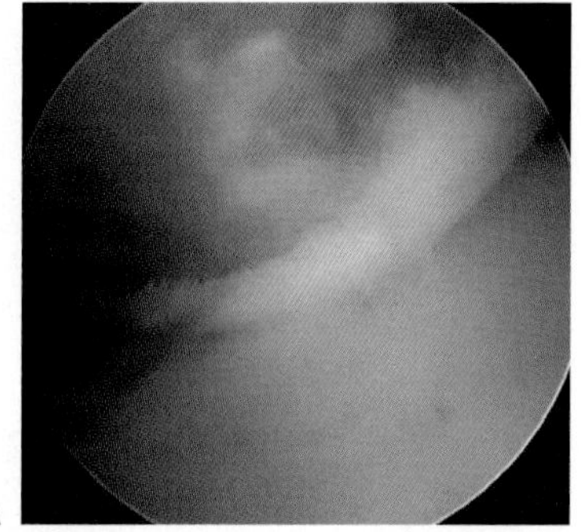

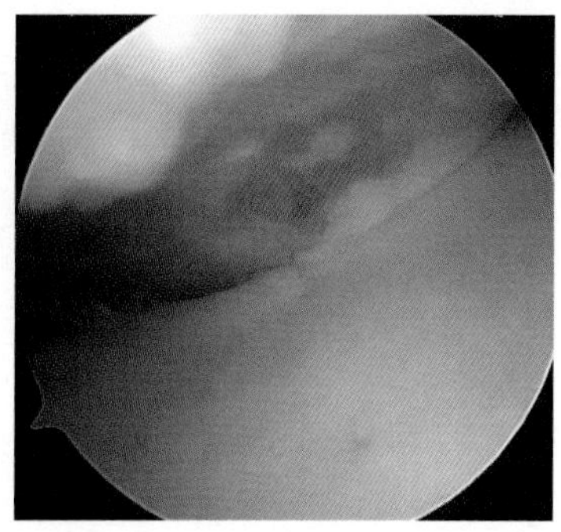

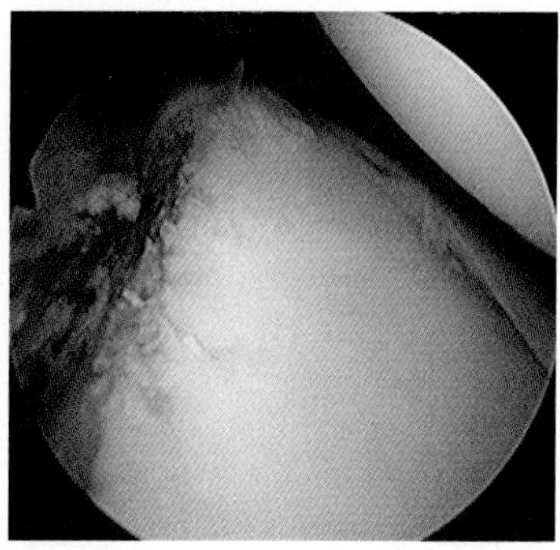

FIG 5 • **A.** Hill-Sachs lesion on glenoid face. **B.** Hill-Sachs lesion engaged, with humeral head locked over anterior glenoid. **C.** Arthroscopic view (right shoulder) of inverted pear: camera anterosuperior, showing anterior glenoid bone loss.

- In the senior author's experience with traumatic anterior instability, a Bankart lesion will typically extend from the 2 o'clock to the 6 o'clock position. To restore anatomy appropriately, the surgeon should be able to instrument and place suture anchors at the inferior aspect of the joint in the 6 o'clock position.
- Arthroscopic knots may be sliding, sliding-locking, or simple. Knot selection is less important than the ability to reproduce the desired knot security and tissue tension consistently.

Preoperative Planning

- The indications for arthroscopic stabilization include:
  - Primary anterior dislocation in young, high-demand patients
  - Recurrent, traumatic anterior instability without bone loss
  - Overhead athletes, especially throwing athletes, where preserving motion is important
- Contraindications to arthroscopic stabilization include a large Hill-Sachs lesion (the "engaging" Hill-Sachs) and bony deficiencies of the glenoid that represent more than 20% (the "inverted pear"[4]) (**FIG 5**).
- Arthroscopic stabilization for collision athletes and patients with osseous Bankart lesions is controversial.
  - However, several recent reports describe favorable results with arthroscopic repair in these groups.[3,5,21,22,31]
  - The decision to do arthroscopic versus open repair continues to be debated as arthroscopic results are reported (see Table 1).[34]
- All pertinent radiographic studies should be reviewed to confirm prior hardware, expected soft tissue injuries, and potential bony injuries.
- An examination under anesthesia should confirm anteroinferior instability in the operative shoulder and verify range of motion. It is important to note the normal range of motion in the contralateral shoulder before final positioning.

Positioning

- Both the beach-chair position and the lateral decubitus position may be used for instability surgery. We prefer the lateral decubitus position to allow greater access to the inferior portions of the joint.
- For the lateral decubitus position the patient is stabilized with a beanbag in a 30-degree backward tilt to place the glenoid face parallel to the floor.
  - A three-point distraction device that applies longitudinal and vertical traction allows distraction of the humerus.
  - Typically 5 pounds of longitudinal traction is combined with 7 pounds of lateral traction or distraction.
- In most cases an interscalene block provides excellent operative and postoperative pain control.
  - For the beach-chair position, this may be all that is required.
  - For the lateral decubitus position, it is prudent to add general anesthesia for comfort.
- Preoperative antibiotics are administered before the skin incision (**FIG 6**).

Approach

- A standard posterior portal should be placed in the soft spot at midglenoid level, taking care to be just lateral to the glenoid.
- The blunt arthroscopic trocar and sheath are then inserted into the space between the glenoid rim and the humeral head.
- Using needle localization, the surgeon places the anterior portals. The anterosuperior portal should be as high as possible while staying just inferior to the biceps tendon.
- The anteroinferior portal should enter just above the superior border of the subscapularis.
  - The needle used for portal placement should first be navigated throughout the joint to ensure that instrumentation with suture shuttling devices and anchor insertion equipment is feasible.
- The anterosuperior portal is instrumented with a 7.0-mm cannula and the anteroinferior portal is instrumented with an 8.25-mm cannula (**FIG 7A–C**).

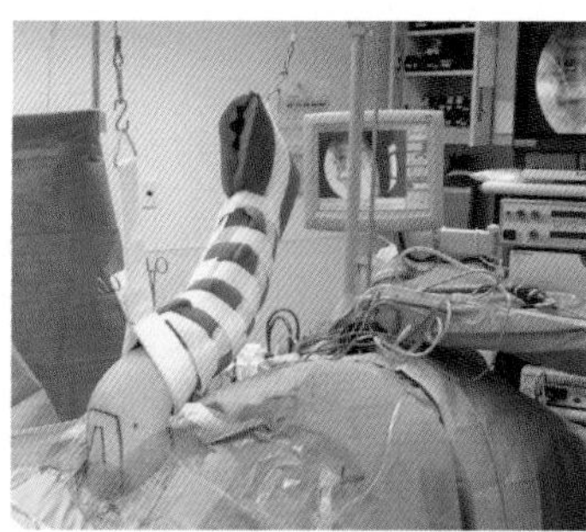

FIG 6 • Setup for the lateral decubitus position with arm traction device.

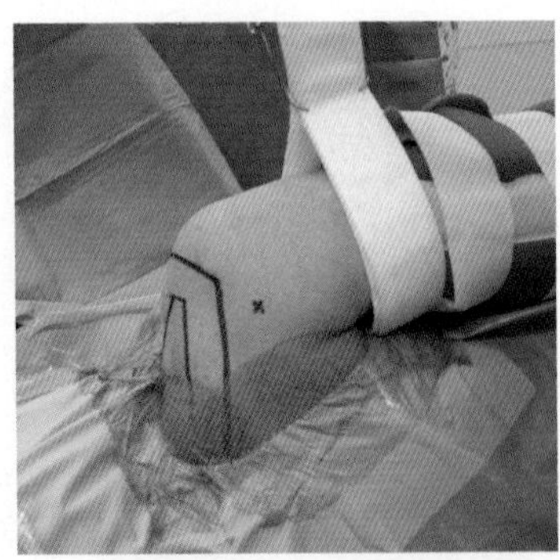

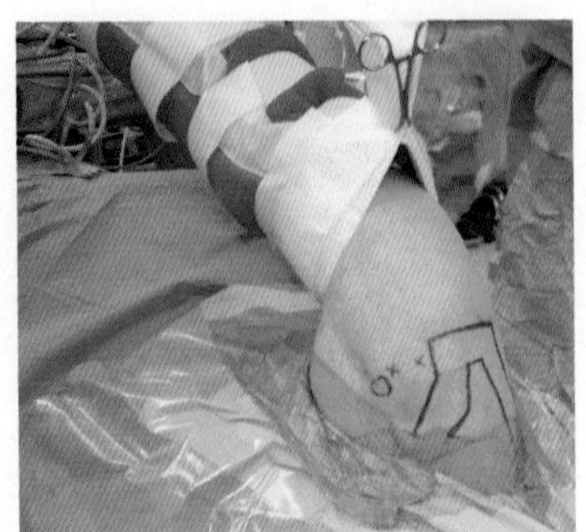

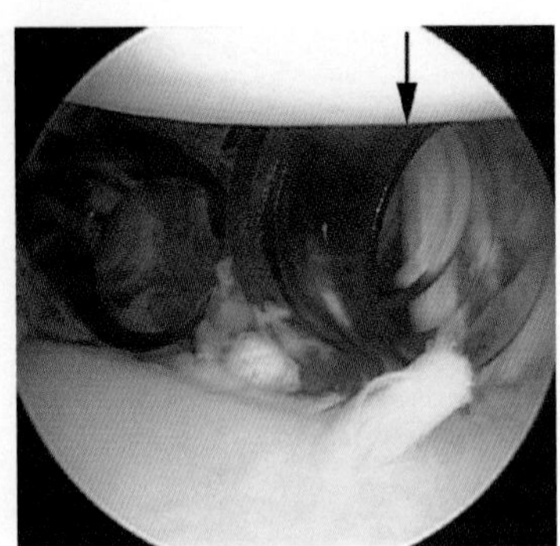

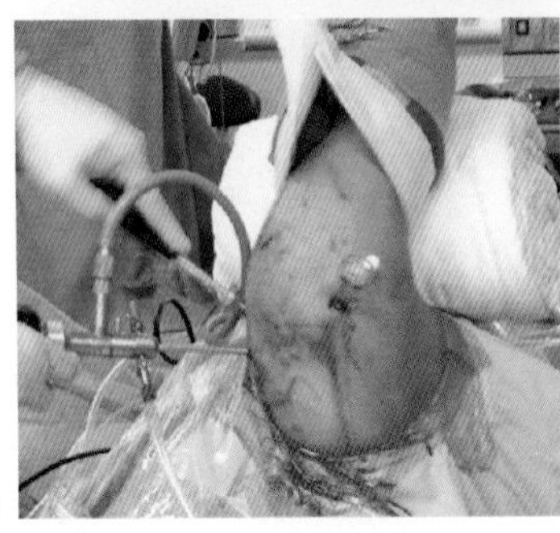

FIG 7 • **A.** View of posterior portal position. **B.** View of anterior portal positions. **C.** View of dual anterior portals. Note spread between cannulas to allow instrument passage. **D.** View of rolled blanket "bump" positioned in axilla to improve visualization.

- Before beginning the surgical procedure, a through diagnostic arthroscopy is performed.
- After diagnostic arthroscopy, the arthroscope is brought to the anterosuperior portal and another 8.25-mm cannula is placed in the posterior portal.
- With the arthroscope in the anterosuperior portal, visualization of the inferior glenohumeral ligament and labrum is optimized.
- A rolled blanket "bump" placed into the axilla provides further gentle distraction and improves exposure of the inferior aspect of the joint (**FIG 7D**).

SUTURE FIRST (AUTHORS' PREFERRED TECHNIQUE)

Arthroscopy and Glenoid Preparation

- First, the labral and ligamentous complex must be released off the face of the glenoid.
  - Care should be taken to maintain the tissue as one unit, using elevators to adequately release to at least the 6 o'clock position.
  - When muscle fibers of the subscapularis are visible, the release is adequate (**TECH FIG 1A**).
- The glenoid neck must be prepared by either a burr or a shaver to decorticate down to bleeding bone. A meniscal rasp can be a helpful adjunct.
  - The bone preparation must be as inferior as the soft tissue release on the glenoid.
- It is critical to begin the repair at the low 6 o'clock position in the capsule.
- Various techniques may be used to ensure that the initial shuttling suture can be placed inferior at the 6 o'clock position. Options include:
  - Arthroscope in anterosuperior portal (our preferred method): suture-passing instrument inserted through posterior cannula (**TECH FIG 1B**)
  - Arthroscope in anterosuperior portal: suture-passing instrument inserted through anteroinferior cannula (**TECH FIG 1C,D**)
  - Arthroscope in posterior portal: suture-passing instrument inserted through anteroinferior cannula to capture tissue (**TECH FIG 1D**). Arthroscope in anterosuperior portal with shuttling instrument brought in from anteroinferior portal

"Pinch and Tuck"

- Capsular retensioning and labral repair may be accomplished by the "pinch and tuck" method (**TECH FIG 2**).
- Using a curved suture-passing device, the capsule is pierced 5 to 10 mm lateral to the labrum.
- The device exits the capsule and pierces the capsule again to re-enter at the lateral base of the labral complex and emerge at the articular margin.
- A monofilament suture is inserted to be used as a shuttle suture. The shuttling suture or device will eventually be used to shuttle the nonabsorbable suture housed in the anchor. Or it may be used to shuttle a nonabsorbable suture being used purely as a plication suture.
- With the introduction of newer ultrastrong suture, subsequent knot tying will combine capsular plication and labral repair.
- All shuttling should be done from the articular side of the labrum out to the soft tissue side and through a cannula.

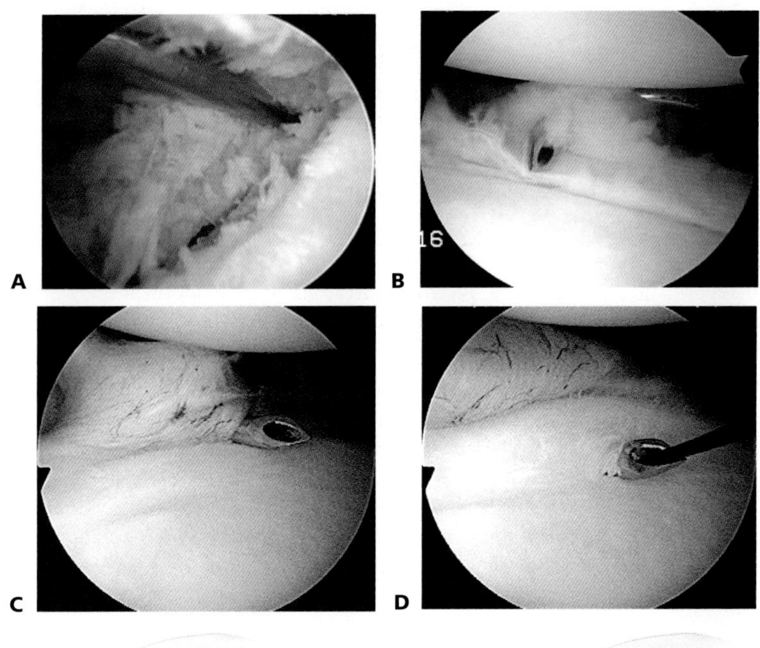

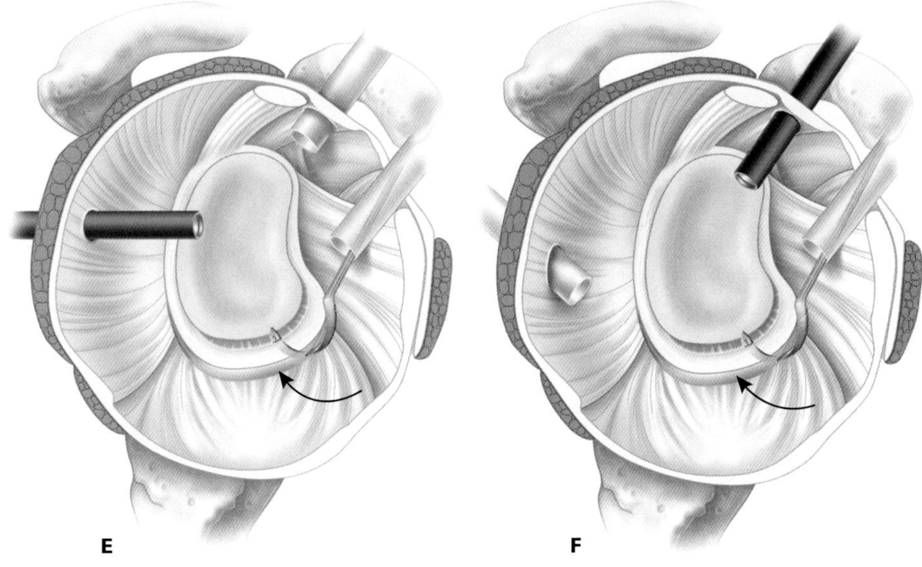

TECH FIG 1 • Right shoulder. **A.** Elevator releasing labral and capsular tissue off face of glenoid. **B.** Pinch of capsular and ligamentous tissue with shuttling instrument coming from posterior portal to place at inferior aspect. **C.** Shuttling instrument brought through anteroinferior portal and taking tuck of inferior capsule. **D.** After piercing capsule the needle of the shuttling instrument pierces the labrum. **E.** Camera in posterior portal with suture passer in anteroinferior cannula. **F.** Camera in anterosuperior portal with suture passer in anteroinferior cannula.

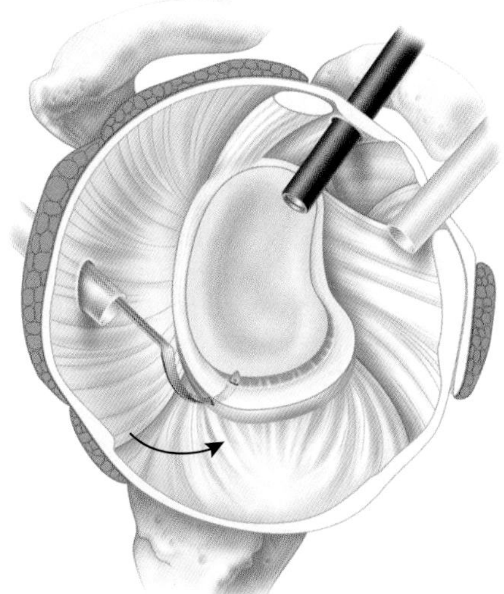

TECH FIG 2 • Camera in anterosuperior portal with suture passer in posterior cannula.

Anchor Placement

- The initial suture anchor is placed inferiorly on the glenoid, close to the 6 o'clock position.
  - Suture anchors should be placed on to the articular face of the glenoid to recreate the "bumper" effect of the normal labrum.
  - It is critical to place anchors 5 to 10 mm cephalad to the shuttle suture to accomplish the "superior shift" portion of the procedure (TECH FIG 3A). Subsequent knot-tying will combine capsular re-tensioning and labral repair.
- If appropriate access for anchor placement cannot be gained from the anteroinferior portal, a percutaneous transsubscapular entry may be used.
  - In this case, a stab incision is made just inferior to the anteroinferior portal.
  - Using needle localization the surgeon confirms appropriate access, and a small trocar may be inserted to place the anchor onto the glenoid (TECH FIG 3B,C).

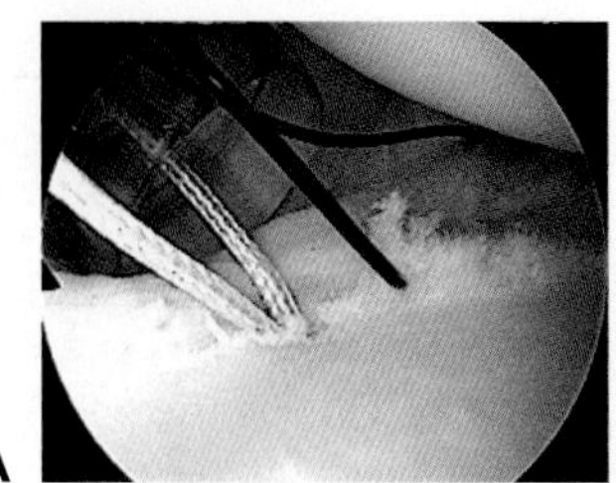
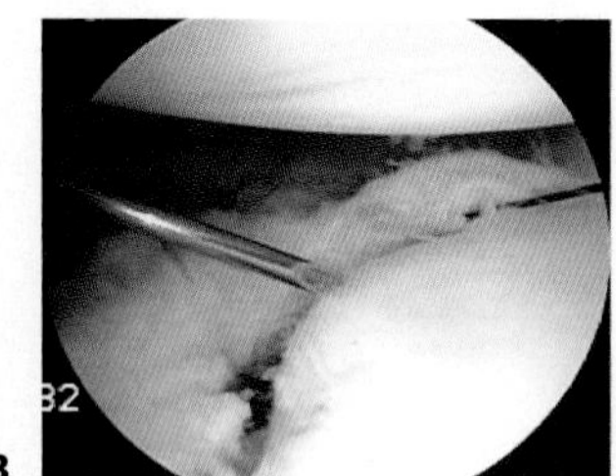
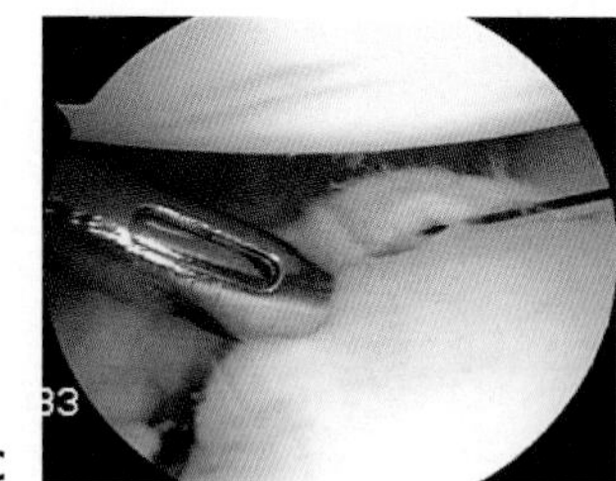

TECH FIG 3 • A. Anchor placed superior to shuttle suture. **B.** Transsubscapular needle localization for inferior anchor. **C.** Placement of transsubscapular trocar for inferior anchor.

Capsular Plication

- The process of capsular plication and anchoring is repeated, moving in a superior direction to restore labral anatomy and retension the inferior glenohumeral ligament.
  - Typically at least four anchors are used in the final construct.
- It may be necessary to return the arthroscope to the posterior portal for placement of the most cephalad anchor (2 o'clock position for the right shoulder) to avoid anterior instrument crowding. A 7.0-mm cannula may be reinserted in the anterosuperior portal for instrumentation. The final repair should re-establish normal positioning of the glenoid labrum over the glenoid rim and retension the inferior glenohumeral ligament (**TECH FIG 4A,B**)

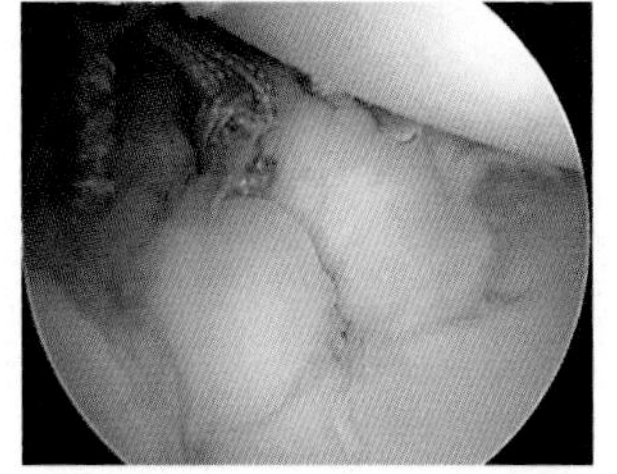
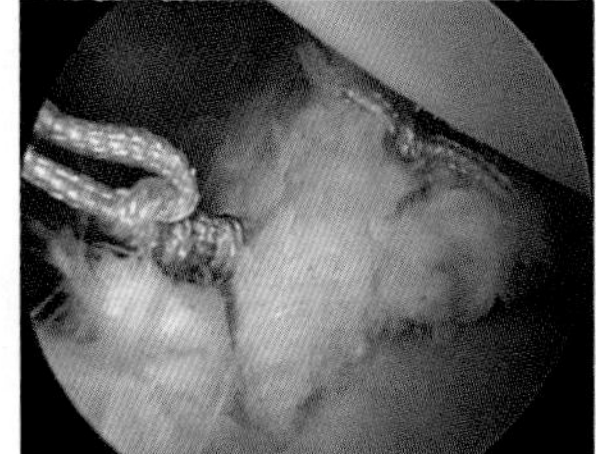

TECH FIG 4 • A. Finished repair with labral "bumper" re-established. **B.** Finished repair with inferior glenohumeral ligament tension re-established.

ANCHOR FIRST

- The same general techniques and principles from the suture-first technique apply.
- An anchor is inserted onto the face of the glenoid in an appropriate location.
- Both limbs of the anchor suture are pulled out of a cannula for suture management.
- A tissue penetrator or suture-shuttling device is used to gather the inferior tissue and place a shuttle suture.
- The suture is grasped in the joint and pulled out the anterosuperior cannula.
- A standard suture-shuttle technique is used to pass the anchor suture.

ADDITIONAL ENHANCING TECHNIQUES

Traction Suture

- If access to the inferior capsule and labrum is difficult, a "traction suture" can be used.
- The initial stitch can be placed in the inferior capsule and then brought out the anterosuperior portal.
- Traction on this stitch may allow a more inferior grasp of tissue in the early stages of a repair.

Mattress Suture

- In addition to simple sutures, a mattress suture can be used to position the tissue on the glenoid face.
- For a mattress suture, the process of capsular plication with a suture-passing device and subsequent suture shuttling is repeated so that both limbs of the suture exit the tissue on the tissue side.
- As the arthroscopic knot is tied, a mattress stitch is created to enhance capsular plication and gather additional capsular tissue on the glenoid rim.
- This is particularly useful with a degenerative atrophic labrum or with poor-quality capsular tissue (**TECH FIG 5**).

Posterior Anchors

- Should the Bankart lesion extend posteriorly past the 6 o'clock point, posterior anchors may be required.
- A percutaneous technique for anchor insertion can be employed using needle localization and a trocar and anchor guide through a posteroinferior stab incision.
- Alternatively, a posteroinferior portal may be established using needle localization and gradually increasing dilators to place an additional cannula for posterior and inferior access.

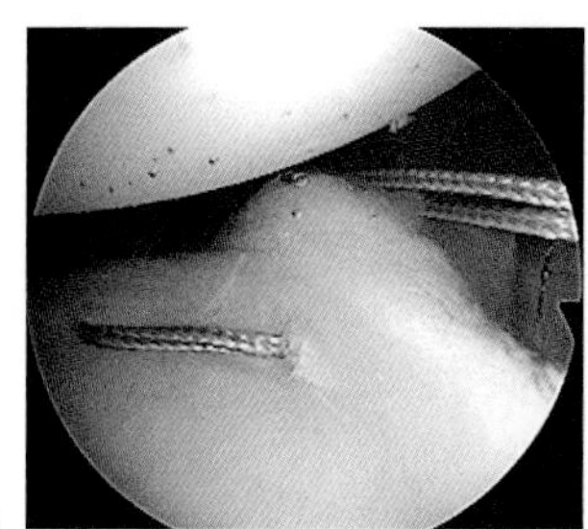

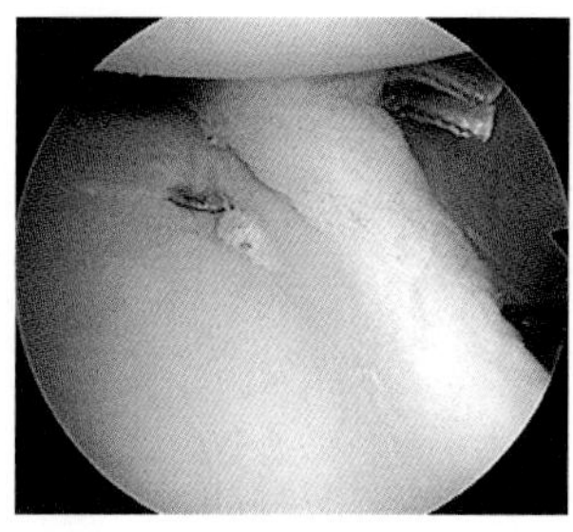

TECH FIG 5 • A. Mattress posteroinferior plication suture placed in a right shoulder viewed from anterosuperior portal. **B.** Final mattress stitch with gathered tissue.

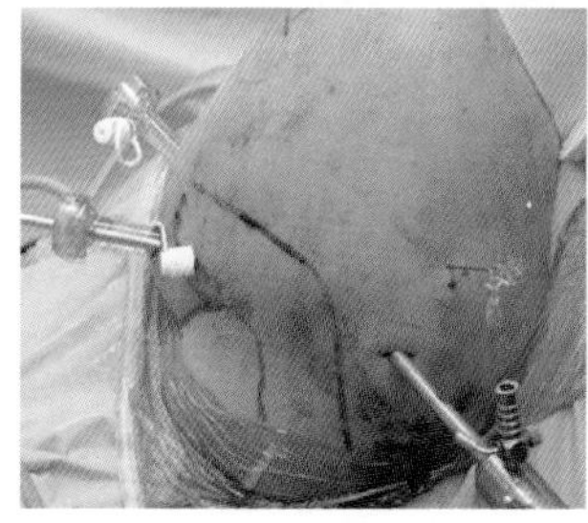

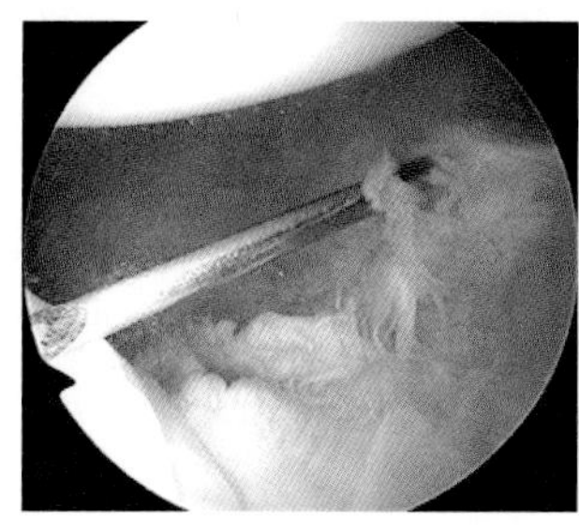

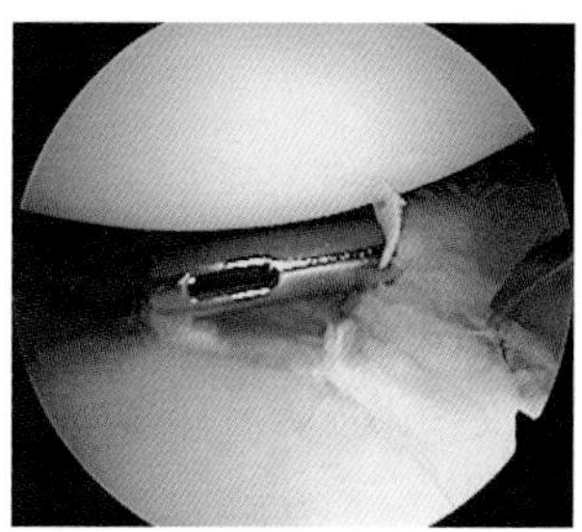

TECH FIG 6 • A,B. Needle localization of posterior stab to ensure access to glenoid. **C.** Protective trocar for anchor inserted for posterior anchor placement.

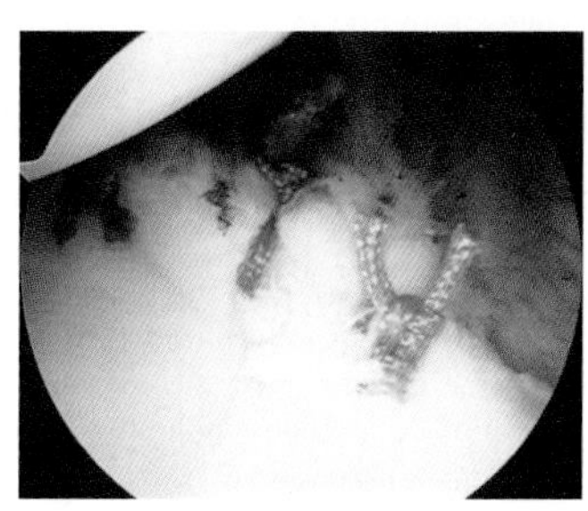

TECH FIG 7 • Posterior capsular plication.

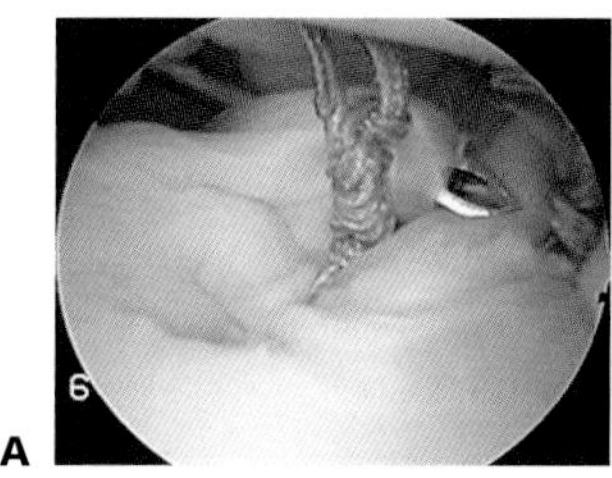

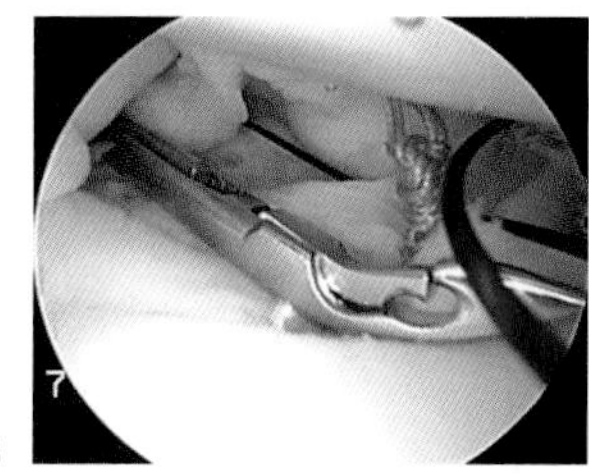

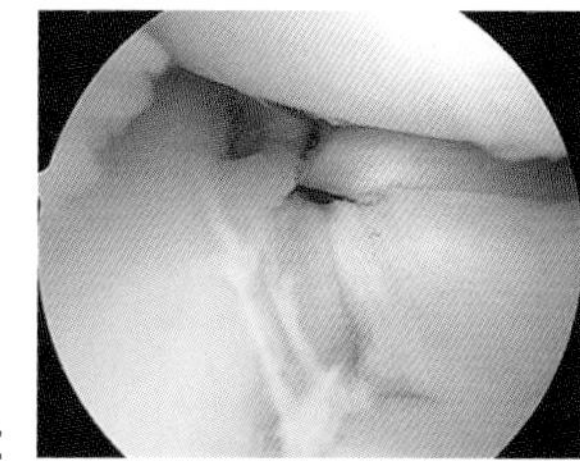

TECH FIG 8 • A. Suture passer penetrating middle glenohumeral ligament to deliver suture. **B.** Tissue penetrator piercing superior portion of rotator interval (superior glenohumeral and coracohumeral ligament) and just anterior to biceps tendon to grasp suture. **C.** Completed stitch.

- This accessory posterior portal is typically located more laterally on the shoulder (TECH FIG 6).

Plication Stitches

- If the posterior labrum is intact but posterior laxity remains, plication stitches can be placed to better balance the anterior and posterior tension on the inferior glenohumeral ligament.
- Using the pinch-tuck technique, the capsule and ligament can be grasped and connected to the labrum (TECH FIG 7).

Closure of Rotator Interval

- When additional stability is required, the rotator interval can be closed.
- Current recommendations for rotator interval closure include greater then 1+ sulcus sign, laxity with a posterior component, and a collision athlete.[9]
- A stitch is passed through a suture passer placed in the anterosuperior cannula through the superior border of the subscapularis or the middle glenohumeral ligament.
- The superior glenohumeral and coracohumeral complex is then pierced with a tissue penetrator to grasp the suture. The suture is then tied and cut with a guillotine knot cutter (TECH FIG 8).

PEARLS AND PITFALLS

Patient selection	■ Major reported reasons for failure of arthroscopic stability procedures include[2]: ■ Failure to appreciate and address excess capsular laxity ■ Failure to evaluate and address bone loss adequately
Portal placement pearls	■ The posterior portal should be placed so that the camera angle replicates the angle of the glenoid face. ■ The anterosuperior portal should be placed far enough from the anteroinferior portal to maintain a skin bridge and working room. ■ The anteroinferior portal should enter just above the subscapularis so instruments and cannula are not blocked by the subscapularis and may reach the inferior glenoid and pouch.
Technical considerations	■ The labrum and the inferior glenohumeral ligament complex must be adequately released to at least the 6 o'clock position. The surgeon should visualize muscle fibers of the subscapularis. ■ Soft tissues must be mobilized superiorly on the glenoid to re-establish tension of the inferior glenohumeral ligament complex and decrease inferior capsule space. ■ Suture anchors must be placed 1 to 2 mm on the articular surface to recreate the soft tissue "bumper." ■ Adequate fixation requires at least four stabilization points. ■ Suture management must be consistent and simple. Sliding, sliding-locking, and simple knots are all acceptable, provided the surgeon can consistently replicate a solid repair.

POSTOPERATIVE CARE

- Goals of postoperative care include controlled mobilization to allow adequate soft tissue healing, adequate motion (external rotation), and successful return to activities.
- Postoperative protocols must respect the biologic repair process.
- Our postoperative protocol includes:
  - Immediate postoperative immobilization in an abduction orthosis
  - Codman exercises and pendulum exercises immediately with assistance
  - Active assisted range-of-motion exercises, including external rotation (0 to 30 degrees) and forward elevation (0 to 90 degrees), for 6 weeks
  - Weeks 6 to 12 include active assisted and active range of motion with the goal of establishing full range of motion.
  - Strengthening exercises begin only after full motion is restored.
  - Sports-specific exercises are begun at 16 to 20 weeks.
  - Final release to full activity is 20 to 24 weeks.

OUTCOMES

- Multiple recent studies using a suture anchor technique similar to the open method have documented clinical success, with recurrent instability rates of 4% to 10%.[5,8,10,18,34]
- As arthroscopic techniques and equipment have evolved, the literature indicates decreasing rates of recurrence and results approaching open instability procedures.
- Careful patient selection remains critical for arthroscopic instability procedures and may vary with surgeon experience.

COMPLICATIONS

- The overall rate of recurrent instability from arthroscopic stabilization can safely be placed at 10% to 15%.
- Postoperative glenohumeral noise or squeaking can occur if arthroscopic knots are captured in the glenohumeral joint. This may require later débridement of the knots.
- Loss of external rotation from overtightening can occur.
- Rupture of the repair can occur with aggressive early activities or rehabilitation.
- Injury to the axillary nerve is possible with electrical or mechanical damage.

REFERENCES

1. Arciero RA, Wheeler JH, Ryan JB, et al. Arthroscopic Bankart repair versus nonoperative treatment for acute, initial anterior shoulder dislocations. Am J Sports Med 1994;22:589–594.
2. Boileau P, Villalba M, Hery JY, et al. Risk factors for recurrence of shoulder instability after arthroscopic Bankart repair. J Bone Joint Surg Am 2006;88A:1755–1763.
3. Bottoni CR, Smith EL, Berkowitz MJ, et al. Arthroscopic versus open shoulder stabilization for recurrent anterior instability: a prospective randomized clinical trial. Am J Sports Med 2006;34: 1730–1737.
4. Burkhart SS, De Beer JF. Traumatic glenohumeral bone defects and their relationship to failure of arthroscopic Bankart repairs: significance of the inverted-pear glenoid and the humeral engaging Hill-Sachs lesion. Arthroscopy 2000;16:677–694.
5. Carreira DS, Mazzocca AD, Oryhon J, et al. A prospective outcome evaluation of arthroscopic Bankart repairs: minimum 2-year follow-up. Am J Sports Med 2006;34:771–777.
6. Cole BJ, Millett PJ, Romeo AA, et al. Arthroscopic treatment of anterior glenohumeral instability: indications and techniques. AAOS Instr Course Lect 2004;53:545–558.
7. Cooper DE, Arnoczky SP, O'Brien SJ, et al. Anatomy, histology, and vascularity of the glenoid labrum. An anatomical study. J Bone Joint Surg Am 1992;74A:46–52.
8. Fabbriciani C, Milano G, Demontis A, et al. Arthroscopic versus open treatment of Bankart lesion of the shoulder: a prospective randomized study. Arthroscopy 2004;20:456–462.
9. Fitzpatrick MJ, Powell SE, Tibone JE, et al. The anatomy, pathology, and definitive treatment of rotator interval lesions: current concepts. Arthroscopy 2003;19(Suppl 1):70–79.
10. Gartsman GM, Roddey TS, Hammerman SM. Arthroscopic treatment of anterior-inferior glenohumeral instability: two- to five-year follow-up. J Bone Joint Surg Am 2000;82A:991–1003.
11. Hovelius L. Incidence of shoulder dislocation in Sweden. Clin Orthop Relat Res 1982:127–131.
12. Hovelius L, Augustini BG, Fredin H, et al. Primary anterior dislocation of the shoulder in young patients: a ten-year prospective study. J Bone Joint Surg Am 1996;78A:1677–1684.
13. Hovelius L, Olofsson A, Sandström B, et al. Nonoperative treatment of primary anterior shoulder dislocation in patients forty years of age and younger. A prospective twenty-five-year follow-up. J Bone Joint Surg Am 2008;90(5):945–952.
14. Itoi E, Hatakeyama Y, Kido T, et al. A new method of immobilization after traumatic anterior dislocation of the shoulder: a preliminary study. J Shoulder Elbow Surg 2003;12:413–415.
15. Itoi E, Hatakeyama Y, Sato T, et al. Immobilization in external rotation after shoulder dislocation reduces the risk of recurrence. A randomized controlled trial. J Bone Joint Surg Am 2007;89(10): 2124–2131.

16. Itoi E, Lee SB, Amrami KK, et al. Quantitative assessment of classic anteroinferior bony Bankart lesions by radiography and computed tomography. Am J Sports Med 2003;31:112–118.
17. Itoi E, Sashi R, Minagawa H, et al. Position of immobilization after dislocation of the glenohumeral joint: a study with use of magnetic resonance imaging. J Bone Joint Surg Am 2001;83A: 661–667.
18. Kim SH, Ha KI, Cho YB, et al. Arthroscopic anterior stabilization of the shoulder: two- to six-year follow-up. J Bone Joint Surg Am 2003; 85A:1511–1518.
19. Kirkley A, Griffin S, Richards C, et al. Prospective randomized clinical trial comparing the effectiveness of immediate arthroscopic stabilization versus immobilization and rehabilitation in first traumatic anterior dislocations of the shoulder. Arthroscopy 1999;15: 507–514.
20. Kirkley A, Werstine R, Ratjek A, et al. Prospective randomized clinical trial comparing the effectiveness of immediate arthroscopic stabilization versus immobilization and rehabilitation in first traumatic anterior dislocations of the shoulder: long-term evaluation. Arthroscopy 2005;21:55–63.
21. Larrain MV, Botto GJ, Montenegro HJ, et al. Arthroscopic repair of acute traumatic anterior shoulder dislocation in young athletes. Arthroscopy 2001;17:373–377.
22. Mazzocca AD, Brown FM Jr, Carreira DS, et al. Arthroscopic anterior shoulder stabilization of collision and contact athletes. Am J Sports Med 2005;33:52–60.
23. McLaughlin HL, MacLellan DI. Recurrent anterior dislocation of the shoulder. II. A comparative study. J Trauma 1967;7:191–201.
24. Mizuno N, Yoneda M, Hayashida K, et al. Recurrent anterior shoulder dislocation caused by a midsubstance complete capsular tear. J Bone Joint Surg Am 2005;87A:2717–2723.
25. Neviaser TJ. The anterior labroligamentous periosteal sleeve avulsion lesion: a cause of anterior instability of the shoulder. Arthroscopy 1993;9:17–21.
26. Robinson CM, Jenkins PJ, White TO, et al. Primary arthroscopic stabilization for a first-time anterior dislocation of the shoulder. A randomized, double-blind trial. J Bone Joint Surg Am 2008;90(4): 708–721.
27. Rowe CR. Recurrent dislocation of the shoulder. Lancet 1956;270: 428–429.
28. Rowe CR, Sakellarides HT. Factors related to recurrences of anterior dislocations of the shoulder. Clin Orthop 1961;20:40–48.
29. Sachs RA, Lin D, Stone ML, et al. Can the need for future surgery for acute traumatic anterior shoulder dislocation be predicted? J Bone Joint Surg Am 2007;89(8):1665–1674.
30. Soslowsky LJ, Flatow EL, Bigliani LU, et al. Articular geometry of the glenohumeral joint. Clin Orthop Relat Res 1992:181–190.
31. Sugaya H, Moriishi J, Kanisawa I, et al. Arthroscopic osseous Bankart repair for chronic recurrent traumatic anterior glenohumeral instability. J Bone Joint Surg Am 2005;87A:1752–1760.
32. Tauber M, Resch H, Forstner R, et al. Reasons for failure after surgical repair of anterior shoulder instability. J Shoulder Elbow Surg 2004;13:279–285.
33. te Slaa RL, Wijffels MP, Brand R, et al. The prognosis following acute primary glenohumeral dislocation. J Bone Joint Surg Br 2004; 86B:58–64.
34. Westerheide KJ, Dopirak RM, Snyder SJ. Arthroscopic anterior stabilization and posterior capsular plication for anterior glenohumeral instability: a report of 71 cases. Arthroscopy 2006;22:539–547.
35. Wheeler JH, Ryan JB, Arciero RA, et al. Arthroscopic versus nonoperative treatment of acute shoulder dislocations in young athletes. Arthroscopy 1989;5:213–217.

Chapter **3**

Arthroscopic Treatment of Posterior Shoulder Instability

Fotios P. Tjoumakaris and James P. Bradley

DEFINITION

- Posterior shoulder instability results in pathologic glenohumeral translation ranging from mild subluxation to traumatic dislocation. Most patients with this pathologic entity report pain in provocative positions of the glenohumeral joint, a condition referred to as recurrent posterior subluxation.
- Posterior shoulder instability is much less common than anterior instability, representing about 5% to 10% of all patients with pathologic shoulder instability.[2,5,10]
- A decision must be made regarding surgical treatment of this condition when an extended trial of conservative measures, such as physical therapy, has failed.

ANATOMY

- The important stabilizing structures of the glenohumeral joint are the articular surfaces and congruity of the humerus and glenoid of the scapula, the capsular structures, the glenoid labrum, the intra-articular portion of the biceps tendon, and the rotator cuff muscles.
- Pathologies of the posterior capsule and labral complex are believed to be the main contributors to posterior instability.
- With the arm forward-flexed to 90 degrees, the subscapularis provides significant stability against posterior translation, and as the arm is placed in neutral, the coracohumeral ligament resists this force. With internal rotation of the shoulder (follow-through phase of throwing), the inferior glenohumeral ligament complex is the main restraint to posterior translation.[1]
- Histologic evaluation of the posterior capsule shows it to be relatively thin and composed of only radial and circular fibers, with minimal cross-linking.

PATHOGENESIS

- Posterior instability can be the result of trauma in the form of a direct blow to the anterior shoulder or may occur as the result of indirect forces acting on the shoulder, causing the combined movements of shoulder flexion, adduction, and internal rotation.[13]
- Electrocution and seizures are the most common causes of an indirect mechanism resulting in posterior dislocation.
- Patients with recurrent posterior subluxation may present with more vague symptoms, with pain being the chief complaint. Athletes may report that velocity with throwing is diminished, and a sharp pain may accompany the follow-through phase of throwing.
- Other associated injuries such as superior labrum anterior posterior (SLAP) lesions, rotator cuff tears, reverse Hill-Sachs defects, and chondral injuries may be present and contribute to the pathology.[4]

NATURAL HISTORY

- Patients with a history of a chronically locked posterior dislocation are at increased risk for the development of chondral injury and subsequent degenerative arthritis.[6]
- Static posterior subluxations of the humeral head have been correlated with the presence of arthritis in young adults whose instability was left untreated.[14]
- No long-term studies on the arthroscopic treatment of shoulder instability have documented a reduction in the development of osteoarthritis.

PATIENT HISTORY AND PHYSICAL FINDINGS

- A thorough history is obtained, documenting whether a dislocation has occurred (as well as the need for closed reduction) or if the primary symptoms are pain.
- The circumstances regarding pain are documented, namely onset (provocations), severity, ability to participate in sports, and whether symptoms are present at rest.
- Any response to conservative treatment (ie, physical therapy, rest, anti-inflammatory medication) should be noted.
- As with the examination of any joint, the shoulder is palpated to elicit tenderness and range of motion is documented. Any restriction in motion should be compared to the contralateral extremity, and differences between active and passive motion may indicate pain or capsular contracture.
- Impingement signs are tested to determine whether any associated rotator cuff tendinitis is present.
- Other examinations for posterior instability are:
  - Strength testing. Weakness may be the result of deconditioning or may indicate underlying rotator cuff or deltoid pathology.
  - Load and shift test. The degree of pathologic subluxation is assessed, as well as any apprehension or pain experienced by the patient during provocative testing.
  - Jerk test. A positive jerk test indicates pathologic posterior subluxation.
  - Kim test. A positive Kim test suggests a posteroinferior labral tear or subluxation.
  - Circumduction test. A positive test result is highly suspicious of posterior subluxation or dislocation.
  - Sulcus sign evaluation. A positive sulcus sign suggests multidirectional instability.

IMAGING AND OTHER DIAGNOSTIC STUDIES

- Plain radiographs, including a glenohumeral anteroposterior view, scapular Y view, axillary lateral view, and supraspinatus outlet view, should be obtained to rule out associated injuries, bone defects (either humeral or glenoid), or degenerative changes (**FIG 1A**).
- Magnetic resonance (MR) arthrography is currently the best method for imaging the posterior capsulolabral structures.
- Findings on MR suggestive of posterior instability are posterior humeral head translation, posterior labral injury, posterior labrocapsular avulsion, humeral avulsion of the posterior band of the inferior glenohumeral ligament, posterior glenoid bone defects, and anterior humeral head bone defects (**FIG 1B**).

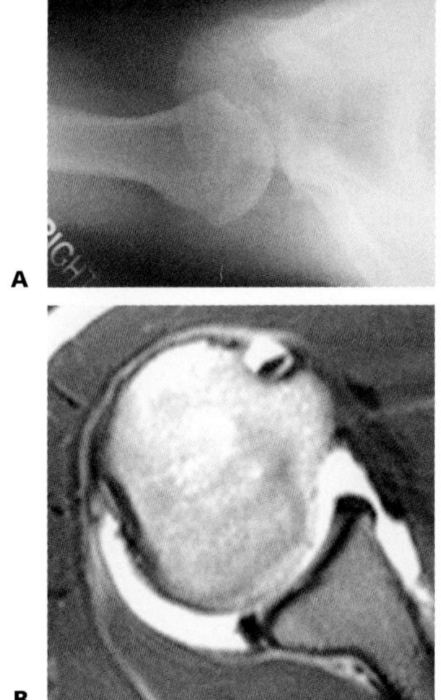

FIG 1 • **A.** Axillary lateral radiograph that demonstrates glenoid hypoplasia, which predisposes to posterior instability of the shoulder. **B.** Axial image from an MR arthrogram that demonstrates a posterior labral lesion. Contrast can be seen between the posterior labrum and the articular margin of the glenoid, indicating a labral tear or avulsion.

DIFFERENTIAL DIAGNOSIS

- Posterior shoulder dislocation (may be locked)
- Recurrent posterior subluxation
- Multidirectional instability
- Internal impingement
- SLAP tear
- Rotator cuff tear
- Acromioclavicular joint injury
- Fracture (eg, glenoid, greater tuberosity)

NONOPERATIVE MANAGEMENT

- An extended period of nonoperative management is warranted in most cases of posterior shoulder instability.
- Nonoperative therapy constitutes physical therapy to regain a full and symmetric shoulder range of motion, with later emphasis placed on strengthening the rotator cuff and scapular stabilizing muscles.
- The premise of a conditioning program is to enable the dynamic stabilizers of the shoulder to compensate for the deficient static stabilizers (eg, capsule, labrum).
- Once full motion and strength are achieved, return to sport is gradually introduced.

SURGICAL MANAGEMENT

- Surgical management of posterior instability is considered when an exhaustive rehabilitation program has failed to alleviate disabling posterior subluxation, or when instability is the result of a macrotraumatic event.

Preoperative Planning

- All imaging studies are again reviewed and the pathology is determined.
- Any bone deficiencies, loose bodies, and concomitant rotator cuff and SLAP tears should be evaluated and treatment determined before arrival in the operating room.
- An examination under anesthesia is performed before positioning to confirm the diagnosis. This examination should consist of sulcus test, load and shift test, and manual circumduction test or jerk test.

Positioning

- We prefer lateral decubitus positioning because this offers greater exposure than the beach-chair position for evaluating the posterior labrum and capsule.
- An inflatable beanbag and kidney rests hold the patient in the lateral position.
- Foam cushions are used to pad the axilla and all bony prominences, including the fibular head (protection of the peroneal nerve).
- The operative extremity is placed in 10 pounds of traction in 45 degrees of abduction and 20 degrees of forward flexion (**FIG 2**).

Approach

- We use an all-arthroscopic technique for this procedure, with a posterior portal that is used as the main working portal (through the posterior deltoid) and an anterior portal (placed through the rotator interval) that is used for arthroscopic visualization.

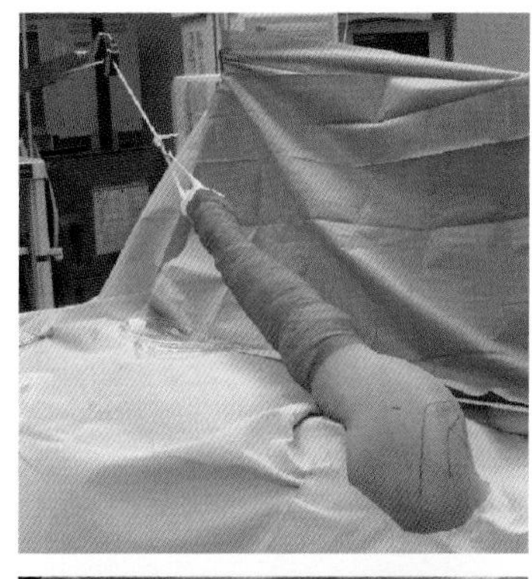

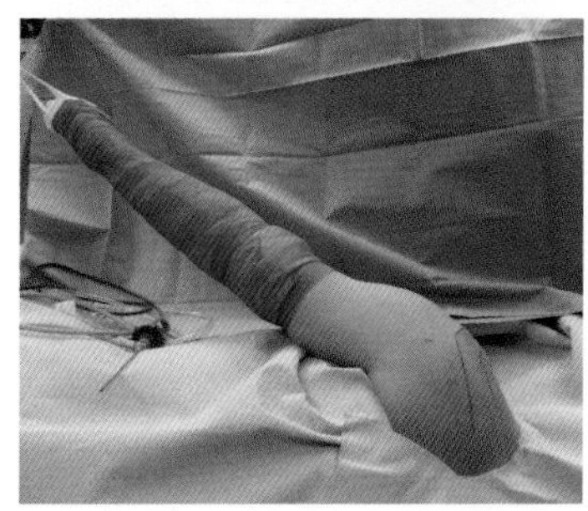

FIG 2 • **A.** Lateral decubitus is the preferred position for arthroscopic surgery of the posterior capsule and labrum. **B.** The arm is placed in 10 to 15 pounds of traction and slightly abducted and forward flexed.

TECHNIQUES

PORTAL PLACEMENT

- The glenohumeral joint is first injected (posteriorly) with 50 mL of sterile saline through an 18-gauge spinal needle.
- A posterior portal is established 1 cm distal and 1 cm lateral to the standard posterior portal that is used for routine shoulder arthroscopy. This portal is often in line with the lateral border of the acromion (**TECH FIG 1A**).
- Placement of this portal more laterally than typical allows adequate access to the posterior glenoid rim for later anchor placement.
- An anterior portal is established high in the rotator interval via an inside-out technique with a switching stick. As an alternative, this portal can be established with a spinal needle via an outside-in technique (**TECH FIG 1B**).
- The anterior switching stick is then replaced with an 8.25-mm distally threaded clear cannula.

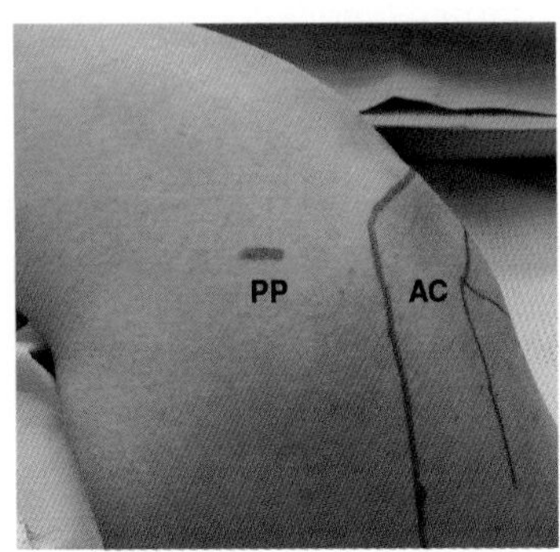

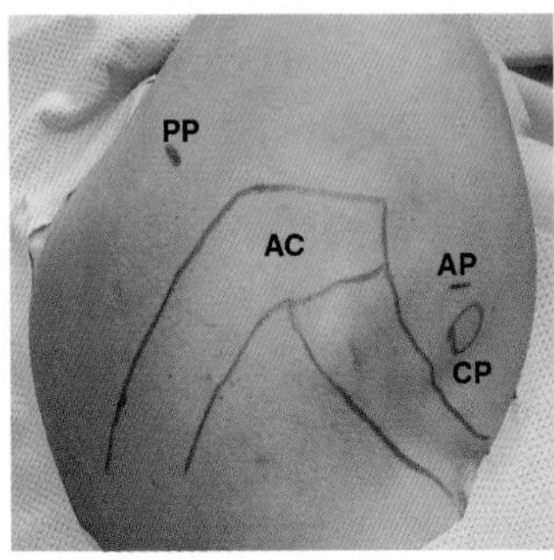

TECH FIG 1 • **A.** The posterior portal (*PP*) is marked in line with the lateral border of the acromion (*AC*). **B.** Surface landmarks identify the posterior portal (*PP*), acromion (*AC*), anterior portal (*AP*), and coracoid process (*CP*).

DIAGNOSTIC ARTHROSCOPY

- With the arthroscope in the posterior portal, a diagnostic arthroscopy is performed.
- The articular surfaces of the glenohumeral joint are inspected for chondral damage. The posterolateral aspect of the humeral head is inspected for any Hill-Sachs lesions (which may indicate combined anterior instability).
- The anterior and inferior labrum is inspected and the glenohumeral ligaments are visualized.
- The biceps tendon and superior labrum are probed to detect any pathology. Concomitant SLAP tears are common with posterior instability.
- The rotator cuff is inspected (including the subscapularis tendon).
- A switching stick is then placed in the posterior portal and replaced with an additional 8.25-mm distally threaded clear cannula. The arthroscope is then replaced into the anterior cannula for viewing; it remains there for the rest of the operation.
- The posterior capsule and labrum are inspected and probed (**TECH FIG 2**).
- The anterior humeral head surface is inspected for any reverse Hill-Sachs lesions, which may indicate macroinstability.

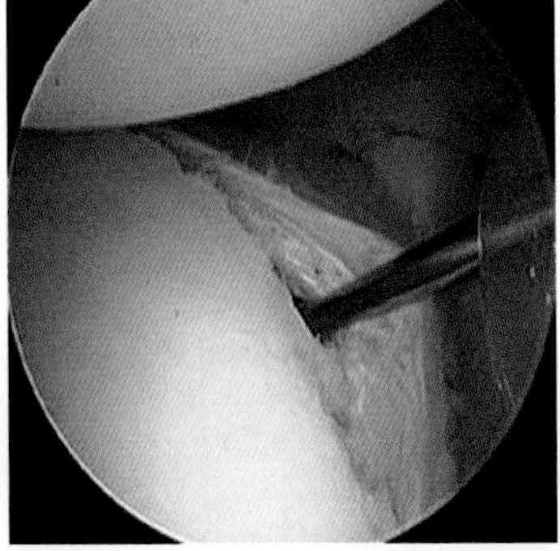

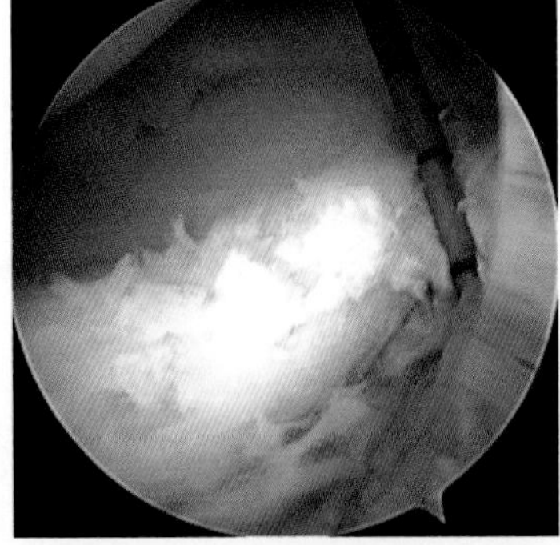

TECH FIG 2 • **A.** Arthroscopic view from the posterior portal showing an avulsed posterior labrum. **B.** A complete avulsion of the labrum off the posterior glenoid is visualized from the posterior portal.

PREPARATION OF THE GLENOID AND PLACEMENT OF SUTURE ANCHORS

- Typically the posterior labrum is detached and the capsule attenuated, requiring the placement of suture anchors.
- An arthroscopic rasp or chisel is used to mobilize the labrum from the glenoid rim.
- The rasp is then used to débride the capsule to create an optimal environment for healing.
- A motorized shaver or burr can be used on the glenoid rim to achieve a bleeding surface for healing.
- Suture anchors are placed along the articular margin, not the glenoid neck, for the repair and capsular plication (**TECH FIG 3A**).
- Typically we use three, 3-mm Bio-Suture Tak suture anchors with no. 2 FiberWire (Arthrex Inc., Naples, FL). A number of other commercially available anchors can be used in a similar fashion.
- The anchor pilot holes are predrilled and the anchor is inserted with a mallet.
- The anchor is placed so that the sutures are perpendicular to the glenoid rim. This facilitates passage of the most posterior suture through the torn labrum.
- The anchors are evenly spaced on the posterior glenoid rim for a symmetric repair (**TECH FIG 3B**).

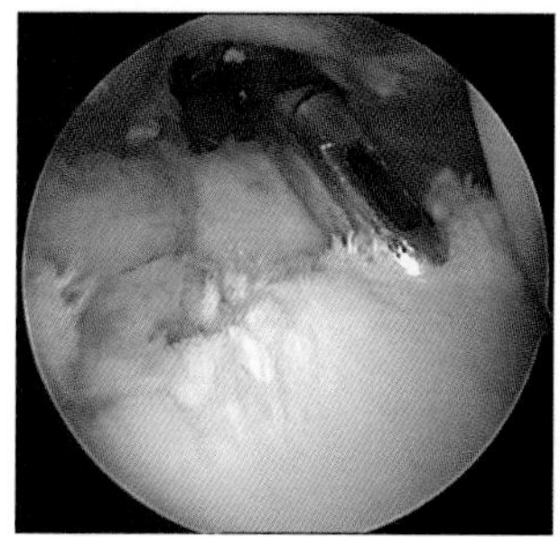

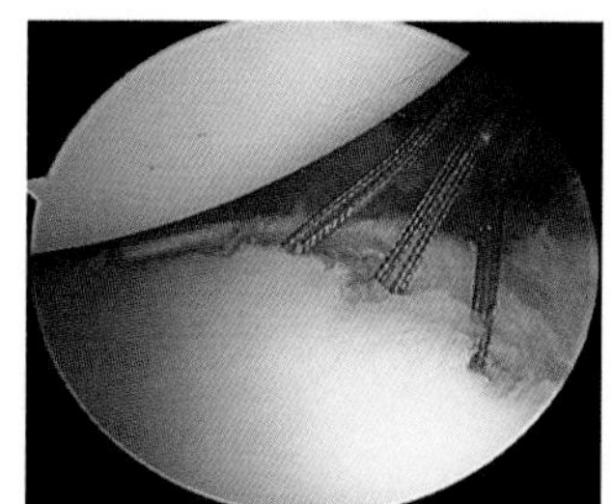

TECH FIG 3 • **A.** The anchor is placed on the glenoid margin. A drill is used to place a pilot hole before insertion of the anchor. **B.** The anchors are evenly spaced on the posterior glenoid margin to provide a symmetric and balanced repair.

LABRAL AND CAPSULAR REPAIR

- A 45-degree Spectrum Hook (Linvatec Corp., Largo, FL) loaded with number 0 PDS suture (Ethicon, Somerville, NJ) is used to shuttle the suture through the capsule and labrum (**TECH FIG 4A**).
- The suture hook is delivered through the capsule (if a plication is warranted) and under the torn labrum at the articular margin of the glenoid.
  - An inferior-to-superior direction is used for this maneuver to achieve a small capsular plication.
- This direction of suture passage is aimed at restoring tension to the posterior band of the inferior glenohumeral ligament.
  - Patients with significant instability clinically may require a more aggressive plication than those with isolated pathology to the glenoid labrum.
- The PDS is fed into the glenohumeral joint and the passer is withdrawn.

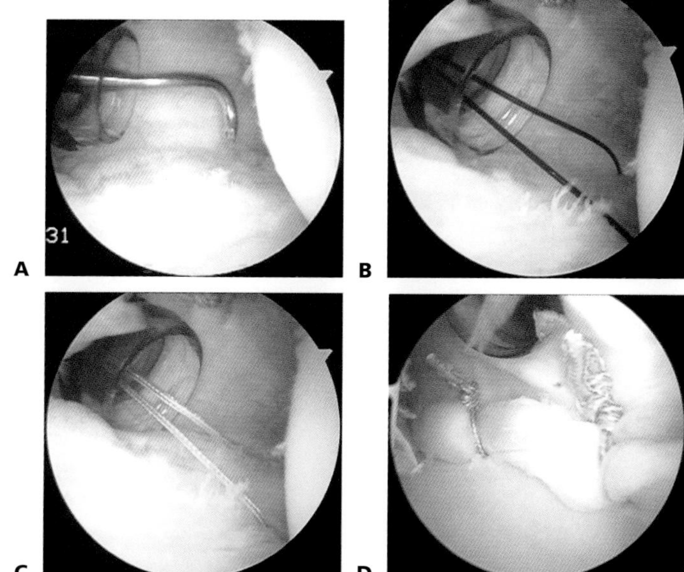

TECH FIG 4 • **A.** A suture hook is used to shuttle the anchor limb through the capsulolabral complex. **B.** The PDS suture has been passed through the capsule and posterior labrum. **C.** The anchor limb suture is then shuttled via the PDS suture. **D.** The sutures are tied using arthroscopic knot-tying techniques through the posterior portal, and the capsulolabral plication is finished.

TECHNIQUES

- A suture grasper is then used to withdraw the most posterior suture in the anchor and the PDS that has been delivered through the capsulolabral complex.
  - Grabbing the more posterior suture helps to ensure that the suture limbs do not become entangled.
- The PDS is then fashioned into a single loop and tied over the braided FiberWire suture.
- The opposite limb of the PDS is then pulled and the FiberWire is delivered through the labrum and capsule (**TECH FIG 4B,C**).
- Additional sutures are then shuttled in similar fashion to complete the repair.
- After each suture has been shuttled through the capsule and labral complex, it is tied using arthroscopic knot-tying techniques (**TECH FIG 4D**).
- We prefer to begin our repair inferiorly and advance superiorly up the posterior glenoid rim. In this way, the tension achieved with each advancing stitch can be assessed.

REPAIR COMPLETION

- An arthroscopic awl is used to penetrate the posterior bare area of the humerus in an effort to achieve punctate bleeding to augment the healing response.
- The posterior cannula is then withdrawn to just posterior to the level of the capsule and the posterior capsular incision is closed with a PDS suture.
- A crescent Spectrum suture passer is used to penetrate one side of the capsule by the posterior capsular incision, and the suture is threaded into the joint.
- The suture is retrieved through the opposite side of the incision with a penetrator and an arthroscopic knot is tied down to close the portal (**TECH FIG 5**).
- Varying the distance of the suture from the portal incision allows additional tension to be applied to the posterior capsule.
- If additional plication is warranted (such as in multidirectional instability), additional sutures can be placed in the rotator interval or anterior capsule as described elsewhere in this text.
- The skin portals are closed with interrupted nylon suture and the patient is placed in a sling that allows slight abduction.

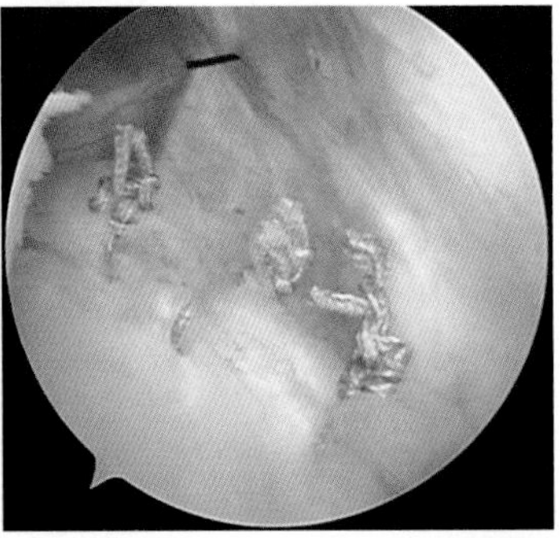

TECH FIG 5 • The repair is completed after closure of the posterior portal (suture shown in black).

PEARLS AND PITFALLS

Indications	■ A thorough history and examination with correlating radiographic studies help in determining the correct diagnosis. ■ Patients should be counseled extensively on nonoperative therapy.
Patient positioning	■ Debate exists as to which position allows better exposure of the posterior glenoid. ■ The surgeon should feel comfortable with whichever position is chosen; however, we feel that the lateral decubitus position offers better visualization.
Portal placement	■ Placing the posterior portal slightly lateral to the standard portal allows for easier placement of the anchors. ■ Placing the anterior portal superior in the rotator interval allows better visualization.
Anchor placement	■ Placing the anchors perpendicular to the glenoid margin and shuttling the posterior suture is paramount in preventing suture entanglement.
Repair	■ The repair should be tailored to the precise pathology of the patient as determined by the history, physical examination, and imaging studies. Patients without labral pathology may require an isolated plication. ■ We prefer suture anchors regardless of which type of repair is necessary (capsule plication, capsulolabral plication, or labral repair).
Knot tying	■ The surgeon should feel comfortable with both sliding and nonsliding knots before attempting arthroscopic repair techniques.

POSTOPERATIVE CARE

- The patient leaves the operating room in an abduction sling that can be removed for passive range-of-motion exercises at home.
  - We allow 90 degrees of forward elevation and external rotation to 0 degrees by 4 weeks after surgery.
- The sling is discontinued 6 weeks after surgery and active-assisted range-of-motion exercises and gentle passive range-of-motion exercises are progressed.
- Pain-free, gentle internal rotation exercises are instituted at 6 weeks.
- At 2 to 3 months after surgery, range of motion is progressed to achieve full passive and active range of motion.
  - Stretching exercises can be instituted for any deficiency in motion at this point.
- After 4 months, the shoulder is often pain-free and eccentric rotator cuff strengthening is begun.
- At 5 months, isotonic and isokinetic exercises are advanced.
- At 6 months, throwing athletes undergo isokinetic strength testing.
  - If 80% of the strength and endurance of the contralateral extremity is attained, a throwing program is begun.
  - Full, competitive throwing is typically not attained until 12 months after surgery.
- Nonthrowing athletes are often released to a sport-specific program by 6 months, when 80% of their strength has returned.

OUTCOMES

- Arthroscopic posterior stabilization has achieved good results with respect to recurrence of instability and return to sport in athletes.
- Studies have shown rates of recurrence of 0% to 8% and rates of return to sport of 89% to 100%.[3,7,15]

COMPLICATIONS

- Recurrent instability
- Stiffness
- Infection
- Neurovascular injury

REFERENCES

1. Blasier RB, Soslowsky LJ, Malicky DM, et al. Posterior glenohumeral subluxation: active and passive stabilization in a biomechanical model. J Bone Joint Surg Am 1997;79A:433–440.
2. Boyd HB, Sisk TD. Recurrent posterior dislocation of the shoulder. J Bone Joint Surg Am 1972;54A:779.
3. Bradley JP, Baker CL 3rd, Kline AJ, et al. Arthroscopic capsulolabral reconstruction for posterior instability of the shoulder: a prospective study of 100 shoulders. Am J Sports Med 2006;34: 1061–1071.
4. Gartsman GM, Hammerman SM. Superior labrum anterior and posterior lesions: when and how to treat them. Clin Sports Med 2000; 19:115–124.
5. Hawkins RJ, Koppert G, Johnston G. Recurrent posterior instability (subluxation) of the shoulder. J Bone Joint Surg Am 1984;66A: 169.
6. Keppler P, Holz U, Thielemann FW, et al. Locked posterior dislocation of the shoulder: treatment using rotational osteotomy of the humerus. J Orthop Trauma 1994;8:286–292.
7. Kim SH, Ha KI, Park JH, et al. Arthroscopic posterior labral repair and capsular shift for traumatic unidirectional recurrent posterior subluxation of the shoulder. J Bone Joint Surg Am 2003;85A: 1479–1487.
8. Kim SH, Park JC, Jeong WK, et al. The Kim test: a novel test for posteroinferior labral lesion of the shoulder: a comparison to the jerk test. Am J Sports Med 2005;33:1188–1192.
9. Kim SH, Park JC, Park JS, et al. Painful jerk test: a predictor of success in nonoperative treatment of posteroinferior instability of the shoulder. Am J Sports Med 2004;32:1849–1855.
10. McLaughlin HL. Posterior dislocation of the shoulder. J Bone Joint Surg Am 1952;34A:584.
11. Pollock RG, Bigliani LU. Recurrent posterior shoulder instability. Diagnosis and treatment. Clin Orthop Relat Res 1993;291:85–96.
12. Silliman JF, Hawkins RJ. Classification and physical diagnosis of instability of the shoulder. Clin Orthop Relat Res 1993;291:7–19.
13. Tibone JE, Bradley JP. The treatment of posterior subluxation in athletes. Clin Orthop 1993;291:124–137.
14. Walch G, Ascani C, Boulahia A, et al. Static posterior subluxation of the humeral head: an unrecognized entity responsible for glenohumeral osteoarthritis in the young adult. J Shoulder Elbow Surg 2002;11:309–314.
15. Williams RJ III, Strickland S, Cohen M, et al. Arthroscopic repair for traumatic posterior shoulder instability. Am J Sports Med 2003; 31:203–209.

Chapter 4

Arthroscopic Treatment of Multidirectional Shoulder Instability

Steven B. Cohen and Jon K. Sekiya

DEFINITION

- Neer and colleagues[14] described the concept of multidirectional instability of the shoulder in detail in 1980.
  - This established the difference between unidirectional instability and global laxity of the capsule inferiorly, posteriorly, and anteriorly.
- Subjective complaints of pain and global shoulder instability
- Subluxation or dislocation from traumatic, microtraumatic, or atraumatic injury

ANATOMY

- Stability of the shoulder relies on dynamic and static restraints.
- Static restraints:
  - Inferior glenohumeral ligament
    - Anterior band resists anterior translation in 90 degrees of abduction and external rotation.
    - Posterior band resists posterior translation in forward flexion, adduction, and internal rotation.
  - Middle glenohumeral ligament
    - Resists anterior translation in 45 degrees of abduction
  - Superior glenohumeral ligament
    - Resists posterior and inferior translation with arm at side
  - Rotator interval and coracohumeral ligament
    - Resists posterior and inferior translation with arm at side
- Dynamic restraints
  - Rotator cuff muscles
  - Deltoid
  - Effects of concavity and compression
- Shoulder instability has been found to be a result of several pathologic processes:
  - Capsular laxity
  - Labral detachment and Bankart lesion
  - Rotator interval defects

PATHOGENESIS

- Typically, there is not a history of a traumatic shoulder dislocation, but it may be the inciting event. Most commonly, the instability is due to microtrauma resulting in global capsular laxity.
- There may be a history of recurrent dislocations or repetitive subluxation events.
- Patients are typically young and active and present with the following:
  - Pain
  - Complaints of shoulder shifting
  - Difficulty with overhead activity
  - Inability to do sports
  - Instability while sleeping
  - Trouble with activities of daily living
  - Episodes of "dead arm" sensation
  - Failed prior attempts at physical therapy

NATURAL HISTORY

- Unable to change static restraints
- Stability can be achieved by restoring neuromuscular control through rehabilitation.
- Recurrent dislocations may lead to Hill-Sachs lesions, glenoid erosion, or chondral injury, which may predispose to early degenerative arthritis of the glenohumeral joint.
- Recurrent instability affecting daily activities despite formal physical therapy generally requires surgical treatment.

PHYSICAL FINDINGS

- Infrequent atrophy
- Symmetric range of motion
  - Possible scapulothoracic winging
  - Loss of active motion may be related to pain.
  - Loss of passive motion may be from capsular contracture.
- Normal strength testing
  - Loss of strength can indicate rotator cuff pathology or nerve injury.
- Evaluation for ligamentous laxity
  - Frequently positive for generalized ligamentous laxity
  - Predisposed to shoulder instability
- Evaluation for impingement. Impingement may be a sign of rotator cuff tendinitis or internal impingement in throwers.
- Stability testing
  - Positive increased load and shift test for anterior and posterior translation
  - Positive sulcus sign (both in neutral and external rotation) for inferior translation
  - A sulcus sign graded as 3+ that remains 2+ in external rotation is pathognomonic for multidirectional instability.
- Specific tests
  - Apprehension test: Positive result indicates anterior instability.
  - Relocation test: Positive result indicates anterior instability.
  - O'Brien sign: Pain or click indicates a superior labrum anterior posterior (SLAP) tear; anterosuperior pain indicates acromioclavicular joint pathology.
  - Jerk test: Positive result indicates posteroinferior instability.
  - Kim test: Positive result indicates posteroinferior instability.
  - Circumduction test: Positive result indicates posterior instability.
  - Speed's test: Positive result indicates biceps tendinitis or SLAP tear.

IMAGING AND DIAGNOSTIC STUDIES

- Plain radiographs
  - Anteroposterior view

Table 1 MRI Findings

Structure	MRI Finding
Anterior labrum	+/– Bankart tear
Posterior labrum	+/– Labral tear
Superior labrum	+/– Superior labrum anterior posterior (SLAP) tear
Inferior capsule	+/– Capsular laxity, enlarged axillary pouch
Humeral head	+/– Hill-Sachs or reverse Hill-Sachs lesion
Glenoid	+/– Bony Bankart or glenoid erosion

- Axillary lateral or West Point axillary view
- Outlet view
- Stryker notch view
- Evaluate for:
  - Hill-Sachs or reverse Hill-Sachs lesion
  - Glenoid pathology
  - Bony humeral avulsion of the glenohumeral ligaments

- Magnetic resonance (MR) arthrogram (Table 1): Evaluate for:
  - Capsular laxity
  - Labral pathology
  - Biceps tendon pathology
  - Rotator cuff lesions (rare)
- Computed tomography
  - Evaluate for proximal humeral and glenoid bony pathology.

NONOPERATIVE TREATMENT

- In many patients with atraumatic multidirectional instability, proper neuromuscular control of dynamic glenohumeral stability has been lost.
- The goal is to restore shoulder function through training and exercise.
- Patients with loose shoulders may not necessarily be unstable, as evidenced by examining the contralateral asymptomatic shoulder in patients with symptomatic multidirectional instability.
- The mainstay of treatment is nonoperative, with attempts to achieve stability using scapular and glenohumeral strengthening exercises.

SURGICAL TREATMENT

Indications

- Patients who have attempted a dedicated program of physical therapy, have functional problems, and remain unstable may then be candidates for surgical treatment.
- Patients with a history of multidirectional instability who sustain fractures of the glenoid or humeral head with a dislocation generally require surgical treatment.
- Patients with significant defects in the humeral head associated with multiple dislocations consistent with Hill-Sachs lesions may require earlier surgical treatment.
- Glenoid erosion or lip fractures, if significant, can also necessitate surgical intervention if associated with recurrent instability.

Contraindications

- Patients with voluntary or habitual instability
- Patients who have not attempted a formal physiotherapy program should avoid initial surgical treatment.
- Any patient unable or unwilling to comply with the postoperative rehabilitation regimen

Surgical Planning

- Patient education is critical in planning surgical treatment for the patient with an unstable shoulder.
- Patients should have failed a trial at nonoperative treatment and have persistent instability with functional deficits.
- The goal of surgical treatment is to reduce capsular volume and restore glenoid concavity with capsulolabral augmentation.
- Decreasing capsular volume may lead to decreased range of motion.
  - It is important to discuss this possibility with the patient because some more active athletic patients such as throwers, gymnasts, and volleyball players may not tolerate losses of motion to maintain participation in their sport.
- Additional risks should be discussed, including infection, recurrence of instability, pain, neurovascular injury, persistent functional limitations, and implant complications.
- The surgical planning continues with the evaluation under anesthesia and diagnostic arthroscopy.
  - This may alter the plan to include any combination of the following: capsular plication (anterior, posterior, or inferior), rotator interval closure, anteroposterior labral repair, SLAP repair, biceps tenodesis or tenotomy, and possible conversion to an open capsular shift.
- Arthroscopic techniques have evolved from capsular shift via transglenoid sutures, Bankart repair and shift with biodegradable tacks or suture anchors, thermal capsulorrhaphy, rotator interval repair, and capsular plication.
  - Standard portals are listed in Table 2.
- Our current method of treatment for patients with multidirectional shoulder instability who have failed to respond to nonoperative attempts is to perform an arthroscopic capsular shift by reducing capsular volume using capsular plication with a multipleated repair.[18]

Table 2 Arthroscopic Portals

Portal	Location
Standard	
Posterior	2 cm inferior and medial to posterolateral border of acromion
Anterosuperior	Lateral to coracoid (external) and just inferior to biceps tendon (internal) in the rotator interval
Anteroinferior	Lateral to coracoid (external) and just superior to subscapularis tendon (internal)
Accessory	
Superior	1 cm lateral and anterior to posterolateral border of acromion
Inferoposterior	2 cm inferior to standard posterior portal
Neviaser	In the notch between posterior acromioclavicular joint and spine of scapula

Anesthesia and Patient Positioning

- The procedure can be performed under interscalene block or general endotracheal anesthesia with an interscalene block for postoperative pain control.
- The patient is then placed in the lateral decubitus position with the affected shoulder positioned superior.
  - An inflatable beanbag holds the patient in position.
  - Foam cushions are placed to protect the peroneal nerve at the neck of the fibula on the down leg.
  - An axillary roll is placed.
  - The operating table is placed in a slight reverse-Trendelenburg position.
  - The full upper extremity is prepared to the level of the sternum anteriorly and the medial border of the scapula posteriorly.
  - The operative shoulder is placed in 10 pounds of traction and is positioned in 45 degrees of abduction and 20 degrees of forward flexion.
- Alternatively, the beach-chair position can be used. In our experience, however, this position gives limited exposure of the posterior inferior capsule.
  - The head of the bed is raised to about 70 degrees with the affected shoulder off the side of the bed with support medial to the scapula.
  - The head should be well supported and all bony prominences padded.
  - The entire arm, shoulder, and trapezial region are prepared into the surgical field.

TECHNIQUES

ESTABLISHING LANDMARKS AND PORTALS

- The bony landmarks, including the acromion, distal clavicle, acromioclavicular joint, and coracoid process, are demarcated with a marking pen (**TECH FIG 1**).
- After prepping and draping the patient, the glenohumeral joint is injected with 50 mL of sterile saline through an 18-gauge spinal needle to inflate the joint.
- A posterior portal can be established 1 cm proximal (high) and 1 cm lateral (humeral) to the standard posterior portal to allow access to the rim of the posterior glenoid for anchor placement if a posterior labral or capsular repair is necessary.
- An anterior portal is then established in the rotator interval via an outside-in technique using a spinal needle.
  - Care should be taken using the switching stick to verify that the low anterior inferior 5 o'clock anchor can be placed through this portal.
  - If two anterior portals are desired, this portal should be placed "high" in the interval to make room for the second "low" portal.
- Typically, an additional anteroinferior portal is unnecessary using our multipleated technique.
  - If a second portal is desired, it is created using a spinal needle at the level just superior to the subscapularis tendon lateral to the coracoid and at least 1 cm inferior to the anterior portal.

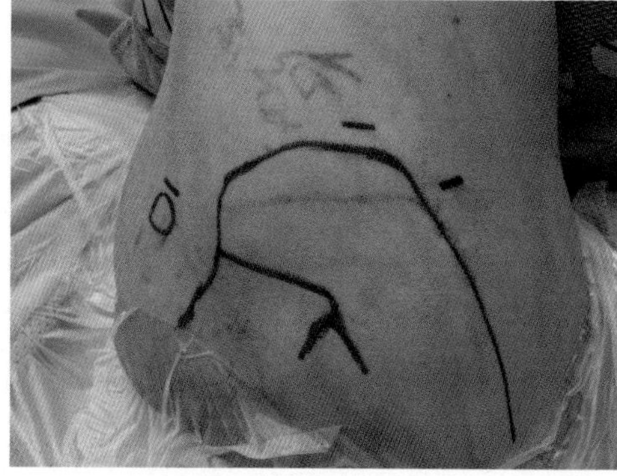

TECH FIG 1 • Arthroscopic portals.

DIAGNOSTIC ARTHROSCOPY

- The examination under anesthesia is performed on a firm surface with the scapula relatively fixed and the humeral head free to rotate.
  - A "load and shift" maneuver, as described by Murrell and Warren,[13] is performed with the patient supine.
  - The arm is held in 90 degrees of abduction and neutral rotation while an anterior or posterior force is applied in an attempt to translate the humeral head over the anterior or posterior glenoid.
  - A "sulcus sign" is performed with the arm adducted and in neutral rotation to assess whether the instability has an inferior component.
  - A 3+ sulcus sign that remains 2+ or greater in external rotation is considered pathognomonic for multidirectional instability.
  - Testing is completed on both the affected and unaffected shoulders, and differences between the two are documented.
- Diagnostic arthroscopy of the glenohumeral joint
  - The labrum, capsule, biceps tendon, subscapularis, rotator interval, rotator cuff, and articular surfaces are visualized in systematic fashion.
    - This ensures that no associated lesions will be overlooked.
  - Lesions typically seen in multidirectional instability include:
    - Patulous inferior capsule
    - Labral tears (**TECH FIG 2**) or fraying and splitting
    - Widening of the rotator interval
    - Articular partial-thickness rotator cuff tears

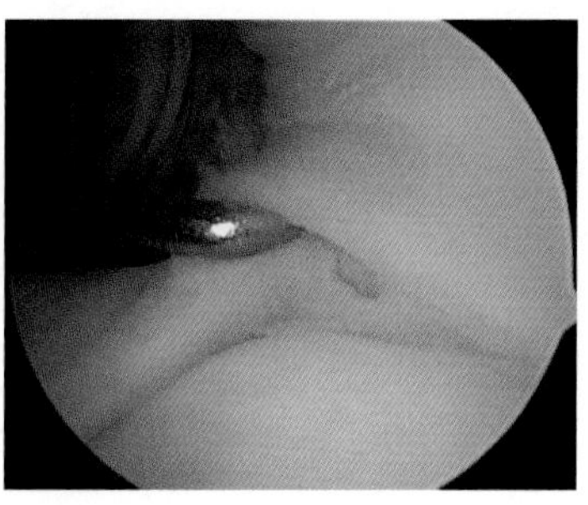

TECH FIG 2 • Labral tear.

- After viewing the glenohumeral joint from the posterior portal, the arthroscope is switched to the anterior portal to allow improved visualization of the posterior capsule and labrum.
- A switching stick can then be used in replacing the posterior cannula with an 8.25-mm distally threaded or fully threaded clear cannula (Arthrex Inc., Naples, FL), thus allowing passage of an arthroscopic probe and other instruments through the clear cannula to explore the posterior labrum for evidence of tears.

PREPARATION FOR REPAIR

- The arthroscope remains in the posterior portal and the anterior portals serve as the working portal for the anterior repair and vice versa for the posterior repair.
- The side (anterior or posterior) that is least unstable is fixed first. For example, if posterior instability is the most severe direction, the anterior and inferior sides are fixed first and the posterior capsule and labrum is addressed last.
- An arthroscopic rasp or chisel is used to mobilize any torn labrum from the glenoid rim (TECH FIG 3A).
- A motorized synovial shaver or meniscal rasp is used to abrade the capsule adjacent to a labral tear and to débride and decorticate the glenoid rim to achieve a bleeding surface for capsular plication (TECH FIG 3B).

A 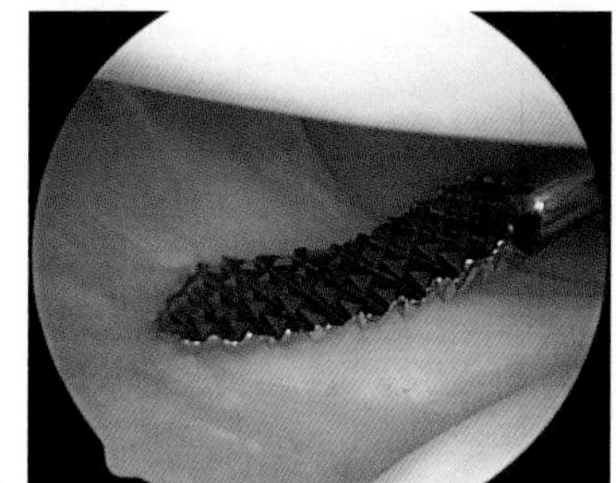

B 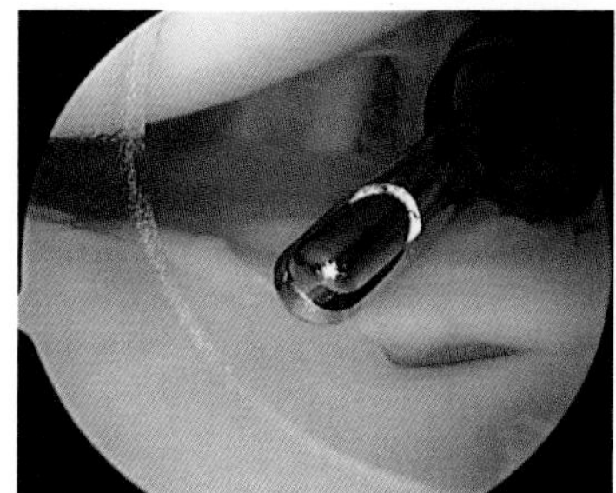

TECH FIG 3 • **A.** Rasping capsule to stimulate healing after capsular plication. **B.** Capsular and glenoid abrasion with a motorized shaver.

MULTIPLEATED PLICATION

- A 3.0-mm Bio-Suture Tak anchor loaded with no. 2 FiberWire (Arthrex, Naples, FL) is placed in the 5 o'clock position (right shoulder) for the anterior repair and the 7 o'clock position for the posterior repair and the sutures are brought out through the working portal (TECH FIG 4A,B).[19]
- A soft tissue penetrator (Spectrum Suture Hook, Linvatec, Largo, FL) or crescent suture passer is passed through the labrum directly adjacent to the anchor and the inferior FiberWire on the anchor is pulled through the labrum (TECH FIG 4C).
- The penetrator is then used to pierce the inferior capsule in the most anteroinferior (5 o'clock anchor) and lateral point or posteroinferior (7 o'clock anchor) and lateral point.
- Once through the capsule, a no. 1 PDS suture (Ethicon, Johnson & Johnson, Somerville, NJ) is shuttled into the joint and the penetrator is removed (TECH FIG 4D).
- A suture grasper is then used to grab both the passed PDS suture and the labral suture and pull them out of the same portal, or the working portal if two portals are used.
- The PDS suture is tied with a simple knot to the FiberWire and then used to shuttle the working suture through the inferior tuck of capsule (TECH FIG 4E).
- This simple process is repeated while moving superiorly up the capsule until adequate capsular tension is restored (TECH FIG 4F). This can be done multiple times until adequate capsular tension is achieved with each suture.
- The suture is checked to ensure it will still slide, and then a locking sliding knot backed with three half-hitches is tied. The remaining suture is then cut (TECH FIG 4G).
- This is begun posteriorly and inferiorly (7 o'clock anchor), working posterior with additional anchors as necessary (TECH FIG 4H), and then anterior and inferiorly (5 o'clock anchor), working up anterior, again using additional anchors as necessary (TECH FIG 4I). This would be the case if anterior instability is the most severe direction. If posterior instability is predominant, then the plication would begin anteriorly and inferiorly and then finish posteriorly.
- The completed multipleated capsular plication reduces volume and improves stability (TECH FIG 4J).

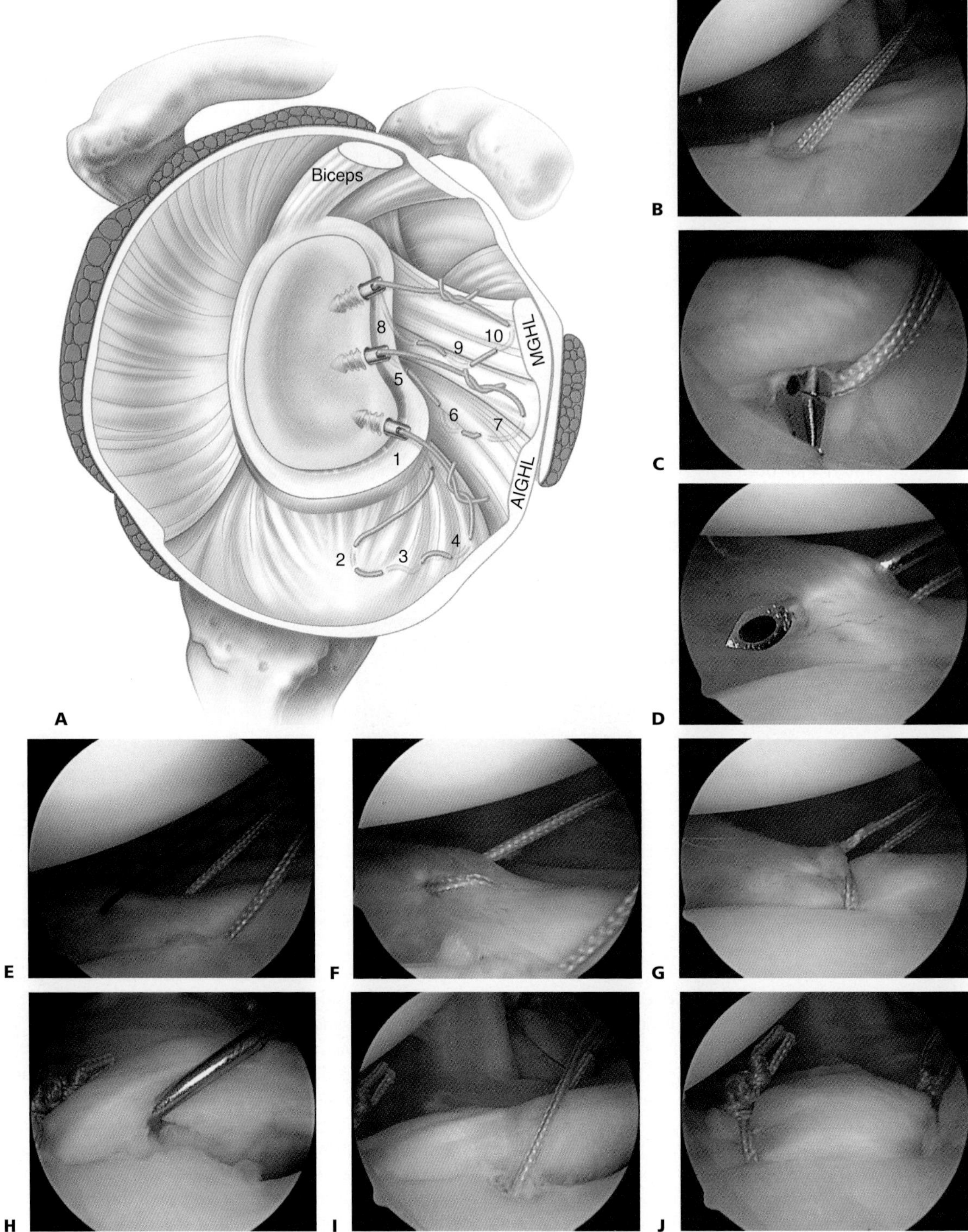

TECH FIG 4 • A. Multipleated plication. **B.** Placing anchor on the rim of the glenoid. **C.** Passing suture through labrum using a suture passer. **D.** Passing Spectrum suture passer in the capsular tissue and placing no. 1 PDS suture. **E**. Passing PDS suture into joint through capsular tissue. **F.** Passing FiberWire suture through capsulolabral tissue after multipleat passage. **G.** Completed tied knot after first anchor and capsular plication. **H.** Residual labral tear remaining after first anchor placed and capsule plicated. **I.** Placing second anchor as necessary for the capsulolabral repair and plication. **J.** Completed plication with multiple anchors.

ARTHROSCOPIC KNOT TYING

- We prefer the sliding, locking Weston knot, but a number of arthroscopic knot-tying techniques work well.
- What is most important is that the surgeon is familiar with the knot used and skilled in its use.
- The posterior braided suture exiting through the capsule is threaded through a knot-pusher and the end is secured with a hemostat.
- This suture serves as the post, which in effect will advance the capsule and labrum to the glenoid rim when the knot is tightened.
- The knot should be secured posteriorly on the capsule, not on the rim of the glenoid, to prevent humeral head abrasion from the knot.
- Each half-hitch must be completely seated before the next half-hitch is thrown.
- Placing tension on the non-post suture and advancing the knot-pusher "past point" will lock the Weston knot.
- A total of three alternating half-hitches are placed to secure the Weston knot.
- This knot has been found to be biomechanically similar to an open square knot.[4]

ROTATOR INTERVAL CLOSURE

- In the setting of multidirectional instability, the rotator interval may not require closure (defined by a 2+ or greater sulcus sign that does not improve in external rotation) if a multipleated repair is performed both anteriorly and posteriorly to bring up the entire axillary pouch.[16]
- However, if rotator interval closure is required, it is viewed with the arthroscope in the posterior portal.
- A crescent suture passer is advanced from the anterior portal through the anterior capsule just above the superior border of the subscapularis tendon 1 cm lateral to the glenoid.
- It is then passed through the middle glenohumeral ligament at the inferior border of the rotator interval. This makes up the inferior aspect of the rotator interval closure.
- A no. 0 PDS suture is then fed into the joint and retrieved with a penetrator through the superior glenohumeral ligament.
- The PDS suture is then withdrawn out the anterior cannula and exchanged for a no. 2 FiberWire. The knot is then tied blindly in the cannula on the outside of the anterior capsule as the closure is visualized through the posterior portal.

POSTERIOR PORTAL CLOSURE

- A crescent suture passer is advanced from the posterior portal through the posterior capsule just above the superior border of the capsular opening of the posterior portal (TECH FIG 5A).
- A no. 0 PDS suture is then fed into the joint and retrieved with a penetrator through the inferior border of the capsular opening in the posterior portal (TECH FIG 5B).
- The PDS suture is then withdrawn out the posterior cannula and exchanged for a no. 2 FiberWire. The knot is tied blindly in the cannula on the outside of the posterior capsule as the closure is visualized through the anterior portal (TECH FIG 5C).

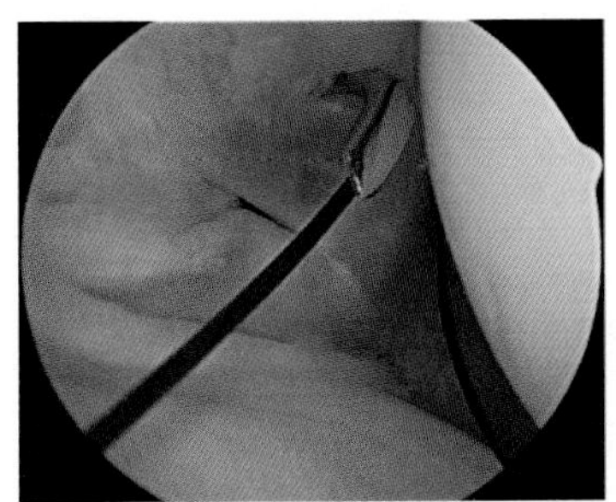

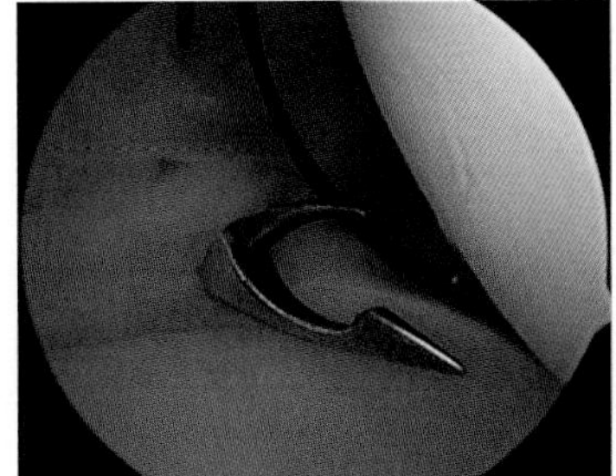

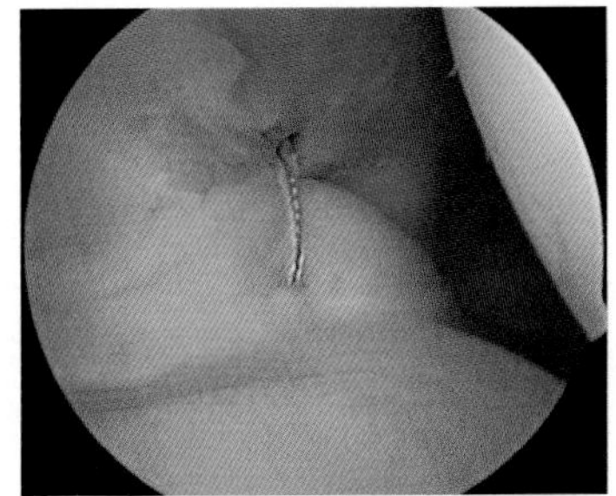

TECH FIG 5 • **A.** Placing crescent suture passer through posterior capsular and passing PDS suture into the joint. **B.** Passing suture grasper through posterior capsule for closure of posterior portal. **C.** Completed closure of the posterior portal after capsular plication.

PEARLS AND PITFALLS

Indications	▪ Persistent pain and functional disability despite appropriate aggressive rehabilitation program
Contraindications	▪ Voluntary dislocators or failure to comply with postoperative rehabilitation program
Multipleated plication technique	▪ Multiple passage of same suture through capsule allows varied amount of volume reduction to address capsular laxity.
Posterior portal closure	▪ Posterior portal closure allows added capsular volume reduction and prevents potential posterior capsule tear from portal location.
Axillary nerve injury	▪ Aggressive passage of Spectrum suture hook in the inferior capsule places axillary nerve at risk. ▪ Shallow capsular penetration prevents injury to axillary nerve.
Recurrent instability	▪ Inadequate capsular volume reduction may allow recurrent instability. ▪ Multipleated technique allows greater capsular volume reduction and restoration of normal tension.

POSTOPERATIVE CARE

- The patient is discharged home on the day of surgery.
- The sutures are removed 6 to 8 days later.
- The arm is immobilized in an Ultrasling (DonJoy, Carlsbad, CA) for 6 weeks (30 degrees abduction in neutral rotation).
- The sling is removed for bathing and for gentle pendulum and elbow, wrist, and hand range-of-motion exercises.
- Isometric exercises are started at week 3, passive and active-assisted range-of-motion exercises at week 3.
- Sling is discontinued at week 6.
- Active range of motion is started at week 6.
- Sport-specific exercises are started at 4 months.
- Overhead sports are started at 6 months.
- The patient can return to contact sports at 6 to 8 months.

OUTCOMES

- Table 3 summarizes outcomes of clinical studies.
- Several studies have investigated the effect of surgical intervention on capsular volume.
- Comparisons have been made between open capsular shifts using numerous techniques, arthroscopic thermal plications, and arthroscopic suture capsular plications by testing capsular volume in cadaveric specimens before and after procedures.
- Table 4 summarizes the results and type of shift performed in these studies.

Table 3 Summary of Clinical Studies of Arthroscopic Treatment of Multidirectional Shoulder Instability

Study	Procedure Performed	Follow-up (mo) Average	Follow-up (mo) Range	Outcome
Duncan & Savoie, 1993[3]	Scope inferior capsular shift		12–36	100% satisfactory
Pagnani et al, 1996[15]	Scope stabilization using transglenoid sutures	55	48–120	74% good or excellent
McIntyre et al, 1997[11]	Scope capsular shift	34		95% good or excellent
Treacy et al, 1999[22]	Scope capsular shift	60		88% satisfactory
Gartsman et al, 2000[8]	Scope labral repair + laser capsulorrhaphy	33	26–63	92% good or excellent
Tauro, 2000[21]	Scope inferior capsular split and advancement		24–60	88% satisfactory
Fitzgerald et al, 2002[6]	Scope thermal capsulorrhaphy	36	24–40	76% satisfactory
Favorito et al, 2002[5]	Scope laser-assisted capsular shift	28		81.5% success
Frostick et al, 2003[7]	Scope laser capsular shrinkage	26	24–33	83% satisfactory
D'Alessandro et al, 2004[2]	Scope thermal capsulorrhaphy	38	24–60	63% satisfactory

Table 4 Summary of Results of In Vitro Capsular Volume Studies

Study	Type of Capsular Shift	Amount of Volume Reduction
Miller et al, 2003[12]	Three open (medial, lateral, vertical)	Medial = 37% Lateral = 50% Vertical = 40%
Karas et al, 2004[9]	Three arthroscopic (thermal, suture plication, combined)	Scope thermal = 33% Scope plication = 19% Scope combined = 41%
Victoroff et al, 2004[23]	Arthroscopic thermal	Scope thermal = 37%
Luke et al, 2004[10]	Open inferior vs. arthroscopic thermal	Open inferior = 50% Scope thermal = 30%
Cohen et al, 2005[1]	Open lateral vs. arthroscopic plication	Open lateral = 50% Scope plication = 23%
Sekiya et al, 2007[17]	Open inferior vs. arthroscopic multipleated plication	Open inferior = 45% Scope multipleated = 58%

COMPLICATIONS

- Loss of motion
- Recurrence of instability
- Neurovascular injury
- Failure to address missed causes of instability
  - Large Hill-Sachs lesions that cause instability and are not addressed at surgery may lead to recurrence.[20]

REFERENCES

1. Cohen SB, Wiley W, Goradia VK, et al. Anterior capsulorrhaphy: an in vitro comparison of volume reduction—arthroscopic plication versus open capsular shift. Arthroscopy 2005;21:659–664.
2. D'Alessandro DF, Bradley JP, Fleischli JE, et al. Prospective evaluation of thermal capsulorrhaphy for shoulder instability: indications and results, two- to five-year follow-up. Am J Sports Med 2004;32:21–33.
3. Duncan R, Savoie FH III. Arthroscopic inferior capsular shift for multidirectional instability of the shoulder: a preliminary report. Arthroscopy 1993;9:24–27.
4. Elkousy HA, Sekiya JK, Stabile KJ, et al. A biomechanical comparison of arthroscopic sliding and sliding-locking knots. Arthroscopy 2005;21:204–210.
5. Favorito PJ, Langenderfer MA, Colosimo AJ, et al. Arthroscopic laser-assisted capsular shift in the treatment of patients with multidirectional shoulder instability. Am J Sports Med 2002;30:322–328.
6. Fitzgerald BT, Watson BT, Lapoint JM. The use of thermal capsulorrhaphy in the treatment of multidirectional instability. J Shoulder Elbow Surg 2002;11:108–113.
7. Frostick SP, Sinopidis C, Al Maskari S, et al. Arthroscopic capsular shrinkage of the shoulder for the treatment of patients with multidirectional instability: minimum 2-year follow-up. Arthroscopy 2003;19:227–233.
8. Gartsman GM, Roddey TS, Hammerman SM. Arthroscopic treatment of anterior-inferior glenohumeral instability: two- to five-year follow-up. J Bone Joint Surg Am 2000;82A:991–1003.
9. Karas SG, Creighton RA, DeMorat GJ. Glenohumeral volume reduction in arthroscopic shoulder reconstruction: a cadaveric analysis of suture plication and thermal capsulorrhaphy. Arthroscopy 2004;20: 179–184.
10. Luke TA, Rovner AD, Karas SG, et al. Volumetric change in the shoulder capsule after open inferior capsular shift versus arthroscopic thermal capsular shrinkage: a cadaveric model. J Shoulder Elbow Surg 2004;13:146–149.
11. McIntyre LF, Caspari RB, Savoie FH III. The arthroscopic treatment of multidirectional shoulder instability: two-year results of a multiple suture technique. Arthroscopy 1997;13:418–425.
12. Miller MD, Larsen KM, Luke T, et al. Anterior capsular shift volume reduction: an in vitro comparison of 3 techniques. J Shoulder Elbow Surg 2003;12:350–354.
13. Murrell GA, Warren RF. The surgical treatment of posterior shoulder instability. Clin Sports Med 1995;14:903.
14. Neer CS II, Foster CR. Inferior capsular shift for involuntary inferior and multidirectional instability of the shoulder: a preliminary report. J Bone Joint Surg Am 1980;62:897–908.
15. Pagnani MJ, Warren RF, Altchek DW, et al. Arthroscopic shoulder stabilization using transglenoid sutures. A four-year minimum follow-up. Am J Sports Med 1996;24:459–467.
16. Sekiya JK, Ong BC, Bradley JP. Thermal capsulorrhaphy for shoulder instability. AAOS Instr Course Lect 2003;52:65–80.
17. Sekiya JK, Willobee JA, Miller MD, et al. Arthroscopic multi-pleated capsular plication compared with open inferior capsular shift for multidirectional instability. Arthroscopy 2007;23:1145–1151.
18. Sekiya JK, Zehms CT. Arthroscopic management of recurrent shoulder instability. Op Tech Sports Med 2006;13:189–195.
19. Sekiya JK. Arthroscopic labral repair and capsular shift of the glenohumeral joint: Technical pearls for a multiple pleated plication through a single working portal. Arthroscopy 2005;21:766.
20. Stehle J, Wickwire AC, Debski RE, et al. A technique to reduce Hill-Sachs lesions after acute anterior dislocation of the shoulder. Tech Shoulder Elbow Surg 2005;6:230–235.
21. Tauro JC. Arthroscopic inferior capsular split and advancement for anterior and inferior shoulder instability: technique and results at 2- to 5-year follow-up. Arthroscopy 2000;16:451–456.
22. Treacy SH, Savoie FH III, Field LD. Arthroscopic treatment of multidirectional instability. J Shoulder Elbow Surg 1999;8: 345–350.
23. Victoroff BN, Deutsch A, Protomastro P, et al. The effect of radiofrequency thermal capsulorrhaphy on glenohumeral translation, rotation, and volume. J Shoulder Elbow Surg 2004;13:138–145.

Chapter 5

Arthroscopic Treatment of Superior Labral (SLAP) Tears

Brian Cole and John-Paul Rue

DEFINITION

- Superior labral (SLAP) tears represent injury to the superior aspect of the glenoid labrum, extending from anterior to posterior, including the biceps anchor.[14]

ANATOMY

- The superior glenoid labrum is composed of fibrocartilaginous tissue between the hyaline cartilage of the glenoid surface and the joint capsule fibrous tissue.[13]
- The vascular supply of the glenoid labrum does not come from the underlying glenoid, but rather from penetrating branches of the suprascapular, circumflex scapular, and posterior humeral circumflex arteries in the surrounding capsule and periosteal tissue.
- There is histologic evidence that vascularity is decreased in the anterior, anterosuperior, and superior aspects of the glenoid labrum.[2]

PATHOGENESIS

- The long head of the biceps functions to depress the humeral head and serves as an adjunct anterior stabilizer of the shoulder.[5,6]
- Disruption of the biceps anchor and the superior labrum, as seen in type II SLAP tears, can result in glenohumeral instability.
- Although SLAP tears are commonly associated with trauma such as traction or compression injuries, up to one third of patients with SLAP lesions have no history of trauma.[10]
- SLAP tears are commonly classified according to Snyder[14] as type I (fraying of superior labrum with intact biceps anchor), type II (detached superior labrum and biceps anchor), type III (bucket-handle tear of the superior labrum with intact biceps anchor), and type IV (bucket-handle tear of the superior labrum with extension into the biceps tendon).
- Other variations have been described that reflect associated injury to the anterior labrum and other structures.[8]

NATURAL HISTORY

- Conservative nonoperative treatment of SLAP tears is usually unsuccessful.
- Simple débridement of unstable SLAP tears (type II and IV) is generally not recommended because the results are poor.[3]

PATIENT HISTORY AND PHYSICAL FINDINGS

- Traction and compression are the two primary mechanisms of injury for SLAP tears.
- A SLAP tear should be considered in a patient with a history of a traction or compression injury with persistent mechanical symptoms such as catching or locking.
- Several clinical tests have been described that focus on the examination of the biceps tendon anchor on the superior glenoid. The Speed, Yergason, O'Brien, and load-compression tests are commonly used.
  - Speed and Yergason tests: Pain with the maneuvers suggests a SLAP tear.
  - O'Brien test: Pain with downward pressure applied to the internally rotated arm that is relieved with supination suggests a SLAP tear.
  - Load-compression test: Painful clicking or popping suggests a SLAP tear.
- Type II SLAP tears found in younger patients are commonly associated with instability and a Bankart lesion, whereas type II SLAP tears found in patients older than 40 are often associated with rotator cuff pathology.[7]
- Although no single clinical test can predictably be used to diagnose a SLAP tear, the examiner should use all of these tests, along with the history and a high clinical index of suspicion, to make the diagnosis of a SLAP tear.

IMAGING AND OTHER DIAGNOSTIC STUDIES

- Although conventional radiographs (anteroposterior and supraspinatus outlet and axillary views) are the standard for initial evaluation of a patient with shoulder complaints, magnetic resonance imaging (MRI) is the most sensitive imaging tool for evaluating the superior glenoid labrum, with a sensitivity and specificity of about 90%.[1]
- The use of contrast arthrography MRI may improve the overall accuracy of MR for diagnosing SLAP tears.[9]
- Despite advances in imaging techniques, the gold standard for the diagnosis of a SLAP tear is arthroscopy.

DIFFERENTIAL DIAGNOSIS

- Glenohumeral instability
- Rotator cuff pathology
- Acromioclavicular joint pathology

NONOPERATIVE MANAGEMENT

- Physical therapy is the mainstay of nonoperative treatment of most shoulder injuries.
- Selective intra-articular injections with local anesthetic and corticosteroids can be diagnostic and occasionally therapeutic.
- The rehabilitation program should focus on achieving and maintaining a full range of motion and strengthening the rotator cuff and scapula stabilizers.
- Although physical therapy may be useful for regaining range of motion and strength, most patients with SLAP tears will continue to have symptoms despite physical therapy.

SURGICAL MANAGEMENT

- Surgical treatment of SLAP tears should be considered for patients who have persistent symptoms despite appropriate conservative management.

- Contraindications for SLAP repair include patients who are high-risk surgical candidates (ie, the risk of anesthetic complications outweighs the possible benefits of successful repair).

Preoperative Planning

- Preoperative assessment of glenohumeral instability is paramount to understanding the pathophysiology of a patient's shoulder complaints.
- Associated instability and any other coexisting pathology must also be addressed at the time of SLAP repair.

Positioning

- Beach-chair position
- Lateral decubitus position
  - May be preferred for cases of suspected labral pathology, especially if associated with posterior instability, because this position allows improved visualization and access with distraction.
  - No more than 10 to 15 pounds of traction should be used owing to increased risk of brachial plexus injuries.

Approach

- The primary goal of any SLAP repair is to stabilize the biceps anchor and address any coexisting pathology.
- After a thorough diagnostic evaluation, SLAP lesions are treated according to Snyder[14] (see the Techniques section).
  - Standard anterosuperior and anteroinferior portals are established.
  - Accessory portals may also be established depending on the location of the SLAP tear.

TECHNIQUES

TYPE I SLAP TEARS

- Type I SLAP tears may be treated using a motorized shaver to simply débride the degenerative or frayed tissue.
- Care must be taken not to detach the biceps anchor from the superior glenoid.

TYPE II SLAP TEARS

- Type II SLAP tears are the most commonly encountered SLAP tears (TECH FIG 1).
  - They represent detachment of the biceps anchor from the superior glenoid labrum.
  - As such, the primary goal of any repair should be to securely reattach the superior labral tissue to the superior glenoid.

Glenoid Preparation

- After identifying the detachment by direct probing, a 4.5-mm motorized shaver is used to gently débride any frayed or degenerative tissue.
- A motorized burr is used to débride the superior glenoid to exposed, bleeding bone (TECH FIG 2).

Accessory Portal Placement

- An accessory trans-rotar cuff portal is made using an outside-in technique. No cannula is inserted because this portal will be used only to insert the anchor.
  - This portal may be adjusted anteriorly or posteriorly depending on the location of the SLAP tear.
  - A spinal needle is used to ensure that the correct trajectory is achieved to place the anchor at about a 45-degree angle to the glenoid face.
  - A no. 11 blade knife is used to make the skin incision, but a cannula is not inserted because this portal will be used only to insert the suture anchor drill guide and anchor after drilling.

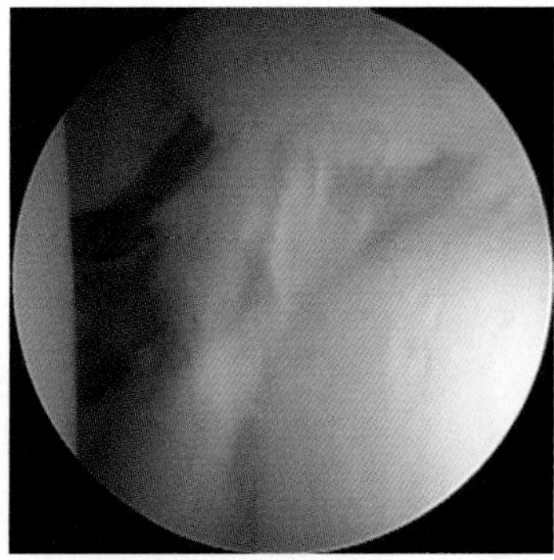

TECH FIG 1 • Arthroscopic view of type II superior labral anterior posterior (SLAP) lesion.

Suture Anchor Placement

- The suture anchor drill guide is placed on the glenoid face at about a 45-degree angle to the face, ensuring that the anchor will be solidly in bone (TECH FIG 3).
  - The suture anchor may be single- or double-loaded with nonabsorbable no. 2 braided suture, depending on preference.
  - If more than one suture anchor is to be used, the surgeon starts the repair posteriorly and works anteriorly to aid in visualization.
- The anchor is placed in the same trajectory as the drill, ensuring that the drill guide is maintained in its proper orientation and position.

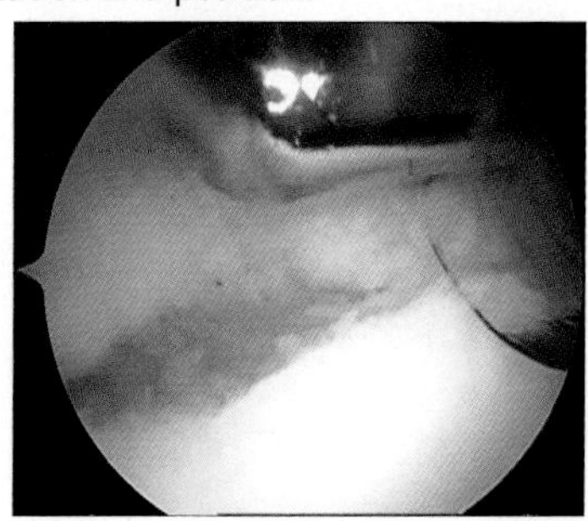

TECH FIG 2 • Preparing superior glenoid with burr.

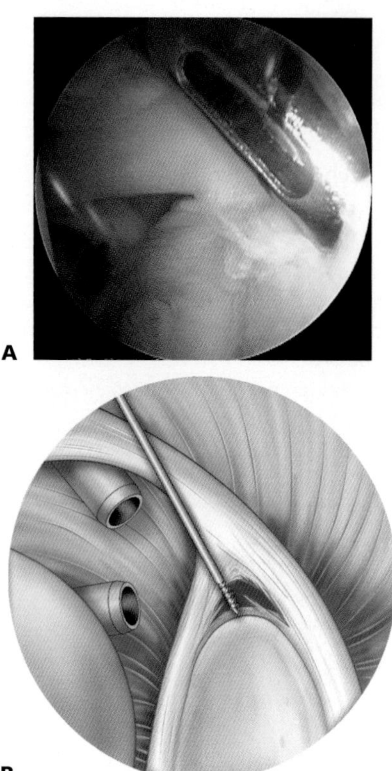

TECH FIG 3 • Drilling suture anchor through lateral portal.

Suture Management

- One limb (limb a) of the suture is retrieved out through the anterior superior cannula, using either a crochet hook or suture grasper.
- A crochet hook is used to capture the other limb (limb b) of the anchor suture and bring it out the anterior inferior cannula (TECH FIG 4).

Suture Passage

- Through the anterosuperior cannula and starting at the posterior edge of the tear superiorly, the surgeon passes a tissue penetrator (Spectrum, ConMed Linvatec, Largo, FL) through the labrum (TECH FIG 5A,B).
  - A 45-degree left-curved tissue penetrator is used for a right shoulder SLAP tear (45-degree right-curved for the left shoulder) loaded with a no. 1 monofilament or Shuttle Relay suture passer (ConMed Linvatec, Largo, FL) as a pull-through suture.
- An arthroscopic grasper inserted through the anteroinferior cannula is used to grasp the monofilament passing suture as it penetrates the superior labrum, and the free end is pulled out through the anteroinferior cannula (TECH FIG 5C,D).
- A simple knot is tied in the passing suture (see Tech Fig 5D, inset) and the free end of limb b from the suture an-

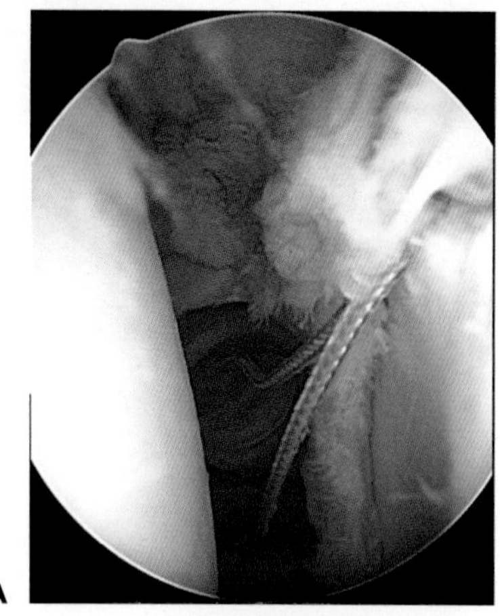

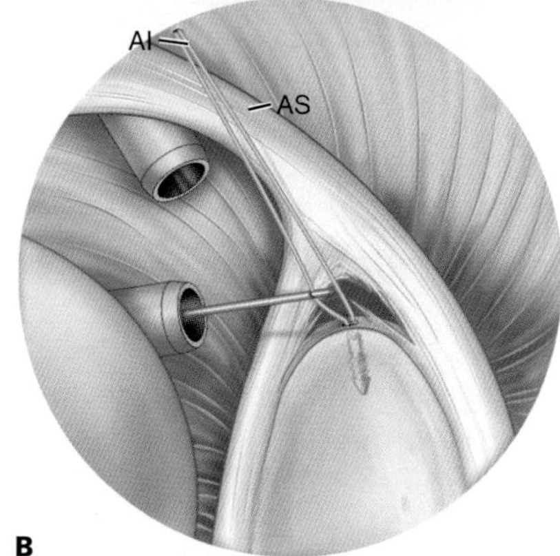

TECH FIG 4 • The surgeon retrieves one limb of the anchor suture out the anterosuperior cannula (*AS*) and one limb out the anteroinferior cannula (*AI*).

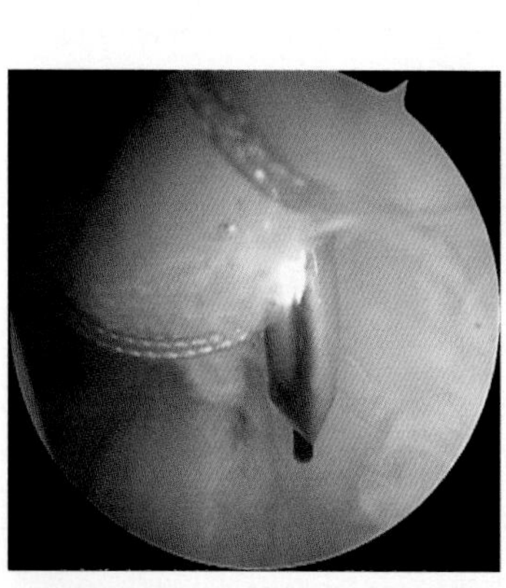

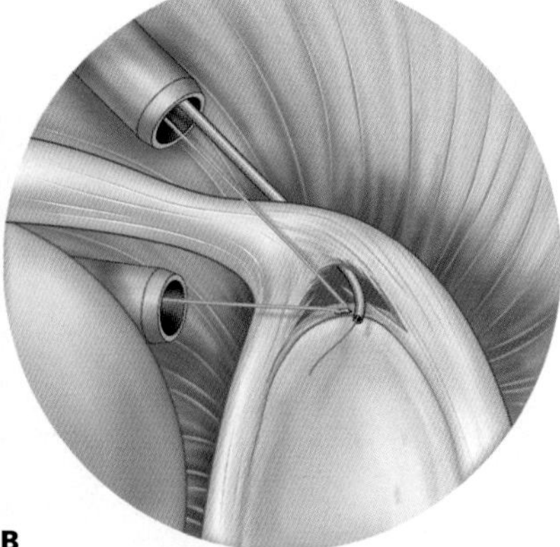

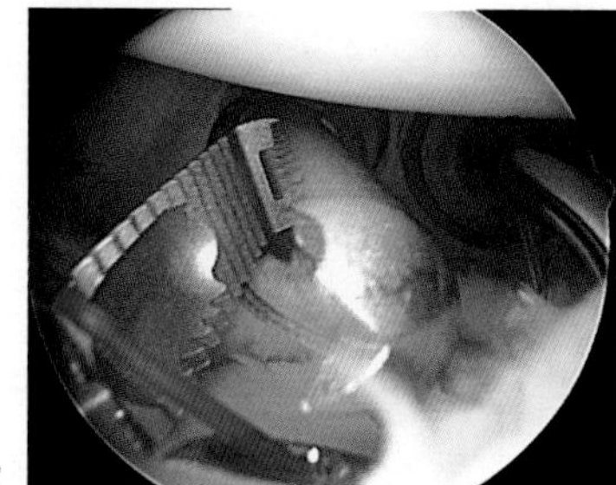

TECH FIG 5 • **A,B.** Spectrum tissue penetrator loaded with monofilament passing suture through superior labrum. **C,D.** Shuttle relay passing suture retrieved through the anteroinferior cannula. *(continued)*

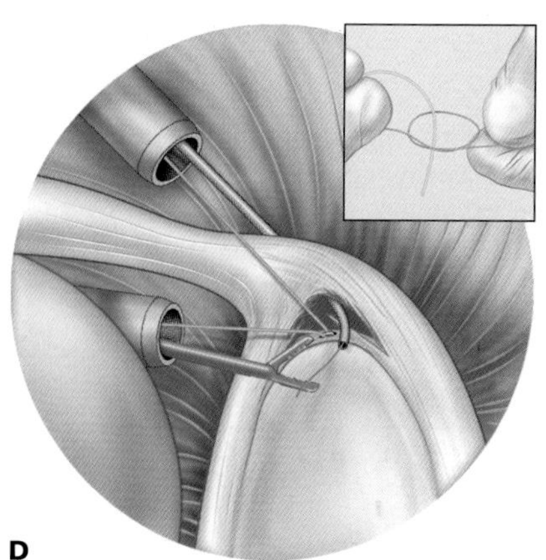

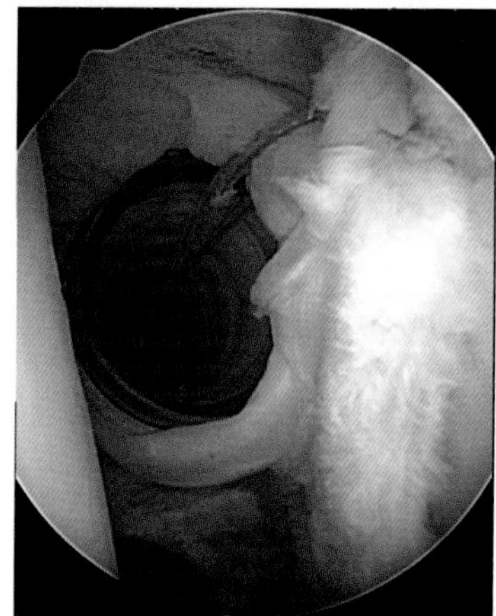

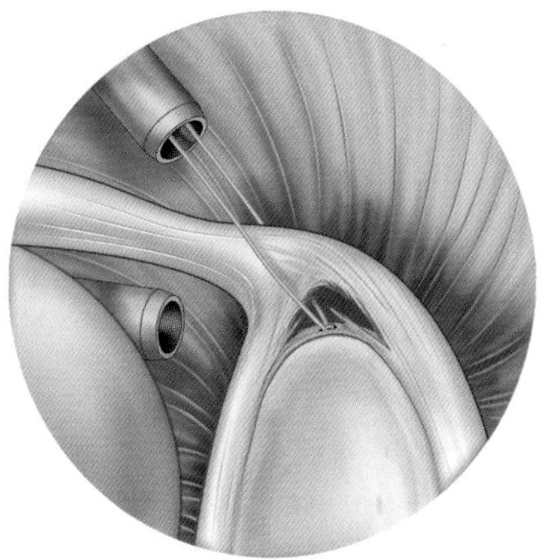

TECH FIG 5 • *(continued)* **E,F.** The surgeon firmly pulls the shuttle relay suture through the anterosuperior cannula so that the two ends of the anchor suture are together in the anterosuperior cannula.

chor is inserted through the loop. The suture is pulled gently but firmly through the anterosuperior portal so that the two ends of the anchor suture are together out of the anterosuperior portal (TECH FIG 5E,F). (If a Shuttle Relay suture passer is being used, the free end of the anchor suture is placed through the wire loop and the same steps are followed.)

- The surgeon should ensure that the anchor is not unloaded of its suture during this process by maintaining continuous arthroscopic visualization of the anchor.
- There should be no movement of the suture at the anchor eyelet.

Knot Tying

- Making sure that the post limb is off the glenoid surface, the surgeon ties the suture using either a sliding knot or a series of half-hitches, taking care to switch posts and alternate directions of the loops.
- The excess suture is cut using an arthroscopic suture cutter.

Additional Suture Anchor Placement

- This procedure is repeated until the biceps anchor has been securely reattached to the superior glenoid (TECH FIG 6).
- The surgeon should take care when securing the anterior aspect of the SLAP tears so that a normal labral foramen or an anterosuperior labral variant is not incorrectly identified as a SLAP tear, causing inadvertent tightness and resulting in decreased range of motion.

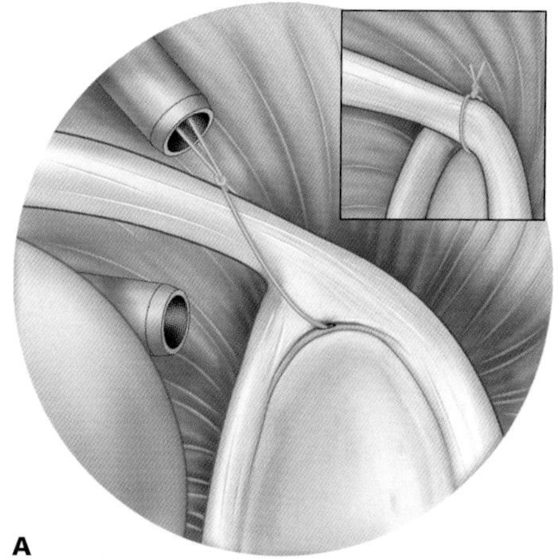

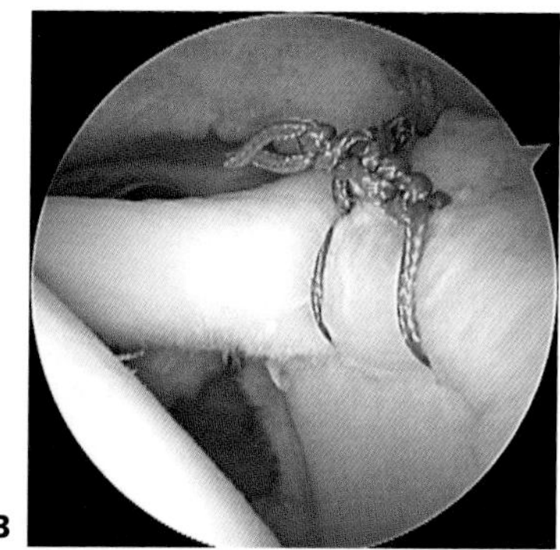

TECH FIG 6 • Completed superior labral anterior posterior (SLAP) lesion repair.

TYPE III SLAP TEARS

- Simple débridement of the labral bucket-handle tear is the preferred surgical technique for type III SLAP tears because the biceps anchor is intact.

TECHNIQUES

TYPE IV SLAP TEARS

- Type IV SLAP tears involve a bucket-handle tear of the superior labrum with a tear of the biceps tendon.
  - The biceps anchor may be detached as well.
- Treatment is débridement of the labral tear and biceps tendon tear, with repair of the biceps anchor if needed, essentially converting the tear to a type II and then repairing the anchor detachment.
- In an older patient with significant biceps tendon degeneration, biceps tenodesis should be considered.
- Similarly, in a younger patient with a tear extending into the biceps tendon, repair of any tendon tears should be considered.

PEARLS AND PITFALLS

Indications	▪ All associated pathology is identified and addressed (eg, instability, rotator cuff pathology, acromioclavicular joint disorders).
Planning	▪ Lateral decubitus positioning is considered if posterior labral pathology is suspected.
Portal placement	▪ Proper technique must be used in placing portals at the beginning of the case, with attention to positioning of the portals both in the superoinferior plane and the medial-lateral plane. Improperly placed portals can greatly increase the difficulty of this operation. A spinal needle is used to judge the angle of approach for each portal before making the portal to ensure that the correct trajectory is obtained.
Suture management	▪ When retrieving and handling anchor sutures, the surgeon should not place tension on either limb and should maintain continuous visualization of the anchor–suture interface to ensure that the anchor is not unloaded. The surgeon should take care to avoid twists because these can place increased stress on a suture or knot and lead to breakage. The surgeon should place one anchor at a time and tie each suture or remove and replace the cannula and place the suture outside the cannula for suture storage to prevent tangles during tying.
Other	▪ Articular cartilage damage is avoided by firmly seating the drill guide on the edge of the glenoid and avoiding skiving onto the glenoid face.

POSTOPERATIVE CARE

- 0 to 4 weeks: Sling at all times except for hygiene and exercises. (Active range of motion allowed in all planes except external rotation in abduction starting at 2 weeks.)
- 4 weeks: Discontinue sling. Start passive range of motion with emphasis on posterior capsule stretching.
- 6 weeks: External rotation in abduction allowed. Start strengthening.
- 3 months: Sports allowed except throwing (4 months)

OUTCOMES

- Table 1 summarizes outcomes from studies of SLAP tear repairs.

COMPLICATIONS

- Infection (rare)
- Brachial plexus neuropathy secondary to traction of the arm in the lateral decubitus position
  - Care must be taken to ensure that the smallest amount of traction and distraction necessary is used, with close monitoring of the tension applied to neurovascular structures.
- Persistent pain
  - Healed repair: Biceps tenodesis should be considered for pain relief.

Table 1 Results of Arthroscopic Superior Labral Anterior Posterior (SLAP) Lesion Repair

Study	Surgical Procedure	No. of Patients	Average Follow-up	Results
Cordasco et al, 1993[3]	Débridement only	27		89% good or excellent results at 1-year follow-up; 63% excellent results at 2-year follow-up; only 44% return to competition at 2-year follow-up
Field & Savoie, 1993[4]	Arthroscopic suture repair	20	21 mo	Rowe scale: 100% good or excellent results ASES scores: statistically significant increase in function score, decrease in pain score
Morgan et al, 1998[11]	Arthroscopic suture repair	102	1 year	97% good or excellent results 4% return to competition among overhead throwers
O'Brien et al, 2002[12]	Arthroscopic suture repair (transrotator cuff portal)	31 (type II)	3.7 yr	71% good or excellent, 19% fair results Average postoperative ASES score: 87.2

ASES, American Shoulder and Elbow Society.

- Failed repair
  - Repeat arthroscopy should be considered with revision repair.
  - Biceps tenodesis should be considered for severely degenerative or intractable cases.

REFERENCES

1. Chandnani V, Yeager T, Deberardino T, et al. Glenoid labral tears: prospective evaluation with MR imaging, MR arthrography, and CT arthrography. AJR Am J Roentgenol 1993;161:1229–1235.
2. Cooper D, Arnoczky S, O'Brien S, et al. Anatomy, histology, and vascularity of the glenoid labrum: an anatomical study. J Bone Joint Surg Am 1992;74A:46–52.
3. Cordasco F, Steinman S, Flatow E, et al. Arthroscopic treatment of glenoid labral tears. Am J Sports Med 1993;21:425–431.
4. Field L, Savoie F. Arthroscopic suture repair of superior labral detachment lesions of the shoulder. Am J Sports Med 1993;21: 783–790.
5. Healey J, Barton S, Noble P, et al. Biomechanical evaluation of the origin of the long head of the biceps tendon. Arthroscopy 2001; 17:378–382.
6. Itoi E, Kuechle D, Newman S, et al. Stabilising function of the biceps in stable and unstable shoulders. J Bone Joint Surg Br 1993;75B: 546–550.
7. Kim T, Quaele W, Cosgarea A, et al. Clinical features of the different types of SLAP lesions: an analysis of one hundred and thirty-nine cases. J Bone Joint Surg Am 2003;85A:66–71.
8. Maffet M, Gartsman G, Moseley B. Superior labrum-biceps tendon complex lesions of the shoulder. Am J Sports Med 1995;23:93–98.
9. Magee T, Williams D, Mani N. Shoulder MR arthrography; which patient group benefits most? AJR Am J Roentgenol 2004;183: 969–974.
10. Mileski R, Snyder S. Superior labral lesions in the shoulder: pathoanatomy and surgical management. J Am Acad Orthop Surg 1998;6:121–131.
11. Morgan C, Burkhard S, Palmeri M, et al. Type II SLAP lesions: three subtypes and their relationships to superior instability and rotator cuff tears. Arthroscopy 1998;14:553–565.
12. O'Brien S, Allen A, Coleman S, et al. The trans-rotator cuff approach to SLAP lesions: technical aspects for repair and a clinical follow-up of 31 patients at a minimum of 2 years. Arthroscopy 2002;18:372–377.
13. Prodromos C, Ferry J, Schiller A, et al. Histological studies of the glenoid labrum from fetal life to old age. J Bone Joint Surg Am 1990;72A:1344–1348.
14. Snyder S, Karzel R, Del Pizzo W, et al. SLAP lesions of the shoulder. Arthroscopy 1990;6:274–279.
15. Verma NN, Cole BJ, Romeo AA. Arthroscopic repair of SLAP lesions. In: Miller MD, Cole BJ, eds. Textbook of Arthroscopy. Philadelphia: Saunders, 2004:159–168.

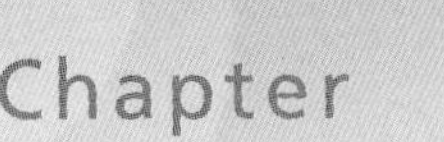

Chapter 6 Management of Shoulder Throwing Injuries

Matthew T. Boes and Craig D. Morgan

DEFINITION

- Throwers place unique stress on their shoulder girdles due to the repetitive nature and magnitude of force associated with the activity.
- Throwing athletes are prone to shoulder dysfunction due to chronic fatigue and weakening of the posterior shoulder musculature that over time leads to maladaptive contracture of the posteroinferior glenohumeral joint capsule.[5]
- Posteroinferior capsular contracture alters the biomechanics of the glenohumeral joint during the throwing motion and produces a predictable constellation of injuries in disabled throwers, including superior labral and biceps anchor disruption, undersurface progressing to full-thickness rotator cuff tears, and disruption of the anteroinferior capsule or labrum.[3]
- Symptoms resulting from these injuries have commonly been referred to as the "dead arm syndrome," where the athlete cannot compete at the premorbid level due to shoulder discomfort with throwing and resultant loss of pitch velocity and control.[3]
- Although most often seen in pitchers, similar shoulder dysfunction may occur in baseball position players as well as athletes in other sports requiring forceful and repetitive overhead activity.

ANATOMY

- Eighteen muscles attach to the scapula and control its position on the chest wall.
  - Scapular position dictates glenoid position and orientation and is critical for normal glenohumeral function.
- A force of up to 1.5 times body weight is generated during the throwing cycle. The scapular stabilizers and posterior rotator cuff muscles contract violently at ball release and protect the glenohumeral joint from the deceleration force of the arm.
- The relative position of the glenohumeral ligaments changes with different arm positions. As the arm is brought into full abduction and external rotation (late cocking phase), the posterior band of the inferior glenohumeral ligament complex (PIGHL) moves from a posteroinferior position to a position directly inferior (6 o'clock) in relation to the glenoid.[3]

PATHOGENESIS

- Posterior shoulder muscle weakness due to chronic, repetitive loading is the inciting lesion causing disability in throwers.
- Posterior muscle weakness leads to shoulder dysfunction as a result of both scapular dyskinesis and PIGHL contracture. One of these pathologic entities may predominate in the disabled thrower, but they are generally intimately related.[5]
- In scapular dyskinesis, the position of the scapula on the chest wall (or "scapular attitude") is altered owing to loss of scapular elevation and retraction control. The scapula drops (infera), moves lateral from the midline (protraction), and abducts from the midline. The inferior scapular angle may also lift off the chest wall and pitch toward the front of the body (antetilt).
  - The predominant direction of these positional changes will vary depending on which scapular muscles are predominantly affected.
  - Altered scapular position causes abnormal tension on the insertion of scapular stabilizer muscles and over time leads to inflammation and pain ("traction tendinopathy").[5]
- PIGHL contracture involves failure of the weakened posterior shoulder muscles to counteract the distraction force of the arm after ball release exposes the PIGHL to abnormal stress due to the forward-flexed and adducted position of the arm at follow-through. Fibroblastic thickening and contracture of the PIGHL occur as a maladaptive response to greater stress (Wolf's law of collagen).
  - PIGHL contracture can be identified clinically as a scapular-stabilized glenohumeral internal rotation deficit (GIRD) in the throwing shoulder (designated by subscript "ts") versus nonthrowing shoulder (subscript "nts").[3]
- The thickened PIGHL alters the normal biomechanics of the glenohumeral joint, particularly as the arm is brought into abduction and external rotation (late cocking phase). The normal glenohumeral contact point is shifted posteriorly and superiorly due to the thickened and contracted PIGHL occupying a position directly inferior to the humeral head in this arm position (**FIG 1A,B**).[6]
- Alteration of the glenohumeral contact point leads to a predictable pathologic cascade with continued throwing.[3]
  - Posterosuperior shift allows greater clearance of the tuberosity over the posterosuperior glenoid rim, enabling pathologic hyperexternal rotation of the arm in the late cocking phase.
  - Increased external rotation of the throwing shoulder is adaptive in these athletes to some extent (used to maximize throwing arc and angular velocity at ball release).[3] However, pathologic hyperexternal rotation leads to:
    - An abnormal posteriorly directed force vector and torsion on the biceps anchor. The biceps anchor ultimately fails and "peels back" medially along the posterosuperior glenoid neck (the "SLAP event"). SLAP tears are typically anterior and posterior or posterior subtypes of type II tears (the "thrower's SLAP").[8]
    - Rotator cuff tears occur because of abrasion and torsion of tendon fibers. Torsion failure is most pronounced on the articular side of the tendons, resulting in partial undersurface tears most commonly seen in throwers. These tears may at times progress to full thickness with continued throwing.
    - Posterosuperior shift of the glenohumeral contact point causes relative relaxation and "pseudo-laxity" in the anterior capsule (**FIG 1C,D**). With continued hyperexternal rotation, tension may ultimately cause anteroinferior capsular fiber attenuation, leading to tertiary anterior glenohumeral instability, which occurs in about 10% of

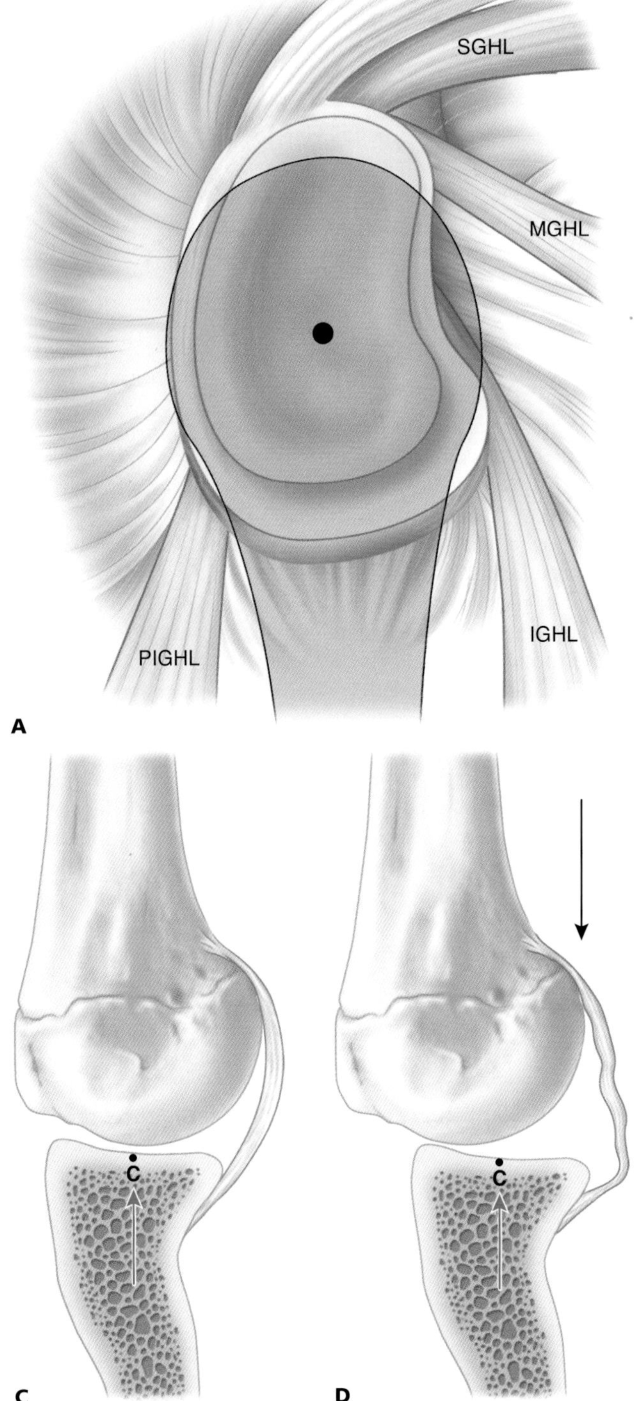

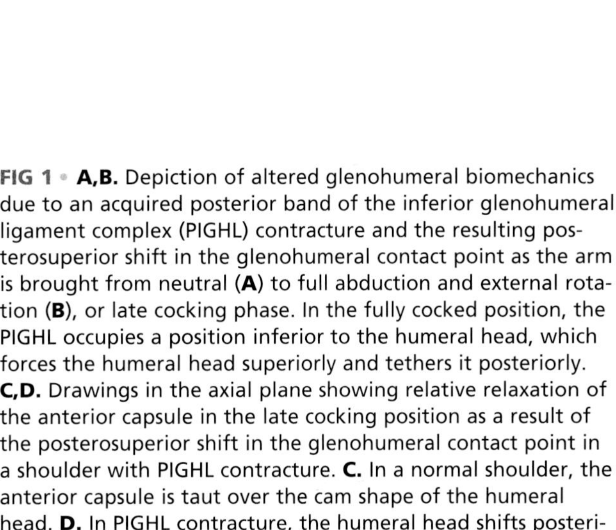

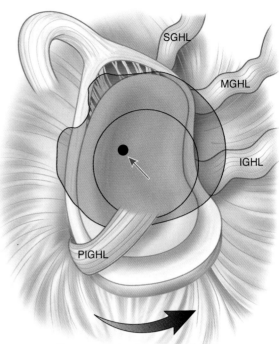

FIG 1 • **A,B.** Depiction of altered glenohumeral biomechanics due to an acquired posterior band of the inferior glenohumeral ligament complex (PIGHL) contracture and the resulting posterosuperior shift in the glenohumeral contact point as the arm is brought from neutral (**A**) to full abduction and external rotation (**B**), or late cocking phase. In the fully cocked position, the PIGHL occupies a position inferior to the humeral head, which forces the humeral head superiorly and tethers it posteriorly. **C,D.** Drawings in the axial plane showing relative relaxation of the anterior capsule in the late cocking position as a result of the posterosuperior shift in the glenohumeral contact point in a shoulder with PIGHL contracture. **C.** In a normal shoulder, the anterior capsule is taut over the cam shape of the humeral head. **D.** In PIGHL contracture, the humeral head shifts posteriorly, which decreases tension in the anterior capsule, creating relative laxity. *C*, center of glenoid.

affected athletes. Discrete "Bankart-type" lesions of the labrum occasionally occur in this group. Anterior instability is a later event in the pathologic cascade, not the primary lesion as previously described.[7]

NATURAL HISTORY

- Athletes manifesting clinical findings of posterior muscle weakness and scapular asymmetry without signs of labral or rotator cuff pathology may correct their shoulder dysfunction with a progressive scapular muscle strengthening program and return to normal function when asymmetry resolves.
- Throwers who have vague shoulder discomfort and demonstrate an internal rotation deficit (GIRD) are started on focused internal rotation stretches ("sleeper" stretches) to alleviate PIGHL contracture and restore normal glenohumeral biomechanics. GIRD reduction to less than 20 degrees removes the athlete from being at risk for shoulder injury and generally allows return to premorbid function.

- Pain with throwing is indicative of injury to glenohumeral structures.
  - Once actual injury to glenohumeral structures, particularly the labrum, has occurred, mechanical symptoms ensue and the thrower will not be able to return to normal function without surgical repair.

PATIENT HISTORY AND PHYSICAL FINDINGS

- Common early complaints include vague tightness in the shoulder and a difficulty or inability to "get loose" during a warm-up period.
- Pitchers describe a loss of control and decrease in throwing velocity, which early on may be pain-free.
- Pain is most prominent during the late cocking phase of throwing when the peel-back phenomenon of the superior labrum occurs, caused by the posterosuperior glenohumeral shift.[4]
  - Pain is localized to the posterosuperior shoulder and is described as "deep."
  - Mechanical symptoms, such as painful popping or clicking, may occur after injury to the superior labrum, particularly during late cocking and early acceleration.
- The surgeon should check for tenderness in the coracoid, the acromioclavicular joint, and the superomedial scapular angle.
- Both shoulder girdles must be completely exposed or subtle asymmetry will be overlooked.
  - Inspection is done with the patient standing in front of fixed vertical and horizontal references (such as window blinds or door frames) so that affected and nonaffected shoulders can be compared for scapular height and malposition (**FIG 2**).
  - Superior and inferior angles as well as the medial scapular border are marked as a visual reference. Spinous processes are marked for a midline reference.
  - Asymmetry from the unaffected side when in protraction or infera indicates scapular stabilizer muscle weakness.
  - When in abduction or antetilt, increasing magnitude compared to opposite side signifies scapular muscle weakness.
- Range-of-motion measurements are performed in the supine position with the scapula stabilized by anterior pressure over the glenohumeral joint directed into the examination table, which prevents contribution of scapulothoracic motion. Nonstabilized measurements will be erroneously high and will not reveal the true magnitude of glenohumeral pathology.
  - Measurements are made using a special goniometer that incorporates a carpenter's bubble level to provide a vertical reference point (perpendicular to floor) from which measurements are made.
  - External rotation (ER) + internal rotation (IR) = total mobility arch (TMA)
  - $IR_{nts} - IR_{ts}$ = glenohumeral internal rotation deficit (GIRD)
  - $TMA_{ts} \approx TMA_{nts}$ in healthy throwers
  - $GIRD_{ts} > 20$ degrees seen in "shoulders at risk" for injury; generally $GIRD_{ts} \approx$ loss of TMA_{ts} vs. TMA_{nts}
- Scapular relocation tests are performed in the supine position with the arm maximally forward-flexed. A positive test is indicated by pectoralis minor tension that is accentuated with the arm forward-flexed; traction at the coracoid insertion is relieved by scapular repositioning.
- The specificity of tests for type II SLAP lesions in throwers has been determined as follows[8]:
  - The modified Jobe relocation test is specific for posterior subtype. In throwers with SLAP tears, their usual pain is reproduced and they will localize to the posterosuperior joint line ("deep"). Pain in the abduction and external rotation (ABER) position is due to an unstable labrum; anterior pressure reduces the labrum and relieves pain.
  - O'Brien's test is specific for anterior subtype. A positive result is defined as pain with resisted forward flexion and pronation; pain is diminished or relieved with supination.
  - The Speed test is specific for anterior subtype. A positive result is defined as pain with resisted forward flexion.

IMAGING AND OTHER DIAGNOSTIC STUDIES

- Plain radiographs: anteroposterior (AP), scapular lateral, and axillary views to detect bone or joint space abnormalities
- Magnetic resonance (MR) arthrography: We routinely order intra-articular contrast material because it improves the ability to detect labral and capsular abnormalities as well as partial-thickness rotator cuff tears (**FIG 3**).

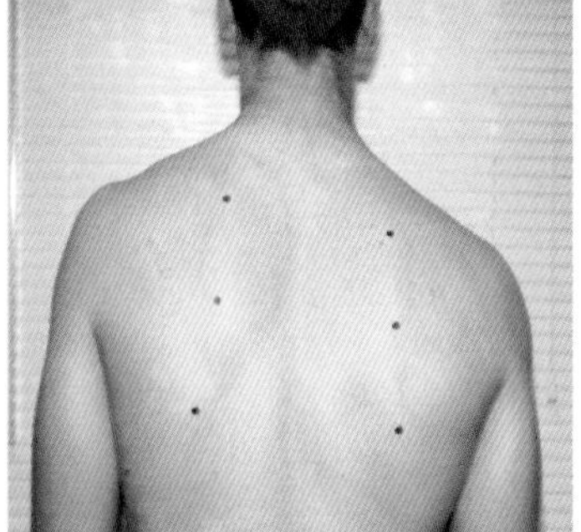

FIG 2 • Thrower with right scapular dyskinesis. Scapular asymmetry is highlighted by marking the superior and inferior scapular angles as well as the midpoint of the medial border. Affected right side shows scapular infera and protraction compared to the unaffected left side.

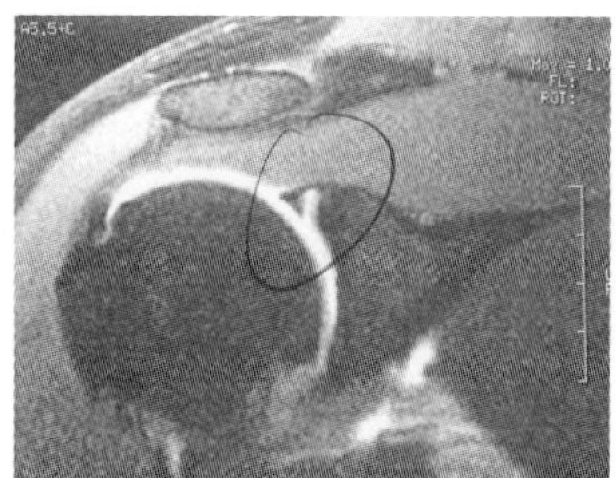

FIG 3 • Coronal MRI arthrogram study. The vertically oriented high-signal lesion in the substance of the biceps anchor (*circle*) suggests a superior labrum anterior-to-posterior (SLAP) tear. In addition, there is evidence of partial undersurface tearing of the supraspinatus tendon.

DIFFERENTIAL DIAGNOSIS

- Subacromial irritation secondary to rotator cuff weakness and dysfunction
- Various forms of anterior shoulder pain, acromioclavicular joint dysfunction, and posterior periscapular pain secondary to scapular dyskinesis and the SICK scapula syndrome (Scapular malposition, Inferior medial scapular winging, Coracoid tenderness, and scapular dysKinesis).[5]
- Pain with throwing may occur with rare conditions such as bone tumors, stress fractures, and growth plate abnormalities.

NONOPERATIVE MANAGEMENT

- Symptomatic athletes are begun on a scapular reconditioning program combined with internal rotation posteroinferior capsular "sleeper" stretches.
- Scapular reconditioning focuses on regaining scapular elevation and retraction control; progress is assessed by repeat examination for normalization of scapular symmetry.
  - Initially bilateral shoulder shrugs and rolls are combined with retraction "no money" exercises.
  - The patient progresses to closed-chain "table top" movements and wall-washing motions.
  - Finally, prone "Blackburn"-type exercises are instituted.
- "Sleeper" stretches focus on the posteroinferior capsular contracture that initiates the internal derangement in the glenohumeral joint (**FIG 4**). Response to a course of internal rotation stretching will determine the extent of the PIGHL contracture.
  - 90% of athletes will decrease their GIRD to an acceptable magnitude with 10 to 14 days of focused stretching (less than 20 degrees) with near-normalization of TMA_{ts} and TMA_{nts}.
  - The remaining 10% have recalcitrant PIGHL contracture and will show little or no decrease in GIRD after a period of stretching; they are termed stretch nonresponders. These are generally veteran athletes with longstanding GIRD and may require posteroinferior quadrant capsulotomy to regain internal rotation.

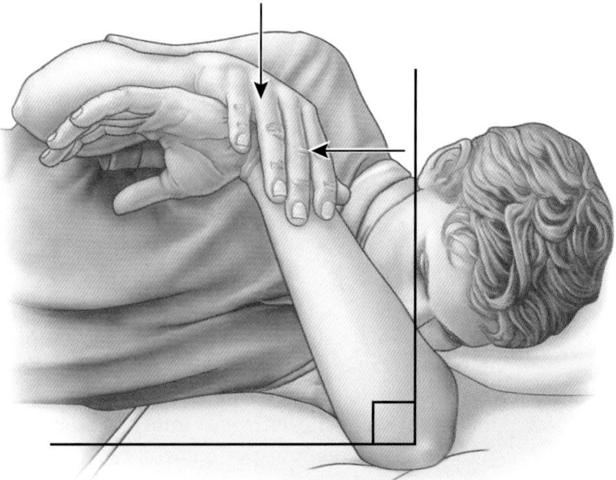

FIG 4 • "Sleeper" stretch of the posteroinferior capsule of the left shoulder. Patient lies on the affected side to stabilize the scapula and isolate stretch to the glenohumeral capsule. Affected shoulder and elbow are flexed 90 degrees. The opposite hand is used to exert a downward force on the affected arm to stretch the shoulder in internal rotation and decrease posterior band of the inferior glenohumeral ligament complex (PIGHL) contracture.

SURGICAL MANAGEMENT

- Athletes presenting with pain and mechanical symptoms during throwing as well as findings suggestive of intra-articular pathology on MR arthrogram are indicated for arthroscopic evaluation and treatment.
- Rarely, posteroinferior capsulotomy is indicated in throwers unresponsive to internal rotation stretching to decrease GIRD. This portion of the procedure is almost never necessary in a young thrower, however.
- Contraindications to the surgical technique below include those similar to other elective arthroscopic shoulder procedures.

Preoperative Planning

- Surgical treatment of the throwing shoulder may involve repair of the superior labrum as well as associated injuries to the rotator cuff and anterior capsulolabral structures, as well as contracture of the posteroinferior capsule.
  - All pathology must be anticipated before beginning the case, and all necessary instruments and materials need to be present on the back table to prevent intraoperative delays.
- A fluid pump is used during the procedure to distend the joint and limit bleeding to improve visualization (set at 60 mm Hg). Prolonged procedures increase the risk of having to perform the surgery through distended tissue, which makes instrument manipulation in the joint difficult and can severely compromise the procedure.
- The following order of possible intra-articular repairs is recommended to ease visualization and prevent loss of access to various locations in the joint:
  - Anteroinferior labral repair (if required)
  - Posterior SLAP repair
  - Anterior SLAP repair
  - Anterior capsular redundancy (if present)
  - Posteroinferior capsulotomy (if required)
  - Rotator cuff tear (if present)

Treatment of Associated Injury

- We débride partial-thickness rotator cuff tears that represent less than 50% of the diameter and repair those larger than 50% of the diameter as described in Chapter SM-10.
  - Given the young age and high-level activity of these athletes, strong consideration should be given to repair in borderline cases.
- Anteroinferior capsulolabral injury
  - Throwers may develop stretching and attenuation of the anteroinferior capsule, separation of the anteroinferior labrum from the glenoid rim, or a combination of the two.
- We perform mini-plication of the anterior capsule in the following circumstances:
  - Evidence of frayed or attenuated anterior capsule with intact anterior labrum
  - A persistent drive-through sign after superior labral repair, or more than 120 degrees of external rotation at 90 degrees of abduction noted during the preoperative examination
- Posterior capsular release is rarely indicated (about 10% of cases).
  - Response to internal rotation stretching is assessed preoperatively.

- Patients displaying little to no response to stretching (unable to attain GIRD less than 20 degrees) are indicated for capsulotomy to allow restoration of full motion and normal glenohumeral biomechanics.

Positioning

- A preoperative intrascalene nerve block is recommended to improve pain control postoperatively.
- Antibiotics for skin flora are administered.
- The patient is in the lateral decubitus position using an inflatable beanbag.
  - The arm is secured to a rope and pulley system that is attached to 10 pounds of weight.
  - A spring-gated, carabiner-type device is added between the end of the traction cord and the suspension pulley so that an unscrubbed assistant can remove the arm from traction during the procedure for dynamic diagnostic maneuvers (see below).
- Advantages of the lateral decubitus position include:
  - Better visualization of the superior labrum and widening of the superior recess due to gravity for easier anchor placement and knot tying
  - Secure position of the arm, which negates the need for an assistant to hold the arm

Approach

- The following arthroscopic portals are used to varying extents in the surgical treatment of disabled throwers:
  - Posterior: established first; main viewing portal
  - Anterior: main working portal: knot tying; anchor placement in anterosuperior glenoid rim
  - Posterolateral ("portal of Wilmington"): anchor placement in the posterosuperior glenoid; passage of sutures through the posterosuperior labrum. No cannulas are used in this percutaneous portal. Only small-diameter anchor insertion devices and suture passers are used to minimize injury to the cuff musculature because this portal traverses the muscular portion of the posterosuperior rotator cuff.
  - Anterosuperior: accessory portal added depending on the nature of the intra-articular pathology; may be used to view the anteroinferior labrum and capsule, or to assist in shuttling sutures through the anteroinferior capsule

TECHNIQUES

ESTABLISHING PORTALS

- The posterior portal is established by identifying the posterolateral acromial border and making a 5-mm skin incision about 2 cm medial and 2 to 3 cm inferior to the posterior corner of the acromion in the palpated soft spot between the infraspinatus and teres minor portions of the rotator cuff.
  - A blunt trocar is directed from this incision anteriorly with gentle pressure to palpate the space between the rounded humeral head laterally and the glenoid rim medially.
  - The coracoid process is palpated with the opposite index finger and is used as a guide to direct the trocar to the correct plane into the glenohumeral joint.
- The remaining portals are established after arthroscopic examination of the joint using an "outside-in" technique with an 18-gauge spinal needle.
  - The spinal needle creates minimal soft tissue trauma, and multiple passes can be made as needed to determine the proper location of secondary portals to yield unimpeded trajectories to areas of the joint requiring repair (**TECH FIG 1**).

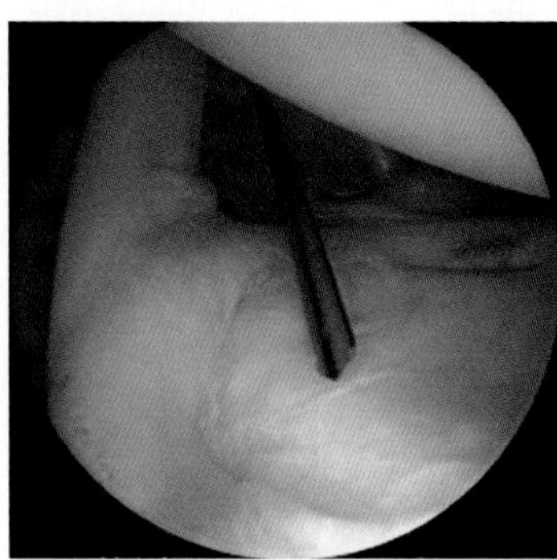

TECH FIG 1 • 18-gauge spinal needle is used to localize the anterosuperior portal.

DIAGNOSTIC ARTHROSCOPY

- The joint is systematically inspected to ensure that all areas are examined and no pathology is overlooked.
  - Areas requiring particular attention in disabled throwers include superior labrum and biceps anchor, rotator cuff insertion, posterior capsule and recess, and anteroinferior labrum and capsule.
- We routinely perform provocative tests to assess both superior labral integrity and overall stability in the joint.
  - Peel-back test: The posterosuperior labrum is assessed dynamically for evidence of instability in the abducted and externally rotated position (late cocking position). The arm is released from traction and is brought into the full cocking position; an unstable labrum will fall off the glenoid rim and shift medially along the glenoid neck (**TECH FIG 2A–D**).
  - Drive-through test: Normally, intact capsular and labral restraints appose the humeral head into the glenoid such that easy passage of the arthroscope from posterior to anterior at the midpoint of the glenoid or sweeping of the scope from superior to inferior along the anterior glenoid rim is not possible. When these maneuvers are possible, they are nonspecific evidence of disruption of the labrum or capsular ligaments according to the "circle concept" of glenohumeral stability.[3,9]

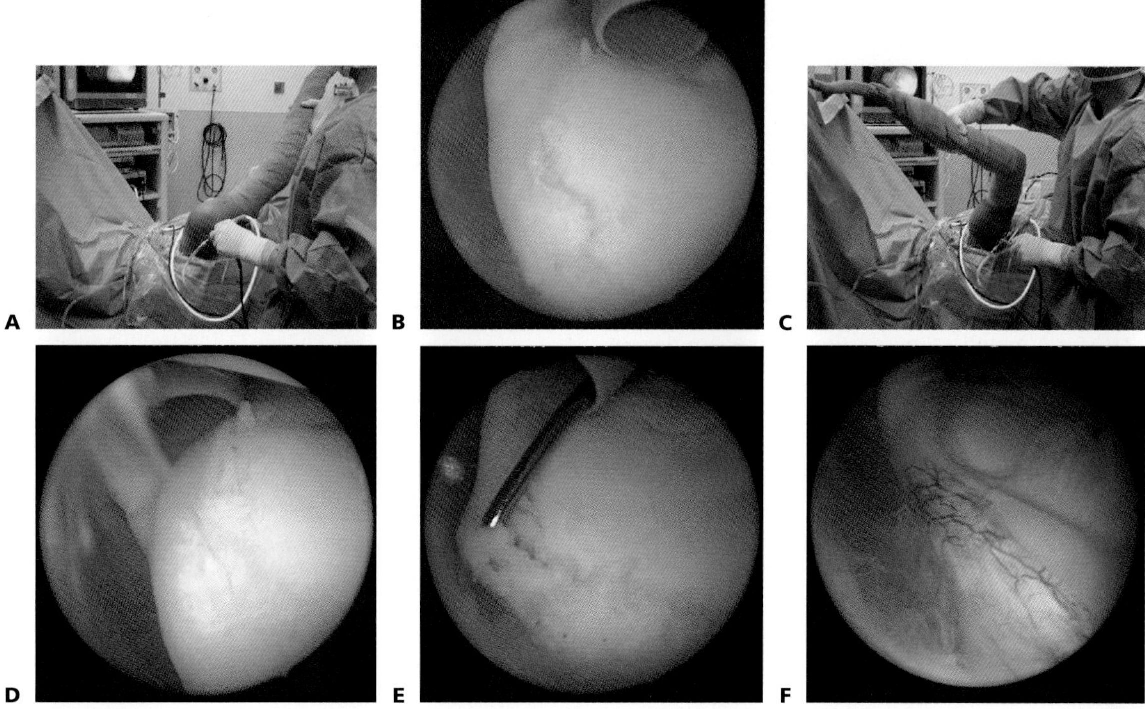

TECH FIG 2 • **A–D.** Peel-back test performed intraoperatively to detect an unstable superior labrum. **A.** The arm is removed from the traction apparatus and is shown in the neutral position. **B.** Corresponding arthroscopic image to **A.** The biceps anchor is reduced to its normal anatomic position on the superior labrum in the neutral arm position. **C.** The arm is then brought into abduction and full external rotation to dynamically assess the stability of the biceps anchor. **D.** Corresponding arthroscopic image to **C.** An unstable labrum will fall medially off the superior glenoid and "peel back" along the glenoid neck with full cocking of the arm. **E.** A probe is introduced through the anterosuperior portal to palpate the stability of the labrum. **F.** Evidence of capsular irritation adjacent to a posterosuperior labral detachment. There is also adjacent fraying of the labrum.

- After provocative tests, secondary portals are established depending on the pathology requiring repair as outlined above.
- A probe is introduced to palpate structures and confirm visual findings (TECH FIG 2E).
- Signs of labral injury may be subtle.[4] Careful inspection and probing are often required to detect:
    - Fraying and disruption of superior labral fibers inserting into the glenoid
    - Adjacent irritation of the capsule (TECH FIG 2F)
    - Disruption of the smooth contour of the articular cartilage at the glenoid rim
    - Superior labral sulcus more than 5 mm or a biceps root that can be displaced medially along the glenoid neck

INTRA-ARTICULAR DÉBRIDEMENT

- A full-radius motorized shaver (Stryker Endoscopy, San Jose, CA) is used to gently remove frayed or flaplike tissue and loose debris from the joint.
- Careful control of suction pressure on the shaver will ensure that only loose tissue is removed and the bulk of the repairable labrum is retained.

SUPERIOR LABRAL REPAIR

Site Preparation

- We briefly outline our steps for SLAP repair because they may differ slightly from elsewhere in this text.
    - Regardless of the specific techniques used, the goal is secure fixation of the biceps anchor to the glenoid rim and obliteration of the peel-back phenomenon.
- An arthroscopic rasp (Arthrex, Naples, FL) is used to separate any loose attachments of the labrum to the glenoid rim to mobilize the lesion and free it from medialized scar (similar to a medialized Bankart lesion).
    - A rasp is preferred over a sharp elevator, which can skive and injure normal labral tissue.

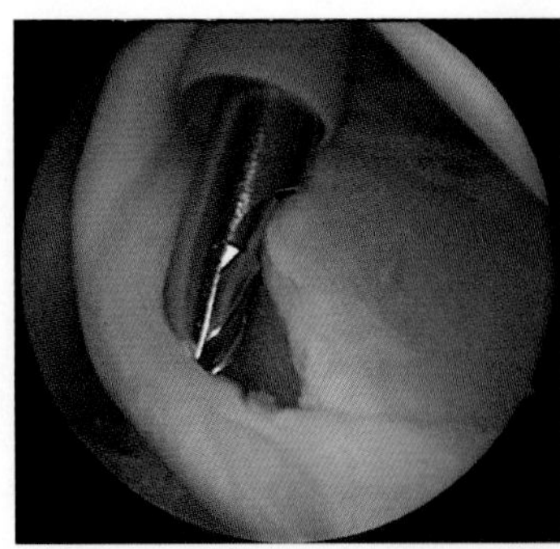

TECH FIG 3 • A motorized burr is used to prepare the glenoid bone bed before labral repair. Care is taken to prevent inadvertent damage to the labrum.

- A motorized burr is used to remove cartilage from the rim and lateral glenoid neck, yielding a punctate-bleeding cortical bone bed to accept the repaired labrum (TECH FIG 3). This step is crucial to ultimate healing of the repair.
  - We prefer a burr with protective hood that prevents injury to labral tissue (SLAP burr; Stryker).
  - No suction is used while the burr is operating to prevent inadvertent injury to labral tissue.
- Loose tissue and debris created by the rasp and burr are removed with the shaver.

Posterior Anchor Insertion

- Evaluation is made for appropriate anchor location. The number of anchors used is arbitrary but must be sufficient to negate peel-back forces and stabilize the biceps anchor.
  - We prefer bioabsorbable, tap-in anchors for SLAP repair (3.0-mm BioSutureTack; Arthrex) because they are easier to control during insertion than the screw-in type of anchors.
- The previously established anterior portal used for probing is used for anterior anchor insertion.
  - For posterosuperior anchors, we prefer the percutaneous portal of Wilmington.
  - The approximate location of the skin incision for this portal is usually 1 cm anterior and 1 cm lateral to the posterolateral corner of the acromion (TECH FIG 4A).
  - A spinal needle is used to locate this portal to allow proper insertion angle for anchor placement in the glenoid rim at 45 degrees relative to the glenoid face to ensure secure fixation in bone and prevent skiving under the glenoid articular cartilage or along the glenoid neck (TECH FIG 4B).
- A 4-mm skin incision is made and the Spear guide (3.5 mm; Arthrex) with sharp trocar is used to pierce the muscular portion of the posterior rotator cuff as it is advanced into the joint.
  - Penetration of the Spear guide is done under direct arthroscopic visualization to ensure that the guide enters the joint medial to the rotator cable, which marks the intra-articular location of the musculotendinous junction of the rotator cuff (TECH FIG 4C). Because of its small diameter and passage in the muscular portion of the cuff, there is minimal iatrogenic injury with this approach.
  - The sharp trocar is removed, and the Spear guide is brought immediately onto the glenoid rim adjacent to the previously prepared bone bed and held firmly in the proper orientation as described above (TECH FIG 4D).
- An assistant passes the power drill into the guide and carefully advances the drill bit to the hilt.
- Position of the Spear guide is carefully maintained as the drill is removed and the anchor is introduced in the guide and tapped into a fully seated position in the bone.
  - We insert these anchors to the hilt of the handle of the insertion device.
  - Gentle twisting inline with the anchor is often needed to remove it in dense bone.
    - Alternatively, gentle tapping with a mallet inline can be used to remove the inserter.
  - The Spear guide is removed and the anchor fixation is tested with gentle pulling on the sutures (TECH FIG 4E).

Suture Passage

- Both suture limbs are brought out the anterior cannula using a looped suture retriever (Arthrex) (TECH FIG 5A).
  - The medial suture (closest to labrum) is designated for passage through the labrum.

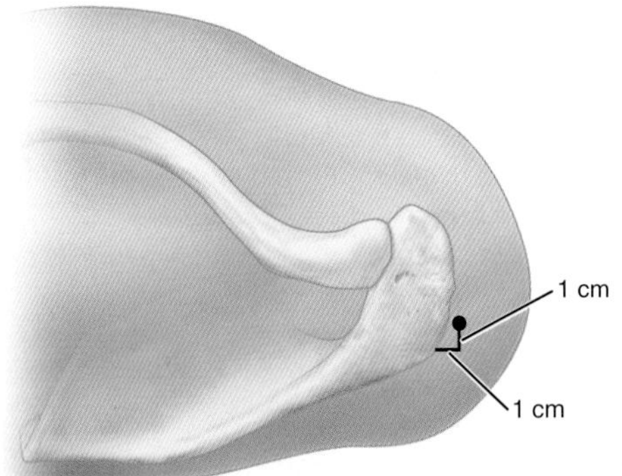

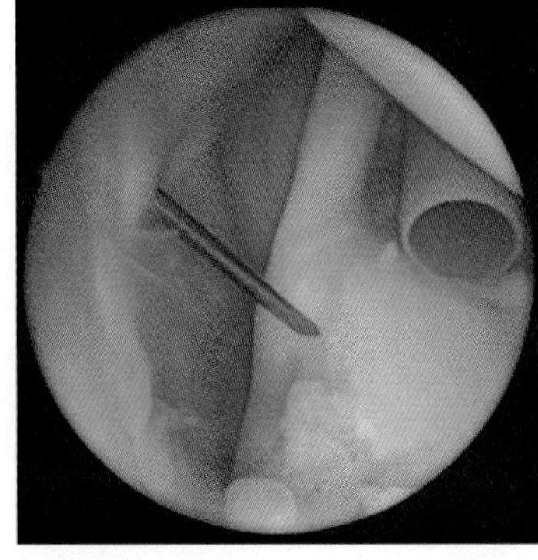

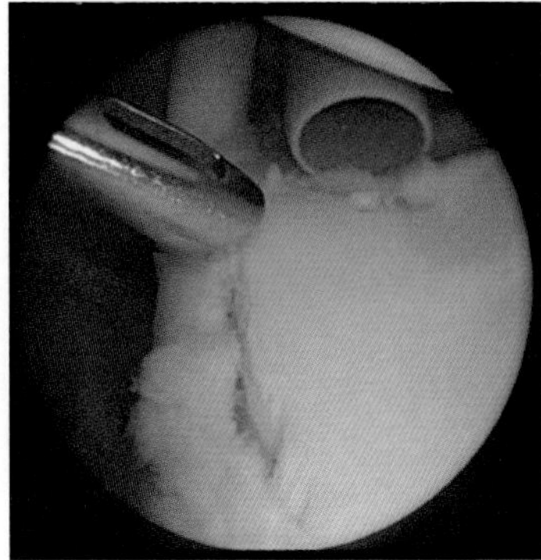

TECH FIG 4 • **A.** Approximate location for the skin incision for the "portal of Wilmington." **B.** 18-gauge spinal needle is used to accurately locate the portal of Wilmington to allow proper position and angle of insertion of suture anchors in the superior glenoid depending on the extent of the superior labral tear. **C.** The Spear guide pierces the joint capsule along the same trajectory determined by the spinal needle and medial to the rotator cable as described in the text. (The sharp obturator used to pierce the capsule for entry into the joint has been removed.) *(continued)*

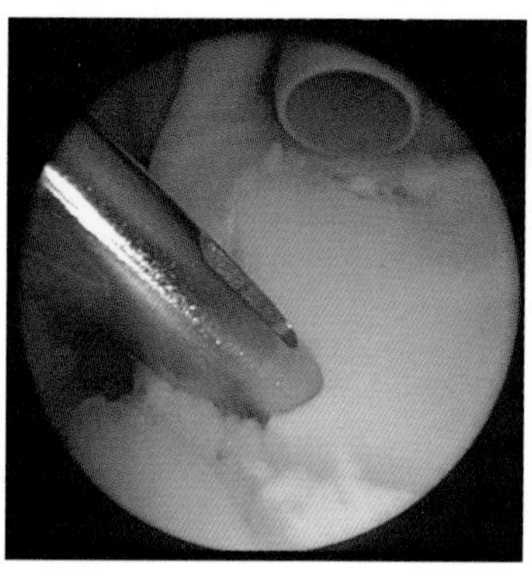

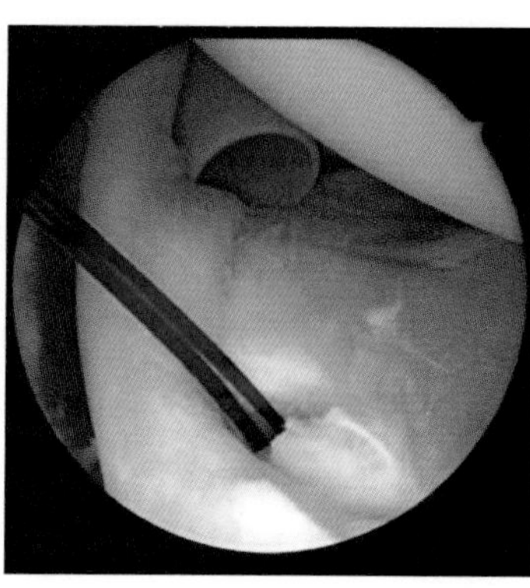

TECH FIG 4 • *(continued)* **D.** Spear guide is carefully positioned on the glenoid rim and held firmly in place during drilling and anchor insertion. Proper insertion angle (45 degrees to the glenoid face) is critical for firm fixation of the suture anchor in bone. **E.** Spear guide is removed. The suture anchor has been fully inserted in the glenoid rim, and fixation is tested with a steady pull on the sutures. (In this image, the anchor has been rethreaded with no. 1 PDS suture before the start of the case [see text]).

- A small-diameter suture-passer device with a retrievable wire loop (Lasso SuturePasser; Arthrex) is used to shuttle the suture through the labrum.
  - The suture-passer device is brought into the joint via the same incision and trajectory as the Spear guide (TECH FIG 5B).
  - It is used to pierce the labrum from superior to inferior at the location of the anchor to achieve a solid bite of labral tissue (TECH FIG 5C).
- The wire loop is advanced over the glenoid rim and retrieved through the anterior portal (TECH FIG 5D).
- The previously identified suture is threaded into the loop and the suture-passer device is gently removed from the portal of Wilmington while shuttling the "post-limb" suture through the superior labrum.
- Suture passage is done slowly and under visualization so that tangles may be identified and corrected from the anterior portal using the suture retriever (TECH FIG 5E,F).

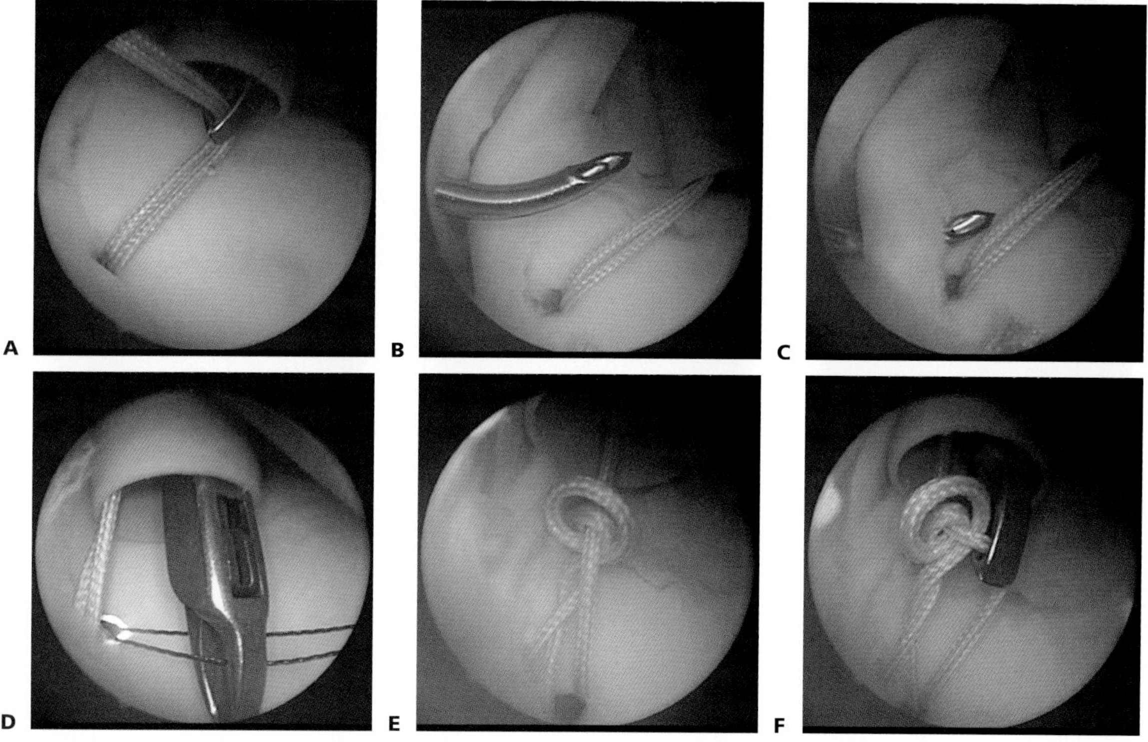

TECH FIG 5 • **A.** Both suture limbs are retrieved through the anterosuperior portal. In this image, the suture anchor has been used with the FiberWire suture that the anchor is normally packaged with (see text). **B.** The suture-passing device is brought into the joint through the same trajectory as the Spear guide in the previous steps, minimizing the risk of inadvertent damage to the rotator cuff and capsule. **C.** The suture-passing device is advanced through the superior labrum from superior to inferior to capture the bulk of the labrum and is carefully advanced over the glenoid rim to prevent damage to the articular surface. The wire loop is advanced for retrieval from the anterosuperior portal. **D.** The wire loop is retrieved from the anterosuperior portal using a gated suture retriever. The previously identified "post-limb" suture (the suture closest to the labrum as they exit the fully seated anchor) is threaded into the wire loop. The suture-passing device and wire loop are then carefully withdrawn out the portal of Wilmington, shuttling the "post-limb" suture through the labrum. **E.** Passing suture limbs slowly allows for identification of suture tangling, which may occur during suture passage through the labrum. **F.** Slack sutures are easily untangled using a gated suture retriever to identify and untangle sutures from the anterosuperior portal. *(continued)*

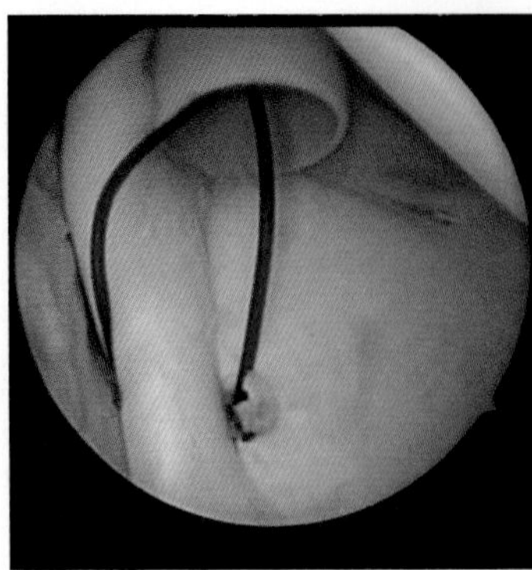

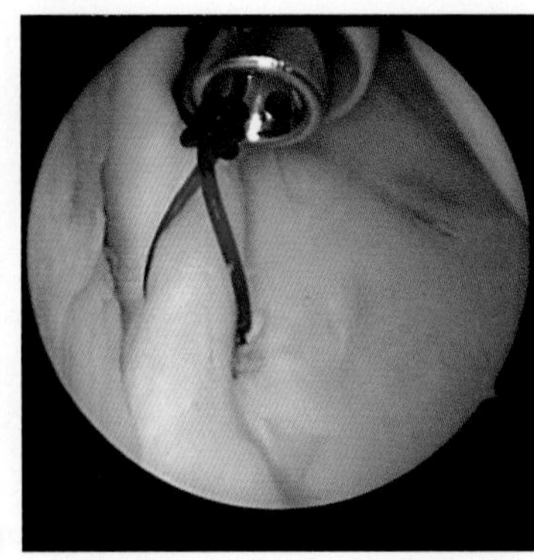

G H

TECH FIG 5 • *(continued)* **G.** The "post-limb" suture (now through the labrum and exiting portal of Wilmington) is retrieved through the anterosuperior portal for knot tying. **H.** The knot is tied either anterior or posterior to the biceps tendon, depending on ease of approach. (This image shows a suture anchor that has been rethreaded with no. 1 PDS suture before the start of the case and is a different case example than the one in **A–G**.)

- The post-limb suture is retrieved from the portal of Wilmington back to the anterior portal for knot tying either anterior or posterior to the biceps anchor, depending on ease of approach (TECH FIG 5G,H).
- The above steps are repeated as needed for additional posterior anchors in the superior labrum.

Anterosuperior Repair

- Anterosuperior anchors are placed through the anterior cannula with the same orientation concerns and technique as described for posterior anchors.
- Anterior suture limbs are passed and retrieved through the same anchor, which can create tangling of sutures. In addition, given the orientation of passage and retrieval of anterior sutures through the anterior cannula, a "sawing" effect can be created as the suture is drawn through the tissue, which may damage the anterosuperior labrum.
  - To minimize this risk, we use a tissue-penetrating device with a gated suture-retriever loop (eg, BirdBeak; Arthrex) to retrieve the post-limb suture through the anterosuperior labrum.

Dynamic Assessment of Repair

- Peel-back test: The peel-back phenomenon should be obliterated and the labrum should remain firmly fixed to the superior glenoid during full cocking of the arm (TECH FIG 6).
- Drive-through test: Advancement through the joint at mid-glenoid should not be possible after SLAP repair; if this test continues to be positive, then additional anteroinferior capsular redundancy is likely (see below).

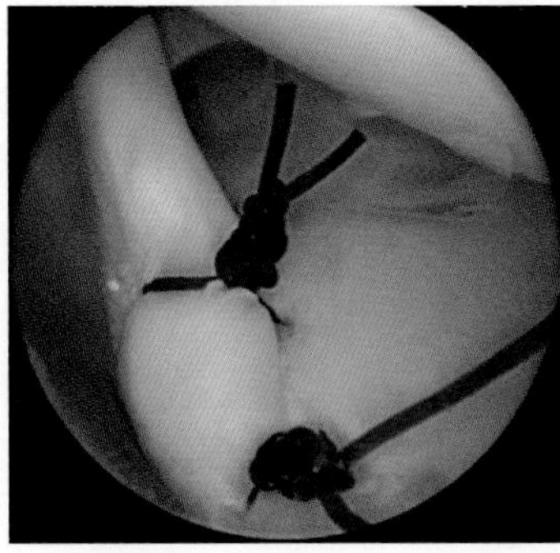

TECH FIG 6 • Completed repair after an additional suture anchor has been placed in the posterosuperior labrum. The peel-back test shows no instability of the biceps anchor and firm fixation of the superior labrum to the glenoid rim.

MINI-PLICATION OF THE ANTERIOR CAPSULE

- The extent of capsular plication is subjective. The goal is to obliterate redundant capsule by placing sutures sequentially from inferior to superior to eliminate anterior instability while preventing inadvertent restriction to full external rotation (TECH FIG 7A,B).
- A rasp or "whisker" shaver (Arthrex) is used to abrade the capsule to aid in healing of the plication (TECH FIG 7C,D).
- no. 1 PDS sutures are placed beginning anteroinferiorly with pointed suture advancement instruments of varying curvatures (Spectrum; Linvatec, Key Largo, FL).
  - A "bite" capsule is taken laterally and advanced and sutured to the anteroinferior labrum, obliterating a redundant anterior recess (TECH FIG 7E,F).
- Placement of sequential sutures allows for repeat examination to ensure anterior stability is restored without creating motion restriction (TECH FIG 7G).
- Rarely, a discrete anteroinferior labral avulsion from the glenoid is present that is repaired as described elsewhere in the text. This is most easily accomplished before superior labral repair.
- An additional anteroinferior portal may be required to achieve an appropriate anchor insertion angle onto the glenoid rim and to ease suture passage and management.

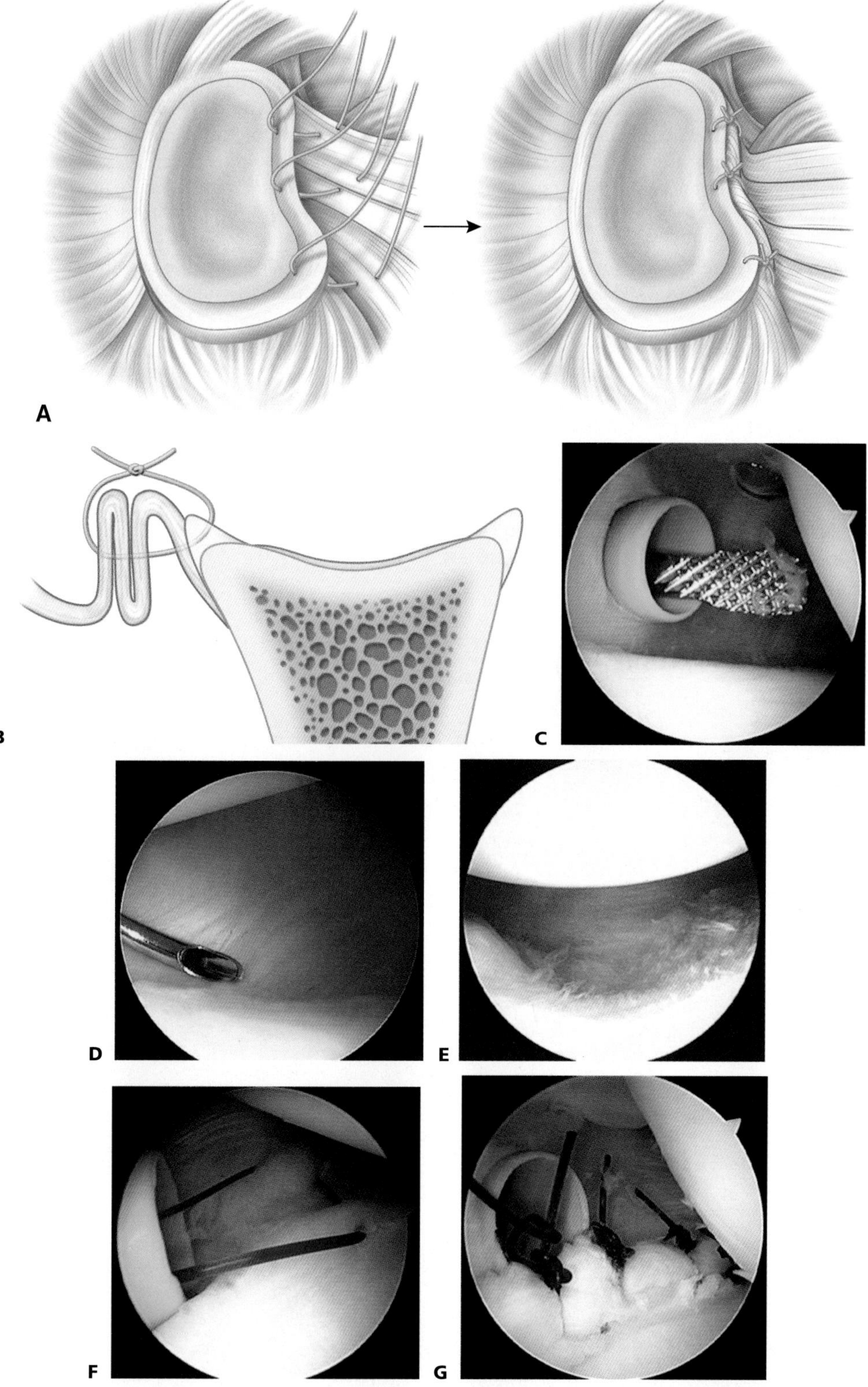

TECH FIG 7 • **A.** Multiple anterior plication sutures are used to obliterate redundant anteroinferior capsular tissue. **B.** Diagram in axial orientation to the glenoid showing accordion-like plication and shortening of the anterior capsule as it is sutured to the labrum. **C.** An arthroscopic rasp is used through the anterosuperior portal to abrade the capsular tissue and generate a healing response in the tissue after plication. **D.** Anterior capsule after abrasion and before suture placement. **E.** Starting anteroinferiorly, a pointed suture-passing device is used to suture a bite of lateral capsule to the labrum, as shown in **F.** As the knot is tied, this suture effectively shortens and reduces the anterior capsule. **G.** Multiple no. 1 PDS anteroinferior capsular plication sutures after tying of the final and most superior plication stitch.

POSTEROINFERIOR CAPSULOTOMY

- As stated earlier, a posterior capsulotomy is indicated only in patients unable to attain a GIRD of less than 20 degrees to allow restoration of full motion and normal glenohumeral biomechanics (TECH FIG 8A).
- Arthroscopic findings in these recalcitrant cases include inferior recess restriction and a thickened PIGHL (more than 6 mm thick).
- Two techniques can be used:
  - Arthroscope in anterior portal and instrumentation in standard posterior portal
  - Arthroscope in standard posterior portal and instrumentation in portal of Wilmington. We prefer this method because it allows more direct visualization of the capsular tissue as it is released (TECH FIG 8B). A small-diameter cannula (5.5 mm) may be needed to allow easy passage of the cautery through the portal of Wilmington.
- A hooked-tip arthroscopic electrocautery with long shaft (Meniscal Bovie; Linvatec) is used to create a full-thickness capsulotomy from the 6 o'clock to the 3 or 9 o'clock position in the posteroinferior quadrant.
- The capsulotomy is made approximately a quarter-inch from the labrum.
- Gentle sweeping motions are used to successively divide tissue under direct visualization (TECH FIG 8C–E).
- It is critical to perform the procedure without chemical paralysis induced by the anesthesia staff.
  - Muscular twitching will alert the surgeon that the electrocautery is too close to the axillary nerve and causing injury.
  - If this occurs, the capsulotomy should be shifted to a more superior and medial position or abandoned altogether if no safe zone is found.
- Posteroinferior capsulotomy typically results in a 50- to 60-degree increase in internal rotation immediately postoperatively.

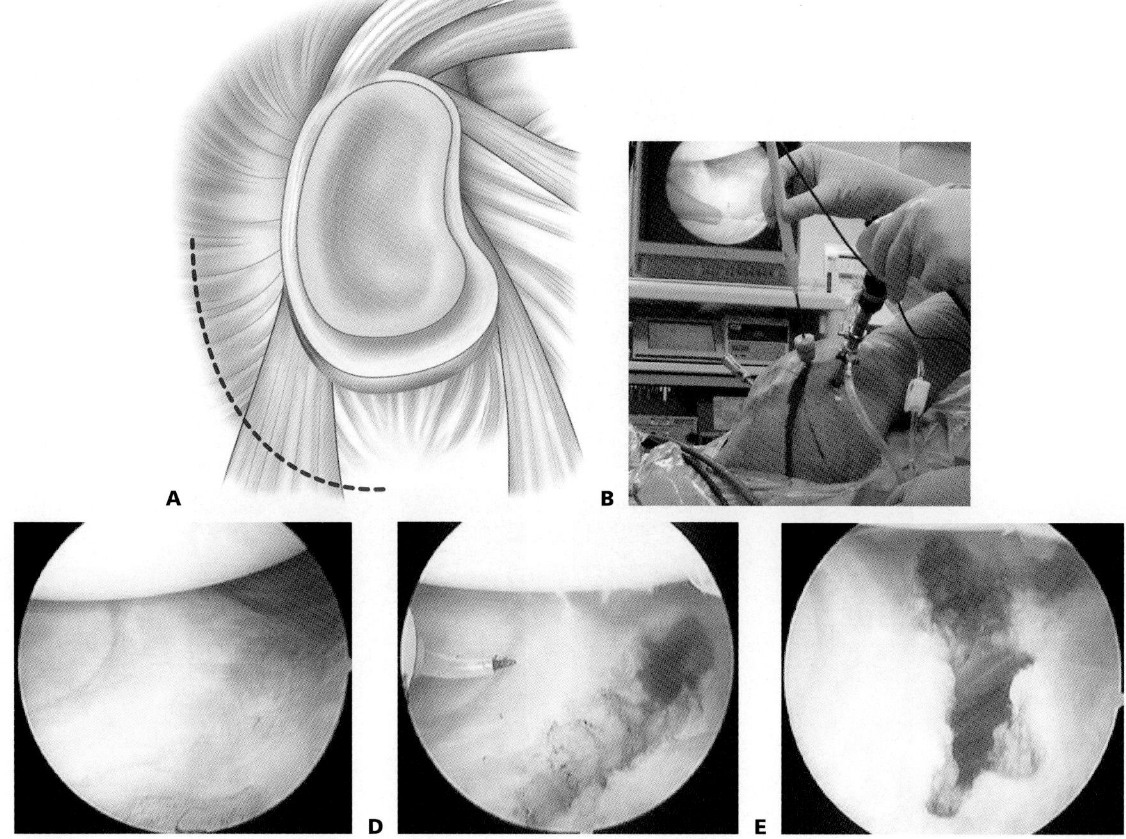

TECH FIG 8 • **A.** Location of the posteroinferior quadrant capsulotomy. **B.** Intraoperative view showing the instrument placement for posteroinferior quadrant capsulotomy. The arthroscope is in the standard posterior viewing portal and the cautery is in the portal of Wilmington. A small-diameter cannula (5.5 mm) may be required for passage of the hook-tipped cautery device through the portal of Wilmington. **C.** View of the posteroinferior capsule showing thickening and restriction of the inferior recess. **D.** The hook-tipped cautery is used to successively divide the capsule about 3 to 5 mm from the labrum under direct visualization. **E.** Completed capsulotomy. Muscle fibers just posterior to the capsule are visible between the divided edges of the capsule.

PEARLS AND PITFALLS

Physical examination	■ Examiner must stabilize the shoulder girdle with anterior pressure over the glenohumeral joint to negate scapulothoracic motion while performing range-of-motion measurements and determining total mobility arch and glenohumeral internal rotation deficit. Failure to measure isolated glenohumeral motion will yield erroneously high values that are useless in diagnosing the pathology and monitoring treatment.
Positioning	■ The lateral decubitus position offers a better view of the superior labrum and approach for suture passage because gravity causes superior recess tissue to fall away from the biceps anchor and widen the surgical field.
Steps to avoid shoulder distention when using a fluid pump	■ An efficient surgical plan should be developed before the case; it is modified as needed after diagnostic arthroscopy. The surgeon should work expeditiously; sufficient arthroscopic skills, including suture passage and knot tying, are required. ■ All anticipated instruments should be open on the back table at the start of the procedure. ■ The pump should be turned off if a pause in the procedure is needed. ■ An assistant should hold cannulas in the joint once they are passed through the capsule, particularly during suture passage and knot tying, or the cannulas will back out and allow distention of superficial tissues.
Suture anchors	■ For fixation of the superior labrum, we now rethread anchors with absorbable suture (#1 PDS) to avoid pain from prominent knots, as has been our observation with permanent suture material in the superior labrum.
Suture passage	■ Tangling of sutures during suture passage can easily occur. It is also easily corrected when there is slack in the sutures. Suture limbs should be passed slowly and under visualization to allow for corrections. ■ A looped suture-passing device is best used with two cannulas: one to pass the loop and a second to retrieve the loop and thread the intended "post-limb" suture. Passing and retrieving sutures through the same cannula will result in tangling. ■ If one cannula has the best angle of approach for suture passage, a tissue-penetrating retriever is used to pierce the tissue and retrieve the suture through the same cannula to avoid tangling.
Knot tying	■ The surgeon should not attempt to tie knots percutaneously because tissue will interfere with sliding and tightening of the knot. Suture limbs should be transferred to a cannula for knot tying. ■ An assistant should point and stabilize the cannula at the anchor to simplify tying. ■ The surgeon should learn and become proficient with one sliding and one nonsliding knot. A two-hole knot pusher (Arthrex) is useful for cinching the limbs down and untwisting the limbs during successive throws.

POSTOPERATIVE CARE

- Follow-up
  - Procedures are performed on an outpatient basis.
  - Return for dressing change postoperative day 1.
  - Ice or cooling pad is encouraged for first 48 hours.
  - Sutures are removed at 1 week.
  - Starting at 1 week, self-directed range-of-motion exercises are begun under specific guidelines (see below). Patients are seen regularly to assess progress and modify rehabilitation as needed.

Rehabilitation Time Table

- Immediate
  - Passive external rotation with arm at side (not abduction) within specific parameters
  - Elbow flexion and extension
  - Capsulotomy patients are started on "sleeper" stretches on postoperative day 1.
- Weeks 1 to 3
  - Pendulum exercises
  - Passive range of motion using pulley device in forward flexion and abduction to 90 degrees only
  - Start shoulder shrugs and scapular retraction exercises in sling.
  - Sling should be worn when not out for exercises.
- Weeks 3 to 6
  - Sling is discontinued at 3 weeks.
  - Passive range of motion is advanced to full motion in forward flexion and abduction.
  - "Sleeper" stretches are started in patients not having capsulotomy.
- Weeks 6 to 16
  - Stretching and flexibility exercises are continued.
  - Passive external rotation stretching in 90 degrees of abduction is begun.
  - Strengthening for rotator cuff, scapular stabilizers, and deltoid is started at 6 weeks.
  - Biceps strengthening is delayed until 8 weeks.
  - Daily "sleeper" stretches are continued.
- 4 months
  - Interval throwing program on level surface
  - Stretching and strengthening is continued (internal rotation stretches are emphasized).
- 6 months
  - Pitchers begin throwing full speed depending on pain-free progression through interval throwing program.
  - Continue daily internal rotation stretches.
- 7 months
  - Full-velocity throwing from mound
  - "Sleeper" stretches and scapular conditioning are

performed daily indefinitely while the patient continues throwing competitively.

OUTCOMES

- SLAP repair in high-level throwers: 182 pitchers treated over 8 years (one third professional, one third college, one third high school)[2]
  - 92% returned to premorbid performance or better.
  - Average UCLA score was 92% excellent at 1 year and 87% excellent at 3 years.
  - 164 pitchers undergoing SLAP repair and posteroinferior capsular stretching:
    - Average GIRD = 46 degrees preoperatively, 15 degrees at 2 years
  - Eight pitchers undergoing SLAP repair and posteroinferior quadrant capsulotomy:
    - Average GIRD = 42 degrees preoperatively, 12 degrees at 2 years
    - Average fastball velocity = 11-mph increase at 1 year

COMPLICATIONS

- Similar to other arthroscopic shoulder reconstructions: rare incidence of infection; failed repair; painful adhesion formation; subacromial irritation; stiffness
- Physicians and therapists must be vigilant about development of postoperative stiffness in overhead athletes. Stiffness can be addressed effectively with modification of the rehabilitation program if it is identified early with regular follow-up and directed therapy.

REFERENCES

1. Burkhart SS. Arthroscopically-observed dynamic pathoanatomy in the Jobe relocation test. Presented at Symposium on SLAP Lesions. 18th Open Meeting of the American Shoulder and Elbow Surgeons, Dallas, TX, Feb. 16, 2002.
2. Burkhart SS, Morgan CD. SLAP lesions in the overhead athlete. Orthop Clin North Am 2001;32:431–441.
3. Burkhart SS, Morgan CD, Kibler WB. The disabled throwing shoulder: spectrum of pathology, part I: pathoanatomy and biomechanics. Arthroscopy 2003;19:404–420.
4. Burkhart SS, Morgan CD, Kibler WB. The disabled throwing shoulder: spectrum of pathology, part II: evaluation and treatment of SLAP lesions in throwers. Arthroscopy 2003;19:531–539.
5. Burkhart SS, Morgan CD, Kibler WB. The disabled throwing shoulder: spectrum of pathology, part III: the SICK scapula, scapular dyskinesis, the kinetic chain, and rehabilitation. Arthroscopy 2003;19: 641–661.
6. Grossman MG, Tibone JE, McGarry MH, et al. A cadaveric model of the throwing shoulder: a possible etiology of superior labrum anterior-to-posterior lesions. J Bone Joint Surg Am 2005;87A:824–831.
7. Jobe CM. Posterior superior glenoid impingement: expanded spectrum. Arthroscopy 1995;11:530–537.
8. Morgan CD, Burkhart SS, Palmeri M, et al. Type II SLAP lesions: three subtypes and their relationship to superior instability and rotator cuff tears. Arthroscopy 1998;14:553–565.
9. Panossian VR, Mihata T, Tibone JE, et al. Biomechanical analysis of isolated type II SLAP lesions and repair. J Shoulder Elbow Surg 2005;14:529–534.

Chapter 7

Arthroscopic Treatment of Biceps Tendonopathy

J. R. Rudzki and Benjamin S. Shaffer

DEFINITION

- The long head of the biceps tendon has long been recognized as a potential source of pain and cause of shoulder impairment.[1,19,20,33]
- Although biceps tendon pathology can occur in isolation, it more frequently occurs concomitantly with rotator cuff disease, and its neglect may account for a subset of patients who fail to respond to rotator cuff repair.
- Pathology of the long head of the biceps tendon presents in a spectrum from subtle tendinopathy observed on diagnostic imaging studies to frank tearing or subluxation appreciated intraoperatively.
- Because the functional significance of the biceps tendon long head has been the subject of considerable debate, treatment has often been tailored more to patient symptoms, activity levels, and expectations rather than strict operative criteria.
- The ideal indications and optimal operative technique remain controversial, although recent advances in arthroscopic technology have led to an evolution of surgical strategies.

ANATOMY

- The long head of the biceps brachii originates from the supraglenoid tubercle and the superior aspect of the glenoid labrum.
- Multiple anatomic variants of the long head biceps tendon origin have been described, the most common of which involves an equal contribution from the anterior and posterior labrum.[32]
- The tendon travels intra-articularly (but extrasynovially) an average of 35 ± 5 mm toward the intertubercular (bicipital) groove between the greater and lesser tuberosities.[28]
  - The mean tendon length is 9.2 cm, with greatest width at its origin (about 8.5 × 7.8 mm).[23]
- At the site of intra-articular exit lies the annular reflection or biceps pulley, whose fibers are derived from the superior glenohumeral, the coracohumeral ligament, and the superficial or anterior aspect of the subscapularis tendon (**FIG 1**). Externally this structure's counterpart is the transverse humeral ligament.
- The bicipital groove has been a topic of significant study in the literature for its relevance to arthroplasty and it has been implicated as a contributing factor to tendinopathy involving the long head of the biceps.[6,26]
  - The dimensions of the bicipital groove vary along its mean 5-cm length. At its entrance, the width ranges from 9 to 12 mm, and the depth is about 2.2 mm. In its midportion, the groove narrows to a mean width of 6.2 mm and depth of about 2.4 mm, which may contribute to the entrapment of a hypertrophic intra-articular component; this has been referred to as the "hourglass biceps."[6,15,26]
  - The bicipital groove internally rotates from proximal to distal with a mean change in rotation of the lateral lip estimated at about 16 degrees.[15]
- The biomechanical significance of the biceps tendon long head is controversial. Some authors have advocated a role of the long head of the biceps in contributing to shoulder stability in overhead athletes.[12,25] Other authors, in separate studies,

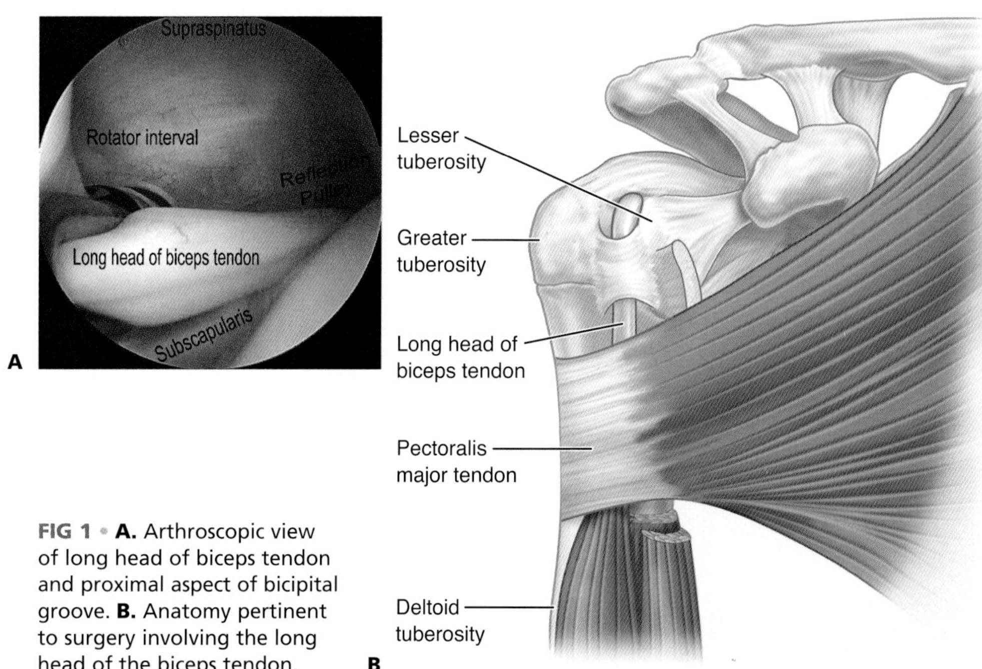

FIG 1 • **A.** Arthroscopic view of long head of biceps tendon and proximal aspect of bicipital groove. **B.** Anatomy pertinent to surgery involving the long head of the biceps tendon.

have used electromyographic analysis to conclude that the long head of the biceps tendon does not contribute to shoulder stability.[18,36]

- The extent of functional loss of supination and elbow flexion strength after biceps tenotomy has not been clearly established and is a source of controversy in the literature but may be estimated at 10%.[34]

PATHOGENESIS

- Long head of biceps tendinopathy encompasses a spectrum of pathology, including intratendinous signal change, synovitis of the sheath, partial tearing, and frank tendon rupture (**FIG 2**).
- The etiology of long head biceps tendinopathy is thought to be multifactorial.
- Identifiable causes include degenerative changes (usually in association with rotator cuff disease),[19,33,34] degenerative osteophyte spurring and stenosis within the bicipital groove,[6,26] inflammatory disease, traumatic injury, lesions of the biceps pulley complex or subscapularis tendon, and subtle forms of glenohumeral instability or superior labral anterior posterior (SLAP) tears.
- Lesions of the pulley complex (which contributes to stability of the tendon within the intertubercular groove) or tears of the upper subscapularis tendon may permit intra-articular subluxation and mechanical symptoms.
- "Hidden" cuff tears within the rotator interval or compromise of the annular reflection pulley may permit extra-articular long head biceps subluxation, which can lead to pathologic changes to the long head biceps tendon.
- Tears of the superior labrum such as type II SLAP tears and more subtle patterns of instability such as the peel-back mechanism in throwing athletes can also cause bicipital tendinopathy.

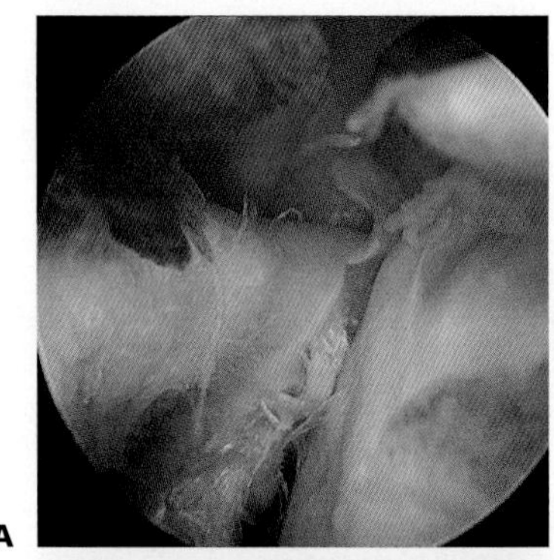

A

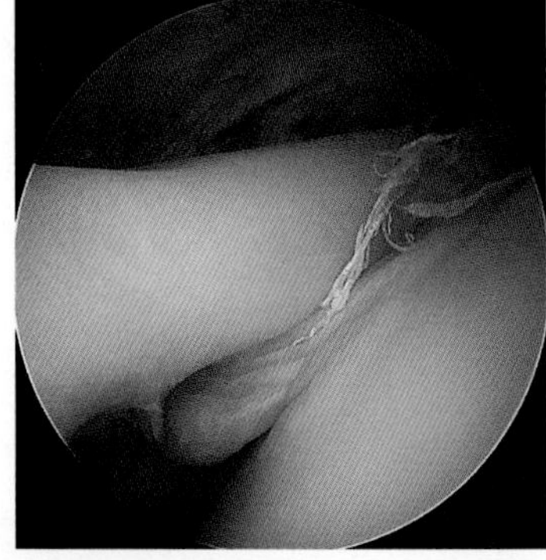

B

FIG 2 • Arthroscopic images of tendinopathy and tearing of the long head of the biceps tendon.

NATURAL HISTORY

- Little is known about the natural history of biceps tendinopathy, so prediction of a patient's clinical course is difficult.
- Patients with high-grade tendinopathy, either in isolation or in association with cuff tears, seem to be at risk of subsequent rupture.
- Spontaneous rupture often alleviates the chronic pain preceding the event.[34]

PATIENT HISTORY AND PHYSICAL FINDINGS

- As for bicipital tendinopathy, patients' historical presentations vary.
  - Patients may complain of anterior shoulder pain exacerbated by resisted elbow flexion and supination.
  - The history and character of shoulder pain is less helpful in making the diagnosis than the appropriate physical examination and diagnostic imaging findings in a relevant context.
- Biceps tendon disorders can present either in isolation or in association with other pathology, typically tears of the rotator cuff.
- Pain due to biceps pathology is often referred to the bicipital groove area.
- Physical examination findings are variable but typically include focal tenderness to palpation over the course of the biceps long head in the bicipital groove.
- Examinations and tests to perform include:
  - Speed's test: low sensitivity and specificity (estimated 32% to 68% and 56% to 75%); may be indicative of biceps tendinopathy in appropriate clinical setting
  - Yergason's test: A positive result suggests biceps tendinopathy in the appropriate clinical context.
  - Active compression test: Primarily assists in differentiating between symptomatic superior labral pathology and acromioclavicular joint pathology. A positive result may suggest biceps tendinopathy in the appropriate clinical context.
- Despite these recommendations, few studies have corroborated the sensitivity, reliability, or accuracy of these findings.

IMAGING AND OTHER DIAGNOSTIC STUDIES

- Magnetic resonance imaging (MRI) and ultrasound are the primary methods by which biceps tendinopathy is diagnosed.
- For the diagnosis of subluxation or dislocation of the long head of the biceps, ultrasound has a reported sensitivity of 96% to 100% and specificity of 100%.[2] For the assessment of complete rupture or the determination of a normal tendon, ultrasound has a sensitivity of 50% to 75% and specificity of 100%. Ultrasound is most useful to demonstrate pathology in the intertubercular groove and has been shown to be highly operator-dependent.
- MRI can identify intratendinous tendon abnormality, bicipital sheath hypertrophy, concomitant superior labral and rotator cuff pathology, the intra-articular course of the tendon, and the relationship of the biceps to the structures of the annular reflection pulley that stabilize it (**FIG 3**).

DIFFERENTIAL DIAGNOSIS

- Long head biceps brachii tendinitis or tenosynovitis
- Long head biceps brachii partial tear
- Long head biceps brachii rupture
- Long head biceps brachii instability or subluxation

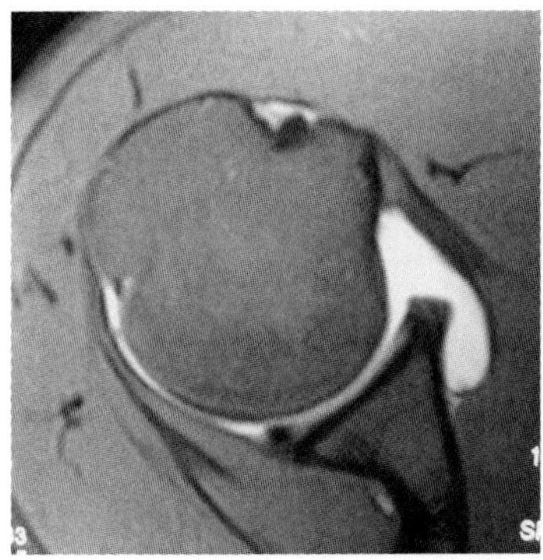

FIG 3 • Coronal MR image showing a normal-appearing biceps tendon in the bicipital groove adjacent to a normal subscapularis tendon and overlying annular reflection pulley.

- SLAP tear
- Acromioclavicular joint pathology
- Anterosuperior rotator cuff tear
- Subcoracoid impingement
- Subscapularis pathology

NONOPERATIVE MANAGEMENT

- Treatment of biceps tendinopathy depends in part on whether it presents in isolation as a primary problem or is associated with other pathology.
- Alternative nonoperative management of suspected biceps pathology includes activity modification, a course of nonsteroidal anti-inflammatory medication, and corticosteroid injections targeted directly into the biceps sheath within the intertubercular groove. Such an injection can be both therapeutic and diagnostic.[4]
- Some authors have advocated injection under ultrasound guidance.
- Long head biceps ruptures traditionally have been treated with nonoperative management, based on the perception that this problem rarely results in any significant impairment.
  - Patients may object, however, to the presence of a "Popeye" deformity (bulge in the volar aspect of the midportion of the brachium) (**FIG 4**) and possible fatigue-related cramping.

SURGICAL MANAGEMENT

- Surgical decision making includes patient factors, biceps tendon structural compromise, and concomitant shoulder pathology.

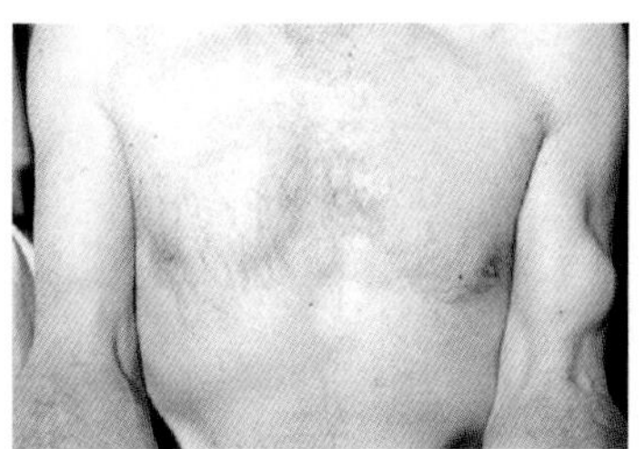

FIG 4 • "Popeye" deformity of the left arm.

- With respect to tendon involvement, nonscientific relative surgical indications include symptomatic partial-thickness tearing or fraying greater than 25% to 50% of its diameter, or tendon subluxation or dislocation from its normal position within the bicipital groove.
- Patient factors influencing treatment include the patient's age and activity level, occupation, desired recreational activities, and expectations.
- Because the biceps tendon is a known "pain generator," its evaluation and inclusion in treatment of cuff disorders is particularly important.
  - Preoperative consideration must be given to anticipate operative strategies if encountered.
- Operative alternatives in treating biceps tendon disorders include débridement, tenolysis (release of the biceps tendon long head), and tenodesis, in which the biceps is reattached to either bone or soft tissue of the proximal humerus. Each has advantages and disadvantages (Table 1).
- The selected surgical approach should take into consideration patient factors, intraoperative findings, and surgeon preference and comfort.
  - Patient factors include age, work, recreational and activity demands, expectations, and perspective on influence of cosmesis.
  - Intraoperative findings influence decision making in a number of ways, including bone quality, soft tissue quality, the presence of injury to the biceps sling or subscapularis, and the presence of instability.
  - Surgeon factors include arthroscopic proficiency and experience and concomitant surgical procedures that may influence the treatment approach (eg, swelling in the subacromial space during concomitant arthroscopic rotator cuff repair).
- Few studies have compared surgical alternatives within the same population of patients. Most such comparative studies

Table 1 Indications for Tenodesis and Tenotomy

Procedure	Advantages	Disadvantages
Tenodesis	Better cosmesis Maintenance of length–tension relationship of biceps Decreased risk of fatigue-related cramping Maintenance of forearm supination and elbow flexion strength	Potential pain at tenodesis site Potential failure of tenodesis to heal Potential persistent tenosynovitis
Tenotomy	Typically minimal discomfort No need for placement of implants into proximal humerus or bone–tendon healing High rate of success for pain relief Minimal risk of persistent tenosynovitis	Potential fatigue-related cramping Significant potential for Popeye sign and undesirable cosmetic result Potential for slight to mild forearm supination and elbow flexion deficit

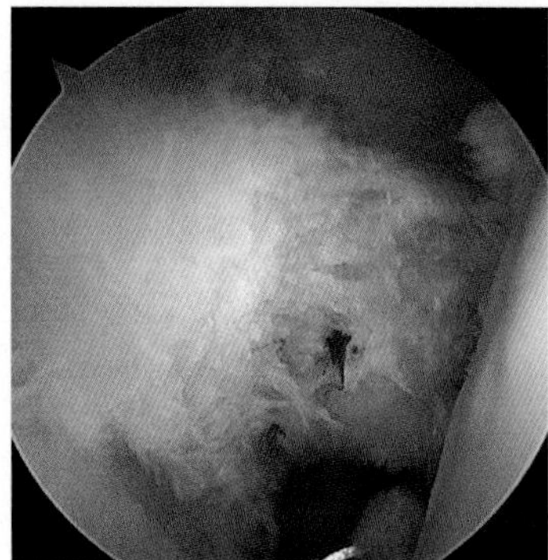

FIG 5 • Arthroscopic débridement of a partial-thickness tear.

have design flaws due to patient and pathology heterogeneity, in addition to procedures addressing frequent concomitant pathology.

- The ideal indications for débridement versus tenolysis versus tenodesis (soft tissue or bone) remain unclear at this time.
- Arthroscopic débridement is an initial component of nearly every biceps tendon surgical procedure.
  - In cases of fraying or partial tearing, débridement alone may be adequate to eliminate its contribution as a pain generator (**FIG 5**).
  - This is particularly true in cases in which the preoperative workup did not suggest the biceps as a significant component of patient symptoms, and when concomitant pathology may otherwise explain the patient's presentation.
- The degree of tendon involvement requiring definite surgical management with either tenolysis or tenodesis has not been scientifically established in the literature and varies depending on concomitant pathology.
  - Some authors have advocated consideration of addressing the biceps tendon surgically with débridement alone when less than 50% of the tendon's diameter appears involved (in addition to addressing any concomitant pathology), but assessing the percentage of tendon involvement is an inexact science.
  - When the biceps is thought to be the predominant cause of symptoms or occurs in isolation, débridement alone may fail to adequately address the pathology and relieve the patient's symptoms.
- With regard to tenodesis studies, biomechanical analysis has focused on construct strength.
  - Several tenodesis techniques provide sufficient construct strength, based on load-to-failure and cyclic displacement data.
  - One such study found that one particular interference screw tenodesis had a statistically significant greater resistance to pullout than a double suture anchor technique.[28]
  - Despite biomechanical testing, the actual amount of fixation strength necessary (and whether there is clear superiority of bone or soft tissue reattachment) is unknown.

Preoperative Planning

- Clinical evaluation to determine the contribution of the biceps tendon to patient symptoms is an important component of decision making and helps when encountering biceps pathology.
- Examinations for cuff pathology, particularly in the rotator interval ("hidden lesions" of the cuff) and for subscapularis integrity (belly press or lift-off test) are necessary components of the preoperative workup.
- Accurate preoperative evaluation should include appropriate radiographs to assess bicipital and acromial (outlet view) morphology.
  - The bicipital groove view permits assessment of groove depth and the presence of osteophytes but may be unnecessary given the typical quality of routine axial MR images.[8]
- MR images can be viewed to assess for biceps continuity (sagittal and coronal views) and intratendinous signal change (axial views) as well as tendon subluxation (axial and coronal views).
  - Attention must be paid when examining MR films to evaluate the appearance of the adjacent subscapularis, whose upper border is an important restraint against inferior biceps subluxation.

Positioning

- Positioning is a matter of surgeon preference.
  - When biceps tendon pathology is perceived to be isolated or a significant component of the patient's presentation, we have found that beach-chair positioning affords optimal orientation.
  - Biceps tenodesis or tenolysis can also be easily performed in the lateral decubitus position.
- All bony prominences are carefully padded and the neck is maintained in a neutral position, ensuring adequate circumferential exposure to the scapula (posteriorly) and medial to the coracoid (anteriorly).
- Alternatively, depending on surgeon preference, the patient may be placed in the lateral position.

Approach

- Standard arthroscopic portals for this procedure include the posterolateral portal for initial viewing, an anterior "operative" rotator interval portal, and the direct lateral subacromial portal (operative and viewing).
- Additional accessory portals within the antero-supero-lateral aspect of the rotator interval may facilitate work in the subdeltoid space during tenodesis.
- On initial arthroscopic examination, the biceps is carefully inspected along its course from the posterosuperior glenoid labral attachment to its exit within the bicipital sheath.[32]
  - Examination should include both visualization along the course and down the sheath (enhanced by use of a 70-degree lens) and palpation.
- Because only a portion of the biceps tendon long head is visualized within the joint, the biceps tendon must be translated into the joint using a probe, switching stick, or some tissue-safe tool. This enhances the surgeon's ability to visualize tendinopathic changes that may otherwise go unrecognized.
  - Meticulous examination of the proximate annular reflection pulley and subscapularis tendon insertion is obligatory.
- Biceps long head abnormalities can include:
  - Hyperemia, seen in patients with adhesive capsulitis or in biceps instability
  - Overt subluxation: Most commonly subluxation is inferior due to injury to its inferior restraints, composed of the upper subscapularis tendon, or bicipital sling, composed of

the intra-articular extension of the coracoacromial and coracohumeral ligaments.

- Subtle subluxation: Some authors have described a subtle instability pattern in which biceps tendon excursion within the otherwise normal-appearing sheath is greater than normal and deserves "stabilization."
- Biceps "incarceration": Some authors advocate the arthroscopic active compression test to assess for this uncommon entity. This test is performed intraoperatively with the arm positioned in forward elevation, slight adduction, and internal rotation.

BONY TENODESIS

Arthroscopic Interference Screws

- Before release at the superior labral attachment, the biceps long head must be controlled.
  - This is best achieved by the securing suture about 1 to 2 cm distal to the attachment.
  - This can be done either via spinal needle and PDS percutaneously, or by suture passage using a variety of available suture-shuttling instruments.
  - The biceps tendon attachment is then released at the anterosuperior glenoid using a bipolar cautery, arthroscopic scissors or basket, or retractable knife.
- The suture tagging the long head of the biceps tendon is then retrieved though an anterior skin incision just outside the arthroscopic cannula and secured with a Kelly clamp.
- The arthroscope is redirected into the subacromial space. Using the direct lateral portal, an arthroscopic bursectomy facilitates adequate visualization within the subdeltoid space and selection of the site of tenodesis.
- Visualization of the anterosuperior proximal humerus in the subdeltoid space may be facilitated by placing the traditional lateral portal slightly more anteriorly, as advocated by Romeo et al.[29]
  - With the camera repositioned in this lateral portal, the long head of the biceps tendon is identified in the sheath within the intertubercular groove (just lateral to the lesser tuberosity); this can be facilitated by a spinal needle.
- Using the small incision through which the biceps has been retrieved, the bicipital sheath is now incised with an arthroscopic scissors, electrocautery device, or retractable arthroscopic knife.
- The release is performed along the lateral aspect of the sheath to minimize any risk to the subscapularis tendon's insertion.
- The release should also be deep enough only to visualize the groove and tendon within it, because the ascending branch of the anterior humeral circumflex artery (the primary blood supply to the humeral head) lies beneath.
- This incision in the bicipital sheath is carried proximally to the lateral aspect of the rotator interval and the tendon is then retrieved through either the anterior or accessory anterolateral portal and secured with a clamp.
- The proximal end of the tendon is then resected after first placing a nonabsorbable whipstitch just distal to the site of intended tenotomy.
  - Because the interference screw can cause fraying of conventional first-generation sutures, the whipstitch is better composed of a newer second-generation material such as FiberWire or Herculine.
- The suture should be placed 10 to 20 mm distal to the exposed proximal portion, depending on how much diseased tendon is present, how much was resected intraoperatively, and the intended location of the tenodesis.
- When using an interference screw, the surgeon must ensure that the length of the suture is sufficient to pass through the cannulated interference screwdriver (**TECH FIG 1**).
  - Attention to suture management by use of cannulas is critical at this point. They ensure optimal visualization and soft tissue and suture management and minimize iatrogenic trauma to adjacent soft tissues.
- A guidewire for the tenodesis screw is driven into the intertubercular groove about 15 mm distal to the superior aspect of the groove (at the leading edge of the supraspinatus insertion).[29] The guidewire is inserted perpendicular to the groove to a depth of 30 mm.
- The scope is repositioned within the lateral (or most anterior lateral) portal and a cannulated 8-mm reamer is drilled to a depth of about 30 mm under direct arthroscopic visualization.
- The guidewire is removed and a screw is selected for tenodesis. Usually an 8-mm bioabsorbable implant is chosen, but this varies depending on bone quality.
- The proximal tendon is then retrieved with its previously placed whipstitch from the subdeltoid space out through the anterolateral portal.
- One limb of the whipstitch is loaded to the tenodesis screwdriver, and the bioabsorbable screw is loaded.
- The suture limb within the screwdriver is secured with a clamp at the top of the driver, thereby fixing the tendon at the tip of the insertion device for delivery to the base of the tunnel.
- The tendon and driver are inserted the full depth of the tunnel, and the interference screw is advanced while maintaining the driver position and suture tension. It should be advanced such that it is flush with the cortical surface of the intertubercular groove.
- The two remaining suture limbs (one exiting the cannulated screw, the other trailing between the screw and the bone tunnel) are arthroscopically tied on the top of the interference screw, providing further reinforcement.
- The arthroscopic portals and subacromial space are irrigated thoroughly and injected with local anesthetic with epinephrine.

Arthroscopic Suture Anchors

- Before being released at the superior labral attachment, the biceps long head must be controlled. This is best achieved by securing the suture about 1 to 2 cm distal to the attachment.

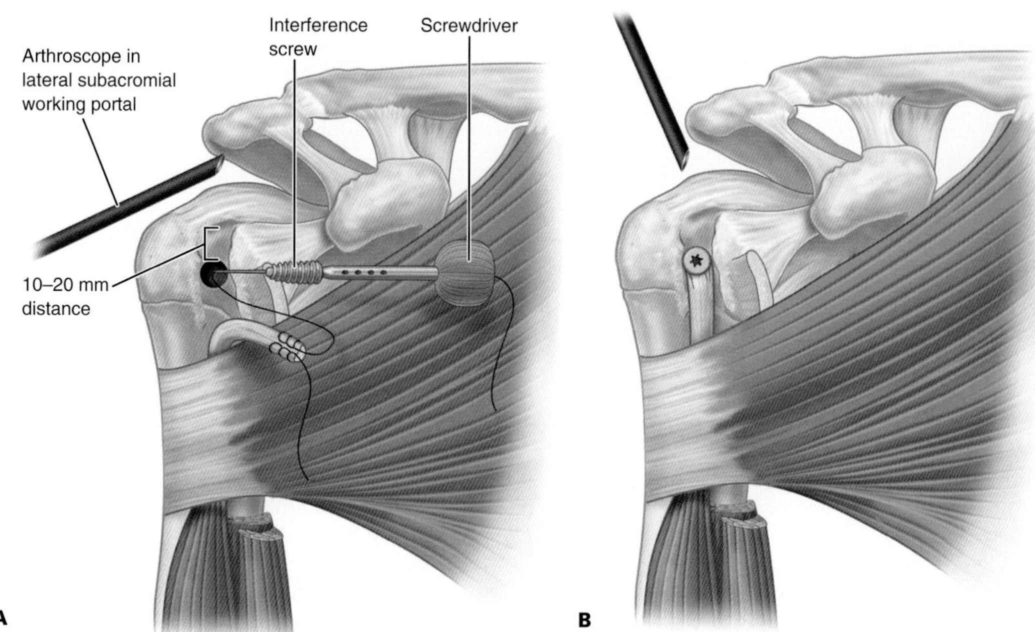

TECH FIG 1 • Arthroscopic interference screw method of tenodesis of the long head of the biceps tendon. The arthroscope is in the lateral subacromial working portal. **A.** The tendon is placed into the recipient hole in the bicipital groove and securely fixed with an interference screw. **B.** Completed tenodesis.

- This can be achieved either via spinal needle and PDS percutaneously or by suture passage using a variety of available suture-shuttling instruments.
- The biceps tendon attachment is then released at the anterosuperior glenoid using a bipolar cautery, arthroscopic scissors or basket, or retractable knife.
- The tagging 0 PDS suture controlling the proximal aspect of the tendon is pulled through the anterior portal skin incision outside of the cannula and secured with a Kelly clamp.
- The arthroscope is redirected into the subacromial space, where a bursectomy is performed from a direct lateral portal for adequate visualization within the subdeltoid space. The site of tenodesis is then selected based on surgeon preference.
- The intertubercular groove is identified by incising the annular reflection pulley as described above, and an arthroscopic burr is used to prepare the intertubercular groove by generating a bleeding bony bed.
- Next, two suture anchors are inserted (one proximal and one about 1 to 1.5 cm distal) within the prepared intertubercular groove, and sutures from these anchors are shuttled through the long head of the biceps tendon using a spinal needle and 0 PDS suture or a penetrating grasper device to securely fix the biceps into the groove.
- Although simple mattress sutures may be effective at achieving fixation, compromised tissue quality may lend to gradual suture–tissue failure, with pulling out of the tendon and failure.
  - An alternative locking knot configuration can be achieved using multiple percutaneous shuttling sutures, retrieved through the anterior interval cannula (**TECH FIG 2**).
  - Alternatively, the Mahalik biceps hitch, as described by Mahalik and Snyder, affords excellent fixation of the biceps tendon for tenodesis.
- An alternative technique involves an intra-articular tenodesis. Advantages include the ability to perform the procedure without requiring movement of the scope from the joint to the subacromial space, or subacromial bursectomy.
  - In this procedure, a stay suture is placed at the origin of the biceps sheath just at the anterior margin of the supraspinatus.
  - Flexion of the shoulder and use of a 70-degree lens facilitate identification of the most superior aspect of the bicipital groove. This will be the site of tenodesis.
  - The biceps tendon is released from its origin, with the stay sutures percutaneous (at the site of spinal needle penetration).
  - The anterosuperior portal is used to target the proximal humeral tenodesis site, generating a healing response along the proximal centimeter of the bicipital groove. By rotating and flexing the shoulder, the biceps tendon can be translated to permit good visualization of the tenodesis site and to facilitate subsequent targeting for anchor placement.
  - Several alternative fixation techniques exist, the most common of which is anchor insertion, followed by suture passage and knot tying through the proximal tendon stump.
  - Alternatively, the surgeon may make multiple passes through the biceps tendon (using a locking stitch of nonabsorbable suture such as FiberWire) and then use a knotless-type anchor (such as the Arthrex "push-lock" or "swivel-lock") to perform a secure tenodesis in a percutaneous fashion over a previously placed small-diameter cannula. This latter technique is particular good in cases with cuff tears, in which the proximal bicipital groove is so readily accessible.

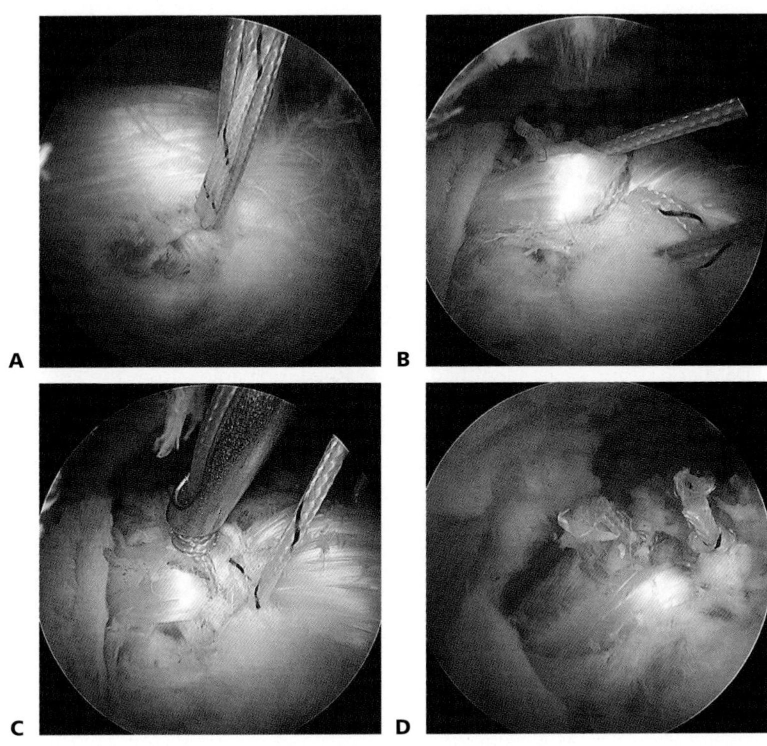

TECH FIG 2 • Arthroscopic images showing intra-articular tenodesis of the long head of the biceps tendon at the proximal aspect of the bicipital groove. **A.** Anchor placement. **B.** Suture passage. **C.** Knot tying. **D.** Completed tenodesis.

SOFT TISSUE TENODESIS

Arthroscopic Fixation

- This technique, in which the biceps tendon is secured to the soft tissues in the rotator interval, is based on the percutaneous intra-articular transtendon (PITT) technique described by Sekiya[30] and Rodosky[10] (**TECH FIG 3**).
- A spinal needle is placed percutaneously through the lateral aspect of the rotator interval proximate to the annular reflection pulley and then through the biceps tendon, about 1 to 2 cm distal to its supraglenoid origin.

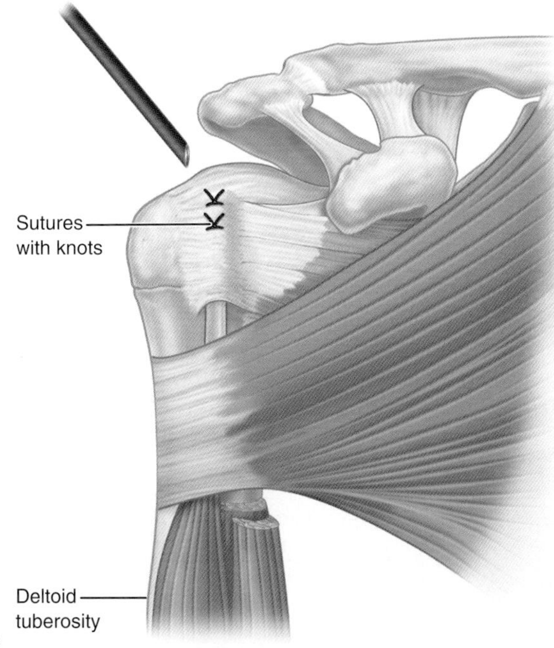

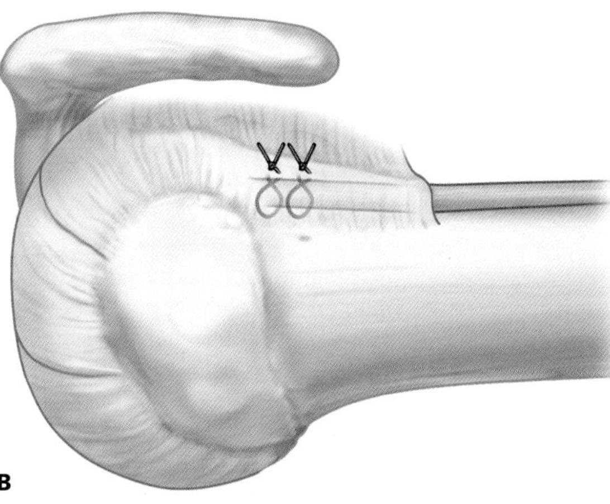

TECH FIG 3 • Percutaneous transtendinous or soft tissue tenodesis of the long head of the biceps tendon. **A.** Coronal plane view of suture fixation to secure the long head of the biceps tendon to the adjacent soft tissue structures in the proximal portion of the bicipital groove. **B.** Sagittal view showing the fixation with the arm in forward elevation and the knots secured in the subdeltoid space.

- A 0 PDS suture is then shuttled through the tendon; it is retrieved through the anterior interval portal using a grasper.
- This suture is then replaced by shuttling a nonabsorbable suture (such as no. 2 FiberWire or other comparable suture).
- This process is repeated 5 to 6 mm distally along the biceps tendon's course just proximal to the superior aspect of the intertubercular groove. Ideally, this second suture is of a different color so that the first set of suture limbs can be distinguished from the second.
- Next, the limb of the no. 2 nonabsorbable suture exiting the cannula is shuttled with the second PDS back through the biceps and annular reflection pulley. A mattress suture is placed in these structures. It exits the skin through two separate punctures made by the spinal needle passages.
- A tenotomy is performed via the anterior interval portal using an Arthrocare wand, needle-tip Bovie, arthroscopic scissors, or up-biting narrow meniscal basket.
- The intervening residual stump is excised and the arthroscope repositioned within the subacromial space, which is carefully débrided to enhance visualization and retrieval of the two suture sets.
  - Retrieval of the percutaneous suture pairs is facilitated with an arthroscopic "crochet hook."
  - An alternative technique for retrieving hard-to-find sutures involves making a small incision directly over the percutaneous suture exit sites and loading the suture limb within a single-loop knot pusher, which is then pushed through the skin and into the cleared anterior subacromial space. The sutures are then easily identified and grasped, unloading from the knot pusher, which is withdrawn without difficulty.
- Upon retrieval, which can be done one at a time, mattress sutures are tied under direct arthroscopic visualization in the anterior subacromial space.
- After thorough irrigation, the joint, subacromial space, and arthroscopic portals are infiltrated with 0.25% Marcaine with epinephrine.

ARTHROSCOPIC BICEPS TENOTOMY

- In the appropriately selected patient, the procedure is carried out by simply releasing the biceps tendon at its attachment site from a rotator interval portal while viewing from posteriorly.
- The intervening segment of diseased biceps tendon (in cases of tendinopathy) can be resected.
- Distal migration of the tendon can be discouraged by either leaving a residual wider portion of the diseased tendon just proximal to the proximal bicipital groove or by including a small piece of the anterior superior labrum at the time of tenotomy.
- Either of these strategies may preclude the tendency for distal translation and formation of a "Popeye" muscle.

PEARLS AND PITFALLS

Indications	▪ Careful assimilation of the preoperative history, physical examination, and imaging data with the findings at surgery is essential to determine which symptomatic lesions require treatment. ▪ A thorough discussion with patients about the goals, expectations, and potential complications of tenotomy and tenodesis is a key component of obtaining successful patient-based outcomes.
Portal placement	▪ The location of the rotator interval portal will greatly influence the ease with which an arthroscopic tenodesis can be performed. If the initial portal is too medial, establishing an accessory anterolateral portal over the intertubercular groove about 2 cm distal and 1 cm medial to the anterolateral aspect of the acromion will facilitate instrument passage and visualization. ▪ The location of the direct lateral portal along the anterior half of the acromion in the sagittal plane will aid in visualization when working in the subdeltoid space. ▪ Portal placement can be optimized by localization and triangulation using a spinal needle.
Diagnostic arthroscopy	▪ A key component of the arthroscopic examination is using a probe, switching device, or other instrument to displace the intertubercular portion of the tendon into the glenohumeral joint for adequate assessment. In addition, a careful examination of the fibers of the annular reflection pulley and the subscapularis insertion is essential. When viewing from the standard posterior portal, using a 70-degree lens can enhance visualization of the proximal intertubercular groove when performing an intra-articular tenodesis.
Visualization	▪ An adequate bursectomy facilitated by the use of electrocautery for hemostasis will significantly assist in visualization during arthroscopic tenodesis. ▪ Attention to accurate portal placement, fluid management (pump pressure), and procedure duration will help limit soft tissue extravasation, which can impair visualization and lead to performing the tenodesis open.
Arm position	▪ Manipulating the arm in flexion and extension, as well as rotation, can help in visualization as well as anchor targeting.
Suture management	▪ Careful suture management during tenodesis is key to avoid inadvertent soft tissue interposition, leading to inadequate fixation, skin dimpling, or unnecessary soft tissue dissection.

POSTOPERATIVE CARE

- The postoperative protocols for long head biceps tendon surgery vary according to the specific technique (débridement, tenotomy, or tenodesis).
  - Often the protocol will depend on the concomitant procedures, such as rotator cuff repair, performed.
- In general, after tenotomy, sling immobilization is used for 4 to 6 weeks, with passive elbow flexion and extension as dictated by the surgeon's preference and comfort level.
  - Forceful, active elbow flexion is prohibited for 6 weeks, by which time it is expected that the biceps tendon will have scarred into the groove or "autotenodesed" sufficiently to begin active motion.[23]
    - This period of protection also serves to minimize the potential for a Popeye deformity and fatigue-related cramping.
  - To further minimize the risk of distal retraction, some surgeons have described the use of a compressive wrap around the arm.
    - If too tight, however, the effect may be that of a tourniquet, leading to pain, swelling, and ecchymoses.
- After biceps tenodesis, patients are immobilized in a sling for 4 to 6 weeks, with the amount of active-assisted elbow flexion and extension dictated by surgeon preference and comfort.
  - Active elbow flexion is prohibited for about 6 to 8 weeks to allow tenodesis healing.
  - Some surgeons favor limiting the last 15 to 20 degrees of terminal extension for 4 to 6 weeks after surgery to minimize stress at the tenodesis site.
  - Active elbow flexion exercises are then slowly incorporated into the rehabilitation program after 6 to 8 weeks, with strengthening delayed until the third postoperative month.

OUTCOMES

- Outcome interpretation is challenging because of the limited number of studies and the lack of homogeneous patient populations. Surgical procedures to the biceps are typically only one component of surgically treated shoulder pathology in most studies.
- Arthroscopic tenodesis
  - Checchia et al[7] reported 93% good and excellent results in 14 of 15 patients, as determined by UCLA scores, who underwent arthroscopic rotator cuff repair and transtendinous soft tissue tenodesis at a mean follow-up of 32 months.
  - Boileau et al[5] reported their results of arthroscopic biceps tenodesis with interference screw fixation at mean follow-up of 17 months with a Constant score improvement from 43 preoperatively to 79 at latest follow-up ($P < 0.005$).
  - The historical literature regarding biceps tenodesis defines a range of unacceptable or poor results ranging from 6% to 40%.[16]
  - The results of open biceps tenodesis have been variable and are summarized in Table 2. Briefly, the results of arthroscopic tenodesis to date indicate that the procedure is an effective treatment for refractory biceps tendinopathy in appropriately indicated patients and may be more favorable for patients under 60 years of age.
- Arthroscopic tenotomy
  - Outcomes of arthroscopic tenotomy suggest that in the appropriately selected patient, this procedure can reliably provide pain relief, with minimal functional limitations or functional improvement.
  - Gill et al[11] in 2001 reported their results of tenotomy in 30 patients at a mean follow-up of 19 months. These patients scored an average of 82 by the American Shoulder and

Table 2 Outcomes of Arthroscopic Treatment of Biceps Tendinopathy

Author	No. Cases	Technique	Outcome Measure	Outcome
Checchia et al, 2005	15	Arthroscopic transtendon tenodesis	UCLA; mean 32-month follow-up	93% good and excellent results
Elkousy et al, 2005[10]	12	Arthroscopic transtendon tenodesis	Subjective telephone interview; 6-month follow-up	100% subjective assessment of benefit from procedure; 0% incidence of cramping or "Popeye" deformity
Kelly et al, 2005[16]	54	Arthroscopic tenotomy	American Shoulder and Elbow Surgeons (ASES) scale, UCLA, L'Insalata, cramping, Popeye, pain; mean 2.7-year follow-up	68% good to excellent results; 38% complained of fatigue discomfort after resisted elbow flexion; 70% Popeye sign
Walch et al, 2005[34]	307	Arthroscopic tenotomy	Constant score; mean 57-month follow-up	87% satisfied or very satisfied; mean Constant score improvement from 48 preop to 68 postop
Boileau et al, 2004[5]	43	Arthroscopic interference screw tenodesis	Constant score; mean 17-month follow-up	Mean Constant score improvement from 43 preop to 79 postop
Gill et al, 2001[11]	30	Arthroscopic tenotomy	ASES; mean 19-month follow-up	Mean ASES score at follow-up was 82 points; 87% satisfactory results
Berlemann et al, 1995[4]	15	Open keyhole tenodesis	Subjective assessment; mean 7-year follow-up	64% good and excellent results, 29% fair results
Walch et al, 2005	86	Open tenodesis	Subjective assessment	99% satisfied or very satisfied
Becker et al, 1989[3]	51	Open tenodesis	Subjective assessment; mean 7-year follow-up	About 48% had moderate to severe pain at mean 7-year follow-up.

Elbow Surgeons (ASES) grading scale (but no preoperative comparison data were available) and a significant reduction in pain and improvement in function. They reported 87% satisfactory results and a complication rate of 13%, including one patient with a painless cosmetic deformity, two patients with loss of overhead function and subacromial impingement, and one patient with persistent pain.

- Kelly et al[16] reported the results of 54 arthroscopic tenotomies at a mean of 2.7 years of follow-up, with 68% good to excellent results. However, 70% had a Popeye sign, and 38% of patients reported fatigue-related discomfort. They found minimal loss of elbow strength as assessed by biceps curls, and 0% loss for individuals over 60. Fatigue-related discomfort was not present in the patients over 60.
- Walch et al[33] in 1998 reported the results of 307 arthroscopic tenotomies of the long head of the biceps in conjunction with cuff tear treatment. They found a statistically significant improvement in the mean Constant score from 48 to 68 points and reported 87% satisfactory results.
- In summary, the results of arthroscopic tenotomy to date indicate that the procedure is an effective treatment for refractory biceps tendinopathy in appropriately selected patients and may be more favorable for patients over 50 to 60 years of age.

COMPLICATIONS

- The primary complications of tenodesis include persistent pain, failure of the tenodesis, and refractory tenosynovitis.
  - Failure of the tenodesis to heal may result in rupture of the tendon with distal retraction. In such cases, as often occurs in patients with spontaneous biceps tendon rupture, symptoms usually resolve with time.
  - One study has suggested that the quality of remaining tendon available for tenodesis can significantly affect the success of the procedure.[5]
  - Recent evidence suggests that oral nonsteroidal anti-inflammatory medication may inhibit healing, so this may be a suboptimal postoperative analgesic option.
- The primary complications of tenotomy are:
  - Cosmetic deformity in the form of a Popeye sign
  - Fatigue-related cramping
  - Potential slight decrease in elbow supination and flexion strength

REFERENCES

1. Alpantaki K, McLaughlin D, Karagogeos D, et al. Sympathetic and sensory neural elements in the tendon of the long head of the biceps. J Bone Joint Surg Am 2005;87:1580–1583.
2. Armstrong A, Teefey SA, Wu T, et al. The efficacy of ultrasound in the diagnosis of long head of the biceps tendon pathology. J Shoulder Elbow Surg 2006;15:7–11.
3. Becker DA, Cofield RH. Tenodesis of the long head of the biceps brachii for chronic bicipital tendinitis: long-term results. J Bone Joint Surg Am 1989;71A:376–381.
4. Berlemann U, Bayley I. Tenodesis of the long head of biceps brachii in the painful shoulder: Improving results in the long term. J Shoulder Elbow Surg 1995;4:429–435.
5. Boileau P, Krishnan SG, Coste JS, et al. Arthroscopic biceps tenodesis: a new technique using bioabsorbable interference screw fixation. Tech Shoulder Elbow Surg 2001;2:153–165.
6. Boileau P, Ahrens PM, Hatzidakis AM. Entrapment of the long head of the biceps tendon: the hourglass biceps—a cause of pain and locking of the shoulder. J Shoulder Elbow Surg 2004;13:249–257.
7. Checchia SL, Doneux PS, Miyazaki AN, et al. Biceps tenodesis associated with arthroscopic repair of rotator cuff tears. J Shoulder Elbow Surg 2005;14:138–144.
8. Cone RO, Danzig L, Resnick D, et al. The bicipital groove: radiographic, anatomic, and pathologic study. AJR Am J Roentgenol 1983;141:781–788.
9. Eakin CL, Faber KJ, Hawkins RJ, et al. Biceps tendon disorders in athletes. J Am Acad Orthop Surg 1999;7:300–310.
10. Elkousy HA, Fluhme DJ, O'Connor DP, et al. Arthroscopic biceps tenodesis using the percutaneous, intra-articular trans-tendon technique: preliminary results. Orthopedics 2005;28:1316–1319.
11. Gill TJ, McIrvin E, Mair SD, et al. Results of biceps tenotomy for treatment of pathology of the long head of the biceps brachii. J Shoulder Elbow Surg 2001;10:247–249.
12. Glousman R, Jobe F, Tibone J, et al. Dynamic electromyographic analysis of the throwing shoulder with glenohumeral instability. J Bone Joint Surg Am 1988A;70:220–226.
13. Goldfarb C, Yamaguchi K. The biceps tendon: dogma and controversies. In: Cannon WD, De Haben KE, eds. Sports Medicine and Arthroscopy Review. Philadelphia: Lippincott Williams & Wilkins, Inc; 1999:93–103.
14. Holtby R, Razmjou H. Accuracy of the Speed's and Yergason's tests in detecting biceps pathology and SLAP lesions: comparison with arthroscopic findings. Arthroscopy 2004;20:231–236.
15. Itamura J, Dietrick T, Roidis N, et al. Analysis of the bicipital groove as a landmark for humeral head replacement. J Shoulder Elbow Surg 2002;11:322–326.
16. Kelly AM, Drakos MC, Fealy S, et al. Arthroscopic release of the long head of the biceps tendon: functional outcome and clinical results. Am J Sports Med 2005;33:208–213.
17. Kim SH, Yoo JC. Arthroscopic biceps tenodesis using interference screw: end-tunnel technique. Arthroscopy 2005;21:1405.
18. Levy AS, Kelly BT, Lintner SA, et al. Function of the long head of the biceps at the shoulder: electromyographic analysis. J Shoulder Elbow Surg 2001;10:250–255.
19. Murthi AM, Vosburgh CL, Neviaser TJ. The incidence of pathologic changes of the long head of the biceps tendon. J Shoulder Elbow Surg 2000;9:382–385.
20. Neer CS II. Anterior acromioplasty for chronic impingement syndrome of the shoulder. A preliminary report. J Bone Joint Surg Am 1972;54A:41–50.
21. Nord KD, Smith GB, Mauck BM. Arthroscopic biceps tenodesis using suture anchors through the subclavian portal. Arthroscopy 2005;21:248–252.
22. O'Brien SJ, Pagnani MJ, Fealy S, et al. The active compression test: a new and effective test for diagnosing labral tears and acromioclavicular joint abnormality. Am J Sports Med 1998;26:610–613.
23. Osbahr DC, Diamond AB, Speer KP. The cosmetic appearance of the biceps muscle after long-head tenotomy versus tenodesis. Arthroscopy 2002;18:483–487.
24. Ozalay M, Akpinar S, Karaeminogullari O, et al. Mechanical strength of four different biceps tenodesis techniques. Arthroscopy 2005; 21:992–998.
25. Pagnani MJ, Deng XH, Warren RF, et al. Role of the long head of the biceps brachii in glenohumeral stability: a biomechanical study in cadavera. J Shoulder Elbow Surg 1996;5:255–262.
26. Pfahler M, Branner S, Refior HJ. The role of the bicipital groove in tendinopathy of the long biceps tendon. J Shoulder Elbow Surg 1999;8:419–424.
27. Richards DP, Burkhart SS. A biomechanical analysis of two biceps tenodesis fixation techniques. Arthroscopy 2005;21:861–866.
28. Rodosky MW, Harner CD, Fu FH. The role of the long head of the biceps muscle and superior glenoid labrum in anterior stability of the shoulder. Am J Sports Med 1994;22:121–130.
29. Romeo AA, Mazzocca AD, Tauro JC. Arthroscopic biceps tenodesis. Arthroscopy 2004;20:206–213.
30. Sekiya JK, Elkousy HA, Rodosky MW. Arthroscopic biceps tenodesis using the percutaneous intra-articular transtendon technique. Arthroscopy 2003;19:1137–1141.
31. Tuoheti Y, Itoi E, Minagawa H, et al. Attachment types of the long head of the biceps tendon to the glenoid labrum and their relation-

ships with the glenohumeral ligaments. Arthroscopy 2005;21: 1242–1249.

32. Vangsness CT Jr, Jorgenson SS, Watson T, et al. The origin of the long head of the biceps from the scapula and glenoid labrum. An anatomical study of 100 shoulders. J Bone Joint Surg Br 1994;76B: 951–954.
33. Walch G, Nové-Josserand L, Boileau P, et al. Subluxations and dislocations of the tendon of the long head of the biceps. J Shoulder Elbow Surg 1998;7:100–108.
34. Walch G, Edwards TB, Boulahia A, et al. Arthroscopic tenotomy of the long head of the biceps in the treatment of rotator cuff tears: clinical and radiographic results of 307 cases. J Shoulder Elbow Surg 2005;14:238–246.
35. Warner JJ, McMahon PJ. The role of the long head of the biceps brachii in superior stability of the glenohumeral joint. J Bone Joint Surg Am 1995;77A:366–372.
36. Yamaguchi K, Riew KD, Galatz LM, et al. Biceps activity during shoulder motion: an electromyographic analysis. Clin Orthop Relat Res 1997;336:122.

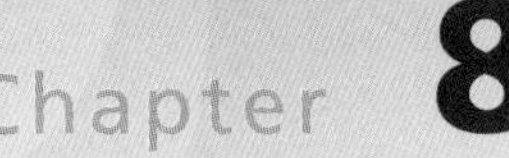

Chapter 8 Arthroscopic Treatment of Subacromial Impingement

R. Timothy Greene and Spero G. Karas

DEFINITION

- Impingement syndrome was originally described by Neer[19] in 1972 as a chronic impingement of the rotator cuff beneath the coracoacromial arch resulting in shoulder pain, weakness, and dysfunction.
- Repetitive microtrauma of the supraspinatus tendon's hypovascular area causes progressive inflammation and degeneration of the tendon, resulting in tendinopathy and rotator cuff tear.
- Extrinsic compression of the rotator cuff may occur against the undersurface of the anterior third of the acromion, the coracoacromial ligament, or the acromioclavicular (AC) joint.
- In a study of cadaveric scapulae, Neer[19] observed a characteristic ridge of proliferative spurs and excrescences on the undersurface of the anterior acromion overlying areas with evidence of rotator cuff impingement.

ANATOMY

- The scapula is a thin sheet of bone from which the coracoid, acromion, spine, and glenoid processes arise.
- The acromion, together with the coracoid process and the coracoacromial ligament, form the coracoacromial arch. The arch is a rigid structure through which the rotator cuff tendons, subacromial bursa, and humeral head must pass.
- The supraspinatus tendon is confined above by the subacromial bursa and the coracoacromial arch and below by the humeral head in an area referred to as the supraspinatus outlet. There is an average of 9 to 10 mm of space between the acromion and humerus in the supraspinatus outlet.[11] This space is narrowed by abnormalities of the coracoacromial arch. Internal rotation or forward flexion of the arm also decreases the distance between the coracoacromial arch and the humeral head.
- The subacromial and subdeltoid bursa overlie the supraspinatus and the humeral head. These bursae serve to cushion and lubricate the interface between the rotator cuff and the overlying acromion and AC joint. The bursa may become thick and fibrotic in response to progressive inflammation, further decreasing the volume of the subacromial space.
- The supraspinatus tendon has a watershed area of hypovascularity located 1 cm medial to the insertion of the rotator cuff. This area may predispose the supraspinatus tendon to degeneration, tendinopathy, and tears from overuse, repetitive microtrauma, or outlet impingement.

PATHOGENESIS

- Extrinsic impingement of the rotator cuff is caused by abnormalities of the coracoacromial arch, resulting in an overall decreased area for the rotator cuff tendons within the supraspinatus outlet.
- Acromial morphology most commonly accounts for narrowing of the supraspinatus outlet.
  - Bigliani et al[4] described three types of acromial morphology: the type I acromion is flat, type II is curved, and type III is hooked. They noted that 73% of cadaver shoulders with rotator cuff tears had a type III acromion.
  - A type I acromion with an increased angle of anterior inclination may cause impingement of the rotator cuff by narrowing the supraspinatus outlet.
- Other processes that narrow the supraspinatus outlet include osteophytes of the AC joint; hypertrophy of the coracoacromial ligament, os acromiale; malunion of the greater tuberosity, clavicle, or acromion; inflammatory bursitis; calcific rotator cuff tendinitis; or a flap from a bursal-sided rotator cuff tear.

NATURAL HISTORY

- Neer[20] classified impingement into three progressive stages:
  - Stage I impingement lesions occur initially with excessive overhead use in sports or work. A reversible process of edema and hemorrhage is found in the subacromial bursa and rotator cuff. This typically occurs in patients less than 25 years old.
  - With repeated episodes of mechanical impingement and inflammation, stage II lesions develop. The bursa may become irreversibly fibrotic and thickened, and tendinitis develops in the supraspinatus tendon. Classically, this lesion is found in patients 25 to 40 years of age.
  - As impingement progresses, stage III lesions may occur, with partial or complete tears of the rotator cuff. Biceps lesions and alterations in bone at the anterior acromion and greater tuberosity may also develop. These lesions are found almost exclusively in patients older than 40.
- Stage I and II lesions typically respond to nonoperative modalities if the offending activity is limited for a sufficient amount of time.
- Refractory stage II lesions and stage III lesions require operative intervention.

PATIENT HISTORY AND PHYSICAL FINDINGS

- Patients with impingement syndrome typically complain of the insidious onset of shoulder pain that primarily occurs with overhead activities. Pain is typically localized to the lateral aspect of the acromion, extending distally into the deltoid.
- Patients may experience pain at night, especially when lying on the affected side.
- Typically, patients with impingement syndrome do not complain of diminished shoulder motion.
- Physical examination methods to identify subacromial impingement include:
  - Palpation of the point of Codman: Tenderness is frequently a sign of supraspinatus tendinitis, tendinopathy, or acute tear of supraspinatus tendon.
  - Range of motion: Patients with impingement may have limited internal rotation from posterior capsular tightness. Active motion is typically more painful than passive motion, especially in the descending phase of elevation.

- Painful abduction arc: Pain from 60 to 120 degrees (maximally at 90) suggests impingement. Patients may externally rotate at 90 to clear the greater tuberosity from the acromion and increase motion.
- Neer's Imingement Sign: This maneuver compresses the critical area of the supraspinatus tendon against the anterior inferior acromion, reproducing impingement pain.
- Hawkins' Sign: This maneuver compresses the supraspinatus tendon against the coracoacromial ligament, reproducing the pain of impingement. It has high sensitivity but low specificity.
- Impingement test: This test has greatly improved specificity for making the diagnosis of subacromial impingement. A positive test is also a predictor of satisfactory outcome after subacromial decompression.[14]

- A complete physical examination of the shoulder should be performed to evaluate for associated pathology or other processes in the differential diagnosis.
  - AC arthritis: This may be clinically asymptomatic, but an inferior AC joint osteophyte can contribute to or cause impingement syndrome. If symptomatic, tenderness may be elicited at the AC joint with palpation and the cross-arm adduction test.
  - Rotator cuff tear: The history of traumatic injury is variable. Patients complain of deep shoulder pain at night and may complain of weakness in the affected shoulder. Strength testing will evaluate for rotator cuff tear and tear size. Evaluation for supraspinatus tendon tear is performed at 90 degrees of abduction in the scapular plane with maximally pronated forearms (Jobe test). Infraspinatus and teres minor weakness is assessed with resistance of external rotation. Inability to hold an externally rotated position is indicative of a massive tear (external rotation lag sign). Weakness of the subscapularis tendon is evaluated with resisted internal rotation. Inability to lift the dorsum of the hand from the ipsilateral sacrum (lift-off test) suggests a subscapularis rupture.
  - Glenohumeral instability: Subluxating or dislocating the humeral head anteriorly, posteriorly, or inferiorly while stabilizing the scapula (load and shift test) helps confirm the diagnosis of glenohumeral instability. Throwing athletes may have a complex pattern of pathology that includes anterior laxity and posterior capsular tightness, which may result in internal impingement. Internal impingement occurs during the late cocking phase of throwing and stems from contact of the articular side of the supraspinatus on the posterosuperior glenoid rim. These patients typically have posterior pain with apprehension testing. Internal impingement must be differentiated from extrinsic outlet impingement caused by coracoacromial arch narrowing. Although a posterior capsule contracture can predispose patients to outlet impingement, classic extrinsic outlet impingement is believed to be rare in throwing athletes.
  - Biceps pathology: Pain is typically in the anterior shoulder. Tenderness may be elicited in the area of the bicipital groove. Pain during resisted flexion of the arm with the elbow in extension and the forearm supinated (Speed's test) indicates biceps pathology.
  - Glenohumeral arthritis: Pain is associated with movement below 90 degrees of elevation. Patients complain of pain at night. Cogwheel crepitus may be present when loading the glenohumeral joint during resisted arm abduction.

IMAGING AND OTHER DIAGNOSTIC STUDIES

- Standard anteroposterior (AP) radiographs in internal and external rotation and a supraspinatus outlet view should be taken for the evaluation of impingement syndrome.
  - A supraspinatus or acromial outlet view is a transscapular view taken with the radiographic beam angled 15 to 20 degrees caudally (**FIG 1**).
  - The outlet view is the best plain radiographic technique to evaluate acromial morphology. With this information, the surgeon may accurately plan the amount of osseous resection required to convert the acromion to type I morphology.
- Additional views or diagnostic tests may be used to further evaluate the painful shoulder.
  - Axillary lateral radiographs may be helpful in showing an os acromiale.
  - Magnetic resonance imaging, computed tomography scan, arthrography, and ultrasonography should be used for patients whose diagnosis of impingement syndrome is not completely clear from the history, physical examination, and radiographs. These other modalities will also help diagnose biceps, labral, and rotator cuff pathology.

DIFFERENTIAL DIAGNOSIS

- Rotator cuff pathology
- AC osteoarthritis
- Glenohumeral instability
- Posterior glenoid and rotator cuff (internal) impingement
- Glenohumeral osteoarthritis
- Biceps tendon pathology
- Adhesive capsulitis
- Cervical spine disease
- Viral brachial plexopathy
- Thoracic outlet syndrome
- Visceral problems (eg, cholecystitis, coronary insufficiency)
- Neoplasm of the proximal humerus or shoulder girdle

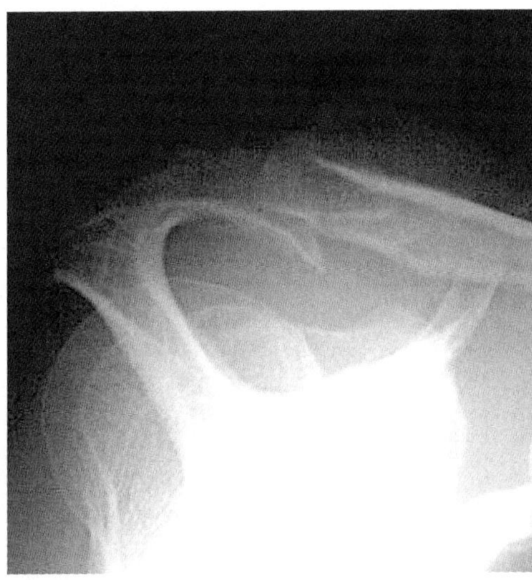

FIG 1 • Supraspinatus outlet view. This view helps the surgeon assess acromial morphology and facilitates preoperative planning for the amount of acromial resection.

NONOPERATIVE MANAGEMENT

- All patients with subacromial impingement syndrome should undergo a course of nonoperative management for 3 to 6 months. In the short term, a graduated physiotherapy program has been shown to be as effective as arthroscopic subacromial decompression.[5]
- Most patients can be successfully treated within 3 to 6 months. Large retrospective studies show that about 70% of patients with impingement syndrome will respond to conservative management.[18]
- The rehabilitation program should start by preventing overuse or reinjury with relative rest and activity modification. Subacromial bursal inflammation may be controlled with nonsteroidal anti-inflammatory medication, hot and cold therapy, ultrasound, and corticosteroid injection when appropriate.
- Therapy is advanced as pain and inflammation subside and is directed at regaining full range of motion and eliminating capsular contractures. In particular, posterior capsular contracture is addressed with progressive adduction and internal rotation stretching.
- As pain continues to decrease and range of motion improves, strengthening of the rotator cuff and periscapular musculature is initiated. This is achieved through progressive resistance exercises with elastic bands or free weights.
  - Patients should avoid overhead weight training (military press, latissimus pulldowns) and long lever arms (straight arm lateral raises) because these maneuvers can exacerbate impingement and place undue torque on the glenohumeral joint.

SURGICAL MANAGEMENT

- Operative intervention is indicated if patients continue to have symptoms of impingement syndrome that are refractory to a progressive rehabilitation program of stretching and strengthening over a minimum 3- to 6-month period.
- If the diagnosis is not completely clear, a more extensive diagnostic workup is warranted before surgical intervention.
  - The most common cause of failure for arthroscopic subacromial decompression and anterior acromioplasty is error in diagnosis.[1]

Preoperative Planning

- Imaging studies are reviewed to make sure that the preoperative diagnosis is correct.
- Particular attention should be paid to acromial morphology, the status of the AC joint, and evidence of rotator cuff pathology because these disease processes often coexist.
  - The preoperative supraspinatus or acromial outlet view gives the surgeon an accurate measurement of the amount of bone that must be resected from the anterior acromion to convert the acromial morphology to type I.[16]
  - If the AC joint has developed osteoarthritic changes, the presence of an inferior AC joint osteophyte may contribute to subacromial impingement. The presence of AC arthritis may not be clinically symptomatic; thus, coplaning of the inferior AC joint should be performed with the subacromial decompression. If the AC arthritis is symptomatic, distal clavicle resection should be performed in conjunction with subacromial decompression.
  - Preoperative knowledge of a rotator cuff tear is important for surgical planning of equipment, resources, and operative time as well as patient informed consent, recovery time, and time lost from work.
- Failure to recognize associated pathology is a common source of surgical failure.
- Examination under anesthesia of the affected shoulder is done before positioning. Passive range of motion is documented. The patient should be evaluated for a posterior capsule contracture, which can exacerbate impingement symptoms. Release of the posterior capsule with manipulation or arthroscopic cautery can improve a significant posterior capsule contracture.
- Anterior and posterior glenohumeral translation is examined using a modified load and shift test. Inferior translation is evaluated with the sulcus test.

Positioning

- The patient may be positioned in the beach-chair or lateral position.
- Advantages of the beach-chair position include a more customary setup for conversion to open cases such as biceps tenodesis.
- Advantages of the lateral position include better joint distraction for concomitant intra-articular arthroscopic procedures such as labral repair.

Approach

- Standard anterior, posterior, and lateral arthroscopic shoulder portals are used to perform the diagnostic arthroscopy and subacromial decompression.
- The details of these procedures are outlined in the Techniques section.

TECHNIQUES

ARTHROSCOPY

- The bony anatomy of the acromial borders, clavicle, AC joint, and coracoid process is outlined with a skin marker. The proposed site of the posterior, anterior, and lateral portals are marked (**TECH FIG 1**).
  - The posterior portal is located 2 cm medial and 2 to 3 cm distal to the posterolateral aspect of the acromion. This is the "soft spot" in the posterior triangular region of the humeral head, glenoid, and acromion.
  - The anterior portal is marked 1 cm lateral and 1 to 2 cm cephalad to the coracoid process.
  - The lateral portal is marked 2 to 3 cm distal to the lateral border of the acromion at the junction of the anterior and middle thirds of the acromion.
- The portal sites are infused with a mixture of 1% lidocaine and 1:300,000 diluted epinephrine solution.
- The glenohumeral joint is infused with 50 mL of the dilute lidocaine and epinephrine solution.
- The posterior portal is established with a 5-mm skin incision and a trocar is placed into the glenohumeral joint. Return of the previously injected solution confirms intra-articular placement.

- The trocar is removed and the arthroscope is placed. Inflow is established through the arthroscope.
- An 18-gauge spinal needle is used to confirm the anterior portal that was marked preoperatively. A 5-mm skin incision is placed over the site of the needle entry point and a probe is placed through the anterior portal.
- A diagnostic arthroscopy is performed. All surfaces of the glenohumeral joint, the glenoid labrum, glenohumeral ligaments, biceps tendon, rotator interval, and rotator cuff are thoroughly inspected.
- Particular attention is paid to the presence of glenohumeral arthritis, labral pathology associated with glenohumeral instability, and rotator cuff tears because they can mimic an impingement syndrome.

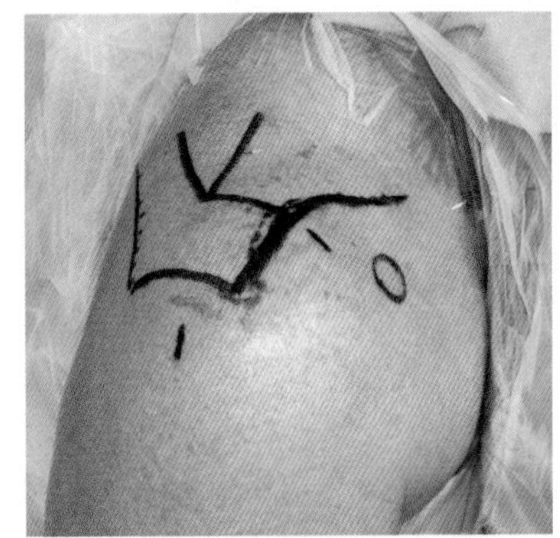

TECH FIG 1 • Acromioclavicular anatomy is outlined and the portal sites are marked.

SUBACROMIAL DECOMPRESSION

- Twenty milliliters of 1% lidocaine and 1:300,000 diluted epinephrine are injected into the subacromial space before intra-articular diagnostic arthroscopy.
- A blunt trocar is used to redirect the posterior portal from the intra-articular position to the subacromial space. The correct position is confirmed by palpating the hard undersurface of the acromion with the trocar tip.
- Once the trocar is felt to be in the subacromial space, it is swept laterally through the subdeltoid bursa to open the subacromial space. Care should be taken to avoid sweeping the trocar medial to the AC joint, which could injure the acromial branch of the thoracoacromial artery.
- The arthroscope is introduced and an initial assessment of the subacromial bursa and acromial spur is done.
- A 5-mm skin incision is used to establish the lateral portal 2 to 3 cm distal to the midlateral border of the acromion.
- A 5.5-mm full-radius resector is introduced through the lateral portal.
  - Visualization is often difficult because of the thickened and inflamed subacromial bursa. Therefore, triangulation of the arthroscope and full-radius resector must be done by palpation.
  - Bursectomy cannot be initiated until the cutting flutes of the resector are visualized.
- The tip of the anterolateral aspect of the acromion is palpated with the resector to confirm the correct subacromial orientation. Bursal resection is completed in an anterior-to-posterior and lateral-to-medial direction (TECH FIG 2A). Care must be taken not to resect the highly vascular bursal tissue medial to the musculotendinous junction of the rotator cuff.
- A radiofrequency electrocautery device is used to coagulate any bleeding and remove the remaining soft tissue from the undersurface of the acromion, starting at the anterolateral corner of the acromion (TECH FIG 2B).
- The electrocautery device is used to peel the coracoacromial ligament from the undersurface of the acromion and completely excise the remaining ligament stump. A complete resection of the coracoacromial ligament is confirmed when the undersurface of the deltoid is visualized as it drapes over the acromial edge (TECH FIG 2C).

A 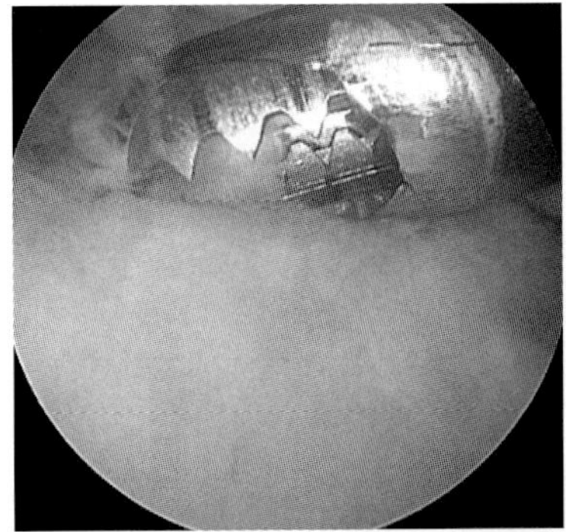
B 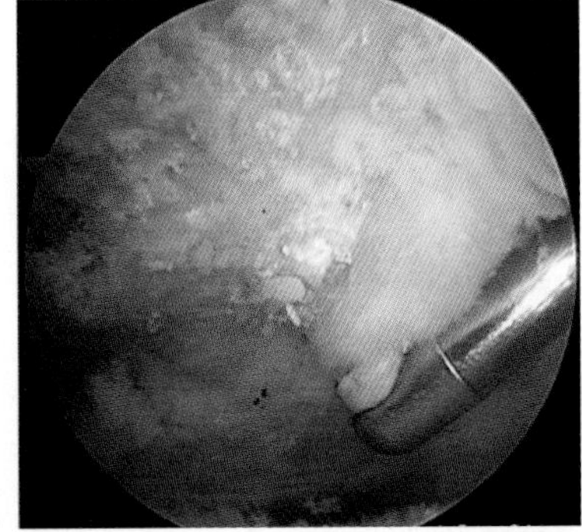
C 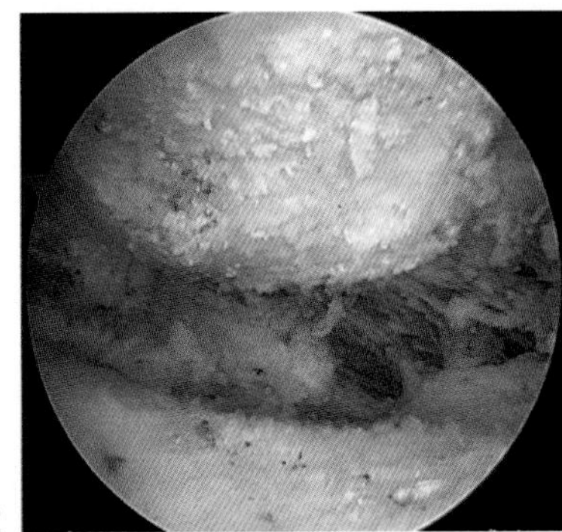

TECH FIG 2 • **A.** Arthroscopic bursectomy. The bursa overlying the tendinous portion of the rotator cuff must be thoroughly resected to evaluate the tendons for bursal-side rotator cuff tear. **B.** Soft tissue on the undersurface of the acromion is denuded with a radiofrequency electrocautery. Removing the soft tissue will expose the bony undersurface of the acromion and facilitate acromioplasty by the burr's cutting flutes. **C.** The acromial spur is now completely visualized. The coracoacromial (CA) ligament must be completely resected from the anterolateral acromion. Failure to do so may result in residual impingement by the CA ligament. Visualization of the undersurface fibers of the deltoid indicates a complete CA ligament resection. *(continued)*

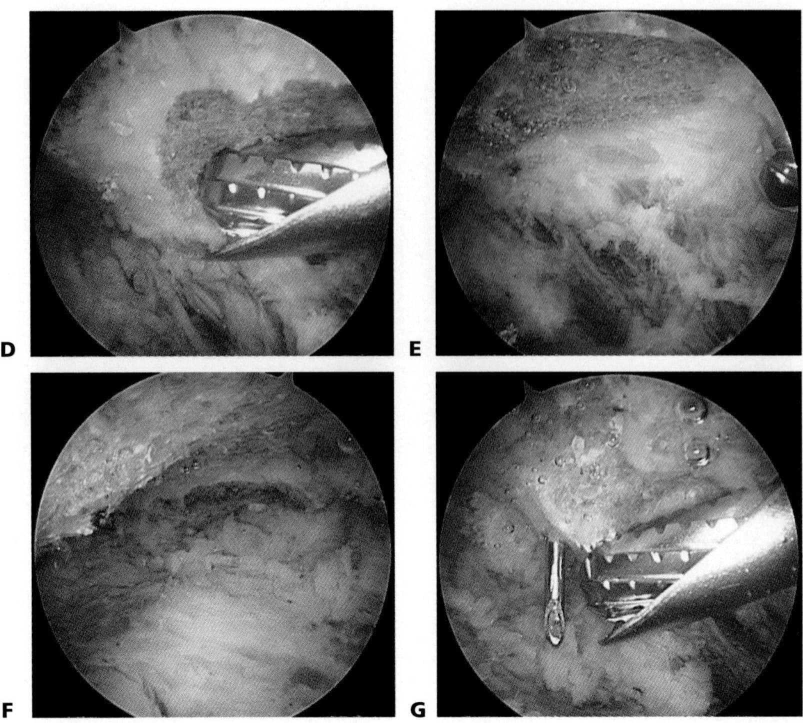

TECH FIG 2 • *(continued)* **D.** The acromioplasty begins at the far anterolateral tip of the acromion. The burr's diameter, usually 5 to 6 mm, is used to assess the initial depth of the acromial resection. The acromioplasty proceeds in 5- to 6-mm strips from anterior to posterior and lateral to medial. **E.** Completed acromioplasty. The undersurface of the acromion is converted to a type I morphology. Any residual ridges or rough edges can be safely smoothed with the burr in the reverse cutting position. **F.** View of the acromioplasty from the lateral portal. At the procedure's completion, the arthroscope should be placed in the lateral portal to assess the acromion for any residual downslope or unresected bone. The acromioclavicular joint is also well visualized from this portal and may be resected or coplaned via the anterior portal. **G.** Coplaning of the acromioclavicular joint. The posterior or lateral portal is used for arthroscopic visualization. Coplaning is performed with the burr in the anterior or lateral portal.

- Anterior acromioplasty is performed with a 5.5-mm burr via the lateral portal.
  - Resection begins in the anterolateral corner of the acromion. The desired depth of resection, estimated from the preoperative films, is obtained by measuring with the diameter of the burr (TECH FIG 2D).
  - This depth of resection is achieved anteriorly from the anterolateral corner of the acromion to the medial acromial facet of the AC joint.
  - The depth of resection is then progressively thinned posteriorly to the midportion of the acromion such that there is a smooth zone of transition from the anterior to the midportion of the acromion (TECH FIG 2E).
- Any ridges or rough edges may be smoothed with the burr in the "reverse cutting" position. The reverse position provides a much less aggressive bone resection, which is ideal for smoothing the bone once the acromioplasty is completed.
- The arthroscope is placed in the lateral portal to check the adequacy of resection (TECH FIG 2F). Any residual unresected acromion or impinging osteophytes from the undersurface of the AC joint should be resected.
  - Radiofrequency electrocautery should be used to resect the highly vascular soft tissue on the undersurface of the AC joint.
  - From the anterior or lateral portal, the 5.5-mm burr is used to coplane the distal portion of the clavicle flush with the acromion (TECH FIG 2G).

CUTTING BLOCK TECHNIQUE

- Anterior acromioplasty may be carried out using the cutting block technique.
- The arthroscope is placed in the lateral portal and a 5.5-mm burr is placed in the posterior portal.
- The tip of the burr is placed on the undersurface of the anterior acromion. If type I acromial morphology is present, the burr will lie flush with the undersurface of the posterior acromion.
- The undersurface of the posterior acromion is used as a guide for resection of the anterior acromion.
- The anterior acromion is resected until the burr is flush with the undersurface of the posterior acromion, producing type I acromial morphology (TECH FIG 3).

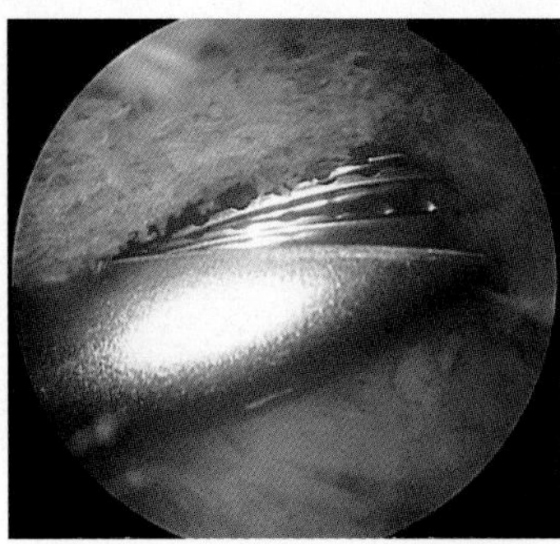

TECH FIG 3 • Completed acromioplasty via the "cutting block" technique. The acromion is viewed from the lateral portal while the burr is used to approach the acromion from the posterior portal. The burr sits flush with the undersurface of the acromion, indicating a type I acromial morphology.

WOUND CLOSURE

- As much fluid as possible is drained from the subacromial and intra-articular space. With the fluid inflow turned off, the suction tubing may be placed on the arthroscope's outflow portal to completely drain the subacromial space.
- Wounds are closed subcutaneously with 3.0 Monocryl suture.
- Steri-Strips and a sterile dressing are applied.

PEARLS AND PITFALLS

Error in diagnosis	■ This is the most common cause of failure of subacromial decompression. A detailed history and physical examination are essential. When the diagnosis is in doubt, MRI or additional imaging tests are indicated. Acromioclavicular arthritis, instability, glenohumeral arthritis, biceps lesions, and rotator cuff tears commonly coexist with impingement or may mimic impingement.
Hemostasis	■ Excessive intraoperative bleeding obscures adequate visualization and may lead to inadequate bony resection. ■ Twenty milliliters of a 1:300,000 diluted epinephrine and saline solution may be injected into the subacromial space before decompression to limit bleeding. ■ Hypotensive anesthesia is effective in controlling bleeding if not medically contraindicated. ■ Bleeders encountered during the decompression may be cauterized. The origin of bleeding is followed with the arthroscope until the inflow tamponades the bleeder. Cautery may then be used to stop the hemorrhage. Alternatively, the inflow pump pressure may be turned up to match the patient's mean arterial pressure. Inflow pressure tamponade is effective in limiting bleeding but should not be used for more than a few minutes, as the shoulder will swell quickly with this technique.
Inadequate bone resection	■ Inadequate bone resection may be a cause of surgical failure and may be avoided by preoperative knowledge of the appropriate amount of bone to resect from the supraspinatus outlet view. ■ The key to adequate osseous resection is clear biplanar visualization through the posterior and lateral portals.
Inadequate bursectomy and subacromial débridement	■ These may compromise surgical outcome by affecting visualization of a bursal-sided rotator cuff tear or continued mass effect from a retained thickened subacromial bursa. ■ Bursectomy should be complete such that the bursal surface of the rotator cuff is clearly exposed and the undersurface of the acromion is skeletonized.
Retained coracoacromial ligament	■ Incomplete resection may lead to ongoing impingement from the coracoacromial ligament. ■ Complete excision of the coracoacromial ligament is confirmed by visualizing the undersurface of the deltoid across the anterior aspect of the acromion. ■ The coracoacromial ligament extends at least 15 mm along the lateral acromial edge. The surgeon should resect the coracoacromial ligament completely and visualize the undersurface of the deltoid at least 15 mm posterior to the anterolateral corner of the acromion.

POSTOPERATIVE CARE

- Patients are placed in a sling for comfort postoperatively but are encouraged to discontinue the sling immediately when the interscalene block wears off.
- Patients are initially started on passive range-of-motion exercises. Therapy is advanced to active range of motion with terminal stretching as comfort allows. A rotator cuff and periscapular strengthening program is initiated once full range of motion is achieved. Terminal stretching, especially the posterior capsule, is continued for the next several months postoperatively.
- The therapy regimen is advanced as rapidly as motion and pain allow.
- Patients may return to work or sport as pain resolves and motion and strength normalize. This can take anywhere from 6 weeks to 6 months.
- Patients with classic outlet impingement from a type III acromion typically improve quickly.
- Patients with a significant component of tendinopathy or a bursal-sided rotator cuff tear may take much longer to improve.

OUTCOMES

- The success rate for arthroscopic subacromial decompression ranges from 73% to 95%.[2,7,8,9,21–24]
- The clinical results and predictability of bony resection for arthroscopic subacromial decompression have been shown to be equivalent to those of the open decompression.[13]

- The advantages of the arthroscopic procedure far surpass those of the open procedure and include less surgical morbidity, preservation of the deltoid attachment, allowing rapid advancement of rehabilitation, and direct visualization of the glenohumeral joint. It is the senior author's opinion that open decompression surgery for routine impingement is a dated technique that should be relegated to the status of historical interest.

- Hawkins et al[10] found a significant increase in satisfactory outcomes after arthroscopic subacromial decompression by extending the lateral portal 1.5 to 2 cm and assessing the adequacy of decompression by digital palpation.
  - This technique is especially effective for surgeons early in their arthroscopic experience, where confirmation by digital palpation can give tactile as well as visual feedback on the adequacy of acromial resection.
- Coplaning impinging osteophytes from the AC joint after subacromial decompression has shown uniformly good results.[3,6]
  - Beveling the inferior 25% to 50% of the distal clavicle and medial acromion has resulted in neither significant AC joint hypermobility nor compromise in the outcome of subacromial decompression.[3,6]
- With appropriate patient selection, combined arthroscopic subacromial decompression and distal clavicle resection for coexisting impingement syndrome and AC joint symptoms has shown excellent results with long-term follow-up.[12,15]

COMPLICATIONS

- Infection
- Bleeding
- Neurovascular injury
- Fistula formation from excessive drainage
- Acromial fracture[17]

REFERENCES

1. Altchek DW, Carson EW. Arthroscopic acromioplasty: indications and technique. AAOS Instr Course Lect 1998;47:21–28.
2. Altchek DW, Warren RF, Wickiewicz TL, et al. Arthroscopic acromioplasty: techniques and results. J Bone Joint Surg Am 1990;72A:1198–1207.
3. Barber FA. Long-term results of acromioclavicular joint coplaning. Arthroscopy 2006;22:125–129.
4. Bigliani LU, Morrison DS, April EW. The morphology of the acromion and its relationship to rotator cuff tears. Orthop Trans 1986;10:228.
5. Braman J, Flatow E. Arthroscopic decompression and physiotherapy have similar effectiveness for subacromial impingement. J Bone Joint Surg Am 2005;87A:11:2595.
6. Buford D, Mologne T, McGrath S, et al. Midterm results of arthroscopic co-planing of the acromioclavicular joint. J Shoulder Elbow Surg 2000;9:498–501.
7. Esch JC. Arthroscopic subacromial decompression: a clinical review. Orthop Clin North Am 1993;24:161–171.
8. Esch JC, Ozerkis LR, Helgager JA, et al. Arthroscopic subacromial decompression: results according to the degree of rotator cuff tear. Arthroscopy 1988;4:241–249.
9. Gartsman GM. Arthroscopic acromioplasty for lesions of the rotator cuff. J Bone Joint Surg Am 1990;72A:169–180.
10. Hawkins RJ, Plancher KD, Saddemi SR, et al. Arthroscopic subacromial decompression. J Shoulder Elbow Surg 2001;10:225–230.
11. Jobe CM, Coen MJ. Gross anatomy of the shoulder. In: Rockwood CA, Matsen FA, Wirth MA, et al, eds. The Shoulder, ed 6. Philadelphia: Saunders, 2004:33–95.
12. Kay SP, Dragoo JL, Lee R. Long-term results of arthroscopic resection of the distal clavicle with concomitant subacromial decompression. Arthroscopy 2003;8:805–809.
13. Lindh M, Norlin R. Arthroscopic subacromial decompression versus open acromioplasty: a two-year follow-up study. Clin Orthop Relat Res 1993;290:174–176.
14. Mair SD, Viola RW, Gill TJ, et al. Can the impingement test predict outcome after arthroscopic subacromial decompression? J Shoulder Elbow Surg 2004;13:150–153.
15. Martin SD, Baumgarten TE, Andrews J. Arthroscopic resection of the distal aspect of the clavicle with concomitant subacromial decompression. J Bone Joint Surg Am 2001;83A:328–335.
16. Matthews LS, Blue JM. Arthroscopic subacromial decompression: avoidance of complications and enhancement of results. AAOS Instr Course Lect 1998;47:29–33.
17. Matthews LS, Burkhead WZ, Gordon S, et al. Acromial fracture: A complication of arthroscopic subacromial decompression. J Shoulder Elbow Surg 1994;3:256–261.
18. Morrison DS, Frogameni AD, Woodworth P. Non-operative treatment of subacromial impingement. J Bone Joint Surg Am 1997;79A:5:732–737.
19. Neer CS. Anterior acromioplasty for the chronic impingement syndrome in the shoulder: a preliminary report. J Bone Joint Surg Am 1972;54A:1:41–50.
20. Neer CS. Impingement lesions. Clin Orthop Relat Res 1983;173:70–77.
21. Patel VR, Singh D, Calvert PT, et al. Arthroscopic subacromial decompression: results and factors affecting outcome. J Shoulder Elbow Surg 1999;8:231–237.
22. Paulos LE, Franklin JL. Arthroscopic shoulder decompression development and application: a five-year experience. Am J Sports Med 1990;18:235–244.
23. Roye RP, Grana WA, Yates CK. Arthroscopic subacromial decompression: two- to seven-year follow-up. Am J Sports Med 1995;11:301–306.
24. Ryu RK. Arthroscopic subacromial decompression: a clinical review. Arthroscopy 1992;8:141–147.
25. Speer KP, Lohnes J, Garrett WE. Arthroscopic subacromial decompression: results in advanced impingement syndrome. Arthroscopy 1991;7:291–296.

Chapter 9 Acromioclavicular Disorders

R. Timothy Greene and Spero G. Karas

DEFINITION

- A number of pathologic processes may affect the acromioclavicular (AC) joint, altering anatomy, biomechanics, and normal function.
- The most common of these are primary osteoarthritis, posttraumatic arthritis, and distal clavicle osteolysis.

ANATOMY

- The AC articulation is a diarthrodial joint composed of the medial end of the acromion and the distal end of the clavicle. The joint supports the shoulder girdle through the clavicular strut.
- A fibrocartilaginous intra-articular disc is present in variable shape and size.
- The average size of the AC joint is 9 × 19 mm.[11] The sagittal orientation of the joint surface varies, ranging from an almost vertical orientation to a downsloping medial angulation of 50 degrees.[11]
- The stability of the AC joint is provided by capsular (AC) ligaments, the extracapsular (coracoclavicular) ligaments, and the fascial attachments of the overlying deltoid and trapezius.
  - The AC ligaments are the primary restraint to anteroposterior translation.
  - The superior AC ligament, reinforced by attachments of the deltoid and trapezius fascia, resists vertical translation at small physiologic loads. However, the coracoclavicular ligaments are the primary restraint to superior displacement under large loads.

PATHOGENESIS

- Degeneration of the AC joint is a natural part of aging.
  - DePalma[11] has shown degeneration of the fibrocartilaginous disc as early as the second decade of life and degenerative changes in the AC joint commonly by the fourth decade.
- The superficial location of the joint may predispose it to traumatic injury.
- The clavicle acts as a supporting strut for the scapula, helping maintain its orientation and biomechanical advantage for glenohumeral motion. Large forces may be transmitted from the extremity to the axial skeleton through the small surface area (9 × 19 mm) of the AC joint.
  - Repetitive transmission of large forces, such as weightlifting or heavy labor, may result in degeneration of the joint.
  - Repetitive microtrauma to the AC joint may cause subchondral fatigue fractures that undergo a subsequent hypervascular response, resulting in reabsorption and osteolysis (distal clavicular osteolysis).

NATURAL HISTORY

- Despite the frequency of radiographically evident AC joint degeneration, symptomatic arthritis of the AC joint is relatively uncommon.
- Studies have shown that 8% to 42% of patients with type I and II AC joint injuries develop chronic AC symptoms from posttraumatic arthritis.[2,3]
- Distal clavicle fractures may also result in posttraumatic arthritis.
- Patients with symptomatic AC joint degeneration have been successfully treated nonoperatively with activity modification.[12]

PATIENT HISTORY AND PHYSICAL FINDINGS

- Patients with isolated AC pathology typically experience pain over the anterior or superior aspect of the shoulder in an area between the midpart of the clavicle and the deltoid insertion.
- Pain occurs with activities of daily living that involve internal rotation and adduction such as putting on a coat sleeve, hooking a brassiere, or washing the opposite axilla.
  - Younger patients may complain of pain with weightlifting, golf swing follow-through, swimming, or throwing.
- Physical examination of the AC joint includes:
  - Palpation: Tenderness on direct palpation suggests AC pathology.
  - Cross-arm adduction test: This test is highly sensitive but not specific for AC pathology; it is often positive with impingement syndrome. Pain should be confirmed anteriorly because this maneuver will cause posterior pain if posterior capsular tightness is present.
  - Paxinos test: Combined with a bone scan, this test was found to be the most predictive factor for AC joint pathology.[16]
  - Diagnostic AC injection: Elimination of symptoms is diagnostic of AC pathology and prognostic for successful distal clavicle resection.
- A complete physical examination of the shoulder should be done to evaluate associated pathology and to rule out other differential diagnoses (as described below).
- Impingement syndrome commonly coexists with or may mimic AC pathology, and awareness of this possibility should be used to rule out its existence.

IMAGING AND OTHER DIAGNOSTIC STUDIES

- The AC joint is best evaluated radiologically with a Zanca view. This provides an unobstructed view of the AC joint by tilting the x-ray beam 10 to 15 degrees cephalad of the normal shoulder AP (**FIG 1A**).
  - Characteristic radiographic changes of primary and posttraumatic arthritis of the AC joint include osteophyte formation with trumpeting of the distal clavicle, sclerosis, and subchondral cyst formation. Narrowing of the AC joint will also be present; however, this occurs as a normal part of aging.

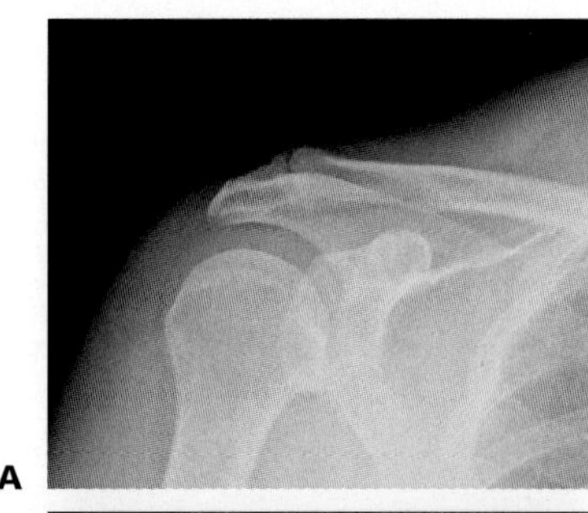

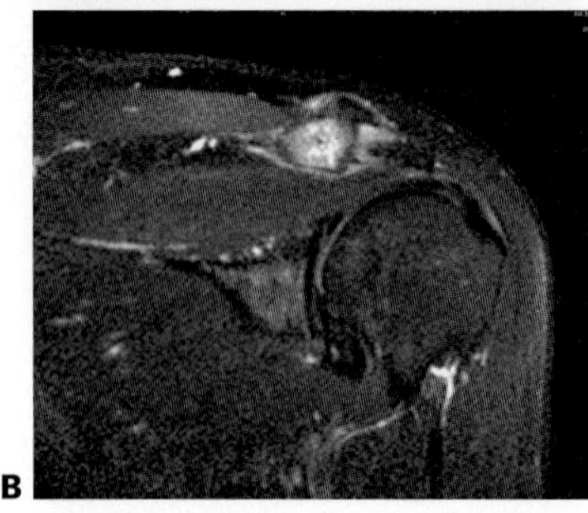

FIG 1 • **A.** Dedicated AC joint view of the shoulder best shows AC joint arthropathy or subluxation. Patients with degenerative changes on plain film or MRI, however, frequently have no symptoms. **B.** Edema in the AC joint. AC joint edema is a common finding in patients with symptomatic AC joint disease. Capsular distention and hypertrophy are also present.

  - Rheumatoid arthritis affecting the AC joint would typically show periarticular erosions and osteopenia with less spurring than osteoarthritis.
  - Distal clavicle osteolysis characteristically shows osteopenia, cystic changes of the distal clavicle, and widening of the joint space with narrowing of the distal clavicle.
- The supraspinatus outlet view may show inferior clavicular osteophytes, which may contribute to an impingement syndrome.
- The axillary lateral view of the shoulder may show anterior or posterior displacement of the clavicle, indicative of trauma to the AC joint.
- Three-phase technetium bone scan is highly sensitive and specific for AC joint pathology.
  - Bone scan is especially useful in diagnosing AC pathology that is not evident with conventional radiography.
- Magnetic resonance imaging (MRI) is sensitive in identifying AC pathology but has poor specificity, as AC abnormalities are frequently observed in clinically asymptomatic patients. Reactive edema in the AC joint is more predictive of clinical symptoms than are MRI findings of degenerative changes in the AC joint (**FIG 1B**).[13]

DIFFERENTIAL DIAGNOSIS

- Intrinsic AC pathology
  - Primary osteoarthritis
  - Posttraumatic arthritis
  - Inflammatory arthritis
  - Crystal-induced arthritis
  - Septic arthritis
  - Distal clavicle osteolysis
- Intrinsic shoulder pathology
  - Impingement syndrome
  - Rotator cuff tears
  - Biceps lesions
  - Glenohumeral arthritis
  - Early adhesive capsulitis
- Musculoskeletal tumors of the distal clavicle and proximal acromion
- Extrinsic conditions
  - Cervical spine disorder
  - Referred visceral problems (cardiac, pulmonary, or gastrointestinal disorders)

NONOPERATIVE MANAGEMENT

- The initial management of painful AC pathology should be conservative and should include a combination of activity modification, ice or heat therapy, nonsteroidal anti-inflammatory medications, corticosteroid injection, and physical therapy.
- Activity modification should focus on avoiding the inciting painful activities. Some patients may be successfully treated nonoperatively with activity modification.
- Intra-articular corticosteroid injection with 1 mL of 1% lidocaine and 1 mL of corticosteroid is effective in relieving AC joint pain, but the duration of relief is variable. Patients may receive multiple injections.
- Physical therapy consisting of terminal stretching and rotator cuff strengthening may be effective if a concomitant impingement syndrome exists. Isolated AC pathology typically does not respond to physical therapy.
- Patients should undergo 3 to 6 months of conservative management before operative intervention.

SURGICAL MANAGEMENT

- Patients with continued AC joint symptoms despite adequate conservative management over a 3- to 6-month period are appropriate candidates for surgical intervention.
- Significant pain relief from an AC joint injection should be documented before surgery, as this is prognostic for a good result after distal clavicle excision.

Preoperative Planning

- Preoperative history, physical examination, and imaging studies should be reviewed before operative intervention.
- A lidocaine injection test should be completed preoperatively and the patient should experience significant pain relief.
- If the diagnosis is in doubt and the patient does not receive significant pain relief from the lidocaine injection, a more detailed workup should be completed before surgery.
  - Error in diagnosis accounts for a significant number of failures of distal clavicle resections.[12]

Positioning

- The patient may be placed in the beach-chair or lateral decubitus position.
- We prefer the beach-chair position, as it facilitates conversion to an open procedure such as biceps tenodesis. The beach-chair position also places the AC joint in its more customary in vivo orientation, which may aid the surgeon during arthroscopy.

Approach

- There are two methods to resect the distal clavicle: the indirect (subacromial) approach and the direct (superior) approach.

- The choice of approach depends on the presence of concomitant shoulder pathology and the status of the AC joint.
  - The indirect approach is used when there is coexisting shoulder pathology, such as an impingement syndrome or a rotator cuff tear, allowing the patient to undergo simultaneous subacromial decompression and rotator cuff repair. The indirect approach is also helpful for markedly narrow AC joints, allowing wider exposure and thus better visualization of the AC joint surfaces.
  - The direct approach may be used for patients with isolated AC pathology or if there is adequate joint space to place the burr.
- We prefer the indirect (subacromial) approach to resect the distal clavicle because associated pathology can be addressed, fewer incisions are made, and the joint can be easily and adequately resected from this approach.

INDIRECT (SUBACROMIAL) DISTAL CLAVICLE RESECTION

- A complete diagnostic arthroscopy of the glenohumeral joint is performed.
- The arthroscope is redirected into the subacromial space through the posterior portal.
- A complete bursectomy and diagnostic subacromial arthroscopy is performed, as described in the previous section on subacromial decompression.
  - If an impinging spur from the acromion or an osteophyte from the inferior AC joint is present, subacromial decompression and coplaning of the AC joint are performed, as previously described.
- The AC joint may be difficult to orient due to variations in patient anatomy. An 18-gauge spinal needle may be placed percutaneously into the AC joint to facilitate orientation (TECH FIG 1A).
- If coplaning of the AC joint has not been previously performed with the subacromial decompression, an electrocautery device is used to remove the soft tissue from the undersurface of the AC joint.
- A 5- to 6-mm burr is then inserted in the lateral portal and the acromial side of the AC joint is resected. This will expose the distal aspect of the clavicle (TECH FIG 1B).
  - Both the acromial and clavicular sides of the AC joint should be beveled. This maneuver will create more working space and will allow easier access to the AC joint once the burr is introduced into the anterior

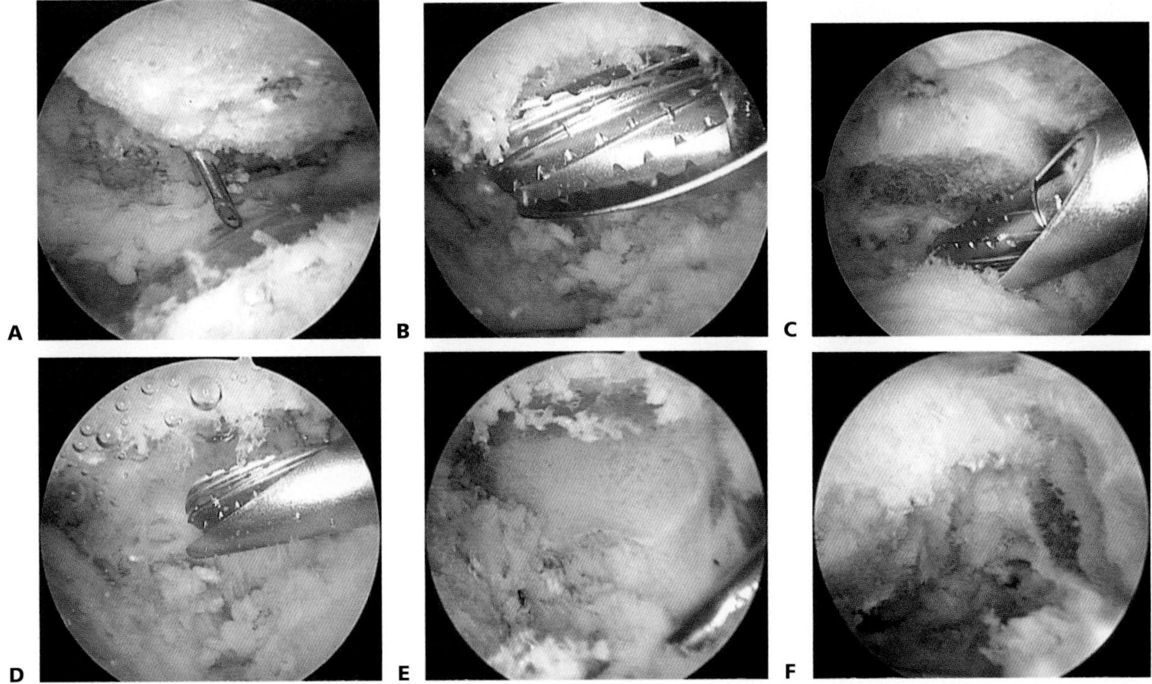

TECH FIG 1 • **A.** A spinal needle may be placed in the AC joint to help orient the surgeon. **B.** View of the AC joint from the posterior portal. The burr is in the lateral portal and is used to take down the acromial side of the AC joint. This maneuver will decompress the subacromial space and help expose the distal clavicle. **C.** Beveling the distal clavicle. With the burr in the lateral portal, the undersurface of the distal clavicle is scored. The surgeon can base the amount of clavicular resection on the length of the burr. **D.** The arthroscope is placed in the lateral portal and the burr is introduced into the AC joint via the anterior portal. The resection is completed using the landmarks established when previously beveling the distal clavicle. **E.** The completed AC joint resection is viewed "end on" from the lateral portal. **F.** The arthroscope is introduced into the anterior portal to view the adequacy of the posterior AC resection. The resection is adequate. The posterior AC joint capsule is left intact.

portal. Inferiorly directed pressure over the distal clavicle will also enhance its visualization.
  - The burr tip is about 10 to 12 mm long. Thus, when approaching the distal clavicle from the lateral portal, the length of the burr tip can be used to measure the length of distal clavicle to be resected, typically 8 to 10 mm (TECH FIG 1C).
  - Care should be taken to preserve the anterior and posterior AC ligaments if possible. The inferior joint capsule will be resected with the indirect approach.
- The arthroscope is now placed in the lateral portal and the 5.5-mm burr is placed in the anterior portal (TECH FIG 1D).
  - The burr is placed in the beveled area previously established via the lateral portal.
  - Resection of the remaining dorsal two thirds of the distal clavicle is accomplished starting at the anteroinferior aspect of the distal clavicle and working in a posterosuperior direction.
  - Again, care is taken to preserve the superior and posterior AC ligaments and superior joint capsule.
- About 1 cm of the distal clavicle is resected. Again, this can be estimated by comparing the size of the resection with the size of the burr (TECH FIG 1E).
- The arthroscope is then placed in the anterior portal to evaluate the adequacy of resection (TECH FIG 1F).
  - The arm may be placed in maximal cross-body adduction with the arthroscope in the anterior portal to confirm that the ends of the acromion and clavicle do not touch.

DIRECT (SUPERIOR) DISTAL CLAVICLE RESECTION

- A portal for the arthroscope is placed superiorly, 1 cm posterior to the AC joint. A 5-mm incision is made to introduce the trocar for the arthroscope.
- Once the arthroscope is introduced, the anterior working portal is placed under direct visualization starting superior and 1 cm anterior to the AC joint (TECH FIG 2A).
- A smaller arthroscope (2.7 mm) and soft tissue resector (2.0 mm) may be needed initially if the AC joint is significantly narrowed (TECH FIG 2B).
- An electrocautery device is used to remove the soft tissue on the AC joint undersurface.
- The AC joint is progressively resected until a larger burr (5.5 mm) will fit into the joint space.
- The anterior distal clavicle is resected first starting inferior and working superiorly.
  - Again, care is taken to preserve the anterior, posterior, and superior AC ligaments and capsule.
- When the anterior resection is completed, the arthroscope is placed in the anterior portal and the burr is placed in the posterior portal.
  - Resection of the posterior distal clavicle is completed from inferior to superior (TECH FIG 2C).
- The arthroscope is then placed in the anterior portal and the adequacy of resection is assessed.
  - A cross-body adduction maneuver may be performed to ensure that no contact remains between the clavicle and acromion.

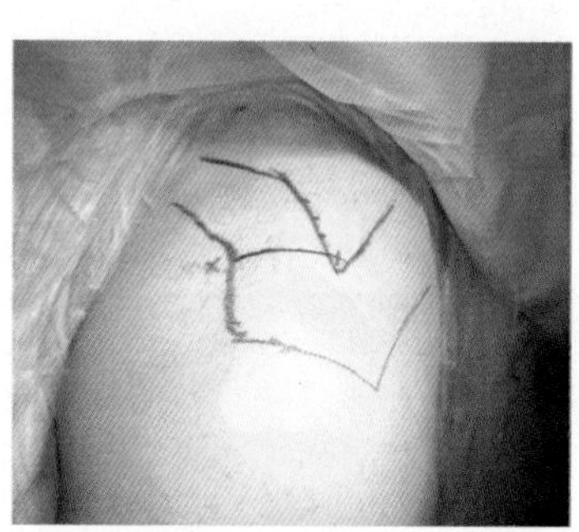
A

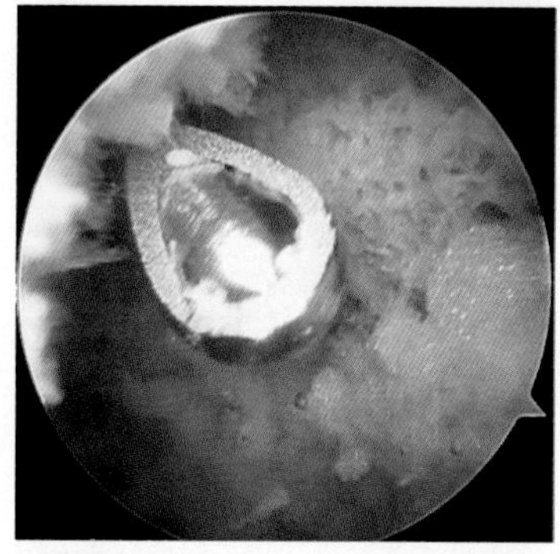
B

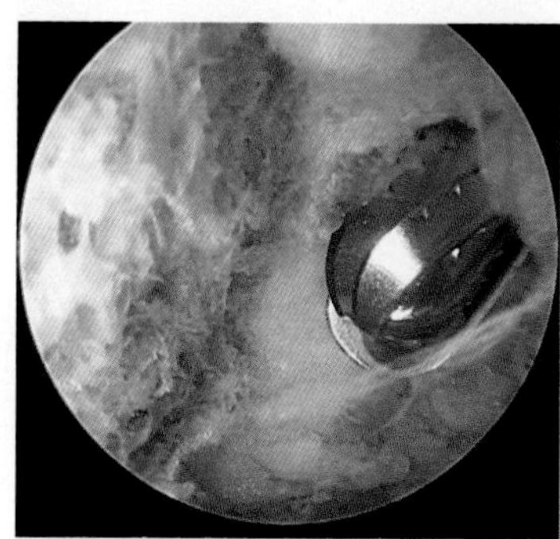
C

TECH FIG 2 • A. Portals for the direct technique of AC joint resection. **B.** A 2.7-mm shaver in the anterior AC joint. The arthroscope is in the posterior portal. Narrowing of a degenerative AC joint frequently precludes the use of a larger burr for the initial resection. **C.** Completion of the posterior clavicular resection with the direct technique. The initial resection is completed with small joint instruments, and a 5.5-mm burr may then be introduced into the posterior portal to complete the resection. Again, the posterior AC joint capsule is preserved.

WOUND CLOSURE

- As much fluid as possible is drained from the subacromial and intra-articular space. Suction may be placed on the arthroscopic cannula's outflow port to speed the extrication of superfluous fluid.
- Wounds are closed subcutaneously with 3.0 Monocryl suture.
- Steri-Strips and a sterile dressing are applied.

PEARLS AND PITFALLS

Diagnostic error	■ Diagnostic error is a common cause of failure of distal clavicle resection. A careful history and physical examination must be done before operative intervention. Patients must have significant relief of acromioclavicular (AC) symptoms after the intra-articular lidocaine injection test. A positive injection test is also prognostic for a good outcome after distal clavicle resection. ■ Many patients may have radiographic evidence of AC degeneration, but often these patients have no clinical symptoms. Symptomatic patients frequently have osseous edema on MRI evaluation of the AC joint.
AC joint orientation	■ It may be difficult to discern the orientation of the AC joint from subacromial space. Eighteen-gauge needles may be placed at the anterior and posterior aspects of the AC joint to aid in orientation. Visualization of the distal clavicle may be enhanced by resecting the medial aspect of the acromion and using inferior-directed pressure over the distal end of the clavicle.
Inadequate distal clavicle resection	■ This is a common technical error resulting in surgical failure. ■ Inadequate resection of the posterior and superior cortical ridge commonly causes residual abutment against the acromion. ■ One centimeter of distal clavicle resection is adequate for successful operative treatment; however, the adequacy of resection should be assessed in each case by dynamic cross-arm adduction with the arthroscope in the anterior portal. ■ If there is any question regarding the adequacy of resection, the anterior portal may be extended 1 cm superiorly and the resection may be assessed by direct digital palpation.
AC joint instability	■ Care should be taken to preserve as much of the AC capsular ligaments as possible, especially the superior ligament, which provides the primary resistance to posteriorly directed forces. Inadvertent release of the coracoclavicular ligaments should also be avoided because they resist axial compression of the AC joint. Thus, loss of coracoclavicular ligament function may cause abutment between the distal clavicle and acromion despite adequate bony resection.

POSTOPERATIVE CARE

- Patients are placed in a sling for comfort postoperatively but are encouraged to discontinue the sling immediately when the interscalene block wears off.
- Patients are started on passive range-of-motion exercises for the first postoperative week. Therapy is advanced to active range of motion with terminal stretching in the second postoperative week. A resisted rotator cuff and periscapular strengthening program is initiated the third week postoperatively. Terminal stretching is continued for the next several months postoperatively, especially posterior capsule stretches.
- The therapy regimen is advanced as rapidly as motion and pain allow.
- Patients can typically return to sport in 2 to 3 months. Graduated return is advised. For example, golfers should only chip and putt for the first month postoperatively. Weightlifters can begin training with lighter weights and avoid pressing motions until comfortable.

OUTCOMES

- The published success rates of arthroscopic distal clavicle resection are generally good and parallel the results of open distal clavicle resection.
  - Good or excellent outcomes have been reported in 83% to 100% of patients undergoing arthroscopic distal clavicle resection for primary osteoarthritis, posttraumatic osteoarthritis, or distal clavicle osteolysis.[1,5,7–10,14,15,17]
- The results of open versus arthroscopic distal clavicle resection have been retrospectively reviewed in the literature.
  - Several authors have found equivalent long-term results of open and arthroscopic distal clavicle resections; however, a significantly quicker recovery time has been observed with the arthroscopic resection.[4,6]
  - The quicker recovery time is a result of deltoid attachment preservation, which eliminates postoperative protection of the deltoid and allows for rapid advancement of physical therapy.

COMPLICATIONS

- Infection
- Bleeding
- Neurovascular injury
- AC joint instability
- Painful scar formation
- Heterotopic ossification at the resection site

REFERENCES

1. Auge WK, Fischer RA. Arthroscopic distal clavicle resection for isolated atraumatic osteolysis in weight lifters. Am J Sports Med 1998; 2:189–192.
2. Bergfeld JA, Andrish JT, Clancy WG. Evaluation of the acromioclavicular joint following first-and second-degree sprains. Am J Sports Med 1978;6:153–159.
3. Cox JS. The fate of the acromioclavicular joint in athletic injuries. Am J Sports Med 1981;9:50–53.
4. Flatow EL, Cordasco FA, Bigliani LU. Arthroscopic resection of the outer end of the clavicle from a superior approach: a critical, quantitative, radiographic assessment of bone removal. Arthroscopy 1992; 1:55–64.
5. Flatow EL, Duralde XA, Nicholson GP, et al. Arthroscopic resection of the distal clavicle with a superior approach. J Shoulder Elbow Surg 1995;4:41–50.
6. Gaenslen ES, Satterlee CC, Schlehr FJ. Comparison of open versus arthroscopic distal clavicle excision with acromioplasty. Othrop Trans 1996;19:258.

7. Gartsman GM. Arthroscopic resection of the acromioclavicular joint. Am J Sports Med 1993;21:71–77.
8. Jerosch J, Steinbeck J, Schroder M, et al. Arthroscopic resection of the acromioclavicular joint. Knee Surg Sports Traumatol Arthrosc 1993;1:209–215.
9. Kay SP, Ellman H, Harris E. Arthroscopic distal clavicle excision: technique and early results. Clin Orthop 1994;301:181–184.
10. Martin SD, Baumgarten TE, Andrews JR. Arthroscopic resection of the distal clavicle with simultaneous subacromial decompression. Orthop Trans 1996;20:19–20.
11. Depalma AF. Surgical anatomy of acromioclavicular and sternoclavicular joints. Surg Clin North Am 1963;43:1541–1550.
12. Shaffer BS. Painful conditions of the acromioclavicular joint. J Am Acad Orthop Surg 1999;7:176–188.
13. Shubin Stein BE, Ahmad CS, Pfaff CH, et al. A comparison of magnetic resonance imaging findings of the acromioclavicular joint in symptomatic versus asymptomatic patients. J Shoulder Elbow Surg 2006;1:56–59.
14. Snyder SJ, Banas MP, Karzel RP. The arthroscopic Mumford procedure: an analysis of results. Arthroscopy 1995;11:157–164.
15. Tolin BS, Synder SJ. Our technique for the arthroscopic Mumford procedure. Orthop Clin North Am 1993;24:143–151.
16. Walton J, Mahajan S, Paxinos A, et al. Diagnostic values of tests for acromioclavicular joint pain. J Bone Joint Surg Am 2004;86A: 807–811.
17. Zawadsky M, Marra G, Wiater M, et al. Osteolysis of the distal clavicle: long-term results of arthroscopic resection. Arthroscopy 2000;6: 600–605.

Chapter 10 Arthroscopic Treatment of Rotator Cuff Tears

Robert Z. Tashjian, Jay D. Keener, and Ken Yamaguchi

DEFINITION

- Rotator cuff disease encompasses a spectrum of disorders ranging from tendinitis to partial and full-thickness tendon tearing.
- It is the most common shoulder disorder treated by an orthopedic surgeon, with over 17 million U.S. individuals at risk for the disabilities caused by the disease.
- The prevalence of full-thickness tearing of the rotator cuff ranges from 7% to 40% across multiple studies.[17,20]
- Age-related degenerative change is a primary factor in the development of rotator cuff tears.[24]
  - Asymptomatic full-thickness tears have been found in 13% of the population between age 50 and 59 and in over 50% of people older than 80 years old.[20]
- The risks and benefits of both nonoperative and operative treatment must be considered for each individual patient.
  - A number of factors are critical in deciding how to treat full-thickness tears, including a history of trauma, patient age, tear size, degenerative muscle and tendon changes, and functional disability.
- Traditionally, open rotator cuff repair was the standard of care for symptomatic full-thickness rotator cuff tears.
  - Several disadvantages are inherent to open rotator cuff repairs. These include the need for deltoid detachment, difficult visualization of associated glenohumeral joint pathology, larger incisions, more extensive surgical dissection, and potentially a higher infection rate.
- The surgical treatment of full-thickness rotator cuff tears has been revolutionized by the advent of arthroscopic surgery.
  - With the introduction of arthroscopy, rotator cuff repair has moved from mini-open repairs to complete arthroscopic repairs.
- As techniques of complete arthroscopic rotator cuff repair have advanced, attempts have been made to treat larger tears arthroscopically. To do this, stronger fixation constructs must be used.
  - Single-row suture anchor repairs have been reported with good overall clinical results, but healing rates decrease as tear size increases.[5,6]
  - Double-row repair constructs with a medial and lateral row have been shown to provide improved initial biomechanical strength and restoration of the normal anatomic rotator cuff insertion.[14–16]
  - In the setting of a full-thickness rotator cuff tear, we now perform a double-row suture anchor repair if technically possible. While the double-row repair is more technically demanding, the potential advantages of anatomic restoration of the tendon insertion, improved biomechanical fixation, and improved healing may lead to improved functional outcomes.

ANATOMY

- The rotator cuff is a complex of four muscles arising from the scapula and inserting onto the tuberosities of the proximal humerus.
- The supraspinatus and infraspinatus muscles make up two thirds of the posterior cuff. The two tendons fuse together and have a direct bony insertion.
- When performing a double-row rotator cuff repair, knowledge of the dimensions of the rotator cuff insertion or "footprint" is critical.
  - The supraspinatus averages 25 mm wide and has a medial-to-lateral footprint (tendon attachment) of 12.1 mm at the midtendon (**FIG 1**).
  - There is a normal sulcus between the articular cartilage and the medial aspect of the supraspinatus footprint; it averages 1.5 mm in width.
  - The infraspinatus has been shown to average 29 mm wide, with a mean medial-to-lateral width of 19 mm.
- Suture anchor repair constructs using a single row of anchors have been shown to restore only 67% of the original footprint of the rotator cuff.[2]
  - Adding a second row of anchors increases the contact area of the repair 60%.[21]
  - The biomechanical properties of the double-row repair are improved compared to single-row repairs and include decreased strain over the footprint area, increased stiffness, and increased ultimate failure load.[14]

PATHOGENESIS

- The etiology of rotator cuff tears is multifactorial.
- The major factors are age-related degenerative changes of the tendon and physiologic loading.
  - The theory of age-related accumulative damage is supported by histologic findings of decreased fibrocartilage at the cuff insertion, decreased vascularity, fragmentation of the tendon with cellular loss, and disruption of Sharpey fiber attachments to bone.
  - Clinical studies support the aging theory as a primary cause of rotator cuff disorders.[24]
    - In a recent review of 586 consecutive patients with unilateral shoulder pain, rotator cuff tears were found to be correlated with increasing age, with an almost perfect 10-year difference between patients with no tear, a unilateral tear, and bilateral tears.
    - The average age of patients presenting with rotator cuff-derived pain with no tear was 48.7 years old; unilateral tear, 58.7 years old; and bilateral tears, 67.8 years old.
- Physiologic loading of the tendon has also been postulated as a mechanism for cuff tearing.
  - Localized degeneration of the articular region of the tendon, most commonly in the supraspinatus, is indicative of a tendon loading etiology.

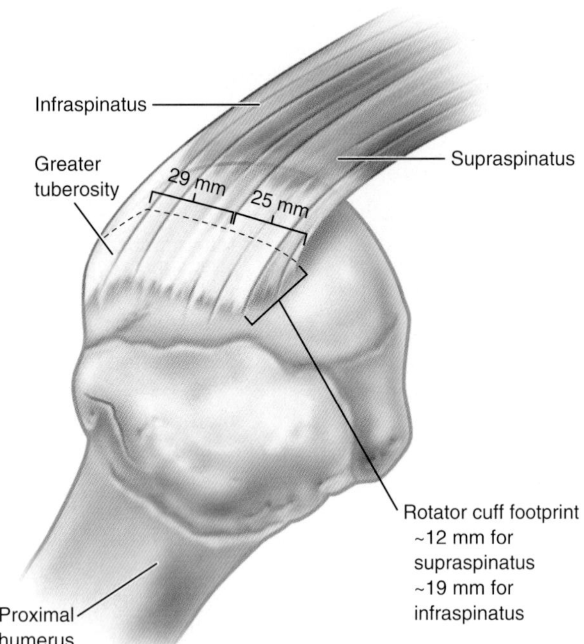

FIG 1 • Anatomy of the rotator cuff footprint.

- Uniform changes throughout the entire tendon, which are not commonly found, would be more suggestive of an age-related degenerative process.
- Age and loading likely have a multiplicative effect, with tendons in an older person both being more susceptible to damage from normal physiologic loading and exhibiting a worse healing response.

- Genetics may also have a significant role in the predisposition for rotator cuff tears.
  - A strong relationship between rotator cuff tearing and family history has been shown.
  - One study found a relative risk of 2.42 for full-thickness rotator cuff tears in siblings of patients with cuff tears versus controls.[10]
  - This increased risk in siblings implies that genetic factors may play a role in the development of rotator cuff tears.

NATURAL HISTORY

- Information about the natural history of rotator cuff disease is fundamental to understanding treatment indications.
- Because symptomatic tears are often treated, our understanding of the natural history of rotator cuff disease is based on the study of asymptomatic rotator cuff tears.
- Asymptomatic tears are extremely common in the population, and many of these are at risk for the development of symptoms over time.
  - In one study, over 51% of patients with a previously asymptomatic rotator cuff tear and a contralateral symptomatic tear will develop symptoms in the asymptomatic tear over an average of 2.8 years.[25]
  - Once a tear becomes symptomatic, 50% will progress in size. Only 20% of those remaining asymptomatic will progress.
  - No tears were found to decrease in size over time, suggesting that a significant percentage of patients with asymptomatic tears are at risk for symptom development.
  - Symptom development was also correlated with enlargement of the tear. Therefore, there is a limited intrinsic healing potential for the rotator cuff.
  - Just as importantly, there is a significant risk for tear progression, which will likely lead to significant functional deterioration and symptoms.
  - In addition, the potential for healing after surgery may be influenced by the irreversible muscle and tendon changes that occur in delayed repairs.
- Clinical evidence of spontaneous healing of partial-thickness tears also appears limited.
  - Partial-thickness tears are likely to progress to full-thickness tears over time.
  - At an average of 8.4 years postoperatively, 35% of partial-thickness rotator cuff tears treated with arthroscopic acromioplasty and débridement without repair progressed to full-thickness tears.[13]
  - Although both partial-thickness and full-thickness tears tend to progress, the rate of progression in partial-thickness tears appears to be much slower.

PATIENT HISTORY AND PHYSICAL FINDINGS

- Patients with rotator cuff disorders often complain of pain, weakness, or both in the shoulder.
- The development of symptoms is often insidious.
  - There may be a recollection of minor trauma (eg, episode of heavy lifting, catching a heavy object).
  - Pain is usually localized to the anterior or anterolateral aspect of the shoulder, often extending down the front or side of the shoulder to the elbow.
  - Pain exacerbated with use, especially with overhead activities, is common.
  - Sleep disruption is also common in patients with symptomatic rotator cuff disease.
- Weakness is a complaint for patients with large full-thickness rotator cuff tears.
  - Pain from tendinitis or small tears may simulate lack of strength, however. Therefore, weakness alone is not diagnostic of a large tear.
  - Similarly, patients with large or massive tears may have very reasonable function.
  - More commonly, however, these patients report overhead weakness and fatigue.
  - If gross weakness is recognized suddenly after a trauma, a rotator cuff injury should be suspected and investigated.
- In the setting of chronic rotator cuff tears, inspection of the shoulder will often reveal atrophy of the supraspinatus and infraspinatus.
  - Prior surgical incisions should be noted. If previous open rotator cuff repair with deltoid detachment was performed, deltoid repair integrity should be assessed, along with axillary nerve function.
  - Range-of-motion testing should be performed both actively and passively.
  - Passive range of motion is often preserved except in the setting of chronic large tears, where static superior head migration leads to limited forward elevation with inferior capsule contracture.
  - Posterior capsular contracture is also a common finding with both small and large tears.

- Active motion is often limited in scapular plane elevation. This may be due to either weakness or pain.
- Shoulder strength should be evaluated with manual muscle testing.
  - Various arm positions will isolate the rotator cuff and specifically test these muscles for dysfunction.
  - The supraspinatus, infraspinatus, and teres minor can be isolated with resisted scapular plane elevation at 90 degrees in neutral rotation, resisted external rotation in full adduction and slight internal rotation, and external rotation in 90 degrees of abduction and 90 degrees of adduction, respectively.
  - Either the belly-press or lift-off test can be used to test subscapularis function.
    - Belly-press test: Inability to maintain maximum internal rotation without the elbow dropping posterior to the midsagittal plane of the trunk indicates impaired subscapularis function.
    - Lift-off test: Inability to maintain *active* maximal internal rotation with hand off the lumbar spine without extending the elbow indicates impaired subscapularis function.
  - Electromyographic analysis has shown that the belly-press activates the upper subscapularis while the lift-off activates the lower subscapularis.
  - Painful limitation of motion may limit the usefulness of the lift-off test.
  - This information may improve our ability to determine the extent of subscapularis dysfunction.
- Special tests have been developed to aid in diagnosis:
  - The Neer impingement test (forward elevation in internal rotation) and the Hawkins impingement test (elevation to 90 degrees, cross-body adduction and internal rotation) were designed to elicit symptoms by impinging the rotator cuff on the undersurface of the acromion and coracoacromial ligament.
  - The Hornblower sign indicates teres minor dysfunction or tearing if there is weakness or inability to achieve full external rotation in an abducted position.
  - A positive result (weakness or pain) in the empty can test (Jobes sign) indicates dysfunction of the supraspinatus tendon.
  - Weakness with resisted external rotation in adduction represents dysfunction or tearing of the infraspinatus tendon.
  - External rotation lag sign: Inability to maintain the shoulder in a fully externally rotated position indicates significant dysfunction or tearing of the infraspinatus muscle.
  - Variable accuracy of these tests has been shown when used in isolation, but accuracy may be improved when used in combination with other provocative examinations.[18]
  - We do not routinely use these examinations, however. Instead, we base our findings on pain or weakness with resisted strength testing.

IMAGING AND OTHER DIAGNOSTIC STUDIES

- Four standard shoulder radiographs should be taken of every patient evaluated for shoulder pain: anteroposterior (AP), true AP with active shoulder abduction, axillary lateral, and scapular-Y views.
  - The decision to obtain further imaging studies is based on radiographic findings along with data obtained from the history and physical examination.
  - In a patient with a small full-thickness rotator cuff tear, radiographs are usually normal.
  - With increasing tear chronicity, sclerotic and cystic changes of the greater tuberosity are often noted.
  - With increasing tear size, proximal humeral migration can be found on the AP and true AP views.
  - Proximal migration is best identified on the true AP view as loss of a concentric reduction of the proximal humeral and glenoid centers of rotation.
  - Humeral elevation may be static or dynamic depending on the chronicity of the tear. Static elevation occurs with contracture of the inferior capsule.
  - Narrowing of the acromiohumeral interval on the AP view has also been used to identify large tears.
- MRI of the shoulder in patients with rotator cuff tears evaluates both the tendon and muscle quality.
  - Full-thickness tears show increased signal intensity at the tendon insertion on T2-weighted images.
  - MRI has been shown to have over 90% sensitivity and specificity in detecting tears without previous surgery.
  - Fatty infiltration and atrophy of the rotator cuff musculature can also be identified on MRI.
  - Increased fatty infiltration of the rotator cuff muscles has been correlated with poorer tendon healing and worse final postoperative outcomes after repair.
- In the hands of a skilled ultrasonographer, ultrasound has a sensitivity and specificity similar to that of MRI.
  - Benefits of ultrasound include limited radiation, ability to routinely perform bilateral examinations, and a dynamic component of the examination, which can significantly aid in differentiating scar from tendon.
  - The most significant limitation of ultrasound is the need for an experienced ultrasonographer.
- CT and CT arthrography has been widely used in Europe for the diagnosis of rotator cuff tears.
  - In patients with pacemakers or aneurysm clips, CT arthrography is a good alternative to MRI. Limitations of CT include increased radiation exposure and poorer soft tissue resolution compared to MRI.
  - Similar to MRI, muscle quality, including atrophy and fatty infiltration, can be examined and has been shown to be predictive of tendon healing and outcomes after surgery.

DIFFERENTIAL DIAGNOSIS

- Rotator cuff tendinitis
- Partial-thickness rotator cuff tear
- Rotator cuff contusion
- Adhesive capsulitis
- Arthritis or chondral injury
- Calcific tendinitis
- Biceps tendon pathology (tendinitis or tearing)
- Suprascapular nerve entrapment or spinoglenoid notch cyst
- Internal impingement

NONOPERATIVE MANAGEMENT

- The decision to pursue nonoperative management in the setting of a full-thickness rotator cuff tear depends on both patient and tear characteristics. Asymptomatic tears are extremely common, with MRI, ultrasound, and arthrography studies showing a 4% to 13% incidence in subjects 40 to 60 years old and over 50% in subjects older than 80.[20] All asymptomatic tears should be treated nonoperatively. In subjects younger than 65, serial monitoring with sequential MRI or ultrasounds is reasonable, given that over 51% of patients with a previously asymptomatic tear and a contralateral symptomatic tear will develop symptoms in the asymptomatic shoulder over an average of 2.8 years.[25]

- For symptomatic tears, nonoperative treatment has shown moderate success, with 45% to 82% satisfactory results.[3,11,22] Nonoperative treatment includes anti-inflammatory medications, shoulder stretching, and rotator cuff and scapular stabilizer strengthening exercises. A limited number of subacromial cortisone injections may be performed, especially in patients who are not surgical candidates. Chronic large or massive rotator cuff tears in any age group or any chronic full-thickness tear in patients older than age 70 should undergo an initial trial (at least 3 months) of nonoperative management. Because irreversible changes have already occurred to the cuff or the articular cartilage in most of these patients, it is safe to attempt nonoperative treatment for a period of time. Failure of nonsurgical treatment is an indication for arthroscopic repair.

SURGICAL MANAGEMENT

- The decision to proceed with operative treatment of rotator cuff disease requires an evaluation of the risks and benefits associated with both surgical and nonsurgical treatment.
- While the risks of surgical management are well known, the risks of nonoperative treatment may not be so obvious.
  - Tear progression, muscle fatty infiltration and atrophy, and arthritis are potential irreversible risks of nonoperative treatment of rotator cuff tears.
  - Knowledge about these risks can help guide treatment.
- Early surgical repair should be considered in all acute tears and any chronic small or medium-sized tears in patients younger than age 65.
  - These patients are at significant risk for developing the irreversible changes previously mentioned with prolonged nonoperative treatment.
  - These patients also have the greatest potential for healing. Consequently, the benefits of early surgical treatment combined with the inherent risks of prolonged nonoperative treatment guide us to early surgical repair.

Preoperative Planning

- Tear size and chronicity will determine the difficulty of the repair, so careful preoperative imaging evaluation is important in surgical preparation.
  - If a tear is very large, the surgeon should make sure that a variety of different suture-passing devices are available to assist in the repair.
  - A Banana Suture Lasso (Arthrex, Naples, FL) can be passed through the Neviaser portal in large, medially retracted tears to shuttle suture through the tendon.
  - Angled Suture Lassos (Arthrex) can be placed through accessory portals to pass sutures from difficult angles not easily approached through the lateral working cannulas.
  - Larger anchors should be available if bone quality is poor.
- Assess preoperative motion after the patient is anesthetized but before initiating the surgical procedure. Fixed superior humeral migration in the setting of a large rotator cuff tear will lead to inferior capsular contracture. In these patients, perform preoperative manipulation under anesthesia in forward elevation to increase the subacromial space available, thus facilitating the repair.

Positioning

- Beach-chair position advantages
  - This is an anatomic position that permits better orientation and understanding of shoulder anatomy while performing the repair.
  - Examination under anesthesia is facilitated by stabilizing the scapula in the beach-chair position compared with the lateral position.
  - The arm can be easily manipulated in surgery without the need to unhook it from a traction unit.
  - Traction is not required but can be added in an inferior direction to increase the subacromial working space.
  - Humeral rotational control is easily accomplished. This can be critical when working on different regions (anterior vs. posterior) of the greater tuberosity.
  - Conversion to an open procedure is easily performed without redraping.
- Lateral decubitus position advantages
  - Many surgeons believe that the lateral position improves visualization and maneuverability of the scope due to traction.
  - It significantly improves inferior access to the glenohumeral joint, which makes it less difficult to perform glenohumeral procedures but has little impact on subacromial procedures.
- Transient and permanent nerve damage has been reported due to traction in the lateral position. Consequently, we prefer to perform all subacromial procedures, including rotator cuff repair, in the beach-chair position.

TECHNIQUES

DOUBLE-ROW ROTATOR CUFF REPAIR WITH "MASON-ALLEN"-TYPE CONSTRUCT USING SCREW-IN SUTURE ANCHORS

Portal Placement and Cannula Insertion

- The camera is placed in the subacromial space through a posterior portal.
- Our preferred starting posterior portal is slightly more lateral than a standard posterior portal. This is done to gain better visualization of the lateral greater tuberosity during repair. Also, a slightly inferior position is preferred, since portals will migrate superiorly with shoulder swelling.
- A lateral working portal is developed under spinal needle localization. Portals should be placed low enough so that cannulas are introduced parallel to the rotator cuff tendon. This allows for easier subacromial instrumentation. The portal should be placed at about the midpoint of the tear in small or medium-sized tears.
  - A second lateral portal can be placed in larger tears with cannulas separated by several centimeters. Clear fully threaded 8.25–mm cannulas are placed in these portal sites.

- Another large threaded cannula is placed through an anterolateral portal, anterior to the acromion, at the same level as the lateral and posterior portals. Again, maintaining low portal placement is critical so instruments will be passed parallel to the tendon, allowing the greatest excursion of instruments in the subacromial space. The anterolateral portal is mainly used as an accessory portal for suture retrieval and storage.

Repair Site Preparation

- A soft tissue ablation device is used through the lateral portal to clear all the soft tissue on the undersurface of the acromion extending posteriorly, including the soft tissue and fat around the scapular spine. This will significantly improve the mobility of the tear. Soft tissue is removed from the greater tuberosity with a shaver, exposing cortical bone.
- Mobility of the torn tendon is assessed with a tissue grasper through the lateral portal.

Anchor and Suture Placement

- Once the tear has been determined to be repairable, a medial row of suture anchors (5.5-mm metal screw-in style) is placed. Anchors are loaded with two no. 2 Fiberwire sutures (Arthrex).
  - For small and medium-sized tears, we routinely place two medial anchors at the level of the anatomic neck. Each anchor is separated by 1 to 1.5 cm. Anchors are placed through small stab incisions just off the lateral border of the acromion.
  - For large and massive tears, we place three medial anchors.
- Sutures from the medial row of anchors are next passed through the tendon. Starting with the most anterior anchor, both strands from one suture are passed through the tendon at the anterior aspect of the tear in a horizontal mattress fashion. Sutures are passed approximately 1 cm medial to the lateral edge of the tear. One strand of the second suture is passed adjacent to the most posterior strand of the first suture. This strand is retrieved out the anterolateral portal along with the two strands of the first suture.
- The steps are repeated for the posterior anchor of the medial row. Two strands of one suture are passed at the posterior aspect of the tear in a mattress fashion. One strand of the second suture is placed just anterior to the previously placed mattress suture and retrieved out the anterolateral portal.
- Both strands of the posterior mattress stitch are retrieved out the lateral portal, tied arthroscopically, and cut. Similarly, both strands of the anterior mattress stitch are retrieved out the lateral portal, tied, and cut.
- The remaining strands passed through the tendon are in the anterolateral cannula and tied to one another outside the shoulder. The tails are cut and the knot is then advanced into the shoulder by pulling on the opposite two strands of the two sutures, creating a large horizontal mattress stitch between the anterior and posterior anchors (**TECH FIG 1A**).
- A single lateral suture anchor is then placed at the lateral aspect of the rotator cuff footprint on the greater

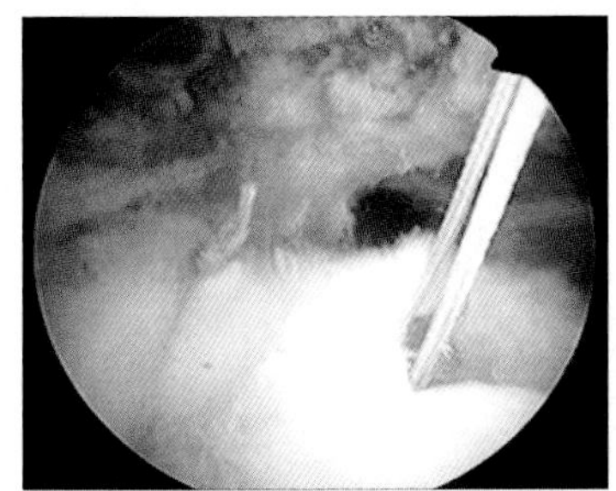

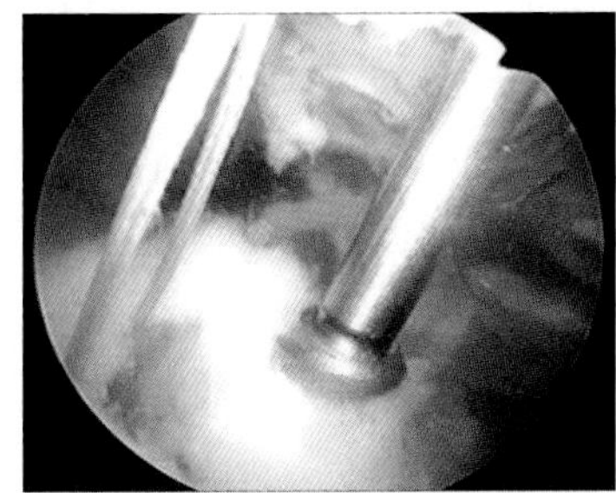

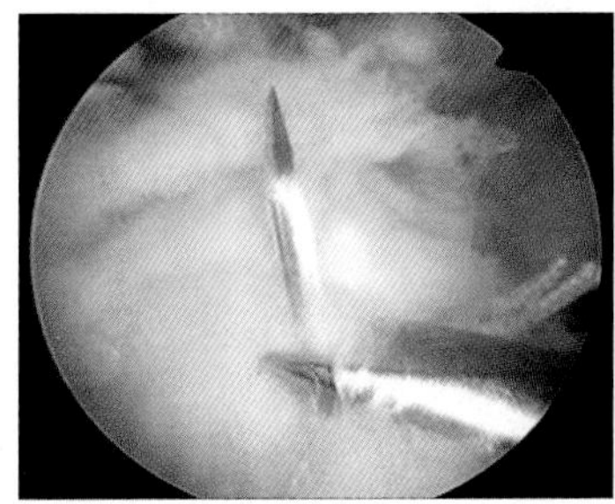

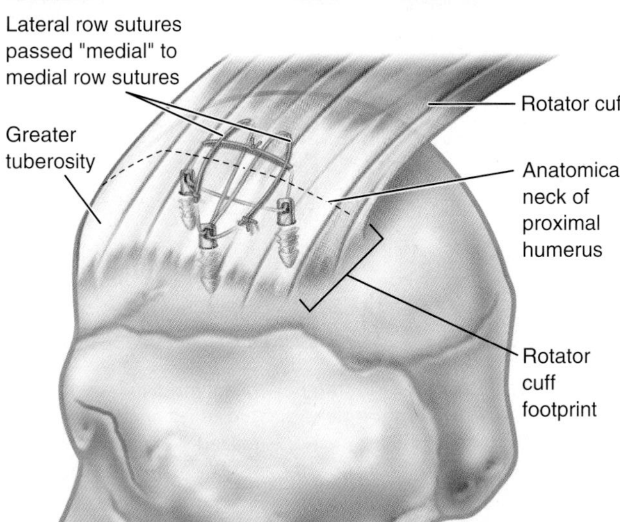

TECH FIG 1 • **A.** Arthroscopic picture showing the bridging horizontal mattress stitch between two medial-row anchors. Suture strands on right are the other limbs of the horizontal mattress stitch, which will be tied arthroscopically after the lateral-row stitches have been passed and tied. **B.** Lateral-row suture anchor placed at the lateral aspect of the greater tuberosity between the two medial-row anchors. **C.** Passage of lateral-row stitches medial to the bridging medial-row horizontal mattress stitch with a Scorpion suture passer. **D.** Final repair construct of a double-row repair using two medial and one lateral screw-in suture anchors.

tuberosity, halfway between the medial anchors (TECH FIG 1B). One strand of one suture is retrieved out the lateral portal and passed medial to the horizontal stitch between the anterior and posterior medial anchors.

- This step is repeated with the second suture from the lateral anchor. These stitches are passed using a Scorpion suture passer (Arthrex) (TECH FIG 1C).

- Once the lateral anchor sutures are passed, the remaining strands from the medial sutures are pulled on by an assistant to tension the medial horizontal mattress stitch between the medial anchors while the lateral-row sutures are tied. While tension is applied to the medial row, the lateral simple stitches are tied arthroscopically and cut.
- Finally, the remaining two strands from the medial row anchors are retrieved out the lateral portal and tied arthroscopically.
- The final construct has two medial-row anchors with a mattress stitch between the anchors and one lateral anchor with two simple stitches passed medial to the horizontal mattress between the medial anchors. This creates a "Mason-Allen" type of construct with the lateral simple stitches passed medial to the bridging medial horizontal mattress stitch (TECH FIG 1D).

DOUBLE-ROW ROTATOR CUFF TEAR WITH "MASON-ALLEN"-TYPE CONSTRUCT USING MEDIAL SCREW-IN SUTURE ANCHORS AND LATERAL PUSHLOCK ANCHORS

- This repair technique follows the previous repair technique. After the anterior and posterior medial-row mattress sutures are tied, the tails of these sutures are not cut. Instead, they are retrieved out the anterolateral portal and stored. The bridging horizontal mattress stitch between the two medial anchors is created as described in the previous technique.
- The untied suture strands (one from the anterior anchor and one from the posterior anchor) from the bridging mattress stitch between the anterior and posterior anchors (TECH FIG 2A) are retrieved out the lateral portal.
- Both suture strands are then passed simultaneously medial to the horizontal mattress bridging mattress stitch with the Scorpion suture passer (Arthrex). This creates a Mason-Allen type of locking stitch construct.
- Through one of the accessory lateral portals where the medial-row anchors were placed, a suture retriever is placed. Three strands are grabbed with the retriever: one strand from the tied posterior mattress stitch, one strand from the tied anterior mattress stitch, and one of the strands passed medial to the bridging horizontal mattress stitch.
- All three strands are placed in a PEEK 3.5-mm PushLock knotless suture anchor (Arthrex). The PushLock awl is placed through the same lateral accessory portal and an anchor hole is tapped along the lateral aspect of the greater tuberosity at the posterior aspect of the tear (TECH FIG 2B). After a hole is tapped, the anchor is introduced into the joint through the same portal and impacted into the hole. The PushLock anchor has three strands (one strand from the tied posterior mattress stitch, one strand from the tied anterior mattress stitch, and one of the strands passed medial to the bridging horizontal mattress stitch) (TECH FIG 2C). As the anchor is impacted, all three strands should be tensioned to reduce the rotator cuff to the footprint. All three strands are then cut after final impaction of the PushLock anchor.
- The previous steps are repeated, grabbing the second suture strand from the anterior and posterior mattress stitches and the second strand passed medial to the bridging mattress stitch. All three are placed in a second PushLock anchor and an anchor pilot hole is created at the anterior aspect of the tear along the lateral aspect of the greater tuberosity footprint.

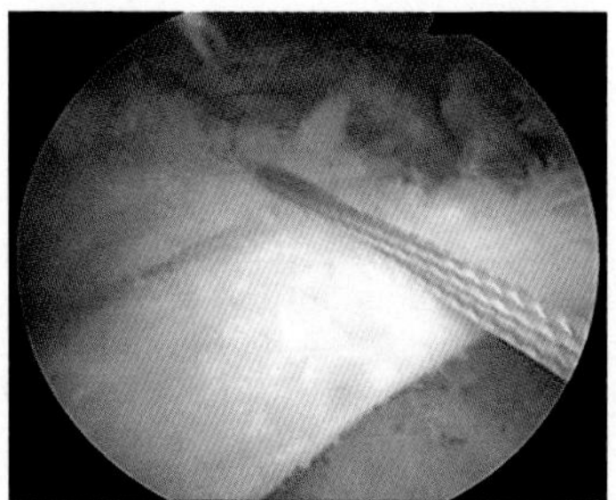
A

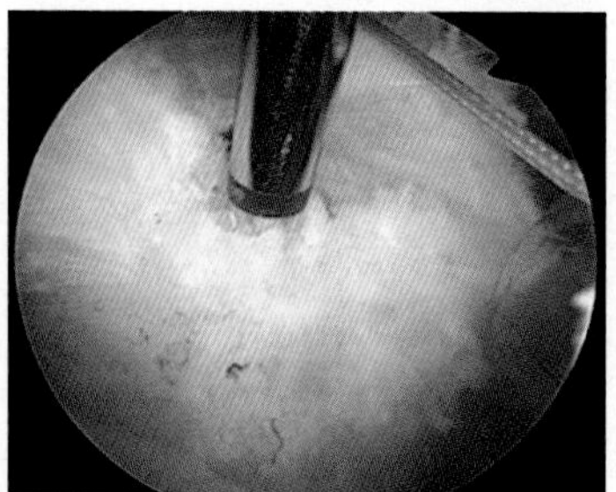
B

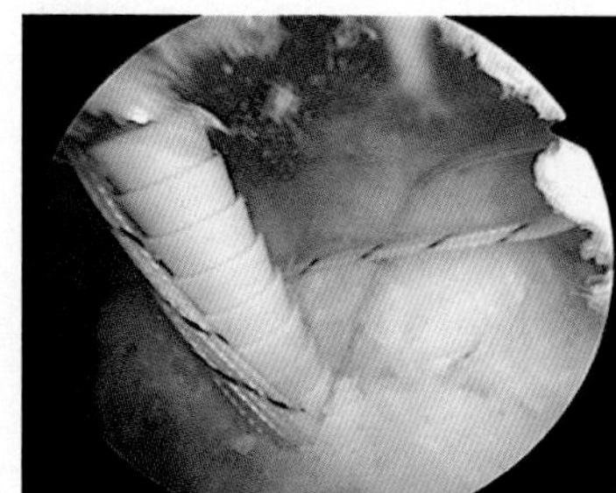
C

TECH FIG 2 • **A.** Arthroscopic picture showing the opposite ends of the bridging horizontal mattress stitch shuttled through the cuff tendon medial to the bridging mattress stitch. **B.** A pilot hole is created using an awl for the posterior PushLock anchor as part of the lateral row. **C.** The posterior PushLock anchor is placed with one strand of suture from the anterior horizontal mattress stitch, one strand from the posterior horizontal mattress stitch, and one limb of the sutures from the bridging mattress stitch. *(continued)*

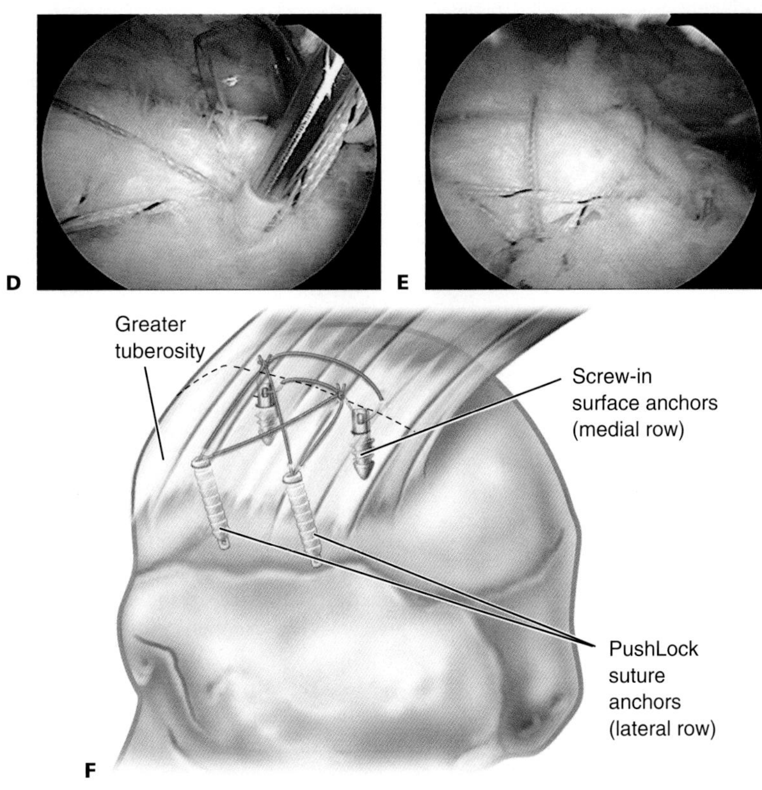

TECH FIG 2 • *(continued)* **D.** The anterior PushLock anchor is placed, finishing the lateral row. **E.** Arthroscopic picture showing the final double-row construct using two lateral PushLock anchors and two medial screw-in anchors. **F.** Diagram showing the final double-row repair using two medial screw-in anchors and two lateral PushLock anchors.

- After pilot hole creation, the anchor is introduced into the joint. With all three suture strands and while the strands are tensioned, the anchor is impacted (TECH FIG 2D). The tails of all three strands are then cut flush with the PushLock anchor, completing the repair.
- The final construct consists of two medial-row anchors and two lateral-row PushLock anchors (TECH FIG 2E,F). Only two arthroscopic knots are required to complete this double-row repair.

PEARLS AND PITFALLS

Portal placement	▪ The posterior portal should be placed more lateral than the standard portal site (standard portal site: 2 cm medial and 2 cm inferior to the posterolateral corner of the acromion) for improved access to the lateral aspect of the greater tuberosity. ▪ Portal placement should err low to facilitate instrumentation after shoulder swelling.
Surgical anatomy	▪ Landmarks should be precisely drawn on the shoulder before arthroscopy to ensure accurate portal placement.
Preoperative examination under anesthesia and manipulation	▪ With large, chronic rotator cuff tears, fixed superior humeral migration is often present. Preoperative manipulation in forward elevation will assist in releasing the inferior capsule, thereby allowing improved access to the subacromial space with inferior traction during surgery.
Hemostasis	▪ Preoperative (5 to 10 minutes) subacromial injection of local anesthetic with epinephrine in the subacromial space will significantly reduce bleeding during repair. ▪ During soft tissue removal around the scapular spine and coracoacromial ligament release along the anteroinferior acromion, the surgeon must watch for vessels that require coagulation.
Passage of lateral low stitches medial to medial horizontal mattress	▪ During passage of the lateral stitches, any resistance to suture passage may mean impalement of previously placed medial-row sutures. If resistance is met, the suture passer should be removed and reloaded without forcing suture passage.
Lateral row PushLock anchor placement	▪ After PushLock anchors are loaded with suture outside the shoulder, they should be placed through the same fascial defect through which sutures were retrieved, thereby preventing suture entanglement in the deltoid fascia.

POSTOPERATIVE CARE

- All patients are initially placed in a sling, which is removed only for elbow range-of-motion exercises three or four times per day to limit elbow stiffness and for bathing.
  - We use a subacromial pain catheter, infiltrating 0.5% bupivacaine (Marcaine) during the first 48 hours postoperatively.
  - Patients remain on antibiotics (cephalexin) while the pain catheter is still in place.
  - Dressings are removed on the second postoperative day and showering is allowed the following day.
  - Patients are seen at 10 days postoperatively for suture removal.
- When to start physical therapy after rotator cuff repair is debated among orthopedic surgeons. The decision is based on the perceived risks and benefits of early motion.
  - The major benefit of early motion is the potential limitation of postoperative shoulder stiffness. The main risks include repair disruption and limited healing.
- Early passive motion has historically been recommended after open rotator cuff repair. With the advent of arthroscopic repairs, scarring from soft tissue dissection is minimized, so limiting early motion is possible.
  - Limited early motion may improve tendon healing.
  - Several factors, including tear size, tendon and bone quality, and preoperative motion, should be considered in this decision.
  - With osteoporotic bone or extremely poor tendon quality, limiting motion initially after repair is recommended.
  - Preoperative shoulder motion is an important factor in determining the initiation of motion. Earlier motion may be initiated if preoperative motion is limited and requires manipulation or release at the time of repair.
  - In general, tear size is the most important factor in determining the timing of postoperative rehabilitation.
    - Limiting early motion in patients with larger tears may provide improved healing potential, given that their overall healing rates are much lower than smaller tears.[5–7]
- Patients with small or medium-sized tears remain in a sling for the first 6 weeks after surgery.
  - Elbow and hand range-of-motion exercises are started immediately.
  - No shoulder motion is allowed during the first 6 postoperative weeks.
  - If there was a significant preoperative motion deficit requiring surgical release or manipulation at the time of repair, early passive motion is allowed.
  - After 6 weeks, the sling is removed and patients are started on passive and active assisted range-of-motion exercises, including forward elevation in the scapular plane, external rotation in full adduction, and pendulum and pulley exercises.
  - Internal rotation and shoulder extension is limited and patients are instructed not to perform any lifting, pushing, pulling, or overhead activity.
  - At 3 months after surgery, strengthening exercises are initiated. These begin with isometric exercises and progress to isotonic exercises, with a stretching program maintained throughout.
  - Return to sports and full unrestricted activity is allowed at 4 to 5 months.
- For large or massive tears, patients remain in a sling with no shoulder motion for 6 weeks.
  - At 6 weeks, the sling is removed and patients are allowed to lift the arm to shoulder height only.
  - Formal physical therapy is not initiated at this time. Instead, a shoulder continuous passive motion (CPM) device (Breg Flexmate S500, Breg, Inc., Vista, CA) is used to regain forward elevation in the scapular plane. CPM use is continued until 3 months postoperatively.
  - At this time, formal physical therapy is initiated, including passive and active motion and strengthening as per the protocol for small and medium-sized tears.
  - Return to sports and unrestricted activities is allowed at 6 months postoperatively.

OUTCOMES

- Functional outcomes after both open and arthroscopic rotator cuff repair have been reported to be durable at long-term follow-up.[7,23] A number of factors have been correlated with outcomes after repair, including patient age, tear size, tear acuity, workers' compensation status, preoperative smoking status, muscle quality, and tendon healing.
- Most series reporting outcomes after complete arthroscopic rotator cuff repair are in single-row repairs. The potential advantage of a double-row repair is improved initial repair fixation strength and restoration of the normal anatomic rotator cuff footprint.[14–16] Improved initial fixation strength and footprint restoration should lead to improved healing rates. In both open and arthroscopic repairs, tendon healing is correlated with improved outcomes.[5,8,9] Therefore, double-row repairs may lead to improved clinical outcomes.
- There are limited series reporting the outcomes of complete arthroscopic double-row rotator cuff repairs.
  - Suguya et al[19] compared healing rates and outcomes between single- and double-row repairs in 78 patients at an average of 35 months after surgery using MRI. There were significant improvements in UCLA and American Shoulder and Elbow Surgeons (ASES) scores in both repair groups, with no significant difference found between techniques. There was a significant increase in retear rates with single-row repairs.
  - Anderson et al[1] recently evaluated 48 patients at a mean of 30 months after double-row repair with ultrasonography. There was a significant improvement in active motion, strength, and outcomes when compared to preoperative values. The overall retear rate was 17%, with no significant difference in outcomes between healed and retorn tendons. Healed shoulders were significantly stronger in elevation and external rotation.
  - Overall, double row-repairs appear to have improved healing rates compared to single-row repairs, although functional results are very similar.

COMPLICATIONS

- Several factors can be directly correlated with persistent pain and limited function after repair.
  - These factors are broken down into three categories: surgeon-controlled, non-surgeon-controlled, and patient-related factors.
  - They include incorrect or incomplete diagnosis, surgical technical error, stiffness, infection, and anesthesia-related complications.

- Continued pain after rotator cuff repair can often occur if a second pathology is not identified and treated.
  - Conditions often confused with rotator cuff disease include cervical spine disorders, suprascapular neuropathy, acromioclavicular joint arthritis, biceps tendonopathy, glenohumeral instability or arthritis, labral tears, and frozen shoulder.
  - A complete history and physical examination can prevent missing several of these problems, which can often be treated concomitantly at the time of rotator cuff repair.
- Technical problems leading to persistent pain and dysfunction after repair can be grouped into repair failures, deltoid detachment, neurologic injury, excess fluid extravasation, and patient positioning injuries.
  - The most likely reason for failure of tendon healing after repair is patient age.
  - Poor surgical technique, including poor knot-tying, limited fixation (number of anchors), and poor anchor insertion technique, can all lead to a weak biomechanical construct.
  - Deltoid detachment is avoided in the setting of complete arthroscopic repair, but if a mini-open approach is performed, then excess detachment without bony repair can lead to failure of healing.
  - Transient neurologic injury can occur secondary to excess traction when the lateral position is used.
  - Proper portal placement is critical to avoid axillary (posterior and lateral portals) and musculocutaneous (anterior portal) nerve injury.
  - Excess swelling due to fluid extravasation into the deltoid can significantly raise intramuscular pressures. Therefore, pump pressures should be kept below 50 mm Hg, with procedure times less than 2 hours.
  - Proper padding around the knees (lateral position) and flexing the hips and knees (beach-chair position) can avoid iatrogenic problems secondary to positioning.
- Postoperative stiffness is another potential complication.
  - With limited surgical dissection associated with complete arthroscopic repairs, the risk of stiffness may be significantly reduced when compared with open repairs.
  - While overall rates of postoperative stiffness have not been clearly reported, more than 5% to 10% of open repairs are complicated by either adhesions in the humeral scapular interface or capsular contracture.
  - We now routinely hold all shoulder motion after arthroscopic repairs for several weeks in an attempt to improve healing rates, with limited concern for developing postoperative stiffness.
  - If significant stiffness does develop that is resistant to therapy, arthroscopic lysis of adhesions in the subacromial space along with capsular release is recommended.
- Infection after rotator cuff repair is uncommon.
  - Most series report infection rates of 1% to 2% after open or mini-open rotator cuff repairs.
  - While there are few reported studies of infection rates after complete arthroscopic repairs, it appears that infection is less common than after open or mini-open repairs.
  - Diagnosis is often delayed in cases of postoperative infection, and persistent wound drainage is the most consistent examination finding.
  - Cultures will often grow *Propionibacterium acnes, Staphylococcus aureus*, and coagulase-negative *Staphylococcus aureus.*
    - *P. acnes* often takes 7 to 10 days to grow on cultures. Therefore, cultures should be held in the setting of postoperative infections for at least 1 week.
  - Treatment consists of multiple débridements and intravenous antibiotics for usually 6 weeks.
  - Outcomes after infection are satisfactory, although significant delays in diagnosis or treatment can lead to inferior results.
- Anesthetic complications can occur after rotator cuff repair.
  - If general anesthesia is used, major complications occur less than 1% of the time.[4]
  - More commonly, nausea, inability to void, and severe pain are the complications seen in the setting of outpatient elective shoulder surgery.
  - If an interscalene block is used, inadequate anesthesia is the most common complication.
  - Temporary Horner syndrome, phrenic nerve paralysis, and recurrent laryngeal nerve block are common but usually without significant consequence.
  - Intraneural injection or needle injury to the nerve roots can occur.
  - Symptoms such as persistent paresthesias or numbness can be irritating but usually resolve with time (possibly several months).

REFERENCES

1. Anderson K, Boothby M, Aschenbrener D, et al. Outcome and structural integrity after arthroscopic rotator cuff repair using 2 rows of fixation: minimum 2-year follow-up. Am J Sports Med 2006;34: 1899–1905.
2. Apreleva M, Ozbaydar M, Fitzgibbons PJ, et al. Rotator cuff tears: the effect of the reconstruction method on the three-dimensional repair site area. Arthroscopy 2002;18:519–526.
3. Bartolozzi A, Andreychik D, Ahmad S. Determinants of outcome in the treatment of rotator cuff disease. Clin Orthop Relat Res 1994; 308:90–97.
4. Bishop J, Klepps S, Lo IK, et al. Cuff integrity after arthroscopic versus open repair: a prospective study. J Shoulder Elbow Surg 2006;15: 290–299.
5. Boileau P, Brassart N, Watkinson DJ, et al. Arthroscopic repairs of full-thickness tears of the supraspinatus: does the tendon really heal? J Bone Joint Surg Am 2005;87A:1229–1240.
6. Galatz LM, Ball CM, Teefey SA, et al. The outcomes and repair integrity of completely arthroscopically repaired large and massive rotator cuff tears. J Bone Joint Surg Am 2004;86A:219–224.
7. Galatz LM, Griggs S, Cameron BD, et al. Prospective longitudinal analysis of postoperative shoulder function: a ten-year follow-up study of full-thickness rotator cuff tears. J Bone Joint Surg Am 2001; 83A:1052–1056.
8. Gazielly DF, Gleyze P, Montagnon C. Functional and anatomic results after rotator cuff repair. Clin Orthop Relat Res 1994; 304:43–53.
9. Harryman DT, Mack LA, Wang KY, et al. Repairs of the rotator cuff. Correlation of functional results with integrity of the rotator cuff. J Bone Joint Surg Am 1991;73A:982–989.
10. Harvie P, Ostlere SJ, The J, et al. Genetic influences in the aetiology of tears of the rotator cuff: sibling risk of a full-thickness tear. J Bone Joint Surg Br 2004;86B:696–700.
11. Itoi E, Tabata S. Conservative treatment of rotator cuff tears. Clin Orthop Relat Res 1992;275:165–173.
12. Jobe FW, Moynes DR. Delineation of diagnostic criteria and a rehabilitation program for rotator cuff injuries. Am J Sports Med 1982; 10:336–339.
13. Kartus J, Kartus C, Rostgard-Christensen L, et al. Long-term clinical and ultrasound evaluation after arthroscopic acromioplasty in patients with partial rotator cuff tears. Arthroscopy 2006;22: 44–49.

14. Kim DH, Ellatrache NS, Tibone JE, et al. Biomechanical comparison of a single-row versus double-row suture anchor technique for rotator cuff repair. Am J Sports Med 2006;34:407–414.
15. Ma CB, Comerford L, Wilson J, et al. Biomechanical evaluation of arthroscopic rotator cuff repairs: double-row compared with single-row fixation. J Bone Joint Surg Am 2006;88A:403–410.
16. Mazzocca AD, Millett PJ, Guanche CA, et al. Arthroscopic single-row versus double-row suture anchor rotator cuff repair. Am J Sports Med 2005;33:1861–1868.
17. Miniaci A, Dowdy PA, Willits KR, et al. Magnetic resonance imaging evaluation of the rotator cuff tendons in the asymptomatic shoulder. Am J Sports Med 1995;23:142–145.
18. Park HB, Yokota A, Gill HS, et al. Diagnostic accuracy of clinical tests for the different degrees of subacromial impingement. J Bone Joint Surg Am 2005;87A:1446–1455.
19. Suguya H, Maeda K, Matsuki K, et al. Functional and structural outcome after arthroscopic full-thickness rotator cuff repair: single-row versus dual-row fixation. Arthroscopy 2005;21:1307–1316.
20. Tempelhof S, Rupp S, Seil R. Age-related prevalence of rotator cuff tears in asymptomatic shoulders. J Shoulder Elbow Surg 1999;8:296–299.
21. Tuoheti Y, Itoi E, Yamamoto N, et al. Contact area, contact pressure, and pressure patterns of the tendon–bone interface after rotator cuff repair. Am J Sports Med 2005;33:1869–1874.
22. Wirth MA, Basamania C, Rockwood CA. Nonoperative management of full-thickness tears of the rotator cuff. Orthop Clin North Am 1997;28:59–67.
23. Wolf EM, Pennington WT, Agrawal V. Arthroscopic side-to-side rotator cuff repair. Arthroscopy 2005;21:881–887.
24. Yamaguchi K, Ditsios K, Middleton WD, et al. The demographic and morphologic features of rotator cuff disease: a comparison of symptomatic and asymptomatic shoulders. J Bone Joint Surg Am 2006;88A:1699–1704.
25. Yamaguchi K, Tetro AM, Blam O, et al. Natural history of asymptomatic rotator cuff tears: a longitudinal analysis of asymptomatic tears detected sonographically. J Shoulder Elbow Surg 2001;10:199–203.

Chapter 11

Arthroscopic Treatment of Subscapularis Tears, Including Coracoid Impingement

Christopher R. Adams and Stephen S. Burkhart

DEFINITION

- A subscapularis tendon tear typically occurs at its insertion into the lesser tuberosity of the proximal humerus.
- Although the subscapularis is the largest of the rotator cuff muscles, historically it has received little attention.
- Subscapularis tendon tears are often overlooked and underdiagnosed; therefore, a proper evaluation of the shoulder is of paramount importance.
- Treatment of subscapularis tendon tears can restore the functional stability of the shoulder.

ANATOMY

- The subscapularis muscle originates from the medial two thirds of the anterior scapular fossa.[4] The muscle courses laterally beneath the coracoid and becomes tendinous at the glenoid rim. The subscapularis tendon becomes confluent with the glenohumeral joint capsule deep to it and inserts into the lesser tuberosity of the proximal humerus (**FIG 1**).
- The normal subscapularis tendon not only intermingles with the fibers of the glenohumeral joint capsule deep to it, but at its insertion it also intermingles with the fibers of the medial sling of the long head of the biceps tendon. The medial sling is composed of fibers from the superior glenohumeral ligament and the coracohumeral ligament complex.
- The tendon insertion is about 2.5 cm long (range 1.5 to 3.0 cm) and is trapezoidal, with the widest portion at its most superior (cephalad) aspect.[17]
- The superior aspect also happens to be the strongest part of the subscapularis insertion.[8]

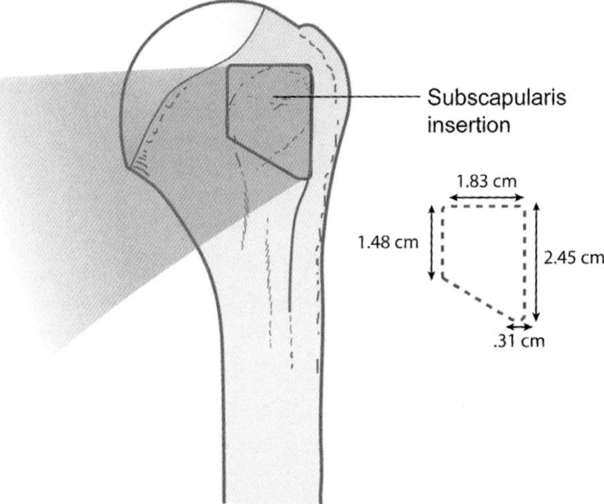

FIG 1 • Subscapularis insertion. The subscapularis insertion is wider at its superior aspect and tapers at its most inferior aspect. The insertion resembles the shape of the state of Nevada.

- The subscapularis muscle is innervated by the upper and lower subscapular nerves, and its blood supply is primarily derived from the subscapular artery.[4]
- The main functions of the subscapularis muscle are to internally rotate and adduct the humerus and to provide an anterior restraint to humeral head translation. The subscapularis also acts in concert with the remaining rotator cuff muscles and deltoid to balance both the coronal- and transverse-plane force couples of the glenohumeral joint.
  - This results in dynamic stabilization to centralize the humeral head on the glenoid ("maintain the golf ball on the golf tee"), providing a stable fulcrum for glenohumeral motion.

PATHOGENESIS

- As with the other rotator cuff tendons, intrinsic factors may play a role in the development of a subscapularis tendon tear. Furthermore, extrinsic mechanical factors have also been implicated in the process.
- The normal subcoracoid space (coracohumeral interval) represents the distance from the coracoid tip to the proximal humerus. If this space is stenotic, the coracoid tip will impinge against the insertion of the subscapularis, causing damage to the tendon insertion.
- Anatomic and imaging studies have defined the normal coracohumeral interval to be between 8.4 mm and 11 mm.[5,7,14]
- Subcoracoid stenosis is defined as less than 6 mm of space between the coracoid and the proximal humerus (either by magnetic resonance imaging [MRI] or arthroscopy).[14]
- Patients with subscapularis tears often have a significantly reduced coracohumeral interval (5 mm with subscapularis tears vs. 10 mm without subscapularis tears).[16]
- In subcoracoid impingement, the coracoid abuts against the anterior surface of the subscapularis, causing increased articular (under) surface tensile forces that can cause tendon fiber failure (**FIG 2**).
- Two separate cadaveric studies found that subscapularis tendon tears are often partial-thickness articular tears. Furthermore, they usually begin at the superior aspect of the insertion and are common in the elderly population.[18,19]
- However, complete tears of the subscapularis tendon often result in medial retraction of the tendon edge to the level of the glenoid.
- The retracted tendon often pulls with it the adjacent medial sling of the biceps tendon (composed of fibers from the superior glenohumeral ligament and coracohumeral ligament).
- The fibers of the medial sling are oriented approximately perpendicular to the fibers of the subscapularis tendon and arthroscopically appear as a comma-shaped soft tissue structure that we refer to as the "comma sign" (**FIG 3**).[13]

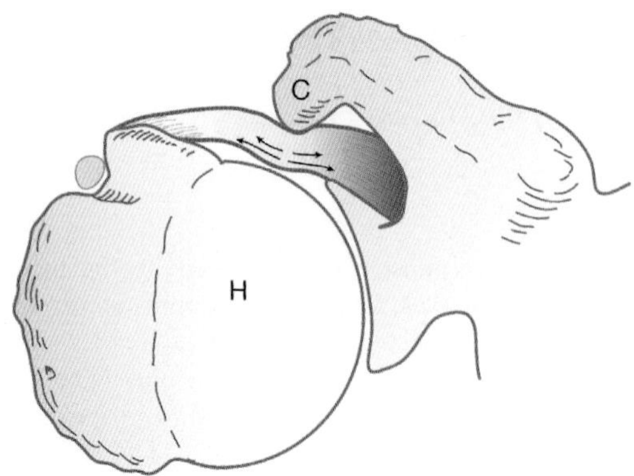

FIG 2 • Schematic drawing of the roller-wringer effect. In patients with subcoracoid impingement, the prominent coracoid tip indents the superficial surface of the subscapularis tendon. This creates tensile forces on the convex, articular surface of the subscapularis tendon and can lead to failure of the subscapularis fibers. *C*, coracoid; *H*, humerus. (From Burkhart SS, Lo IKY, Brady PC. A Cowboy's Guide to Advanced Shoulder Arthroscopy. Philadelphia: Lippincott Williams & Wilkins, 2006.)

- We have found the "comma sign" to be a useful guide for identifying the retracted superolateral edge of the subscapularis tendon.
- The loss of the subscapularis tendon results in an unstable glenohumeral fulcrum and abnormal glenohumeral arthrokinematics.[12]
- Chronic tears of the subscapularis should be repaired (even if there is fatty degeneration and significant muscle atrophy) because the subscapularis may have the capacity to function through a tenodesis effect.[17]

NATURAL HISTORY

- There is little available information on the natural history of subscapularis tendon tears.
- In some patients (especially those with massive rotator cuff tears) the tears can be disabling. Some patients with massive rotator cuff tears never regain functional overhead use of their arms without surgical intervention.

PATIENT HISTORY AND PHYSICAL FINDINGS

- Although most subscapularis tears in the community are degenerative in nature, the classic scenario for a traumatic tear is forced external rotation.
- Forced external rotation results in an eccentric tensile load, which can be particularly dangerous to a "tendon at risk."
- In contrast to patients with the typical posterosuperior rotator cuff tear, who have difficulty with overhead tasks, patients with subscapularis tears often have the burden of diminished function with tasks in front of the body and below the level of the shoulder.
- The typical patient complains of chronic pain and loss of arm strength with activities of daily living in front of the body.
- A complete physical examination is necessary, including evaluation of the cervical spine and both upper extremities. Examinations to perform are:

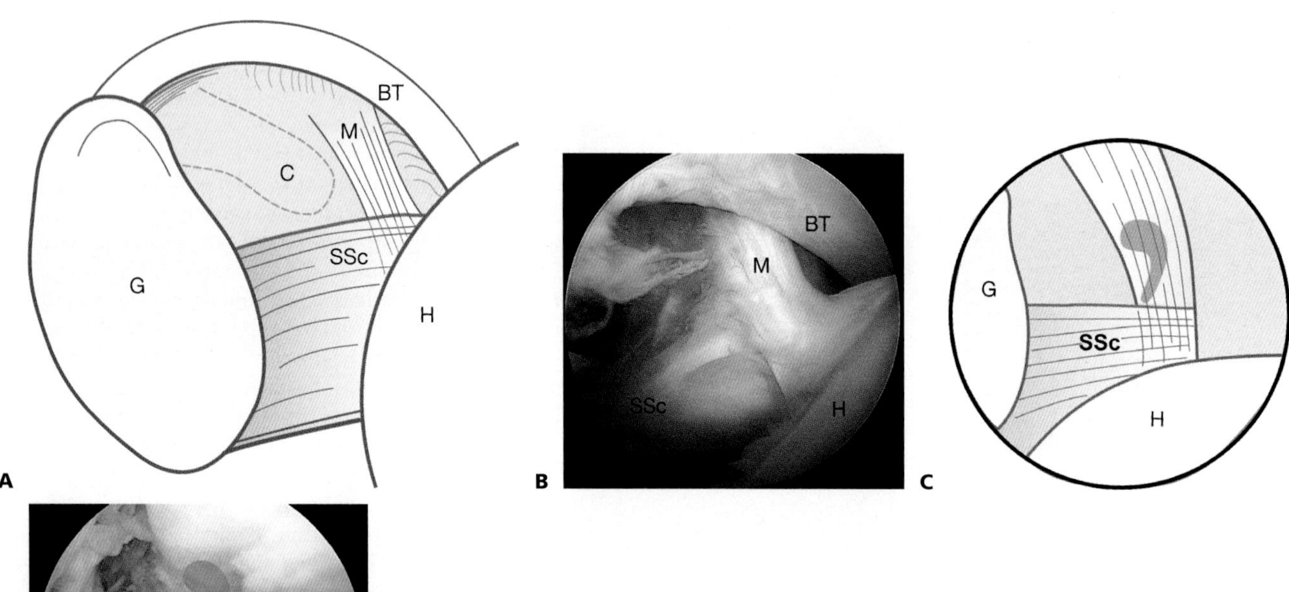

FIG 3 • **A,B.** Anterior structures from a posterior viewing portal of a right shoulder. The medial sling (*M*) of the biceps tendon (*BT*) inserts into the lesser tuberosity of the humerus (*H*) along with the superolateral margin of the subscapularis (*SSc*). **C,D.** Complete subscapularis tendon tear. In this situation, the comma sign (,) leads to the superolateral border of the subscapularis tendon. *G*, glenoid; *C*, coracoid. (From Burkhart SS, Lo IKY, Brady PC. A Cowboy's Guide to Advanced Shoulder Arthroscopy. Philadelphia: Lippincott Williams & Wilkins, 2006.)

- Lift-off test: The test is positive when the patient cannot actively hold the hand away from the lower back; it is positive only when at least 75% of the subscapularis tendon is torn.[1] The test is also difficult to perform for some patients with restricted shoulder motion.
- Napoleon test, also known as modified belly press: Wrist flexed 90 degrees and elbow posteriorly positioned indicates a positive test; the entire subscapularis tendon is torn. An intermediate test is indicated by wrist flexed 30 to 60 degrees; more than 50% of the subscapularis tendon is torn. A negative test occurs when the patient is able to "strike the pose"; less than 50% of the subscapularis tendon is torn.
  - With a significant subscapularis tendon tear the patient flexes the wrist, the elbow drops backward, and the posterior deltoid acts to pull the hand against the belly.
- Bear hug test: A positive test is indicated when the physician can pull the patient's hand off the shoulder.[1] This is the most sensitive test for an upper subscapularis injury (eg, a partial tear involving the superior aspect of the subscapularis tendon).[1]

- A patient with a subscapularis tear often has diminished internal rotation strength and increased passive external rotation (compared to the opposite extremity).
- A patient with a subscapularis tear may also have additional pathology in his or her shoulder.
  - This again emphasizes the importance of a good physical examination that also evaluates the other rotator cuff tendons, the biceps tendon, glenoid labrum, and so forth.
- Patients with a posterosuperior rotator cuff tear often have pain, weakness, or limited elevation and external rotation.
- A significant tear of the subscapularis tendon may result in disruption of the medial sling of the long head of the biceps tendon. This can lead to either partial or complete tears of the biceps tendon with or without medial subluxation.
- A tear of the glenoid labrum often results in "catching" pain that occurs with certain positions of the shoulder, depending on the location of the tear.

IMAGING AND OTHER DIAGNOSTIC STUDIES

- We routinely obtain five views of the shoulder: anteroposterior (AP) internal rotation, AP external rotation, AP with 30-degree caudal tilt, outlet view, and axillary plain films.
  - Evaluation of the plain films may reveal proximal humeral migration (especially with longstanding massive rotator cuff tears), acromial morphology, glenohumeral or acromioclavicular joint degenerative changes, anterior humeral translation (seen with subscapularis tendon disruptions on the axillary view), and so forth.
- We also routinely obtain an MRI of the affected shoulder.
  - The MRI can provide important information on the location and extent of the subscapularis tendon tear.
  - It can also determine whether additional pathology in the shoulder coexists (eg, additional rotator cuff tears, medial subluxation or tears of the long head of the biceps tendon, ganglion cysts, labral tears).
  - Tears of the subscapularis tendon are best appreciated on the axillary images of the MRI (**FIG 4**).

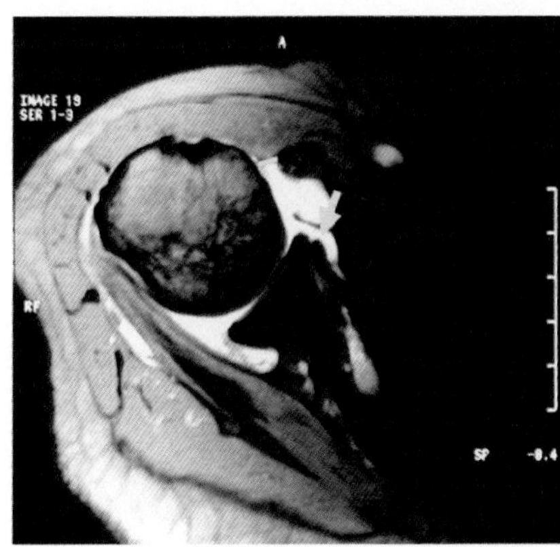

FIG 4 • T2-weighted axial MRI showing a decreased coracohumeral space (*yellow line*) and complete tear of the subscapularis tendon. *Yellow arrow* indicates the edge of the retracted subscapularis tendon. (From Burkhart SS, Lo IKY, Brady PC. A Cowboy's Guide to Advanced Shoulder Arthroscopy. Philadelphia: Lippincott Williams & Wilkins, 2006.)

  - Signal characteristics consistent with fluid may be seen with partial-thickness tears, whereas a loss of part or all of the normal tendon will be seen with full-thickness tears.

DIFFERENTIAL DIAGNOSIS

- Subscapularis tendinitis or bursitis
- Posterosuperior rotator cuff tear
- Biceps tendinitis
- Labral tear
- Neurologic impairment

NONOPERATIVE MANAGEMENT

- The role of nonoperative treatment in patients with symptomatic subscapularis tears is very limited.
- Most patients who present to orthopedic surgeons with subscapularis tears have had the tear for a long time.[3]
- Furthermore, most have attempted and failed nonoperative treatment.
- However, for patients who are not good surgical candidates (eg, very old, ill), nonoperative treatment is warranted.
- Nonoperative treatment typically consists of activities as tolerated with gentle stretching and progressive strengthening of the shoulder.

SURGICAL MANAGEMENT

Preoperative Planning

- The history, physical examination, plain films, and MRI should all be reviewed before operative intervention.

Positioning

- The anesthesiologist administers general anesthesia with endotracheal intubation and applies protective eyewear to the patient.
- The patient is rotated into the lateral decubitus position and an axillary roll is placed.
  - The patient is well padded with pillows beneath and between the legs.

- The patient is secured in place with a vacuum beanbag and is tilted back approximately 10 degrees.
- A warming blanket is applied to prevent hypothermia.
- The sterile field must extend posteriorly to a position medial to the scapula and anteriorly just lateral to the nipple.
- After the patient is properly protected, positioned, padded, and draped, the surgeon performs an examination under anesthesia.
- The assistant prepares the operative extremity with a sterile scrub.
- The arm is then placed in 5 to 10 pounds of balanced suspension (Star Sleeve Traction System; Arthrex Inc., Naples, FL) with the shoulder in 20 to 30 degrees of abduction and 20 degrees of forward flexion (**FIG 5**).

Approach

- Successful treatment of subscapularis tears has been documented with both open and arthroscopic techniques.
- We prefer and will present our arthroscopic technique for treatment of a subscapularis tendon tear.

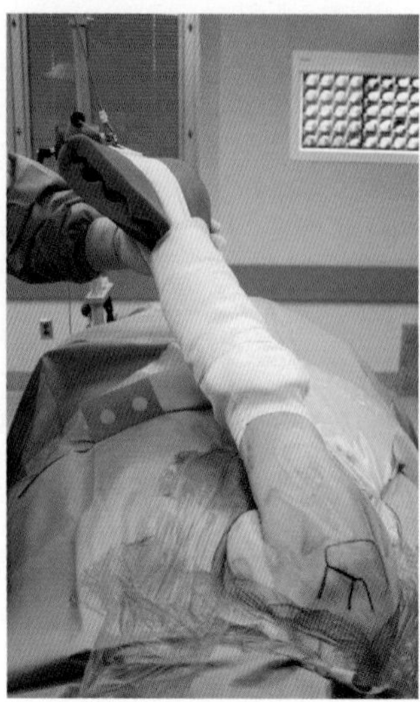

FIG 5 • Positioning in the lateral decubitus position. Photograph from the head looking downward showing the arm suspended in 20 to 30 degrees of abduction and 20 degrees of forward flexion.

TECHNIQUES

PORTALS AND VISUALIZATION

- The surgeon should remember the "6 Ps" for arthroscopic portals: "Proper portal placement prevents poor performance."
- Our standard posterior viewing portal is placed 4 to 5 cm inferior (caudal) to the posterior border of the acromion and 3 to 4 cm medial to the posterolateral corner of the acromion (**TECH FIG 1A**).
- A standard diagnostic arthroscopy of the entire glenohumeral joint is performed.
- To fix the tear one must be able to see the tear. This point cannot be emphasized enough, and throughout the procedure special attention is paid to optimize visualization by controlling bleeding.
  - Key factors include minimizing the pressure differential between the patient's blood pressure and the arthroscopic pump pressure; making use of the Bernoulli principle to achieve turbulence control; and using electrocautery as needed to cauterize specific bleeding points.
- The subscapularis tendon presents a unique problem to visualization. The tendon tear is often in a very confined space that may be unfamiliar to the surgeon (**TECH FIG 1B**). This space can become even more constricted with soft tissue swelling as the case proceeds, so we recommend repairing the subscapularis tendon before addressing any other problems in the shoulder.
- We have found that examination of the subscapularis tendon for a partial tear is optimized with shoulder flexion and internal rotation (lifts the subscapularis tendon off its footprint on the lesser tuberosity; **TECH FIG 1C**).
  - Visualization is further enhanced with a "posterior lever push" in which an assistant pushes the proximal humerus posteriorly while pulling the distal humerus anteriorly (**TECH FIG 1D**).
- A 70-degree arthroscope is an extremely helpful additional tool that can improve visualization by providing an "aerial view."
  - The initial identification and orientation should be done with a 30-degree arthroscope, however, because it is easy to get lost and stray dangerously inferior into the vicinity of neurovascular structures if the 70-degree arthroscope is used initially.
- The primary working portal is the anterosuperolateral portal, which is 1 to 2 cm lateral to the anterolateral corner of the acromion.
  - An 18-gauge spinal needle is introduced into the glenohumeral joint to make a 10-degree angle of approach to the lesser tuberosity.
  - Advantages of the anterosuperolateral portal include a good angle of approach to prepare the lesser tuberosity bone bed; a near-parallel angle of approach to the subscapularis for mobilization and antegrade suture passage; and an angle of approach to the coracoid tip that will allow a coracoplasty to be made in a plane that is parallel to the subscapularis tendon.
- The next portal created is the anterior portal, which is 4 to 5 cm inferior to the anterior acromion, just lateral to the coracoid tip.
  - An 18-gauge spinal needle is introduced into the glenohumeral joint to determine a 45-degree angle of approach to the lesser tuberosity, and then the portal is established in that line of approach.
  - Advantages of the anterior portal include an optimal angle of approach for anchor placement, suture management, and on occasion retrograde suture passage (although we almost always do antegrade suture passage through the subscapularis tendon via an anterosuperolateral portal).

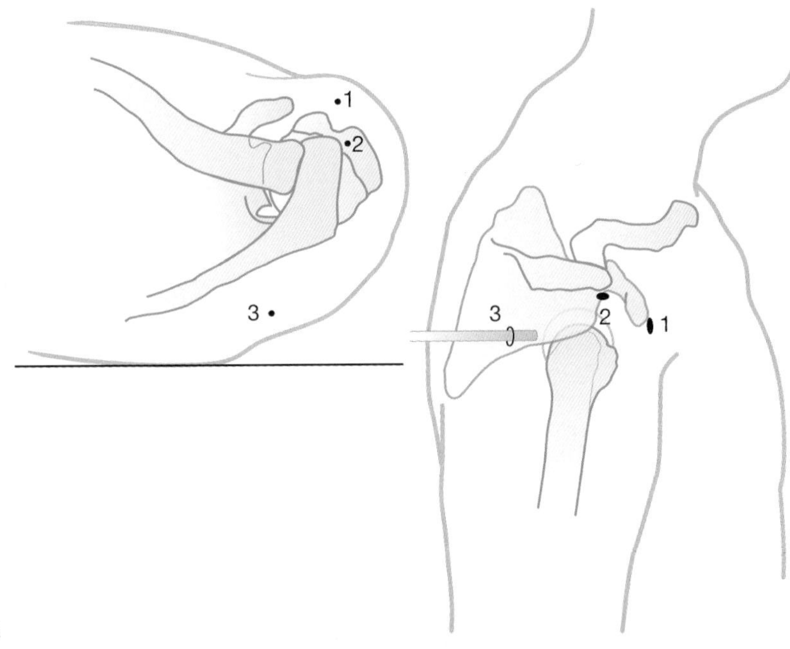

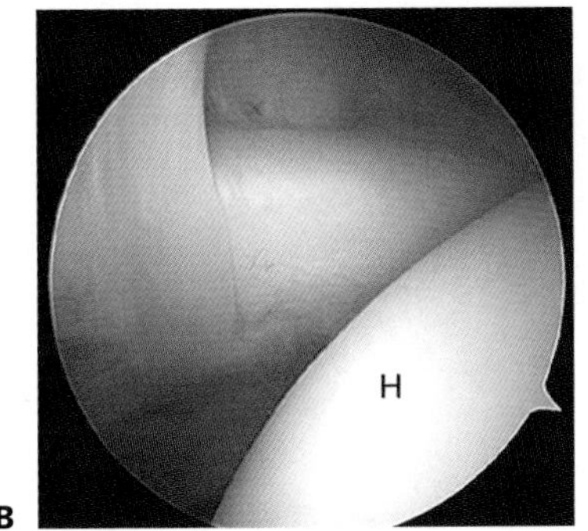

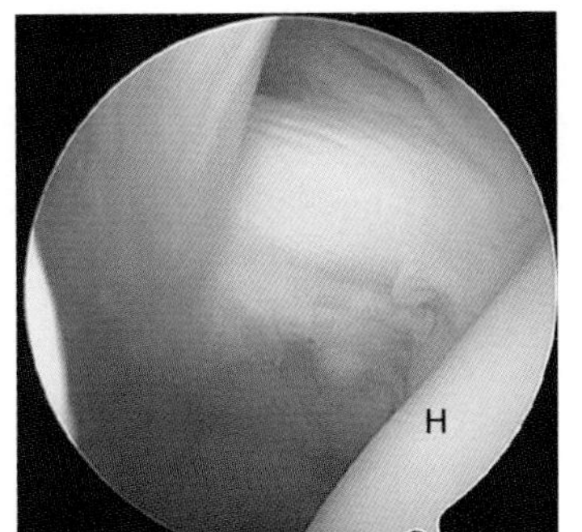

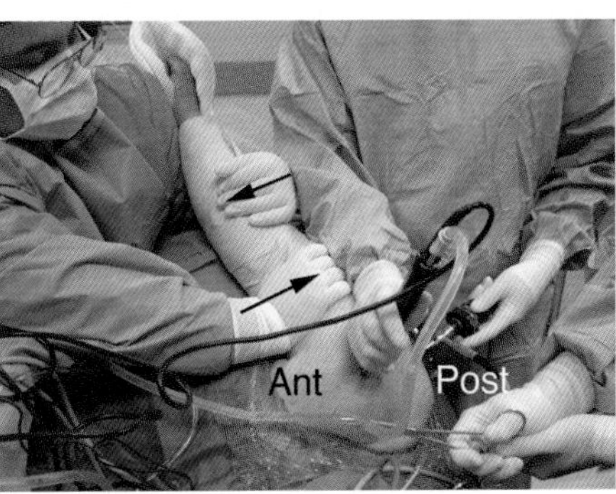

TECH FIG 1 • Portals and visualization. **A.** The anterior (*1*), anterosuperolateral (*2*), and posterior (*3*) portals for arthroscopic subscapularis tendon repair. **B,C.** Arthroscopic view of the subscapularis insertion of a right shoulder from the posterior portal using a 30-degree arthroscope with the arm in 30 degrees of abduction and neutral rotation (**B**) and in internal rotation (**C**). **D**. The posterior lever push. *H*, humeral head. (From Burkhart SS, Lo IKY, Brady PC. A Cowboy's Guide to Advanced Shoulder Arthroscopy. Philadelphia: Lippincott Williams & Wilkins, 2006.)

BICEPS TENDON

- Subscapularis tendon tears are often associated with tearing or medial subluxation of the long head of the biceps tendon.
- The long head of the biceps tendon should be inspected from its base to the intertubercular groove. It is often helpful to pull the tendon into the glenohumeral joint and to pay particular attention to the medial surface of the tendon for partial tearing.
- Also, internal and external rotation of the humerus may reveal subluxation of the tendon. The biceps tendon should never pass posterior to the plane of the subscapularis with rotation of the humerus.
- Most of our patients with biceps tendon tearing or subluxation in association with a torn subscapularis receive a biceps tenodesis.
- In our view the alternatives are suboptimal:
  - Biceps tendon subluxation left alone will result in increased stress to the subscapularis repair and may ultimately cause it to fail.
  - Significant biceps tendon degeneration may result in continued shoulder pain and dysfunction.
  - Biceps tenotomy has been shown in the literature to result in decreased elbow flexion and forearm supination strength, and some patients consider it aesthetically undesirable.[15] Therefore, we perform a biceps tenotomy only in elderly patients with low demands and poorly defined arm musculature.
- The initial step in the tenotomy is to place two half-racking stitches 1 to 2 cm distal to the base of the long head of the biceps tendon (**TECH FIG 2**). These sutures tighten and lock against the tendon to securely hold it after it is tenotomized (in preparation for tenodesis).
- The tenotomy is made at the base of the biceps with electrocautery or scissors. Care is taken not to damage the superior labrum.
- The biceps tendon is then extracted extracorporeally through the anterosuperolateral portal. Pushing on the skin around the tendon's exit point and flexing the elbow and shoulder aid in presenting the tendon out of the portal.
- A no. 2 FiberWire (Arthrex) whipstitch is run with three or four passes on each side of the tendon.

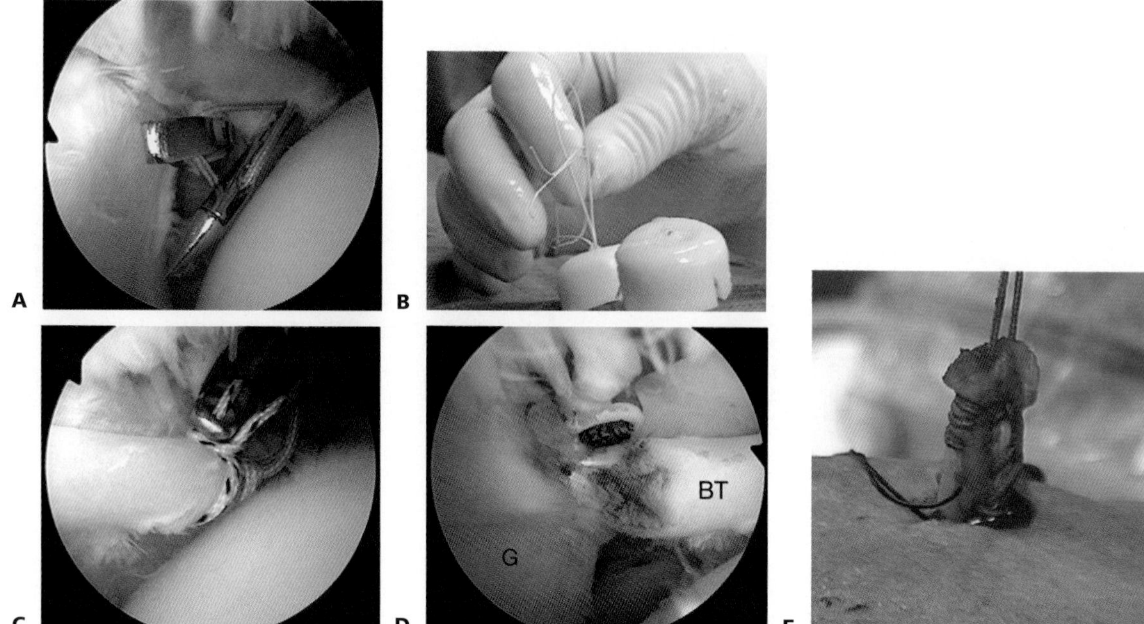

TECH FIG 2 • Biceps tendon. Two half-racking sutures are placed to secure the biceps tendon before tenotomy. **A.** A Penetrator (Arthrex) hands off a FiberWire suture (Arthrex) to a suture retriever. **B.** The FiberWire loop is then exteriorized and the free ends of the suture are passed through the loop. **C.** The free ends of the suture are tensioned to bring the suture loop down to the tendon. **D.** The biceps tendon is released close to its insertion on the superior labrum using an electrocautery Bovie. **E.** The biceps tendon is pulled out through the anterosuperolateral portal using the two half-racking sutures and a locking whipstitch is placed in the biceps, four throws on each side of the tendon. *BT*, biceps tendon; *G*, glenoid. (From Burkhart SS, Lo IKY, Brady PC. A Cowboy's Guide to Advanced Shoulder Arthroscopy. Philadelphia: Lippincott Williams & Wilkins, 2006.)

- The whipstitch sutures are temporarily pulled through the anterosuperolateral portal outside the cannula so that it will be out of the way until it is time to do the biceps tenodesis.
- This temporary tenotomy improves subscapularis visualization and working space. At the end of the case, after the subscapularis tendon has been repaired, we prefer to anchor the biceps tendon to bone using the BioTenodesis screw system (Arthrex) to obtain a secure interference fit of tendon against bone.

SUBCORACOID SPACE

- The first step in defining the subcoracoid space is to identify the coracoid tip.
  - If the subscapularis tendon is intact or partially torn, the coracoid tip is located just anterior to the upper border of the subscapularis tendon. With internal and external rotation of the humerus the coracoid tip can be seen as a moving bulge in the rotator interval.
  - Through the anterosuperolateral portal the electrocautery can be used to create a window in the rotator interval tissue to expose the coracoid tip (the surgeon must take care to preserve the medial sling of the biceps tendon).
- If the subscapularis tendon is completely torn and retracted, the coracoacromial ligament is a useful guide to the coracoid tip.
  - The surgeon should use an instrument to palpate and confirm the location of the coracoid tip.
- We have found that the best method of measuring the coracohumeral interval is direct visualization during arthroscopy with an instrument of known size through the anterosuperolateral portal (eg, the diameter of a shaver blade). Gentle axial distraction may be necessary to obtain an accurate measurement if there is any proximal humeral migration.
- We also routinely place the shoulder in the provocative position of flexion, horizontal adduction, and internal rotation to arthroscopically evaluate if there is any impingement between the coracoid tip and the subscapularis tendon and proximal humerus.
- If there is any evidence of subcoracoid stenosis (coracohumeral interval less than 6 mm) or impingement, we perform a coracoplasty with a goal of creating a coracohumeral interval of 8 to 10 mm.

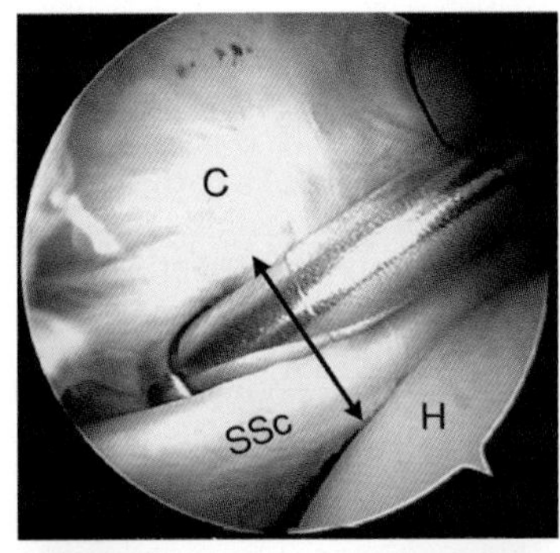

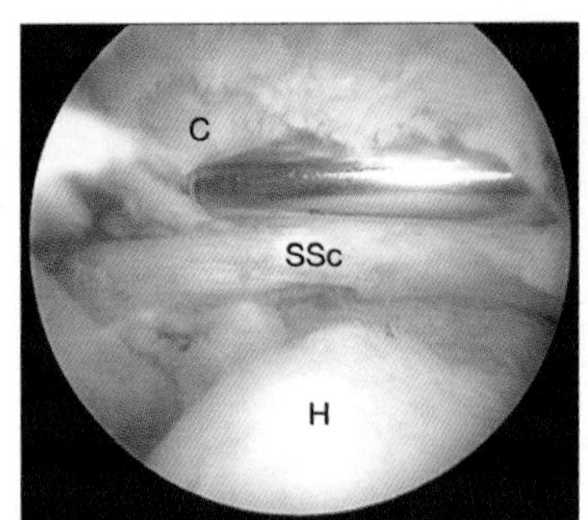

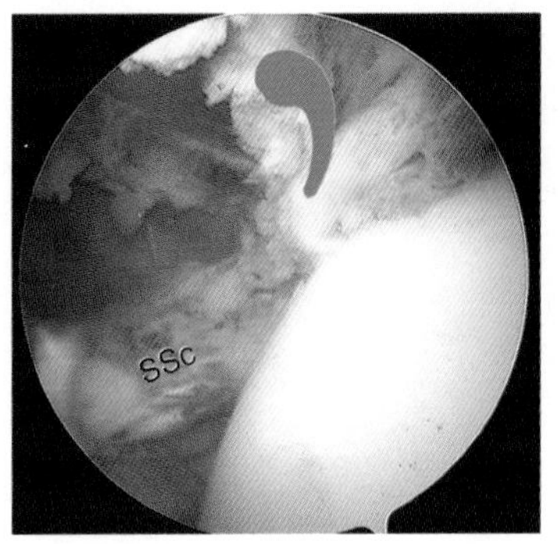

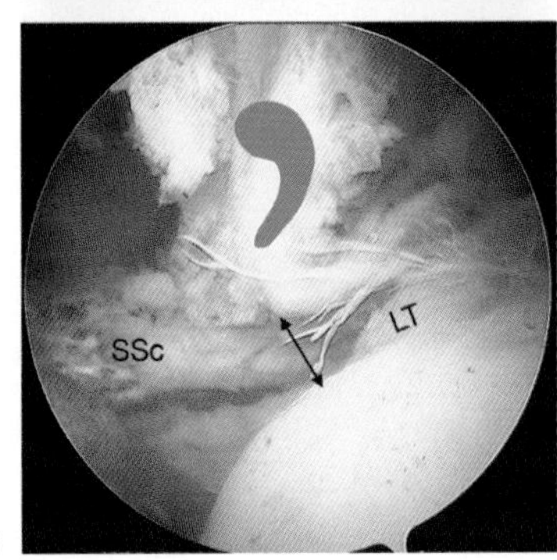

TECH FIG 3 • The subcoracoid space. **A.** A shaver is introduced through an anterolateral portal. The coracohumeral distance is measured (↔), and there is minimal space for the subscapularis tendon, signifying coracohumeral stenosis. **B.** A shaver placed through the anterosuperolateral portal has an approach angle that is essentially parallel to the subscapularis tendon. **C,D.** Arthroscopic pictures of a right shoulder with a posterior viewing portal, 70-degree arthroscope, and no lever push (**C**); with a posterior lever push (**D**). *H*, humerus; *SSc*, subscapularis tendon; *C*, coracoid; (,), comma tissue; *LT*, lesser tuberosity. (From Burkhart SS, Lo IKY, Brady PC. A Cowboy's Guide to Advanced Shoulder Arthroscopy. Philadelphia: Lippincott Williams & Wilkins, 2006.)

- The soft tissues on the posterolateral surface of the coracoid are removed ("skeletonizing" the coracoid) with electrocautery and a motorized shaver (the surgeon must be careful not to release the conjoint tendon from the undersurface of the coracoid tip; **TECH FIG 3A,B**).
- The fibers of the coracoacromial ligament may be released for improved visualization.
- The anterosuperolateral portal provides a great angle of approach for the high-speed burr to be parallel to the subscapularis tendon for the coracoplasty.
- A "posterior lever push" may improve the anterior working space by 5 to 10 mm (**TECH FIG 3C,D**). A second assistant who is anterior to the patient in a lateral decubitus position provides a posterior force to the proximal humerus with a simultaneous anterior force to the distal humerus.
- Alternating between the 30- and 70-degree arthroscopes as needed optimizes visualization.
- The coracoplasty improves the anterior working space for the subscapularis repair and prevents future abrasion to protect the repair.

SUBSCAPULARIS MOBILIZATION

- We routinely perform a three-sided release for complete, retracted subscapularis tendon tears.
- The three-sided release can be difficult secondary to retraction, scarring, and working in a constricted space.
- The surgeon may be concerned about the proximity of neurovascular structures; however, a cadaveric study found that the axillary nerve, axillary artery, musculocutaneous nerve, and lateral cord of the brachial plexus are all more than 25 mm from the coracoid base.[10]
  - The key is to stay on the posterolateral aspect of the coracoid.
- The first step to mobilizing the subscapularis is to place a traction suture at the junction of the superolateral tendon and "comma tissue" (**TECH FIG 4A**).
  - The comma tissue is a comma-shaped fibrous band of tissue at the superolateral border of the subscapularis tendon; its fibers are oriented at right angles to those of the subscapularis. It is the remnant of the medial sling of the biceps after it pulls loose from its footprint on the lesser tuberosity directly adjacent to the footprint of the upper subscapularis.
  - This can be done through the anterosuperolateral portal with a Viper or Scorpion suture passer (Arthrex) loaded with a free no. 2 FiberWire suture (Arthrex). The traction suture can then be held outside the cannula to allow continued use of the anterosuperolateral portal.
- The anterior release (subscapularis from the posterolateral coracoid and deltoid fascia) may be done by alternating the electrocautery with the shaver.
  - If a coracoplasty was not performed earlier, the soft tissues are removed from the coracoid ("skeletonizing" the posterolateral coracoid; **TECH FIG 4B**).
  - The release is continued medial along the posterolateral coracoid until the subscapularis muscle belly is visible beneath the arch of the coracoid neck and base.

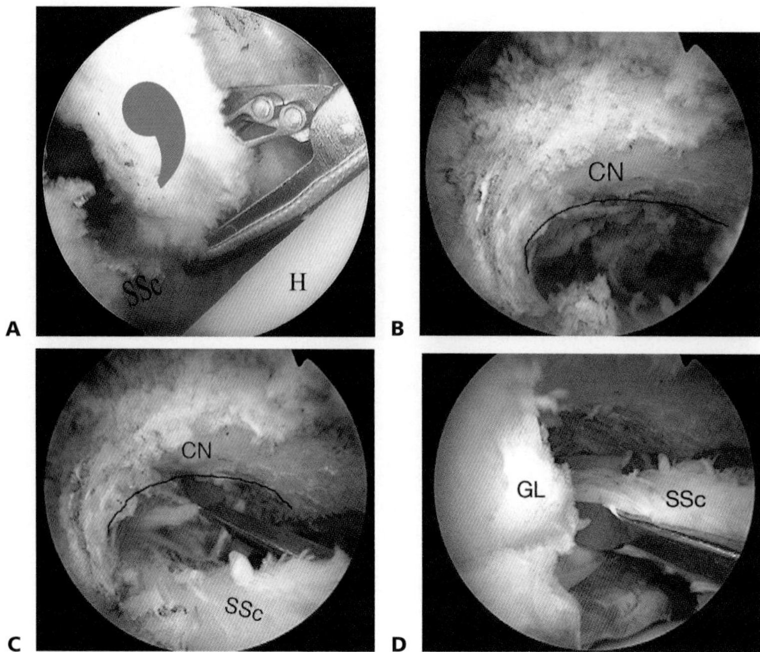

TECH FIG 4 • Subscapularis mobilization. **A.** A traction suture is placed at the junction of the comma (,) and the subscapularis tendon (*SSc*) in a right shoulder seen through a posterior viewing portal. **B.** The coracoid dissection (*solid line*) has skeletonized the posterolateral coracoid to the level of the coracoid neck (*CN*) during the anterior release. **C.** A 30-degree arthroscopic elevator, introduced through an anterosuperolateral portal, is used to perform the superior release, lysing adhesions between the subscapularis and the coracoid neck and base. **D.** A 15-degree arthroscopic elevator is used to develop the plane between the posterior aspect of the subscapularis tendon (*SSc*) and the anterior glenoid neck and glenoid labrum (*GL*) during the posterior release. *H*, humerus. (From Burkhart SS, Lo IKY, Brady PC. A Cowboy's Guide to Advanced Shoulder Arthroscopy. Philadelphia: Lippincott Williams & Wilkins, 2006.)

- The superior release (subscapularis from the undersurface of the coracoid neck and base) may then be done with a 30-degree arthroscopic elevator (**TECH FIG 4C**).
  - The release is done only to the midpoint of the undersurface of the coracoid neck (to prevent damage to the neurovascular structures medial to the coracoid neck).
- The posterior release (subscapularis from the glenoid neck) may then be done with a 15-degree arthroscopic elevator (**TECH FIG 4D**). The release is continued medial until the subscapularis is freely mobile.
  - The posterior release is the safest release (because it is in a very safe plane between the subscapularis and the anterior glenoid neck). The inferior release is the most dangerous and has not been necessary in our experience.

BONE BED PREPARATION AND ANCHOR PLACEMENT

- The anterosuperolateral portal has a great angle of approach for removing the soft tissues off the subscapularis footprint of the lesser tuberosity.
- A ring curette may be used to precisely remove the soft tissues up to the articular margin. Then electrocautery is used to ablate any soft tissue on the footprint (**TECH FIG 5A**).
- The high-speed burr then removes the "charcoal" (residual of electrocauterization) to a bleeding bone bed without decorticating the bone (**TECH FIG 5B**).
- To decrease the tension at the repair site, we have found that the subscapularis footprint may be medialized up to 5 mm with no detriment to its function.

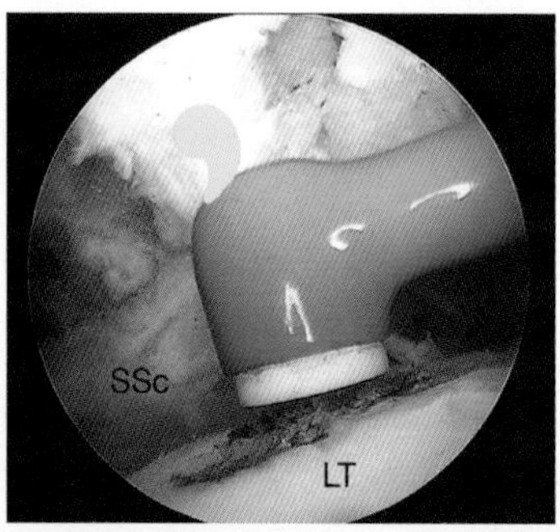

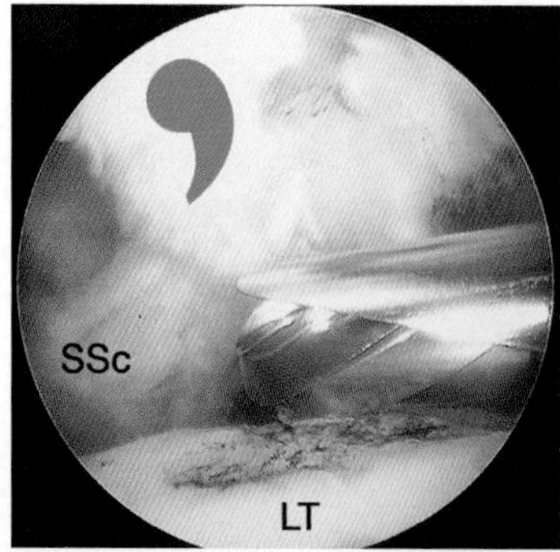

TECH FIG 5 • Bone bed preparation and anchor placement. **A,B.** An electrocautery probe is used to delineate a medialized footprint on the lesser tuberosity (**A**), and a power burr burrs off the "charcoal" down to bleeding bone (**B**). *(continued)*

C 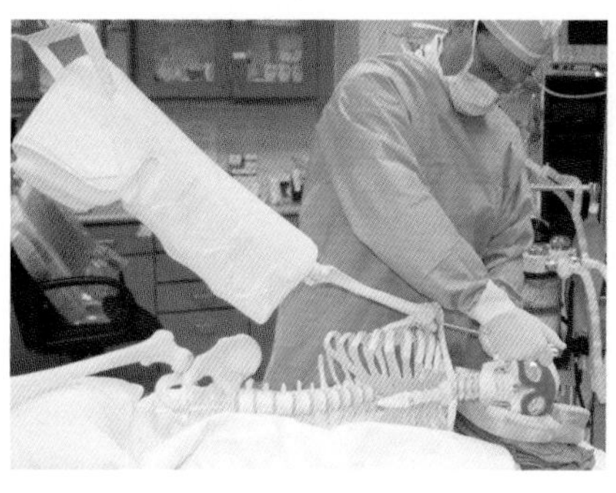

D 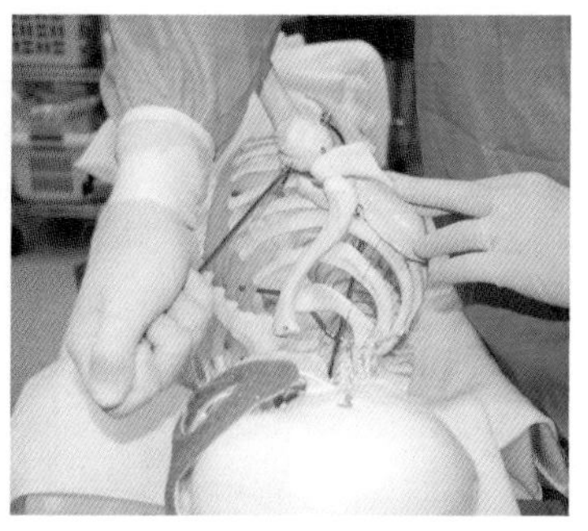

E 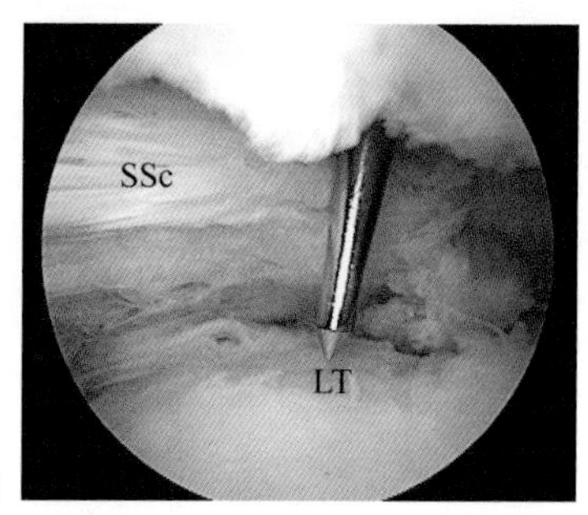

TECH FIG 5 • *(continued)* **C.** This skeleton shows how the arm is held in 20 to 30 degrees of abduction and 20 degrees of forward flexion during shoulder arthroscopy in the lateral decubitus position. **D.** Photograph from the head looking downward shows how the combination of abduction, forward flexion, and normal humeral retroversion necessitates a "hand on face" position during anchor insertion into the lesser tuberosity. This highlights the need for protective goggles on the patient. **E.** This "hand on face" position allows the surgeon to achieve an appropriate "deadman" angle to insert suture anchors into the lesser tuberosity. *LT*, lesser tuberosity; *SSc*, subscapularis. (From Burkhart SS, Lo IKY, Brady PC. A Cowboy's Guide to Advanced Shoulder Arthroscopy. Philadelphia: Lippincott Williams & Wilkins, 2006.)

- One anchor should be placed every centimeter, which typically results in one anchor for a partial tear and two anchors for a complete tear (if a single-row repair is done).
  - The anchors should be placed in order from inferior (caudal) to superior (cephalad).
- We use double-loaded anchors to reduce the load on each suture.
- The best angle of approach for anchor placement is typically through the anterior portal (TECH FIG 5C).
  - The surgeon's hand and instruments (eg, punch and anchor inserter) are often close to the patient's face, which is one reason we place protective eyewear on every patient (TECH FIG 5D,E).

SUTURE PASSAGE AND KNOT TYING

- We prefer the Viper or Scorpion suture passers (Arthrex) because they allow antegrade suture passage and retrieval (retrograde suture passage is difficult because the coracoid often blocks a good angle of approach).
- One strand of suture is retrieved from the anchor, pulled out the anterosuperolateral cannula, and loaded in the suture passer.
- Tension is placed on the traction suture (which is inside the anterosuperolateral portal but outside its cannula) and the suture is passed about 10 mm from the lateral edge of the subscapularis tendon (TECH FIG 6A).
  - For the superior anchor, the sutures should be passed over the top of the superolateral border of the subscapularis, just medial to the "comma tissue." This will provide a "ripstop" to prevent lateral cutout of the sutures.
- The process is repeated for the second suture of the same anchor.
- Both the sutures are tied through a clear cannula with a double-diameter knot pusher (Surgeon's Sixth Finger, Arthrex; TECH FIG 6B).
- We use a six-throw arthroscopic surgeon's knot, which is composed of a static base knot of three stacked half-hitches followed by three reversing half-hitches on alternating posts (TECH FIG 6C).
  - The arthroscopic surgeon's knot with a double-diameter knot pusher has been found in the laboratory to have the best combination of loop and knot security.[11]
- To maximize efficiency and visualization, we tie the sutures of the inferior anchor before working on the superior anchor (TECH FIG 6D).
- After completing the subscapularis tendon repair we internally and externally rotate the humerus to be sure that we have achieved secure apposition of the tendon against the bone.

A 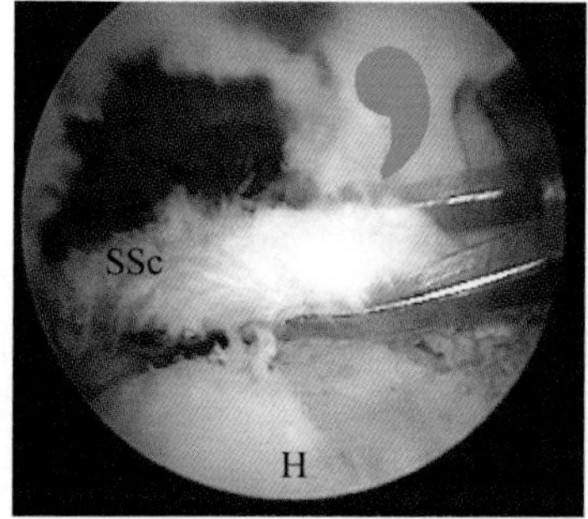

B 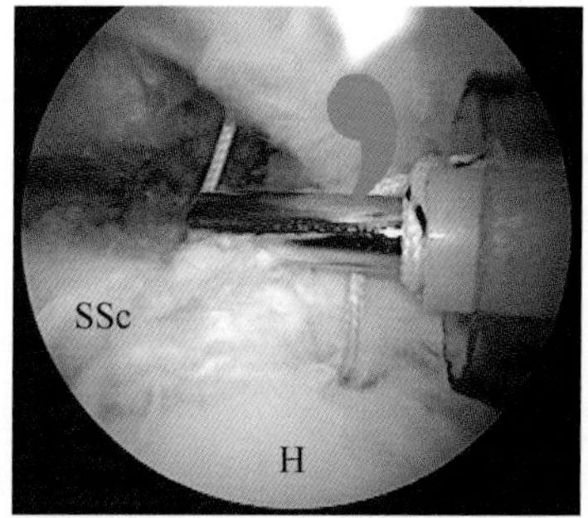

TECH FIG 6 • Suture passage and knot tying. **A.** During suture passage into the upper subscapularis tendon, the tendon is grasped and the suture passed at the junction of the subscapularis (*SSc*) and the comma (,). **B.** The double-diameter knot pusher allows the subscapularis tendon to be manipulated and held in the appropriate position while each half-hitch of the knot is tied. *(continued)*

TECHNIQUES

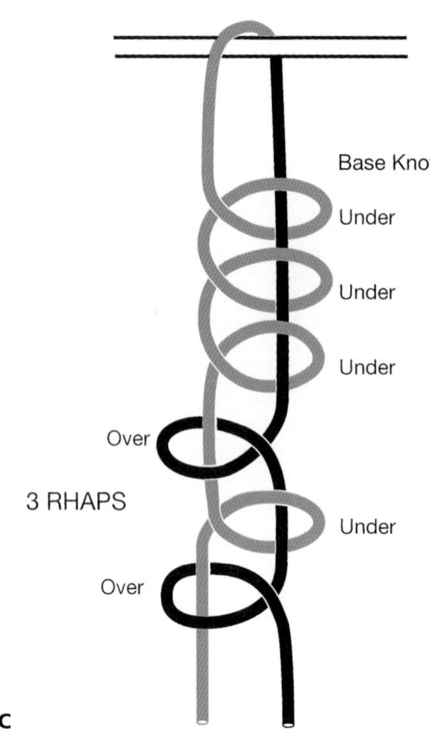

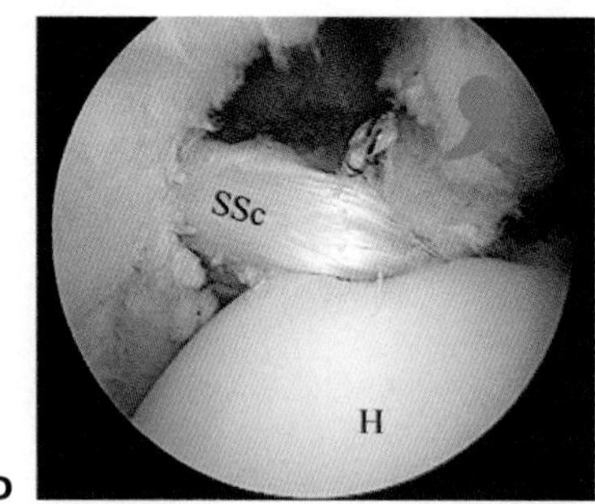

TECH FIG 6 • *(continued)* **C.** Drawing of base arthroscopic knot locked with three reversing half-hitches on alternating posts (RHAP). **D.** Sutures from the upper anchor have been placed at the junction of the vertically oriented comma tissue and the upper border of subscapularis tendon. *H*, humerus. (From Burkhart SS, Lo IKY, Brady PC. A Cowboy's Guide to Advanced Shoulder Arthroscopy. Philadelphia: Lippincott Williams & Wilkins, 2006.)

PEARLS AND PITFALLS

Diagnosis	■ A complete history, a proper physical examination, full evaluation of the diagnostic studies, and a thorough arthroscopic evaluation of the shoulder are necessary.
Portal placement	■ Proper portal placement is imperative to achieve the correct angle of approach to work in the subcoracoid space.
Visualization	■ The key principles include minimizing pressure differentials (hypotensive anesthesia with adequate arthroscopic pump pressure), avoiding turbulence, using the posterior lever push, and using both the 30- and 70-degree arthroscopes freely.
Secure fixation	■ The subscapularis tendon must be securely apposed to the bone to optimize healing. Important biomechanical principles include the proper angle of insertion of the suture anchors; use of double-loaded anchors to reduce the load on each suture; use of strong sutures; proper suture placement in the tendon; and optimized loop and knot security.
Rehabilitation	■ The patient must clearly understand what he or she can do to protect and optimize healing of the subscapularis tendon repair.

POSTOPERATIVE CARE

- An arthroscopic subscapularis tendon repair is usually an outpatient procedure.
- After the arthroscopic portals are closed, a sterile dressing is applied over the shoulder.
- A sling with a small pillow is applied with the arm at the side. The sling is worn full-time for 6 weeks, except when bathing or eating.
- During the first 6 weeks the patient should perform daily active wrist and elbow motion.
  - The patient must not externally rotate past neutral (straight-ahead position) for 6 weeks.
  - There is no overhead motion in the first 6 weeks.
- At 6 weeks from the operation the sling is discontinued.
  - The patient is started on a passive stretching program that includes passive external rotation with a cane up to 45 degrees and overhead stretches with a rope and pulley.
- At 12 weeks from the operation the patient is started on a strengthening program with elastic bands.
  - If the subscapularis tear is part of a massive anterosuperior rotator cuff tear, then strengthening is delayed until 16 weeks postoperatively.
  - Progression to light weights is based on the patient's progress.
  - Rehabilitation focuses on strengthening the scapular stabilizers and deltoid and rotator cuff muscles.

- Return to full, unrestricted activities is usually at 6 to 12 months and is based on the patient, the size of the tear, the strength of the repair, and the patient's rehabilitation progress.

OUTCOMES

- The results after arthroscopic subscapularis tendon repair have been quite favorable.[2,3,9]
- The senior author (SSB)[3] published his preliminary results in 2002.
  - In this series of 25 consecutive patients with a mean follow-up of 11 months, 92% had good or excellent results by the UCLA criteria.
  - There was a significant improvement in pain and functional motion.
  - Eight of ten patients who had proximal humeral migration preoperatively had reversal of the migration and functional overhead use of their arm.
- Bennett[2] also found encouraging results in his prospective cohort with 2- to 4-year follow-up.
  - The patients had a mean American Shoulder and Elbow Surgeons (ASES) score improvement from 16 preoperatively to 74 postoperatively.
  - Visual analogue pain scores improved from 9 preoperatively to 2 postoperatively.
- Kim et al,[9] in a recent report of patients who had an arthroscopic repair of isolated partial articular-sided tears, found similar improvements in pain and function.
  - At a mean follow-up of 27 months, UCLA scores improved from 23 preoperatively to 33 postoperatively, ASES scores improved from 67 to 96, and visual analogue pain scores improved from 5 to 0.3.

COMPLICATIONS

- Stiffness
- Retear
- Neuropraxia
- Infection

REFERENCES

1. Barth JRH, Burkhart SS, DeBeer JF. The bear hug test: a new and sensitive test for diagnosing a subscapularis tear. Arthroscopy 2006;22:1076–1084.
2. Bennett WF. Arthroscopic repair of isolated subscapularis tears: a prospective cohort with 2- to 4-year follow-up. Arthroscopy 2003;19:131–143.
3. Burkhart SS, Tehrany AM. Arthroscopic subscapularis tendon repair: technique and preliminary results. Arthroscopy 2002;18:454–463.
4. Dick TP, Howden R. Gray's Anatomy: The Classic Collector's Edition. London: Crown Publishers, 1977.
5. Friedman RJ, Bonutti PM, Genez B. Cine magnetic resonance imaging of the subcoracoid region. Orthopedics 1998;21:545–548.
6. Gerber C, Hersche O, Farron A. Isolated rupture of the subscapularis tendon: results of operative repair. J Bone Joint Surg Am 1996;78A:1015–1023.
7. Gerber C, Terrier F, Zehnder R, et al. The subcoracoid space: an anatomic study. Clin Orthop 1987;215:132–138.
8. Halder A, Zobitz ME, Schultz E, et al. Structural properties of the subscapularis tendon. J Orthop Res 2000;18:829–834.
9. Kim SH, Oh I, Park J, et al. Intra-articular repair of an isolated partial articular-surface tear of the subscapularis tendon. Am J Sports Med 2005;33:1825–1830.
10. Lo IK, Burkhart SS. Arthroscopic coracoplasty through the rotator interval. Arthroscopy 2003;19:667–671.
11. Lo IK, Burkhart SS. Arthroscopic knots: determining the optimal balance of loop and knot security. Arthroscopy 2004;20:489–502.
12. Lo IK, Burkhart SS. Subscapularis tears: arthroscopic repair of the forgotten rotator cuff tendon. Tech Shoulder Elbow Surg 2002;3:282–291.
13. Lo IK, Burkhart SS. The comma sign: an arthroscopic guide to the torn subscapularis tendon. Arthroscopy 2003;19:334–337.
14. Lo IK, Burkhart SS. The etiology and assessment of subscapularis tendon tears: a case for subcoracoid impingement, the roller-wringer effect, and TUFF lesions of the subscapularis. Arthroscopy 2003;19:1142–1150.
15. Mariani EM, Cofield RH, Askew LJ, et al. Rupture of the tendon of the long head of the biceps brachii: surgical versus nonsurgical treatment. Clinic Orthop Relat Res 1988;228:233–239.
16. Richards DP, Burkhart SS, Campbell SE. Relation between narrowed coracohumeral distance and subscapularis tears. Arthroscopy 2005;21:1223–1228.
17. Richards DP, Burkhart SS, Lo IK. Subscapularis tears: arthroscopic repair techniques. Orthop Clin North Am 2003;34:485–498.
18. Sakurai G, Ozaki J, Tomita Y, et al. Incomplete tears of the subscapularis tendon associated with tears of the supraspinatus tendon: cadaveric and clinical studies. J Shoulder Elbow Surg 1998;7:510–515.
19. Sano H, Ishii H, Trudel G, et al. Histologic evidence of degeneration at the insertion of 3 rotator cuff tendons: a comparative study with human cadaveric shoulders. J Shoulder Elbow Surg 1999;8:574–579.
20. Schwamborn T, Imhoff AB. Diagnostik und klassifikation der rotatorenmanschettenlasionen. In: Imhoff AB, Konig U, eds. Schulterinstabilitat-Rotatorenmanschette. Darmstadt: Steinkopff Verlag, 1999:193–195.

Chapter 12 Repair and Reconstruction of Acromioclavicular Injuries

Amir Mostofi, Augustus D. Mazzocca, and Robert A. Arciero

DEFINITION

- About 9% of shoulder girdle injuries involve damage to the acromioclavicular (AC) joint.
- This is a sequential injury beginning with the AC ligaments, progressing to the coracoclavicular ligaments, and finally involving the deltoid and trapezial muscles and fascia.
- Patients usually report direct trauma to the lateral shoulder or a fall on an outstretched arm driving the humeral head into the AC joint, resulting in a dislocation with pain at the AC joint, in particular with cross-arm adduction.
- Dislocations are classified by severity of injury, radiographic findings, and position of the clavicle[12] (Table 1).

ANATOMY

- The AC joint is a diarthrodial joint that primarily rotates as well as translates in the anteroposterior as well the superoinferior plane.
- The scapula (acromion) can protract and retract, using the AC joint as a pivot point.
- Normal scapular motion consists of substantial rotations around three axes and plays a major role in the motion at the AC joint.
- The articular surface is made up of hyaline cartilage containing an intra-articular meniscus type of structure, all surrounded by a joint capsule with a synovial lining.
- The AC joint static stabilizers include the acromioclavicular ligaments (superior, inferior, anterior, and posterior), the coracoclavicular ligaments (trapezoid and conoid), and the coracoacromial (CA) ligament.
- The AC joint dynamic stabilizers consist of the deltoid and trapezius muscles.
- Appreciating the location of the coracoclavicular ligament attachment on the clavicle is important. The trapezoid attaches on the undersurface of the clavicle at an anterolateral position. The conoid is a broad stout ligament located in a posterior and medial position. Both the trapezoid and conoid are posterior to the pectoralis minor attachment on the coracoid (**FIG 1**).
- The AC joint capsule and the capsular ligaments are the primary restraints of the distal clavicle to anterior-to-posterior translation. More specifically, the superior and posterior AC capsular ligaments prevent posterior displacement of the clavicle and abutment against the scapular spine.[5]
- The trapezoid and conoid span the coracoclavicular space (1.1 to 1.3 cm) and contribute to vertical stability, preventing superior and inferior translation of the clavicle.
- The AC and coracoclavicular ligaments all contribute to the prevention of motion in all planes. The conoid ligament has the highest in situ forces with superior loads, regardless of the integrity of the AC ligaments. The AC ligaments are the main restraints to posterior and anterior translation. However, when the AC ligaments are transected, the conoid is the primary restraint to anterior loads and the trapezoid is the primary restraint to posterior loads.[3]
- The AC joint is innervated by the lateral pectoral nerve and the suprascapular nerve.

PATHOGENESIS

- The mechanism of most AC joint injuries is a direct blow to the lateral acromion with the arm adducted.
- Indirect injury occurs by falling on an adducted outstretched hand or elbow, causing the humeral head to translocate superiorly and drive the humeral head into the acromion.

NATURAL HISTORY

- Most patients with type I or II AC joint separations typically have full recovery with no long-term sequelae. However, some patients continue to be symptomatic. In one study, up to 27% of patients with type I and II injuries had persistent pain and required a surgical procedure. Some patients treated nonoperatively continued to have instability and pain with provocative tests (level IV evidence).[7]
- Most patients with type III separations do well with conservative treatment. In a survey of Major League Baseball team physicians, 80% of athletes treated nonoperatively had complete pain relief and normal function (level IV evidence).[6] Studies have failed to show a statistical difference in the return to activity (level IV evidence).[8]
- Type IV, V, and VI AC joint separations do poorly without operative intervention (level V evidence).[2] Persistent pain is attributed to a chronically dislocated AC joint with severe soft tissue disruption.

PATIENT HISTORY AND PHYSICAL FINDINGS

- The mechanism of injury is an important history finding that clues one into a possible AC joint injury.
- Pain at the AC joint is difficult to differentiate from glenohumeral pathology because of the dual innervation of the AC joint by the lateral pectoral nerve and suprascapular nerve.
  - Because of the innervation by the lateral pectoral nerve, some patients may present with anteromedial pain, further complicating the picture.
- Pain in the trapezius region and anterolateral deltoid is more specific for AC joint injury, whereas pain located only in the lateral deltoid is more indicative of a subacromial process.
- Pathology of the AC joint is identified by a triad of point tenderness, positive pain at the AC joint with cross-arm adduction, and relief of symptoms by injection of a local anesthetic.
- Methods for examining the AC joint include the following:
  - AC joint compression (shear) test: Isolated painful movement at the AC joint in conjunction with a history of direct trauma indicates AC joint pathology.
  - Cross-arm adduction test: Look for pain specifically at the AC joint. Pain at posterior aspect of shoulder or lateral shoulder might indicate other pathology.

Table 1 Classification of Acromioclavicular (AC) Joint Injuries

Type	Description	Illustration	Examination Findings	Radiographic Findings
I	Sprain of the AC joint with all ligaments intact Mechanism of injury consistent with AC joint injury No evidence of instability		Point tenderness at the AC joint and positive provocative tests	Radiographs are normal.
II	Rupture of AC ligaments Sprain of coracoclavicular (CC) ligaments		Mild subluxation of the AC joint can be observed with stress examination.	Radiographs of the lateral end of the clavicle may be slightly elevated, but stress views fail to show a 100% separation of the clavicle and acromion.
III	Complete disruption of both the AC and CC ligaments without significant disruption of the deltoid or trapezial fascia. The clavicle is unstable in both the horizontal and vertical planes.		The upper extremity is usually held in an adducted position with the acromion depressed while the clavicle appears high-riding, but in reality the acromion and the rest of the upper extremity is displaced inferior to the horizontal plane of the lateral clavicle.	Radiographs show up to 100% increase in the CC interspace.
IV	Complete disruption of both the AC and CC ligaments		The distal clavicle is posteriorly displaced into the trapezius muscle and may tent the posterior skin. Evaluation of the sternoclavicular (SC) joint is necessary to rule out anterior SC joint dislocation.	Posteriorly displaced clavicle can be seen on axillary view, which is always obtained in the standard radiographic evaluation of the AC joint.
V	AC and CC ligaments are disrupted		Severe droop secondary to anteroinferior translation of the scapula around the thorax, due to the weight of the arm and the geometry of the chest wall. This is considered the third translation of the scapula with loss of the clavicular strut. Reduction of the distal clavicle with shoulder shrug differentiates type III from type V (distal clavicle buttonhole through soft tissue sleeve).	Trapezial and deltoid fascia disrupted. Two to three times increase in the CC distance or a 100% to 300% increase in the clavicle-to-acromion radiographic distance.
VI	Inferior dislocation of distal clavicle. Reduction may be blocked from interposition of the intact posterosuperior AC ligaments within the AC interval. Mechanism is thought to be severe hyperabduction and external rotation of the arm combined with retraction of the scapula.		The distal clavicle is found in two orientations, either subacromial or subcoracoid, behind the intact conjoined tendon.	

- Paxinos test[16] is sometimes done in conjunction with bone scan to assess damage to AC joint.
- O'Brien test: Symptoms at the top of the joint must be confirmed by examiner palpating the AC joint. Anterior glenohumeral joint pain suggests labral or biceps pathology.
- Local point tenderness at the AC joint while keeping the glenohumeral joint still is suspicious for localized AC joint pathology.

IMAGING AND OTHER DIAGNOSTIC STUDIES

- Standard radiographs include AP, supraspinatus outlet view (**FIG 2A**), and axillary and Zanca views.
- A Zanca view is made by tilting the x-ray beam 10 to 15 degrees toward the cephalic direction (**FIG 2B,C**).
  - The AC joint is more superficial and surrounded by less soft tissue than the glenohumeral joint.

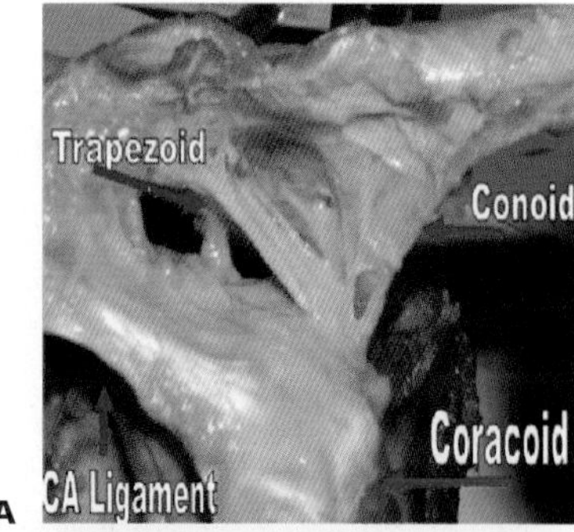

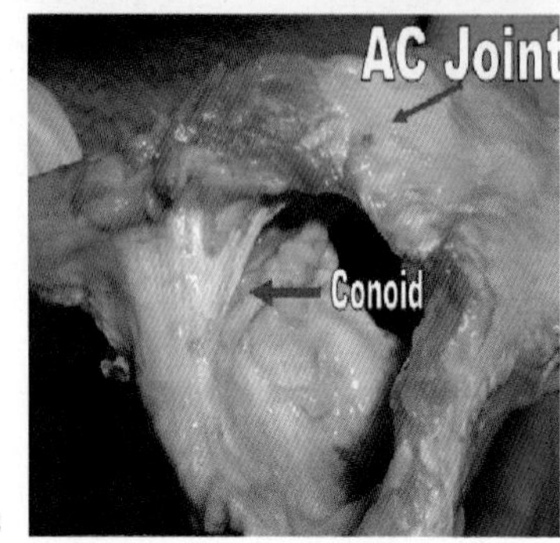

FIG 1 • **A.** Anterior view. The trapezoid is anterolateral, whereas the conoid is a posteromedial structure. **B.** Posterior view. The conoid can be seen as a broad ligament that fans out, attaching to the clavicle in a posteromedial position.

- The AC joint may be better visualized if a reduced penetration strength is used compared to standard radiographs of the glenohumeral joint.
- An axial view of the shoulder is important in differentiating a type III from a type IV AC joint injury.
  - Coracoid base fractures can also be identified on this view.
- A normal coracoclavicular interspace, in conjunction with a complete dislocation of the AC joint, may indicate a coracoid fracture, in which case a Stryker notch view is helpful (**FIG 2D**).
- The AC joint width is normally 1 to 3 mm and decreases with age. The width seen on radiographs is influenced by the individual variability of obliquity of the joint in relation to the x-ray beam.
- An increase in the coracoclavicular distance (usually 1.3 cm) of 25% to 50% over the normal side indicates complete coracoclavicular ligament disruption.
- Although seldom necessary and mainly a historical practice, stress views (5 to 10 pounds placed in the ipsilateral hand) with increased coracoclavicular interspace on the AP view may help differentiate between type II and type III injuries.
- Bone scan may help confirm subtle AC joint pathology and arthrosis.

DIFFERENTIAL DIAGNOSIS

- Cervical spine pathology
- Trapezial spasm
- Scapular dyskinesia
- Hyperlaxity
- Distal clavicle or acromion fracture
- Coracoid fracture

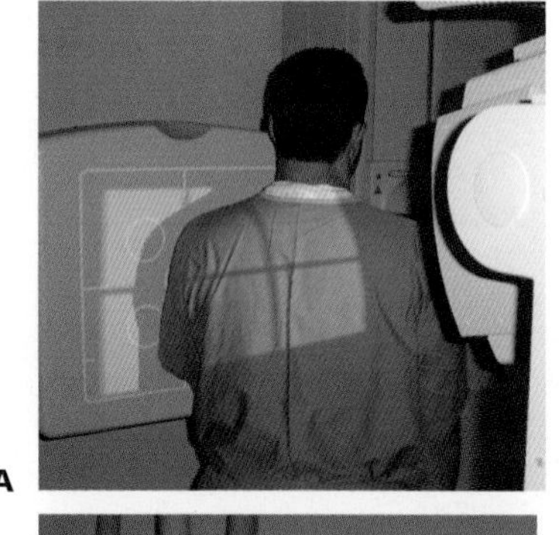

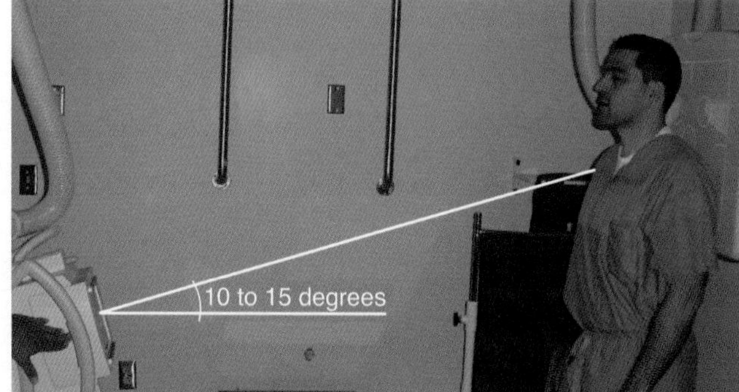

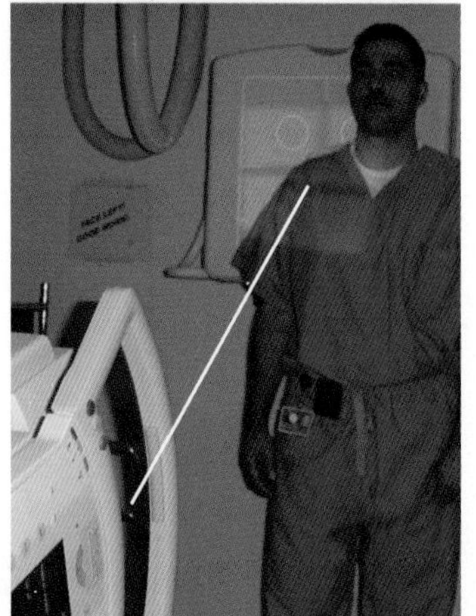

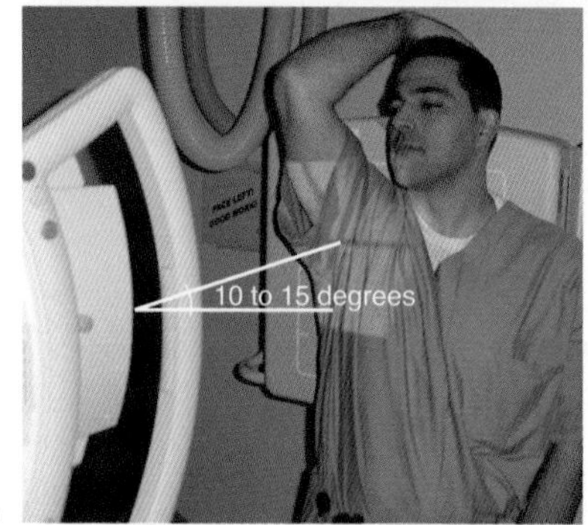

FIG 2 • Positioning for radiographic studies. **A.** Supraspinatus outlet view. **B,C.** Zanca view. For optimal visualization of the acromioclavicular joint, the x-ray source is directed 10 degrees cephalad with reduced penetration strength compared to a standard radiograph. **D.** Stryker notch view. This view helps rule out concomitant injuries. It is helpful when a coracoid fracture is suspected with a normal coracoclavicular interspace.

- Glenohumeral pathology (impingement, rotator cuff, Hill-Sachs, Bankart, superior labral anterior posterior [SLAP] lesion, biceps)
- Ulnar paresthesias
- Thoracic outlet syndrome

NONOPERATIVE MANAGEMENT

- The main goals of treatment, whether surgical or nonsurgical, are to achieve a pain-free shoulder with full range of motion and strength and no limitations in activities.
- Most type I and type II AC joint separations are treated in a nonoperative fashion.
- Treatment begins with a sling, ice, and a brief period of immobilization only for pain control. Rehabilitation is started as soon as tolerated.
- The rehabilitation program consists of four phases:[4]
  - Pain control, immediate protective range of motion and isometric exercises
  - Strengthening exercises using isotonic contractions
  - Unrestricted functional participation with the goal of increasing strength, power, endurance, and neuromuscular control
  - Return to activity with sports-specific functional drills
- Surgical intervention should be considered after rehabilitation if pain persists for greater than 3 months.
- Type III injuries:
  - These patients are usually evaluated on a case-by-case basis, taking into account hand dominance, occupation, heavy labor, position and sport requirements (quarterbacks, pitchers), scapulothoracic dysfunction, and risk for re-injury.
  - In a meta-analysis of 1172 patients, 88% of those treated with surgery and 87% of those treated without surgery had satisfactory outcomes (level IV evidence).[8]
    - In patients with type III injuries treated nonoperatively versus operatively, there was no difference in strength at 2 years of follow-up (level IV evidence).[14]
  - Schlegel and Burks[13] found that only 20% of patients reported a suboptimal outcome with conservative care. Objective studies showed that patients had no limitation of shoulder motion in the injured extremity and no difference compared with the unaffected extremity in rotational shoulder muscle strength. A finding that may affect heavy laborers was a decrease of 17% in bench press strength at the 1-year follow-up (level IV evidence).
  - If symptoms persist for greater than 3 months, including increased pain, impingement due to scapular dyskinesia, decreased strength, inability to get the arm into a cocking position in throwing, and painful instability, especially posterior instability with the clavicle abutting the anterior portion of the spine of the scapula, then operative intervention may be indicated.

SURGICAL MANAGEMENT

- Again, the main goals of treatment, whether surgical or nonsurgical, are to achieve a pain-free shoulder with full range of motion and strength and no limitations in activities.
- Complete AC joint injuries (type IV, V, and VI) are usually treated operatively because of the significant morbidity associated with persistently dislocated joints and severe soft tissue disruption.
- Most surgeons will treat type III injuries conservatively for 12 weeks and consider surgical stabilization if persistent pain and instability exist. In an attempt to return an athlete or high-demand patient to work more rapidly, some will stabilize a type III separation, hoping to decrease painful instability.
- Some patients treated nonoperatively will have persistent pain and an inability to return to their sport or job and will require surgical stabilization.
- Operative choices:
  - AC ligament repair
  - Dynamic muscle transfer
  - CA ligament transfer
  - Coracoclavicular ligament repair
  - Distal clavicle resection with coracoclavicular reconstruction
  - Distal clavicle resection without coracoclavicular reconstruction
  - Anatomic reconstruction of the coracoclavicular ligament
  - Arthroscopic variations of the above
- In the treatment of chronic AC joint pain with distal clavicle resection, arthroscopy of the glenohumeral joint can be undertaken to rule out concomitant injuries. Missed SLAP lesions and labral pathology have been reported as a cause of failed distal clavicle resection.[1]
- The modified CA ligament transfer (Weaver-Dunn) is the gold standard of treatment for the reconstruction of the AC joint and is presented here.
- Anatomic reconstruction of the coracoclavicular ligaments (ACCR) attempts to recreate the normal anatomy and biomechanics of the AC joint. This technique has been studied in our biomechanics laboratory and is in clinical trials. The ACCR is our procedure of choice and is also presented here.
- Various arthroscopic techniques have been described for fixation of AC separations.
  - A description of an arthroscopic procedure using a high-strength suture and endobutton device is provided.
  - Although our preferred treatment of acute type III injuries is conservative, this technique may be helpful for surgeons who decide to stabilize and splint acute type III injuries in high-demand patients.

Preoperative Planning

- A successful outcome depends on reasonable patient expectations and compliance with the postoperative regimen, including postoperative sling immobilization for 6 weeks.
- All radiographs are reviewed.
- Reports indicate that concomitant injuries such as SLAP lesions and labral tears are a cause of failure after distal clavicle resection.[1]
- Magnetic resonance imaging (MRI) may be obtained to rule out concomitant injuries that also need to be addressed.
- If using a modified Weaver-Dunn or ACCR, the surgeon should discuss with the patient the options for autograft or allograft.

Positioning

- The patient is placed in the beach-chair position after induction of general anesthesia (**FIG 3**).
- A specialized shoulder table is not used. We prefer a standard table that provides posterior support and stabilization of the scapula.
- A small bump is placed on the medial scapular edge to stabilize it and elevate the coracoid anteriorly.

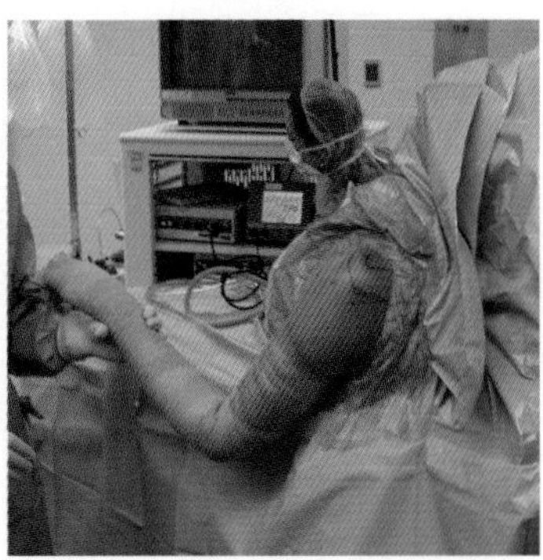

FIG 3 • The beach-chair position is used, with a small bump placed on the medial scapular edge to bring the coracoid anteriorly and to secure the scapula. The head should be mobile to allow repositioning if needed during clavicle reaming. The arm is free draped from the sternoclavicular joint laterally.

- The head is mobile because repositioning is sometimes necessary during medial clavicle drilling.
- Wide draping is done to expose the sternoclavicular joint and posterior clavicle for complete visualization of the shoulder girdle.
- The arm is free draped to allow free motion and reduction.

Approach

- The mean length from the end of the clavicle, or the AC joint, to the coracoclavicular ligaments is 46.3 ± 5 mm; the distance between the trapezoid laterally and the conoid medially is 21.4 ± 4.2 mm.[11]
- In both the Weaver-Dunn and ACCR procedures, the incision is made to allow exposure of the AC joint and coracoid.
- The incision for the Weaver-Dunn is more lateral compared to the ACCR because of the exposure necessary for CA ligament acquisition and because the ACCR clavicle preparation is performed slightly more medially.
  - Again, full exposure of the AC joint and coracoid is necessary in both procedures, and the incision can be extended or curved to allow the necessary exposure.
- Although the AC joint and clavicle are superficial structures with little subcutaneous tissue, in our experience large skin flaps can be used to improve visualization without compromising the vascularity of the skin.
- Full-thickness flaps of the deltotrapezial fascia during the approach are critical for closure. Tagging sutures can be placed during the approach to allow for quick and effective soft tissue coverage over the repair.
- Gelpi retractors are low profile and help retract the deltotrapezial flaps.

TECHNIQUES

ANATOMIC CORACOCLAVICULAR LIGAMENT RECONSTRUCTION

Exposure

- Arthroscopy of the glenohumeral joint can be performed to look for concomitant injuries.
- An incision is made 3.5 cm from the AC joint starting at the posterior clavicle in a curvilinear fashion toward the coracoid along the lines of Langer.
  - The incision is sometimes angled because the key is to have full visualization of the AC joint laterally and the coracoid process medially (**TECH FIG 1**).
- Superficial skin bleeders are controlled down to the fascia of the deltoid with a needle-tip Bovie.
- Full-thickness flaps are made from the midline of the clavicle both posteriorly and anteriorly, skeletonizing the clavicle.
- Tagging sutures are placed in the deltotrapezial fascia.
  - Traction on the tagging sutures or a Gelpi retractor under the flaps is used for visualization.
  - The tagging sutures are used for easy and precise closure of the fascia at the end of the procedure.
- Once the approach is complete, a trial reduction is attempted.
  - The distal end of the clavicle may need to be freed from the trapezius muscle, under the acromion, or coracoid.
  - Interposition of soft tissue may prevent anatomic reduction of the AC joint.

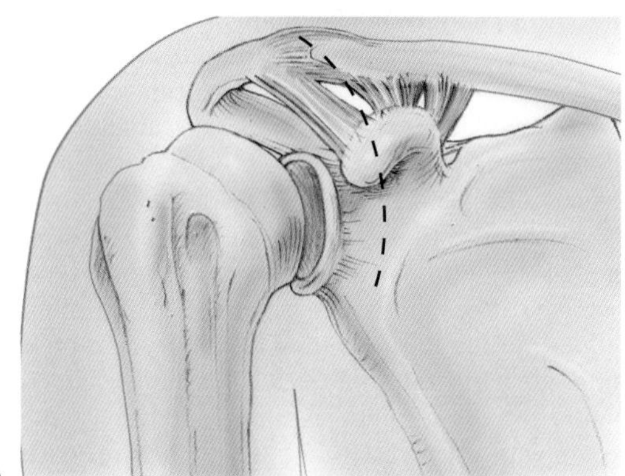

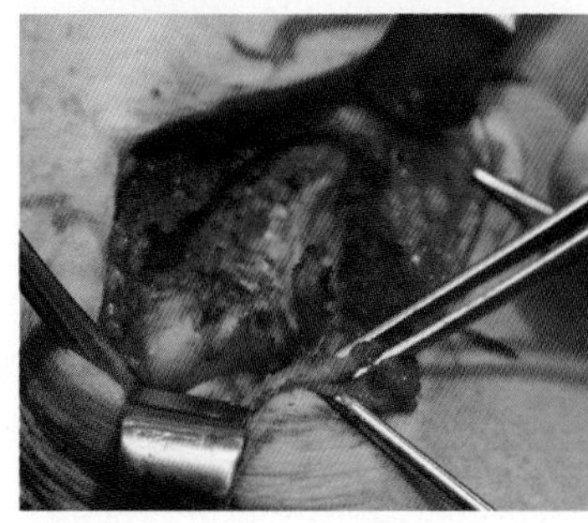

TECH FIG 1 • A curvilinear incision is made 3.5 cm medial to the acromioclavicular joint along the lines of Langer. Visualization of the acromioclavicular joint as well as the coracoid is possible. The deltotrapezial fascia is split along the midline of the clavicle and elevated as two full-thickness flaps.

Graft Preparation

- A semitendinosus allograft or autograft or an anterior tibialis allograft can be used for this procedure (**TECH FIG 2A**). (See the Techniques section of Chap. SM-32 for a description of obtaining a semitendinosus autograft.)

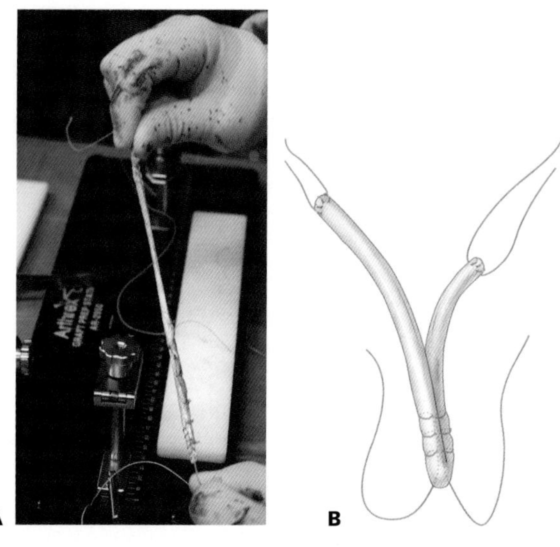

TECH FIG 2 • **A.** Grafts need tendon-grasping sutures at both ends for ease of passage around the coracoid and through bone tunnels. **B.** In our alternative method, grafts that are to be fixed to the coracoid are folded so that there is one short limb and one long limb. A no. 2 nonabsorbable suture is placed through the doubled-over tendon graft in a Krakow manner. Tendon ends are bulleted for ease of passage through bone tunnels.

- Tendon ends are bulleted for easy passage through bone tunnels.
- A whipstitch or grasping suture is placed in the two free ends of the tendon for graft passage through bone tunnels.
- The graft is ready for use if the surgeon is performing our preferred looping method. However, an alternative method is interference screw fixation to the coracoid process.
  - In this option, the graft is folded with one short limb (about 3 inches) and a limb containing the remaining length of the tendon. A no. 2 ultra-high-strength nonabsorbable suture is placed through the doubled-over tendon graft in a Krakow manner (TECH FIG 2B).

Coracoid Preparation

- Standard looping technique
  - A graft can be looped around the base of the coracoid process using an aortic cross-clamp (Stanitsky clamp) or a suture-passing device (Arthrex, Inc., Naples, FL) for biologic fixation.
  - A heavy no. 2 ultra-strength nonabsorbable suture is also placed around the coracoid for use as a nonbiologic form fixation (TECH FIG 3A,B).
- Alternative technique: interference screw fixation to coracoid (TECH FIG 3C)

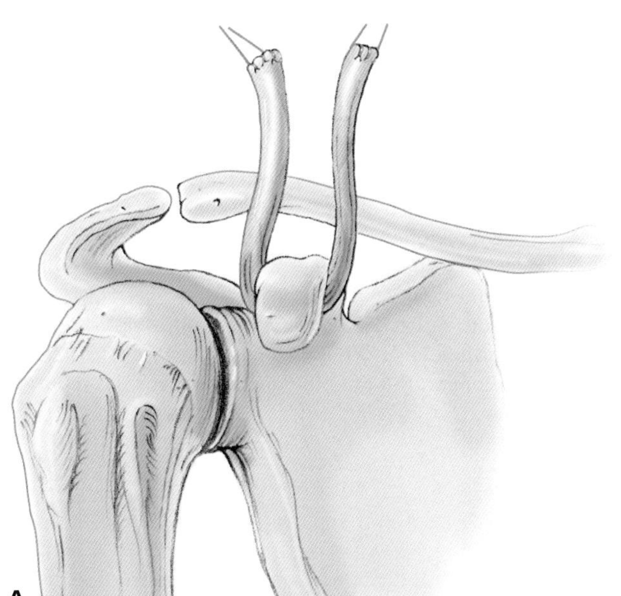

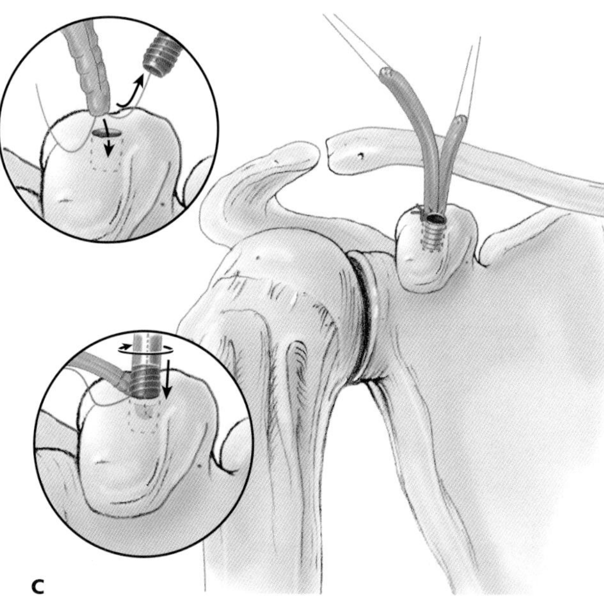

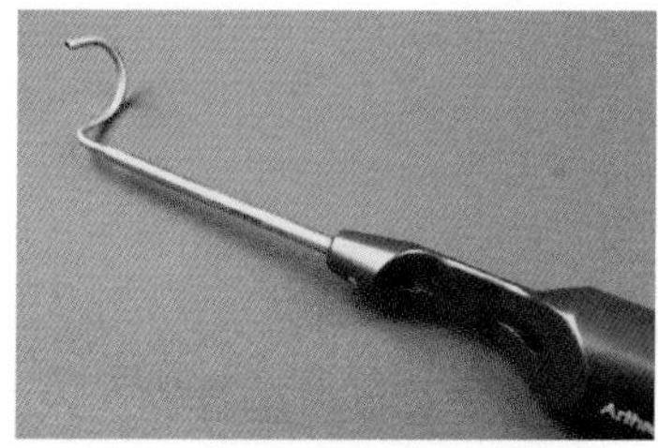

TECH FIG 3 • **A.** The graft is looped around the coracoid. **B.** A suture passer can be used to safely loop the graft and a nonabsorbable suture around the coracoid base. **C.** In the alternative technique, a bone tunnel that approximates the diameter of the graft (usually 6 to 7 mm) is made in the coracoid. One limb of the Krakow suture is placed, and the doubled-over tendon is passed through the PEEK screw and driver (*top inset*). While traction is held with this suture, the tenodesis driver is advanced to touch the tendon graft (*bottom inset*), and the entire tendon, driver, and screw complex is placed into the coracoid bone tunnel.

- Although we currently do not use this method, some may choose to anchor the tendon into the base of the coracoid.
- The diameter of the doubled-over portion of the graft is measured with a standard tendon-measuring device. Using this number, the appropriate cannulated reamer is chosen (6 or 7 mm).
    - The surgeon should use a smaller reamer diameter first and ream up in size if necessary.
- Finger palpation of both lateral and medial portions of the coracoid process and drilling into the coracoid base under direct visualization with a cannulated reamer guide pin are completed.
- One limb of the Krakow suture is passed through a 5.5 × 8-mm nonabsorbable radiolucent tenodesis screw and driver using a Nitinol wire.
- The tenodesis driver is advanced to touch the tendon graft, and the entire tendon, driver, and screw complex is placed into the coracoid bone tunnel until 15 mm of the Krakow suture disappears.
- The sutures from the graft are tied together over the existing interference screw, giving both interference screw and suture anchor advantages.

Clavicle Preparation

- To recreate the conoid ligament, a cannulated guide pin is placed 45 mm away from the distal end of the clavicle and as posterior as possible, taking into consideration the space needed to not "blow out" the posterior cortical rim during reaming.
- A 6-mm cannulated reamer is used to create the tunnel (**TECH FIG 4**).
    - If there is a question of what size reamer to use, starting with the smallest reamer necessary is always a good technique; if necessary the surgeon can ream up.
    - The surgeon reams in under power.
    - The surgeon disconnects the power driver and pulls the reamer out manually to ensure that the tunnel is a perfect circle and not widened by uneven reaming.
- The same procedure is repeated for the trapezoid ligament, which is a more anterior structure than the conoid.
    - This tunnel is centered on the clavicle, approximately 15 mm lateral of the center portion of the previous tunnel.

Graft Fixation and Reconstruction

- The limbs of the graft are crossed over the coracoid and one limb of the biologic graft is placed through the posterior bone tunnel, recreating the conoid ligament.
- The other limb is passed through the anterior bone tunnel in the same fashion, recreating the trapezoid ligament (**TECH FIG 5**).
- The no. 2 ultra-high-strength nonabsorbable suture placed around the coracoid is also passed through the tunnels for nonbiologic augmentation of the repair.
- Upper displacement of the scapulohumeral complex and the use of a large point-of-reduction forceps placed on the coracoid process and the clavicle by the assistant are used to reduce the AC joint.
- Fluoroscopy is used to confirm proper placement of the grafts and reduction of the AC joint.
- The graft is pulled on cyclically multiple times and passed through the tunnels back and forth to reduce any displacement that might occur after fixation.
    - This step is critical to ensure that there is no migration or movement after the fixation is complete.
    - Nevertheless, we often overreduce the AC joint by 2 to 3 mm with the knowledge that a few millimeters of displacement still occurs.
- The graft is positioned so that the graft tail representing the conoid ligament is left 2 cm proud from the superior margin of the clavicle. The long tail of the graft exits the trapezoid tunnel and will later be used to augment the AC joint repair if indicated (see Tech Fig 5).
- With traction placed on the graft, ensuring its tautness, a 5.5 × 8-mm nonabsorbable radiolucent screw is placed in the posteromedial tunnel anterior to the conoid ligament graft.
- Again, the graft is cyclically loaded multiple times. While holding reduction and tension on the ligament, another 5.5 × 8-mm nonabsorbable radiolucent screw is placed in the lateral trapezoid tunnel anterior to the trapezoid ligament graft.
- With both grafts secured, the no. 2 ultra-high-strength nonabsorbable suture is tied over the top of the clavicle, becoming the nonbiologic fixation for the reduced AC joint.

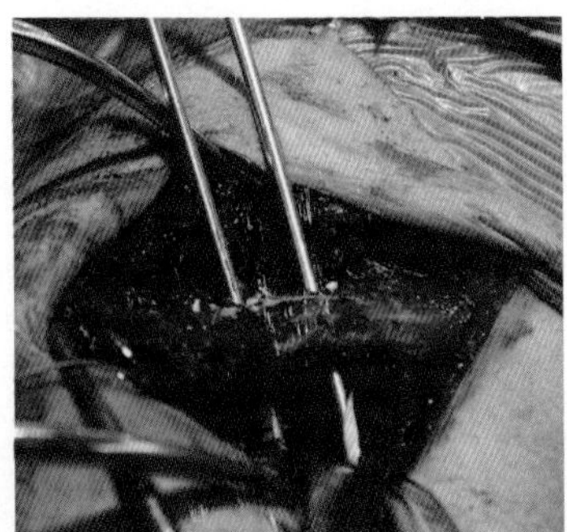

A

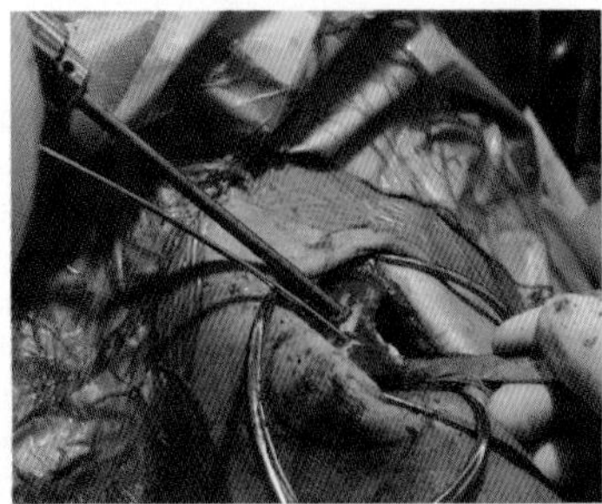

B

TECH FIG 4 • A. Anatomic reconstruction of the coracoclavicular ligaments. For conoid ligament reconstruction, a guide pin is placed in the clavicle 45 mm from the acromioclavicular joint in a posteromedial position. For trapezoid ligament reconstruction, a guide pin is placed 30 mm from the acromioclavicular joint centered on the clavicle. **B.** After confirming the positions of the pins, a 5.5-mm cannulated drill is used to drill the clavicle. Care should be taken to place the conoid tunnel as far posterior as possible without violating the posterior cortex during reaming.

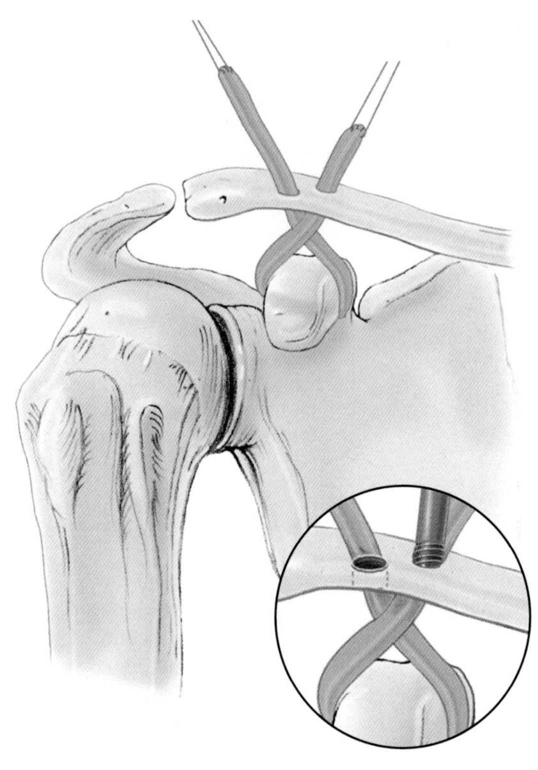

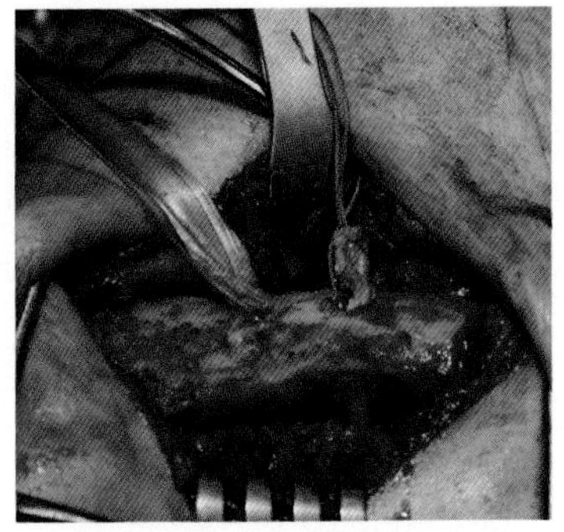

TECH FIG 5 • The free ends of the graft are crossed and passed through the clavicle. The graft is pulled back and forth through the tunnels and cyclic loading is placed on the graft. A short tail is left superior to the clavicle for the conoid ligament while the remainder of the graft exits the trapezoid tunnel, with one end left longer than the other. A 5.5 × 8-mm nonabsorbable radiolucent screw is used for interference fixation of the graft to the conoid tunnel in the clavicle. Cyclic tension is again placed on the graft. While holding reduction and the graft under tension, another 5.5 × 8-mm nonabsorbable radiolucent screw is placed in the anterolateral trapezoid tunnel.

DISTAL CLAVICLE EXCISION VERSUS ACROMIOCLAVICULAR JOINT REPAIR

- For acute injuries, we perform an AC joint repair.
  - The AC joint is exposed. Simple or figure 8 sutures using a no. 0 nonabsorbable suture are used to repair the AC joint capsule and ligaments primarily.
    - The posterior and superior ligaments are key in preventing posterior displacement of the clavicle.
  - The repair can be augmented by using the limbs of the graft used for the coracoclavicular ligament repair.
  - The short limb of the graft exiting the medial tunnel is folded laterally and sewn to the base of the graft exiting the trapezoid tunnel in series (TECH FIG 6A).
    - The long limb exiting the lateral (trapezoid) tunnel is taken laterally and looped on top of the AC joint and used for augmentation of the AC joint capsule repair (TECH FIG 6B,C).
- In chronic dislocations, two options exist.
  - One is to repair the AC joint as detailed above for acute AC joint injuries.
  - Alternatively, if arthrosis is a concern, a distal clavicle excision can be performed.
    - An oscillating osteotome is used to remove 1 cm of the distal clavicle.
    - The posterior cortical rim is beveled.
- The deltotrapezial fascia is meticulously closed using interrupted nonabsorbable sutures, taking care to leave the knots on the posterior aspect of the trapezius.
  - A simple suture can be used to bury the knot if it is prominent.
  - Making clear full-thickness flaps during the approach and using tagging sutures allows for secure coverage of the grafts and clavicle.

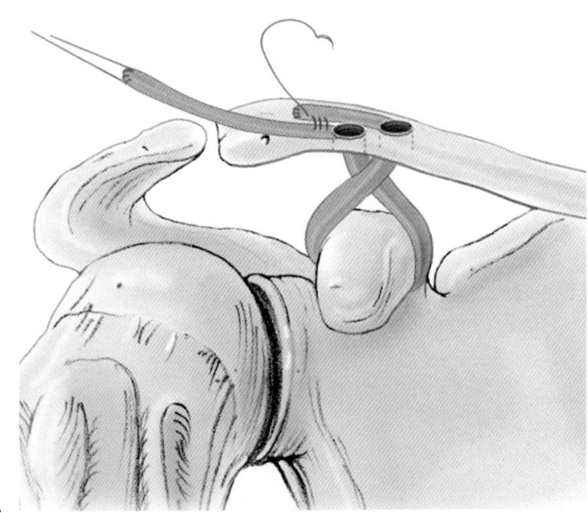

TECH FIG 6 • **A.** The short limb of the graft representing the conoid ligament is folded laterally and sewn to the graft base representing the trapezoid ligament. *(continued)*

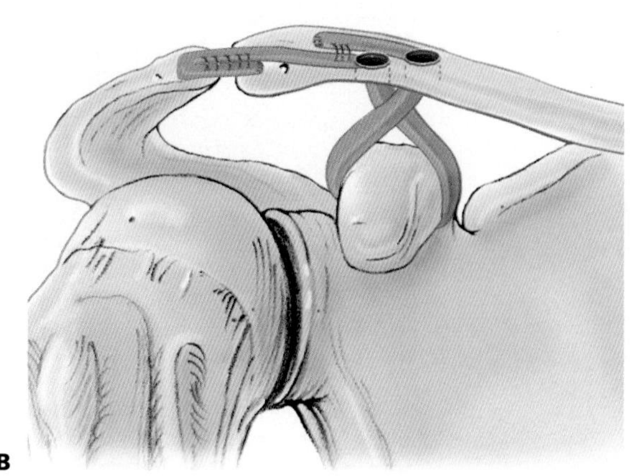

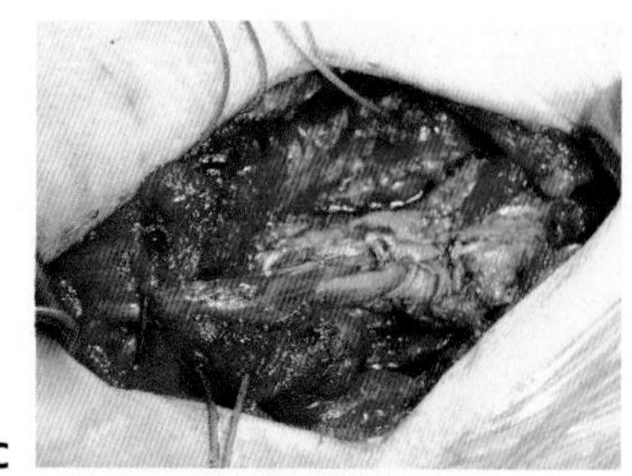

TECH FIG 6 • *(continued)* **B,C.** The long limb representing the trapezoid ligament can be taken laterally and used to augment the acromioclavicular ligament fixation.

MODIFIED WEAVER-DUNN PROCEDURE

- Diagnostic arthroscopy is done if concomitant injuries are suspected.[9]
- An incision is made 1.5 cm from the AC joint starting at the posterior clavicle in a curvilinear fashion toward the coracoid along the lines of Langer.
  - The incision is sometimes angled because the key is to have full visualization of the AC joint laterally and coracoid process medially.
- Superficial skin bleeders are controlled down to the fascia of the deltoid with a needle-tip Bovie.
- Full-thickness flaps are made from the midline of the clavicle both posteriorly and anteriorly, skeletonizing the clavicle (**TECH FIG 7**).
- Alternatively, a "hockey stick" incision can be made laterally from the acromion along the midportion of the clavicle, ending in a hockey stick fashion down toward the corocoid.
  - Periosteal flaps are elevated and a tagging suture can be placed at the medialmost aspect of the flap for accurate closure.

Biologic Fixation: Coracoacromial Ligament Transfer

- The CA ligament is dissected out, especially laterally.
- The CA ligament is detached from its footprint that extends posteriorly on the acromion (**TECH FIG 8A**).
- Two heavy nonabsorbable sutures are placed at the end of the ligament using a whipstitch.
- The CA ligament is held directly superiorly and the corresponding area is marked on the clavicle.
  - This marks the amount of clavicle that needs to be resected to allow easy passage of the CA ligament without sharp turns.
- If adequate arthroscopic resection has not already been performed, an oscillating saw is used to make an oblique cut on the clavicle, leaving more bone superiorly rather than inferiorly, at the level of the previously marked site.
- An intramedullary pocket is curetted inside the clavicle for the CA.
- The AC intra-articular disc is resected, leaving the AC ligaments undisturbed.
- A 2.0-mm drill is used to make two drill holes in a cruciate fashion (lateral clavicle anteriorly, medial clavicle posteriorly) 20 mm medial to the distal cut end of the clavicle (**TECH FIG 8B**).
- A wire-loop is used to pass each limb of the CA ligament suture through the end of the clavicle and out the drill hole made superiorly.
- For augmentation of CA ligament transfer, a 3.5-mm drill hole is made into the clavicle medial to the previously made drill holes for the CA ligament.

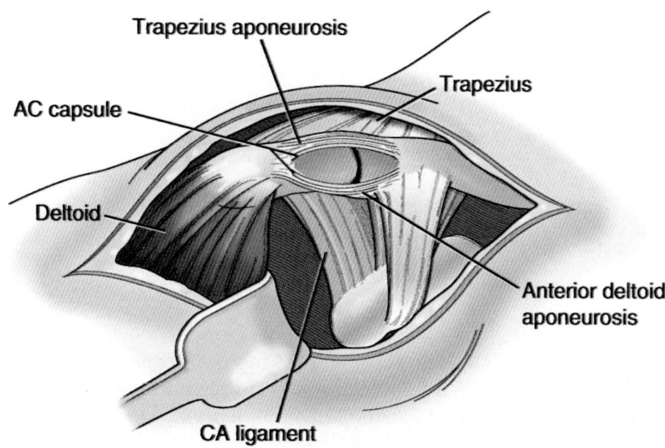

TECH FIG 7 • Transfer of the acromial attachment of the coracoacromial (CA) ligament, the modified Weaver-Dunn procedure. Full-thickness flaps are made from the midline of the clavicle both posteriorly and anteriorly, skeletonizing the clavicle. Periosteal flaps are elevated and a tagging suture can be placed at the medialmost aspect of the flap for accurate closure. A small portion of the anterior deltoid is reflected from the anterior acromion to expose the CA ligament. (Adapted from Galatz LM, Williams GR Jr. Acromioclavicular joint injuries. In: Bucholz RW, Heckman JD, Court-Brown C, eds. Rockwood and Green's Fractures in Adults, vol 2. Philadelphia: Lippincott Williams & Wilkins, 2006:1354.)

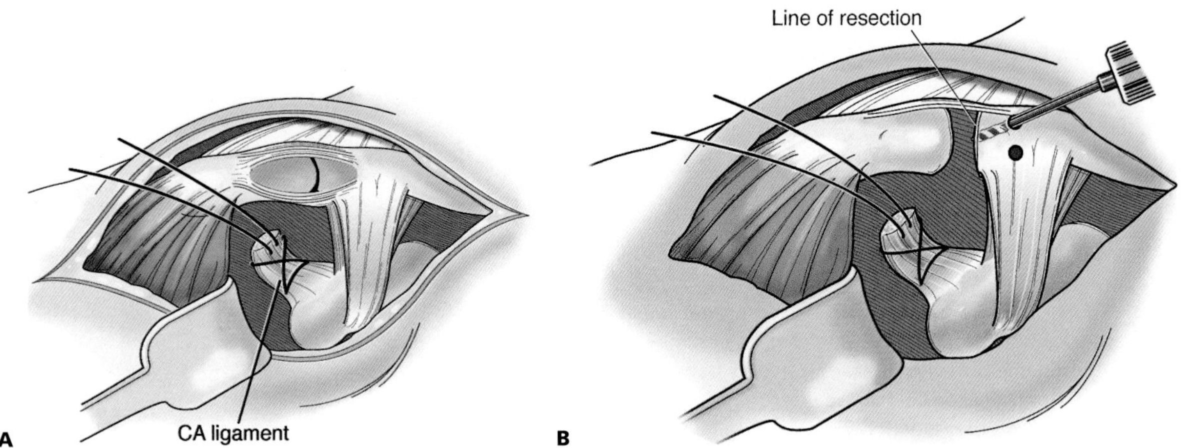

TECH FIG 8 • **A.** The ligament is released from the acromion and sutures are placed in the end. **B.** After a distal clavicle resection, two 2-mm unicortical drill holes are placed in the posterosuperior surface of the distal clavicle, exiting through the intramedullary canal. (Adapted from Galatz LM, Williams GR Jr. Acromioclavicular joint injuries. In: Bucholz RW, Heckman JD, Court-Brown C, eds. Rockwood and Green's Fractures in Adults, vol 2. Philadelphia: Lippincott Williams & Wilkins, 2006:1354.)

- For nonbiologic augmentation, a suture cord is constructed.
  - The surgeon takes three no. 1 absorbable sutures clamped at both ends. One clamp is turned clockwise while holding the other end until the sutures are intertwined together for the entire length of the sutures.
  - This is done with two other sets of three sutures.
  - The three sets are intertwined counterclockwise in the same fashion, resulting in a cord of nine total sutures. The suture cord is passed around the coracoid and through the 3.5-mm drill hole in the clavicle.
- For biologic augmentation an autograft or allograft can be used.

Reduction and Fixation

- Upper displacement of the scapulohumeral complex and the use of a large point-of-reduction forceps placed on the coracoid process and the clavicle by the assistant are used to reduce the AC joint.
  - Slight overreduction during fixation is recommended.
- After reduction is achieved, the surgeon pulls the suture limbs of the CA ligament reconstruction, exiting the bone tunnels, and ties them on the superior surface of the clavicle (TECH FIG 9).
  - The pocket for the CA ligament must be long enough so that after anatomic reduction, the graft is nice and taut.
- If the suture cord was used, the suture cord that was passed around the coracoid and through the clavicle is tied.
  - The surgeon should attempt to place the knot in the least prominent area.
  - The ends of the suture cord are unraveled and each individual suture limb is tied to prevent unraveling of the cable.
  - Finally, all free suture ends are cut.
- If ligament augmentation was used, the ligament is wrapped in a figure 8 fashion and sutured to itself using heavy nonabsorbable sutures.
- Closure is the same as the ACCR technique (see Tech Fig 6C).

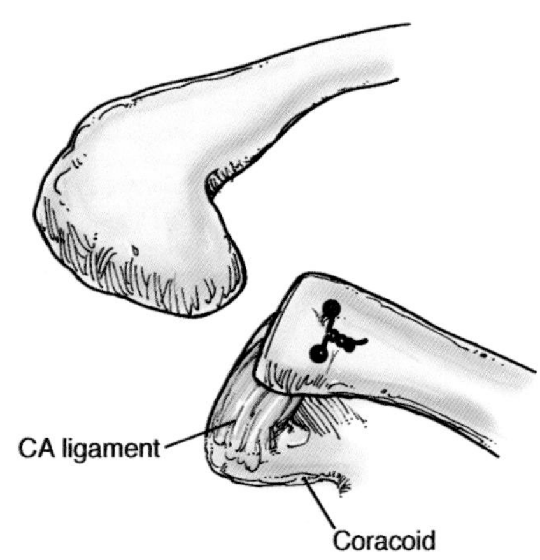

TECH FIG 9 • Using a curette, a pocket is made inside the clavicle for the coracoacromial (CA) ligament. The CA ligament is transferred to the intramedullary canal. The sutures are placed through the drill holes and tied over the top of the clavicle. This pocket has to be large enough so that after reduction of the joint, the CA ligament can be pulled inside without any impediment. If this is done correctly, the ligament should be taut and not overstuffed inside the pocket. (Adapted from Galatz LM, Williams GR Jr. Acromioclavicular joint injuries. In: Bucholz RW, Heckman JD, Court-Brown C, eds. Rockwood and Green's Fractures in Adults, vol 2. Philadelphia: Lippincott Williams & Wilkins, 2006:1354.)

ARTHROSCOPIC STABILIZATION

- The patient is placed in a beach-chair position. Draping is similar to the open procedures, with wide exposure and the arm draped free.

Establishing Portals

- A standard posterior portal is made, followed by two anterior portals (TECH FIG 10).
  - An anterosuperior portal is made using an outside-in technique, using a spinal needle to confirm positioning.
    - Débridement of the rotator interval is done until the tip of the coracoid is visualized.
    - Release of the superior glenohumeral ligament and partial release of the middle glenohumeral ligament may be required for adequate exposure.
    - A 7-mm partially threaded cannula is used for the anterosuperior portal.
  - An anteroinferior portal is made near the tip of the coracoid, again with the outside-in technique, using a spinal needle to confirm positioning and ensuring that the base of the coracoid can be reached using this portal. An 8.25-mm twist-in cannula is inserted for this portal.
- A 70-degree scope may improve visualization of the coracoid base.
- If the 30-degree arthroscope is used, the arthroscope position is changed to the anterosuperior portal.
  - The coracoid base is exposed using mechanical shavers and radiofrequency devices.
  - Any bursa or periosteum is stripped to obtain a full view of the coracoid base.

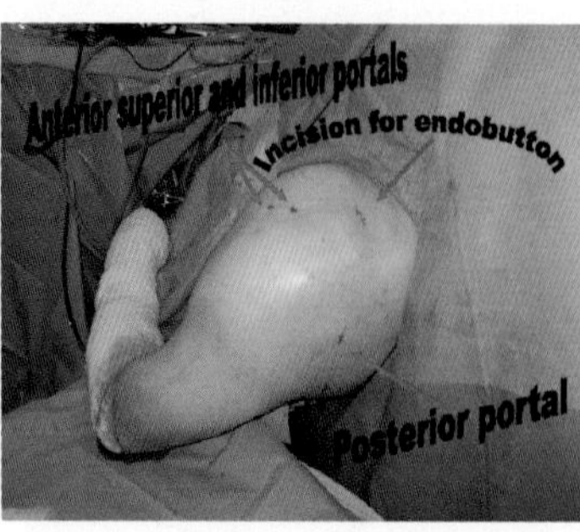

TECH FIG 10 • Three portals are used for arthroscopic repair—the standard posterior portal, an anterosuperior portal, and an anteroinferior portal.

Drilling

- The assembled "Adapteur Drill Guide C-Ring with the Coracoid Drill Stop and Graduated Guide Pin Sleeve" (Arthrex, Inc., Naples, FL) is inserted through the anteroinferior portal (TECH FIG 11A).
- With the drill stop placed at the base of the coracoid (as close to the scapula as possible), the corresponding area is marked on the superior aspect of the clavicle for the guide pin sleeve.
  - This area should be centered on the clavicle and approximately 25 mm from the AC joint.
- A 1.5-cm incision is made over the clavicle in the lines of Langer, and the surgeon dissects down through the deltopectoral fascia.

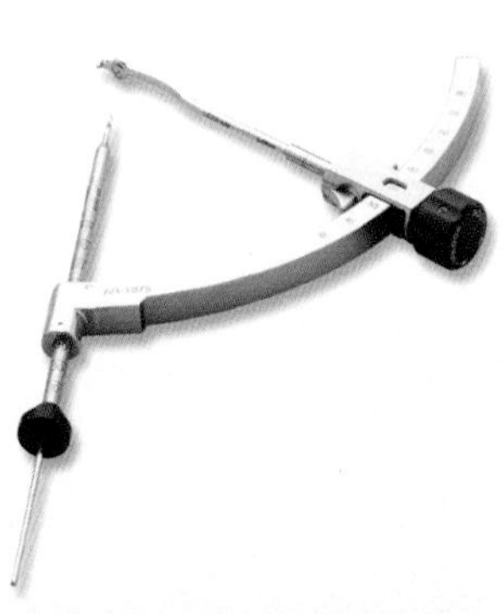
A

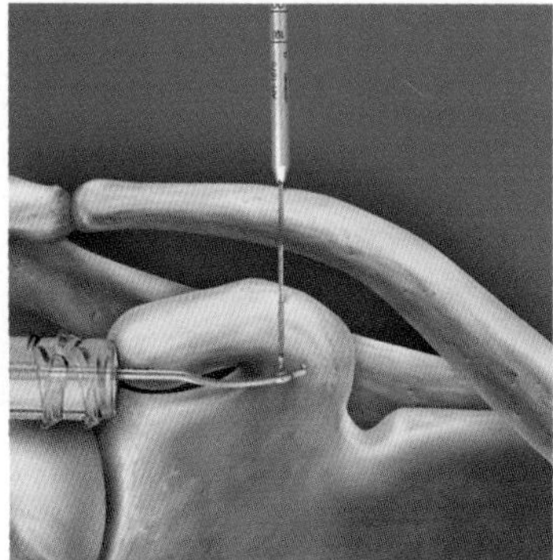
B

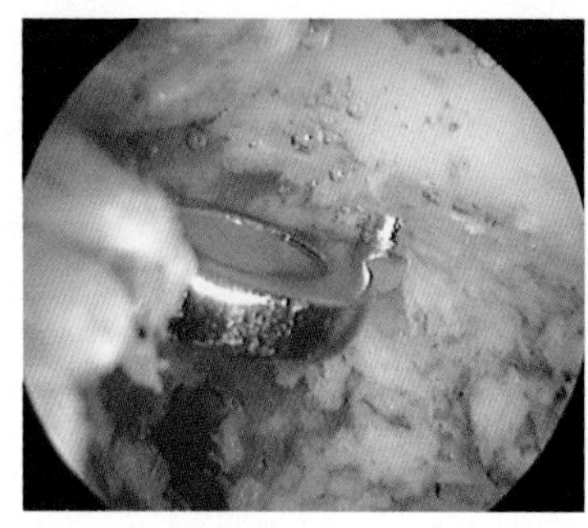
C

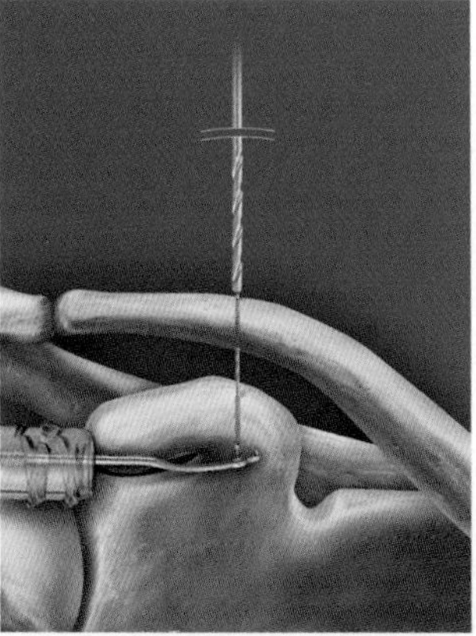
D

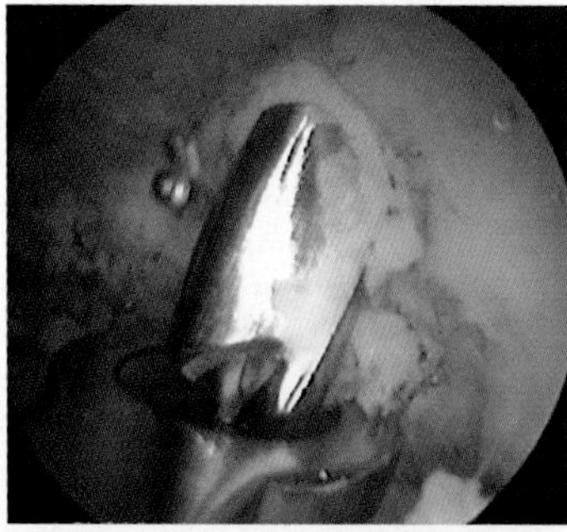
E

TECH FIG 11 • **A.** Adapteur Drill Guide C-Ring (Arthrex Inc., Naples, FL). **B,C.** Using the Adapteur Drill Guide C-Ring with the Coracoid Drill Stop under direct visualization, a guide pin is placed through the clavicle and coracoid, engaging the drill stop. The pin should be centered on the clavicle and the coracoid and should exit the coracoid base as close to the scapula as possible. **D,E.** Once positioning has been confirmed, a 4.0-mm drill is used to drill the clavicle and coracoid. The surgeon should take care to stop at the drill stop and not advance past the coracoid base. (A,B,D: Courtesy of Arthrex, Inc.)

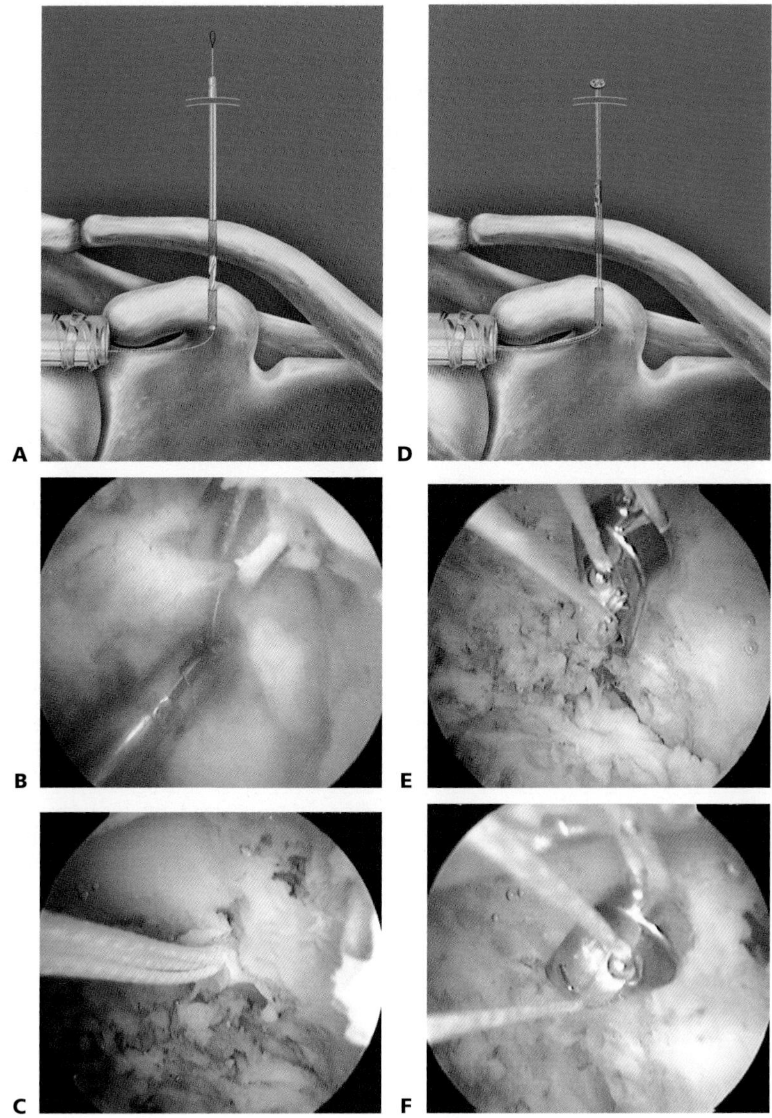

TECH FIG 12 • **A.** The power drill is detached and the cannulated drill is used as a portal to pass an 18-inch Nitinol suture passing wire. **B.** A grasper is used to hold the Nitinol suture while the drill bit is removed. The limb of the Nitinol passing wire is brought out of the anteroinferior portal, leaving the loop superior to the clavicle. **C.** The Nitinol suture passing wire is used to deliver the white traction sutures through the clavicle and coracoid and out of the anteroinferior portal. **D,E.** While holding the blue TightRope suture tails, pulling on one of the white suture tails flips the oblong button to a vertical position, allowing passage of the TightRope through the clavicle and coracoid. **F.** Once past, independent pulling on the white sutures flips the oblong button back to a horizontal position, anchoring it underneath the coracoid. (A,D: Courtesy of Arthrex, Inc.)

- Under direct visualization using the arthroscope, the surgeon places a 2.4-mm guide pin through the drill tip guide, clavicle, and coracoid until the drill stop is engaged (TECH FIG 11B,C).
  - It is important to place the guide pin centered in the base of the coracoid.
- A 4.0-mm cannulated drill is used to drill the clavicle and coracoid while the drill stop prevents migration of the guide pin. The surgeon should always use the arthroscope for direct visualization and avoid drilling beyond the coracoid base (TECH FIG 11D,E).

Suture Passage and Tying

- The power drill is detached, leaving the cannulated drill in place.
- An 18-inch Nitinol suture passing wire is passed down through the cannulated drill and the tip is grasped with the arthroscopic grasper (TECH FIG 12A,B).
  - The drill can now be removed.
- Using the Nitinol passing wire, the two white traction sutures of the oblong button of the TightRope System are

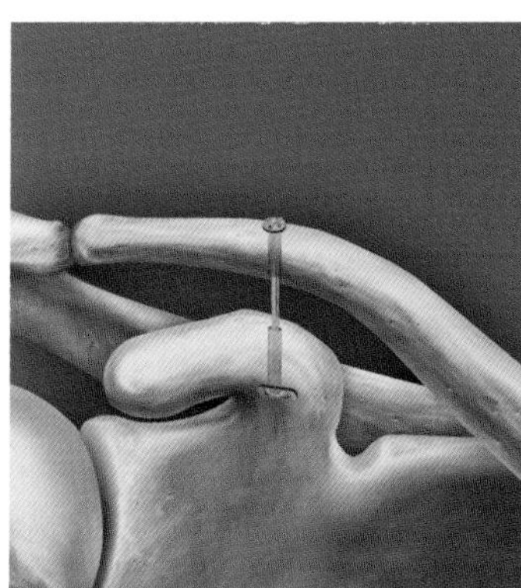

TECH FIG 13 • Placing the arthroscope into the subacromial space via the posterior portal helps to directly visualize the reduction. After reduction of the clavicle, sequential pulling on the blue TightRope suture tails delivers the round button down to the superior clavicle, holding the reduction firmly. The blue sutures are tied securely. (Courtesy of Arthrex, Inc.)

passed through the clavicle, the coracoid, and the anteroinferior portal (**TECH FIG 12C**).

- The blue TightRope suture tails of the round button are held firmly with one hand. The surgeon pulls on the white suture tails attached to the oblong button. This flips the oblong button to a vertical position and allows passage through the drill holes (**TECH FIG 12D,E**).
- The oblong button is pulled through the clavicle and coracoid.
  - Once passed, differential pulling on the white sutures flips the button to a horizontal position, preventing it from retracting through the drill holes (**TECH FIG 12F**).

Clavicle Reduction

- The surgeon pulls on the blue suture tails to advance the round button down to the clavicle. The sutures are tied over the top of the TightRope, making a surgeon's knot and two reverse half-hitches.
  - Leaving the tails long helps the knot to lie flat (**TECH FIG 13**).
- All wounds are irrigated and closed.

PEARLS AND PITFALLS

Positioning and approach	▪ The surgeon should make sure that the patient's head can be repositioned to the side, allowing room for conoid tunnel drilling. ▪ An alternative is to displace the clavicle anteriorly with a towel clip to allow access for conoid tunnel drilling. ▪ The deltoid and trapezial fascia are tagged for good repair.
Graft management	▪ Semitendinosus ends are bulleted to allow for easy graft passage. ▪ Sutures are passed under the coracoid either from medial to lateral or lateral to medial. ▪ If passing lateral to medial, the surgeon should make sure that the medial coracoid base is exposed and should insert a Darrach retractor on the medial base to "catch" the passing device. ▪ Once the graft is passed under the coracoid, the limbs are crossed before they are passed through the clavicle tunnels.
Tunnel preparation and graft fixation	▪ The surgeon should ream in under power. When the power driver is disconnected, the surgeon should pull the reamer out manually to ensure that the tunnel is a perfect circle and not widened by uneven reaming. ▪ Starting with the smallest reamer necessary is always a good technique. The surgeon can ream up at half-millimeter increments if the graft is too large. ▪ The tenodesis screw is inserted anterior to the graft to equally recreate posterior coracoclavicular ligaments.

POSTOPERATIVE CARE

- Postoperative support with a Lerman Shoulder Orthosis (DJO Inc., Vista, CA) or a Gunslinger Shoulder Orthosis (Hanger Prosthetics & Orthotics, Inc., Bethesda, MD) is used for 6 to 8 weeks. These braces are recommended to counter the pull on the shoulder complex by gravity.
- For the first 6 to 8 weeks, the brace may be removed for grooming and supine gentle passive range of motion only.
- Active and passive range-of-motion exercises are started at 8 weeks after surgery.
- If painless range of motion is obtained, strength training is started at 12 weeks.

OUTCOMES

- Anatomic coracoclavicular reconstruction: unpublished data from an ongoing study (level IV evidence) at our institution between 2002 and 2006;
  - 427 cases of AC joint dislocations with a surgical rate of 3.7%
  - 16 cases (two revisions)
  - Mean postoperative months: 28.9
  - One failure (noncompliant)
  - To date, preliminary results show a mean Single Assessment Numeric Evaluation (SANE) score of 98.4/100. Other outcome measures, including American Shoulder and Elbow Surgeons (ASES), Rowe, and Constant scores, are 94.1, 91, and 96, respectively. Patients have a pain rating of less than 1/10 with horizontal adduction and forward elevation and when a posterior force is directed at the AC joint. Postoperative radiographs show that the mean difference in the coracoclavicular distance is 2.1 mm compared to the contralateral side.
- Weaver-Dunn
  - Outcomes are difficult to compare due to the variations in the Weaver-Dunn method used and the makeup of the type of patients and severity of injury within study groups.
  - Rauschning et al[10] reported 12 acute and 5 chronic type III AC joint injuries treated by the Weaver-Dunn procedure. At follow-up 1 to 5 years after the operation, all patients had stable and painless shoulders with resumption of full activities and functionally excellent results (level IV evidence).
  - Tienen et al[15] presented 21 patients with Rockwood type V AC joint dislocations who underwent a modified Weaver-Dunn procedure with clavicle reduction and AC joint fixation using absorbable braided sutures. At a mean follow-up of 35.7 months, 18 patients had returned to their sports without pain within 2.5 months after operation; the average Constant score at last follow-up was 97. Radiographs taken at this time showed residual subluxation in two patients

and, in one patient, redislocation of the joint that occurred because of infection (level IV evidence).

- When chronic and acute repairs of type III AC joint injuries were studied, patients with early repair were significantly better after 3 months. In a study by Weinstein et al,[17] 26 of 27 (96%) patients with early repairs and 13 of 17 (77%) patients with late reconstructions achieved satisfactory results with an average 4-year follow-up (level IV evidence).

- Arthroscopic reconstruction with the TightRope System: preliminary results of an ongoing study:
  - 29 patients with a mean age of 31 years and 6-month follow-up
  - Mean Constant score 91.1
  - Mean ASES score 96.66
  - Return to sports mean of 12 weeks
  - Complications: one hardware failure with revision using TightRope and one patient with transient adhesive capsulitis

COMPLICATIONS

- Loss of reduction
- Excessive distal clavicle resection
- Osteolysis due to nonbiologic fixation material
- Coracoid fracture
- Infection

REFERENCES

1. Berg EE, Ciullo JV. The SLAP lesion: a cause of failure after distal clavicle resection. Arthroscopy 1997;13:85–89.
2. Bradley JP, Elkousy H. Decision making: operative versus nonoperative treatment of acromioclavicular joint injuries. Clin Sports Med 2003;22:277–290.
3. Debski RE, Parsons IM, Woo SL, et al. Effect of capsular injury on acromioclavicular joint mechanics. J Bone Joint Surg Am 2001;83A: 1344–1351.
4. Gladstone J, Wilk K, Andrews J. Nonoperative treatment of acromioclavicular joint injuries. Op Tech Sports Med 1997;5:78–87.
5. Klimkiewicz JJ, Williams GR, Sher JS, et al. The acromioclavicular capsule as a restraint to posterior translation of the clavicle: a biomechanical analysis. J Shoulder Elbow Surg 1999;8:119–124.
6. McFarland EG, Blivin SJ, Doehring CB, et al. Treatment of grade III acromioclavicular separations in professional throwing athletes: results of a survey. Am J Orthop 1997;26:771–774.
7. Mouhsine E, Garofalo R, Crevoisier X, et al. Grade I and II acromioclavicular dislocations: results of conservative treatment. J Shoulder Elbow Surg 2003;12:599–602.
8. Phillips AM, Smart C, Groom AF. Acromioclavicular dislocation. Conservative or surgical therapy. Clin Orthop Relat Res 1998; 10–17.
9. Ponce BA, Millett PJ, Warner JP. Acromioclavicular joint instability: reconstruction indications and techniques. Op Tech Sports Med 2004;12:35–42.
10. Rauschning W, Nordesjo LO, Nordgren B, et al. Resection arthroplasty for repair of complete acromioclavicular separations. Arch Orthop Trauma Surg 1980;97:161–164.
11. Rios C, Arciero R, Mazzocca A. Anatomy of the clavicle and coracoid process for reconstruction of the coracoclavicular ligaments. Am J Sports Med 2007;35:811–817.
12. Rockwood CA, Williams GR, Young DC. Disorders of the acromioclavicular joint. In: Rockwood CA, Matsen F, eds. The Shoulder, ed 2. Philadelphia: WB Saunders, 1990:495–554.
13. Schlegel TF, Burks RT, Marcus RL, et al. A prospective evaluation of untreated acute grade III acromioclavicular separations. Am J Sports Med 2001;29:699–703.
14. Tibone J, Sellers R, Tonino P. Strength testing after third-degree acromioclavicular dislocations. Am J Sports Med 1992;20:328–331.
15. Tienen TG, Oyen J, Eggen PJ. A modified technique of reconstruction for complete acromioclavicular dislocation: a prospective study. Am J Sports Med 2003;31:655–659.
16. Walton J, Mahajan S, Paxinos A, et al. Diagnostic values of tests for the acromioclavicular joint pain. J Bone Joint Surg Am 2006;86A: 807–812.
17. Weinstein DM, McCann PD, McIlveen SJ, et al. Surgical treatment of complete acromioclavicular dislocations. Am J Sports Med 1995;23: 324–331.

Chapter 13

Arthroscopic Acromioclavicular Joint Reduction and Coracoclavicular Stabilization: TightRope Fixation

Michael S. Todd and Winston J. Warme

DEFINITION

- Acromioclavicular (AC) separations are relatively rare injuries that result in disruption of the AC complex.
- Overall incidence of the injury is 3 to 4 per 100,000 in the general population, with up to 52% of cases occurring during sporting events.[5]
- The degree of injury is based on the amount of force transmitted through the acromion to the distal clavicle and the surrounding deltotrapezial fascia.[1,12,19]
- Increased force transmission leads to dissociation of the AC joint and tearing of the coracoclavicular ligaments.
- Determination of the injury type will guide operative versus nonoperative management.[12]

ANATOMY

- The AC joint is a diarthrodial joint composed of the medial acromial margin and the distal clavicle.
- A fibrocartilaginous intra-articular disc between the two bony ends decreases contact stresses.[12]
- Dynamic stability of the AC joint is provided by the trapezial fascia and the overlying anterior deltoid.
- Static stability of the AC joint is provided by:
  - AC ligaments
    - The superior ligament provides the greatest restraint to anterior translation of the distal clavicle.
    - Anterior, posterior, and inferior ligaments add additional horizontal stability to the AC joint.
  - Coracoclavicular ligaments
    - Conoid: arises from the posteromedial aspect of the coracoid and inserts on the posteromedial clavicle
      - Measures about 2.5 cm long and 1 cm wide
      - Provides primary resistance against anterior and superior loading of the clavicle
    - Trapezoid: arises from the anterolateral coracoid just posterior to the pectoralis minor and attaches to the lateral or central clavicle
      - Measures about 2.5 cm long and 2.5 cm wide
      - Provides resistance against posterior loading of the clavicle

PATHOGENESIS

- AC separations are the result of a direct force to the lateral aspect of the shoulder with the arm adducted (ie, fall on point of the shoulder).
- The degree of injury to the AC joint, deltopectoral fascia, and coracoclavicular ligaments will determine the resultant deformity.
- Most low-grade injuries involve only the AC joint and are often self-limited.
- Severe arm abduction during the AC separation can result in subacromial or subcoracoid displacement of the distal clavicle.[12]

PATIENT HISTORY AND PHYSICAL FINDINGS

- A complete physical examination of both upper extremities with the patient appropriately attired and in the upright position is standard.
- Evaluation of the neck and a complete neurologic examination are essential, as higher-grade injuries may manifest with brachial plexus compromise.
- Low-grade injuries will be tender to palpation at the AC joint, with mild elevation possible. Increased deformity is commonly seen as the injury grade increases, but acutely the deformity may be masked by swelling.
- Methods for examining the AC joint include:
  - AC joint compression (shear) test: Isolated painful movement at the AC joint in conjunction with a history of direct trauma indicates AC joint pathology.
  - Cross-arm adduction test: Look for pain specifically at the AC joint. Pain at the posterior aspect of the shoulder or the lateral shoulder might indicate other pathology.
  - Paxino test: sometimes done in conjunction with bone scans to assess damage to AC joint
  - O'Brien test: Symptoms at the top of the joint must be confirmed by the examiner palpating the AC joint. Anterior glenohumeral joint pain suggests labral or biceps pathology.
  - Local point tenderness at the AC joint while the glenohumeral joint is kept still suggests localized AC joint pathology.

IMAGING AND OTHER DIAGNOSTIC STUDIES

- Standard shoulder radiographs can be useful for diagnosis, but overpenetrance may result in poor visualization of the AC joint.
- An axillary view should be included to avoid missing a glenohumeral dislocation and to help assess anteroposterior (AP) translation of the clavicle.

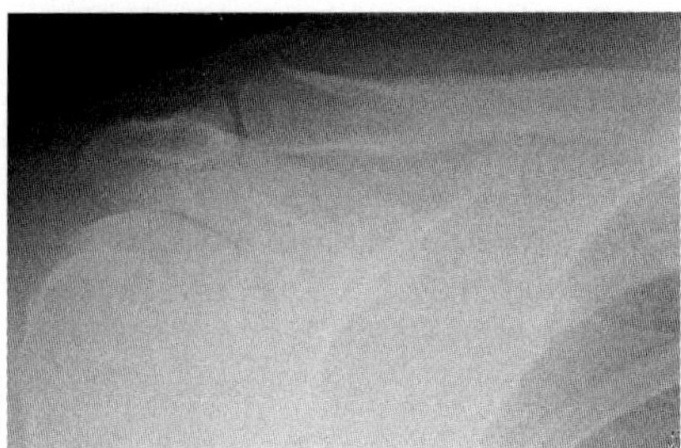

FIG 1 • Zanca view of the acromioclavicular joint.

- A 10- to 15-degree cephalic tilt view (Zanca) avoids superposition of the scapular spine and improves visualization of the AC joint. This also allows evaluation for loose bodies or small fractures that may be missed with standard views of the shoulder (**FIG 1**).[12]
- Stress radiographs
  - Standing views with 10 to 15 pounds of traction applied to the wrists are recommended by some authors to help distinguish the grade of injury because patients may guard with standard standing views.
  - Recent literature does not support the routine use of stress radiographs.[21] They do not affect the decision-making process for operative versus nonoperative management.[12,21] However, one AP view with both AC joints visible is helpful to account for normal variants and determine the degree of displacement.

DIFFERENTIAL DIAGNOSIS

- Distal clavicle fracture
- Acromial fracture
- Glenohumeral dislocation
- Sternoclavicular dislocation
- Scapulothoracic dissociation

CLASSIFICATION

- Rockwood (modification of Allman, Tossey, and Bannister's work) described six types of injuries to the acromioclavicular joint (Table 1).[1,2,12,19]
- This classification scheme has proven to be effective for prognosis and treatment.

Table 1 Rockwood's Six Types of Injuries to the Acromioclavicular Joint

Type	Description
I and II	Incomplete with no or mild subluxation of the acromioclavicular joint
III	Complete disruption of the acromioclavicular ligaments and coracoclavicular ligaments Degree of separation is up to 100% of the coracoclavicular interval.
IV	Posterior displacement of the clavicle through the trapezius muscle
V	Severe displacement with 100% to 300% increase in coracoclavicular interval (Bannister III-C) Involves injury to the deltotrapezial fascia
VI	Inferior displacement of the clavicle to a subacromial or subcoracoid position

NONOPERATIVE MANAGEMENT

- Types I and II
  - Most authors agree that nonoperative management is the treatment of choice for these incomplete injuries.[1,12,16,20]
  - A simple sling for comfort is used, with progression to range of motion as tolerated in 1 to 2 weeks.
  - Return to sports is authorized when the patient has pain-free range of motion and normal strength.
- Type III
  - This is more controversial, although conservative treatment is often successful.
  - Sling for comfort, range-of-motion exercises, and avoidance of contact sports for 6 to 8 weeks may suffice.
  - Padding of the residual deformity for contact athletes may be beneficial. Additional trauma may lead to the development of a higher-grade injury.
- Types IV and VI are routinely treated operatively.

SURGICAL MANAGEMENT

- Indication for surgery is an acute Rockwood type III or VI injury in an active patient unwilling to accept the cosmetic deformity and dysfunction of the affected shoulder.
- The TightRope fixation system (Arthrex, Naples, FL) was originally designed for the treatment of syndesmotic injuries. It has two metal fixation buttons with a continuous loop of no. 5 FiberWire running between them.[17]
  - The technique allows for a quick and relatively simple arthroscopic fixation of acute, high-grade AC separations. Chronic injuries should have the coracoclavicular ligaments reconstructed with autologous or allograft tissue.

Preoperative Planning

- Thorough evaluation of all radiologic studies to rule out associated fractures of the clavicle, coracoid, or glenoid is mandatory.
- Films should be scrutinized and a careful physical examination performed to diagnose sternoclavicular or glenohumeral dislocations.

Positioning

- Standard beach-chair position is used, with all bony and soft tissue prominences well padded.
- The use of an arm positioner (McConnell Orthopaedics, Greenville, TX, or Tenet Medical Engineering, Calgary, Alberta) is optional.
- Preparation is done in standard fashion. An arthroscopy drape is used.

ESTABLISHING ANATOMY AND PORTALS

- Anatomy is identified: coracoid, acromion, clavicle (length and width), AC joint.
- Portals are marked: posterior, anterior inferior, and anterolateral.
- The posterior portal is created for viewing 2 cm inferior and 2 cm medial to the posterolateral edge of the acromion in the "soft spot."
  - Diagnostic arthroscopy with a 30-degree scope of the intra-articular space is routine.[20]
- The subacromial space is entered from this portal using standard technique.
  - We do not find it necessary to move through the rotator interval to identify the coracoid base, although it is recommended in the technique guide.
  - A 70-degree scope may be helpful if the trans-interval technique is used.
- The anterolateral portal is made using an "outside-in technique" in line with the lateral edge of the acromion and the coracoid as a working portal.
- A 5- to 7-mm cannula is introduced to assist with pressure control.

CORACOACROMIAL LIGAMENT AND CORACOID PREPARATION

- With the scope in the posterior portal, the anterolateral acromion and the coracoacromial (CA) ligament are identified. The CA ligament is preserved (TECH FIG 1A).
- The CA ligament is followed to its attachment site on the coracoid (TECH FIG 1B).
- Through the anterolateral portal an arthroscopic ablator or chondrotome is used to resect the subcoracoid bursa and allow better visualization of the inferior aspect of the coracoid and its base.
- There is no need to remove soft tissue from the superior aspect of the coracoid (TECH FIG 1C).
- The surgeon should be cautious when placing instruments medial to the coracoid because the scapular notch lies in close proximity. Injury to the neurovascular bundle is a possibility.
- An 18-gauge spinal needle is used for localization and an "outside-in technique" is used to make the anteroinferior portal just lateral and slightly inferior to the coracoid. An 8.25-mm cannula is inserted.
- The Adapteur Drill Guide C-Ring and Coracoid Drill Stop (Arthrex) is inserted through the anteroinferior portal under the base of the coracoid (TECH FIG 1D).
  - The surgeon should stay as far posterior, near the coracoid base, as possible, and central from a mediolateral standpoint.
- A 1- to 2-cm incision is made over the clavicle in line with the drill guide and the coracoid.

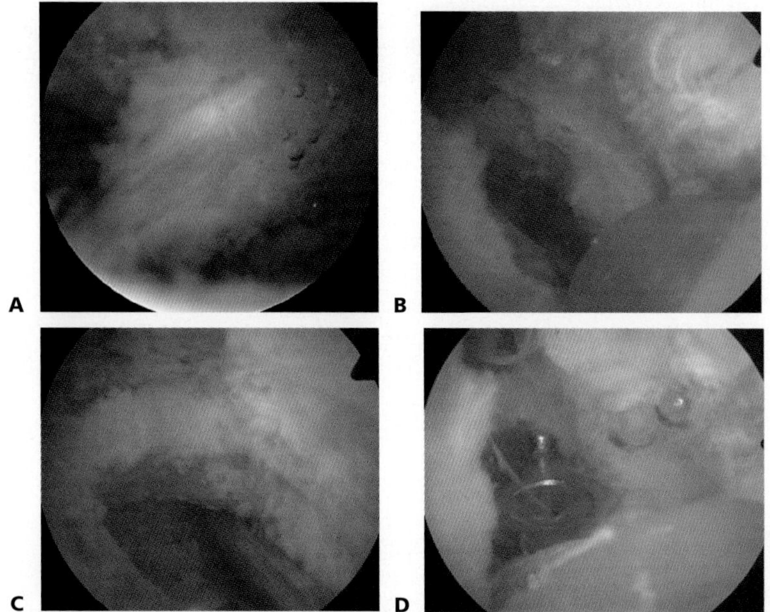

TECH FIG 1 • **A.** Coracoacromial ligament identification. **B.** Coracoid identification. **C.** Soft tissue resection of the coracoid. **D.** Coracoid drill stop placement. The base is hugged posterior.

GUIDE PIN PASSAGE

- Under arthroscopic visualization with the clavicle reduced, a 2.4-mm guide pin is advanced through the center of the clavicle and coracoid. It is captured by the drill stop (**TECH FIG 2A**).
- The guide pin is overreamed with a 4-mm cannulated reamer, using the drill stop to prevent plunging. The scope allows visualization of each step (**TECH FIG 2B**).
- The guide pin is removed and the solid end of the Nitinol wire loop is passed antegrade through the cannulated reamer. It is grasped and removed out the anteroinferior portal with a push-and-pull technique (**TECH FIG 2C,D**).

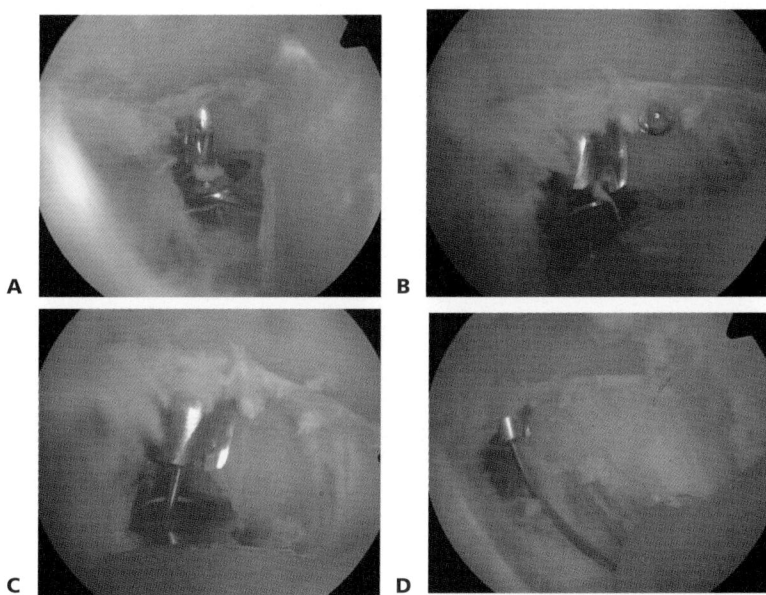

TECH FIG 2 • **A.** Captured 2.4-mm guide pin. **B.** Captured 4-mm drill bit. **C.** Nitinol wire passage. **D.** Retrieval of Nitinol through the anteroinferior portal.

SUTURE PASSAGE

- The TightRope comes fixed with two 2-0 FiberWires to lead the suture button through the bone tunnel and flip accordingly.
- These are passed with the wire loop through the clavicle and coracoid and out the anteroinferior portal.
  - One suture strand should be colored purple with a marking pen for easier differentiation of the "lead" suture from the "flip" suture (**TECH FIG 3A,B**).
- The TightRope button is passed and flipped when visualized with the arthroscope (**TECH FIG 3C,D**).
- The upper extremity is then elevated and the AC joint is overreduced.

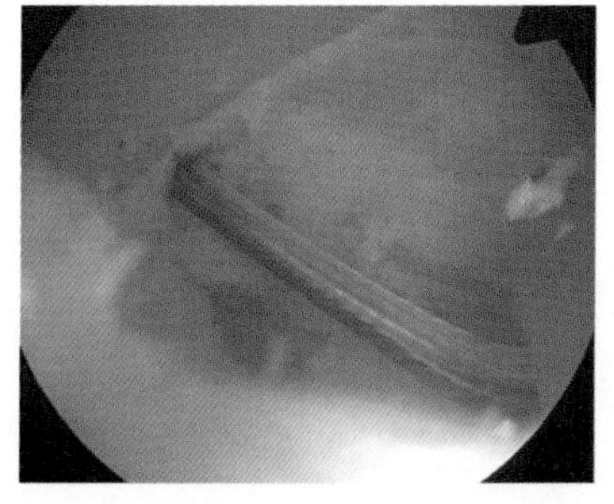

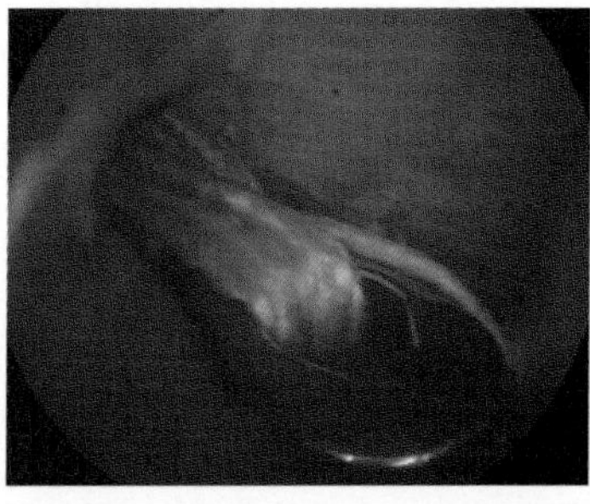

TECH FIG 3 • **A.** Colored "lead" suture. **B.** Suture button exits coracoid base. *(continued)*

TECHNIQUES

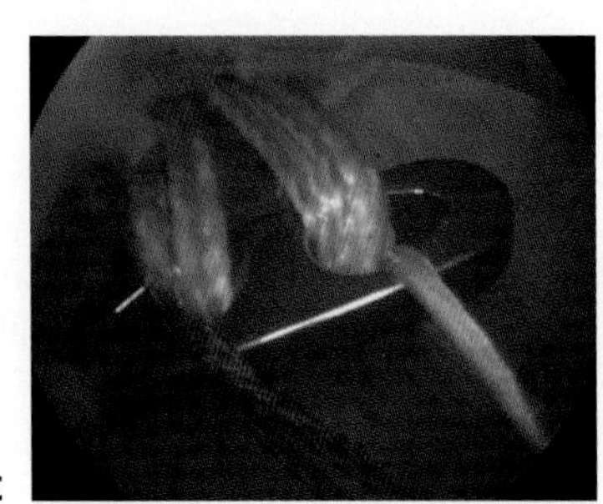
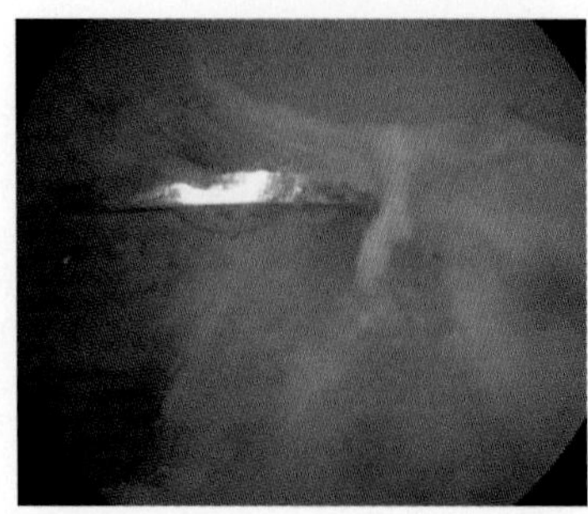

TECH FIG 3 • *(continued)* **C.** Button is flipped by pulling the trailing, uncolored suture. **D.** Reduced button on base of coracoid.

SUTURE TYING

- Two or three square knots are placed over the cephalad suture button (TECH FIG 4A).
- The suture ends should be left about 1 cm long to allow the knot to lie flat under the soft tissues (TECH FIG 4B).
- For additional stability, the soft tissue capsule of the AC joint may be sutured, because this is an important component of AC stability.
- Open versus arthroscopic AC resection should be considered, as the potential exists for the development of painful AC joint arthrosis; however, this is not routinely done.
- The wounds are closed and dressed in the usual fashion.

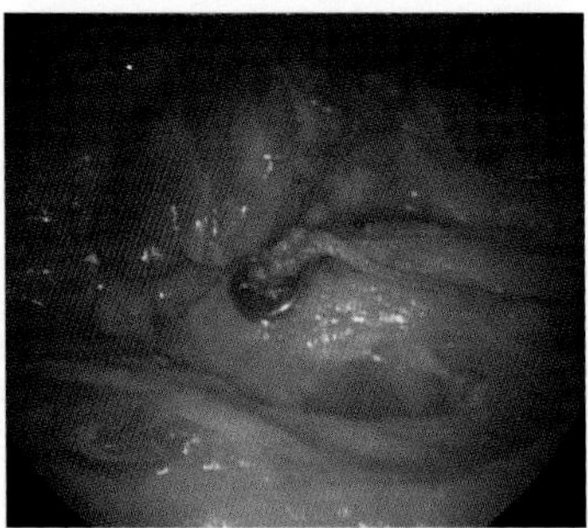
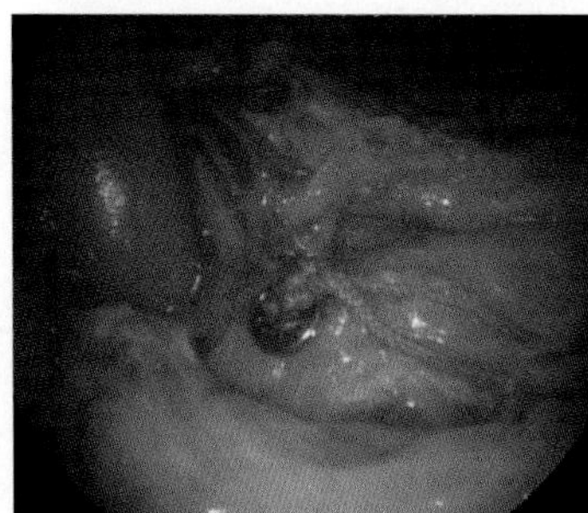

TECH FIG 4 • **A.** Square knot superiorly. **B.** Suture ends are left long.

POSTOPERATIVE CARE

- A sling is used for comfort and to slow down the patient for 4 weeks.
- Range of motion of the elbow is permitted immediately, as are gentle Codman/pendulum exercises.
- Gentle active motion below the shoulder level is permitted until the 6-week mark, at which time progression to full motion is authorized.
- No heavy work or athletics are permitted for 3 months.
- Postoperative radiographs are compared with radiographs made at the 6-week return visit.

COMPLICATIONS

- Infection
- Loss of reduction
- Coracoid fracture[11]
- Clavicle fracture
- Suprascapular neurovascular bundle injury

OUTCOMES

- The TightRope Fixation System is a relatively new system for treatment of acute AC separations. It is not intended for chronic injuries.
- No long-term studies or prospective randomized trials are available.
- Biomechanical data are available only for its syndesmotic use.[18,19]

ACKNOWLEDGMENTS

We thank John Morton, James Willobee, and Jeff Wyman from Arthrex, and the staff of the William Beaumont Army Medical Center Biomedical Research facility.

REFERENCES

1. Allman FL Jr. Fractures and ligamentous injuries of the clavicle and its articulation. J Bone Joint Surg Am 1967;49A:774–784.
2. Bannister GC, Wallace WA, Stableforth PG, et al. The management of acute acromioclavicular dislocation: a randomized prospective controlled trial. J Bone Joint Surg Br 1989;71B:848–850.
3. Chernchujit B, Tischer T, Imhoff AB. Arthroscopic reconstruction of the acromioclavicular joint disruption: surgical technique and preliminary results. Arch Orthop Trauma Surg 2006;126: 575–581.
4. Costic RS, Vangura A Jr, Fenwick JA, et al. Viscoelastic behavior and structural properties of the coracoclavicular ligaments. Scand J Med Sci Sports 2003;13:305–310.

5. Costic RS, Labriola JE, Rodosky MW, et al. Biomechanical rationale for development of anatomical reconstructions of coracoclavicular ligaments after complete acromioclavicular joint dislocations. Am J Sports Med 2004;32:1929–1936.
6. Dimakopoulos P, Panagopoulos A, Syggelos SA, et al. Double-loop suture repair for acute acromioclavicular joint disruption. Am J Sports Med 2006;34:1112–1119.
7. Jari R, Costic RS, Rodosky MW, et al. Biomechanical function of surgical procedures for acromioclavicular joint dislocations. Arthroscopy 2004;20:237–245.
8. Lancaster S, Horowitz M, Alonso J. Complete acromioclavicular separations: a comparison of operative methods. Clin Orthop Relat Res 1987;216:80–88.
9. Lee SJ, Nicholas SJ, Akizuki KH, et al. Reconstruction of the coracoclavicular ligaments with tendon grafts: a comparative biomechanical study. Am J Sports Med 2003;31:648–655.
10. Moneim MS, Balduini FC. Coracoid fracture as a complication of surgical treatment by coracoclavicular tape fixation: a case report. Clin Orthop Relat Res 1982;168:133–135.
11. Pearsall AW IV, Hollis JM, Russell GV Jr, et al. Biomechanical comparison of reconstruction techniques for disruption of the acromioclavicular and coracoclavicular ligaments. J South Orthop Assoc 2002;11:11–17.
12. Rockwood CA Jr, Williams GR Jr, Young DC. Disorders of the acromioclavicular joint. In Rockwood CA Jr, Matsen FA III, eds. The Shoulder. Philadelphia: WB Saunders, 1998:483–553.
13. Salter EG Jr, Nasca RJ, Shelley BS. Anatomical observations on the acromioclavicular joint and supporting ligaments. Am J Sports Med 1987;15:199–206.
14. Schlegel TF, Burks RT, Marcus RL, et al. A prospective evaluation of untreated acute grade III acromioclavicular separations. Am J Sports Med 2001;29:699–703.
15. Taft TN, Wilson FC, Oglesby JW. Dislocation of the acromioclavicular joint: an end-result study. J Bone Joint Surg Am 1987;69A: 1045–1051.
16. Tienen TG, Oyen JF, Eggen PJ. A modified technique of reconstruction for complete acromioclavicular dislocation: a prospective study. Am J Sports Med 2003;31:655–659.
17. Thornes B, Walsh A, Hislop M, et al. Suture-endobutton fixation of ankle tibio-fibular diastasis: a cadaver study. Foot Ankle Int 2003;24:142–146.
18. Thornes B, Shannon F, Guiney AM, et al. Suture-button syndesmosis fixation: accelerated rehabilitation and improved outcomes. Clin Orthop Relat Res 2005;431:207–212.
19. Tossy JD, Mead NC, Sigmond HM. Acromioclavicular separations: useful and practical classification for treatment. Clin Orthop Relat Res 1963;28:111–119.
20. Wolf EM, Pennington WT. Arthroscopic reconstruction for acromioclavicular joint dislocation. Arthroscopy 2001;17:558–563.
21. Yap JJ, Curl LA, Kvitne RS, et al. The value of weighted views of the acromioclavicular joint: results of a survey. Am J Sports Med 1999; 27:806–809.

Chapter 14 Arthroscopic Release of Nerve Entrapment

Felix H. Savoie III and Larry D. Field

DEFINITION

- Suprascapular nerve entrapment may result from constriction within the suprascapular notch, pressure from a ganglion cyst in the floor of the supraspinatus fossa, or a constriction at the spinoglenoid notch.
- The nerve is readily accessible via arthroscopic techniques developed by Thomas Samson and Laurent Lafosse.

ANATOMY

- The suprascapular nerve receives contributions primarily from the C5 root, with additional minor contributions from C4 and C6 nerve roots.
- It exits from the upper trunk of the brachial plexus through the supraclavicular fossa and comes through the suprascapular notch beneath the transverse scapular ligament, dividing into two branches.
  - One branch exits medially to the supraspinatus muscle.
  - The second continues across the floor of the supraspinatus fossa of the scapula toward the junction of the scapular spine and the posterosuperior neck of the glenoid.
- The nerve makes a short turn around the bone junction under the inconsistently present spinoglenoid ligament and travels medially across the superior aspect of the infraspinatus fossa of the scapula, sending branches into this muscle until terminating into the medial aspect of this muscle.[3]

PATHOGENESIS

- Nerve entrapment usually occurs at the suprascapular notch.
  - Trauma, repetitive overhead use requiring hyperretraction and protraction of the scapula (ie, volleyball), and chronic rotator cuff injuries may produce swelling in this area, resulting in pressure on the nerve.
  - Congenital V-shaped suprascapular notch orientation has been implicated as a cause of this entrapment.
- Less common areas of entrapment may occur owing to ganglion cyst compression in the middle or posterior aspect of the fossa, and at the spinoglenoid notch.
  - A thickened spinoglenoid ligament may cause entrapment at the spinoglenoid notch as well.
  - Unusual sources of nerve entrapment include vascular expansion (aneurysm or varices) and tumors.[2]

NATURAL HISTORY

- The natural history of suprascapular nerve entrapment depends on the cause and pathologic changes in the anatomy.
- Spontaneous recovery after rehabilitation treatment has been reported.
- However, if electromyographic nerve conduction studies show evidence of compression, surgical treatment is usually indicated.
- Compression at the suprascapular notch or spinoglenoid area is often the primary problem and is not associated with intra-articular pathology.[6] Compression by ganglion cyst in the supraspinatus fossa is often associated with labral tears that require fixation along with débridement of the cyst. All of these may be managed arthroscopically if nonoperative treatment is ineffective.

PATIENT HISTORY AND PHYSICAL FINDINGS

- The patient often presents with signs and symptoms of impingement and rotator cuff tearing, overhead weakness, pain on forced flexion, and subacromial crepitation.
- Careful inspection may reveal atrophy in the supraspinatus and infraspinatus fossa compared to the opposite side.
- Weakness to supraspinatus isolation, infraspinatus isolation, and Whipple testing is usually present.
- Palpation of the rotator cuff reveals no defect. However, there is usually no, or only minimal, palpable swelling on the distal supraspinatus tendon.

IMAGING AND OTHER DIAGNOSTIC STUDIES

- Most patients will have to undergo magnetic resonance imaging.
  - The test should reveal an intact rotator cuff with atrophy of the supraspinatus and infraspinatus musculature.
  - Occasionally, there will be tearing of the rotator cuff with atrophy that is not in proportion to the size or duration of the tear.
- Electromyographic nerve conduction studies by a neurologist specializing in proximal entrapment lesions of the upper extremity will be definitive in cases of entrapment at the suprascapular or spinoglenoid notch.

DIFFERENTIAL DIAGNOSIS

- The main confusion in this area is with primary impingement and rotator cuff tears.
- The history and physical examination are often similar, but a careful evaluation and physical examination will reveal the differences as delineated in the prior discussion under physical findings.

NONOPERATIVE MANAGEMENT

- There is a limited role for nonoperative treatment of true entrapment neuropathy.
- Pressure from a cyst may be alleviated by aspiration of the cyst.
  - Compression at either the suprascapular or spinoglenoid notch, however, will require release if the nerve conduction study reveals pressure to the nerve in these areas.

SURGICAL MANAGEMENT

- Several approaches to open release have been described (Nicholson, Vastamake, and Post[4,7,8]).
- Recently, Samson and Lafosse have each focused interest on techniques of arthroscopic release.[1–6]

Positioning

- The patient is positioned in the lateral decubitus (preferred) or beach-chair position.

ARTHROSCOPIC RELEASE OF NERVE ENTRAPMENT

- A diagnostic glenohumeral arthroscopy is performed to rule out intra-articular pathology.
- The arthroscope is then positioned in the lateral portal of the subacromial bursa in line with the anterior acromion, providing a picture of the supraspinatus muscle and tendon (TECH FIG 1A).
- It is advanced along the anterior edge of the supraspinatus until the base of the coracoid is visualized (TECH FIG 1B).
- A switching stick is placed in the lateral Neviaser portal and used to palpate along the anterior edge of the supraspinatus fossa medial to the medial aspect of the base of the coracoid (TECH FIG 1C).
- A full-radius shaver can be used from the anterior portal to remove soft tissue as long as it remains lateral to the switching stick, which is functioning as a retractor in addition to a diagnostic tool (TECH FIG 1D).
- On encountering the suprascapular artery, a second medial Neviaser portal is created and the retracting switching stick is removed to this portal and used to pull the artery medially and protect it (TECH FIG 1E).
  - Sliding this retractor along the top of the ligament will also protect any aberrant branches of the nerve that pass superior to the ligament.

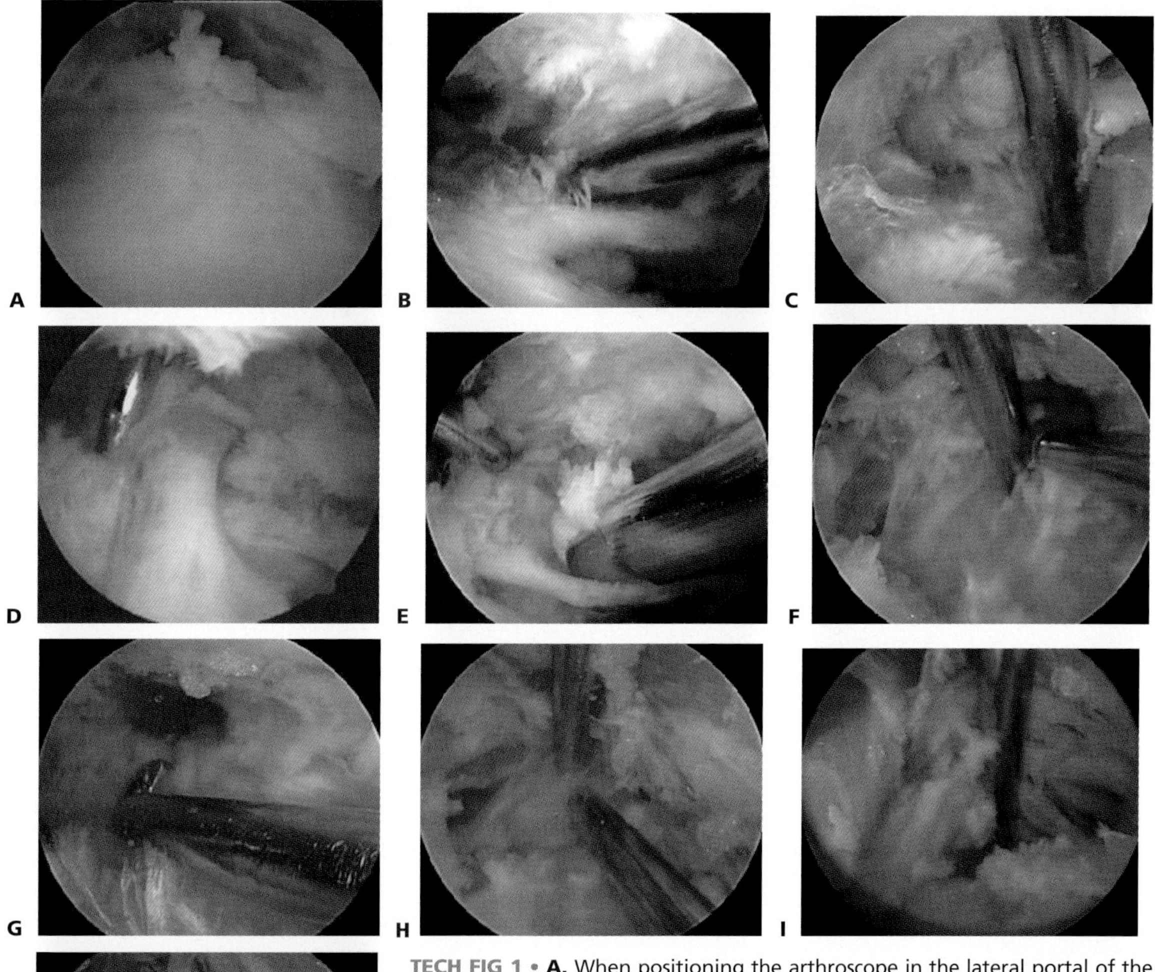

TECH FIG 1 • **A.** When positioning the arthroscope in the lateral portal of the subacromial bursa in line with the anterior acromion, the supraspinatus muscle and tendon can be seen. **B.** Advancing the arthroscope along the anterior edge of supraspinatus allows the surgeon to visualize the coracoid. **C.** Placing a switching stick in the lateral Neviaser portal allows the surgeon to palpate the anterior edge of the supraspinatus fossa medial to the medial aspect of the base of the coracoid. **D.** A shaver can be used from the anterior portal to remove soft tissue; the surgeon must always remain lateral to the switching stick. **E.** A second Neviaser portal is established so that the switching stick can be used to pull the artery medially and protect it. **F.** A blunt probe enters to identify the ligament and protect the underlying nerve. **G,H.** A side biter or shaver can be used to release the ligament. **I.** The exposed nerve. **J.** The suprascapular nerve, artery, and vein are allowed to fall back into a relaxed position.

TECHNIQUES

- A blunt probe is used to identify the ligament and protect the underlying suprascapular nerve (**TECH FIG 1F**).
  - A side biter (**TECH FIG 1G**) or shaver (**TECH FIG 1H**) is then used to release the ligament overlying the notch, exposing the nerve (**TECH FIG 1I**).
- The nerve is retracted medially along with the artery and vein and the ligament resection is completed.
- The suprascapular notch may also be débrided and beveled at this time to resect any sharp edges. An arthroscopic rasp may then be used to complete this process.
- The retractors are removed and the suprascapular nerve, artery, and vein are allowed to fall back into a relaxed position (**TECH FIG 1J**).
  - The nerve can be tracked across the floor of the supraspinatus fossa toward the spinoglenoid notch.
  - The supraspinatus muscle can be evaluated and then retracted anteriorly, exposing the scapular spine, which can then be followed to the spinoglenoid notch if assessment for a constricting spinoglenoid ligament is necessary.
  - This ligament can then be released using a similar retraction technique on the nerve.

PEARLS AND PITFALLS

Pearls	■ The surgeon should maintain the arthroscope in the lateral portal and advance it along the anterior edge of the supraspinatus fossa. ■ The medial aspect of the coracoid base is used as a guide to the suprascapular notch. ■ The medial Neviaser portal is used for a retractor. Using the retractor to protect the artery, vein, and nerve will prevent inadvertent resection when using the shaver or a punch.
Pitfalls	■ The main pitfall is not using a retractor to protect the nerve, artery, and vein. ■ Using too much suction on the shaver pulls the nerve into the shaver owing to a vacuum effect and could cut it. ■ A lack of skilled cadaveric practice in this procedure is a relative contraindication to attempting the operation.

POSTOPERATIVE CARE

- The patient is started on immediate therapy, along with a home neuromuscular stimulator, for the infraspinatus. Correct scapular position is essential to recovery and will facilitate recovering normal strength.
- Although most patients see an immediate decrease in pain and increase in strength, it usually takes 6 to 12 months to regain normal strength in the infraspinatus and supraspinatus musculature.
- Therapy and electrical stimulation are continued until the patient can resume normal activities.

OUTCOMES

- Lafosse has reported more than 90% successful releases using his technique.[9]
- His results are equal to, or better than, most open series reported by other authors.
  - No substantial reports of arthroscopic spinoglenoid ligament release were found during our literature search.
- Nicholson has reported satisfactory results with open release of the spinoglenoid ligament in a series of patients.[7]

COMPLICATIONS

- Few complications have been reported with this technique.
- The primary complication would be inadvertent nerve resection, but this has not been reported to our knowledge.

REFERENCES

1. Bencardino JT, Rosenbert ZS. Entrapment neuropathies of the shoulder and elbow in the athlete. Clin Sports Med 2006;25:1–19.
2. Fabre TH, Piton C, Leclouerec G, et al. Entrapment of the suprascapular nerve: upper limb. J Bone Joint Surg Br 1999;81B:414–419.
3. Goslin KL, Krivickas LS. Proximal neuropathies of the upper extremity. Neurol Clin 1999;17:525–547.
4. Post M. Diagnosis and treatment of suprascapular nerve entrapment. Clin Orthop Relat Res 1999;368:92–100.
5. Sanders TG, Tirman PFJ. Paralabral cyst: an unusual cause of quadrilateral space syndrome. Arthroscopy 1999;15:632–637.
6. Westerheide KJ, Dopirak RM, Karzel RP, et al. Suprascapular nerve palsy secondary to spinoglenoid cysts: results of arthroscopic treatment. Arthroscopy 2006;22:721–727.
7. Nicholson GP, McCarty LP, Wysolcki R: Suprascapular Nerve Entrapment Isolated to the Spinoglenoid Notch. Results of Open Decompression. Presented at 73rd American Academy of Orthopaedic Surgeons Meeting. Chicago Il, March 2006, and at the American Orthopaedic Society for Sports Medicine Specialty Day. Chicago, IL, March 25, 2006.
8. Vastamaki M, Goransson H. Suprascapular nerve entrapment. Clin Orthop Relat Pres 1993;(297):135–143.
9. Lafosse L, Tomasi A, Corbett S, et al. Arthroscopic release of suprascapular nerve entrapment at the suprascapular notch: technique and preliminary results. Arthroscopy 2007;23(1):34–42.

Chapter **15**

Arthroscopic Capsular Releases for Loss of Motion

Ryan W. Simovitch, Laurence D. Higgins, and Jon J.P. Warner

DEFINITION

- Shoulder stiffness can be a function of soft tissue scarring and contracture or osseous changes.
- The stiff or frozen shoulder has been given the name *adhesive capsulitis*.
- There are principally two forms of adhesive capsulitis that result in loss of range of motion and can be safely addressed by arthroscopic releases:
  - Primary adhesive capsulitis (idiopathic)
  - Secondary adhesive capsulitis
    - Associated with metabolic disorder (diabetes mellitus, thyroid disorder)
    - Posttraumatic
    - Postoperative
- Shoulder stiffness can result from intra-articular adhesions, capsular contracture, subacromial adhesions, and subdeltoid adhesions.
- The essential tenet of treating the stiff shoulder is recognizing the anatomic region responsible for the stiffness and releasing the specific structures in this region in a controlled fashion.
  - An adequate appreciation of anatomy is key to restoring motion and avoiding injury to accompanying tendons and nerves.

ANATOMY

- Shoulder motion occurs principally along two interfaces:
  - Glenohumeral articulation
  - Scapulothoracic articulation
- On average, the normal ratio of glenohumeral motion to scapulothoracic motion is 2:1, with the majority of elevation occurring through the glenohumeral joint.
- Capsuloligamentous structures contribute to stability of the shoulder joint and act as check reins at the extremes of motion in their nonpathologic condition.
- Many areas within the capsule are thickened and contain the glenohumeral ligaments (**FIG 1A**):
  - Superior glenohumeral ligament
  - Coracohumeral ligament
  - Middle glenohumeral ligament
  - Inferior glenohumeral ligament complex
    - Anterior band
    - Axillary fold
    - Posterior band
- The rotator interval is a triangular region between the anterior border of the supraspinatus tendon and the superior border of the subscapularis. It contains the superior glenohumeral ligament and the coracohumeral ligament.
- During shoulder motion, tightening and loosening of the glenohumeral ligaments and capsule are accompanied by lengthening and shortening of the rotator cuff and deltoid muscles.
  - A plane between the deltoid and humerus (subdeltoid) exists that, when scarred, can limit glenohumeral motion.
  - A plane between the rotator cuff and acromion exists and is occupied normally by a subacromial bursa.
  - Scar tissue and adhesions in this interface can limit excursion of the rotator cuff and thus glenohumeral joint motion (**FIG 1B**).
- Several structures that are important to preserve are in continuity or proximity to the regions of the capsule that are released arthroscopically in the stiff shoulder.
  - The subscapularis tendon is superficial to the middle glenohumeral ligament. The superior two thirds of the subscapularis is intra-articular.

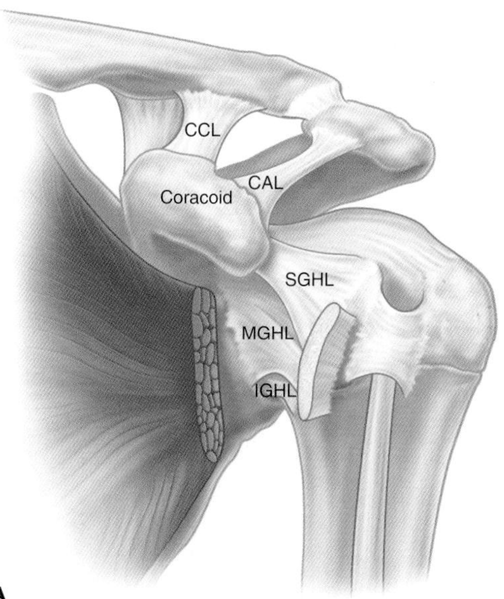

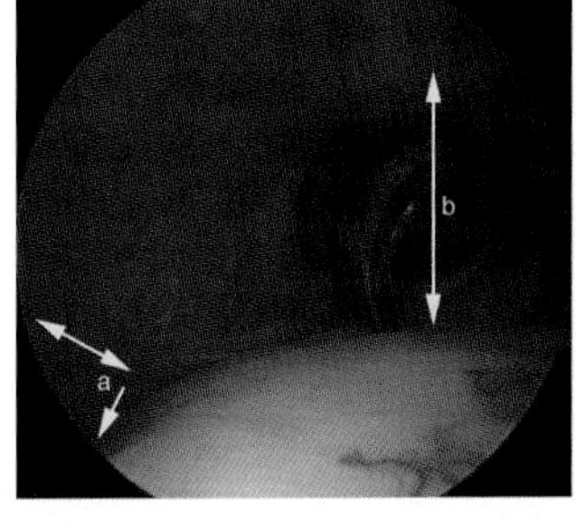

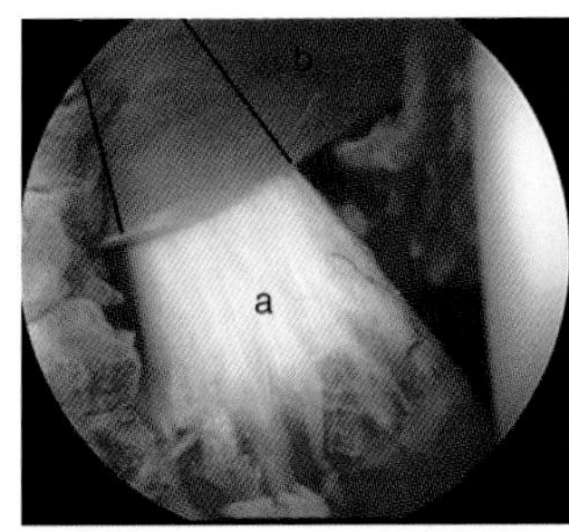

FIG 1 • **A.** Thickenings of the capsule are referred to as the glenohumeral ligaments. In their undiseased state they act as physiologic check reins at extreme ranges of motion. **B.** Fibrous bands can exist in the subacromial space (*a*) between the acromion and rotator cuff as well as in the subdeltoid space (*b*) between the deltoid and rotator cuff or humerus. These can restrict excursion of the rotator cuff and thus active and passive range of motion. **C.** The axillary nerve runs across the superficial surface of the subscapularis and then adjacent to the inferior border of the subscapularis as it heads posteriorly. Anterior capsular release can proceed safely as long as the muscle of the subscapularis is seen inferiorly.

- The biceps tendon courses through the rotator interval.
- The axillary nerve runs adjacent to the inferior border of the subscapularis and then is juxtaposed to the inferior glenohumeral ligament and capsule as it exits the quadrangular space (**FIG 1C**).
- The posterior capsule overlies a distinct layer of rotator cuff muscle posteriorly adjacent to the glenoid.
  - The posterior rotator cuff tendons and capsule are juxtaposed and virtually indistinguishable more laterally.
  - Release of the posterior capsule should be done adjacent to the glenoid to avoid rotator cuff muscle and tendon disruption.
- Contracture of specific capsular regions and ligaments correlates with specific clinical losses of range of motion. This must be determined preoperatively to guide arthroscopic release.
- These anatomic regions and their influence on shoulder motion are as follows:
  - Rotator interval (superior glenohumeral ligament and coracohumeral ligament) restricts external rotation with the shoulder adducted.
  - Middle glenohumeral ligament restricts external rotation at the midranges of abduction.
  - Inferior glenohumeral ligament (anterior band) restricts external rotation at 90 degrees of abduction.
  - Inferior capsule restricts abduction and forward flexion.
  - Posterior capsule and posterior band of the inferior glenohumeral ligament restrict internal rotation.

PATHOGENESIS

- Shoulder stiffness can be primary or secondary.
  - Secondary stiffness occurs as a result of scar formation and adhesions after trauma or surgery of the shoulder as a result of disruption of soft tissue, release of cytokines, and the body's inflammatory response seen after injury.
    - Secondary stiffness can also result iatrogenically, as would be the case after a Putti-Platt or Magnuson-Stack procedure.
  - Primary stiffness is often termed *adhesive capsulitis*.
    - Adhesive capsulitis, also referred to as frozen shoulder, can be idiopathic or associated with a secondary cause that is either intrinsic (eg, rotator cuff tears, biceps tendinitis, or calcific tendinitis) or extrinsic (eg, diabetes, myocardial infarction, thyroid disorders).
- There is no consensus on the definition of frozen shoulder, but it is generally agreed to be a condition with both significant restriction in active and passive range of shoulder motion without an osseous basis for this limitation.
- The pathogenesis of frozen shoulder has been divided into three stages (Table 1). The stages coexist as a continuum and occur over a variable time course in individual patients.

Table 1 Pathogenesis of Frozen Shoulder

Stage	Description	Time Course
Freezing or inflammatory stage	Slow onset of pain, with the shoulder losing motion as the pain worsens	6 weeks to 9 months
Frozen stage	Slow improvement in pain but the stiffness continues	4 to 9 months or more
Thawing stage	Shoulder motion gradually returns to normal	5 to 26 months

NATURAL HISTORY

- Although the natural history of secondary shoulder stiffness is relatively accepted as protracted and refractory to nonoperative treatment, the time course and end result of adhesive capsulitis (primary and secondary) are more controversial.
- In the absence of operative intervention, recent reports have shown measurable restrictions in range of motion at follow-up in 39% to 76%[3,8,10] of patients, in addition to persistent symptoms in up to 50%[2] of patients with adhesive capsulitis.
- Adhesive capsulitis can be protracted, with the mean duration of symptoms 30 months.[10]
- There is a weak correlation between restricted range of motion and pain.
  - Some patients have severe pain but near-normal range of motion.
  - Some patients have very restricted range of motion but no pain.
- In one study, restricted range of motion was found in more than 50% of patients with adhesive capsulitis, but functional deficiency was identified in only 7% of the patients.[10]
- The impact of restricted range of motion or pain on an individual patient's quality of life largely depends on that patient's functional demands.
- Adhesive capsulitis in diabetics tends to be more protracted and more resistant to nonoperative treatment than idiopathic adhesive capsulitis.

PATIENT HISTORY AND PHYSICAL FINDINGS

- Patients with idiopathic adhesive capsulitis often deny a traumatic event but complain of the insidious onset of pain that is refractory to physical therapy and predates the loss of motion.
- Patients with secondary adhesive capsulitis often have a history of trauma, surgery, or medical comorbidities.
  - A history of fracture or extended immobilization should be elicited.
  - Previous surgeries including rotator cuff repair, capsular shift, Putti-Platt, Bristow-Latarjet, open glenoid bone grafting, and open reduction and internal fixation of a fracture should be documented as a potential cause of stiffness.
  - Comorbidities, including diabetes mellitus and thyroid disorders, should be recorded because they are associated with adhesive capsulitis.
- Symptoms expressed by patients with shoulder stiffness include:
  - Loss of range of motion that translates into functional limitations
  - Painful arc of motion
  - Pain often radiating to the deltoid area due to "non-outlet" impingement[5]

- Periscapular pain as a result of transferred pain to the scapulothoracic articulation because of restricted glenohumeral range of motion
- Acromioclavicular joint pain due to increased scapulothoracic motion

- A comprehensive examination of the involved shoulder must be done to note any concomitant pathology. Physical examination methods include:
  - Passive range-of-motion examinations
    - Assessing the anterosuperior capsule: Results are compared to the contralateral shoulder. A loss of passive range of motion in this position suggests contracture of the anterosuperior capsule in the region of the rotator interval. Loss of passive range of motion should always be compared to loss of active range of motion.
    - Assessing the anteroinferior capsule: A loss of passive external rotation in abduction suggests contracture of the anteroinferior capsule.
    - Assessing the inferior capsule: A loss of passive flexion and abduction suggests contracture of the inferior capsule.
    - Assessing the posterior capsule: Cross-chest adduction can be measured in degrees by recording the angle between an imaginary horizontal to the ground and the axis of the arm. A loss of passive internal rotation suggests contracture of the posterior capsule.
  - Lidocaine injection test: Passive and active range of motion in all planes should be recorded before injection. Once pain is alleviated, the postinjection increase in passive and active range of motion is recorded. The recorded increase in range of motion after the injection indicates the extent to which loss of motion is attributable to adhesions and soft tissue contracture as opposed to pain from nonoutlet impingement or a symptomatic acromioclavicular joint.
  - Intra-articular injection: Passive and active range of motion should be recorded in all planes before injection. Passive and active range of motion should be evaluated after the injection to note any improvement after pain relief. A more accurate assessment of range of motion can be made after pain is alleviated. The injection can also be therapeutic in the early stages of adhesive capsulitis when synovitis is present.
- The shoulder should be examined for signs of previous surgery, trauma, deformity, and atrophy.
- Manual motor testing of rotator cuff and deltoid muscles should be done.
- Active and passive range of motion should be noted in all planes both in seated and supine positions. Shoulder motion should be viewed from the front and back of the patient.
  - Assessing range of motion in a supine position controls compensatory scapulothoracic motion and lumbar tilt, yielding a more accurate examination.
  - An equal loss of passive and active range of motion suggests adhesive capsulitis as the cause.
  - Greater loss of active than passive range of motion suggests rotator cuff or nerve injury.
  - Global loss of passive range of motion is typical of adhesive capsulitis, whereas loss of range of motion in one plane is usually attributable to postsurgical scarring or trauma.

IMAGING AND OTHER DIAGNOSTIC STUDIES

- Routine radiographic evaluation should include an anteroposterior (AP) view of the shoulder in neutral, internal, and external rotation, as well as scapular-Y and axillary lateral views.
  - Disuse osteopenia is often noted.
  - Concomitant findings may include osteoarthrosis, calcific tendinitis, or hardware signifying a previous surgical procedure (eg, open reduction and internal fixation, Putti-Platt) (**FIG 2**).
- Magnetic resonance imaging (MRI) is obtained only if a rotator cuff tear or other soft tissue derangement is suspected.
- We do not typically order an arthrogram or laboratory studies to confirm the diagnosis of adhesive capsulitis.

DIFFERENTIAL DIAGNOSIS

- Glenohumeral arthritis
- Acromioclavicular arthritis
- Rotator cuff tendinitis
- Subacromial or subdeltoid bursitis
- Bicipital tendinitis
- Calcific tendinitis
- Septic arthritis
- Rotator cuff tears
- Gout or crystalline arthropathy

NONOPERATIVE MANAGEMENT

- Nonoperative treatment can be attempted but is typically unsuccessful in patients with secondary shoulder stiffness.
- It is indicated in patients with primary and secondary adhesive capsulitis who have had stiffness for less than 4 to 6 months or no previous treatment.
- Nonsteroidal anti-inflammatories are used for pain relief but narcotics are avoided because of dependency issues with long-term use.

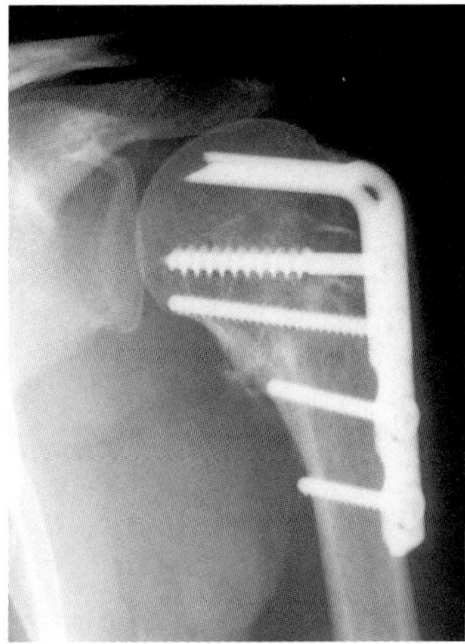

FIG 2 • Hardware on radiographs can be helpful in guiding treatment. In this instance, after treatment of a proximal humerus fracture with a blade plate, adhesions would be expected in the subdeltoid space.

- Injections are helpful in the early stages of adhesive capsulitis to control pain.
  - A series of three intra-articular injections can be given for pain relief. An intra-articular injection is often diagnostic as well, with the alleviation of pain but continued restriction in range of motion.[7,9]
  - Paired injections can be given (a subacromial and intra-articular injection).[11]
- Active-assisted range-of-motion exercises focused on stretching capsular contractures under the supervision of a physical therapist should be done in 5- to 10-minute sessions four or five times a day.[6] Other modalities such as ice and heat can provide comfort before and after exercise but are typically not very effective in the inflammatory or freezing phase.

SURGICAL MANAGEMENT

- Surgical intervention should not be attempted during the early stages of adhesive capsulitis. It may be counterproductive and prohibit an increase in range of motion by abundant scar formation.
- Surgical intervention is indicated for secondary or primary adhesive capsulitis once pain is present only at the extremes of motion and not through the entire arc of motion.
  - We prefer to continue nonoperative management while motion is increasing. We recommend surgery only when patients plateau.

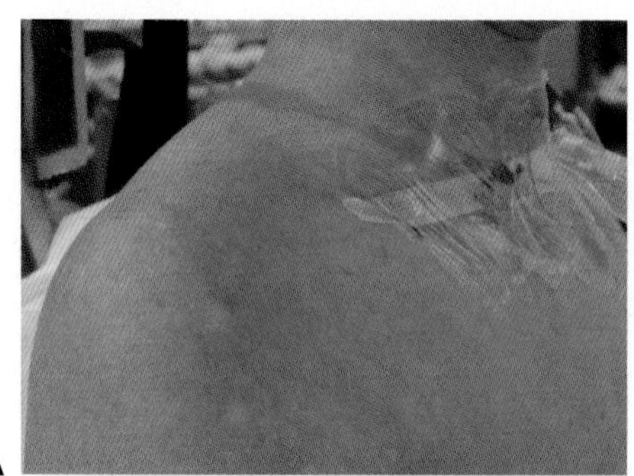

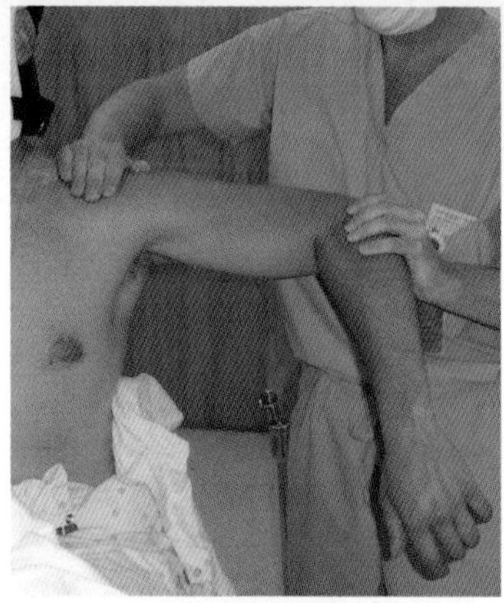

FIG 3 • **A.** An interscalene catheter is established preoperatively to provide muscle paralysis and pain control during the procedure as well as sustained pain control for 48 hours after the arthroscopic release. **B.** Passive range of motion is examined under anesthesia to guide the arthroscopic release. The scapula should be controlled with one of the examiner's hands to avoid scapulothoracic motion.

- We prefer to do a manipulation under anesthesia at the conclusion of an arthroscopic release in a controlled fashion rather than as a stand-alone procedure or before an arthroscopic evaluation and release.

Preoperative Planning

- Imaging is reviewed and concomitant pathology is noted.
  - Rotator cuff tears should be noted because a repair will influence postoperative therapy and the timing of surgery.
  - Glenohumeral arthritis should be noted. These patients may have some benefit from an arthroscopic release, but their results are influenced by the congruity of the glenohumeral joint.
- Unless contraindicated, we use regional anesthesia (30- to 40-cc bolus of a combination of 1.5% mepivacaine and 0.5% bupivacaine) with an indwelling interscalene catheter that provides muscle paralysis and pain control during the procedure as well as up to 48 hours after arthroscopic capsular release (**FIG 3A**).
  - This is essential to postoperative therapy and was shown to be effective and safe.[4,13,14] Patients are admitted for 48 hours of intensive physical therapy under the indwelling interscalene block after surgery.
- An examination under anesthesia is conducted using the range-of-motion principles to assess the anterosuperior, anteroinferior, inferior, and posterior capsules. This guides the emphasis of capsular release (**FIG 3B**).

Positioning

- The patient is placed supine on the operating table in the beach-chair position.
- After an examination under anesthesia, the shoulder is widely prepared and draped well medial to the coracoid anteriorly and to the medial scapular border posteriorly.
- The entire arm is prepared and then placed into a hydraulic arm holder (Spider Limb Positioner, Tenet Medical Engineering, Calgary, Canada) (**FIG 4**). This avoids the need for an assistant to hold the arm.

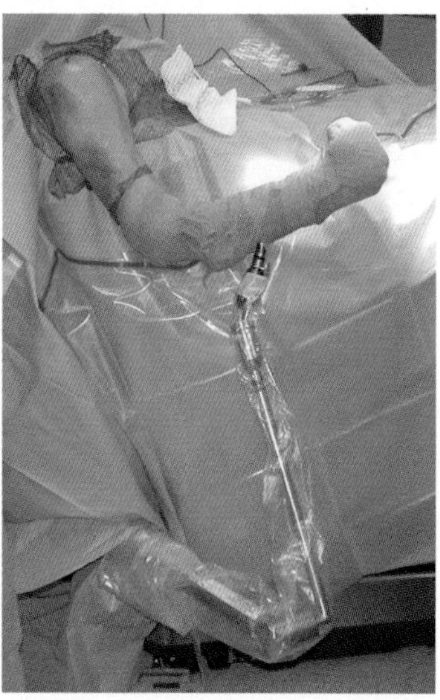

FIG 4 • We use a hydraulic arm holder (Spider Limb Positioner, Tenet Medical Engineering, Calgary, Canada) to secure the arm and avoid the need for an assistant.

ESTABLISHING PORTALS

- The challenging aspect of arthroscopic capsular release is entering the contracted joint while avoiding iatrogenic articular injury (TECH FIG 1A–C).
- We establish the posterior arthroscopic portal slightly higher than normal (TECH FIG 1D).
- An 18-gauge spinal needle is inserted into the joint and insufflated (usually 10 to 15 cc in a contracted joint) with sterile saline.
  - Entry into the joint can be confirmed by noting backflow of saline from the spinal needle.
  - This step ensures proper portal placement and also distends the joint, thus lessening the risk of iatrogenic articular injury (TECH FIG 1E).
- An incision is made where the needle was inserted using a #11 blade and the arthroscope sheath is advanced into the glenohumeral joint.
  - Entry into the joint is confirmed with backflow of saline through the sheath.
- With the arthroscope posteriorly, a spinal needle is inserted lateral to the coracoid through the rotator interval immediately underneath the biceps and above the subscapularis.
- An incision is made with a #11 blade and a 6-mm cannula is then placed through this portal.
- A radiofrequency device is passed through the cannula and used to remove synovium and soft tissue that obscures the view (TECH FIG 1F).

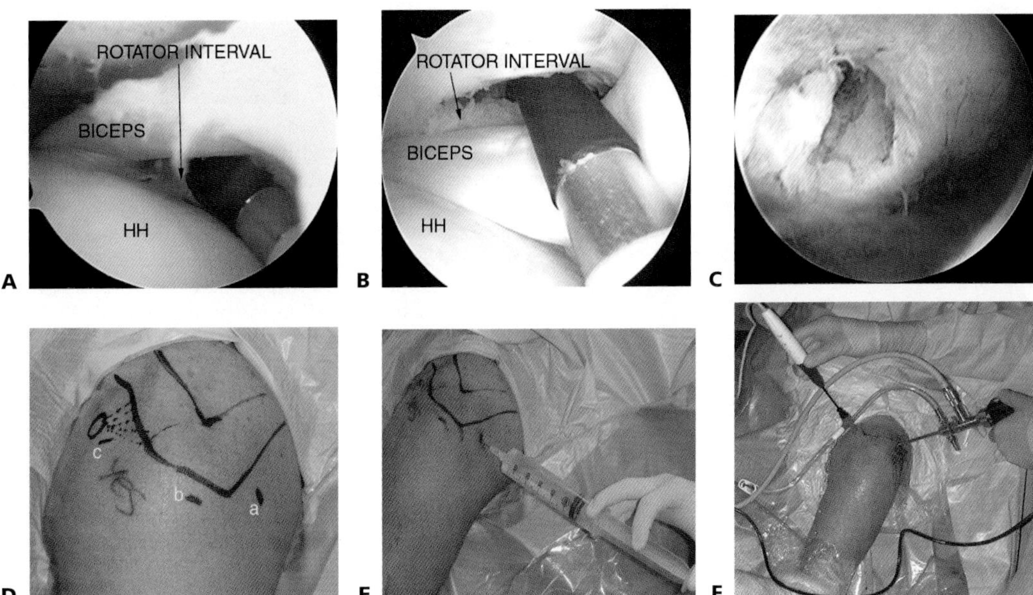

TECH FIG 1 • It is often difficult to enter a shoulder with significant capsular contraction and scarring. **A.** Entering at or above the biceps with the anterior cannula is typically possible. **B.** The biceps can be displaced inferiorly and the rotator interval can be ablated to relax the joint and allow further release inferiorly. **C.** Forced entry with poor visualization can result in significant osteochondral injury, as depicted in this image. *HH*, humeral head. **D.** The posterior portal (*a*) is established higher than normal to lessen the risk of iatrogenic articular damage. The lateral (*b*) and anterior (*c*) portals are established using the outside-in technique with an 18-gauge spinal needle. **E.** Sterile normal saline is injected into the glenohumeral joint. This causes distention, which lessens the risk of iatrogenic articular damage and verifies the portal position. Backflow of saline through the spinal needle ensures entry into the joint as opposed to soft tissue. **F.** The anterior capsule is visualized by the arthroscope from the posterior portal and a radiofrequency device is placed through the cannula anteriorly to remove synovium and create a potential working space.

ANTERIOR CAPSULAR RELEASE

- Resection of contracted and thickened capsule can be done with a radiofrequency device, shaver, or arthroscopic punch.
  - We prefer to use a hook-tipped radiofrequency device to avoid bleeding, resect in a controlled fashion, and benefit from the feedback of electrical stimulation to nearby muscles and nerves.
  - An arthroscopic punch can be used once a leading edge in the capsule has been established (TECH FIG 2A,B).

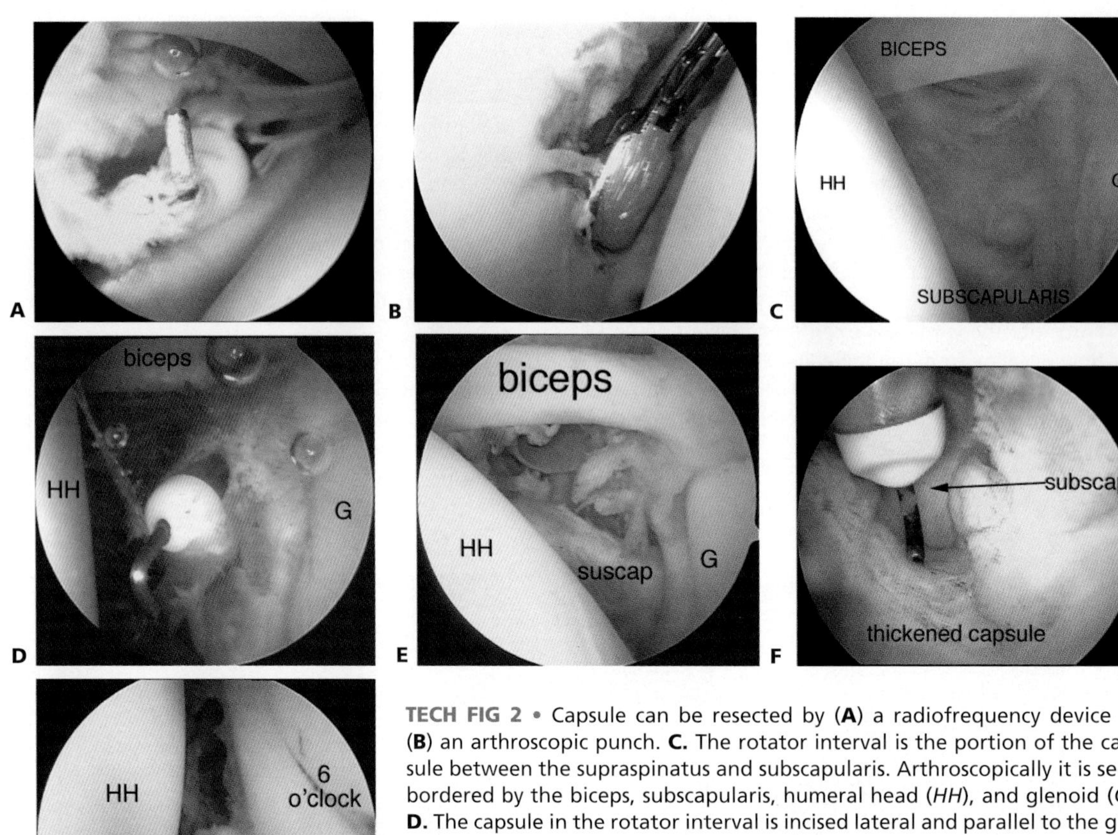

TECH FIG 2 • Capsule can be resected by (**A**) a radiofrequency device or (**B**) an arthroscopic punch. **C.** The rotator interval is the portion of the capsule between the supraspinatus and subscapularis. Arthroscopically it is seen bordered by the biceps, subscapularis, humeral head (*HH*), and glenoid (*G*). **D.** The capsule in the rotator interval is incised lateral and parallel to the glenoid (*G*) starting inferior to the biceps. *HH*, humeral head. **E.** The capsule is incised from just inferior to the biceps up to the leading edge of the subscapularis (*subscap*) tendon. *G*, glenoid; *HH*, humeral head. **F.** A blunt obturator or switching stick can be used to bluntly dissect the deep capsule from the more superficial anterior subscapularis (*subscap*) tendon. This capsule is divided with radiofrequency ablation. **G.** The anterior capsule (*) is divided to the 6 o'clock position. *HH*, humeral head.

- In adhesive capsulitis, the capsule is often up to 1 cm thick compared with the normal 2 mm.
- We resect the anterior capsule systematically.
- The rotator interval capsule is noted between the biceps superiorly and the intra-articular subscapularis inferiorly. This comprises the superior glenohumeral and coracohumeral ligaments (TECH FIG 2C).
- We begin by cutting (ablating) the capsular tissue immediately inferior to the biceps tendon (TECH FIG 2D).
- The capsular tissue is released inferiorly until the superior border of the subscapularis is identified, thus releasing the rotator interval and its contents (TECH FIG 2E).
- A switching stick can then be used to bluntly dissect the capsule from the deep surface of the subscapularis to create a defined interval. This capsule represents the middle glenohumeral ligament (TECH FIG 2F).
- The capsule overlying the subscapularis is then divided to the 6 o'clock position (TECH FIG 2G).
  - Gentle external rotation can place the capsule under additional tension and facilitate its resection.
- The axillary nerve is not at risk as long as the subscapularis muscle is seen (see Fig 1C).
- The shaver is introduced to resect the capsular tissue medially and laterally to provide a generous interval (10 mm) and discourage the healing of capsular tissue in a contracted position.

POSTERIOR CAPSULAR RELEASE

- Release of the posterior capsule is necessary in patients with global capsular contracture or isolated posterior capsular contracture, often seen in patients with "nonoutlet" impingement symptoms as described by Warner.[14]
- The arthroscope is placed through the anterior 6-mm cannula.
  - Inflow is attached to the anterior cannula.
  - A switching stick is placed through the arthroscopic sheath posteriorly into the joint (TECH FIG 3A).
- A 6-mm cannula is exchanged for the arthroscope sheath over a switching stick posteriorly (TECH FIG 3B).
- The hook-tipped radiofrequency device is passed through the cannula and is used to release the posterior

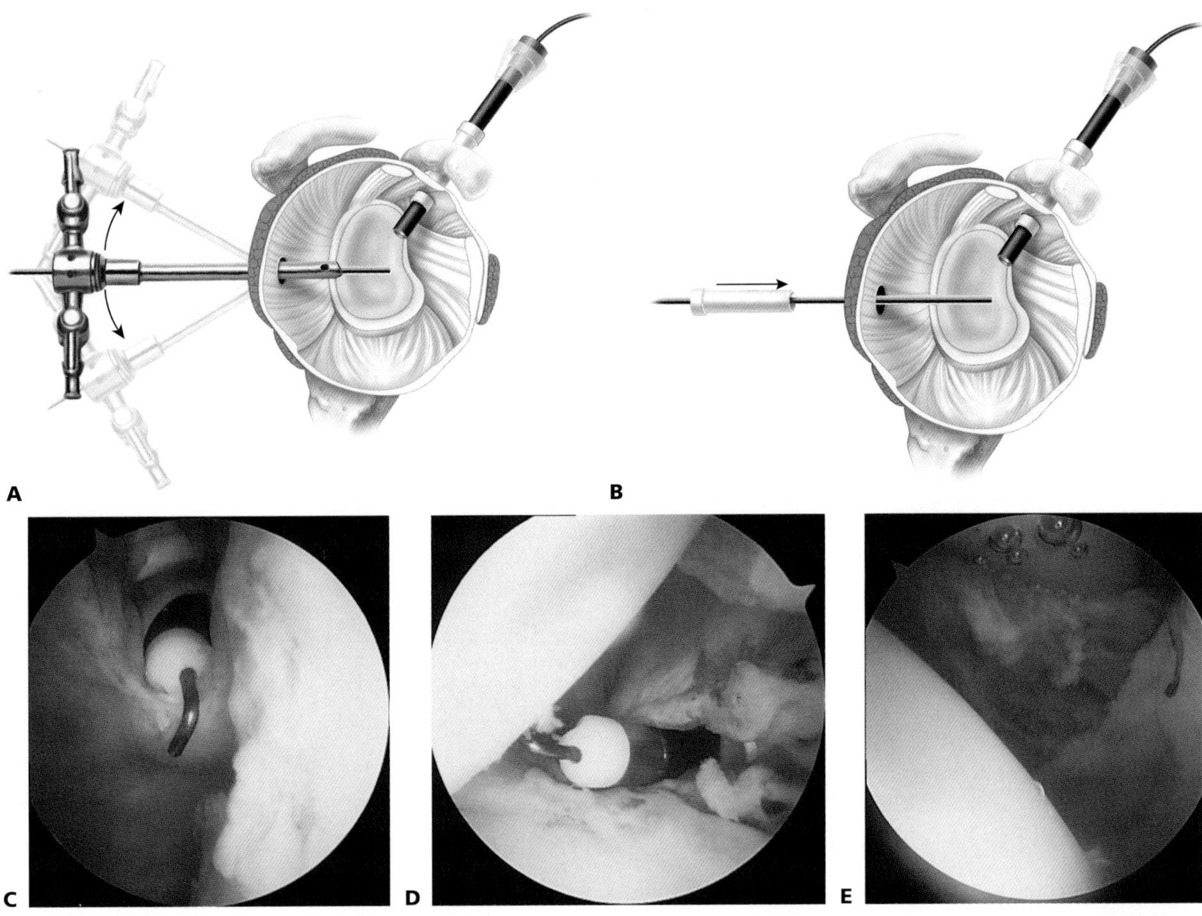

TECH FIG 3 • **A.** The arthroscope is placed through the anterior cannula to view the posterior capsule. A switching stick is placed through the arthroscopic sheath posteriorly. Inflow is attached to the anterior cannula. **B.** A 6-mm smooth cannula is passed over the switching stick posteriorly to facilitate a posterior capsular release. **C.** The posterior capsule is released with the radiofrequency probe through the posterior cannula, noting the increased thickness of the capsule. **D.** The cannula can be retracted if needed to achieve a better angle with the probe. **E.** The capsule is released to the 8 o'clock position.

capsule from just posterior to the long head of the biceps to the 8 o'clock position (TECH FIG 3C–E).

- In our experience, a release of the inferior capsule from 6 o'clock to 8 o'clock is unnecessary.
- A shaver is introduced and used to further resect tissue medially and laterally, leaving a 10-mm capsule-free interval. The capsule is intimate with the infraspinatus and the release should be terminated at the point at which muscle is encountered.

SUBACROMIAL AND SUBDELTOID BURSOSCOPY

- Subacromial and subdeltoid scarring and adhesions are common after prior rotator cuff repair and fracture fixation.
- In cases of adhesive capsulitis there is often a component of subacromial bursitis.
- The subacromial space and subdeltoid space are always evaluated for bursitis as well as dense adhesions.
- The arthroscope is passed into the subacromial space through the posterior portal immediately inferior to the posterior acromion.
- A 6-mm smooth cannula is placed through the anterior portal (TECH FIG 4A).
- A radiofrequency device is passed through the anterior cannula to meet the arthroscopic lens and a subacromial decompression is initiated until the space adjacent to the lateral deltoid is free of adhesions.
- A spinal needle can then be used to locate the position of a lateral portal.
- A lateral portal is made with a #11 blade and a 6-mm cannula is introduced into the subacromial space.
- The anterior and lateral cannulas can alternately be used to achieve an adequate subacromial decompression.
- It is essential to free the interval between the acromion and rotator cuff as well as laterally in the space between the deltoid and proximal humerus (TECH FIG 4B).
- An acromioplasty can be done if indicated, although it is not usually necessary in cases of primary adhesive capsulitis.

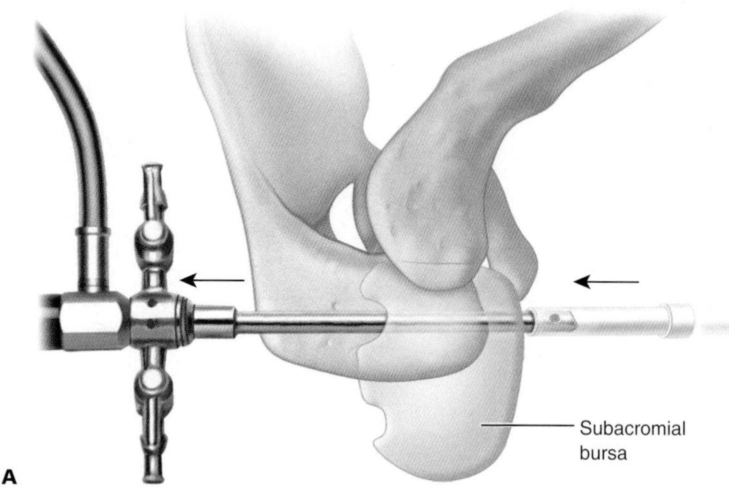

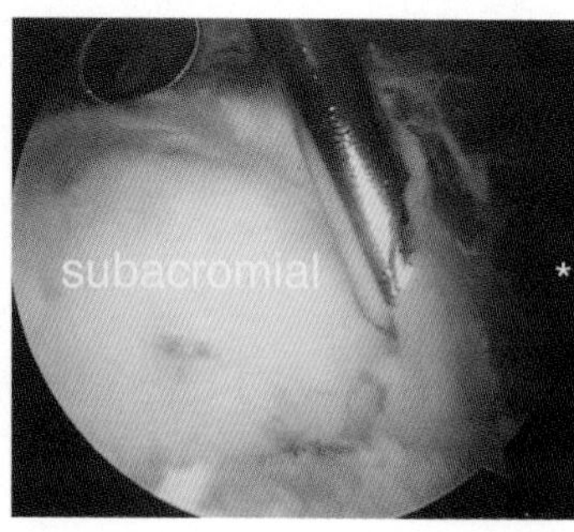

TECH FIG 4 • **A.** The arthroscope sheath and blunt obturator are passed as a unit through the subacromial space and out the previously made anterior portal. The arthroscope is exchanged for the obturator in the sheath and a 6-mm cannula is placed over the sheath and lens tip. Both are withdrawn into the subacromial together, enabling the radiofrequency device to begin work débriding thick soft tissue within view of the arthroscope. **B.** Scar and bursa are removed from the subacromial space and the subdeltoid space (*) using a shaver and radiofrequency device. Adhesions are released between the rotator cuff and the acromion and deltoid.

POSTRELEASE MANIPULATION UNDER ANESTHESIA

- Range of motion is evaluated before manipulation under anesthesia to determine which structures need additional release.
- A sterile dressing is applied and the drapes are removed so that the scapula can be stabilized.
- A manipulation after a capsular release requires far less force and therefore carries a lower risk of fracture.
- The scapula is stabilized with one hand while the surgeon's other hand firmly grasps the humerus above the elbow (TECH FIG 5).
- Sequence of manipulation:
  - External rotation in adduction
  - Abduction
  - External rotation in abduction
  - Internal rotation in abduction
  - Flexion
  - Internal rotation in adduction

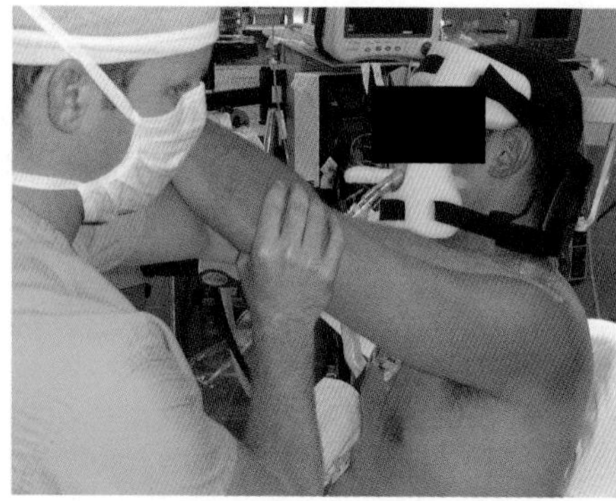

TECH FIG 5 • A gentle manipulation under anesthesia is done after arthroscopic release and once the drapes have been removed.

PEARLS AND PITFALLS

Hemostasis	■ Visualization is essential during a capsular release. We routinely use epinephrine in our bags of saline. In addition, we rely on the use of a radiofrequency device and limit the use of a shaver and arthroscopic punch.
Difficulty entering the glenohumeral joint with the arthroscope	■ Distention of the joint with sterile normal saline through an 18-gauge spinal needle ensures correct position of the portal. ■ Typically the joint can be entered superiorly at the level of the biceps and initial release of the interval should relax the joint, allowing improved visualization.

Difficulty visualizing the subacromial space and establishing portals in the setting of dense scar	▪ The following sequence can help gain access to the subacromial space, which facilitates safe decompression and lysis of adhesions: 1. The arthroscope sheath (with obturator) is passed through the posterior portal adjacent to the posterior acromion toward the anterior portal. 2. With the sheath adjacent to the acromion, the sheath and obturator are passed through the existing anterior portal. 3. The obturator is removed and the arthroscope secured in its sheath (lens and tip of scope exiting out of anterior portal). 4. The 6-mm cannula is placed over the tip of the sheath. 5. In a controlled fashion, the arthroscope is withdrawn into the subacromial space while the cannula is maintained on the tip of the sheath and passed into the subacromial space. 6. A radiofrequency device can be placed in the cannula as it is backed off the sheath by 1 to 2 mm. 7. The arthroscope can now visualize the radiofrequency device in a controlled and reproducible fashion to allow safe decompression instead of relying on blind navigation in dense scar and bursa.

POSTOPERATIVE CARE

- Immediately after surgery, the arm is placed in a simple sling and the shoulder in a cryotherapy sleeve.
- The patient is admitted for 48 hours and a continuous infusion of 0.1% bupivacaine is administered through the previously placed interscalene catheter at 10 to 20 cc per hour based on the pain level.
- Passive range of motion in all planes is initiated on the morning of the first postoperative day by the physical therapists. This is done twice a day.
- The patient is discharged on the afternoon of the second postoperative day after the indwelling catheter is removed.
- A simple sling for comfort is worn on discharge, but the patient is encouraged to use the operative arm for activities of daily living.
- After discharge, the patient immediately begins outpatient physical therapy to include stretching and water therapy whenever possible:
  - Five days a week for 2 weeks
  - Three days a week for 2 weeks
  - At 1 month, therapy regimen is transitioned to home program.
  - Strengthening is initiated with elastic bands and weights only when range of motion is achieved. We prefer no strengthening until full range of motion is achieved.

OUTCOMES

- Multiple studies have shown the efficacy of arthroscopic capsular release for shoulder stiffness.
- In one study with an average of 33 months of follow-up, final motion at latest follow-up was 93% of the opposite side compared to 41% preoperatively, with a significant improvement in reported health status (SF-36) and ability to use the arm functionally.[5]
- Warner et al[13] found significant gains in range of motion (within 7 degrees of the values for the normal contralateral shoulder) in 23 patients with idiopathic adhesive capsulitis treated by arthroscopic release. All patients had either no pain or only occasional mild pain with forceful use of the shoulder.
- Warner et al[14] found significant gains in range of motion in all planes in 11 patients with postsurgical stiffness who underwent either an anterior or combined anterior and posterior arthroscopic capsular release after failed nonoperative treatment.
- "Non-outlet" impingement with an associated posterior capsular contracture has been effectively treated by arthroscopic posterior capsular release with an average improvement of internal rotation at 90 degrees of abduction of 37 degrees and alleviation of pain in all but one of the nine patients studied.[12]
- Beaufils et al[1] showed that arthroscopic capsular release is effective at improving range of motion regardless of the cause of a stiff shoulder, although releases for postsurgical stiffness are less likely to alleviate pain than those done for adhesive capsulitis.

COMPLICATIONS

- Axillary nerve injury
- Rotator cuff tendon disruption
- Iatrogenic chondral injury
- Fracture or dislocation during manipulation under anesthesia
- Recurrence of stiffness

REFERENCES

1. Beaufils P, Prevot N, Boyer T, et al. Arthroscopic release of the glenohumeral joint in shoulder stiffness: a review of 26 cases. Arthroscopy 1999;15:49–55.
2. Binder A, Bulgen DY, Hazelman BL. Frozen shoulder: a long-term prospective study. Ann Rheum Dis 1984;43:361.
3. Bulgen DY, Binder A, Hazelman BL, et al. Frozen shoulder: a prospective clinical study with an evaluation of the three treatment regimens. Ann Rheum Dis 1983;43:353.
4. Cohen NP, Levine WN, Marra G, et al. Indwelling interscalene catheter anesthesia in the surgical management of stiff shoulder: a report of 100 consecutive cases. J Shoulder Elbow Surg 2000;9:268.
5. Harryman DT, Matsen FA III, Sidles JA. Arthroscopic management of refractory shoulder stiffness. Arthroscopy 1997;13:133–147.
6. Holvacs T, Warner JP. Acquired shoulder stiffness: posttraumatic and postsurgical. In: Warner JP, Iannotti J, Flatow W, eds. Complex and Revision Problems in Shoulder Surgery. Philadelphia: Lippincott Williams & Wilkins, 2005:236.
7. Lundber BJ. The frozen shoulder: clinical and radiographical observations. The effect of manipulation under general anesthesia: structure and glycosaminoglycan content of the joint capsule. Acta Orthop Scand Suppl 1969;119.
8. Murnagham JP. Frozen shoulder. In: Rockwood CAJ, Matsen FA, eds. The Shoulder. Philadephia: WB Saunders, 1990:837.
9. Quin CE. "Frozen shoulder": evaluation and treatment with hydrocortisone injections and exercises. Ann Phys Med 1965;8:22.
10. Reeves B. The natural history of the frozen shoulder syndrome. Scand J Rheumatol 1986;4:193.
11. Richardson AT. Ernest Fletcher lecture: the painful shoulder. Proc R Soc Med 1975;68:731.
12. Ticker JB, Beim GM, Warner JP. Recognition and treatment of refractory posterior capsular contracture of the shoulder. Arthroscopy 2000;16:27–34.
13. Warner JP, Allen A, Marks PH, et al. Arthroscopic release for chronic, refractory adhesive capsulitis of the shoulder. J Bone Joint Surg Am 1996;78A:1808–1816.
14. Warner JP, Allen A, Marks P, et al. Arthroscopic release of postoperative capsular contracture of the shoulder. J Bone Joint Surg Am 1997;79A:1151–1158.

Chapter 16 Arthroscopic Treatment of Scapulothoracic Disorders

Michael J. Huang and Peter J. Millett

DEFINITION

- Several terms have been used to describe the elements of scapulothoracic bursitis and crepitus, such as snapping scapula, washboard syndrome, scapulothoracic syndrome, and rolling scapula.
- The first description of scapulothoracic crepitus is credited to Boinet in 1867.[1]
- By 1904, Mauclaire[5] had described three subclasses—*froissement*, *frottement*, and *craquement*—depending on the loudness and character of the sound.
- Milch[6] and then Kuhn et al[4] added to the understanding by differentiating sounds of soft tissues (*frottement*) from those arising from an osseous lesion (*craquement* or crepitus).

ANATOMY

- Major bursae
  - Infraserratus bursa located between the serratus anterior muscle and the chest wall
  - Supraserratus bursa located between the subscapularis and the serratus anterior muscles
- Minor bursae
  - Not consistently identified on cadaveric or clinical studies
  - Adventitial in nature; thought to arise secondary to abnormal biomechanics of the scapulothoracic joint
  - Superomedial angle of the scapula
    - Infraserratus
    - Supraserratus
  - Spine of scapula
    - Trapezoid
  - Inferior angle of scapula
    - Infraserratus

PATHOGENESIS

- Scapulothoracic bursitis can be caused by atrophied or fibrotic muscle, anomalous muscle insertions, or elastofibroma (rare benign soft tissue tumor located on the chest wall).
- Osteochondromas and malunited fractures of the ribs or scapula can also cause pathology in this articulation.
- Infectious causes include tuberculosis or syphilis.
- The tubercle of Luschka is a prominence at the superomedial aspect of the scapula that can be excessively hooked and can cause altered biomechanics.
- Scoliosis or thoracic kyphosis can contribute to scapulothoracic crepitus.
- Unrelated disorders include cervical radiculopathy, glenohumeral pathology, and periscapular strain.

NATURAL HISTORY

- Scapulothoracic disorders are often associated with repetitive overhead activities or with a history of trauma.
- Constant motion leads to inflammation and a cycle of chronic bursitis and scarring.
- Mechanical impingement and pain with motion are a result of tough fibrotic tissue, furthering the inflammatory cycle.

PATIENT HISTORY AND PHYSICAL FINDINGS

- Repetitive overhead activities or trauma
- Palpable or audible crepitus over the involved area
- Occasionally bilateral or positive family history
- Localized tenderness over the inflamed area is most common.
  - Superomedial border is the most commonly affected area.
  - Inferior pole is also a common site of pathology.
- Pseudowinging (nonneurologic etiology) may result from fullness over the involved area and compensation of scapular mechanics due to pain.
- Crepitus alone, without pain, may be physiologic and not warrant treatment.

IMAGING AND OTHER DIAGNOSTIC STUDIES

- Tangential scapular views to identify bony anomalies
- Computed tomography is controversial but can be helpful if osseous lesions are suspected and plain radiographs are normal.
- Magnetic resonance imaging (MRI) is also controversial but can identify the size and location of bursal inflammation.
- Injection of a corticosteroid and local anesthetic is helpful to confirm the diagnosis.

DIFFERENTIAL DIAGNOSIS

- Atrophied, fibrotic muscle or anomalous muscle
- Malunited rib or scapular fracture
- Mass (eg, elastofibroma, osteochondroma)
- Infection (ie, tuberculosis, syphilis)
- Scoliosis or kyphosis
- Cervical spine radiculopathy
- Glenohumeral disease

NONOPERATIVE MANAGEMENT

- Rest
- Nonsteroidal anti-inflammatory
- Activity modification
- Physical therapy
  - Local modalities
  - Periscapular strengthening, emphasizing subscapularis and serratus anterior
  - Postural training
- Figure 8 harness for kyphosis
- Injection may be of benefit for both diagnosis and treatment.

SURGICAL MANAGEMENT

- Indicated for patients who have failed to respond to conservative therapy
- Open treatment

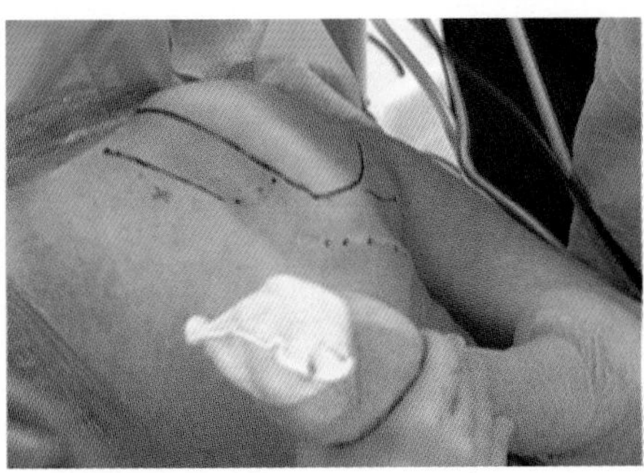

FIG 1 • The arm behind the back in extension and internal rotation: the "chicken wing" position.

- Has been used successfully in treatment of both bursitis[7,9] and crepitus[6,8]
- Requires fairly large exposure and subperiosteal dissection of the medial musculature, with repair back to bone after débridement of pathologic tissue is accomplished
- Arthroscopic treatment
  - Minimizes morbidity of the exposure and facilitates early rehabilitation and return to function

Preoperative Planning

- If a bony mass is detected, computed tomography findings will help guide the planned resection.

Positioning

- The patient is placed in the prone position, with the arm behind the back in extension and internal rotation (the so-called chicken wing position; **FIG 1**).

Approach

- Decisions regarding open versus arthroscopic treatment for these disorders should be based on surgeon experience and comfort level.

POSTOPERATIVE CARE

- Sling for comfort
- Gentle passive motion immediately
- Active and active-assisted motion and isometric exercises are started at 4 weeks postoperatively.
- Periscapular strengthening starts at 8 weeks postoperatively.

OUTCOMES

- No large series of arthroscopic treatment have been published.
- Several smaller series have reported favorable outcomes after arthroscopic surgery.[2,3]

COMPLICATIONS

- Pneumothorax
- Infection
- Inadequate resection, recurrence of symptoms

ARTHROSCOPIC PORTALS

- The initial "safe" portal is 2 cm medial to the medial scapular edge at the level of the scapular spine, between the chest wall and serratus anterior (**TECH FIG 1A**).
  - Avoids dorsal scapular nerve and artery
  - The space is distended with 150 mL saline via spinal needle and then the portal is created.
- After insertion of a 4.0-mm 30-degree arthroscope into the first portal, a second "working" portal is established under direct visualization (**TECH FIGS 1B and 1D**).
  - It is placed about 4 cm inferior to the first portal.
  - A 6-mm cannula is inserted into this portal.
- An additional superior portal can be placed as described by Chan et al[1] (**TECH FIG 1C**).
  - Portals superior to the scapular spine place the dorsal scapular neurovascular structures, accessory spinal nerve, and transverse cervical artery at risk, however.

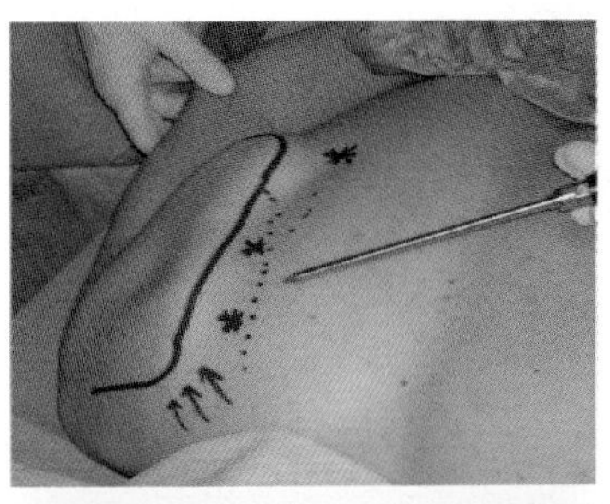
A

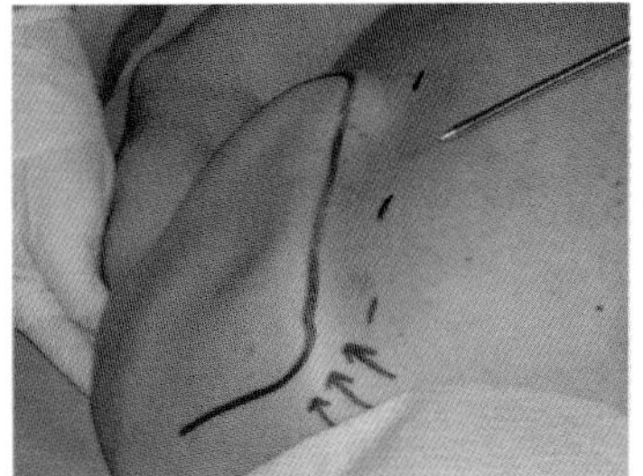
B

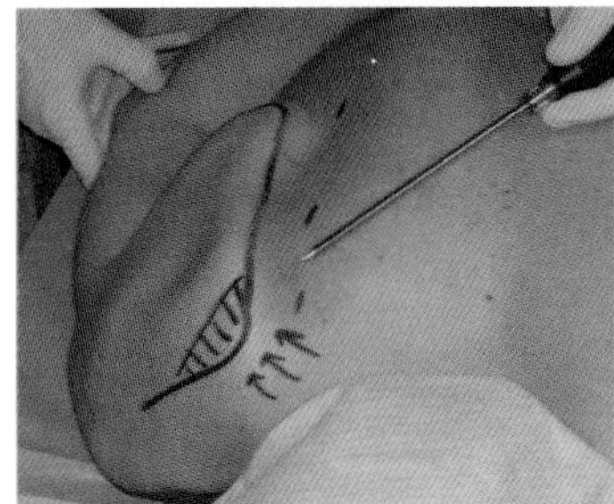
C

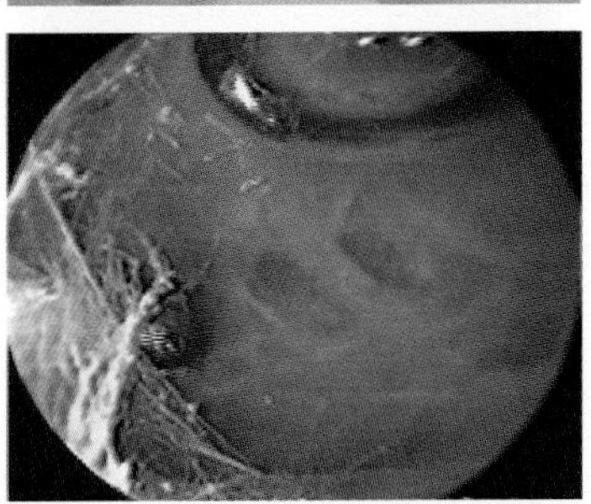
D

TECH FIG 1 • Placement of the first arthroscopic portal (**A**), the second "working" arthroscopic portal (**B**), and the optional superior portal (**C**). **D.** Arthroscopic view from the first portal.

TECHNIQUES

RESECTION

- A methodical approach to resection is needed because there are minimal anatomic landmarks.
- Radiofrequency ablation and motorized shaving are used (TECH FIG 2A,B).
- The surgeon proceeds medial to lateral and inferior to superior.
- Spinal needles can be used to outline the medial border of the scapula (TECH FIG 2C,D).
- Switching portals and the use of a 70-degree arthroscope may be necessary (TECH FIG 2E,F).
- The superomedial angle of the scapula is identified by palpation through the skin.
- Radiofrequency is used to detach the conjoined insertion of the rhomboids, levator scapulae, and supraspinatus from the bone.
- A partial scapulectomy is performed using a motorized shaver and burr.
- The arm should then be placed through a range of motion to assess the resection.

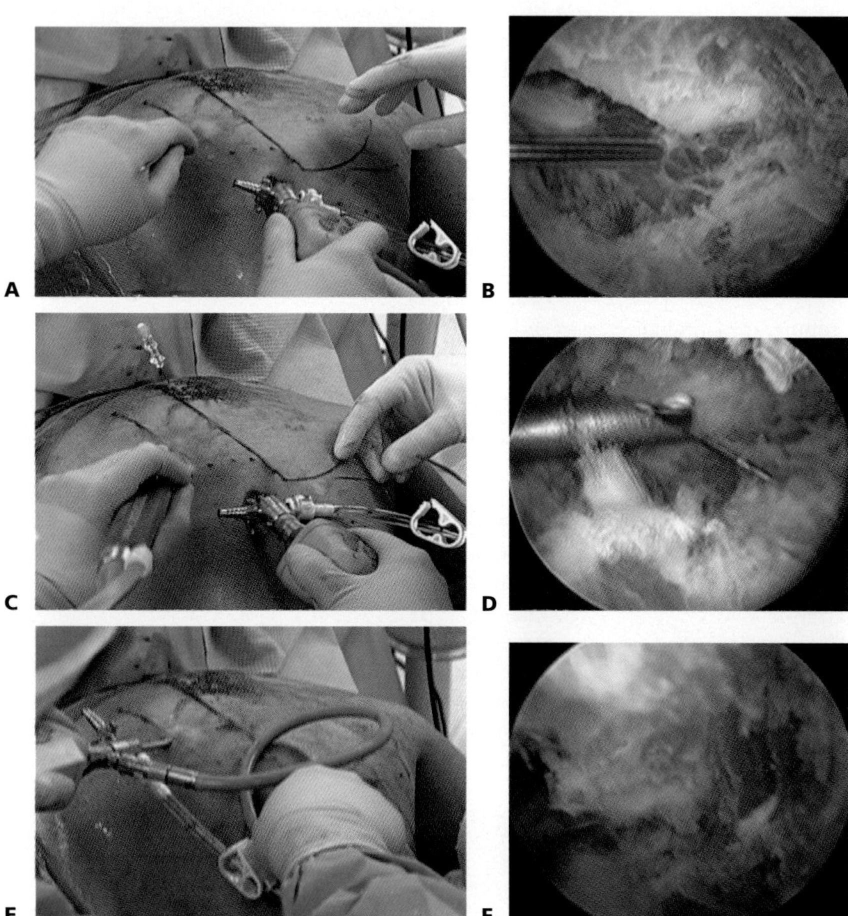

TECH FIG 2 • **A,B.** Resection and débridement of the scapula. **C,D.** The spinal needle is used as a guide to the medial border of the scapula. **E,F.** Final débridement.

PEARLS AND PITFALLS

Portal placement	▪ The surgeon should consider the neurovascular structures and the thoracic structures. ▪ The surgeon should enter parallel to the ribs and use a spinal needle to localize the portals. ▪ More inferiorly placed portals are safer because the dorsal scapular nerve arborizes terminally.
Visualization	▪ Predistention ▪ Epinephrine for vasoconstriction ▪ Appropriate pump pressure ▪ The surgeon should work expeditiously.
Bursectomy	▪ Inadvertent thoracotomy is avoided. ▪ A complete bursectomy is performed. ▪ The surgeon should avoid perforating the subscapularis muscle medially (bleeding).
Partial scapulectomy	▪ Preoperative planning with computed tomography or three-dimensional computed tomography ▪ Anatomy is localized with a spinal needle. ▪ Adequate resection is performed.

REFERENCES

1. Chan BK, Chakrabarti AJ, Bell SN. An alternative portal for scapulothoracic arthroscopy. J Shoulder Elbow Surg 2002;11:235–238.
2. Ciullo J, Jones E. Subscapular bursitis: conservative and endoscopic treatment of "snapping scapula" or "washboard syndrome." Orthop Trans 1993;16:740.
3. Harper GD, McIlroy S, Bayley JI, et al. Arthroscopic partial resection of the scapula for snapping scapula: a new technique. J Shoulder Elbow Surg 1999;8:53–57.
4. Kuhn JE, Plancher KD, Hawkins RJ. Symptomatic scapulothoracic crepitus and bursitis. J Am Acad Orthop Surg 1998;6:267–273.
5. Mauclaire M. Craquements sous-scapulaires pathologiques traits par l'interposition musculaire interscapulothoracique. Bull Mem Soc Chir Paris 1904;30:164–168.
6. Milch H. Partial scapulectomy for snapping of the scapula. J Bone Joint Surg Am 1950;32A:561–566.
7. Nicholson GP, Duckworth MA. Scapulothoracic bursectomy for snapping scapula syndrome. J Shoulder Elbow Surg 2002;11:80–85.
8. Richards RR, McKee MD. Treatment of painful scapulothoracic crepitus by resection of the superomedial angle of the scapula: a report of three cases. Clin Orthop Relat Res 1989;247:111–116.
9. Sisto DJ, Jobe FW. The operative treatment of scapulothoracic bursitis in professional pitchers. Am J Sports Med 1986;14:192–194.

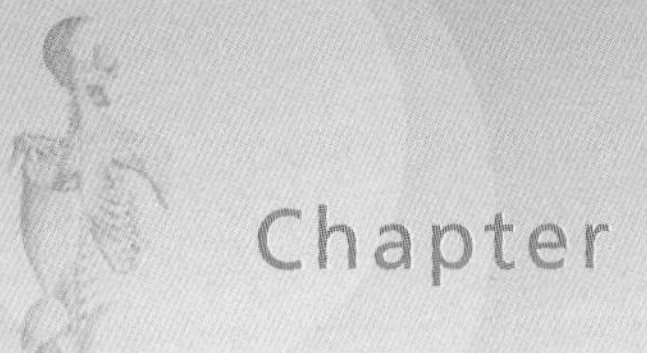

Chapter 17 Arthroscopic Débridement and Glenoidplasty for Shoulder Degenerative Joint Disease

Christian J.H. Veillette and Scott P. Steinmann

DEFINITION

- Osteoarthritis (OA) is a degenerative disorder of synovial joints characterized by focal defects in articular cartilage with reactive involvement in subchondral and marginal bone, synovium, and para-articular structures.[1,10]
- Patients with degenerative joint disease (DJD) of the shoulder often have coexisting pathology, including bursitis, synovitis, loose bodies, labral tears, osteophytes, and articular cartilage defects.[2,3,9]
- Arthroscopic débridement may be a reasonable treatment option in these patients after conservative methods have been unsuccessful and when joint replacement is not desired.
- Historically, patients who have early OA in whom concentric glenohumeral articulation remains with a visible joint space on the axillary radiograph are candidates for arthroscopic débridement.[14]
- Patients with severe glenohumeral arthritis for whom shoulder arthroplasty is not ideal, such as young or middle-aged patients and older patients who subject their shoulders to high loads or impact, remain an unresolved clinical problem and are potential candidates for arthroscopic techniques.
- There are four basic options for arthroscopic treatment in a patient with DJD of the shoulder:
  - Glenohumeral joint débridement
  - Capsular release
  - Subacromial decompression
  - Glenoidplasty
- Choosing which of these four options to perform on a shoulder with DJD depends on the degree of arthritis and the skill, philosophy, and experience of the surgeon.
- The goal of arthroscopic débridement is to provide a period of symptomatic relief rather than reverse or halt the progression of OA.

ANATOMY

- The normal head shaft angle is about 130 degrees, with 30 degrees of retroversion.
- The articular surface area of the humeral head is larger than that of the glenoid, allowing for large normal range of motion.
- Glenoid version, the angle formed between the center of the glenoid and the scapular body, averages 3 degrees and is critical for stability.
- The glenoid fossa provides a shallow socket in which the humeral head articulates. It is composed of the bony glenoid and the glenoid labrum.
- The labrum is a fibrocartilaginous structure surrounding the periphery of the glenoid. The labrum provides a 50% increase in the depth of the concavity and greatly increases the stability of the glenohumeral joint.
- The glenoid had an average depth of 9 mm in the superoinferior direction and 5 mm in the anteroposterior direction with an intact labrum.[6,8]
- Capsuloligamentous structures provide the primary stabilization for the shoulder joint (**FIG 1**).
  - Within this capsule are three distinct thickenings that constitute the superior glenohumeral ligament, middle glenohumeral ligament, and inferior glenohumeral ligament.

PATHOGENESIS

- OA may be classified as primary, when there is no obvious underlying cause, or secondary, when it is preceded by a predisposing disorder.
- Pathology in patients with glenohumeral OA includes a degenerative labrum, loose bodies, osteophytes, and articular cartilage defects in addition to synovitis and soft tissue contractures.
- The disease process in OA of the shoulder parallels that of other joints. Degenerative alterations primarily begin in the articular cartilage as a result of either excessive loading of a healthy joint or relatively normal loading of a previously disturbed joint.[12]
- Progressive asymmetric narrowing of the joint space and fibrillation of the articular cartilage occur with increased cartilage degradation and decreased proteoglycan and collagen synthesis.
- Subchondral sclerosis develops at areas of increased pressure as stresses exceed the yield strength of the bone and the subchondral bone responds with vascular invasion and increased cellularity.

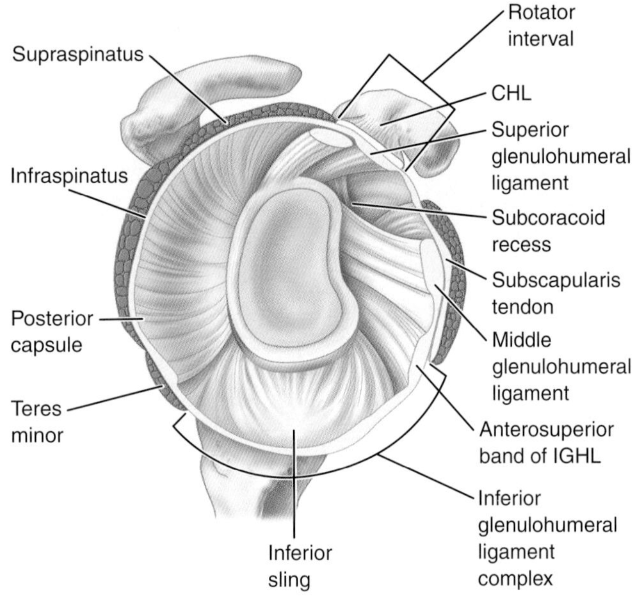

FIG 1 • Glenoid anatomy. The glenoid has an average depth of 9 mm in the superoinferior direction and 5 mm in the AP direction with an intact labrum.

- Cystic degeneration occurs owing to either osseous necrosis secondary to chronic impaction or the intrusion of synovial fluid.
- Osteophyte formation occurs at the articular margin in nonpressure areas by vascularization of subchondral marrow, osseous metaplasia of synovial connective tissue, and ossifying cartilaginous protrusions.
- Fragmentation of these osteophytes or of the articular cartilage itself results in intra-articular loose bodies. In late stages, complete loss of articular cartilage occurs, with subsequent bony erosion.
- Posterior glenoid erosion is predominant, leading to increased retroversion of the glenoid and predisposing to subluxation and reduction of the humeral head, causing symptoms of instability.

NATURAL HISTORY

- Information on the natural history of OA in individuals and its reparative processes is limited.
- Progression of OA is considered generally to be slow (10 to 20 years), with rates varying among joint sites.[10]
- No specific longitudinal studies exist on the progression of shoulder OA.

PATIENT HISTORY AND PHYSICAL FINDINGS

- Typical history for patients with OA is progressive pain with activity over time.
- In early stages, pain is related to strenuous or exertional activities but over time it progresses to activities of daily living. In later stages, pain occurs at rest and at night.
- Pain may be mistaken for impingement syndrome early in the disease process or rotator cuff disease when symptoms occur in the presence of good motion.
- Progression of the disease often leads to secondary capsular and muscular contractures with loss of active and passive motion.
- Mechanical symptoms such as catching and grinding are often reported with use of the shoulder.
- The pain of shoulder OA can be divided into three types:
  - Pain at extremes of motion: due to osteophytes and stretching of the inflamed capsule and synovium
  - Pain at rest: due to synovitis (pain at night is not the same as pain at rest and may be due to awkward positions or increased pressure)
  - Pain in the mid-arc of motion: usually associated with crepitus and represents articular surface damage
- Physical examination should include the following:
  - Range of motion: Loss of both active and passive motion consistent with soft tissue contractures. In patients with preserved passive motion but loss of active motion, rotatory cuff pathology should be ruled out.
  - Compression–rotation test: Pain during mid-arc of motion is a potentially poor prognostic indication.
  - Neer test and Hawkins test: Often patients with OA have positive impingement signs related to articular lesions in the glenohumeral joint or to the synovitis in the joint and subacromial pathology.
  - Supraspinatus evaluation: Weakness may reflect associated supraspinatus tear. Patients with OA may have weakness related to pain inhibition on resistance.
  - Infraspinatus and teres minor evaluation: Weakness may reflect associated posterior rotator cuff tear. Patients with OA may have weakness related to pain inhibition on resistance.
  - Subscapularis evaluation: Weakness may reflect associated subscapularis tear. Patients with OA may have weakness related to pain inhibition on resistance.

IMAGING AND OTHER DIAGNOSTIC STUDIES

- A standard shoulder series consisting of a true anteroposterior view in the scapular plane, a scapular lateral view, and an axillary view should be obtained on all patients before surgical intervention (**FIG 2A,B**).
  - Classic findings of glenohumeral OA are joint space narrowing, subchondral sclerosis, subchondral cysts, and osteophyte formation.
  - Posterior wear of the glenoid is often noted on the axillary view in later stages of the disease.
- Magnetic resonance imaging (MRI) is more sensitive for the diagnosis of early-stage OA than are plain radiographs and can identify concurrent soft tissue pathology.
- Up to 45% of patients with grade IV chondral lesions can have no radiographic (MRI or plain radiograph) evidence of OA on preoperative imaging.[2,13]
- Computed tomography (CT) scanning provides improved visualization of the bony glenoid, osteophytes, and loose bodies (**FIG 2C**).
  - Three-dimensional reconstructions provide an excellent visual representation of the biconcave glenoid to assist in preoperative planning (**FIG 2D**).

DIFFERENTIAL DIAGNOSIS

- Impingement syndrome
- Adhesive capsulitis
- Superior labral anterior to posterior (SLAP) lesions
- Rotator cuff tears
- Instability

NONOPERATIVE MANAGEMENT

- Standard nonoperative modalities, such as nonsteroidal anti-inflammatory medications, steroid injections, and physical therapy, should be explored before arthroscopic techniques.

SURGICAL MANAGEMENT

- Current indications for arthroscopic osteocapsular arthroplasty and glenoidplasty are patients with the following:
  - Moderate to severe glenohumeral OA
  - A biconcave glenoid
  - Moderate to severe pain causing functional impairment that has failed to respond to nonsurgical treatment
  - Painless crepitus with glenohumeral motion during joint compression
- Patient must have a relative contraindication to total shoulder arthroplasty such as age younger than 50 years, excessive physical demands, or unwillingness to consider shoulder replacement.
- Age and prior successful total shoulder arthroplasty on the contralateral shoulder are not contraindications.

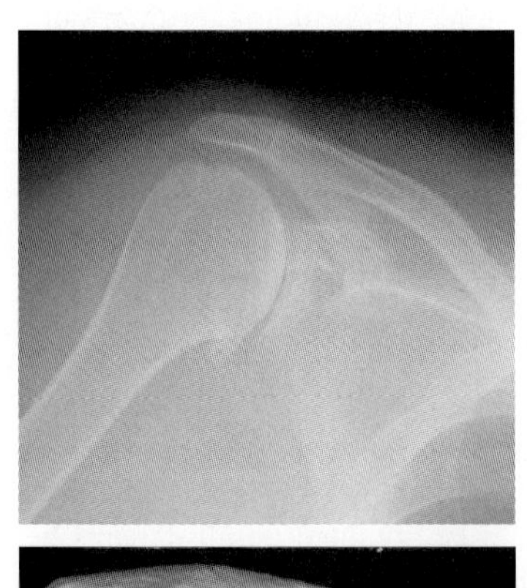

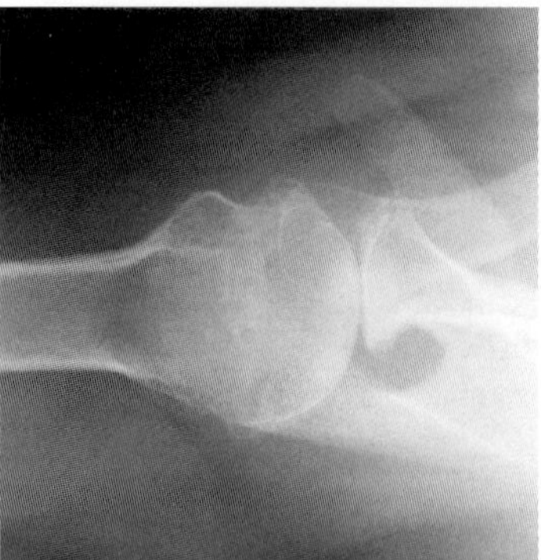

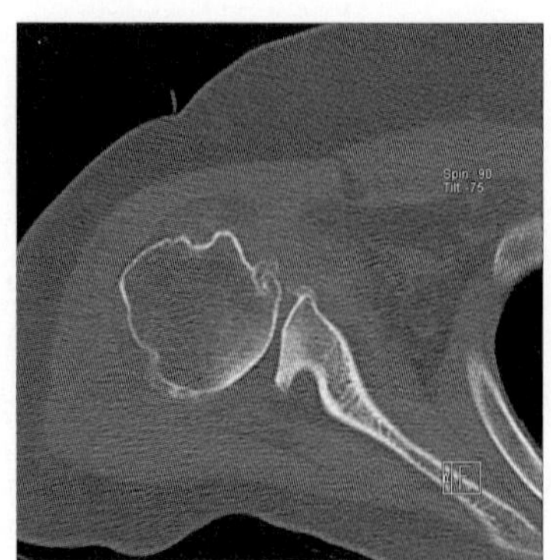

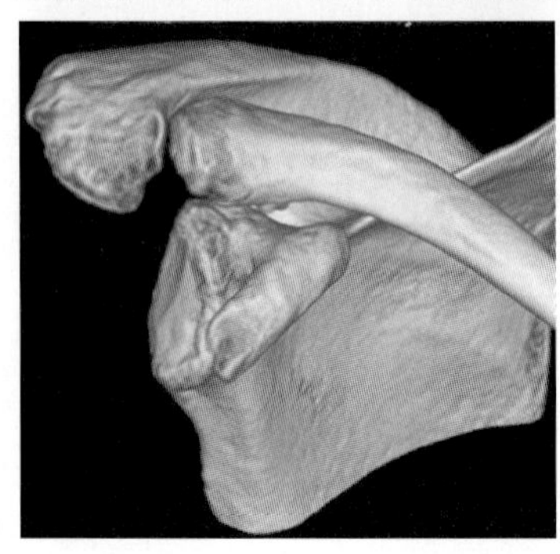

FIG 2 • **A.** AP radiograph shows loss of joint space, subchondral sclerosis, and hypertrophic changes with early inferior osteophyte formation. **B.** Axillary lateral radiograph reveals complete loss of joint space with typical posterior glenoid wear and static posterior subluxation of the humeral head. **C.** Two-dimensional computed tomography scan shows loss of articular cartilage, subchondral sclerosis, osteophytes, and posterior glenoid erosion with static posterior subluxation of humeral head. **D.** Three-dimensional reconstruction view shows biconcave glenoid with humerus subtracted from view as would be anticipated from an anterosuperior arthroscopic portal. These views allow the glenoid and humerus to be rotated to understand exact location of pathology to be seen from different arthroscopic working portals.

- Glenoidplasty is performed if there is a biconcave glenoid from posterior wear and involves recontouring the surface to recreate a single concavity.
  - The rationale is to restore the position of the humeral head, thus reducing posterior subluxation, increasing the surface area of articulation, decreasing joint pressure, and relaxing the anterior soft tissues.
- Subacromial decompression preoperative examination and intraoperative arthroscopic findings implicate the subacromial space as source of pain.
  - A thickened bursa consistent with chronic bursitis has been documented, and several authors advocate a soft tissue decompression, at a minimum.[3,15]
  - Bleeding from the undersurface of the acromion may lead to subacromial fibrosis and loss of motion. Therefore, routine subacromial decompression is not recommended.

Preoperative Planning

- The surgeon should review high-quality radiographs, especially the axillary view if glenoidplasty will be performed, to plan the increase in depth of the glenoid required to convert the biconcave glenoid back to a single concavity.
- The surgeon examines the range of motion under anesthesia and compares it to the opposite side.

Positioning

- The patient is placed in the beach-chair or lateral decubitus position after regional anesthesia (interscalene block) or general anesthesia is obtained.
  - Unobstructed access to the anterior and posterior aspects of the shoulder is imperative (**FIG 3**).
- A potential disadvantage of the lateral decubitus position is the need to take the arm out of traction periodically to check the range of motion after capsular resection.
- If working in the area of the axillary nerve, the semi-abducted position used in the lateral decubitus position tends to bring the axillary nerve closer to the capsule.

Approach

- A standard midposterior arthroscopic portal is established in usual fashion.
- A standard anterior portal is made using an 18-gauge spinal needle under direct arthroscopic vision to locate the position in the rotator interval.
- Additional portals that are often required include a midlevel anterior portal (adjacent to the superior border of the subscapularis) for osteophyte removal and a posteromedial portal for placement of a retractor to clear the axillary pouch from the humeral head and neck.
- It is helpful to place both the posterior and anterior portals a bit more inferior than usual to allow easier access to the inferior aspect of the joint.

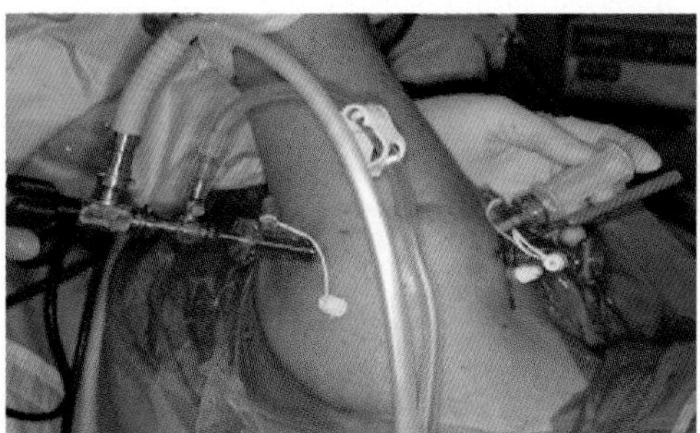

FIG 3 • Patient placed in the lateral decubitus position.

DIAGNOSTIC ARTHROSCOPY

- A standard 15-point assessment of the arthroscopic glenohumeral anatomy as outlined by Snyder[11] is performed.
- Typical findings include extensive synovitis, especially on the undersurface of the rotator cuff, fraying of the labrum, and fibrillation or loss of articular cartilage.

SYNOVECTOMY AND DÉBRIDEMENT

- A complete systematic synovectomy is performed using a combination of an arthroscopic thermal device to minimize bleeding and a full-radius shaver (4.8 or 5.5 mm).
  - The surgeon begins by removing synovium from the anterosuperior aspect of the joint, moving posteriorly and then inferiorly into the axillary recess and finally the posterior inferior synovium.
  - A full-radius shaver is used to débride the fraying labrum and remove loose bodies and unstable chondral flaps.

INFERIOR OSTEOPHYTE EXCISION

- The surgeon removes impinging osteophytes, especially any inferior osteophyte from the humeral head, and performs appropriate capsular or interval releases to regain passive motion.
  - An efficient way to visualize and remove inferior osteophytes is to view from the anterior portal using a standard 30-degree arthroscope and then establish a posterior inferior working portal. The shaver or burr can then be brought in posteriorly to remove capsule or osteophytes.
  - The inferior humeral osteophyte is removed first through the posterior inferior working portal using a 4.0-mm hooded burr (which protects the inferior capsule and the axillary nerve) beginning posteriorly and moving anteriorly.
  - The humerus can be internally rotated to deliver the osteophyte and improve positioning of the instrument.

CAPSULECTOMY AND RELEASE

- The inferior capsular attachment to the humeral head should be identified and used as a landmark to recreate the normal architecture of the humerus.
  - A 5.5-mm full-radius shaver is useful to débride any loose bony fragments and soft tissues from the burr.
  - Suction on the instruments should be avoided to decrease the likelihood of unintentional damage to the axillary nerve from soft tissue drawn into the instrument.
  - A curved curette may be required to reach around and remove the anterior aspect of the inferior osteophyte.
  - Fine contouring may be done with the shaver or hand rasps as necessary.
- Working space in the inferior axillary pouch is markedly increased after removal of the inferior osteophyte and permits improved visibility of the inferior capsule and safer performance of partial capsulectomy.
- A full-radius shaver is placed through the posterior portal and used to create a capsulotomy in the posterior aspect of the inferior capsule (in the right shoulder at the 7 o'clock position) adjacent to the glenoid rim.
- The plane between the inferior capsule and underlying soft tissues is then developed with a wide duck-billed basket punch moving from a posterior to an anterior direction. The shaver is then used to widen the resection.
- The capsulectomy should be performed as close to the glenoid rim as possible to minimize the risk to the axillary nerve, which should be identified and protected with a probe after the 6 o'clock position is reached.
- A partial capsulectomy is then performed anteriorly, anterior osteophytes are removed, and the capsule is removed from the rotator interval (**TECH FIG 1**).

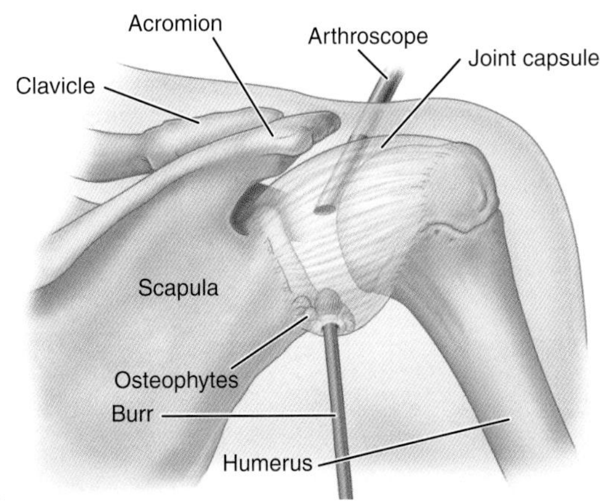

TECH FIG 1 • Osteocapsular arthroplasty. Osteophyte removal is usually best done before resection of the capsule and primarily involves working in the inferior aspect of the glenohumeral joint. **A.** Inferior osteophytes are best viewed from the anterior portal using a standard 30-degree arthroscope, and then the shaver or burr can be brought in from a posterior inferior working portal to remove capsule or osteophytes. *(continued)*

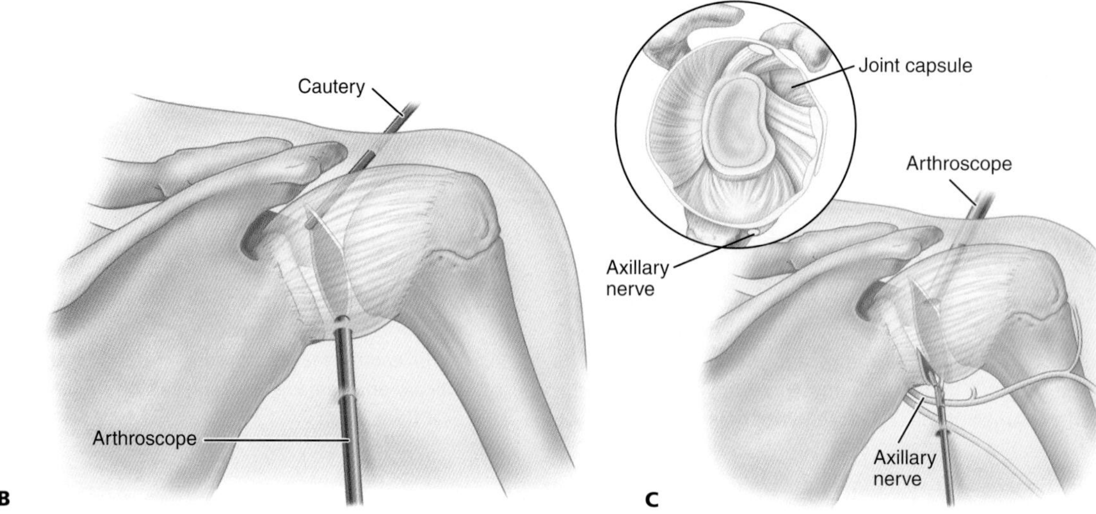

TECH FIG 1 • *(continued)* **B.** Anterior capsulectomy is done viewing from a posterior portal and using an anterior portal to direct a cautery–radiofrequency device or a shaver to release the anterior capsule from the anterior glenoid surface. **C.** Inferior capsulectomy is performed viewing from the anterior portal, and a duck-billed resector is brought into the joint from posterior to remove the inferior capsule.

  - This can be done viewing from a posterior portal and using an anterior portal to direct a cautery–radiofrequency device or a shaver to release the anterior capsule from the anterior glenoid surface.
- Any residual anteroinferior capsule can be resected from the anterior portal to connect with the inferior capsulectomy.
- The direct posterior capsule is not generally removed, just as it is not typically resected during a total shoulder replacement. The posterior capsule is often lax from the posterior subluxation and posterior glenoid wear seen in osteoarthritis.

GLENOIDPLASTY

- Anterior and posterior portals are used to perform the procedure, and the biconcave shape of the glenoid can best be visualized by looking inferiorly from the anterior portal (TECH FIG 2A).
- A full-radius shaver is used to remove the remaining cartilage from the anterior glenoid facet (TECH FIG 2B).
- The central vertical bony ridge is then removed using a 4-mm round burr moving from anterior to posterior in a superior to inferior direction.
- The glenoid is divided into quarters and the superior half is contoured first to allow comparison with the prior biconcave glenoid (TECH FIG 2C).
- The view of the glenoid can be alternated from front to back, and once a single concave surface has been established, a large hemispherical hand rasp can be used to deepen and smooth the surface (TECH FIG 2D).
- The glenoidplasty is assessed intraoperatively by performing a compression–rotation test and palpating for crepitus and assessing the rotation of the humerus on the new glenoid surface arthroscopically.

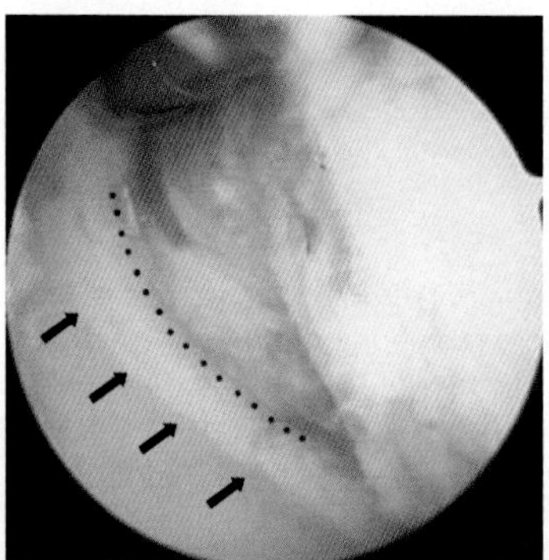

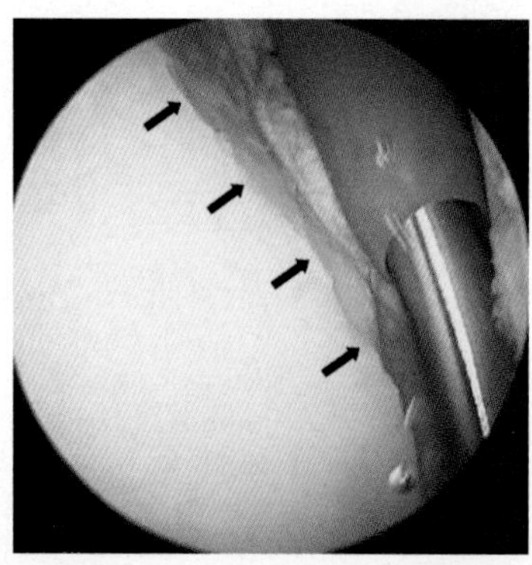

TECH FIG 2 • Arthroscopic images of glenoid with posterior erosion prior to glenoidplasty (**A**) and after removal of anterior cartilage from glenoid (**B**). A bony central ridge separates the anterior and posterior aspects of the glenoid. *(continued)*

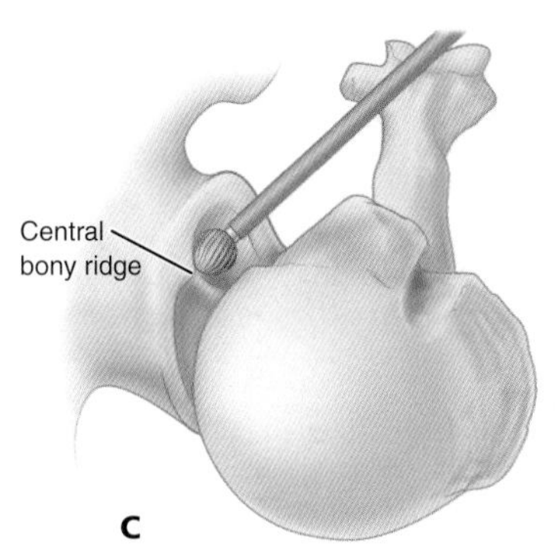

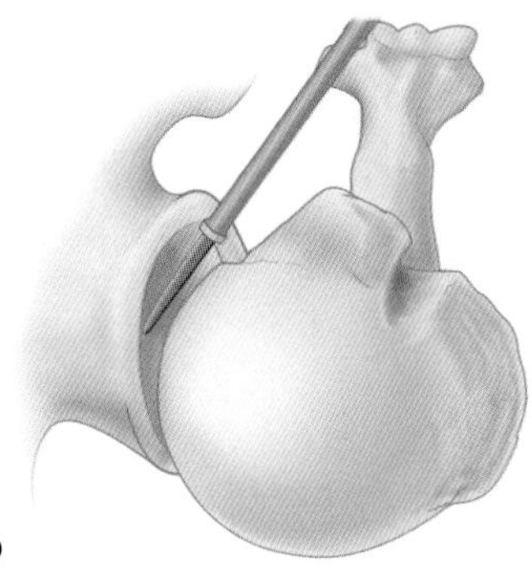

TECH FIG 2 *(continued)* **C,D.** Glenoidplasty is performed with an anterior and a posterior portal. **C.** With the surgeon alternating viewing from the front and the back, the remaining cartilage is first removed from the anterior glenoid facet and then the central vertical bony ridge is resected. A round 4-mm burr is usually sufficient to accomplish this task. **D.** Once a single concave surface is established, a large rasp can be used to smooth the surface.

SUBACROMIAL DECOMPRESSION

- Using standard portals to explore the subacromial space, a shaver or cautery–radiofrequency probe is placed above the rotator cuff, and any thickened bursa is removed.
- Bursal-sided fraying or tearing of the rotator cuff can also be addressed at the same time.
- There is usually no need to perform an acromioplasty, but if a minor spur of the acromion is encountered it can be resected. The corocoacromial ligament should be preserved.

PEARLS AND PITFALLS

Indications	■ Moderate to severe glenohumeral osteoarthritis ■ Painless crepitus during glenohumeral motion in the midrange with joint compression ■ Age younger than 50 years or heavy physical demands on the shoulder
Preoperative planning	■ Computed tomography scan with three-dimensional reconstructions to visualize biconcave glenoid from anticipated arthroscopic views
Débridement	■ Complete, systematic synovectomy with removal of all traces of synovitis ■ Thermal ablation device is helpful for removal of synovitis and simultaneous control of bleeding. ■ Removal of inferior osteophyte on humeral head greatly increases working space for inferior capsulectomy. ■ Anterior capsulectomy is performed with arthroscope posterior and instruments anterior. ■ Inferior capsulectomy is performed with arthroscope anterior and instruments posterior. ■ Capsulectomy should be performed as close to the glenoid rim as possible to minimize the risk to the axillary nerve.
Glenoidplasty	■ The surgeon removes anterior cartilage and defines the central bony ridge. ■ Glenoid is divided into four quadrants. Glenoidplasty starts on the inferior half to allow comparison with the biconcave glenoid. ■ Assistant must translate the humeral head posteriorly when working on the anterior aspect of the glenoid, and vice versa when working posteriorly. ■ A curved hand rasp is used to fine-tune the glenoid contour.

POSTOPERATIVE CARE

- Full, unrestricted passive and active assisted range of motion is initiated on the first postoperative day.
- Patients with an osteocapsular arthroplasty and glenoidplasty have an indwelling glenohumeral catheter for postoperative analgesia and stay in the hospital overnight.
- Most patients benefit from a structured therapy program supervised by a trained therapist to encourage full passive and active motion.
- The patient begins isometric strengthening immediately and progresses to isotonic exercises as tolerated.
- Patients should be allowed to go back to work as soon as they are comfortable.

OUTCOMES

- Ellman et al[3] showed the benefit of arthroscopic débridement of the glenohumeral joint in 18 patients who underwent initial shoulder arthroscopy for impingement syndrome but were shown at operation to have coexisting glenohumeral DJD that was not evident on preoperative clinical and radiographic evaluation.
- Weinstein et al[14] reported an 80% satisfactory improvement in 25 patients with early OA treated with arthroscopic débridement.
- Cameron et al[2] reported on 61 patients with grade IV chondral lesions of the shoulder treated with arthroscopic débridement with or without capsular release. Overall, 88% of patients had a satisfactory outcome.

- Pain relief is not related to the radiographic stage of arthritis or the location of the lesion. However, return of pain and failure are associated with osteochondral lesions greater than 2 cm in diameter.[2]
- Kelly et al[7] presented the results on 14 patients with a mean age of 50 years treated with osteocapsular arthroplasty and glenoidplasty. Early follow-up at 3 years showed an 86% rate of improvement, and 92% agreed that the surgery was worthwhile. No complications were reported and there was no evidence of medial migration of the humerus.

COMPLICATIONS

- None of the previously published studies on arthroscopic treatment of glenohumeral OA reported complications.
- Ogilvie-Harris and Wiley[9] reported 15 complications in 439 patients (3%) treated with arthroscopic surgery of the shoulder.
- Medial migration of the humerus after glenoidplasty and inability to perform glenoid resurfacing during total shoulder replacement has not been encountered.

REFERENCES

1. Altman RD. Overview of osteoarthritis. Am J Med 1987;83:65–69.
2. Cameron BD, Galatz LM, Ramsey ML, et al. Non-prosthetic management of grade IV osteochondral lesions of the glenohumeral joint. J Shoulder Elbow Surg 2002;11:25–32.
3. Ellman H, Harris E, Kay SP. Early degenerative joint disease simulating impingement syndrome: arthroscopic findings. Arthroscopy 1992; 8:482–487.
4. Gachter A, Gubler M. Shoulder arthroscopy in degenerative and inflammatory diseases. Orthopade 1992;21:236–240.
5. Gartsman GM, Taverna E. The incidence of glenohumeral joint abnormalities associated with full-thickness, reparable rotator cuff tears. Arthroscopy 1997;13:450–455.
6. Howell SM, Galinat BJ. The glenoid-labral socket: a constrained articular surface. Clin Orthop Relat Res 1989;243:122–125.
7. Kelly E, O'Driscoll SW, Steinmann S. Arthroscopic glenoidplasty and osteocapsular arthroplasty for advanced glenohumeral arthritis. Presented at Annual Open Meeting of the American Shoulder and Elbow Surgeons, 2001.
8. Lazarus MD, Sidles JA, Harryman DT II, et al. Effect of a chondral-labral defect on glenoid concavity and glenohumeral stability: a cadaveric model. J Bone Joint Surg Am 1996;78A:94–102.
9. Ogilvie-Harris DJ, Wiley AM. Arthroscopic surgery of the shoulder: a general appraisal. J Bone Joint Surg Br 1986;68:201–207.
10. Rottensten K. Monograph Series on Aging-Related Diseases IX: Osteoarthritis. Chron Dis Can 1996;17:92–107.
11. Snyder SJ, Waldherr P. Shoulder arthroscopy techniques: 15-point arthroscopic anatomy. Orthopaedic Knowledge Online. April 7, 2004. Available at: http://www5.aaos.org/oko/shoulder_elbow/arthroscopy/anatomy/anatomy.cfm. Accessed October 30, 2006.
12. Stacy GS, Basu PA. Primary osteoarthritis. eMedicine. Available at: http://www.emedicine.com/radio/topic492.htm. Accessed October 30, 2006.
13. Umans HR, Pavlov H, Berkowitz M, et al. Correlation of radiographic and arthroscopic findings with rotator cuff tears and degenerative joint disease. J Shoulder Elbow Surg 2001;10:428–433.
14. Weinstein DM, Bucchieri JS, Pollock RG, et al. Arthroscopic debridement of the shoulder for osteoarthritis. Arthroscopy 2000;16:471–476.
15. Witwity T, Uhlmann R, Nagy MH, et al. Shoulder rheumatoid arthritis associated with chondromatosis, treated by arthroscopy. Arthroscopy 1991;7:233.

Chapter 18 Elbow Arthroscopy: The Basics

John E. Conway

DEFINITION

- Elbow arthroscopy involves the use of an arthroscope to examine the interior of the elbow joint and provides the opportunity to perform minimally invasive diagnostic and therapeutic procedures.
- Elbow arthroscopy has evolved to allow the definitive care of more than a dozen complex elbow conditions.
- Despite an expanded understanding of the surrounding neurovascular anatomy, essential portal placement for access to the elbow joint continues to present a level of risk for injury that exceeds that seen in other joints.[4,6,7,13]
- The safe application of this treatment modality requires that the surgeon have a solid grasp of the relative anatomy, fellowship or laboratory training in treatment techniques, experience as an arthroscopist, and an objective assessment of his or her own level of skill.

ANATOMY

- Neurovascular injury risk is relatively high and a three-dimensional grasp of elbow anatomy is essential for safe and successful elbow arthroscopy (**FIG 1**).[1,3,5–8,10–12,14]
- Miller et al[8] showed that the bone-to-nerve distances in the 90-degree-flexed elbow increased with joint insufflation an average of 12 mm for the median nerve, 6 mm for the radial nerve, and 1 mm for the ulnar nerve.
  - The capsule-to-nerve distance changes very little with insufflation, however, and the protective effect of insufflation is lost when the elbow is in extension.
- Miller et al[8] also showed that in the insufflated, 90-degree-flexed elbow, both the radial and median nerves passed within 6 mm of the joint capsule and that the radial nerve was on average 3 mm closer to the capsule than the median nerve. The ulnar nerve was essentially on the capsule.
  - Others have also shown the close proximity of the radial nerve to the joint capsule and stressed the greater risk to this nerve during both portal placement and capsular resection.[2,3,6,8,12]
- Stothers et al[11] emphasized the importance of elbow flexion during portal placement and showed that the portal-to-nerve distances decreased an average of 3.5 to 5.1 mm laterally and 1.4 to 5.6 mm medially when the elbow was in extension.
  - For the distal anterolateral portal, the distance from the sheath to the radial nerve averaged 1.4 mm (range 0 to 4 mm) in extension and 4.9 mm (2 to 10 mm) in flexion.
- Field et al[3] compared three anterolateral portals and reported a statistically significant difference in portal-to-radial nerve distance, with greater safety shown with the more proximal locations.
- Anatomic studies suggest three guidelines for neurovascular safety:
  - Portal placement is safer when the elbow is flexed 90 degrees than when it is in extension.[11]
  - Maximal joint distention before portal placement increases the safety during placement by increasing the nerve-to-portal distance.[3,5,6,11]

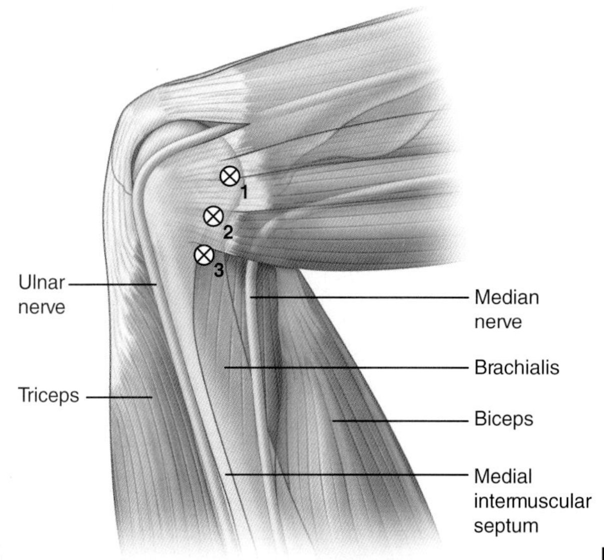

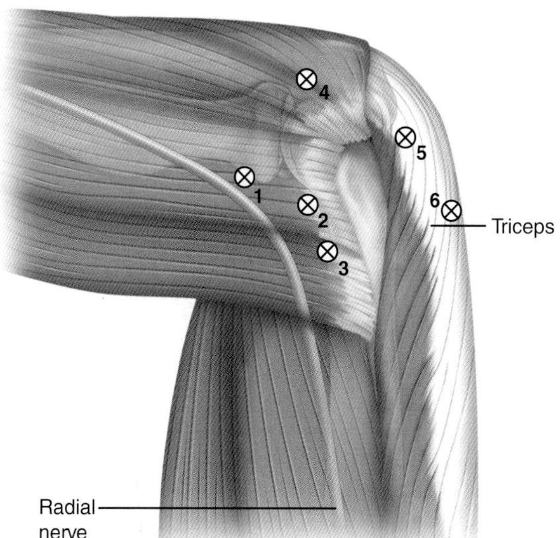

FIG 1 • **A.** Relative anatomy of the medial elbow and the arthroscopic portal sites: *1*, standard anteromedial; *2*, mid-anteromedial; and *3*, proximal anteromedial. **B.** Relative anatomy of the lateral and posterior elbow and the arthroscopic portal sites: *1*, distal anterolateral; *2*, mid-anterolateral; *3*, proximal anterolateral; *4*, direct posterolateral; *5*, posterolateral; and 6, posterior central.

- The nerve-to-portal distance is greater for the more proximal anterior portals than for the more distal anterior portals.

PATIENT HISTORY AND PHYSICAL FINDINGS

- This chapter does not address a specific condition but instead offers a broad view of the basic considerations and setup issues for a surgical treatment that may be applied to many different elbow problems.
- A complete review of the numerous clinical tests described for the diagnostic evaluation of the elbow would exceed the scope of this chapter.

IMAGING AND OTHER DIAGNOSTIC STUDIES

- Routine preoperative elbow radiographs should include a true lateral view, a standard anteroposterior (AP) view, and an AP view of both the distal humerus and proximal forearm when joint motion loss prevents full joint extension.
- Additional radiographic views include the cubital tunnel view, the posterior impingement view, the capitellum view, and the radial head view.
  - The cubital tunnel view, an AP projection of the humerus with the elbow maximally flexed, provides a clear view of the medial epicondyle and cubital tunnel groove.
  - The posterior impingement view is also an AP projection of the humerus with the elbow maximally flexed, but the humerus is rotated into 45 degrees of external rotation. This image offers better assessment of the posteromedial edge of the olecranon tip and the medial epicondyle apophysis.
  - The capitellum view, an AP projection of the ulna with the elbow flexed 45 degrees, provides a tangential view of the capitellum for better evaluation of osteochondritis dissecans lesions.
  - The radial head view is an oblique view of the 90-degree-flexed elbow with the beam passing between the ulna and the radial head. It allows for clear imaging of both the radial head and the radial–ulna interval.
- Although this point is sometimes argued, computed tomography is often useful when resection of intra-articular bone is considered as a part of contracture release arthroscopy.
- Magnetic resonance (MR) imaging in a closed high-field magnet with thin-section, optimized, high-spatial-resolution sequences may provide exceptional detail of the structures surrounding the elbow joint; however, MR arthrography, with either saline or gadolinium, will improve the assessment of intra-articular structures such as loose bodies.

SURGICAL MANAGEMENT

- The indications for elbow arthroscopy include the evaluation and treatment of septic arthritis, lateral synovial plica syndrome, systemic inflammatory arthritis, loose bodies, synovitis, osteochondritis dissecans (OCD), degenerative arthritis, posterior impingement, traumatic arthritis, trochlea chondromalacia, arthrofibrosis, lateral epicondylitis, joint contracture, posterolateral rotatory instability, and olecranon bursitis.
- Treatment options for these conditions include diagnostic evaluation, loose body removal, synovial biopsy, partial or complete synovectomy, plica excision, extensor carpi radialis brevis tendon débridement, capsule release, capsulotomy, capsulectomy, exostosis excision, ulnohumeral arthroplasty, contracture release, chondroplasty, microfracture chondroplasty, percutaneous drilling or fixation of OCD lesions, capitellum osteochondral transplantation, radial head excision, internal fixation of fractures, lateral ulnar collateral ligament plication, ulnar nerve decompression, and finally olecranon bursoscopy and bursectomy.
- The relative contraindications for elbow arthroscopy include recent joint or soft tissue infection, developmental changes, previous trauma or surgery that significantly alters the normal neurovascular, bony, or soft tissue anatomy of the elbow, extensive extracapsular heterotopic ossification, complex regional pain syndrome, and conditions that prevent distention of the elbow capsule.
- Previous ulnar nerve transposition usually requires exposure of the ulnar nerve before the creation of an anteromedial portal.

Preoperative Planning

- As with all medical conditions, the importance of the information gained from a careful and complete history and examination for establishing an accurate diagnosis cannot be overemphasized.
- Plain radiographs are also essential, but some authors suggest that computed tomography and MRI offer little in the preoperative assessment.
  - In contrast, the exact location of intra-articular, capsular, and extra-articular bone, the thickness of the joint capsule, the integrity of the cartilage covering an OCD lesion, and the presence of stress fractures or loose bodies unseen on radiographs are a few examples of how additional imaging may direct or modify care.
- The surgeon should consider how associated procedures to be performed in conjunction with the arthroscopy will affect patient positioning and the possible need to reposition during the case.
- Fluoroscopy should be available when drilling, pinning, or internal fixation is considered.
- In addition to standard arthroscopic instrumentation, the preoperative plan should also consider the need for specialized instruments such as retractors and special biters for contracture release surgery and small-fragment-fixation devices for OCD or fracture care.
- Elbow arthroscopy may be done using either general or regional anesthesia.
  - General anesthesia is typically preferred as it allows for complete muscle relaxation. Regional blockade is reserved for contracture release procedures where repeated manipulation and continuous passive motion is planned during the hospitalization.
  - While regional anesthesia may be given before surgery, many surgeons prefer to wait until the status of the neurovascular structures is established in the recovery setting.
  - Indwelling catheter regional anesthesia is described and sometimes recommended for contracture release procedures, but not all centers are comfortable or experienced with these techniques, and repeated regional anesthesia during the hospitalization appears to be equally effective.
  - The use of ultrasound during injection may decrease the morbidity associated with regional anesthesia.

Positioning

- The four patient positions for elbow arthroscopy are the supine cross-body position, the supine suspended position, the lateral decubitus position, and the prone position.
  - While the latter two positions are most popular today, experience with one of the supine positions still offers advantages. For example, a surgeon who prefers the prone position may elect to use the supine cross-body position when arthroscopic and open procedures are combined, preventing the need for repositioning.
- Supine cross-body position
  - Arthroscopy in this position may be done with one of several commercially available arm-holding devices but is performed equally well with an assistant acting as the arm holder (**FIG 2A**).
  - Because the elbow is not rigidly stabilized in this position, complex procedures may be more challenging and present a greater level of risk for injury.
  - The supine cross-body position is most useful when a less demanding arthroscopic procedure is performed along with an open surgery.
- Supine suspended position
  - This position requires the use of a traction device from which the arm is hung. Capture of the hand or wrist is necessary, and finger traps on the index and long fingers work well in this regard (**FIG 2B**).
  - The elbow is not stabilized against either a post or pad, which allows considerable movement of the elbow beneath the hand.
  - Two potential disadvantages of this position are the unexpected withdrawal of the arthroscope from the freely swinging joint and the almost vertical position of the arthroscope during arthroscopy of the posterior compartment.
- Lateral decubitus position
  - This position for elbow arthroscopy is typically set up the same as for shoulder surgery except that the arm is draped across a padded horizontal post attached to the table (**FIG 2C**).
  - The advantage of this position over the supine positions is that a stable platform is created on which the upper arm rests. There is equal access to the anterior and posterior compartments.
  - The advantage of this position over the prone position becomes apparent when management of the airway is at issue. If prone positioning is a concern, such as in patients with a high body mass index or compromised lung volume, the case is probably best done in the lateral decubitus position.
  - One disadvantage of this position is that small patients, such as gymnasts with OCD lesions, are difficult to position lateral and still maintain full access to the arm.

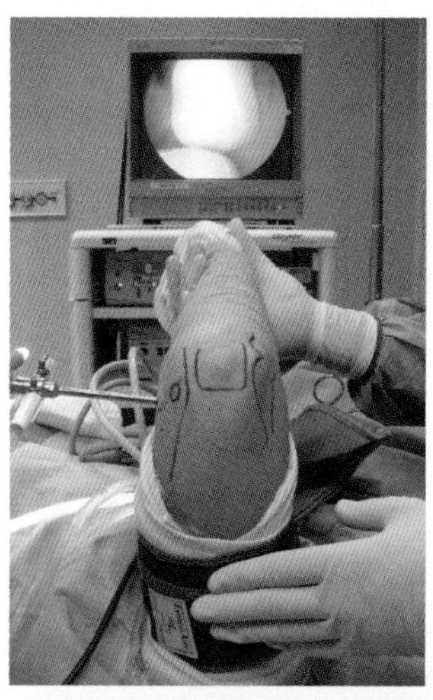
A

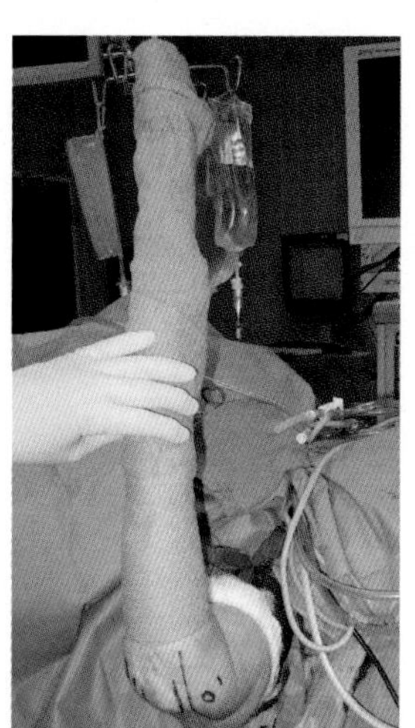
B

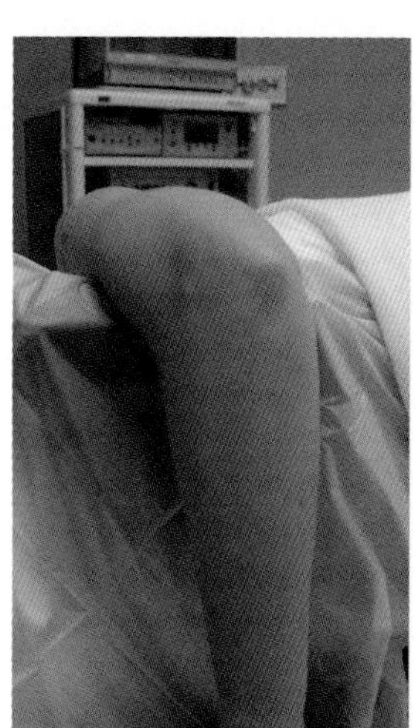
C

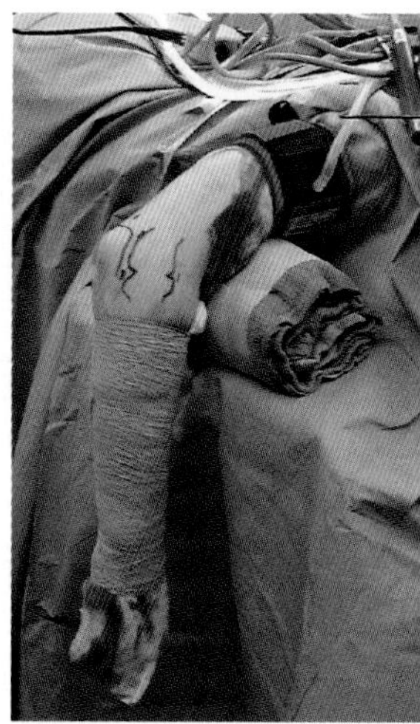
D

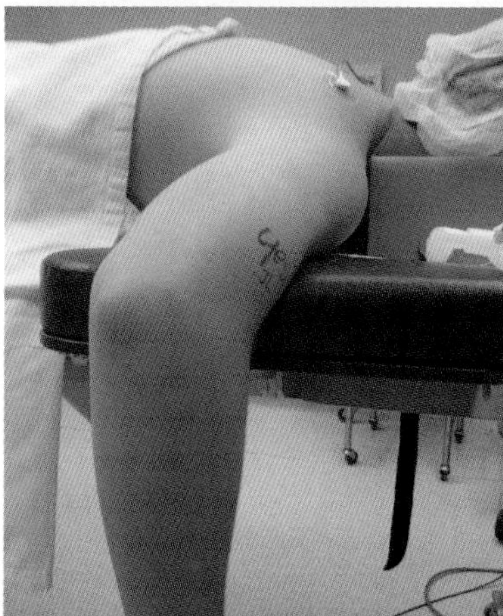
E

FIG 2 • Positioning. **A.** Left elbow draped in the supine cross-body position. An arthroscope is in the proximal anteromedial portal and a loose body is shown on the monitor. **B.** Left elbow draped in the supine suspended position. Sterile towels and elastic wrap are used to cover finger traps attached to the index and long fingers. **C.** Left elbow in the lateral decubitus position. **D.** Right elbow draped in the prone position. A roll of towels is placed between the upper arm and a shortened armboard aligned with the table. **E.** Right elbow draped over a shortened padded armboard.

- Prone position
  - Many surgeons, because of the stability and access provided, prefer the prone position. However, careful attention to positioning is essential to avoiding complications (**FIG 2D**).
  - The airway must be secure and the face should be well padded.
  - Chest rolls are used to lift the chest and abdomen from the table, decreasing the airway pressure required for ventilation.
  - The knees are padded and the feet are elevated.
  - The nonoperative arm is placed on a well-padded arm board, with attention to the ulnar nerve, and the operative arm is allowed to hang over a shortened, padded armboard positioned along the side of the table (**FIG 2E**).
  - Pulses in all four extremities are confirmed.
  - After draping, a small roll of towels is placed beneath the upper arm to align the humerus in the coronal plane of the body and to allow the elbow to flex to 90 degrees.

Approach

- The first arthroscopic portal is anterior except when the entire procedure is accomplished through posterior portals. Occult conditions may exist in the anterior compartment, and a complete diagnostic assessment of the joint requires anterior portals.
- Whether the initial anterior portal should be medial or lateral is debatable but usually determined by surgeon preference and patient diagnosis. Good arguments may be made for either approach.[1,9,13]
- The second anterior portal may then be created with either outside-in or inside-out methods. We prefer to make the medial portal first and then create the lateral portal with an outside-in method.
- Instruments
  - A standard 4.0-mm, 30-degree offset arthroscope may be used for virtually all elbow arthroscopic procedures. On rare occasion, both a 4.0-mm, 70-degree offset arthroscope and a 2.7-mm arthroscope may be helpful. Because it is often necessary to maintain the tip of the arthroscope just a few millimeters through the capsule, an arthroscope sheath without side flow ports is preferred and minimizes fluid extravasation into soft tissues.
  - Essential instruments include an 18-gauge spinal needle, a hemostat, a Wissinger rod, switching rods, and both standard and small mechanical shavers (**FIG 3A,B**).
  - Specialized instruments have recently become available from several sources and include a series of curved and straight arthroscopic retractors, curettes, and osteotomes. Hand biters, designed to resect the anterior capsule more safely, are very useful during contracture release surgery (**FIG 3C**).

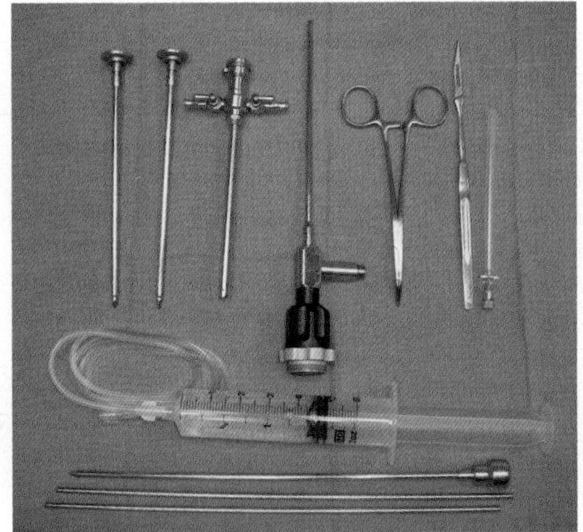
A

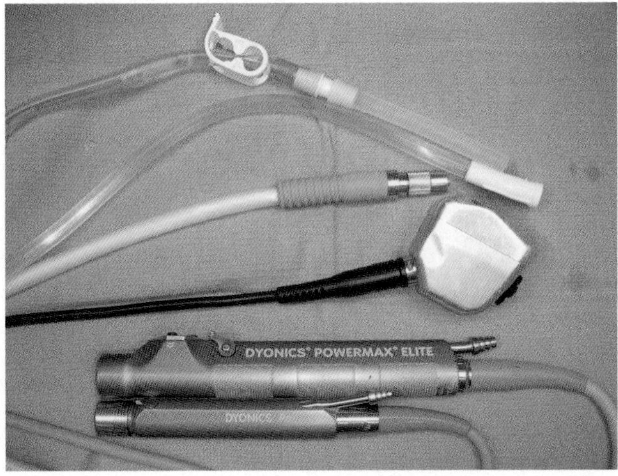

B

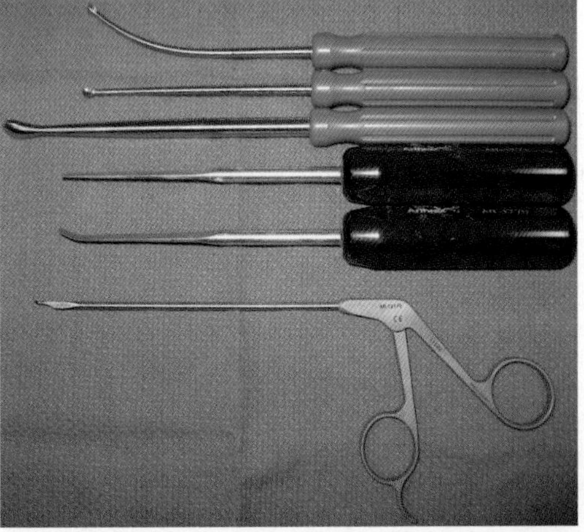
C

FIG 3 • **A,B.** Basic instruments used in elbow arthroscopy. **A.** A standard 4.0-mm, 30-degree offset arthroscope, an arthroscope sheath with sharp and dull trocars, an 18-gauge spinal needle, a 60-cc saline in large syringe with connector tubing, a hemostat, a Wissinger rod, and switching rods. **B.** A standard mechanical shaver, a mini mechanical shaver, an arthroscope camera, a light cord, inflow tubing, and suction tubing. **C.** Specialized instruments for elbow arthroscopy: a hand biter and curved and straight arthroscopic retractors, curettes, awls, and osteotomes.

LIMB PREPARATION

- Setup and portal positions are shown in the supine cross-body position.
- After the administration of general anesthesia, the operative-arm shoulder is relocated to extend just over the edge of the surgical table, affording access to the whole extremity and limiting the reach required for the surgeon.
  - Both the shoulder and the entire arm are prepared and draped and a sterile tourniquet is applied as proximally as possible.
- After limb exsanguination, the tourniquet is elevated and an elastic compression wrap is applied tightly to the forearm, extending from distal to proximal and ending just distal to the radial head.
  - The elastic wrap will limit fluid extravasation into the subcutaneous tissues and the muscle compartments of the forearm and potentially decrease the risk of compartment syndrome.
- Landmarks about the elbow and the proposed arthroscopic portal sites are marked.
- Before portal placement, the joint is distended with saline using an 18-gauge spinal needle passed through the posterolateral "soft spot" (**TECH FIG 1**).
  - The "soft spot" is located at the center of the triangle formed by the olecranon prominence, the lateral epicondyle prominence, and the lateral margin of the radial head.
- Connector tubing attached to a 60-mL syringe allows an assistant to maintain joint distention during the creation of the initial portal without obstructing the surgeon's access.

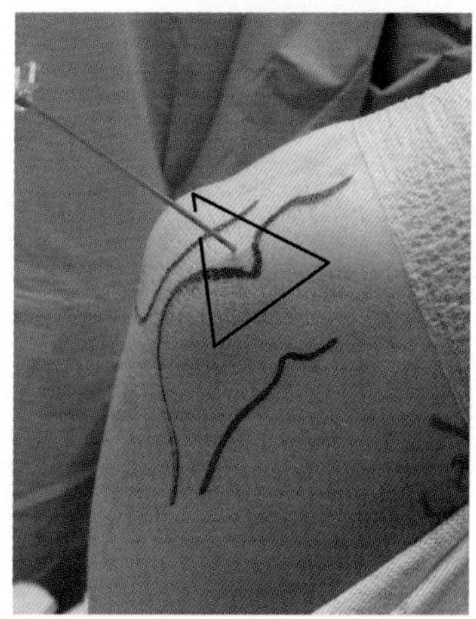

TECH FIG 1 • Left elbow joint in the supine cross-body position being inflated with saline through the posterolateral "soft spot" with an 18-gauge spinal needle. The "soft spot" is found at the center of a triangle formed by the olecranon tip, the lateral epicondyle prominence, and the lateral margin of the radial head.

Order of Portal Placement

- Anterior or posterior
  - Neurovascular risk is the most important factor to be considered when determining the order of portal placement.
  - Soft tissue swelling and loss of the capacity to distend the joint would be expected after the creation of the posterior portals and would place both the median and radial nerves closer to the path of the anterior portals.
  - Most surgeons choose to begin the arthroscopy with the anterior portals.
- Medial or lateral
  - The order is usually determined by surgeon preference and the nature of the conditions requiring treatment.
  - The sheath-to-nerve distance for the mid-anteromedial portal averages 23 mm,[5] that for the distal anterolateral portal averages 3 mm,[5] and that for the proximal anterolateral portal averages 14.2 mm.[3]
  - Because the nerve-to-sheath distance is greater for the anteromedial portals than for the anterolateral portals, it has been argued that the initial approach to the joint is safer when medial.
- Once the medial portal is established, the lateral portal can be made with an outside-in technique and an 18-gauge spinal needle[11,12] or with an inside-out technique and a Wissinger rod.[5]
  - Both methods are relatively safe techniques, but the outside-in method affords greater control of the angle into the joint and potentially greater access to the anterior humerus.

ANTEROMEDIAL PORTALS

- There are three commonly described anteromedial portals: standard, mid, and proximal (**TECH FIG 2A**).
- The nerve at greatest risk for injury is the medial antebrachial cutaneous nerve. This risk diminishes when the depth of the portal incision avoids cutting the subcutaneous tissues.[6]
- Dissection to the flexor fascia with a blunt-tipped hemostat allows mobilization of the cutaneous nerves away from the portal for additional protection.
  - Up to six branches are described crossing the medial elbow, and on average at least one branch is within 1 mm (range 0 to 5 mm) of the portal (**TECH FIG 2B**).
- Both the median nerve and the brachial artery are also at risk during medial portal placement.
  - Continuing the hemostat dissection to the medial joint capsule (**TECH FIG 2C**), introducing the arthroscope sheath with a blunt trocar, and finally penetrating the capsule with a sharp trocar will allow safe medial capsule penetration and avoid extracapsular arthroscope placement.
  - Some authors argue that sharp trocars have no role in elbow arthroscopy; however, blunt trocars are more inclined to penetrate the capsule laterally or, even less desirably, to remain extracapsular. Modifying a sharp trocar by blunting the tip provides a safe and effective compromise.

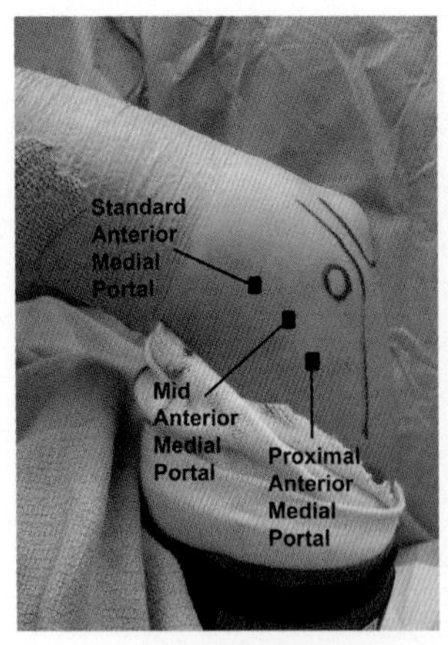

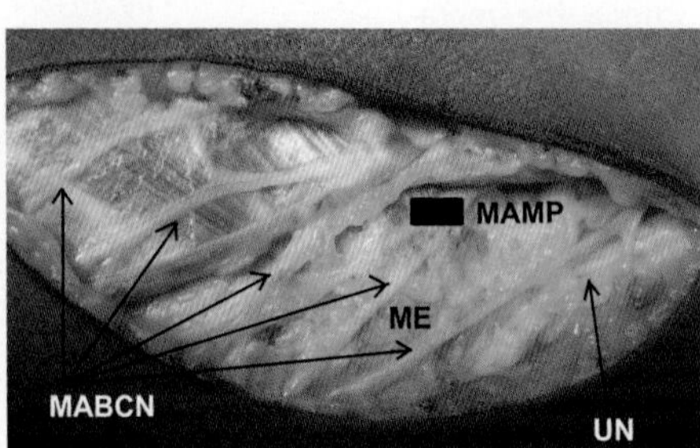

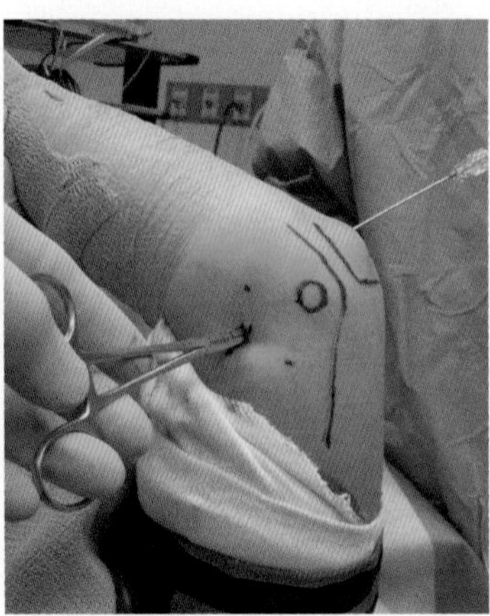

TECH FIG 2 • **A.** Medial surface of the left elbow in the supine cross-body position. Locations of the standard and proximal anteromedial portals are shown. **B.** Medial elbow showing multiple branches of the medial antebrachial cutaneous nerve (*MABCN*). **C.** Anteromedial portal being created with hemostat dissection through the skin, subcutaneous tissues, fascia, and muscle to the medial capsule. *ME*, medial epicondyle; *MAMP*, mid-anteromedial portal; *UN*, ulnar nerve.

Standard Anteromedial Portal

- Andrews and Carson[2] described the standard anteromedial portal as located 2 cm anterior and 2 cm distal to the prominence of the medial epicondyle. They reported that the median nerve-to-sheath distance was 6 mm.
  - The path of the portal penetrates the common flexor origin, as well as the flexor carpi radialis and the pronator muscles.
  - In some patients, the portal also penetrates the medial border of the brachialis muscle.
- Lynch et al[6] showed that with joint distention and 90-degree elbow flexion, this portal averaged 14 mm from the median nerve. However, Stothers et al[11,12] showed that the median nerve-to-sheath distance averaged only 7 mm (range 5 to 13 mm) and that the brachial artery-to-sheath distance was just 15 mm (range 8 to 20 mm).
- The standard anteromedial portal may be created with either medial (outside-in) or lateral (inside-out) methods. Some authors suggest that it is more safely created using the latter method with a rod exchange technique.
- Although this portal offers excellent visualization of the anterolateral contents of the elbow joint, it is now most commonly recommended as an accessory portal for capsular retractors.

Proximal Anteromedial Portal

- The proximal anteromedial portal, popularized by Poehling et al,[10] is described as 2 cm proximal to the prominence of the medial epicondyle and just anterior to the medial intermuscular septum.
  - Others have subsequently described this portal as up to 2 cm anterior to the septum.[9]
- The locations of both the septum and the ulnar nerve must be established before portal placement and the path of the portal must remain anterior to the septum.
- Arthroscope sheath contact with the anterior humerus is advised to further protect the median nerve.[10]
- In this location, at 90 degrees of flexion and with joint distention, the portal averages 12.4 mm (range 7 to 20 mm) from the median nerve, 18 mm from the brachial artery, 12 mm (range 7 to 18 mm) from the ulnar nerve, and 2.3 mm (0 to 9 mm) from the medial antebrachial cutaneous nerves.
- This portal also provides visual access to the lateral elbow joint structures, but viewing the superior capsular structures, the lateral capitellum, and the radiocapitellar joint space is limited compared to the standard anteromedial portal.[11,12]

Mid-Anteromedial Portal

- A modification of the proximal anteromedial portal was described by Lindenfeld[5] as located 1 cm proximal and 1 cm anterior to the prominence to the medial epicondyle.
- The portal is directed distally into the center of the joint to preserve the protection afforded by the proximal location and was shown to average 22 mm from the median nerve.

ANTEROLATERAL PORTALS

- While at less risk for injury than the medial antebrachial cutaneous nerve, the anterior branch of the posterior antebrachial nerve crosses the lateral elbow and may be injured during portal placement. Limiting the depth of the skin incision and using the arthroscope to cast a silhouette of the nerve may provide reasonable protection.
- There are three anterolateral portal locations: distal, mid, and proximal (TECH FIG 3).

Distal Anterolateral Portal

- Andrews and Carson[2] were first to describe an anterolateral portal and recommended placement 3 cm distal and

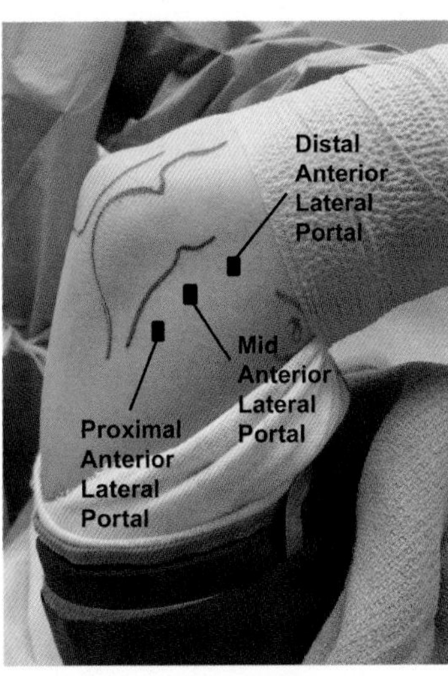

TECH FIG 3 • Lateral surface of the left elbow in the supine cross-body position. Locations of the distal, mid, and proximal anterolateral portals are shown.

1 cm anterior to the prominence of the lateral epicondyle. Their work documented that the radial nerve averaged 7 mm from the arthroscope sheath when the elbow was flexed 90 degrees.

- Others have reported that the nerve-to-sheath distance was less, averaging only 3 to 4.9 mm,[5,11,12] and that in extension this distance was just 1.4 mm.
  - Field et al[3] showed that Andrew and Carson's recommendation located the portal near or directly over the radial head in all specimens studied, and that for smaller patients these measurements would potentially place the portal distal to the radial head.
- To lessen the risk of radial nerve injury, landmarks, rather than measurements, are used to determine that the portal is proximal to the radial head.[3]
- Because of safety concerns, this portal is much less commonly used than the more proximal portals and is typically reserved for a blunt retractor.
- An outside-in method is effective and probably safest.
  - With the elbow at 90 degrees, the forearm in slight pronation, and the joint maximally distended, an 18-gauge spinal needle is placed just anterior to the radial head and directed proximally toward the center of the radiocapitellar joint (TECH FIG 4).
  - A hemostat is then used to dissect through the capsule and a blunt-tipped retractor is introduced to mobilize the anterior capsule.
  - The arthroscope and working instruments are placed in more proximal portals.
- Superficially, the anterior branch of the posterior antebrachial cutaneous nerve was shown to lie on average 7.6 mm (range 0 to 20 mm) from the portal entry and was in contact with the sheath in 43% of elbows studied.[11]

Mid-Anterolateral Portal

- The mid-anterolateral portal is safer and used more commonly than the distal anterolateral portal.

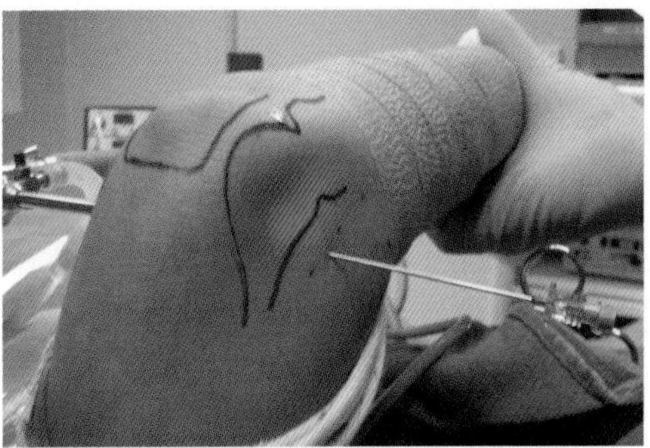

TECH FIG 4 • Lateral surface of the left elbow with a mid-anterolateral portal being created using an outside-in method. The spinal needle defines the path of the portal.

- Field et al[3] compared distal, mid, and proximal anterolateral portals and found that the more proximal portals were statistically farther from the sheath than the distal portal. They described the location of the mid-anterolateral portal as 1 cm anterior to the prominence of the lateral epicondyle and just proximal to the anterior margin of the radiocapitellar joint space.
- At 90 degrees of flexion, the radial nerve-to-sheath distance was reported to average 9.8 mm without joint distention and 10.9 mm with distention. This was more than twice the distance reported for the distal portal.
- Both inside-out and outside-in methods are effective and safe means to establish this portal. This portal is most useful for visualization of the medial elbow and débridement of the anterior radiocapitellar joint surfaces.

Proximal Anterolateral Portal

- Stothers et al[11,12] described the location of the proximal anterolateral portal as 1 to 2 cm proximal to the prominence of the lateral epicondyle, with the path of the portal along the surface of the anterior humerus. The sheath is directed toward the center of the elbow joint, penetrating the brachioradialis, brachialis, and extensor carpi radialis muscles before passing through the joint capsule.
- Several studies have shown that the radial nerve-to-sheath distance averaged 9.9 to 14.2 mm in the 90-degree-flexed and distended elbow.[3,11] This represents a statistically significant increase in the distance from the nerve from the sheath compared to either the mid or the distal portal.
- The anterior branch of the posterior antebrachial cutaneous nerve averaged 6.1 mm from the portal, with the trocar in contact with the nerve 29% of the time.[11]
- The proximal anterolateral portal may be made before or after the anteromedial portal, and an outside-in method is most commonly recommended.
- Although the view of the anteromedial structures was similar for all three anterolateral portals, the proximal anterolateral portal was consistently described as providing a more extensive evaluation of the joint, particularly when viewing the radiocapitellar joint.[11,12,14]

POSTERIOR PORTALS

- Compared with the anterior portals, all posterior portals are relatively safe[11] (TECH FIG 5).
- Laterally, the posterior antebrachial cutaneous nerve is at risk, and there are anecdotal reports of injury to the radial nerve branch to the anconeus muscle.
- The ulnar nerve is the closest major nerve to any posterior portal and has been described as no closer than 15 to 25 mm from the posterior central portal.[11]
  - This nerve is typically at risk only during posteromedial capsule resection for joint contracture release; however, even with safely performed perineural capsulectomy, recovery of flexion for patients with less than 110 degrees of preoperative elbow flexion still exposes the ulnar nerve to traction injury.
  - In this setting, nerve transposition is advised.
- The posterior portals may be established with the elbow between 45 and 90 degrees of flexion.[11,12]
  - Less flexion is recommended and is thought to decrease the tension in the posterior tissues, expand the olecranon fossa, and provide greater access to the medial and lateral recesses.

Posterior Central Portal

- The posterior central portal, also called the straight posterior portal, has been described by many authors and is usually located 2 to 4 cm proximal to the olecranon prominence and halfway between the medial and lateral condyles.
- This is commonly the initial posterior portal and provides good visualization of the olecranon fossa, the olecranon tip, the posterior trochlea, and the medial recess. The lateral recess, the central trochlea, and the radiocapitellar joint are less well seen.

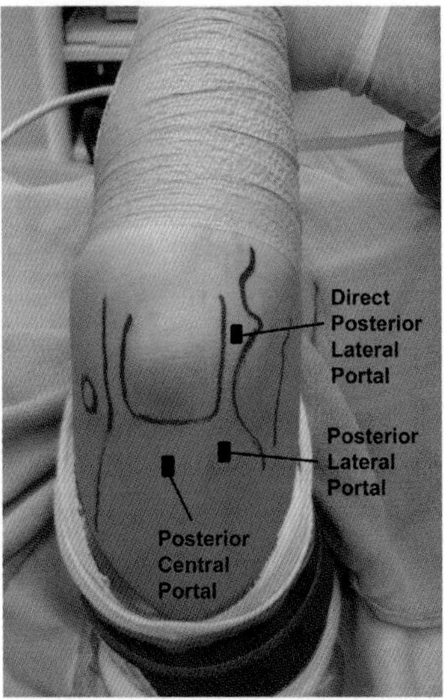

TECH FIG 5 • Posterior surface of the left elbow in the supine cross-body position. Locations of the posterior central, posterolateral, and direct posterolateral portals are shown.

- Although the ulnar nerve-to-sheath distance is consistently described as 15 mm or more,[11] the nerve should always be palpated and outlined before portal placement.
- Sharp dissection and sharp trocars are often discouraged when establishing anterior portals; however, a no. 11 blade may be used safely to create the posterior central portal and probably limits triceps tendon trauma.
  - An 18-gauge needle is first used to confirm the location of the fossa, and the blade is then directed toward the center of the fossa and in line with the tendon fibers.
  - For patients with arthrofibrosis, the portal may be more easily created with a sharp trocar.
- An intercondylar foramen is found in some patients, so caution is advised when establishing this portal.
  - Transhumeral access to the anterior compartment is possible through the foramen.
  - In patients without a foramen, a fenestration technique using a small-headed reamer is described for anterior access.
  - Use of the posterior central portal for anterior compartment visualization is recommended only for those well experienced in elbow arthroscopy, however.

Posterolateral Portal

- Andrews and Carson[2] described the posterolateral portal as 3 cm proximal to the olecranon and through the lateral border of the triceps tendon.
- More distally, accessory portals may be safely placed anywhere between the proximal posterolateral portal and the soft spot.[1,12] The location of the portal is determined by the intended purpose.
  - For procedures performed in the posteromedial region of the elbow, a more proximal portal will provide greater access and visualization.
  - In contrast, a more distal portal will facilitate procedures confined to the posterolateral recess.
- An 18-gauge needle is used to confirm proper access to the olecranon fossa and the lateral gutter.
  - The scope is established in the olecranon fossa while remaining directly on the lateral column of the humerus to avoid capture of the posterior fat pad.
- When properly placed, this portal provides a clear view of the olecranon fossa, the olecranon tip, the posterior and central trochlea, the medial recess, the lateral recess, and the posterior radiocapitellar joint.

Direct Posterolateral Portal

- The direct posterolateral portal is typically the site used for joint inflation before anterior portal placement. The location is defined as the center of a triangle formed by the prominence of the lateral epicondyle, the prominence of the olecranon, and the radial head (see Tech Fig 1).
- Also known as the mid-lateral portal, the dorsal lateral portal, and more commonly the "soft spot" portal, this portal penetrates the anconeus muscle and consistently provides the best view of the radiocapitellar joint.

Lateral Radiocapitellar Portal

- O'Driscoll and Morrey[9] described the standard mid-lateral portal, also called the lateral radiocapitellar portal, and noted that this portal is difficult to create because of limited space.
- This portal is best used when a very small mechanical shaver blade may be employed in the management of OCD capitellum lesions and radiocapitellar chondral injury.
- An 18-gauge needle is used to determine appropriate portal location (TECH FIG 6).

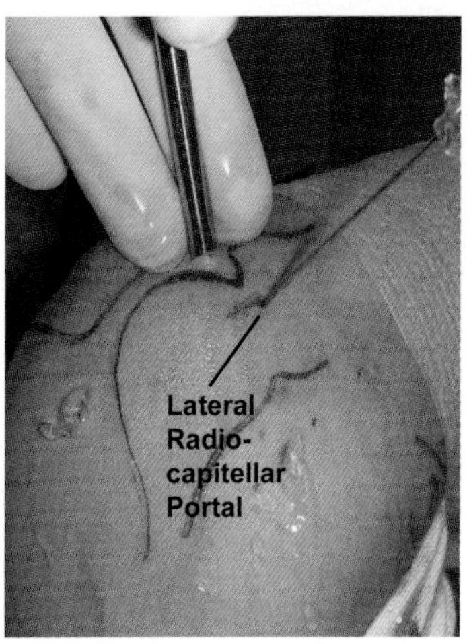

TECH FIG 6 • Posterolateral surface of the left elbow with the arthroscope in the direct posterolateral portal and an 18-gauge spinal needle being used to determine the appropriate location for the accessory direct radiocapitellar portal.

PEARLS AND PITFALLS

Preparation	■ The surgeon should know the structural and neurovascular anatomy of the elbow well. ■ The surgeon should work within his or her experience and acknowledge his or her limitations. ■ A thoroughly considered surgical plan is mandatory.
Neurovascular risk	■ All bony landmarks and portal sites are outlined before starting. ■ Depth of all skin incisions is limited. ■ The elbow joint is maximally distended with fluid before creating the anterior portals. ■ The elbow is maintained at 90 degrees during anterior portal placement and capsular resection. ■ More proximal portal sites should be used for the anterior portals. ■ The location of the medial intermuscular septum must be confirmed, and the surgeon must remain anterior to it while creating the proximal anteromedial portal. ■ Retractors are used for visualization and protection during synovectomy and capsulectomy. ■ Suction is avoided during mechanical resection of the capsule. ■ Previous trauma or surgery may alter the location of neurovascular structures. ■ Ulnar nerve subluxation may reposition the nerve directly beneath the proximal medial portal. ■ Postoperative vascular compromise from either direct vascular injury or compartment syndrome is difficult to assess after regional anesthesia.
Fluid management and tissue swelling	■ The amount of fluid extravasation into the soft tissues is limited with an end-flow arthroscope sheath, low-pressure gravity inflow, and a forearm compression wrap.

POSTOPERATIVE CARE

- Wounds are routinely closed with simple sutures.
- Synovial–subcutaneous and synovial–cutaneous fistulas have been described and most commonly occur in the posterolateral portals along the lateral margin of the triceps tendon.[4]
  - Deep absorbable sutures placed in the fascia of the lateral triceps along with locking mattress sutures in the skin will minimize the risk for this complication.
- Unless contraindicated by the procedure performed, the elbow is splinted near full extension to minimize swelling.
- The arm is elevated overnight and the splint is removed the following day.
- Passive and active range-of-motion exercises are started as soon as the procedure performed will allow.
- For patients undergoing contracture release surgery, an axillary regional block is performed early the next day.
  - The elbow is gently taken through a full arc of motion and then placed into continuous passive motion.
- Based on the extent of the release, the amount of swelling, and the level of pain, the patient is hospitalized for 1 to 3 days.
- Postoperative static progressive range-of-motion braces and physical therapy are also used to recover motion.

COMPLICATIONS

- The incidence of neurologic complications after elbow arthroscopy has been reported to be 0% to 14%.[4]
  - Transient as well as incomplete and complete permanent nerve palsies, including iatrogenic nerve resection injuries, have also been described for the radial, ulnar, and median nerves.
- Kelly et al[4] retrospectively reviewed 473 consecutive arthroscopy procedures and found an overall complication rate of 7%.
  - Transient neuropraxia was the most common immediate minor complication and included radial nerve, ulnar nerve, posterior interosseous nerve, anterior interosseous nerve, and medial antebrachial cutaneous nerve palsies.

- Risk factors include autoimmune disorder, contracture, capsulectomy, and possibly prolonged tourniquet time.

- Prolonged clear or serous drainage from anterolateral and mid-lateral portal sites was the most common minor complication and was reported to occur in 5% of patients.
- Deep infection occurred in 0.8% of patients; all the cases occurred in patients who had received intra-articular corticosteroids at the end of the procedure.
- Mild postsurgical contracture occurred in 1.6% of patients.[1,4]

REFERENCES

1. Abboud JA, Ricchetti ET, Tjoumakaris F, et al. Elbow arthroscopy: basic setup and portal placement. J Am Acad Orthop Surg 2006; 14:312–318.
2. Andrews JR, Carson WG. Arthroscopy of the elbow. Arthroscopy 1985;1:97–107.
3. Field LD, Altchek DW, Warren RF, et al. Arthroscopic anatomy of the lateral elbow: a comparison of three portals. Arthroscopy 1994; 10:602–607.
4. Kelly EW, Morrey BF, O'Driscoll SW. Complications of elbow arthroscopy. J Bone Joint Surg Am 2001;83A:25–34.
5. Lindenfeld TN. Medial approach in elbow arthroscopy. Am J Sports Med 1990;18:413–417.
6. Lynch GJ, Myers JF, Whipple TL, et al. Neurovascular anatomy and elbow arthroscopy: inherent risks. Arthroscopy 1986;2:191–197.
7. Marshall PD, Fairclough JA, Johnson SR, et al. Avoiding nerve damage during elbow arthroscopy. J Bone Joint Surg Br 1993;75B: 129–131.
8. Miller CD, Jobe CM, Wright MH. Neuroanatomy in elbow arthroscopy. J Shoulder Elbow Surg 1995;4:168–174.
9. O'Driscoll SW, Morrey BF. Arthroscopy of the elbow: diagnostic and therapeutic benefits and hazards. J Bone Joint Surg Am 1992;74A: 84–94.
10. Poehling GG, Whipple TL, Sisco L, et al. Elbow arthroscopy, a new technique. Arthroscopy 1989;5:222–281.
11. Stothers K, Day B, Regan W. Arthroscopy of the elbow: anatomy, portal sites, and a description of the proximal lateral portal. Arthroscopy 1995;11:449–457.
12. Stothers K, Day B, Regan W. Arthroscopic anatomy of the elbow: an anatomical study and description of a new portal. Arthroscopy 1993;9:362–363.
13. Verhaar J, van-Mameren H, Brandsma A. Risks of neurovascular injury in elbow arthroscopy: starting anteriomedially or anteriolaterally? Arthroscopy 1991;7:287–290.
14. Woods GW. Elbow arthroscopy. Clin Sports Med 1987;6:557–564.

Chapter 19

Arthroscopic Treatment of Chondral Injuries and Osteochondritis Dissecans

Marc Safran

DEFINITION

- Osteochondritis dissecans (OCD) is a progressive form of osteochondrosis involving focal injury to the subchondral bone or its blood supply. It may occur in many different areas of the adolescent skeleton.
- The knee is the most common location for OCD, but it may occur in several locations of the elbow, including the radial head, the trochlea, and the capitellum (the most common location within the elbow).
- The injury to the subchondral bone results in loss of structural support for the overlying articular cartilage. As a result, degeneration and fragmentation of the articular cartilage and underlying bone occur, often with the formation of loose bodies.
- The histopathology of the subchondral bone in OCD is consistent with osteonecrosis.
- Articular cartilage injury may also occur anywhere in the elbow, especially after trauma. More common locations of nonarthritic chondral injury include the radial head and capitellum.

ANATOMY

Bony Anatomy

- The bony anatomy of the elbow allows for two complex motions: flexion–extension and pronation–supination.
- The ulnohumeral articulation of the elbow is almost a true hinge joint with its constant axis of rotation through the lateral epicondyle and just anterior and inferior to the medial epicondyle. This well-fitted hinge joint allows for little excessive motion or toggle.
- The radius articulates with the proximal ulna and rounded capitellum of the distal humerus. The radiocapitellar joint and the proximal radioulnar joint allow for pronation–supination (**FIG 1A**). The ulnohumeral joint allows for flexion–extension of the elbow.
- The ulnohumeral joint has 11 to 16 degrees of valgus. This results in increased compressive force in the lateral elbow (radiocapitellar joint) with axial loading.

Ligamentous Anatomy

- The ligaments of the elbow are divided into the radial and ulnar collateral ligament complexes.
  - The lateral or radial collateral ligamentous complex provides varus stability. These ligaments are rarely stressed in the athlete.
  - The ulnar or medial collateral ligament complex consists of three ligaments: the anterior oblique, the posterior oblique, and the transverse.
- The ulnar collateral ligament complex, particularly the anterior oblique ligament, resists valgus force, such as occurs with throwing, whereas the radiocapitellar joint is a secondary restraint to valgus force (**FIG 1B**).

Intraosseous Vascular Anatomy

- There are two nutrient vessels in the lateral condyle of the developing elbow.
- Each vessel extends into the lateral aspect of the trochlea, with one entering proximal to the articular cartilage and the other entering posterolaterally at the origin of the capsule.
- Although these two vessels communicate with each other, they do not do so with the metaphyseal vasculature. The rapidly expanding capitellar epiphysis in the developing elbow thus receives its blood supply from one or two isolated trans-chondroepiphyseal vessels that enter the epiphysis posteriorly.

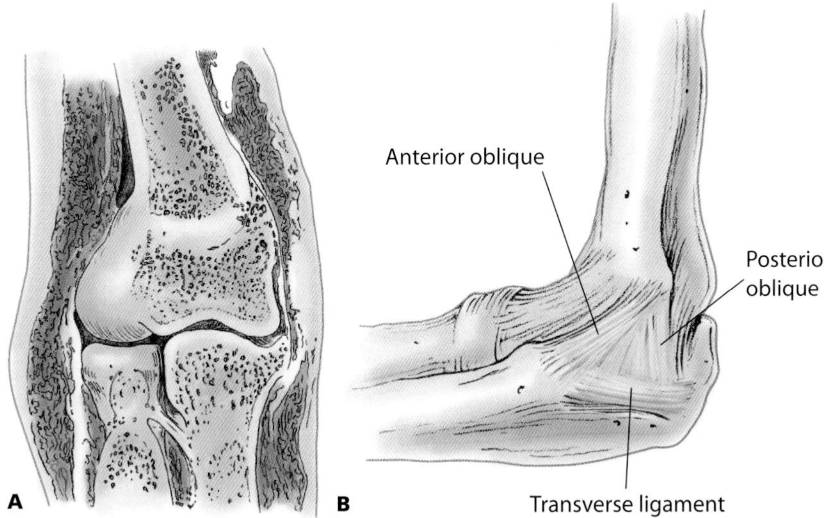

FIG 1 • **A.** Cross-section of the elbow showing the round, convex capitellum and the matching concave radial head. **B.** Anatomy of the medial elbow ligamentous complex. The ulnar collateral ligament complex comprises three ligaments: the anterior oblique, posterior oblique, and transverse ligaments.

- These vessels function as end-arteries passing through the cartilaginous epiphysis to the capitellum.
- Metaphyseal vascular anastomoses do not make significant contributions to the capitellum until approximately 19 years of age, placing this region at risk for vascular injury.

PATHOGENESIS

- The cause of OCD is unclear and controversial.
- OCD typically affects the dominant extremity of adolescents and young adults, with onset of symptoms between 11 to 16 years of age.
- Most cases are seen in high-level athletes who experience repetitive valgus stress and lateral compression across the elbow (eg, overhead throwing athletes, gymnasts, weightlifters).
- The lesion usually affects only a portion of the capitellum.
- Genetic factors, trauma, and ischemia have been proposed as causes.
- Most authors believe that the primary mechanism of injury is repetitive microtrauma in a genetically predisposed individual's developing elbow that results in vascular injury due to the tenuous blood supply.
- The capitellum is softer than the radial head.
- Repeated microtrauma, such as axial loading in the extended elbow or repeated throwing that produces valgus forces on the elbow, results in increased force in the radiocapitellar joint.
  - The repetitive microtrauma caused by these forces has been proposed to weaken the capitellar subchondral bone and result in fatigue fracture.
  - Should failure of bony repair occur, an avascular portion of bone may then undergo resorption with further weakening of the subchondral architecture. This is consistent with the characteristic rarefaction often seen at the periphery of the lesion.
  - The altered subchondral architecture can no longer support the overlying articular cartilage, rendering it vulnerable to shear stresses, which may lead to fragmentation.
- The tenuous blood supply of the end-arterioles in the capitellum may become injured with the repetitive microtrauma, resulting in OCD.
- Although a genetic predisposition to OCD has been proposed in the literature, convincing scientific evidence of OCD as a heritable condition does not currently exist. Some individuals are more susceptible than others, and this may be genetically based.

NATURAL HISTORY

- The natural history of capitellar OCD is unpredictable. No reliable criteria exist for predicting which lesions will collapse with subsequent joint incongruity and which will go on to heal without further sequelae.
- If healing is going to take place, it usually occurs by the time of physeal closure.
- If healing is not going to take place, repetitive microtrauma and shear stresses to the articular surface of a lesion that has lost its subchondral support may result in further subchondral collapse and deformation with joint incongruity as well as articular cartilage injury, fragmentation, and loose body formation.
- In advanced cases, degenerative changes accompanied by a decreased range of motion are likely to develop.

PATIENT HISTORY AND PHYSICAL FINDINGS

- The classic patient with OCD is an adolescent athlete who experiences repetitive valgus stress and lateral compression across the elbow (eg, overhead throwing athletes, gymnasts, weightlifters).
  - The patient usually complains of the insidious onset of poorly localized, progressive lateral elbow pain in the dominant arm.
  - He or she may also note a flexion contracture.
- The throwing athlete may note a reduction in throwing distance or velocity or both.
- Prodromal pain is not always present.
- Typically, pain is exacerbated with activity and relieved by rest.
- In advanced cases in which a fragment has become unstable or loose body formation has occurred, mechanical symptoms of elbow locking, clicking, or catching may be present.
- Physical examination methods
  - On examination, there may be tenderness to palpation and crepitus over the radiocapitellar joint.
  - Effusion indicates intra-articular irritation and may be consistent with a loose or unstable OCD lesion or loose body.
  - Swelling, palpated in the posterolateral gutter (soft spot), may be appreciated.
  - Crepitus may be present on range-of-motion testing.
  - Loss of 10 to 20 degrees of extension is common and mild loss of flexion and forearm rotation may also be seen. Loss of pronation is less common.
  - Provocative testing includes the "active radiocapitellar compression test," which consists of forearm pronation and supination with the elbow in full extension in an attempt to reproduce symptoms.
- The examiner should rule out radiocapitellar overload as the result of ulnar collateral ligament insufficiency using the milking maneuver, modified milking maneuver, valgus stress test, or moving valgus stress test.

IMAGING AND OTHER DIAGNOSTIC STUDIES

- Diagnostic evaluation of the elbow for OCD begins with plain radiographs—an anteroposterior (AP) view, lateral view, oblique views, and a 45-degree flexion AP, which is particularly good at revealing the lesion.
- Radiographs typically show the classic radiolucency (**FIG 2A**) or rarefaction of the capitellum (**FIG 2B**) in addition to irregularity or flattening of the articular surface.
- The lesion frequently appears as a focal rim of sclerotic bone surrounding a radiolucent crater with rarefaction located in the anterolateral aspect of the capitellum.
- Radiographs, however, may not reveal the osteochondral lesions in the earlier stages. They are not of much benefit for truly chondral lesions.
- In advanced cases, articular surface collapse, loose bodies, subchondral cysts, radial head enlargement, and osteophyte formation may be seen.
- Further diagnostic imaging of OCD lesions primarily consists of magnetic resonance imaging (MRI), although ultrasonography and bone scintigraphy have been used.
- MRI is especially valuable in assessing the integrity of the articular cartilage overlying the OCD lesion as well as in

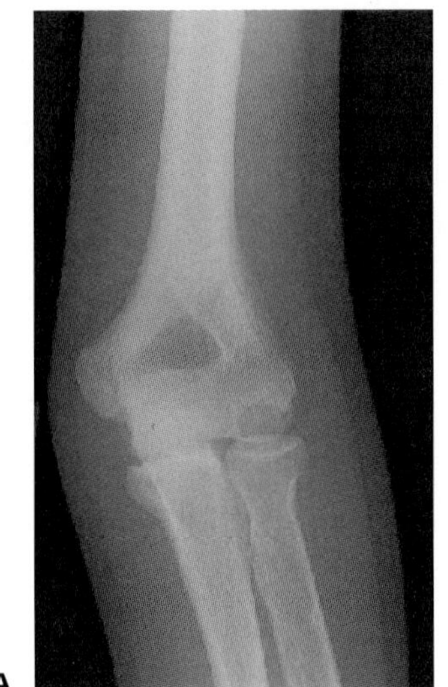
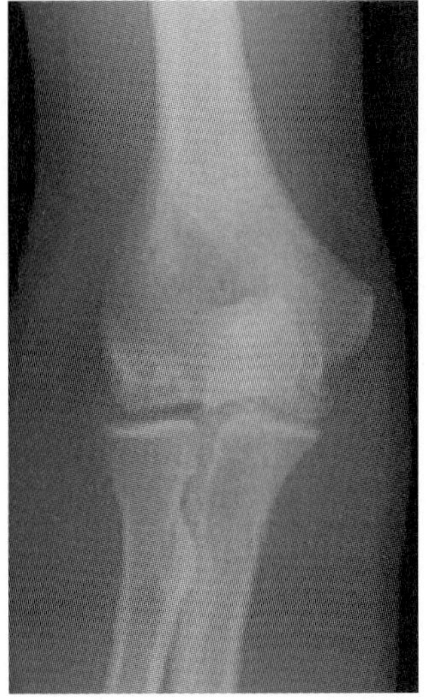
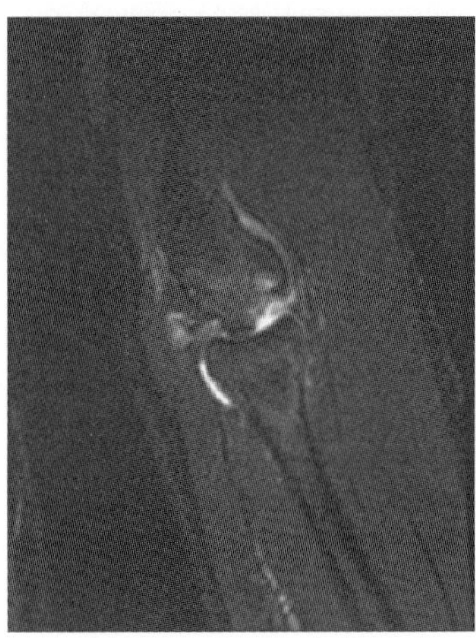

FIG 2 • **A.** Radiograph of a 15-year-old baseball pitcher with osteochondritis dissecans (OCD) of the capitellum of the dominant elbow. Clear lesion and sclerosis of the bony bed are shown. **B.** OCD in a 15-year-old gymnast with rarefaction of the capitellar lesion on oblique radiograph of the elbow. **C.** MRI of the elbow of a baseball pitcher, revealing OCD with loss of overlying articular cartilage and loose body.

diagnosing OCD in its early stages and identifying loose bodies (**FIG 2C**).

- Controversy exists over the utility of contrast-enhanced MR arthrography. This technique, however, can potentially provide additional information regarding the status of the articular cartilage and identification of loose bodies.
- Bone scintigraphy is very sensitive for identifying osteoblastic activity or increased vascularity at the site of an OCD lesion. However, it is nonspecific and has limited usefulness in diagnosis.
- Computed tomography can help define bony anatomy and identify loose bodies.
- Ultrasonography can also help in the assessment of capitellar lesions, including early stages, but ultrasound is technician dependent.

DIFFERENTIAL DIAGNOSIS

- Panner disease
- Infection
- Lateral epicondylosis
- Lateral epicondylar apophysitis
- Radial head osteochondrosis
- Radial head or neck injury
- Radiocapitellar overload and chondromalacia due to ulnar collateral ligament injury
- Posterolateral rotatory instability

NONOPERATIVE MANAGEMENT

- The choice of conservative or surgical management depends on the patient's age, symptoms, size of the lesion, and stage of the lesion, specifically the integrity of the cartilage surface.
- The goal of treatment for OCD of the elbow is to prevent the progression of the disorder, detachment of the osteochondral lesion, and degenerative changes of the articular cartilage.
- Small, nondisplaced lesions with intact overlying articular cartilage in younger (skeletally immature) athletes are best managed conservatively with relative rest and activity modification, ice, and nonsteroidal anti-inflammatories, particularly if the bone scan shows increased bony activity.
- Activity modification consists of avoiding throwing activities and weight bearing on the involved arm.
- Short-term immobilization (less than 2 to 3 weeks, depending on symptoms) may be considered.
- Serial radiographs, at 10- to 12-week intervals, are obtained to monitor healing.
- Activity modification is continued until the radiographic appearance of revascularization and healing.
- Radiographic findings of OCD may persist for several years. As a result, after conservative management, the most important issue in terms of an athlete's ability to return to sports is symptom resolution.
- Most patients can return to full activity after 6 months.

SURGICAL MANAGEMENT

- The indications for surgical treatment include persistent symptoms despite conservative management, symptomatic loose bodies, articular cartilage fracture, displacement of the osetochondral lesion, and cold bone scan.
- The surgeon must assess the size, stability, and viability of the fragment and decide whether to remove the fragment or attempt to surgically reattach it.
- Most fragments cannot be reattached and therefore are excised, followed by local débridement.
- Arthroscopic abrasion chondroplasty or subchondral drilling may be performed to encourage healing.
- Although symptoms usually improve, about half of all patients will continue to have chronic pain or limited range of motion.
- In general, many athletes cannot return to their prior levels of competition.
- Surgical indications for operative management of stable lesions with intact articular cartilage include radiographic evidence of lesion progression and failure of symptom resolution despite a 6-month trial of a conservative, nonoperative regimen.

- Arthroscopic examination, débridement as needed, and drilling or microfracture of the OCD lesion (with or without in situ pinning) are usually the surgical treatments of choice.

- Unstable lesions, characterized by overlying articular cartilage injury and instability as well as collapse or disruption of the subchondral bone architecture, and those with loose bodies are usually managed surgically.
  - These lesions are frequently flap lesions. They characteristically present with more advanced radiographic changes (including a well-demarcated fragment surrounded by a sclerotic margin).
  - There is controversy as to whether simple fragment excision or reduction (open or arthroscopic) and internal fixation is the preferred treatment. Many authors advocate excision of displaced fragments, often augmented by drilling or microfracture.
- Critical considerations in operative planning include the size and integrity (viability) of the fragment, the subchondral architecture on the fragment and the opposing bony bed, the potential for anatomic restoration of the articular surface, and the method of fixation if attempted.
- Internal fixation of the fragment may be performed using metallic screws, bioabsorbable screws or pins, Kirschner wire, bone pegs, and dynamic staple fixation.
- There have been a few reports of osteoarticular autograft or allograft plugs in the treatment of more advanced lesions, but experience with this method is limited. The current recommendations are for lesions that involve the lateral column.

Preoperative Planning

- Before surgery, an MRI, preferably with contrast, can be used to assess the integrity of the articular cartilage to help determine whether débridement, loose body removal, and drilling may be needed or more advanced techniques, such as reduction and internal fixation or osteochondral transfer, may be needed.
  - The MRI of the joint is also inspected for loose bodies—their number and location (anterior vs. posterior elbow) (see Fig 2C).

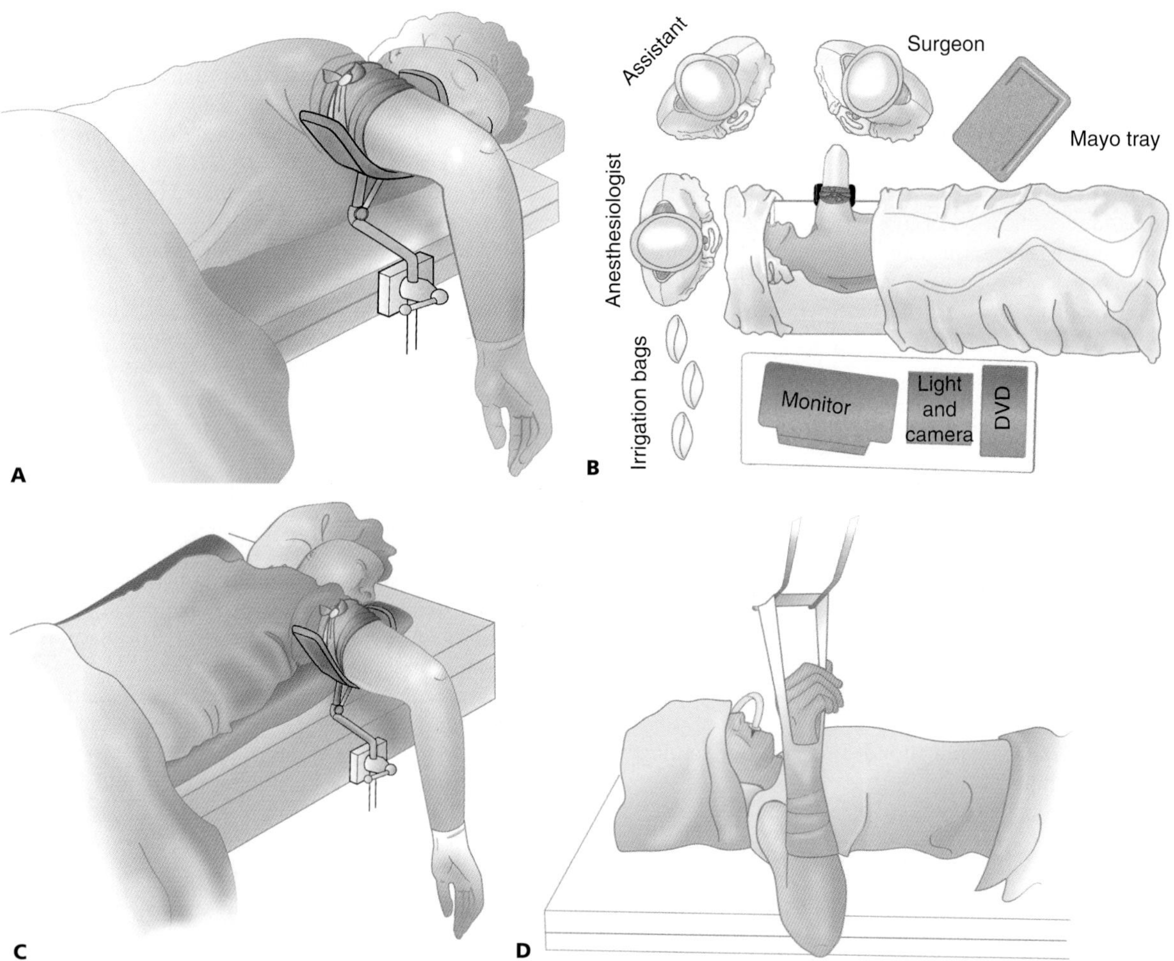

FIG 3 • **A.** Lateral positioning for elbow arthroscopy, including tourniquet placement. **B.** Setup in the operating room for the lateral position. **C.** Prone position of the patient. This is the preferred position, particularly due to the ease of posterior elbow access. The setup of the room is the same and the relative position of the elbow for the surgeon is similar between the prone and lateral positions. **D.** Supine position of the patient. Some surgeons prefer this position because it is easier to convert to open surgery and easier anesthesia management; however, posterior arthroscopic access is more difficult in this position.

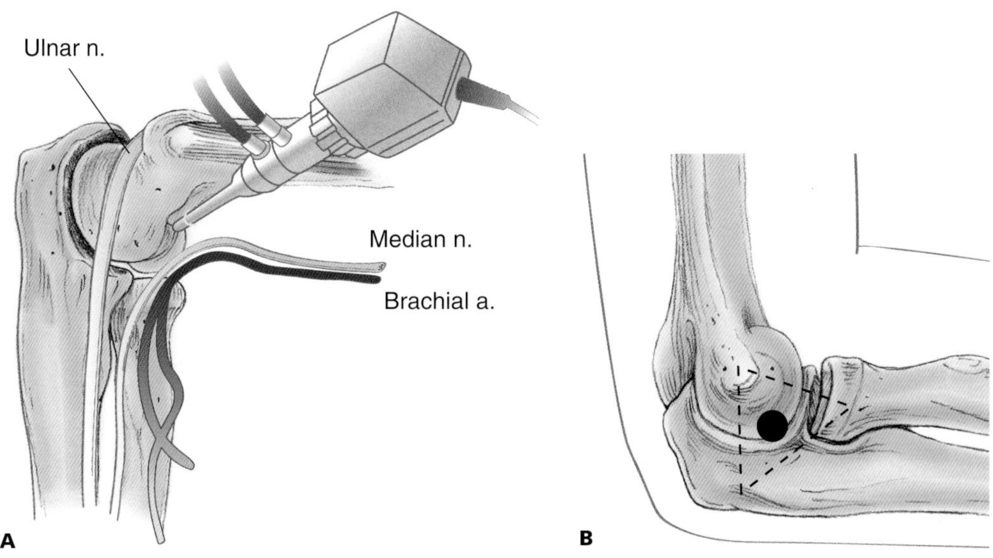

FIG 4 • **A.** The elbow arthroscope is brought in from the proximal anteromedial portal that provides a direct view of the anterior capitellum and radial head. **B.** Position of the direct lateral "soft spot" portal.

- All imaging studies are reviewed.
- Examination under anesthesia is performed to assess range of motion and ligamentous stability, particularly valgus laxity, as injury to the ulnar collateral ligament in the athlete may increase the load on the radiocapitellar joint.

Positioning

- Elbow arthroscopy can be performed in the supine, lateral, or prone position (**FIG 3**).
- Prone positioning is preferred because it allows easy access to the elbow, reduces the risk of sterility breaks if the arm needs to be in a finger-trap device, as needed for supine elbow arthroscopy, and arthroscopy.
- The patient is positioned on chest rolls and padding under the knees and feet and ankles.
- The arm is placed on an arm holder.
- A sterile tourniquet is placed after the arm is prepared and draped.

Approach

- All cases are approached in the same manner initially.
  - Diagnostic arthroscopy of the elbow is carried out, using a proximal anteromedial portal, a proximal anterolateral portal, and two posterior portals. This allows for assessment of the entire joint to ensure that loose bodies are not missed.
- The capitellum may be seen from the proximal anteromedial portal (**FIG 4A**) while the elbow is taken through a full range of motion.
- A direct lateral portal (sometimes called the soft spot portal) is then used to allow direct access to the radiocapitellar joint and is needed to confirm the extent of the OCD or chondral lesion (**FIG 4B**).

TECHNIQUES

ARTHROSCOPIC DÉBRIDEMENT AND LOOSE BODY REMOVAL

- Elbow arthroscopy is begun in the prone (my preference), lateral, or supine position, using the proximal medial portal to visualize the capitellum.
- Complete elbow examination is mandatory to look for loose bodies:
  - Proximal anteromedial portal
  - Proximal anterolateral portal
  - Posterior central portal
  - Posterolateral portal
  - Direct lateral portal
- Loose bodies tend to hide:
  - In the proximal radioulnar joint anteriorly or the gutters
  - In the olecranon fossa or gutters posteriorly, particularly the lateral gutter
- When looking at the capitellum from the proximal anteromedial portal, instrumentation (shavers, burrs, graspers, and curettes) may be accomplished using the proximal anterolateral portal.
- Flexion and extension of the elbow allow for enhanced visualization of the capitellum.
- Loose bodies and chondral fragments may be removed via the anterior portals (**TECH FIG 1A,B**).
- Then the arthroscope is brought in from the posterior portals to look for loose bodies.

- The direct lateral ("soft spot") portal is used for complete evaluation of the capitellum.
  - This portal is mandatory to fully evaluate the extent of the lesion and to allow for adequate débridement of loose cartilage.
  - Often loose bodies will be found using this portal.
- Débridement is performed using shavers, curettes, graspers, and rongeurs to remove loose bodies and any loose, scaly, or fragmented cartilage (**TECH FIG 1C**).

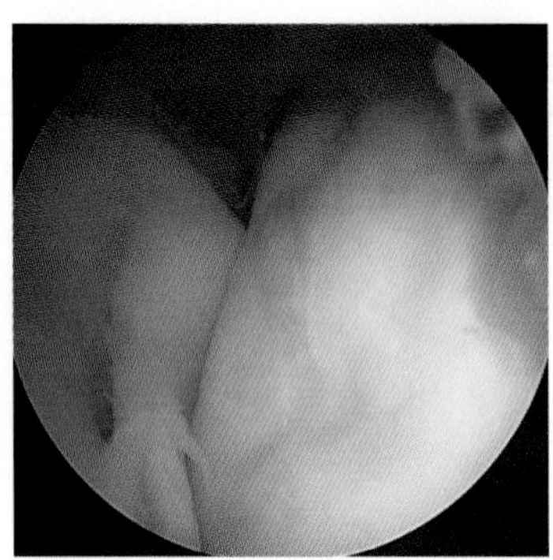
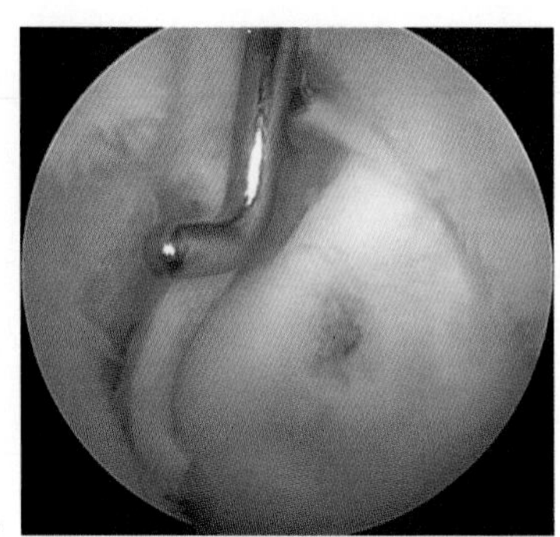
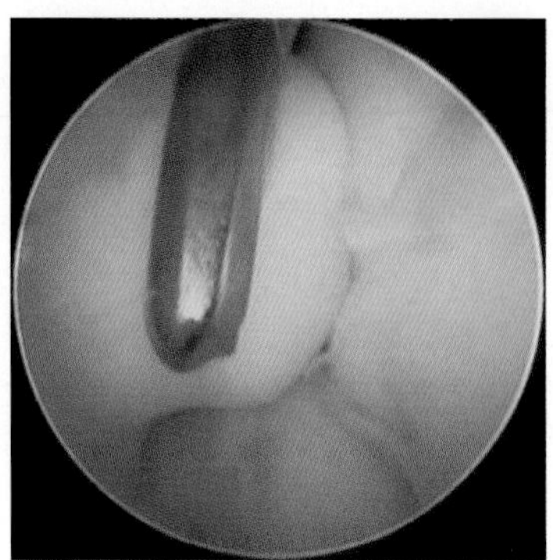

TECH FIG 1 • Osteochondritis dissecans of the capitellum. **A.** View from the proximal anteromedial portal reveals a flap of cartilage from the capitellum (*left*) and a slightly deformed radial head (*to the right*). **B.** Probe on the flap of chondral tissue from the capitellum of this same patient. **C.** Grasper removing a loose body as viewed from the direct lateral portal.

MICROFRACTURE AND ABRASION ARTHROPLASTY

- When the OCD fragment is loose and it is not possible to fix the lesion back to the bony bed, then microfracture or abrasion arthroplasty may be indicated to stimulate a fibrocartilaginous growth in the bony defect.
- The principle is to stimulate cartilage-like regeneration based on the formation of a super-clot that is progressively invaded by multipotent cells from the marrow.
- This is achieved by complete débridement of all unstable and damaged cartilage in the lesion and the preservation of the subchondral layer for chondral lesions, based on experience of the treatment of knee chondral injuries.
- Elbow arthroscopy is begun in the prone (my preference), lateral, or supine position, using the proximal medial portal to visualize the capitellum.
- Complete elbow examination using all four standard and the additional direct lateral arthroscopic portals is mandatory to look for loose bodies.
- When looking at the capitellum from the proximal anteromedial portal, instrumentation (shavers, burrs, graspers, and curettes) may be done using the proximal anterolateral portal.
- Flexion and extension of the elbow allow for enhanced visualization of the capitellum.
- All underlying bone is débrided with an arthroscopic shaver or burr or manually with curettes or pituitary rongeurs.
- Next, the arthroscope is brought in from the posterior portals to look for loose bodies.
- The direct lateral ("soft spot") portal is used for complete evaluation of the capitellum.
  - This portal is mandatory to fully evaluate the extent of the lesion and to allow for adequate débridement of loose cartilage and may allow for a good direction for microfracturing the bed.
- Abrasion is carried out from either anterolateral or direct lateral portals to the complete lesion. This may be done with a shaver on high speed or burr.
- For chondral lesions, abrasion arthroplasty involves removal of the zone of calcified cartilage, then use of a burr to lightly remove only a partial thickness of the subchondral bone to expose subchondral arterioles to bring blood into the lesion. The key is not to go too deep into the cancellous bone.
- For OCD with a cartilage cap that is not intact, abrasion is done lightly to remove only a little bone to allow bleeding into the bony bed.
- Microfracture or drilling can also be used to bring blood into the defect when the OCD or chondral lesion results in an exposed bony bed, with the theoretical benefit of microfracture being that less bone is lost and there is no heat production, which may be seen with drilling.
- The bone is pierced every 3 to 4 mm for a 4-mm depth with an awl for microfracture or 0.062 Kirschner wire for drilling (**TECH FIG 2**).
- If the anterolateral or direct lateral portals do not allow for adequate directionality of the drilling or microfracture, an additional outside-in portal may be made based on the known anatomy and using a spinal needle.

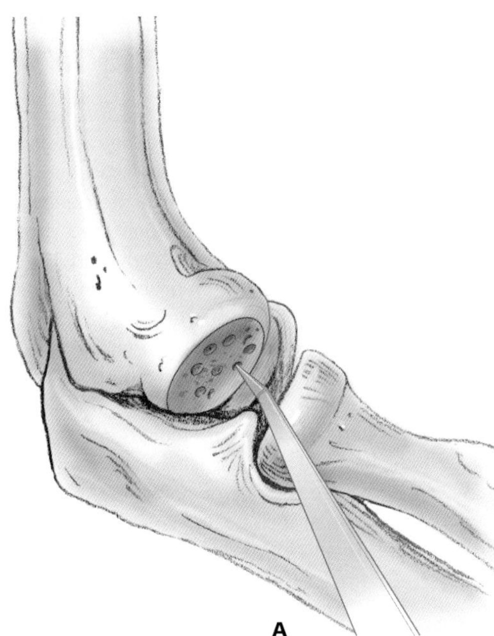

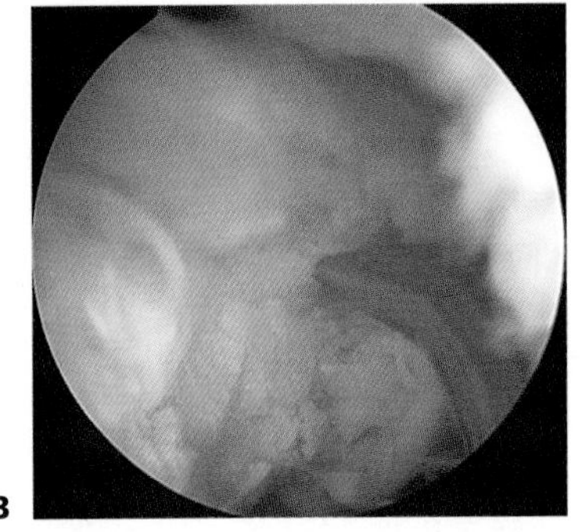

TECH FIG 2 • **A.** Microfracture of the capitellum, making several small perforations within the capitellum about 4 mm apart and 4 mm deep. **B.** Intraoperative arthroscopic photograph from the direct lateral portal with a microfracture awl at the edge of the osteochondritis dissecans lesion after removing the zone of calcified cartilage.

DRILLING FOR INTACT OCD LESIONS

- When the OCD lesion has an intact overlying chondral surface, then drilling may enhance or stimulate a healing response of the lesion, although this is not frequently needed.
- The key is to try to prevent violation of the OCD cartilage cap, although some surgeons drill from outside-in trying to avoid injury to the articular cartilage and some drill from the joint, which will perforate the articular cartilage.
- Elbow arthroscopy is begun in the prone (my preference), lateral, or supine position, using the proximal medial portal to visualize the capitellum.
  - Complete elbow examination using all four standard portals and the additional direct lateral arthroscopic portals is mandatory to look for loose bodies.
- When looking at the capitellum from the proximal anteromedial portal, instrumentation (shavers, burrs, graspers, and curettes) may be done using the proximal anterolateral portal.
- Flexion and extension of the elbow allow for enhanced visualization of the capitellum.
- Next, the arthroscope is brought in from the posterior portals to look for loose bodies.
- The direct lateral ("soft spot") portal is then used for complete evaluation of the capitellum.
- OCD lesions with intact articular cartilage, subchondral softening, fibrillated cartilage, or cartilage character change may be identified visually or palpably using a probe (TECH FIG 3) or alternatively using fluoroscopic imaging.
- Drilling through the cartilage and through the sclerotic subchondral bone is done in an effort to promote healing.
- Attempts are made to limit the number of perforations through the intact cartilage, but the subchondral plate should be penetrated multiple times.
  - This may be accomplished by redirecting the drill in different directions from the same single (or a few) perforations through the articular cartilage.
- The lesion is pierced with an 0.062 Kirschner wire for drilling.
- If the anterolateral or direct lateral portals do not allow for adequate directionality of the drilling, an additional outside-in portal may be made based on the known anatomy and using a spinal needle.

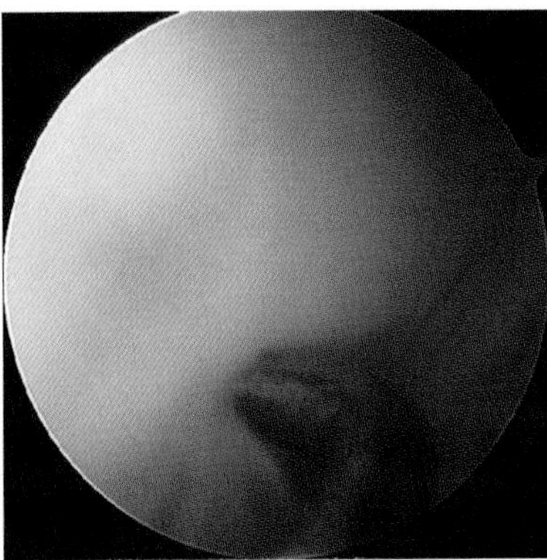

TECH FIG 3 • View from the direct lateral portal of an osteochondritis dissecans lesion with intact articular cartilage. The probe is deforming the intact cartilage owing to the lack of subchondral support.

DRILLING FOR INTACT OCD LESION: OUTSIDE-IN TECHNIQUE

- When the OCD lesion has an intact overlying chondral surface then drilling may enhance or stimulate a healing response of the lesion.
- The key is to try to prevent violation of the OCD cartilage cap, although some surgeons drill from outside in trying to avoid injury to the articular cartilage and some drill from the joint, which will perforate the articular cartilage.
- Elbow arthroscopy is begun in the prone (my preference), lateral, or supine position, using the proximal medial portal to visualize the capitellum.
  - Complete elbow examination using all four standard and the additional direct lateral arthroscopic portals is mandatory to look for loose bodies.
- When looking at the capitellum from the proximal anteromedial portal, instrumentation (shavers, burrs, graspers, and curettes) may be done using the proximal anterolateral portal.
  - Flexion and extension of the elbow allow for enhanced visualization of the capitellum.
- Next, the arthroscope is brought in from the posterior portals to look for loose bodies.
- The direct lateral ("soft spot") portal is then used for complete evaluation of the capitellum.
- OCD lesions with intact articular cartilage, subchondral softening, fibrillation of the cartilage, or cartilage character change may be identified visually or palpably (see Tech Fig 3) or alternatively using fluoroscopy.
- Fluoroscopy is then brought in to identify the lesion.
- Using an anterior cruciate ligament tibial guide or posterior cruciate ligament femoral guide can be useful to help aim the drill bit from outside the elbow toward the lesion.
- Depending on the location of the lesion, the drill is brought from proximal and slightly anterior to the lateral epicondyle or posteriorly on the distal humerus.
- A small incision is made at the proposed drilling entry site and blunt dissection is done to bone.
- The lesion is drilled with a 0.062 Kirschner wire for drilling while watching with fluoroscopy or arthroscopy to ensure the articular cartilage is not violated.
- Multiple passes with the Kirschner wire should be performed to enhance healing throughout the lesion.

INTERNAL FIXATION

- When the OCD fragment is partially detached or completely detached but not malformed and there is significant bone on the cartilage fragment, consideration for reattachment is recommended.
- The principle is to stimulate healing and to stabilize the fragment within the bony bed.
- Elbow arthroscopy is begun in the prone, lateral, or supine position, using the proximal medial portal to visualize the capitellum.
- If it is likely the patient will need internal fixation of a partially detached OCD fragment, and there is a possibility that an arthrotomy is needed, I have found performing the surgery in the lateral position is a bit easier.
- Complete elbow examination using all four standard and the additional direct lateral arthroscopic portals is mandatory to look for loose bodies.
- When looking at the capitellum from the proximal anteromedial portal, instrumentation (shavers, burrs, graspers, and curettes) may be done using the proximal anterolateral portal.
  - Flexion and extension of the elbow allow for enhanced visualization of the capitellum.
- All underlying bone is débrided with an arthroscopic shaver or burr or manually with curettes or pituitary rongeurs.
- Next, the arthroscope is brought in from the posterior portals to look for loose bodies.
- The direct lateral ("soft spot") portal is used for complete evaluation of the capitellum.
  - This portal is mandatory to fully evaluate the extent of the lesion and to allow for adequate débridement and preparation of the bed.
- The osteochondral flap or undersurface of the fragment is elevated and the underlying sclerotic bone is curetted and débrided of fibrous tissue (**TECH FIG 4A**). Drilling of the base is also performed to stimulate healing.
- The abrasion and drilling are carried out from either anterolateral or direct lateral portals to the complete lesion. This may be done with a curette, a shaver on high speed, or a burr and a drill or Kirschner wire to gently débride the bed without removing much bone.
- The flap is then replaced within the bed.
- Retrograde pinning of the lesion with threaded or unthreaded wires can be performed with the wires exiting the lateral epicondyle for later removal (**TECH FIG 4B,C**).
  - The ends of the pins should be positioned below the articular surface so that the wires do not penetrate the joint space.
- Bioabsorbable pins and bioabsorbable screws have been used as an alternative (**TECH FIG 4D**).
- Further, some surgeons will place metallic screws for fixation. These can either be headless variable-pitched screws that are buried beneath the articular surface, or regular-headed screws, which some prefer for better compression but must be removed.
- If the anterolateral or direct lateral portals do not allow for adequate directionality of the drilling or microfracture, an additional outside-in portal may be made based on the known anatomy and using a spinal needle.
- An arthrotomy may be necessary to perform the débridement or internal fixation.

A 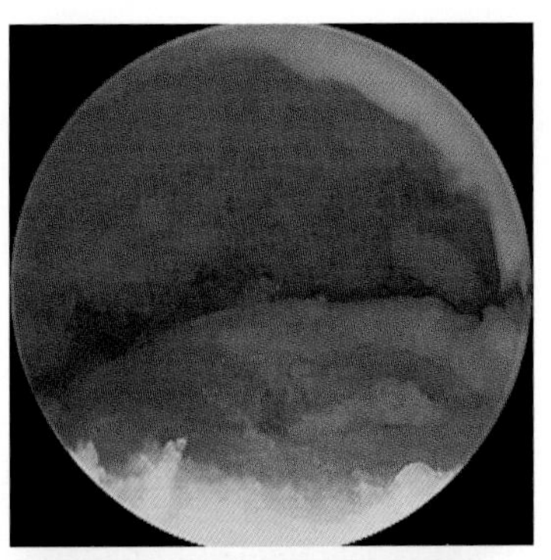
B 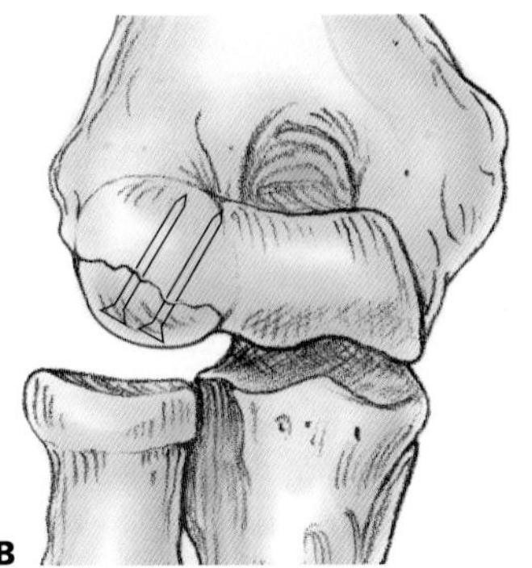
C 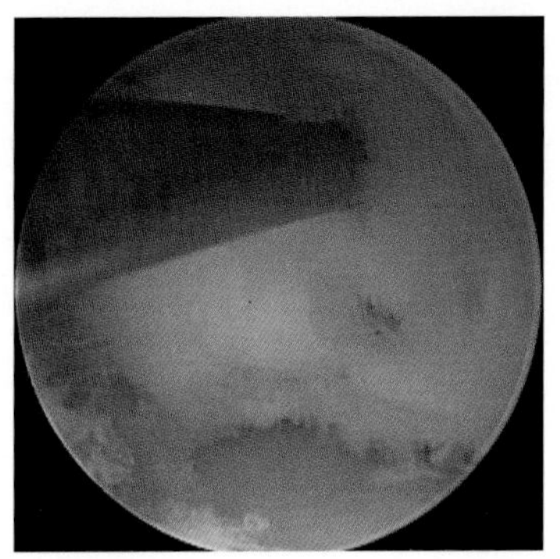
D 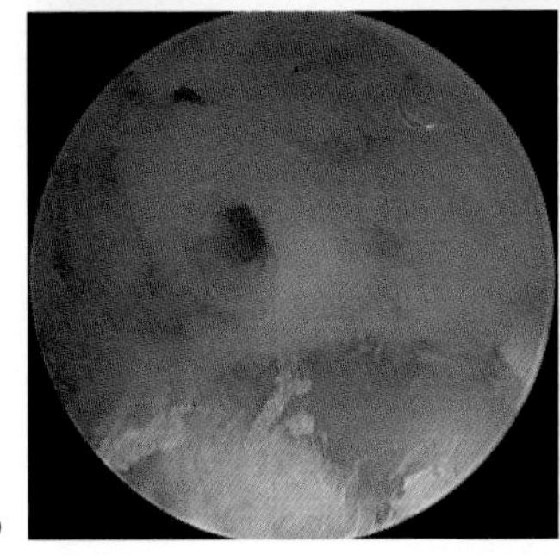

TECH FIG 4 • Osteochondritis dissecans of the capitellum. **A.** The humeral defect is above, and the osteochondral lesion fragment is opened like a trapdoor, inferiorly. This allows for removal of fibrous tissue (already completed) to prepare for repair or fixation of this fragment. **B.** Schematic representation of internal fixation of the lesion with wires or pins. **C.** The lesion is reduced and a Kirschner wire holds the fragment. **D.** The lesion is fixed in place with an absorbable pin (three were used to fix this lesion).

OSTEOCHONDRAL AUTOGRAFT IMPLANTATION

- When the OCD fragment is loose and it is not possible to fix the lesion back to the bony bed, and there is a large crater, particularly if it involves the lateral column, then consideration is given to inserting osteochondral autograft plugs into the defect to eliminate or reduce edge loading and loss of lateral support for the joint.
- This is achieved by taking osteochondral plugs from the knee and implanting them into the capitellum.
- Elbow arthroscopy is begun in the prone, lateral, or supine position, using the proximal medial portal to visualize the capitellum. Because insertion of the plugs often requires an arthrotomy and the grafts must come from the knee, the supine position is preferred.
- Complete elbow examination using all four standard and the additional direct lateral arthroscopic portals is mandatory to look for loose bodies.
- When looking at the capitellum from the proximal anteromedial portal, instrumentation (shavers, burrs, graspers, and curettes) may be done using the proximal anterolateral portal.
- Flexion and extension of the elbow allow for enhanced visualization of the capitellum.
- A posterior or posterolateral approach may be used.
- The radiocapitellar joint is approached anteriorly by splitting the intermuscular plane between the extensor digitorum communis and the extensor carpi radialis longus and brevis, exposing the anterior capsule, which is then incised.
- The posterior approach uses a posterior longitudinal skin incision with the elbow in full flexion. Then the anconeus and posterior capsule are divided, providing direct access to the OCD lesion.
  - The posterolateral Kocher approach uses the interval between the anconeus and extensor carpi ulnaris. The lateral collateral ligament complex is protected and preserved, allowing exposure of the posterior radiocapitellar joint.
- A commercially available osteochondral graft harvesting system is used.
- The size of the lesion is assessed to decide how many grafts and of which size are necessary, although usually less than 100% fill is achieved.
- Recipient sockets are created in the lesion with the recipient graft harvesting tool.
- Occasionally the sclerotic bed makes it difficult to use the recipient harvesting tool and a cannulated drill is needed to make the recipient bed.
- Drilling is carried out at the base of the socket before inserting the graft to allow for marrow stimulation and enhance healing potential.
- Osteochondral grafts about 10 mm long are then harvested arthroscopically or with mini-arthrotomy from the knee intercondylar notch or periphery of the non-weight-bearing portion of the lateral femoral condyle.
- There are only a few case reports of this technique. Some use multiple 3.5-mm plugs and some use single larger osteochondral plugs.
- Depth of the recipient socket is measured with a calibrated depth gauge or alignment stick.
- The length of the osteochondral autograft plug is matched to the depth of the recipient socket.
- The graft is seated flush with the surrounding intact cartilage.
- Complete coverage of the lesion usually is not possible, though coverage of 80% to 90% of the lesion size should be achieved.

PEARLS AND PITFALLS

Nerve injury	■ The greatest risk of elbow arthroscopy, for osteochondritis dissecans or any other diagnosis, is nerve injury. Knowledge of elbow neuroanatomy, particularly as it relates to the arthroscopic portals, is of paramount importance. It is safest to use the proximal medial portal and the proximal lateral portals anteriorly. Distending the joint, using the outside-in technique, and using blunt instruments after skin incision only all help to reduce iatrogenic nerve injury.
Direct lateral portal	■ Familiarity with the direct lateral portal is critical for the evaluation and treatment of chondral and osteochondral lesions of the capitellum. The posterior radial head and capitellum are best seen with this portal, and loose bodies from osteochondritis dissecans occasionally may only be seen from this portal. Full appreciation of the lesion cannot be made without the use of this portal.
Converting to an open procedure	■ Occasionally synovitis or lack of working space makes visualization of the lesion difficult. Further, fixation of the lesion may be difficult arthroscopically. If visualization or fixation is difficult arthroscopically, there should be a low threshold to converting the procedure to open. The threshold of conversion to open should be based on experience and comfort with arthroscopy.

POSTOPERATIVE CARE

- After elbow arthroscopy for débridement or loose body removal:
  - Early range-of-motion exercises are encouraged to prevent loss of elbow motion. Other early goals include reducing swelling, pain, and muscular atrophy.
  - As motion becomes full and the soft tissues are healing with minimal swelling, rehabilitation concentrates on strengthening and endurance of the joint as well as normalization of arthrokinematics of the elbow. This usually begins after 2 weeks.
  - After 4 weeks, the athlete is prepared to return to functional activities with more strengthening, endurance, and flexibility. However, some believe that individuals with OCD lesions who have a defect should not return to sports activities because of the risk of arthritic change in the elbow.
- After in situ drilling, return to sports is usually delayed until 3 to 6 months postoperatively, when there is good radiographic evidence of bony incorporation and healing.
- After microfracture or internal fixation:
  - Range of motion is encouraged, but some clinicians put their patients in a range-of-motion brace positioned in varus to reduce stress over the radiocapitellar joint.
  - Some also consider adding the use of continuous passive motion to help in cartilage nourishment to encourage the microfracture clot or the healing surface of a fixed lesion to reduce adhesions. In these scenarios, strengthening is usually not initiated for at least 6 weeks.
  - Return to gymnastics or throwing sports is delayed until 6 months postoperatively.
- Following the autograft transfer procedure:
  - The joint is immobilized until 2 weeks postoperatively, when the cast or splint is discontinued.
  - Beginning week 3, range-of-motion exercises are started.
  - Strengthening of the elbow and forearm is begun at 3 months postoperatively, and a throwing program is initiated at 6 months, with full return to participation at 10 to 12 months postoperatively.

OUTCOMES

- Reports in the literature on follow-up of the conservative and surgical management of OCD are difficult to compare and interpret because there is a lack of a universally accepted classification system, the numbers of patients in most series is limited, and there are disparities in age at presentation, symptoms, lesion size, location, stability, and viability. Further, there are differences in the method of diagnostic imaging used, surgical technique, and length of follow-up.
- A consensus exists in the literature on the need to limit continual high-stress loading of the radiocapitellar joint in patients treated (even successfully) with OCD to prevent the deterioration of the frequently obtained short-term favorable results. As a result, most pitchers are counseled to move to other positions and gymnasts are advised of the difficulty in returning to continued high-level competitive gymnastics.
- Conservative treatment of OCD does not provide uniformly successful results.
- Takahara et al[6,7] presented the results of nonoperative management of early OCD lesions with an average follow-up of 5.2 years and reported that more than half of these patients had pain with activities, and fewer than half of the lesions showed radiographic improvement.
- Surgery also does not result in uniformly good outcomes.
- In one of the longest follow-up studies available in the elbow OCD literature, Bauer et al[1] presented the results of 31 patients (23 of whom were treated surgically with lesion or loose body excision) with capitellar OCD followed for an average of 23 years. At follow-up, the most common complaints were decreased range of motion (average 9 degrees of flexion loss, 2 degrees of extension loss, and 6 degrees of pronation–supination loss) and pain with activity. Radiographic evidence of degenerative changes involving the elbow joint was present in 61% and radial head enlargement in 58%.
- McManama et al[4] presented data on 14 adolescents with radiocapitellar OCD lesions treated with excision via a lateral arthrotomy with average follow-up of 2 years. Lesions were not sized, but 93% had good or excellent results.
- Jackson et al[3] reported on the roughly 3-year follow-up of OCD lesions in 10 female gymnasts treated primarily with curettage of loose cartilage, drilling, and loose body excision. All of the patients reported symptomatic relief, but only one patient returned to competition, and she did so with discomfort. Average loss of extension at follow-up in this series was 9 degrees, which is consistent with other reports.
- Ruch et al[5] presented the follow-up at an average of 3.2 years after arthroscopic débridement alone for management of elbow

OCD in 12 adolescents. The average flexion contracture improved 13 degrees (23 degrees preoperatively to 10 degrees postoperatively). All patients had capitellar remodeling on follow-up radiographs, and approximately 42% had associated radial head enlargement. Ninety-two percent of the patients in this series were highly satisfied, with minimal symptoms. Of note, five patients (42%) had a triangular lateral capsular avulsion fragment (seen radiographically but not at arthroscopy), which had a statistically significant association with a worse subjective outcome.

- Baumgarten et al[2] presented an average 4-year follow-up (range 24 to 75 months) on 17 elbows with OCD treated in 16 patients. Their results showed that the average flexion contracture improved 14 degrees, approximately 24% had pain, seven of nine (78%) throwers and four of five (80%) gymnasts were able to return to sport, and no patient had demonstrable degenerative joint disease.

COMPLICATIONS

- The complications seen with OCD treated surgically or not include flexion contracture, elbow pain, arthritis, and inability to return to sports.
- Loose bodies may develop in elbows treated nonoperatively.
- Surgical intervention, particularly arthroscopy, has the added risk of nerve injury because the neural structures are so close to the usual elbow arthroscopy portals.

REFERENCES

1. Bauer M, Jonsson K, Josefsson PO, et al. Osteochondritis dissecans of the elbow: a long-term follow-up study. Clin Orthop Relat Res 1992;284:156–160.
2. Baumgarten TE, Andrews JR, Satterwhite YE. The arthroscopic classification and treatment of osteochondritis dissecans of the capitellum. Am J Sports Med 1998;26:520–523.
3. Jackson D, Silvino N, Reimen P. Osteochondritis in the female gymnast's elbow. Arthroscopy 1989;5:129–136.
4. McManama GB Jr, Micheli LJ, Berry MV, et al. The surgical treatment of osteochondritis of the capitellum. Am J Sports Med 1985; 13:11–21.
5. Ruch DS, Cory JW, Poehling GG. The arthroscopic management of osteochondritis dissecans of the adolescent elbow. Arthroscopy 1998;14:797–803.
6. Takehara M, Ogino T, Fukushima S, et al. Nonoperative treatment of osteochondritis dissecans of the humeral capitellum. Am J Sports Med 1999;27:728–732.
7. Takehara M, Ogino T, Sasaki I, et al. Long-term outcome of osteochondritis dissecans of the humeral capitellum. Clin Orthop Relat Res 1999;363:108–115.

Chapter 20 Arthroscopic Treatment of Valgus Extension Overload

Sami O. Khan and Larry D. Field

DEFINITION

- Valgus extension overload of the elbow is commonly seen in the overhead throwing athlete and is associated with medial compartment distraction, lateral compartment compression, and posterior compartment impingement.[4,6]

ANATOMY

- The bony articulation of the elbow joint provides primary stability to varus and valgus force at angles of less than 20 degrees and greater than 120 degrees of flexion.
  - Soft tissues are the chief stabilizers between 20 and 120 degrees, where most athletic activity occurs.
- The ulnar collateral ligament (UCL) is the primary restraint to valgus stress.
  - It is composed of the anterior band, the posterior band, and the transverse ligament.
  - The anterior band is further divided into anterior and posterior bundle, which perform reciprocal functions (**FIG 1**).
- UCL insufficiency can be subtle, with ligament-sectioning studies showing a 3-degree difference when the anterior band of the UCL is cut.[2]

PATHOGENESIS

- Valgus extension overload typically occurs in repetitive overhead athletes, most commonly with pitchers. The repetitive pitching motion imparts a large valgus force on the elbow. Resulting microtrauma and incomplete recovery can lead to attenuation of the UCL.
- Failure of the UCL leads to abnormal valgus rotation of the elbow, affecting the mechanics of the highly constrained articulation of the posterior elbow joint.
- This leads to bony impingement of the posteromedial olecranon and its corresponding fossa.
- Chronic bony impingement can lead to chondral lesions as well as reactive osteophyte formation of the posterior compartment (**FIG 2**).

NATURAL HISTORY

- Thus far, no studies have been performed documenting the natural history of the disease process.
- It is postulated that chronic impingement and valgus extension overload can lead to posteromedial olecranon osteophyte formation that can cause ulnar nerve irritation and loss of elbow extension as well as posterior compartment elbow arthritis.

PATIENT HISTORY AND PHYSICAL FINDINGS

- The patient typically complains of loss of extension with posterior or posteromedial elbow pain.
- Pitchers will report pain during the acceleration and follow-through phases of the throwing motion (**FIG 3**).

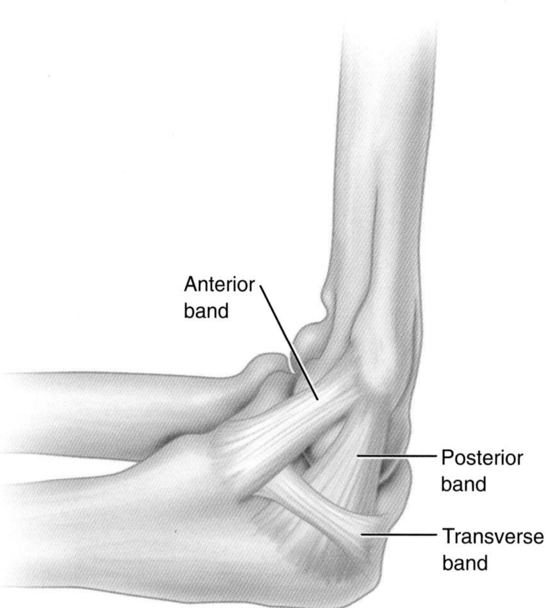

FIG 1 • The ulnar collateral ligament is composed of three bands: anterior, posterior, and transverse. The anterior band is further subdivided into the anterior and posterior bundles.

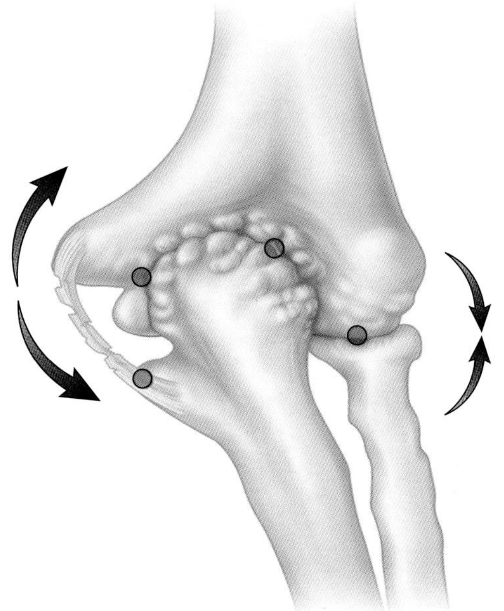

FIG 2 • Valgus extension overload. With ulnar collateral ligament insufficiency, medial compartment distraction and lateral compartment compression ultimately lead to posteromedial olecranon impingement.

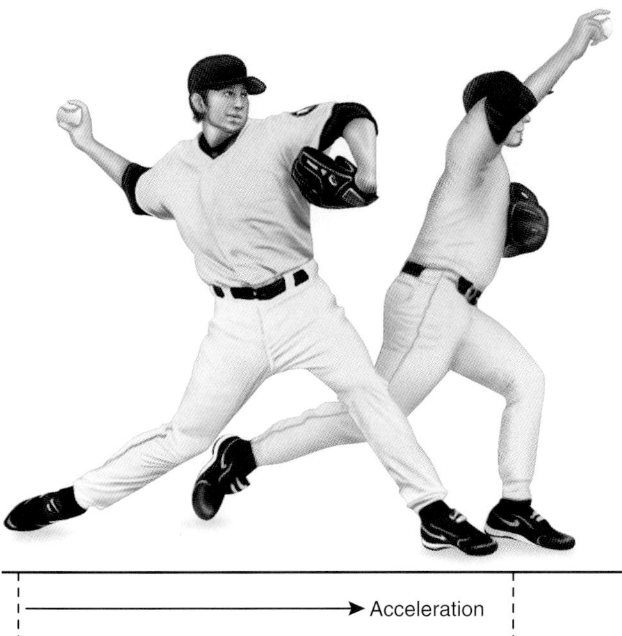

FIG 3 • The pitching athlete with valgus extension overload will often complain of pain during the acceleration and follow-through phases of throwing.

- Physical examination maneuvers relevant to valgus extension overload include:
  - Valgus extension overload test: This maneuver acts to simulate impingement occurring with the throwing motion and to reproduce the symptoms of posterior elbow pain.
  - Valgus stress test: Increased medial joint space opening, loss of end point, or pain elicited is significant for UCL insufficiency.
  - Milking maneuver: Maneuver eliciting pain, apprehension, or instability indicates UCL insufficiency.
  - Posterior olecranon impingement
  - Range of motion of elbow: may reveal loose bodies, chondromalacia, or osteophyte formation; flexion contracture may signify either osteophyte impingement or anterior capsular contracture
- Examination of the elbow should also evaluate for other causes of medial-sided elbow problems, such as isolated UCL insufficiency, ulnar neuropathy, medial epicondylitis, and flexor pronator rupture.

IMAGING AND OTHER DIAGNOSTIC STUDIES

- Radiographs frequently reveal a posterior olecranon osteophyte on standard lateral or anteroposterior views (**FIG 4A**).
  - Some authors also advocate an olecranon axial view (**FIG 4B**).
- Because radiographs cannot predict chondral lesions and soft tissue injuries and often underestimate loose body formation, magnetic resonance (MRI) and computed tomography are frequently used.
  - MRI can also be important in investigating a potential UCL tear (**FIG 4C**).

DIFFERENTIAL DIAGNOSIS

- Isolated UCL insufficiency
- Medial epicondylitis
- Flexor–pronator rupture
- Ulnar neuropathy

NONOPERATIVE MANAGEMENT

- Before recommending surgery, the physician should usually treat the patient nonoperatively for 3 to 6 months.
- Specific goals to be attained during this time are full, nonpainful range of motion; absence of pain and tenderness on physical examination; and satisfactory muscle strength, power, and endurance.
- The patient begins treatment with an initial period of rest (1 to 3 weeks), allowing any synovitis and inflammation to resolve.
- Next, he or she begins wrist and elbow flexor and extensor muscle stretching and strengthening exercises.
- Finally, an interval-throwing program is instituted.

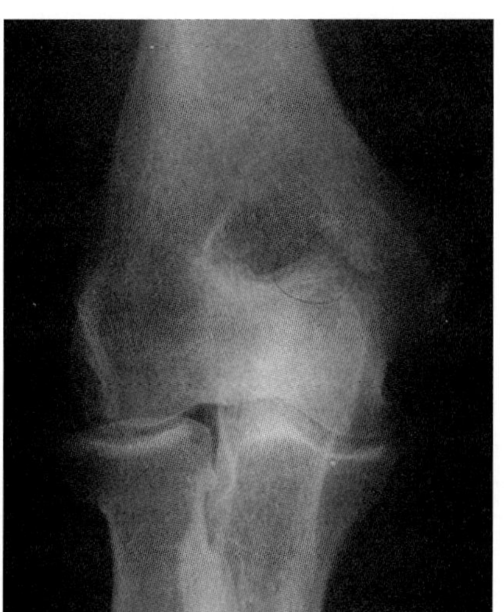

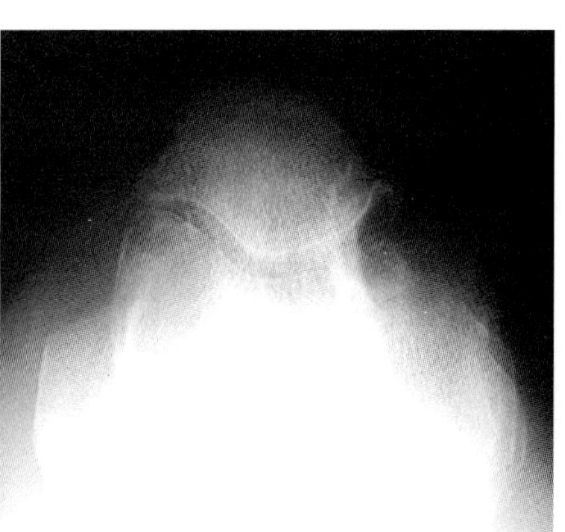

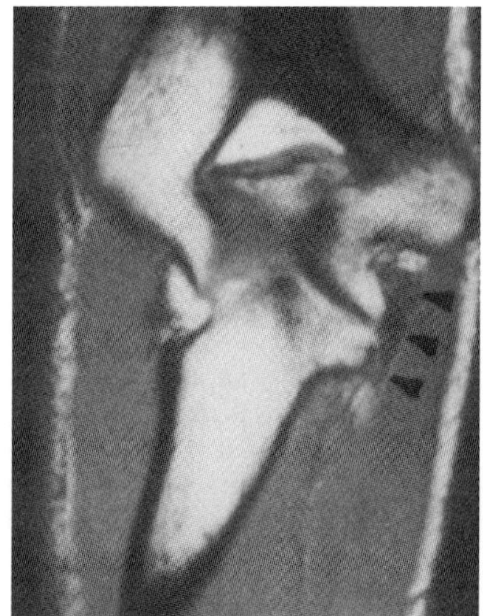

FIG 4 • AP (**A**) and olecranon axial (**B**) radiographs showing spur formation along the posteromedial olecranon. **C.** Coronal section of MRI demonstrating injury to the ulnar collateral ligament.

SURGICAL MANAGEMENT

- Relative contraindications to elbow arthroscopy include severe bony or fibrous ankylosis and previous surgery that has distorted the native anatomy, such as a previous ulnar nerve transposition.

Preoperative Planning

- A thorough history is paramount to planning for arthroscopic elbow surgery.
- The surgeon should confirm that the ulnar nerve is indeed in the groove and cannot be subluxated.
- The surgeon must assess for valgus instability when considering valgus extension overload.
- Failure to address UCL instability in the setting of valgus extension overload may lead to treatment failure.

Positioning

- We prefer the prone position for all elbow arthroscopy because it allows for the elbow to be stabilized as well as giving improved access to the posterior compartment. Posteromedial olecranon spur excision is especially facilitated by the prone position.
- We routinely use a pneumatic tourniquet and a prone arm holder.
- The elbow should be positioned and draped so that the arm is supported by the holder at the proximal upper arm, the elbow rests at 90 degrees of flexion, and the antecubital fossa is free from contact with the holder (**FIG 5**).

Approach

- Elbow arthroscopy has made open resection of olecranon osteophytes primarily a point of historic interest. However, occasions still exist when an open procedure should be performed.
- The determining factor in the decision-making process is whether a contraindication to elbow arthroscopy is present.
- A posteromedial approach to the elbow is used when concomitant UCL reconstruction, ulnar nerve transposition, or exploration of a previously transposed ulnar nerve is to be accomplished in conjunction with removal of posteromedial osteophytes.

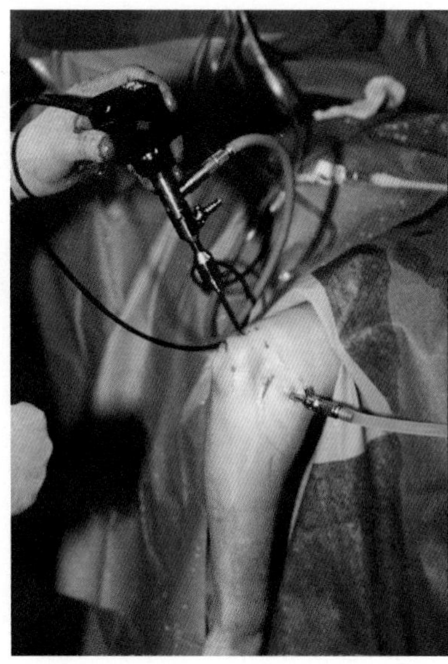

FIG 5 • Intraoperative photograph showing prone positioning for elbow arthroscopy.

Equipment

- General anesthesia is preferred because use of regional anesthesia makes the immediate postoperative motor and sensory examination difficult to interpret.
- A standard 4.0-mm arthroscope, power inflow or pump, standard power débrider, and abraders are required.
- Hand-held instruments as well as only blunt trocars should be used.
- The video monitor is placed on the opposite side of the patient.

Examination Under Anesthesia

- Examination under anesthesia is essential to develop a feel for the character and cause of any extension block.
- A bony block has a hard, sudden stop and a feeling of bony impingement. Anterior capsular contracture often has a slightly softer feel at terminal extension.
- Valgus instability testing throughout the range of motion helps to assess the status of the UCL.

TECHNIQUES

DIAGNOSTIC ARTHROSCOPY

- The medial epicondyle, lateral epicondyle, and ulnar nerve are outlined.
- The surgeon confirms that the ulnar nerve is indeed located within the groove and remains so with range of motion of the elbow.
- The lateral "soft spot" portal location is identified and 20 cc of saline is injected into the elbow joint. Often a slight elbow extension will be seen as the capsule is insufflated.
- Diagnostic arthroscopy must include a complete inspection and evaluation of the elbow.
- An arthroscopic valgus instability test should be performed and medial stability should be documented (**TECH FIG 1A,B**).[3]
- The posterior compartment should be thoroughly evaluated.
  - Examination of the olecranon–olecranon fossa articulation may show osteophyte formation of the posteromedial olecranon (**TECH FIG 1C,D**).
- The olecranon fossa of the humerus should be evaluated for hypertrophy, chondromalacia, and spur formation.
- A systematic examination of the entire elbow joint is necessary to identify and remove any loose bodies present.

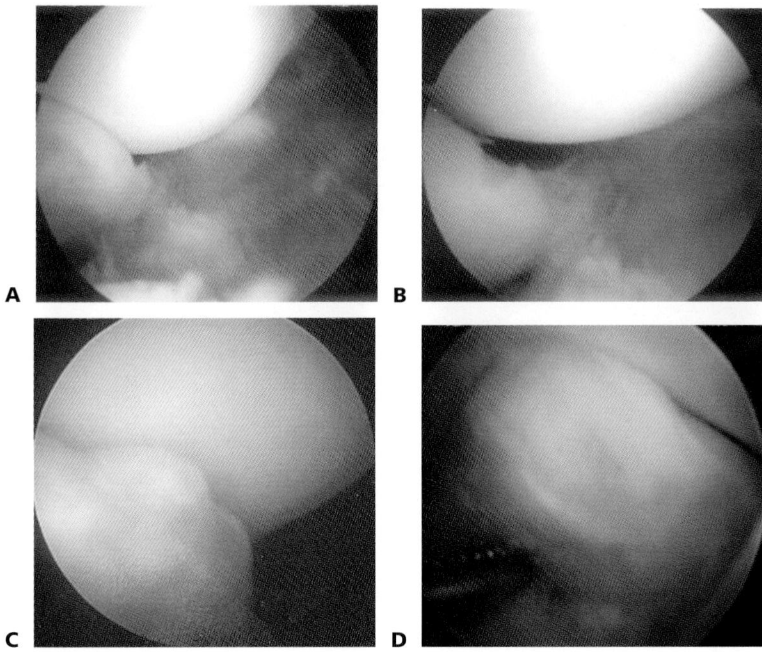

TECH FIG 1 • **A.** The arthroscopic valgus instability test is performed to assess for significant opening in the ulnohumeral articulation. **B.** A diastasis in the medial ulnohumeral articulation is noted. **C,D.** Arthroscopic views of a posteromedial bone spur.

POSTEROMEDIAL OLECRANON SPUR REMOVAL

- First, a viewing portal is established through a posterolateral portal.
- A direct posterior or triceps-splitting portal is established for access of the motorized resector or burr. The posteromedial spur is then resected (TECH FIG 2A,B).
- The ulnar nerve has a close relationship to the medial olecranon. While working medially, the surgeon should minimize the use of suction, use a hooded burr, and always keep the hooded portion oriented toward the ulnar nerve (TECH FIG 2C).

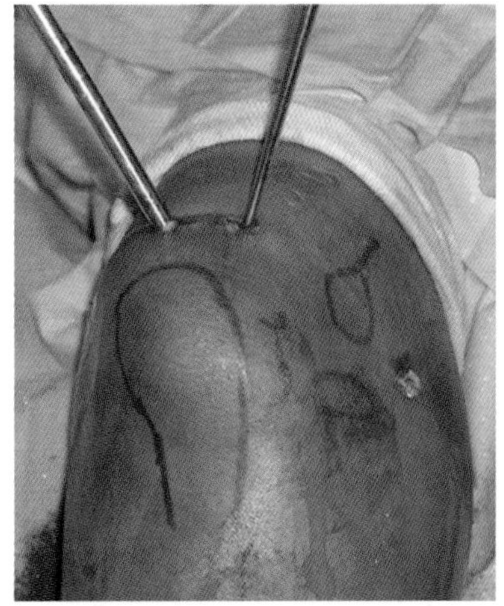

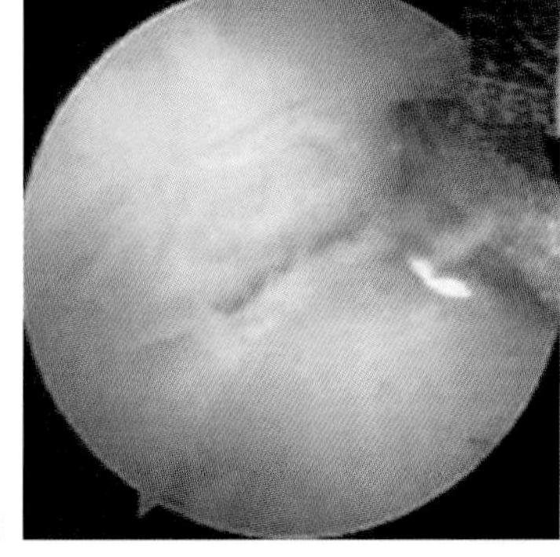

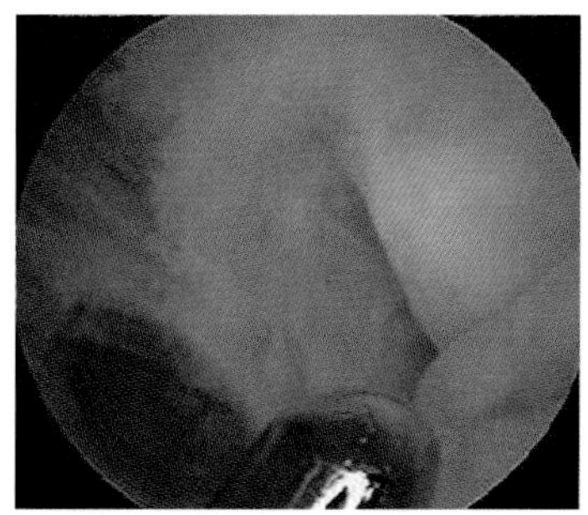

TECH FIG 2 • **A,B.** Posterior compartment olecranon spur excision. **C.** Use of a hooded burr for posteromedial spur resection. The instrument is always pointed away from the ulnar nerve.

EVALUATION AND TREATMENT OF ARTICULAR CARTILAGE

- After clearing out the olecranon fossa, the articular cartilage is carefully inspected.
- Areas of chondromalacia can be treated by the surgeon's choice of microfracture, abrasion chondroplasty, or benign neglect.

TECHNIQUES

DEEPENING OF OLECRANON FOSSA

- Occasionally, hypertrophy of the olecranon fossa necessitates a deepening or fenestration of the olecranon fossa (**TECH FIG 3**).
- This can be performed using the same instruments and positioning.
- When resection is complete, the surgeon should assess elbow extension and valgus instability with a repeat arthroscopic valgus instability test.

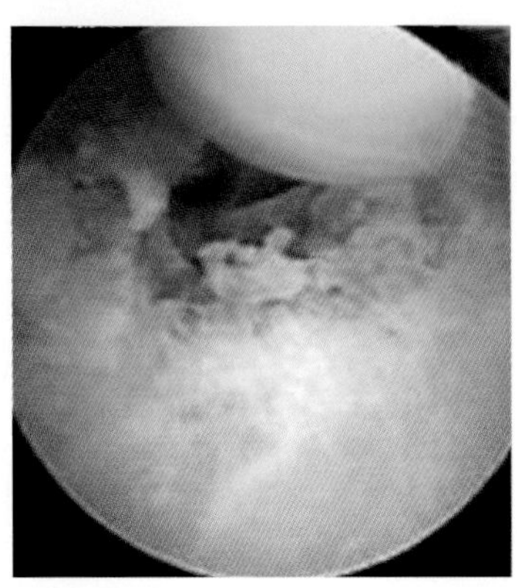

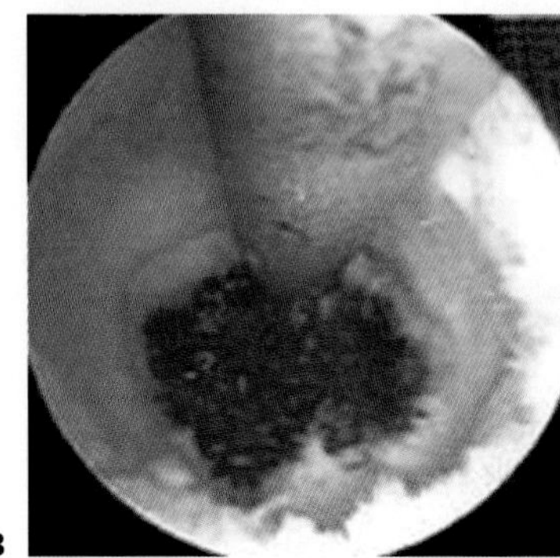

TECH FIG 3 • Arthroscopic views both during (**A**) and after (**B**) olecranon fossa fenestration.

PEARLS AND PITFALLS

Thorough preoperative history and physical examination	▪ Screening for contraindications to elbow arthroscopy can prevent iatrogenic nerve injury. The surgeon should not create a medial portal if the location or orientation of the ulnar nerve is unclear.
Arthroscopic valgus instability test	▪ A careful test before and after spur excision helps prevent unrecognized ulnar collateral ligament instability.
Use of hooded motorized resector	▪ Motorized shavers, even when used properly, present a significant risk of injury to the ulnar nerve.

POSTOPERATIVE CARE

- Patients with valgus extension overload undergoing isolated spur excision are moved rapidly through the rehabilitation process.[5]
- A sling is used sparingly for comfort for the first 7 to 10 days.
- After the first week, patients are encouraged to use the elbow normally for activities of daily living, and they can begin strengthening and range-of-motion exercises.
  - We include flexor–pronator mass strengthening to improve dynamic valgus instability.
- When patients reach a pain-free plateau, they can be advanced through an interval-throwing program.
  - This throwing program typically begins at 6 weeks.
  - A target return to competitive pitching is 3 to 4 months.

OUTCOMES

- The study by Wilson et al[6] included five patients treated with open biplanar spur excision. One reoperation was required in a patient with severe chondromalacia of the olecranon articular surface.
- Bartz et al[1] reported on a series of 24 baseball pitchers treated with a mini-open technique. Nineteen of the 24 obtained complete relief and were able to equal or exceed their preoperative throwing velocity. However, two patients did require reoperation for UCL reconstruction.

COMPLICATIONS

- Thus far, no complications of this diagnosis or procedure have been documented.
- Use of a motorized shaver in the medial gutter to débride olecranon osteophytes in close proximity to the ulnar nerve does warrant extreme caution.
  - In addition, an unrecognized UCL insufficiency has been a documented cause of reoperation.
- Often this diagnosis is difficult to make in the immediate postoperative period; it may become apparent only when the athlete cannot regain his or her pitching velocity and control.

REFERENCES

1. Bartz RL, Lowe WR, Bryan WJ. Posterior elbow impingement. Oper Tech Sports Med 2001;9:245–252.
2. Callaway GH, Field LD, Deng XH, et al. Biomechanical evaluation of the medial collateral ligament of the elbow. J Bone Joint Surg Am 1997;79A:1223–1231.
3. Field LD, Altchek DW. Evaluation of the arthroscopic valgus instability test of the elbow. Am J Sports Med 1996;24:177–181.
4. Miller CD, Savoie FH. Valgus extension injuries of the elbow in the throwing athlete. J Am Acad Orthop Surg 1994;2:261–269.
5. Wilk KE, Arrigo C. Current concepts in the rehabilitation of the athletic shoulder. J Orthop Sports Phys Ther 1993;18:365–378.
6. Wilson FD, Andrews JR, Blackburn TA, et al. Valgus extension overload of the elbow. Am J Sports Med 1993;11:83–88.

Chapter 21

Arthroscopic Treatment of Elbow Loss of Motion

Matthew T. Provencher, Mark S. Cohen, and Anthony A. Romeo

DEFINITION

- Elbow stiffness can cause significant impairment in function of the upper extremity, especially in performance of the activities of daily living (ADLs).
  - A lack of compensatory biomechanical function (ie, the scapula for the shoulder) makes elbow stiffness poorly tolerated.
- A functional arc of 100 degrees (30 to 130 degrees) is required for most ADLs.[13]
- Posttraumatic elbow motion loss is most common, but osteoarthritis, inflammatory conditions, systemic conditions (head injury), and neurologic problems may also cause contractures.
- Flexion loss is less tolerated than extension loss, but loss of extension is more common.[12]
- The key to treatment is to determine the functional and occupational impairment and not base treatment decisions solely on the absolute loss of motion of the elbow.[7]

ANATOMY

- The elbow has a predilection for stiffness based on its anatomy: the close relationship of the capsule to the surrounding ligaments and muscles and the presence of three joints within a synovial-lined joint cavity—a hinge (ginglymus) ulnohumeral articulation and rotatory joint (trochoid) of both the radiohumeral and radioulnar joints.[7]
- The anterior elbow capsule proximally attaches above the coronoid fossa and distally extends to the coronoid (medial) and the annular ligament (lateral). The posterior capsule starts proximally just above the olecranon fossa and inserts at the articular margin of the sigmoid notch and annular ligament (**FIG 1**).
- The anterior capsule is taut in extension and lax in flexion, with the strength of the capsule provided from the cruciate orientation of the fibers of the anterior capsule.
- Greatest capsular capacity is at 80 degrees flexion.[5,15] Normal capacity of 25 mL is reduced significantly in a contracture state to 6 mL.[5,15]

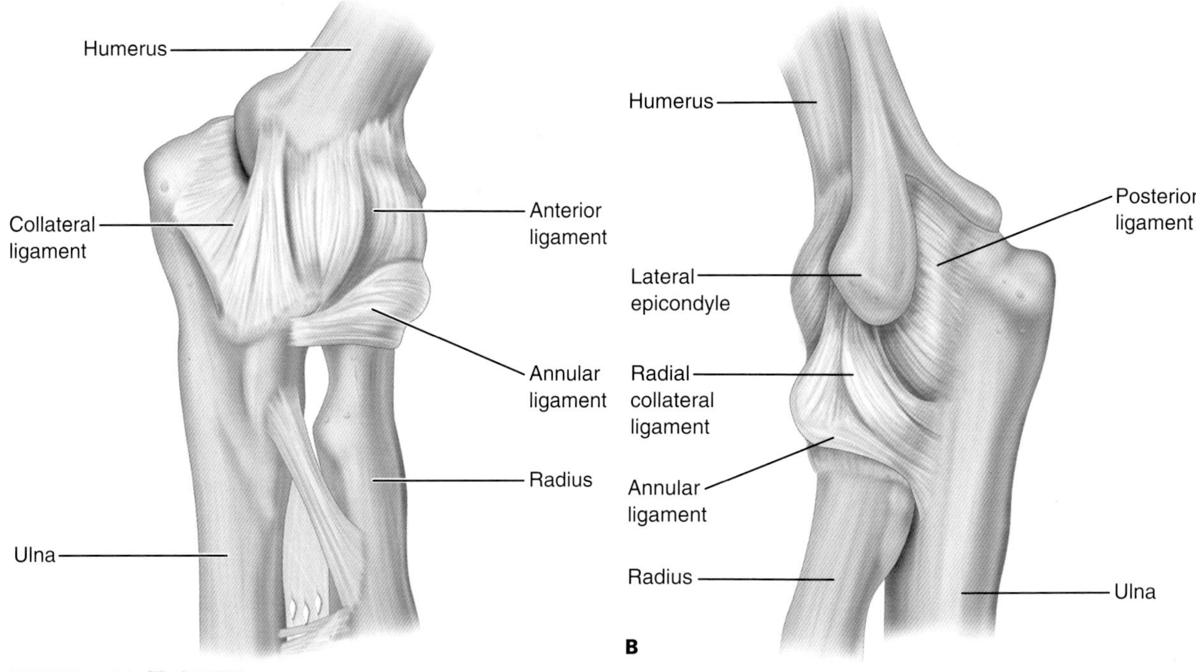

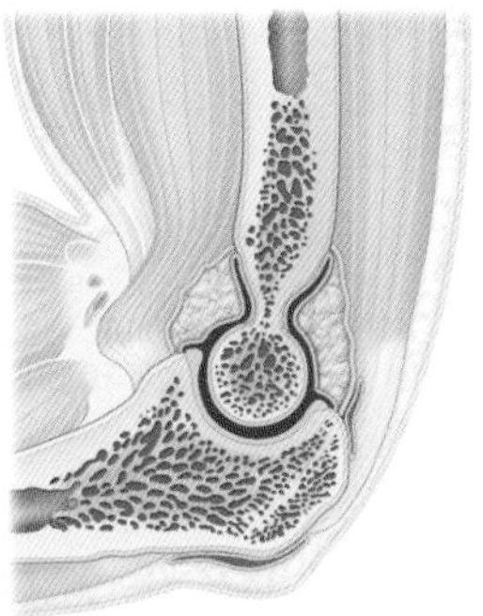

FIG 1 • Anatomic drawing of elbow capsular structures. The anterior (**A**) and posterior capsular areas (**B**) are highlighted. The anterior capsule distally extends to the coronoid medially and annular ligament laterally. **C.** Lateral diagram of the elbow shows the capsular size and fat pad.

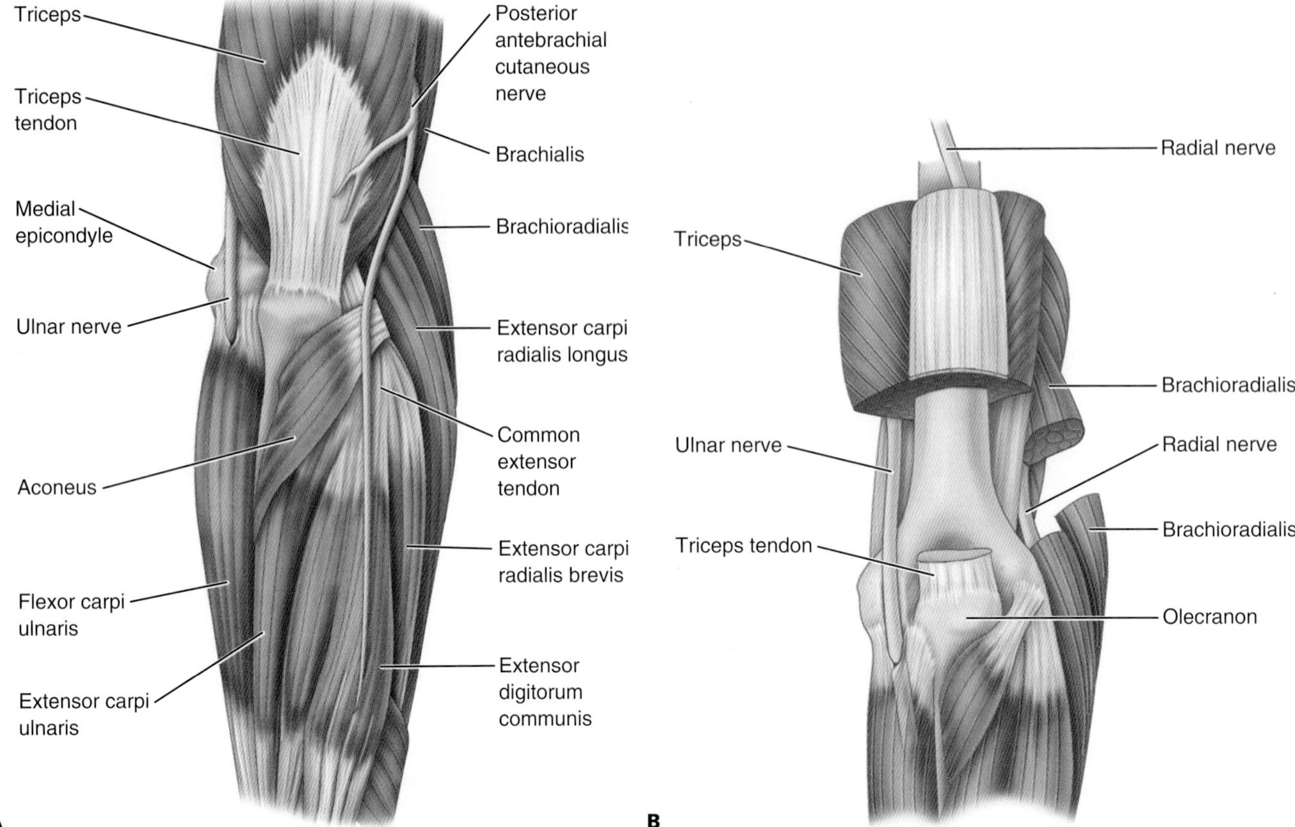

FIG 2 • Anatomic location of the ulnar nerve at the elbow (**A**), which is contained in the cubital tunnel (**B**).

- The joint capsule is innervated by branches from all the major nerves that cross the joint (Hilton's law) and musculocutaneous nerve.[10]
- The cubital tunnel, which houses the ulnar nerve at the elbow, becomes taut in flexion (because the attachment sites of the retinaculum are at maximal distance between the olecranon and medial epicondyle) and lax in extension.
  - Flexion contractures may adversely compress the ulnar nerve (**FIG 2**).

PATHOGENESIS

- The reasons for altered capsular properties are multifactorial and not completely known.
  - Hildebrand et al[6] have found increased numbers of myofibroblasts in the anterior capsule, a cell line that can lead to collagen cell contraction.
  - Increased matrix metalloproteinases and collagen disorganization have also been described in the contracted capsular tissue.
- From a peripheral injury, such as head trauma, a complex chain of events can lead to elbow contracture and heterotopic ossification.
- From a cellular level, there is an increase in the formation of collagen cross-linking, hypertrophy, decreased water content, and decreased proteoglycan content in the contracted elbow tissue.[1]
- Growth factors and other cellular mechanisms may be involved. This is highly variable among individuals.[12]
- There is loss of joint volume (20 mL to 6 mL) and thickened capsular width (from a normal width of approximately 2 mm).[5,10,14]
- Posttraumatic contractures thicken and tighten variable areas of the elbow capsule, especially the anterior aspect.

NATURAL HISTORY

- Elbow contracture is frequently posttraumatic. Heterotopic ossification may occur in conjunction with capsular thickening. Patients most at risk are those with combined head and elbow trauma, burn patients, and those who have undergone surgical approaches to the elbow.[4]
- Classification of the cause of elbow stiffness is important in making treatment decisions (Table 1).[7]
  - Most contractures have mixed elements (both intrinsic and extrinsic factors).[8]
- Morrey[12] characterized elbow stiffness as static or dynamic, based on tissue involvement (Table 2).

PATIENT HISTORY AND PHYSICAL FINDINGS

- It is critical to determine the degree of functional impairment for each patient. Management decisions should be based on subjective impairment, not necessarily the amount of motion loss.[7]
- The surgeon should obtain a history of associated conditions because neurologic, peripheral nerve, or brain injury may influence management decisions.

Table 1 Classification of Elbow Stiffness Based on Location of Structure in Relation to the Elbow Joint

Type	Location	Description
Intrinsic	Within the elbow joint	Articular incongruity after fracture, degenerative changes and loss of cartilage, intra-articular adhesions, loose bodies, synovitis, infection
Extrinsic	Tissues immediately adjacent	Soft tissue and capsular contracture, muscle fibrosis (brachialis especially), collateral ligament stiffness, to the elbow joint heterotopic ossification, skin contractures
Peripheral	Factors anatomically separate from the elbow	Stroke, neurologic problems, peripheral nerve disorder, head injury, cerebral palsy

From Jupiter JB, O'Driscoll SW, Cohen MS. The assessment and management of the stiff elbow. AAOS Instr Course Lect 2003;52:93–111.

- The surgeon should assess the function of the entire ipsilateral and contralateral upper extremity.
- The surgeon should determine hand dominance, the patient's occupation, and the extent of prior therapy, including bracing (both static and dynamic).
- Physical examination should start with the head, including the cranial and cervical nerves.
  - The surgeon palpates the cervical spine and checks the spine range of motion.
  - The surgeon evaluates the shoulder joint to ensure good strength and range of motion.
  - Careful assessment of the ulnar nerve
    - Two-point discrimination: A normal amount of discrimination is less than 6 mm.
    - Froment sign and intrinsic hand muscle function: The patient is asked to grasp a piece of paper between the adducted thumb and index finger. The patient must keep his or her thumb flat against the index finger. If the patient cannot do so, the flexor pollicis longus contributes more to hold paper and indicates weakness of the adductor pollicis and ulnar nerve injury.
    - Decreased grip strength may signify an ulnar nerve problem.
  - Elbow range of motion: Flexion and extension with the humerus flexed to 90 degrees, pronation, and supination can be objectively evaluated with a linear object (pencil) held in a clenched fist and the elbow at the side of the body.
  - Elbow instability examination: The surgeon should check the ligamentous restraints to varus and valgus stress.
  - Ligaments are assessed with varus and valgus stress at 0 and 30 degrees of flexion if amenable.
  - The cubital tunnel is palpated to assess for tenderness or a positive Tinel's sign.

IMAGING AND OTHER DIAGNOSTIC STUDIES

- Plain radiographs (anteroposterior [AP] and lateral) are usually adequate.
  - The AP provides joint line and subchondral bone visualization.
  - If an elbow is contracted more than 45 degrees, the AP view of the joint line is usually distorted,[12] but advanced imaging is rarely necessary unless a fracture or malunion is present.
- The lateral view may show osteophytes on the olecranon or coronoid (**FIG 3A,B**).
  - If there is articular incongruity or other joint abnormalities, the surgeon should consider obtaining a computed tomography scan with reformatted images in the coronal and sagittal planes.
- Radiographs can be used to follow the maturation process of heterotopic ossification.
  - Arthroscopic treatment is usually not recommended in the presence of heterotopic ossification, which usually signifies multiple extrinsic causes of elbow contracture, not amenable to arthroscopic treatment (**FIG 3C**).

DIFFERENTIAL DIAGNOSIS

- Heterotopic ossification
- Closed head injury
- Burns
- Elbow fracture–dislocation
- Dysplastic radial head (congenital)
- Muscular hypotonia
- Stroke

NONOPERATIVE MANAGEMENT

- Nonoperative management should be considered up to 6 months after contracture onset.[8]
- Response is better if there is a soft "spongy" endpoint during range of motion.[8,14]
- The goal is to gain motion gradually without causing additional trauma to the capsule and subsequently development of additional capsular contracture (more pain, inflammation, and swelling leads to more contracture).

Table 2 Characterization of Elbow Stiffness by Tissue Involvement

Classification	Relative Occurrence	Location	Description
Static	Most common	Tissues in and around the elbow joint	Capsule, ligaments, heterotopic ossification, articular and cartilaginous components
Dynamic	Less common	Involves muscles around the joint	Poor muscle tone, nerve injuries, and poor excursion of the muscles that cross the elbow joint

From Morrey BF. The stiff elbow with articular involvement. In: Jupiter JB, ed. The Stiff Elbow. Rosemont, IL: American Academy of Orthopaedic Surgeons; 2006:21–30.

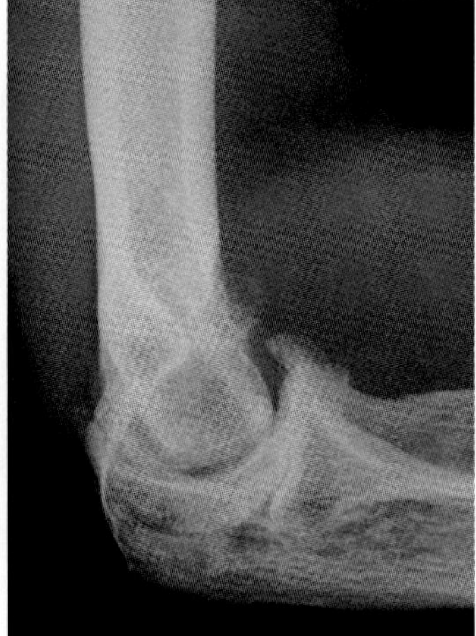

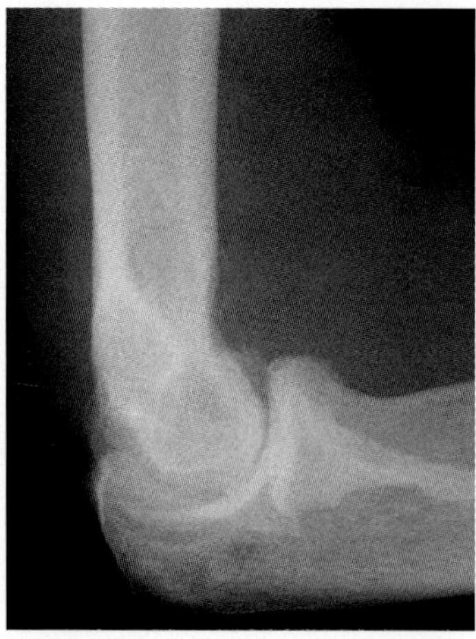

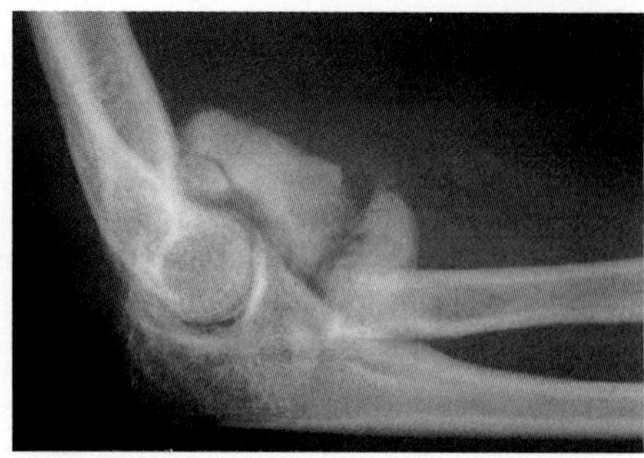

A B C

FIG 3 • **A.** Preoperative lateral radiograph of an elbow before arthroscopic resection of osteophytes at the olecranon and coronoid, with associated anterior capsular contracture. Heterotopic ossification is absent. **B.** Postoperative radiograph after resection of osteophytes. **C.** Lateral radiograph of an elbow with heterotopic ossification. Arthroscopic resection is not recommended in this type of patient.

- Edema control is critical, and therapy should focus on this, not exercises that induce inflammation around the elbow.
- Static and preferably patient-adjusted static progressive splints (turnbuckle splints) have proven valuable and should be used between therapy sessions.[7]
- Dynamic splinting may be helpful, but care should be taken not to incite an inflammatory process because these provide a constant tension over time. Static progressive splints that allow for stress relaxation of the soft tissues are more effective and better tolerated.
- Nonoperative improvements in range of motion vary widely but have been reported anywhere from 10 to 50 degrees or more.[8,10,14]
- O'Driscoll[14] described four stages of elbow stiffness:
  - Bleeding: minutes to hours
  - Edema: hours to days. Both bleeding and edema cause swelling within the joint and surrounding tissues, and the tissues become biomechanically less compliant. Early elbow range of motion through an entire range during stages 1 and 2 can prevent stiffness.
  - Granulation tissue: days to weeks. Splints can be used to regain range of motion.
  - Fibrosis: Maturation of the granulation tissue further decreases compliance. More aggressive splinting is necessary, along with possible surgical management.

SURGICAL MANAGEMENT

- The key is to identify the functional disability of the patient—pain, loss of motion, or both—and what would be most beneficial.
- The indications include a loss of function to preclude the patient from performing ADLs and occupational or vocational activities.
- Arthroscopic treatment of elbow stiffness should be undertaken only if the offending structures can be treated from an arthroscopic approach. Heterotopic ossification is not amenable to arthroscopic treatment.
- Appropriate counseling with the patient should cover realistic expectations of range of motion and functional recovery. Will patients be able to get their hand to their mouth, comb their hair, or reach behind their back, or are more extensive demands required?

Preoperative Planning

- The surgeon should assess for heterotopic ossification on plain radiographs. Arthroscopic treatment is not indicated if this is causing the contracture.
- An examination under anesthesia helps to confirm nonmuscle-related pathology and to assess the static component of contraction, which should mirror the in-office examination.
- If the examination documents irritation or neuropathy, the ulnar nerve should be exposed and released.
  - We recommend that the ulnar nerve be released before the arthroscopic portion for ease of dissection before fluid distention.
  - In patients with elbow flexion of less than 100 degrees and in those with ulnar nerve tension signs or sensitivity to percussion, the nerve should be prophylactically released to prevent compression once flexion is restored postsurgically.[12]
  - The surgeon must ensure that the ulnar nerve cannot be subluxated or transposed.[3]
- Contraindications to arthroscopic release are prior surgery that has altered the neurovascular anatomy, joint deformity that would compromise arthroscopic view, prior ulnar nerve transposition, and malunited elbow fractures.[16]

Positioning

- Either the lateral decubitus or prone position can be used (**FIG 4A,B**).
  - Lateral decubitus: well-padded pillow at edge of beanbag underneath elbow antecubital fossa
  - Prone: adequate chest and arm support, shoulder abducted to 90 degrees
- Well-padded sterile tourniquet for either position

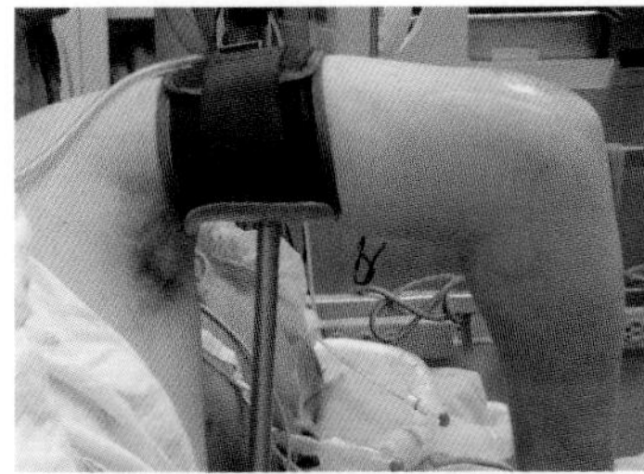

A

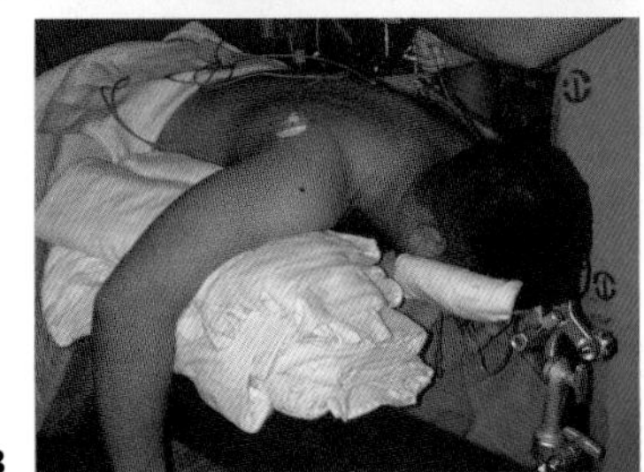

B

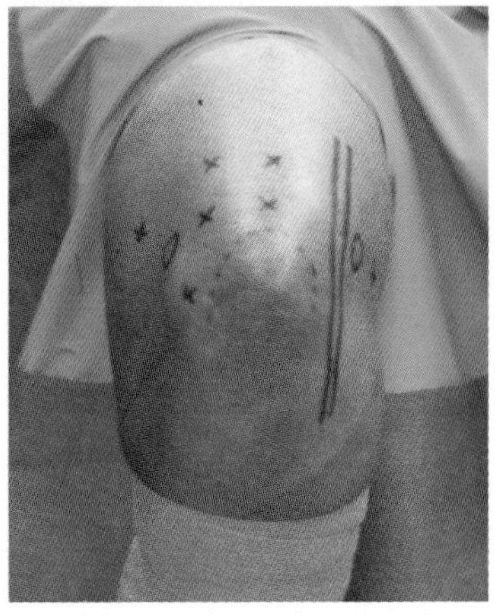

C

FIG 4 • **A,B.** Setup of patient for elbow arthroscopy in lateral (**A**) and prone (**B**) positioning. **C.** Landmarks of the elbow drawn for operative incisions and to identify at-risk structures, including the ulnar nerve, in the prone position.

- The remainder of the arthroscopic setup has been described elsewhere.
- The surgeon should clearly mark the course of the ulnar nerve, portal sites, and bony landmarks with surgical marker (**FIG 4C**).

Approach

- As with any arthroscopy, the surgeon must be able to visualize the joint.
- O'Driscoll states that the single most important factor to improve visualization is the use of arthroscopic retractors.[14]
- Loss of volume makes this difficult, but it can be facilitated with the use of elbow arthroscopic retractors.
- The key is to avoid nerve injury during the approach and during capsular treatment.
- The surgeon should plan for intraoperative ulnar nerve release if indicated. Nerve decompression is performed before arthroscopy because fluid extravasation distorts the surgical tissue planes (**FIG 5**).

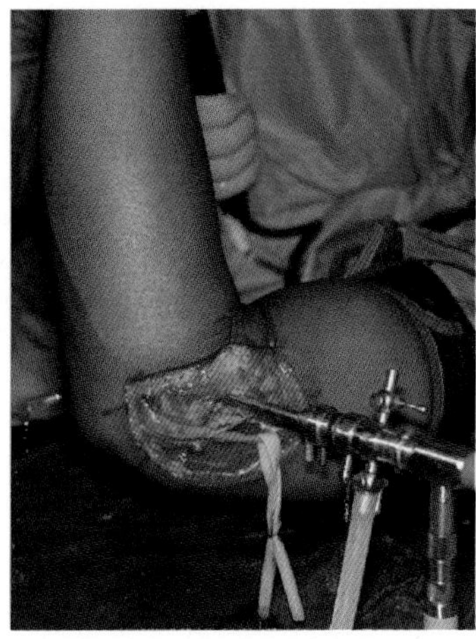

FIG 5 • If the ulnar nerve is thought to be involved, it may be released before starting the arthroscopy to facilitate dissection without the soft tissue changes that occur after fluid extravasation from the elbow joint. The ulnar nerve is marked with a vessel loop.

PORTAL ESTABLISHMENT IN CONTRACTED ELBOW

- The joint is distended with saline through the "soft spot" portal (up to 20 mL, less depending on contracture).
- Portals are established.
  - The 4.5-mm, 30-degree arthroscope is used through a proximomedial portal (about 2 cm proximal to the medial epicondyle and just anterior to the medial intermuscular septum) (**TECH FIG 1A,B**).[2]
  - The proximolateral portal (1.5 to 2 cm proximal to lateral epicondyle) is identified with either a blunt-tipped Wissinger rod or a spinal needle using an outside-in technique. Retractors are used to improve distention and visualization (**TECH FIG 1C**).
- Blunt dissection techniques with the Wissinger rod are used to obtain a working space.
- A 4.5-mm shaver (oscillate function) removes more material from the working space, but not yet the capsule.
- A small radiofrequency device can be used to débride the scar tissue within the joint. Inflow should be increased during the use of thermal energy.
- The capsule is not removed until the tissue planes are better defined to minimize nerve injury risk. The capsule is débrided superficially to define it as a structure.

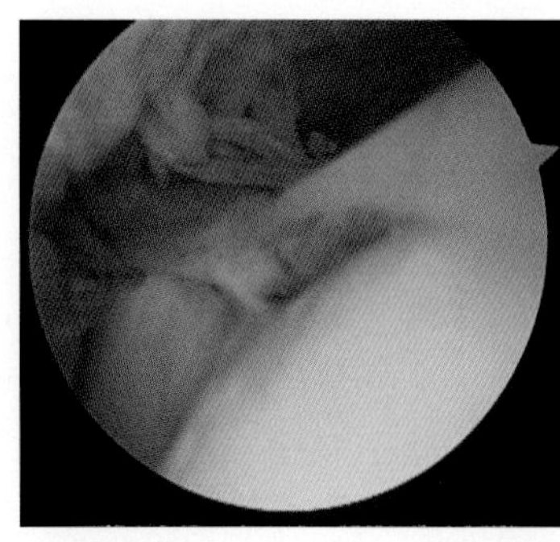

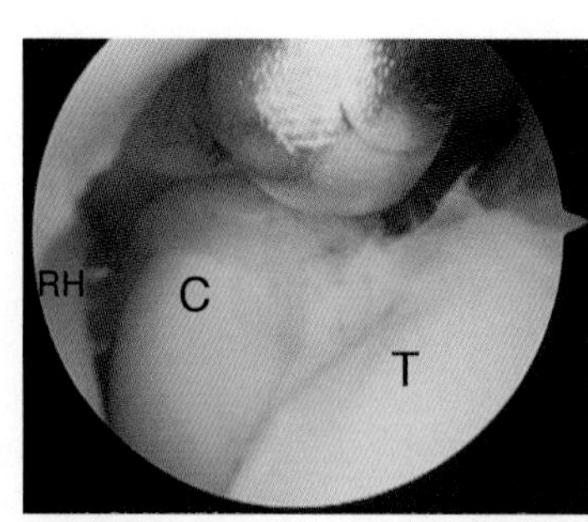

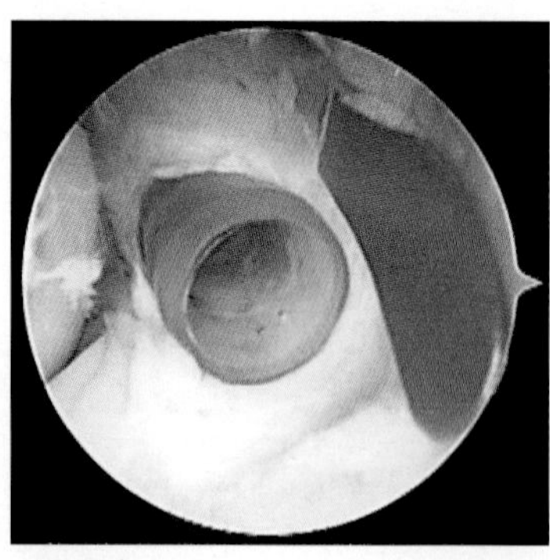

TECH FIG 1 • **A.** Arthroscopic view of a right elbow joint after first obtaining scope entry into the proximomedial portal, looking laterally. There is synovitis in the joint. **B.** After the synovitis is gently débrided with an arthroscopic shaver, the bony overgrowth of the coronoid and radial fossa is revealed. There is a lack of concavity in the trochlea and capitellum area. **C.** Arthroscopic view of elbow joint viewed from the medial portal, showing the increased visualization of the elbow joint that is obtained with the use of intra-articular retractors. *C*, capitellum; *RH*, radial head; *T*, trochlea.

ANTERIOR CAPSULAR RELEASE

- Capsulotomy of the anterior capsule is performed with an arthroscopic basket cutter.
- The brachialis muscle can be visualized and the plane between the capsule and brachialis developed from the lateral working portal (TECH FIG 2A).
  - The brachialis protects the median nerve, so the surgeon should avoid penetrating this muscle.
- The surgeon continues incising the capsule from lateral to medial.
  - The capsulotomy should be continued to the level of the collateral ligaments on each side, but the ligaments are not incised.
- The lateral side is at risk of injuring the radial nerve behind the capsule (just anterior to the radial head).
  - Capsulectomy in this area, although it may improve the results, carries a higher risk for radial nerve injury. It may be safest to remove the capsule well proximal to the joint line on the lateral side to avoid this risk.
  - The posterior interosseous nerve is the most significant nerve at risk during elbow arthroscopy.[16] It is adjacent to the anterolateral capsule (distally).
- The surgeon should view from the lateral portal to ensure adequate medial release (TECH FIG 2B).

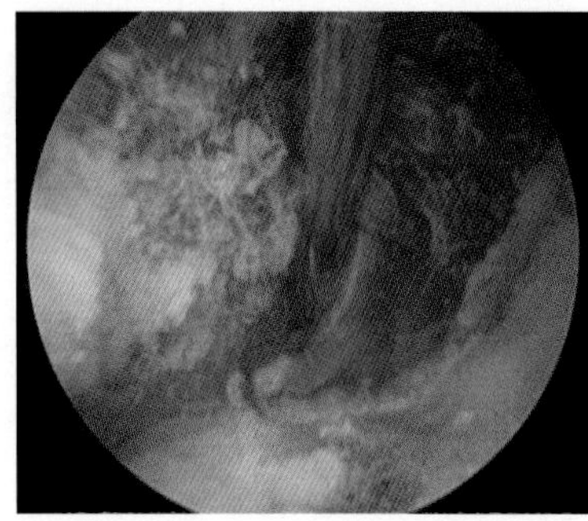

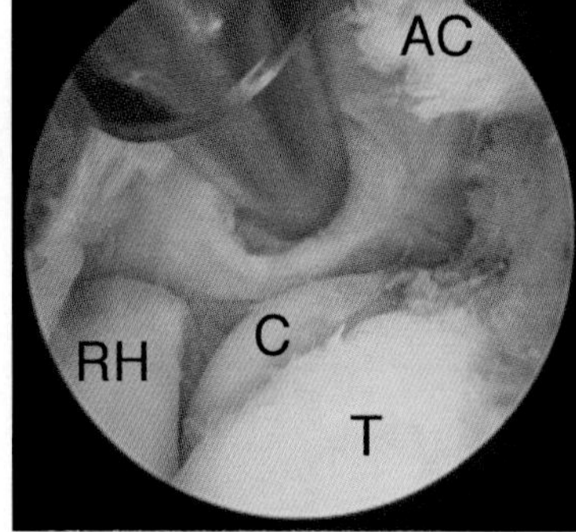

TECH FIG 2 • **A.** Arthroscopic view of the elbow joint after capsulectomy and deepening of the coronoid and radial fossa. The dissection is carried down to the fibers of the brachialis muscle but does not violate the brachialis (retracted structure). **B.** View from the lateral portal shows the partially completed release. Bony work and resection are completed before capsulectomy. The concavity in the coronoid and trochlear fossa areas is formed, but anterior capsulectomy is not yet completed. *AC*, anterior capsule; *C*, capitellum; *RH*, radial head; *T*, trochlea.

POSTERIOR CAPSULAR RELEASE

- The surgeon establishes a posterocentral portal for the arthroscope (4 cm proximal to the olecranon tip through the triceps) and a posterolateral working portal (2 cm proximal to the olecranon tip and lateral to the triceps).
- A shaver is used to débride and open the space and remove loose bodies and osteophytes. Suction is avoided in and along the medial gutter.
- The capsule is elevated from the distal humerus (using a shaver or elevator).

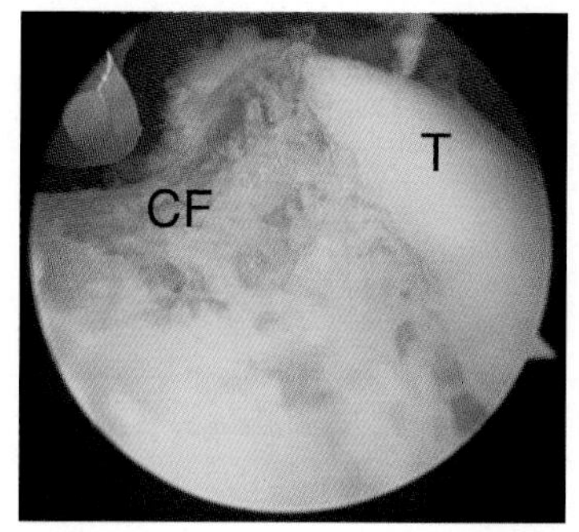

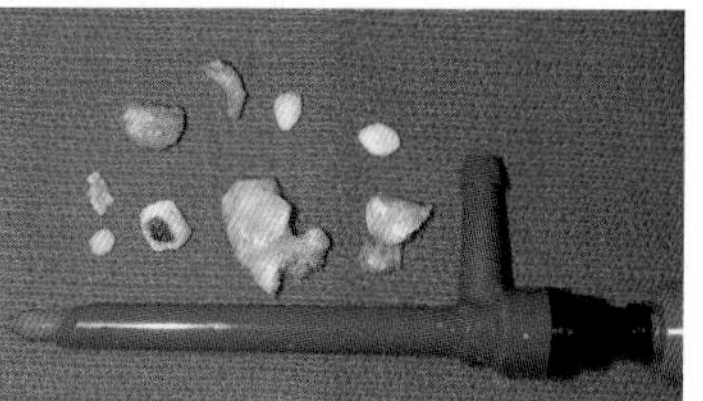

TECH FIG 3 • A. View from the lateral portal after medial release showing completed capsulectomy and bony débridement in the coronoid fossa area. *T*, trochlea; *CF*, coronoid fossa. **B.** Loose bodies are removed during this procedure via a 5-mm smooth cannula.

- The posterior capsule is released with a basket cutter or arthroscopic elevator on the medial and lateral sides; the surgeon stops before the medial aspect of the olecranon fossa (to avoid injury to the ulnar nerve).
- The posteromedial capsule should be resected in the setting of significant flexion loss (posterior band of the medial collateral lateral) and is the floor of the cubital tunnel.
  - The surgeon does the release along the olecranon and retracts the area of capsule near the epicondyle.
- Final inspection from both portals is done to ensure adequate release (TECH FIG 3).
  - Loose bodies are removed via a 5-mm-smooth cannula.

ULNAR NERVE RELEASE AND TRANSPOSITION

- Subcutaneous transposition or in situ decompression of the ulnar nerve can be performed.
- As advocated by O'Driscoll,[14] the ulnar nerve is exposed before performing the arthroscopic release to allow gentle fluid extravasation from the soft tissue posteromedially.
  - Gentle retraction on the nerve can help protect it while performing arthroscopic releases in this area.
- At the end of the case the ulnar nerve can be released using a variety of described techniques.

WOUND CLOSURE AND INTRAOPERATIVE SPLINTING

- A drain is placed through the proximal anterolateral portal because accumulation of fluid will compromise range of motion.
- Our postoperative dressing is a bulky dressing with Webril, Kerlex, and Ace bandage from wrist to shoulder with material cut out in the antecubital fossa to facilitate immediate continuous passive motion (CPM).
  - Alternatively, an anterior plaster slab over the elbow is used with the forearm in full extension (TECH FIG 4).
- Indwelling catheters or a long-acting regional block may be used to facilitate CPM (from full flexion to extension), which should start in the hospital.
- Before starting CPM, the dressing is changed to a soft, noncompressive gauze to prevent skin complications.

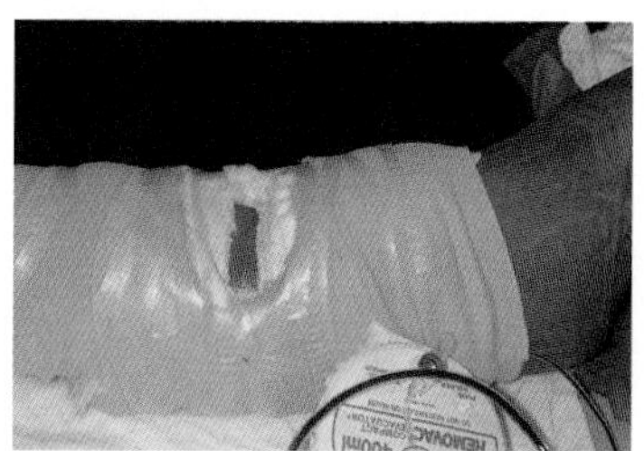

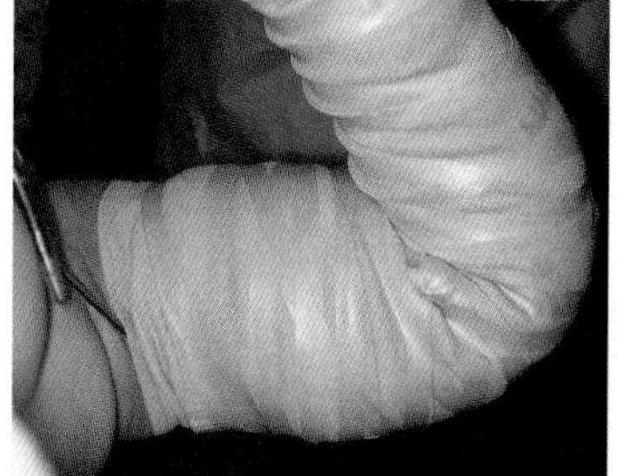

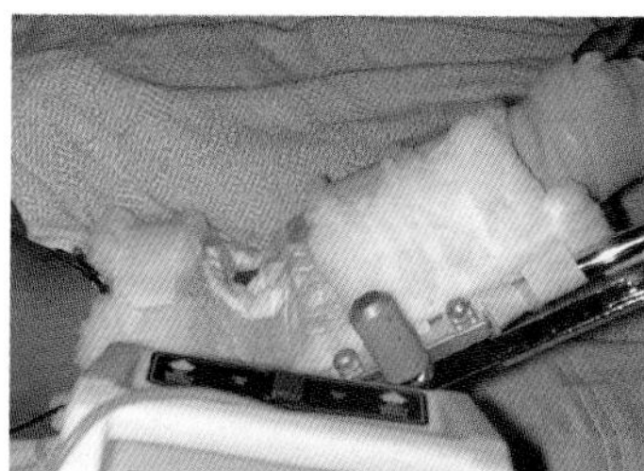

TECH FIG 4 • A. Postoperative dressing is applied to the patient after capsular release in the operating room with a drain. **B.** Flexion obtained after removing splint material from the antecubital fossa. **C.** Immediate continuous passive motion is instituted.

PEARLS AND PITFALLS

Ulnar neuritis	■ Prophylactic release if contracture is significant. The surgeon should err on the aggressive side when in doubt.
Radial nerve and posterior interosseous nerve injury	■ The surgeon should avoid motorized burrs. No suction should be used on the shaver in risk areas. Generous retraction and retractors are used inside the joint.
Posterior interosseous nerve	■ The surgeon should use care with the capsule just anterior to the midline of the radiocapitellar articulation.
Median nerve	■ The surgeon should not penetrate the brachialis muscle.
Ulnar nerve	■ In the medial aspect of elbow joint, the surgeon should retract medially and resect along the olecranon. The ulnar nerve is further from the olecranon.

POSTOPERATIVE CARE

- CPM should be continued at home up to 4 weeks and should be used in full range of motion (0 to 145 degrees) with a bolster behind the elbow.[16]
- Daily physical therapy is instituted, with home CPM continued. Immediate postoperative care and rehabilitation are included.
- The surgeon should consider prophylaxis of heterotopic ossification with indomethacin.

OUTCOMES

- Patients usually regain about 50% of lost motion.[7,14]
- About 80% of patients obtain a functional arc of motion greater than 100 degrees.[7]
- Ball et al[3] reported on 14 patients with mean flexion improvement from 117 degrees to 133 degrees and extension from 35 to 9 degrees; mean arc of motion improved from 69 degrees to 119 degrees (in 10 patients who had motion arc of less than 100 degrees).
- It is difficult to compare arthroscopic versus open capsular releases.
- Compared to open series, Savoie and Field[16] reported on 200 patients with capsular release: there was a mean improvement in extension of −46 degrees to −3 degrees and flexion of 96 degrees to 138 degrees, with a decrease in pain scale score from 6.5 to 1.5.

COMPLICATIONS

- Radial or posterior interosseous nerve palsy
  - Iatrogenic injury can be avoided by avoiding suction in high-risk areas.
  - Retractors of soft tissue are used to improve visualization and distention.
  - The surgeon should use care when anterior to midline of radiocapitellar articulation in the capsule.
- Median nerve
  - Iatrogenic injury is avoided by not penetrating the brachialis muscle.
  - The surgeon should place portals carefully, avoiding anterior.
- Ulnar nerve
  - In the medial aspect of joint, the surgeon should use retractors to move the capsule medially.
  - Transposition before the case may aid in ulnar nerve protection and also allow fluid extravasation.
- Ulnar neuritis
  - If present preoperatively, ulnar nerve release should be ensured.
  - Postoperatively it may be transient; there is a much lower incidence if it is transposed during initial surgery.
- Excessive bone resection, especially of radial head
  - The surgeon should avoid excessive resection.

REFERENCES

1. Akeson W, Amiel AM, Garfin S, et al. Viscoelastic properties of stiff joints: a new approach in analyzing joint contracture. Biomed Materials Engineering 1993;3:67–73.
2. An K, Morrey BF. Biomechanics of the elbow. In: Morrey BF, ed. The Elbow and Its Disorders. Philadelphia: WB Saunders; 2000: 43–74.
3. Ball CM, Meunier M, Galatz LM, et al. Arthroscopic treatment of post-traumatic elbow contracture. J Should Elbow Surg 2002;11: 624–629.
4. Cohen MS. Heterotopic ossification of the elbow. In: Jupiter JB, ed. The Stiff Elbow. Rosemont, IL: American Academy of Orthopaedic Surgeons; 2006:31–40.
5. Gallay S, Richards R, O'Driscoll SW. Intraarticular capacity and compliance of stiff and normal elbows. Arthroscopy 1993;9:9–13.
6. Hildebrand K, Zhang M, van Snellenberg W, et al. Myofibroblast numbers are elevated in human elbow capsules after trauma. Clin Orthop Relat Res 2004;419:189–197.
7. Jupiter JB, O'Driscoll SW, Cohen MS. The assessment and management of the stiff elbow. AAOS Instr Course Lect 2003;52:93–111.
8. King GJ, Faber KJ. Posttraumatic elbow stiffness. Orthop Clin North Am 2000;31:129–143.
9. Mansat P, Morrey BF, Hotchkiss RN. Extrinsic contracture: "the column procedure"—lateral and medial capsular releases. In: Morrey BF, ed. The Elbow and its Disorders. Philadelphia: WB Saunders; 2000:447–467.
10. Morrey BF. Anatomy of the elbow joint. In: Morrey BF, ed. The Elbow and its Disorders. Philadelphia: WB Saunders; 2000:13–42.
11. Morrey BF. The posttraumatic stiff elbow. Clin Orthop Relat Res 2005;431:26–35.
12. Morrey BF. The stiff elbow with articular involvement. In: Jupiter JB, ed. The Stiff Elbow. Rosemont, IL: American Academy of Orthopaedic Surgeons; 2006:21–30.
13. Morrey BF, Askew L, An K, et al. A biomechanical study of normal elbow motion. J Bone Joint Surg Am 1981;63A:872–877.
14. O'Driscoll SW. Clinical assessment and open and arthroscopic treatment of the stiff elbow. In: Jupiter JB, ed. The Stiff Elbow. Rosemont, IL: American Academy of Orthopaedic Surgeons; 2006:9–19.
15. O'Driscoll SW, Morrey BF, An K. Intra-articular pressure and capacity of the elbow. Arthroscopy 1990;6:100–103.
16. Savoie FH III, Field LD. Arthrofibrosis and complications in arthroscopy of the elbow. Clin Sports Med 2001;20(1):123–129.

Chapter 22 Arthroscopic Débridement for Elbow Degenerative Joint Disease

Julie E. Adams and Scott P. Steinmann

DEFINITION

- Primary degenerative arthritis of the elbow joint is a relatively rare condition.[9,18]
- Patients with primary osteoarthritis of the elbow are frequently manual laborers, athletes, and those who rely on wheelchairs or crutches for ambulation.[4,15,18,21]
- Although total elbow arthroplasty provides pain relief and improved range of motion in patients with inflammatory arthritis and or low demands, use in young active patients has been associated with early loosening and is undesirable in this group. Likewise, elbow arthrodesis is undesirable to many patients who do not wish to sacrifice motion in favor of pain relief.[8]
- Open débridement procedures have been described and used with good success.[3,4,6,9,14,16,22,23]
- Arthroscopic procedures have gained acceptance with patients and surgeons for perceived benefits of a minimally invasive nature and better visualization of the joint.
  - More series are confirming results at least equivalent to open procedures, with similar complication rates.
  - Arthroscopic débridement and osteocapsular resection is a procedure that adequately addresses the underlying pathologic processes and is associated with early return to activities, a durable result that does not preclude future reconstructive procedures, and minimal perioperative morbidity.[2,10,11,12,17,20]

ANATOMY

- At the elbow, the coronoid fossa anteriorly, the trochlea, and the olecranon fossa posteriorly articulate with the coronoid and olecranon. Bony osteophytes may develop, leading to impingement in flexion and extension in degenerative conditions.

PATHOGENESIS

- Three main pathologic processes are involved in primary elbow arthritis. Loss and fragmentation of cartilage lead to loose body formation. Osteophytes arise from reactive bone formation.
- These two processes cause impingement and contribute to the third process, progressive joint contractures.[21,22] The capsule becomes abnormally thickened and contracted.
- Symptoms include loss of extension, pain at the end points of motion, and mechanical symptoms such as catching or locking.[4,9]
- Other commonly associated conditions include cubital tunnel syndrome with paresthesias and weakness in the ulnar distribution and decreased grip strength.[4,13]

NATURAL HISTORY

- The natural history is one of slowly progressive joint contracture and discomfort. Ulnar neuritis may develop.

PATIENT HISTORY AND PHYSICAL FINDINGS

- The typical patient is a middle-aged male laborer with a painful dominant elbow, worse with use.
  - Less frequently, patients who depend on wheelchairs or crutches for mobility, and who thus put increased forces across their elbow joints, may be afflicted.
- Progressive loss of motion and pain at the extremes of motion due to impingement of osteophytes are noted.
- Painful crepitus and catching or locking sensations may be noted with range of motion. Usually pain in the mid-arc of motion is absent.
- Patients with contracture of the posterior capsule will lack flexion, whereas those with anterior contractures will lack extension.
- Not infrequently, ulnar nerve irritation is noted. This should be documented and will contribute to decision making regarding the need for decompression or transposition.

IMAGING AND OTHER DIAGNOSTIC STUDIES

- Usually plain film radiographs, clinical examination, and history are sufficient to make the diagnosis (**FIG 1**).
- Radiographs may show joint space narrowing, hypertrophic bony osteophytes, loose bodies, and subchondral sclerosis typical of osteoarthritis.

DIFFERENTIAL DIAGNOSIS

- Usually it is easy to exclude inflammatory arthropathies and posttraumatic arthritis, which may also be treated with this technique.

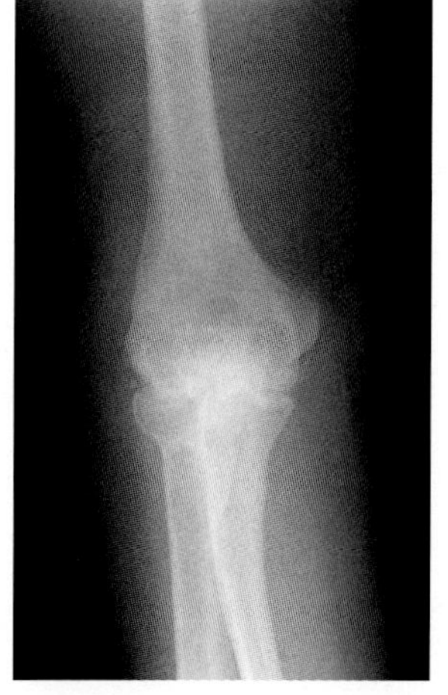

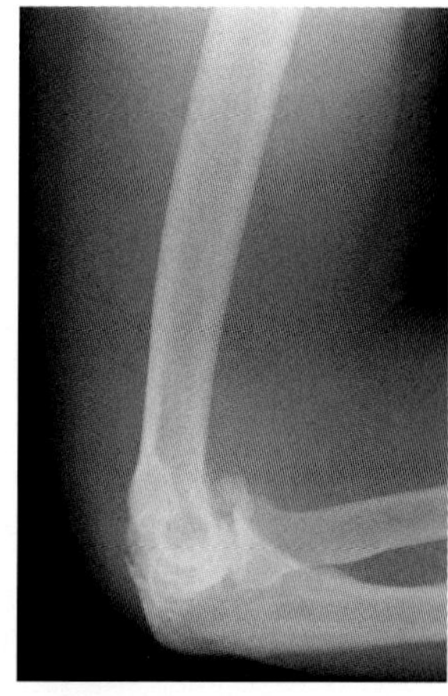

FIG 1 • AP and lateral radiographs of the typical patient with degenerative arthritis of the elbow. Bony osteophytes are noted with loose body formation.

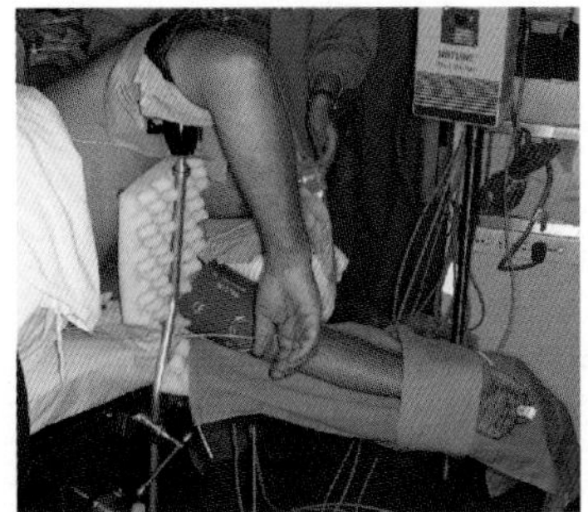

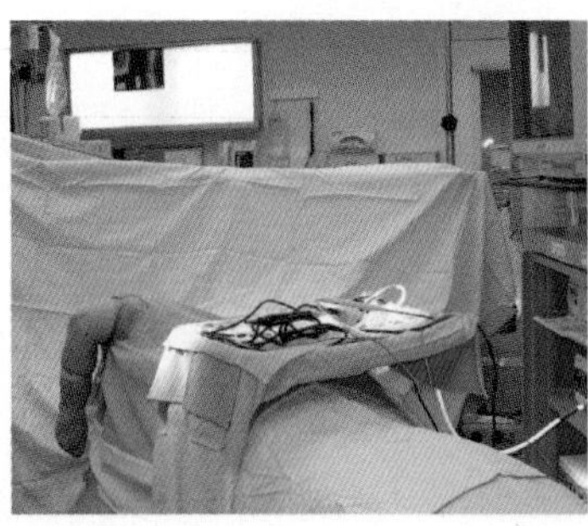

FIG 2 • **A.** The patient is positioned laterally with the arm secured in a dedicated armholder. **B.** Operative setup.

- Physical examination will also exclude other painful elbow conditions, such as tendinitis, instability, or cubital tunnel syndrome.

NONOPERATIVE MANAGEMENT

- Operative treatment should be considered only after exhausting conservative measures, which include activity modification and nonsteroidal anti-inflammatory medications.[17]

SURGICAL MANAGEMENT

- Patients who have failed to respond to nonoperative management and desire improved range of motion and pain relief may be surgical candidates.

Preoperative Planning

- Careful physical examination with attention to neurovascular status should be documented.
- Routine radiographs are usually all that are necessary.

Positioning

- General endotracheal anesthesia is induced and the patient is placed in the lateral decubitus position.
- The arm is secured in a dedicated arm holder, ensuring free access to the elbow with instruments (**FIG 2A**).
  - Positioning the elbow just higher than the shoulder allows free access to the elbow.
- A nonsterile tourniquet is applied and the arm is prepared and draped in the usual fashion (**FIG 2B**).

Approach

- Patients with lack of flexion will need to have the posterior aspect of the joint addressed; patients with lack of extension will require release and débridement anteriorly. Either compartment may be addressed first, depending on the pathology present.
- The standard arthroscopic setup and equipment includes the 4-mm 30-degree arthroscope.
  - A 2.7-mm arthroscope can be used, but in most cases the joint can accommodate a 4-mm arthroscope.
  - A 70-degree arthroscope may likewise be used but is usually not necessary and may be awkward unless the surgeon has experience using this arthroscope.
- Only blunt, not sharp, trocars should be used.
- Retractors such as a Howarth elevator or a large blunt Steinmann pin make the procedure easier and enhance visualization. Commercially available retractors are now available.
- The standard arthroscopic shaver and burr are used.
  - Suction should be placed to gravity only to prevent accidently shaving objects that may be sucked into the shaver (**FIG 3**).
- The portal sites and landmarks, including the radial head, medial and lateral epicondyles, capitellum, and olecranon, should be marked before insufflation of the joint, which may obscure landmarks.
- The ulnar nerve should be examined and its location marked; the surgeon should watch for a subluxating ulnar nerve.
  - If prior surgery has been performed or there is any question of the nerve's location, a small incision may be made to identify and retract the nerve to protect it against inadvertent injury.

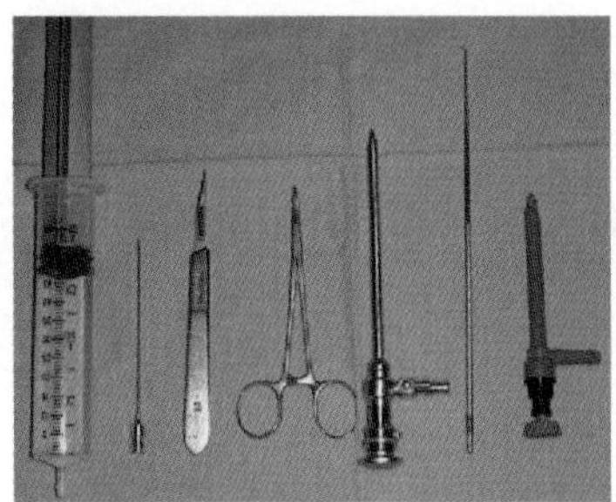

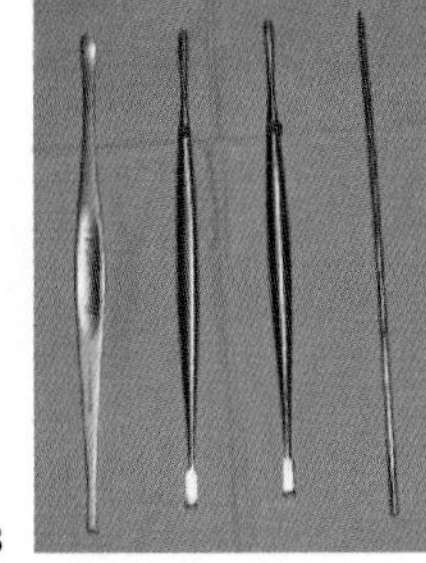

FIG 3 • Standard instruments used for elbow arthroscopy. **A.** From left: syringe for insufflation of the joint, spinal needle, knife, hemostat for spreading to establish portal site, blunt trocar and cannula, switching stick, and blunt trocar and cannula. **B.** Howarth elevators, retractors, and large Steinmann pins are useful for retraction.

ANTERIOR PORTAL PLACEMENT

- The surgical technique for arthroscopic elbow débridement and capsular release involves the standard arthroscopic technique and setup as previously described.[1,19,20]
- The joint is distended with 20 to 30 mL of saline introduced via an 18-gauge needle through the "soft spot" (the center of a triangle formed by the olecranon process, the lateral epicondyle, and the radial head). This makes entry into the joint easier to achieve.
- Portal sites are established according to the order preferred by the surgeon; the procedure described below is our preference.
- Portal sites are made by incising the skin only with a no. 11 blade, and then blunt dissection with a hemostat proceeds to the joint.
  - Capsular entry and joint location is confirmed by sudden egress of fluid.
- The blunt trocar and sleeve are then placed into the joint and exchanged for the arthroscope.
- The anterolateral portal (**TECH FIG 1A**) is established first, with care taken to avoid and protect the radial nerve.
  - This portal is established just anterior to the sulcus between the capitellum and the radial head.
- The anteromedial portal is established using an inside-out technique with direct visualization.
- The arthroscope is removed and replaced with the blunt trocar, which is pushed directly across the joint until it tents the skin overlying the medial side of the elbow.
- The skin is incised over this region and the trocar pushed through the remaining soft tissue.
  - A cannula may be placed over the trocar on the medial side, and the trocar is pulled back into the joint and out the lateral side (**TECH FIG 1B**).
- A proximal anterolateral retraction portal may be established about 2 cm proximal to the lateral epicondyle.

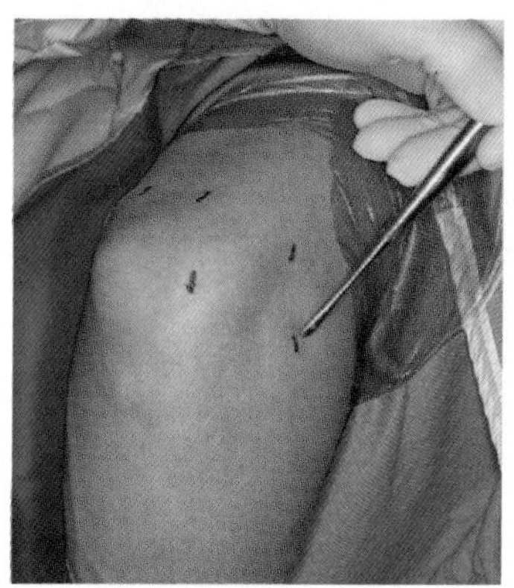

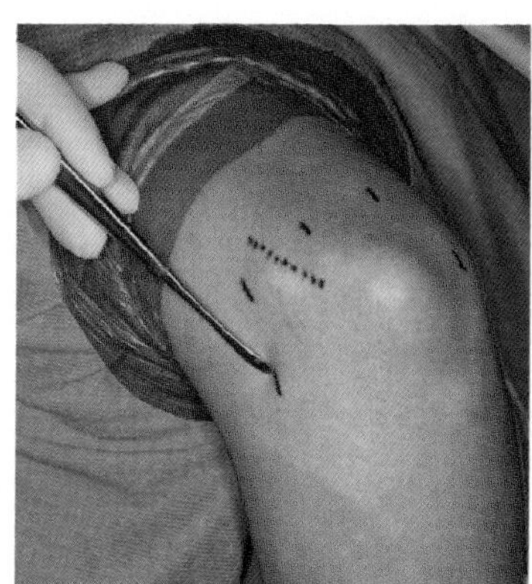

TECH FIG 1 • **A.** Drawing the portal sites and palpable landmarks as well as the ulnar nerve is useful before insufflation of the joint. The anterolateral portal is usually the first portal made. **B.** The anteromedial portal is usually established from inside out. The site of the ulnar nerve is marked.

ANTERIOR CAPSULECTOMY AND ARTHROSCOPIC DÉBRIDEMENT

- A 4.8-mm arthroscopic shaver is introduced through the anteromedial portal with retraction via a proximal anterolateral portal.
- Shaving proceeds to gain visualization.
- The anteromedial capsule is then stripped off the humerus to expand space in the contracted joint.
- Loose bodies are removed as they are identified. Osteophytes are removed with the shaver and burr from the coronoid and radial head fossae.
- After completion of the bony débridement, the anterior capsule is completely resected under direct visualization with the arthroscope in the lateral portal site.
- The biter is used to gain a free edge of the anterior capsule, proceeding from medial to laterally and halting when the fat pad anterior to the radial head is encountered.
- The shaver is used to completely resect the anterior capsule.
- The arthroscope is placed in the medial portal and bony débridement and capsulectomy is completed.

POSTERIOR PORTAL PLACEMENT

- After completing the anterior joint débridement and capsulectomy, attention is turned to the posterior aspect of the joint.
- Again, the location of the ulnar nerve is established and marked (see Tech Fig 1B).
- The posterolateral portal is used for visualization.
  - It is made with the elbow in a 90-degree flexed position and is placed at the lateral joint line at a level with the tip of the olecranon.
- The direct posterior portal is the working portal. It is made 2 to 3 cm proximal to the tip of the olecranon. It penetrates the thick triceps, and a knife should be used to establish this portal.
- Optional posterior retractor portals include one placed 2 cm proximal to the direct posterior portal, situated either slightly medially or laterally.

TECHNIQUES

POSTERIOR DÉBRIDEMENT AND CAPSULAR RELEASE

- After a posterolateral viewing portal and a direct posterior working portal are created, the shaver is placed in the direct posterior portal and osteophytes are removed from the tip and sides of the olecranon and the rim of the olecranon fossa.
- Patients who lack flexion preoperatively should also undergo posterolateral and posteromedial capsular releases.
- When addressing the posteromedial capsule, care should be exercised to identify and protect the ulnar nerve.
- In general, if a large restoration of motion is anticipated postprocedure, if preoperative ulnar nerve symptoms exist, or if preoperative flexion measures less than 90 degrees, the surgeon should consider ulnar nerve decompression or transposition.
  - This may be achieved via arthroscopic decompression if the surgeon has the requisite skill, or an open subcutaneous transposition is done.

PEARLS AND PITFALLS

Joint insufflation	■ Landmarks and structures, including the ulnar nerve, should be palpated and marked before joint distention and beginning the procedure. Joint distention and egress of fluid can distort landmarks. ■ Joint distention allows for ease of entry into the joint; the capsule is expanded and overlying structures are moved away, making joint entry easier and safer.
Portal placement	■ The skin incision for portal placement should proceed through skin only to avoid cutting cutaneous nerves.
Osteophytes	■ Osteophytes should be removed from the radial and coronoid fossae of the humerus as well as the rims of the olecranon; often these are neglected.
Ulnar nerve	■ The ulnar nerve should be examined and its location marked; the surgeon should watch for a subluxating ulnar nerve. If prior surgery has been performed or there is any question of the nerve's location, a small incision may be made to identify and retract the nerve to protect it against inadvertent injury.

POSTOPERATIVE CARE

- After the procedure, motion is assessed (**FIG 4**), the portals are closed in the standard fashion with 3-0 nylon or Prolene sutures, and a sterile compressive dressing applied.
  - A posterior slab of plaster is used to splint the operative extremity in full extension, and the arm is elevated in the "Statue of Liberty" position overnight.
- On postoperative day 1, the splint is removed and the neurovascular status is evaluated, with particular attention to the radial, median, and ulnar nerves.
  - Full active range of motion is initiated. No limitations are placed on use of the arm.
- Heterotopic ossification prophylaxis, consisting of indomethacin 75 mg three times daily for 6 weeks, is initiated.
- Splinting protocols, such as splints that may be adjusted from full extension to full flexion, are useful in most cases. The patient usually alternates hourly between the extremes of motion achieved at the time of surgery.
- Continuous passive motion may be initiated using a continuous passive motion device with or without a nerve block; however, in our experience it is not usually necessary.
  - In patients who cannot practice motion on their own or in those with severe contractures, it may be of benefit, although a consensus regarding the indications and need for continuous passive motion is lacking.

OUTCOMES

- In our series,[2] outcomes after the described procedure in 41 patients and 42 elbows were reviewed after an average follow-up of 176.3 weeks (minimum 2 years of follow-up).
  - Significant improvements in mean flexion (from 117.3 degrees preoperatively to 131.6 degrees, $P < 0.0001$), extension (from 21.4 degrees to 8.4 degrees, $P < 0.0001$), supination (from 70.7 degrees to 78.6 degrees, $P = 0.0056$), and Mayo Elbow Performance Index scores ($P < 0.0001$) were noted, with 81% good to excellent results.

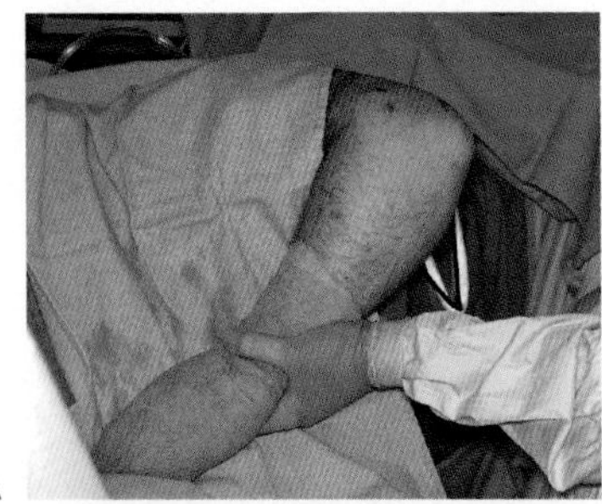

A

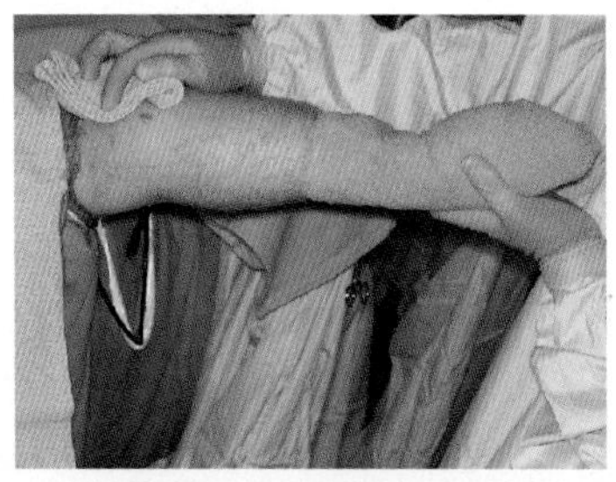

B

FIG 4 • Intraoperatively after release, the range of motion is assessed.

    - Pain decreased significantly (*P* <0.0001).
    - Complications were rare (n = 2; heterotopic ossification and transient ulnar dysthesias).
- Cohen et al[5] compared outcomes after arthroscopic débridement versus open débridement of the elbow for osteoarthritis, using the Outerbridge-Kashiwagi procedure and an arthroscopic modification.
    - Both groups showed improved range of elbow flexion, decrease in pain, and a high level of patient satisfaction.
    - Increases in elbow extension, although improved in both groups, were more modest.
    - Neither procedure included capsular release.
    - Comparison between the open and arthroscopic procedures showed that the open procedure might be more effective in improving flexion, whereas the arthroscopic procedure seemed to provide more pain relief.
    - No differences between overall effectiveness of the two procedures were noted.
- From these series and others in the literature, it appears that arthroscopic débridement and capsular release have similar outcomes with respect to pain relief, improved range of motion, and complications. Although the use of arthroscopic procedures is attractive to decrease morbidity, benefits over open procedures have not been proved.

COMPLICATIONS

- As with any arthroscopic or open procedure about the elbow, the risk of neurovascular injury is a real concern.
- In a series from the Mayo Clinic,[7] 50 complications were observed after 473 elbow arthroscopies for a variety of interventions.
    - Most frequently, this included prolonged wound drainage; other complications included infection, nerve injury, and contractures.
    - No permanent nerve injuries were observed.
- Nevertheless, injuries of each of the susceptible nerves about the elbow joint have been observed.
- Careful attention intraoperatively, appropriate portal placement, and knowledge of anatomy will help prevent injury.

REFERENCES

1. Adams JE, Steinmann SP. Nerve injuries about the elbow. J Hand Surg Am 2006;31A:303–313.
2. Adams JE, Wolff LH III, Merten SM, et al. Primary elbow arthritis: results of arthroscopic debridement and capsulectomy. Presented at American Society for Surgery of the Hand, Sept 6–9, 2006, Washington DC.
3. Allen DM, Devries JP, Nunley JA. Ulnohumeral arthroplasty. Iowa Orthop J 2004;4:49–52.
4. Antuna SA, Morrey BF, Adams RA, et al. Ulnohumeral arthroplasty for primary degenerative arthritis of the elbow: long-term outcome and complications. J Bone Joint Surg Am 2002;84A:2168–2173.
5. Cohen AP, Redden JF, Stanley D. Treatment of osteoarthritis of the elbow: a comparison of open and arthroscopic debridement. Arthroscopy 2000;16:701–706.
6. Kashiwagi D. Osteoarthritis of the elbow joint. In: Kashiwagi D, ed. Elbow Joint. Proceedings of the International Congress, Japan. Amsterdam: Elsevier Science Publishing, 1986:177–188.
7. Kelly EW, Morrey BF, O'Driscoll SW. Complications of elbow arthroscopy. J Bone Joint Surg Am 2001;83A:25–34.
8. McAuliffe JA. Surgical alternatives for elbow arthritis in the young adult. Hand Clin 2002;18:99–111.
9. Morrey BF. Primary degenerative arthritis of the elbow: treatment by ulnohumeral arthroplasty. J Bone Joint Surg Br 1992;74B: 409–413.
10. O'Driscoll SW. Arthroscopic treatment for osteoarthritis of the elbow. Orthop Clin North Am 1995;26:691–706.
11. O'Driscoll SW. Operative treatment of elbow arthritis. Curr Opin Rheumatol 1995;7:103–106.
12. Ogilvie-Harris DJ, Gordon R, MacKay M. Arthroscopic treatment for posterior impingement in degenerative arthritis of the elbow. Arthroscopy 1995;11:437–443.
13. Oka Y, Ohta K, Saitoh I. Debridement arthroplasty for osteoarthritis of the elbow. Clin Orthop 1998;351:127–134.
14. Phillips NJ, Ali A, Stanley D. Treatment of primary degenerative arthritis of the elbow by ulnohumeral arthroplasty: a long-term follow-up. J Bone Joint Surg Br 2003;85B:347–350.
15. Redden JF, Stanley D. Arthroscopic fenestration of the olecranon fossa in the treatment of osteoarthritis of the elbow. Arthroscopy 1993;9:14–16.
16. Sarris I, Riano FA, Goebel F, et al. Ulnohumeral arthroplasty: results in primary degenerative arthritis of the elbow. Clin Orthop 2004; 420:190–193.
17. Savoie FH III, Nunley PD, Field LD. Arthroscopic management of the arthritic elbow: indications, technique, and results. J Shoulder Elbow Surg 1999;8:214–219.
18. Stanley D. Prevalence and etiology of symptomatic elbow osteoarthritis. J Shoulder Elbow Surg 1994;3:386–389.
19. Steinmann SP. Elbow arthroscopy. J Am Soc Surg Hand 2003;3: 199–207.
20. Steinmann SP, King GJ, Savoie FH III. Arthroscopic treatment of the arthritic elbow. J Bone Joint Surg Am 2005;87A:2114–2121.
21. Suvarna SK, Stanley D. The histologic changes of the olecranon fossa membrane in primary osteoarthritis of the elbow. J Shoulder Elbow Surg 2004;13:555–557.
22. Tsuge K, Mizuseki T. Debridement arthroplasty for advanced primary osteoarthritis of the elbow: results of a new technique used for 29 elbows. J Bone Joint Surg Br 1994;76B:641–646.
23. Vingerhoeds B, Degreef I, De Smet L. Debridement arthroplasty for osteoarthritis of the elbow (Outerbridge-Kashiwagi procedure). Acta Orthop Belg 2004;70:306–310.

Chapter 23 Arthroscopic Treatment of Epicondylitis

Kevin P. Murphy, Jeffrey R. Giuliani, and Brett A. Freedman

DEFINITION

- Epicondylitis is overuse tendinosis at the elbow, with pain localized to the origin of the lateral common extensor mass or, much less commonly, the origin of the medial common flexor mass.
- Lateral epicondylitis (LE), also known as tennis elbow, is the most common overuse injury of the elbow, resulting from repetitive microtrauma at the origin of the extensor carpi radialis brevis (ECRB).
  - The hallmark clinical finding is pain localized to the lateral aspect of the elbow reproducible with resisted wrist extension and forearm supination.
- Medial epicondylitis results from repetitive valgus forces at the elbow, with tendinosis commonly localized to the origins of the flexor carpi radialis and pronator teres, with tenderness slightly anterior and distal to the medial epicondyle.
- Nonoperative management is the initial treatment of choice for epicondylitis. It is successful in 90% to 95% of patients.[3,10]
  - Nonetheless, for the 5% to 10% of LE patients who fail to respond to nonoperative management and develop chronic recalcitrant symptoms, the senior author's (KPM) treatment of choice since 1995 has been arthroscopic release.
  - Cadaveric and anatomic studies have shown that elbow arthroscopy and ECRB release is safe, reliable, and reproducible.[7,11]
- The treatment of choice for recalcitrant medial epicondylitis is open débridement of pathologic tissue of the flexor pronator origin. This will not be discussed in this chapter.

ANATOMY

- The common extensor tendon origin represents the confluence of four tendons: ECRB, extensor digitorum communis, extensor digit minimi, and extensor carpi ulnaris.
- The ECRB origin is on the distal anterolateral aspect of the lateral epicondyle. It covers an area of about 1.5 cm and lies deep to the other three muscles of the extensor mass.
- Arthroscopically, the ECRB is the muscle belly and tendon that can be seen lying just superficial to a thinned-out portion of the lateral joint capsule.
- The extensor carpi radialis longus actually originates from the lateral humeral supracondylar ridge, 2 to 3 cm superior to the common extensor tendon, and then passes distally, anterior, and superficial to the ECRB.
- The lateral ulnar collateral ligament is deep to the extensor tendons and originates from the lateral epicondyle, reinforcing the lateral joint capsule as well as inserting onto the annular ligament and supinator ridge of the ulna.

PATHOGENESIS

- The actual pathophysiology of LE is still not completely understood, and minimal advances in our knowledge of the disease process have occurred in the past 2 years.
- Proposed causes include bursitis, synovitis, ligament inflammation, periostitis, tendinitis, tendinosis, and extensor tendon tears.
- It is widely accepted that LE is not an "itis" or inflammatory condition but rather a tendinosis.[6]
  - The most commonly accepted cause today is tendinosis as a result of microscopic tearing of the ECRB muscle with repetitive trauma that causes ingrowth of weakened reparative tissue known as angiofibroblastic hyperplasia or angiofibroblastic tendinosis.
  - The process of repetitive micro- and macrotearing can ultimately lead to a spectrum of ECRB tendinosis ranging from fraying to complete tendon failure if the condition is not addressed early.[6]

NATURAL HISTORY

- Epicondylitis responds to conservative management in 90% to 95% of cases.
  - If treated in the acute setting with activity modification, in conjunction with other conservative modalities, nonsteroidal anti-inflammatory medication may contribute to the alleviation of symptoms experienced with acute LE.
- With progressive repetitive trauma, fraying of the tendon and microtears can progress to macroscopic tears and fibrillations of the ECRB, which ultimately could lead to complete tendon rupture or avulsion.
- If the lateral joint capsule is involved in chronic LE, it can avulse along with the ECRB tendon and create a lateral synovial cyst or a sense of lateral joint instability.
- Chronic refractory LE originates in the ECRB tendon, but it could extend to involve the anterior portion of the extensor digitorum communis, which may ultimately lead to weakness with wrist extension and supination.
- Baker et al[2] have published an arthroscopic classification system for LE that we have found to be reliable (Table 1).
- Rarely, in the chronic setting, treatment may require tendon transfer surgery to restore long extensor function.

Table 1 Arthroscopic Classification of Lateral Epicondylitis

Type	Description
I	Fraying of the undersurface of the ECRB without a definitive tear
II	Linear tears specifically in the undersurface of the ECRB and the lateral capsule
III	Partial or complete avulsions of the ECRB origin

ECRB, extensor carpi radialis brevis.
From Baker CL Jr, Murphy KP, Gottlob CA. Arthroscopic classification and treatment of lateral epicondylitis: two-year clinical results. J Shoulder Elbow Surg 2000;9:475–482.

PATIENT HISTORY AND PHYSICAL FINDINGS

- The pain associated with LE can be secondary to an acute event, but most commonly it is insidious in onset—the result of repetitive microtrauma.
- Patients typically report pain with resisted wrist extension and supination with the elbow extended.
- It is important to ask the patient about length and type of conservative treatment, history of corticosteroid injections, and response to prior therapy.
  - Patients who have had a good or excellent initial response to steroids, followed by reaggravation of symptoms, may have resumed strenuous activities too soon or too abruptly and may respond to an additional trial of nonoperative management.
- A prior surgical history of the involved elbow is extremely important for operative planning and can contribute to the diagnosis. Furthermore, a history of a prior ulnar nerve transposition could place the ulnar nerve at risk when establishing arthroscopic portals and may require an open approach.
- The physical examination should include:
  - Palpation of the lateral epicondyle–common extensor mass; the surgeon should document the exact location of tenderness to palpation, which is critical for differential diagnosis. This is the most predictive examination for LE.
  - Resisted wrist extension: Pain with resisted middle finger extension is commonly present in patients with LE but can also be diagnostic for posterior interosseous nerve (PIN) syndrome.
  - Resisted supination and grip strength: Grip strength is diminished in 78% of patients with LE. Resisted supination elicits pain in 51% of patients. The differential includes bicep tendinitis. Pain with turning a doorknob can also indicate LE.
  - Chair test: The test is positive when a patient refuses or is unable to lift a chair with the arms forward flexed, elbows and wrists in extension, and forearms in pronation.
- The differential diagnosis for lateral elbow pain is long, so it is pertinent to perform a thorough physical examination of both the ipsilateral and contralateral upper extremity, as well as the cervical spine.
- The differential diagnosis of lateral elbow pain includes (but is not limited to) the following:
  - Compressive neuropathy of the radial nerve–radial tunnel syndrome or PIN. The point of maximal tenderness in both radial tunnel syndrome and PIN syndrome is more distal than in LE. PIN syndrome presents with a motor palsy, whereas LE is a diagnosis of pain. Radial tunnel syndrome can be tested for specifically with the resisted middle finger extension test. Selective injections and electrodiagnostics can confirm the diagnosis.
  - Posterolateral rotatory instability is caused by an injury to the lateral ulnar collateral ligament. Although posterolateral rotatory instability can be associated with mechanical symptoms, the lateral pivot shift test can clinically differentiate instability from epicondylitis.[8,10]
  - Osteoarthritis, particularly in the radiocapitellar joint
    - The physical examination usually causes mechanical symptoms and decreased range of motion.
    - Radiographs confirm sclerosis, osteophyte formation, loose bodies, and joint space narrowing of the radiocapitellar joint.

IMAGING AND OTHER DIAGNOSTIC STUDIES

- Radiographs have been of limited benefit in the diagnosis of LE but should be obtained to rule out other causes of pain or coexisting pathology, especially in recalcitrant cases.
  - Radiographic evaluation of the elbow in a patient with lateral elbow pain should be limited to an anteroposterior view in full extension and a lateral view with the elbow flexed at 90 degrees.
  - One study reports an incidence of calcification about the ECRB origin from chronic tendinosis in up to 25% of patients (**FIG 1A**).[9]
- Historically, magnetic resonance imaging (MRI) has had limited utility in the diagnosis of LE.
  - MRI can demonstrate ECRB tendon thickening, increased signal on T1 and T2 images, and in advanced disease high T2-signal cystic areas that correspond to partial or complete ECRB avulsions or large areas of mucoid degeneration, which are nonspecific findings for LE (**FIG 1B**).
  - Despite its limited specificity for LE, MRI can be a useful, noninvasive technique to visualize concomitant intra-articular elbow pathology and soft tissue pathology.

DIFFERENTIAL DIAGNOSIS

- Lateral
  - Radiocapitellar chondromalacia
  - Osteochondral loose bodies
  - Radial head fracture
  - Osteochondritis dissecans lesion
  - PIN entrapment
- Medial
  - Inferior cruciate ligament strains or tears
  - Medial epicondyle avulsion fracture
  - Ulnar neuritis
  - Ulnar subluxation
  - Medial epicondylitis
  - Osteochondral loose bodies
  - Olecranon stress fracture
  - Valgus extension overload syndrome
  - Pronator teres syndrome

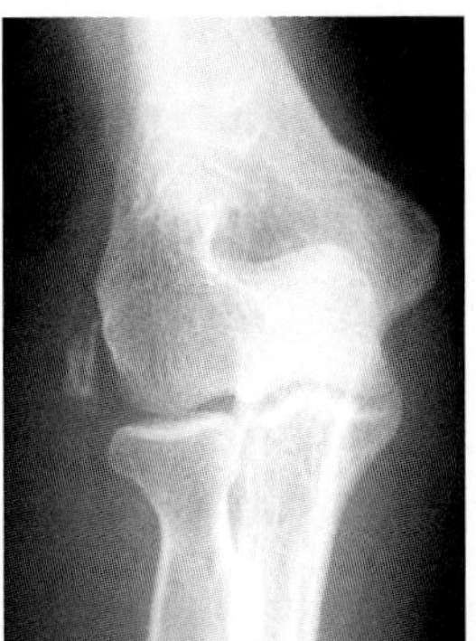
A

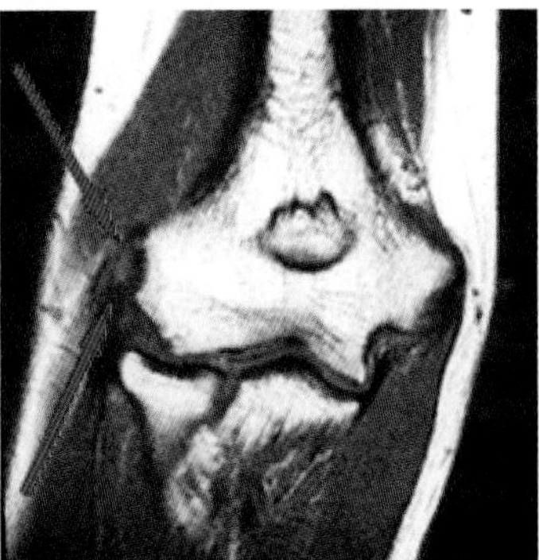
B

FIG 1 • **A.** Standard AP radiograph of the elbow showing calcification of the extensor carpi radialis brevis (ECRB) tendon. **B.** T1-weighted MRI of the elbow. *Arrows* show intermediate or high signal intensity of the ECRB tendon at its insertion site on the lateral epicondylitis.

- Anterior
  - Anterior capsular strain
  - Distal biceps tendon strain
  - Brachialis strain
  - Distal biceps tendon rupture
  - Coronoid osteophyte
- Posterior
  - Valgus extension overload syndrome
  - Triceps tendinitis
  - Triceps tendon avulsion
  - Pronator teres syndrome
  - Olecranon stress fracture
  - Osteochondral loose bodies
  - Olecranon bursitis

NONOPERATIVE MANAGEMENT

- LE responds to conservative management in 90% to 95% of cases.
- Treatment algorithms and modalities are extensive and include rest, activity modification, anti-inflammatory medication, phonophoresis, iontophoresis, massage, stretching, strengthening, counterforce bracing (tennis elbow wraps), sporting equipment modification, acupuncture, extracorporeal shock wave therapy, and corticosteroid injections.
  - No single nonoperative protocol has proved to be the best, and there is a severe paucity in empiric support for any modality.
- Realizing that the natural history of LE appears to be one of spontaneous resolution for most patients within 6 to 12 months, rest and removal of the offending overuse activity is probably the most important component in the initial treatment of LE.
- While steroid injections and nonsteroidal anti-inflammatories have been recommended in the treatment of LE, there is little to no empiric evidence to support their use.
- A three-stage rehabilitation program with the most widespread acceptance entails rest to reduce pain, counterforce bracing followed by progressive wrist extensor strengthening, and a delayed resumption of inciting activities.
- Extracorporeal shock wave therapy has been the most clinically studied nonoperative modality in the past 2 years.
  - It is difficult to clearly define its role in the treatment of LE given the conflicting results in several studies, along with the relatively short-term follow-up data currently available.
  - We believe extracorporeal shock wave therapy should be considered a possible alternative to surgery for refractory cases only. It is not a first-line therapy at this point.

SURGICAL MANAGEMENT

- Despite 3 to 6 months of nonoperative management, approximately 5% to 10% of patients develop recalcitrant symptoms that may require surgical intervention.
- The surgical options include open, percutaneous, and arthroscopic surgical techniques, with success rates that vary from less to 65% to 95% good or excellent outcomes.
- The pervasive move toward minimally invasive surgical techniques and the desire for a quick return to full activity have resulted in research and development of safe and effective means for performing arthroscopic releases for LE.
- In comparison with open procedures, arthroscopy has several distinct advantages, including the ability to address intra-articular pathology, preservation of the superficial common extensor origin and therefore grip strength, faster return to work and sports-related activities, and lower morbidity.
- Arthroscopy appears to combine the best attributes of the earlier return to activity seen with percutaneous procedures and the decreased recurrence rates commonly reported with open procedures.

Preoperative Planning

- The surgeon must review radiographs and imaging studies for concomitant pathology such as osteochondral loose bodies, radiocapitellar arthrosis, fracture, and injury to surrounding soft tissue structures like the lateral collateral ligament complex.
- Under general anesthesia
  - The lateral pivot shift test, described by O'Driscoll, tests the elbow for a lateral ulnar collateral ligament injury by stressing the elbow in supination, and valgus and axial compression as the elbow is moved from full extension over the patient's head to 20 to 40 degrees of flexion.[10]
    - Posterolateral rotatory instability is diagnosed when the radiocapitellar joint subluxes, creating a sulcus proximal to the radial head.
  - In addition, the surgeon must examine the range of motion of the elbow under anesthesia in full flexion and extension, pronation and supination.
  - Examination findings under anesthesia should always be compared with the contralateral extremity.

Positioning

- The patient is placed in the prone position on the operating table in the standard fashion.
- The operative elbow is flexed at 90 degrees and hangs over the bed to gravity. A sandbag may be placed under the operative extremity to maintain elbow flexion.
- The surgeon is seated for the procedure.

Approach

- As stated previously, LE can be treated with a multitude of well-described open or percutaneous procedures with the goal to débride diseased tissue.
- Techniques include partial epicondylectomies, partial resection of the annular ligament, and lengthening (slides) of the extensor tendons.
  - Our bias is toward arthroscopic treatment.
- Numerous arthroscopic portals have been described for elbow arthroscopy, but nine are most commonly used: two medial, four lateral, and three posterior.
- When addressing LE, the surgeon must be able to perform a diagnostic arthroscopy of the anterior compartment of the elbow and be able to visualize, evaluate, and address pathology of the lateral capsule and the undersurface of the ECRB tendon.
- Absolute contraindications to elbow arthroscopy are distortion of normal bony or soft tissue anatomy that precludes safe portal placement, previous ulnar nerve transposition or hardware that interferes with medial portal placement, or local cellulitis.
- Although LE could be addressed through a combination of the different medial and lateral portals, we have had the most success avoiding injury to neurovascular structures and improving visualization with the proximal anteromedial portal as

the standard viewing portal and the proximal lateral portal as the working portal.

- The proximal anterolateral portal pierces the brachioradialis, brachialis, and lateral capsule before entering the anterior compartment with the elbow flexed to 90 degrees.
  - This approach places the radial nerve on average 13.7 mm from the cannula versus 7.2 mm when using the standard anterolateral portal.[1]
- The proximal anteromedial portal passes just anterior to the medial intermuscular septum and stays deep to the brachialis muscle, avoiding injury to the brachial artery and median nerve.
  - On average this portal remains 6 mm proximal to the medial antebrachial cutaneous nerve, 3 to 4 mm anterior to an untransposed ulnar nerve, and 22 mm from the median nerve.[7]

DIAGNOSTIC ELBOW ARTHROSCOPY

- Once the patient is positioned, prepared, and draped and the surgical landmarks are drawn, the joint is distended using an 18-gauge needle to inject 20 mL of saline via the direct lateral approach into the joint (TECH FIG 1).
- The proximal medial portal is established first. This is the viewing portal and allows for the proximal lateral portal to be created under direct arthroscopic visualization.
- The surgeon makes a 2-mm longitudinal skin incision using a no. 11 scalpel blade, 2 cm proximal and 2 cm anterior to the medial epicondyle.
  - This incision should go no deeper than the skin to protect the cutaneous nerves and veins.
  - Alternatively, the arthroscope light can be used to transluminate the skin and identify these structures so that they can be avoided before making the skin incision.
- A hemostat is inserted through the subcutaneous tissue, onto the medial humeral condylar ridge, and down to the medial capsule, using blunt dissection.
  - The capsule is robust and a pop should be felt as it is entered.
  - Some of the normal saline that was previously injected to inflate the joint will now be released through the portal site, further confirming entry into the joint.
  - Staying anterior to the medial intermuscular septum protects the ulnar nerve from danger.
- Next, a blunt trocar is introduced into the joint, followed by the 4-mm, 30-degree arthroscope.
- The anterior compartment of the elbow should be diagnostically inspected for pathology (osteoarthritis, loose bodies, capsuloligamentous flaps or redundancies); these will be addressed once the proximal lateral portal is established.
- After the anterior compartment has been inspected, attention is directed toward the lateral capsule and ECRB tendon.
- An 18-gauge spinal needle is inserted 2 cm proximal and 2 cm anterior to the lateral epicondyle.
- Using techniques for skin and soft tissue management similar to those described for the proximal medial portal placement, the proximal lateral portal is made under direct arthroscopic visualization.
  - The radial nerve is the structure most at risk with this portal.

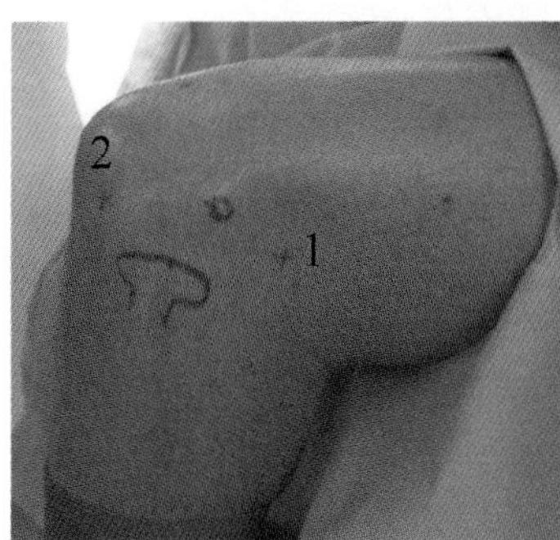

TECH FIG 1 • Lateral intraoperative photograph showing the surgical landmarks with the standard proximal anterolateral working portal (*1*) and the direct lateral portal (*2*). Joint is initially distended with 20 cc of normal saline via the direct lateral portal.

ARTHROSCOPIC LATERAL ELBOW (ECRB) RELEASE

- With the proximal medial portal as the standard viewing portal, the 30-degree scope is advanced just past the radial head to visualize the lateral joint capsule and undersurface of the ECRB origin (TECH FIG 2A).
- The capsule often adheres to the undersurface of the ECRB and can have varying degrees of degeneration, presenting as linear tears (type II lesion), fraying, or yellowish fatty infiltration, or it can have a thin, translucent appearance (TECH FIG 2B).
  - If the capsule is intact, it is débrided using a 4.5-mm synovial shaver inserted in the working portal—the proximal lateral portal.
  - The capsule and tendon may be completely avulsed and retracted; this is classified as a type III lesion (TECH FIG 2C).
- The undersurface of the ECRB is in plain view once the capsule is débrided.
- The release of the muscle should begin at the site of degeneration or tear using a 4.5-mm incisor (TECH FIG 2D).

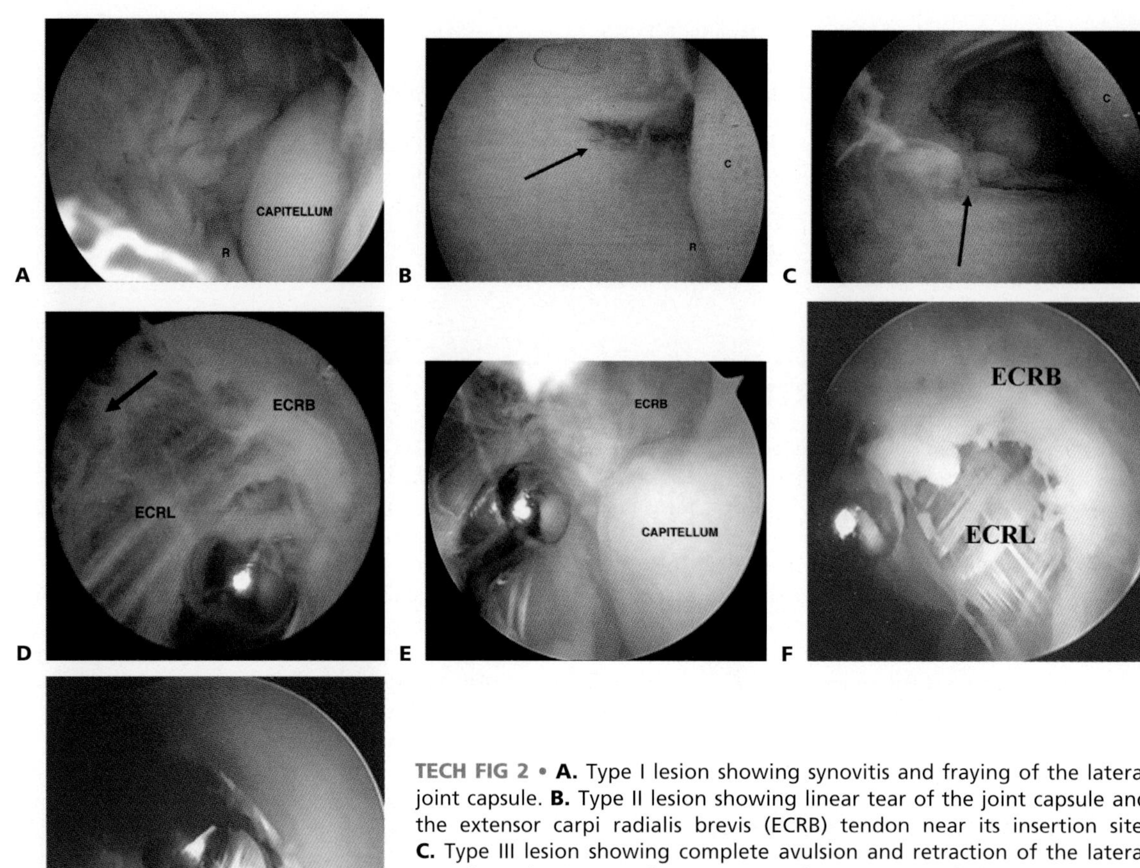

TECH FIG 2 • **A.** Type I lesion showing synovitis and fraying of the lateral joint capsule. **B.** Type II lesion showing linear tear of the joint capsule and the extensor carpi radialis brevis (ECRB) tendon near its insertion site. **C.** Type III lesion showing complete avulsion and retraction of the lateral capsule and ECRB tendon. **D.** Fatty degeneration of the ECRB tendon (*arrow*), which is overlying the ECRL muscle–tendon. **E.** A 4.5-mm shaver is used for the initial débridement of the ECRB, which is in close proximity to the capitellum (*C*) and radial head (*R*). **F.** Débridement of the pathologic ECRB tendon and capsule with healthy-appearing extensor carpi radialis longus superficial. **G.** A 4.0-mm abrader is the final step to decorticate the lateral epicondyle. The ECRB release is complete.

- Next, the surgeon progresses proximally to the ECRB origin on the lateral epicondyle.
  - Care must be taken to avoid injury to the articular surface of the capitellum or radial head during this process (TECH FIG 2E).
- Just superficial to the ECRB the extensor carpi radialis longus will come into view (TECH FIG 2F).
- A 4.0-mm abrader is placed in the proximal lateral portal to débride the remaining origin of the ECRB and to decorticate the lateral epicondyle and distal lateral condylar ridge to promote healing (TECH FIG 2G).
  - The cadaveric model by Kuklo et al[7] showed that using this technique, an average of 23 mm of ECRB tendon and 22 mm of lateral epicondyle can be safely resected.
  - In addition, the 30-degree scope field of visualization avoids injury to the lateral ulnar collateral ligament, which is posterior to an intra-articular line bisecting the head of the radius.[11]
- If needed, a direct lateral portal can be made when the elbow is flexed 90 degrees for access to the posterior compartment.
  - This portal enters the soft tissue triangle created by the radial head, the lateral humeral epicondyle, and the olecranon.
  - The medial antebrachial cutaneous nerve is the structure at risk with this portal.
- Once the arthroscope is introduced into the joint, the elbow is extended and the scope is advanced into the posterior compartment.
- If a working portal is needed, a direct posterior portal can be placed midline between the medial and lateral epicondyles about 3 cm proximal to the olecranon tip.
- The joint is expressed free of all arthroscopic fluid, portals are closed with figure 8 3-0 nylon sutures, and a soft tissue dressing is applied.

PEARLS AND PITFALLS

Indications	■ Indication for arthroscopic release is pain that lasts longer than 3 to 6 months despite a trial of nonoperative methods (rest, counterforce bracing, stretching, and strengthening).
Absolute contraindications	■ Distortion of normal bony or soft tissue anatomy that precludes safe portal placement ■ Previous ulnar nerve transposition or hardware that interferes with medial portal placement ■ Osteomyelitis or local cellulitis
Neurovascular injury	■ Neurovascular injury is avoided by using the "nick and spread" technique: ■ An 11-mm arthroscopic blade placed through the skin is used to pull skin distally for small incision. ■ A hemostat is used to bluntly dissect to the capsule. ■ A 2.7-mm arthroscope is used rather than a 4.0-mm arthroscope. ■ If a 4.0-mm scope is desired, the joint is entered over a switching stick. ■ A postoperative intra-articular injection is not recommended owing to possible extravasation and transient radial nerve palsy.
Complete lateral release	■ The ECRB insertion site spans 1.5 cm of lateral epicondyle. ■ Débridement of the ECRB tendon is carried up the lateral flare of the epicondyle. ■ Lateral epicondyle decortication is best done with an abrader and ensures the entire ECRB tendon is released.
Access to posterior compartment	■ Direct lateral portal for visualization ■ Direct posterior portal as the working portal ■ Surgeon is seated with arthroscope draping across his or her thighs. The patient's wrist should be flexed and the dorsum of the hand should be on the surgeon's thigh. Raising or lowering the bed allows for the elbow to be extended and flexed, respectively.
Iatrogenic lateral collateral ligament complex injury	■ The surgeon should not decorticate posterior to the lateral epicondyle. ■ A 30-degree scope prevents injury to the lateral collateral ligament because it does not allow good posterior visualization.

POSTOPERATIVE CARE

- Postoperatively the patient is placed into a sling for comfort.
- Range of motion is begun immediately with the assistance of a physical therapist.
- Rehabilitation goals include edema control with icing, full active range of motion, gradual strengthening, hand exercises, and ergonomic education.
- Patients return to full activity as tolerated.
- Soldiers undergoing this technique were able to return to full, unrestricted active duty within an average of 6 days (less than 28 days).[11]

OUTCOMES

- Cadaveric and anatomic studies have shown that elbow arthroscopy and ECRB release is safe, reliable, and reproducible.[7,11]
- Two clinical series confirm the long-term subjective and functional improvement, as well as faster return to activity, with arthroscopic treatment.
  - In 16 patients who underwent an arthroscopic release, the average return time to unrestricted work was 6 days, with no complications or need for further surgery.[11]
  - In 2000, we evaluated the clinical results of arthroscopic lateral elbow release. Patients rated 95% of the elbows to be "much better" or "better." Sixty-two percent of the patients were completely pain-free at an average of 2.8 years of follow-up.[2]
- Results from open releases have shown time to return to activity as long as 3 to 6 months, with one study reporting that 60% of patients could not return to high-demand sports participation postoperatively.
- Arthroscopy, unlike open and percutaneous procedures, gives the surgeon the distinct ability to address concurrent intra-articular pathology.
  - This may be particularly important because we have found rates of intra-articular pathology from 11% to 18% in our series, and some have reported rates as high as 40%.[9]

COMPLICATIONS

- Transient nerve palsy versus direct nerve injury[14]
- Superficial infection
- Iatrogenic lateral collateral ligament injury with posterolateral instability[7]
- Hematoma

REFERENCES

1. Adolfsson L. Arthroscopy of the elbow joint: a cadaveric study of portal placement. J Shoulder Elbow Surg 1994;3:53–61.
2. Baker CL Jr, Murphy KP, Gottlob CA. Arthroscopic classification and treatment of lateral epicondylitis: two-year clinical results. J Shoulder Elbow Surg 2000;9:475–482.
3. Boyd HB, McLeod AC. Tennis elbow. J Bone Joint Surg Am 1973; 55A:1183–1187.
4. Field LD, Altchek DW, Warren RF, et al. Arthroscopic anatomy of the lateral elbow: a comparison of three portals. Arthroscopy 1994; 10:602–607.
5. Jerosch J, Schunck J. Arthroscopic treatment of lateral epicondylitis: indication, technique and early results. Knee Surg Sports Traumatol Arthrosc 2006;14:379–382.
6. Kraushaar BS, Nirschl RP. Current concepts review: tendinosis of the elbow (tennis elbow). J Bone Joint Surg Am 1999;81A:259–278.
7. Kuklo TR, Taylor KF, Murphy KP, et al. Arthroscopic release for lateral epicondylitis: a cadaveric model. Arthroscopy 1999;15:259–264.
8. Mehta JA, Bain GI. Posterolateral rotatory instability of the elbow. J Am Acad Orthop Surg 2004;12:405–415.

9. Nirschl RP, Pettrone FA. Tennis elbow: the surgical treatment of lateral epicondylitis. J Bone Joint Surg Am 1979;61A:832–839.
10. O'Driscoll SW, Bell DF, Morrey BF. Posterolateral rotatory instability of the elbow. J Bone Joint Surg Am 1991;73A:440–446.
11. Owens BD, Murphy KP, Kuklo TR. Arthroscopic release for lateral epicondylitis. Arthroscopy 2001;17:582–587.
12. Peart RE, Strickler SS, Schweitzer KM. Lateral epicondylitis: a comparative study of open and arthroscopic lateral release. Am J Orthop 2004;33:565–567.
13. Plancher KD, Halbrecht J, Lourie GM. Medial and lateral epicondylitis in the athlete. Clin Sports Med 1996;15:283–305.
14. Thomas MA, Fast A, Shapiro D. Radial nerve damage as a complication of elbow arthroscopy. Clin Orthop 1987;215:130–131.
15. Verhaar J, Walenkamp G, Kester A, et al. Lateral extensor release for tennis elbow: a prospective long-term follow-up study. J Bone Joint Surg Am 1993;75A:1034–1043.

Chapter 24 Hip Arthroscopy: The Basics

Marc Safran and Matthew A. Stanich

DEFINITION

- The hip is increasingly recognized as a source of pain owing to heightened awareness of pathologies, recent research, enhanced imaging techniques, and greater popularity of hip arthroscopy as a diagnostic and therapeutic tool.
- Hip arthroscopy first was performed on a cadaver in the 1930s by Burman, but it was not performed regularly until the 1980s, serving mostly as a tool for diagnosis and simple treatments, such as loose body removal, synovial biopsy, and partial labrectomy.
- With improvements in instrumentation, indications for hip arthroscopy have expanded, because surgeons now are able to do more in the hip with decreased risk of iatrogenic injury. Further, enhanced imaging techniques have allowed noninvasive diagnosis, and research has led to increased understanding of hip pathologies, furthering interest in this procedure.
- Hip arthroscopy can be performed in the central compartment (femoroacetabular joint) and peripheral compartment (along the femoral neck), which also has expanded the indications and success of hip arthroscopy, propagating the popularity of this procedure.

ANATOMY

- The hip joint is a multiaxial ball-and-socket type of synovial joint in which the head of the femur (ball) articulates with the acetabulum (socket) of the hip.
- Articular cartilage covers the head of the femur and acetabulum but is not present at the fovea.
  - The articular cartilage of the femoral head and acetabulum is relatively thin compared with that of the knee (**FIG 1A**).
- The acetabular labrum is a triangular fibrocartilage that attaches to the rim of the acetabulum at the articular cartilage edge, except at the inferiormost region of the acetabulum, where the transverse acetabular ligament extends the acetabular rim.
- The hip joint is enclosed by a capsule that is formed by an external fibrous layer and internal synovial membrane, and attaches directly to the bony acetabular rim.
- The fibrous layer consists of the iliofemoral, pubofemoral, and ischiofemoral ligaments, which anchor the head of the femur into the acetabulum (**FIG 1B,C**).
- The ligamentum teres is extracapsular and travels from the central acetabulum to the foveal portion of the femoral head (**FIG 1A**).
- The major arteries supplying the hip joint include the medial and lateral circumflex femoral arteries, which branch to provide the retinacular arteries that supply the head and neck of the femur (**FIG 1D**).
- The artery to the head of the femur also supplies blood and transverses the ligament of the head of the femur (ie, the ligamentum teres).
- The labrum has a relatively low healing potential, because vessels penetrate only the outermost layer of the capsular surface.
- Pertinent extra-articular neurovasuclar structures near the hip joint include the lateral femoral cutaneous nerve, femoral nerve, superior gluteal nerve, sciatic nerve, and the ascending branch of the lateral circumflex femoral artery.
- The lateral femoral cutaneous nerve, formed from the posterior divisions of L2 and L3 nerve roots, supplies the skin sensation of the lateral thigh. It travels from the pelvis just distal and medial to the anterosuperior iliac spine (ASIS) and divides into more than three branches distal to the ASIS.
- The femoral nerve and artery run together with the femoral vein. They pass under the inguinal ligament midway between the ASIS and the pubic symphysis, with the nerve being most lateral and the vein most medial but being mostly superficial at the level of the hip.
  - The femoral nerve is 3.2 cm from the anterior hip portal, but slightly closer at the level of the capsule.
- The superior gluteal nerve, formed from the posterior divisions of L4, L5, and S1, passes posterior and lateral to the obturator internus and piriformis muscles, then between the gluteus medius and minimus muscles approximately 4 cm proximal to the hip joint.
- The sciatic nerve, formed when nerves from L4 to S3 come together, passes anterior and inferior to the piriformis and posterior to the deep hip external rotators to supply the hamstrings and lower leg, foot, and ankle.
  - The sciatic nerve is 2.9 cm from the posterior hip arthroscopy portal, but is closest at the level of the capsule.
  - Externally rotating or flexing the hip prior to making the posterior portal brings the nerve dangerously close to the arthroscope.
- The lateral femoral circumflex artery is a branch of the femoral artery that, along with the medial circumflex artery, forms a vascular ring about the neck of the femur, providing arteriole branches to supply the femoral head (**FIG 1D**).
- The lateral femoral circumflex artery is 3.7 cm inferior to the anterior arthroscopy portal; it is much closer at the level of the capsular entry of the arthroscope.

PATHOGENESIS

- Loose bodies can be ossified or nonossified, and can either appear after traumatic hip injury or be associated with conditions such as osteochondritis dissecans and synovial chondromatosis.[18]
- Labral tear often results from hyperextension or external rotation of the hip and is more likely with hip dysplasia.
- Chondral (articular cartilage) damage can result from dislocation or subluxation of the hip or direct impact onto the hip and is associated with labral tears in more than half the cases.[20]
- Femoroacetabular impingement is a major cause of labral tears and chondral damage.
  - It usually occurs when there is loss of femoral head–neck offset (CAM impingement), excessive acetabular coverage (eg, osteophytes, retroversion, overcorrection with pelvic

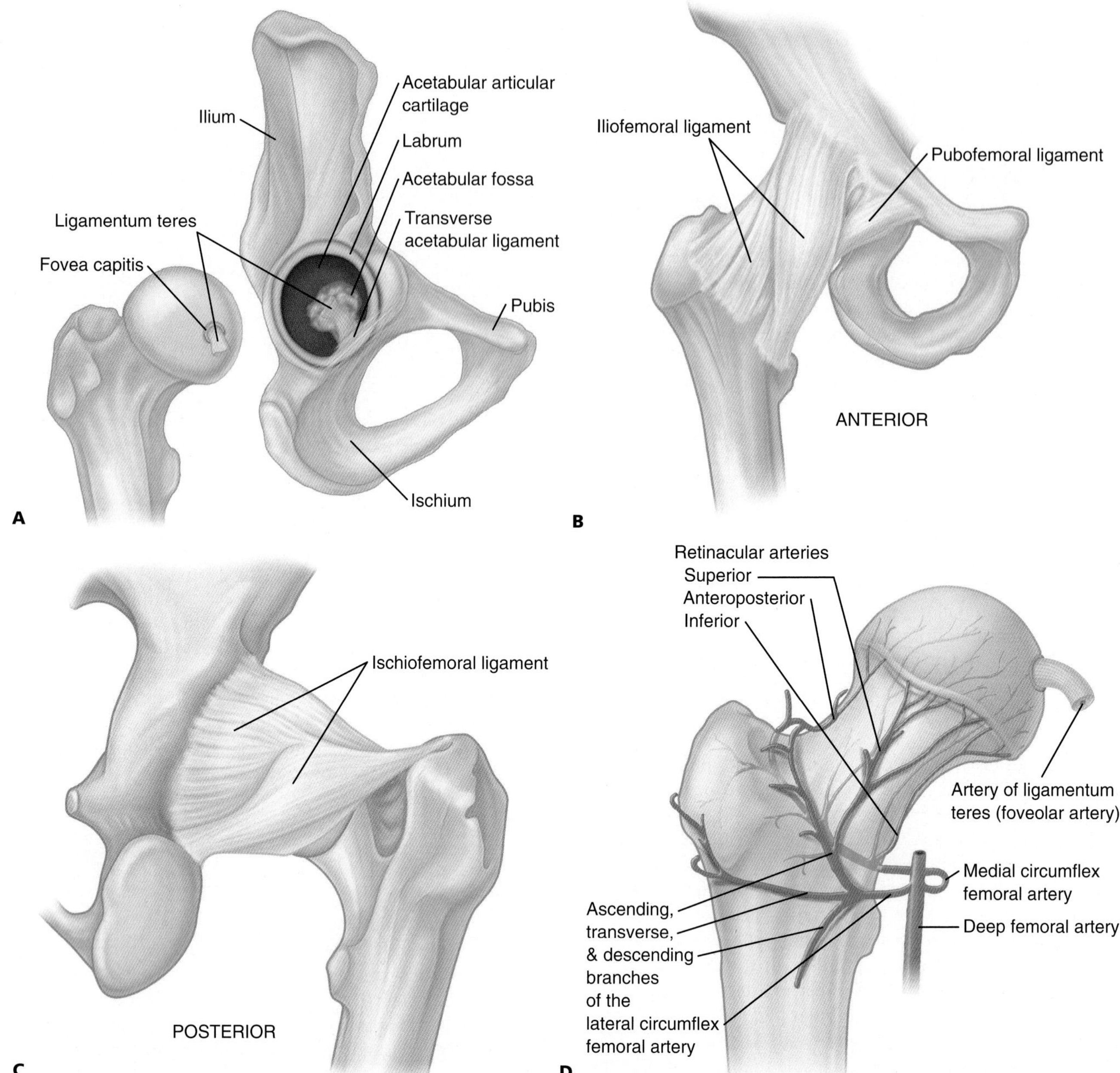

FIG 1 • Anatomy of the hip. **A.** Bony architecture of the hip joint with articular surfaces. Note the fovea and ligamentum teres. Also note the labrum does not continue along the inferior acetabulum and the lack of the articular cartilage on the inferior aspect of the acetabulum. **B,C.** Ligamentous anatomy. The iliofemoral and pubofemoral ligaments anteriorly and the ischiofemoral ligament posteriorly. **D.** Vascular anatomy. Note the medial and lateral circumflex arteries.

osteotomy, protrusio acetabuli, or otto pelvis) (pincer impingement), or both.

- The femoral head–neck junction abuts the acetabulum and labrum, resulting in tearing of the labrum, delamination of the articular cartilage, synovitis, and, eventually, arthritis.

- Ligamentum teres pathology may be due to ligament hypertrophy or partial or complete tearing and may be the result of trauma or degenerative joint disease (DJD).
  - Ligamentum hypertrophy or tearing may result in pain as a result of catching of a thickened or torn edge between the joint surfaces.
- DJD may be associated with loose bodies, labrum tears, chondral damage, ligamentum teres pathology, and synovitis.
- Avascular necrosis of the femoral head is primarily idiopathic, but can be associated with corticosteroid use, alcohol consumption, fracture, and deep sea diving (caisson disease), among others.
- Synovial diseases such as pigmented villonodular synovitis (PVNS), synovial chondromatosis, inflammatory arthritis, and osteochondromatosis can be sources of hip pain and joint damage.

NATURAL HISTORY

- The natural history of most pathologies about the hip has not been studied; much of the purported natural history is conjecture, therefore.

- Removal of loose bodies alleviates mechanical symptoms and reduces articular cartilage damage.
- Labral tears and chondral lesions that are débrided may result in degenerative arthritis.
- Untreated femoroacetabular impingement may result in degenerative arthritis.
- It has been proposed, but not proved, that labral repair or surgery for femoroacetabular impingement may lower the risk of developing DJD or slow the rate of degeneration.

PATIENT HISTORY AND PHYSICAL FINDINGS

- The patient history should include an investigation of the quality and location of pain, timing and precipitating cause of symptoms, and any referred pain.
- Patients with intra-articular pathology may have difficulty with torsional or twisting activities, discomfort with prolonged hip flexion (eg, sitting), pain or catching from flexion to extension (eg, rising from a seated position), and greater difficulty on inclines than on level surfaces.[2]
- Intra-articular pathology may be associated with groin pain extending to the knee and mechanical symptoms such as popping, locking, or restricted range of motion (ROM).[3]
  - The source of intra-articular pathology should be investigated in patients with continous hip pain for longer than 4 weeks.
- Physical examination methods are summarized later.
  - It is important to follow a systemic approach to examination that includes inspection, palpation, ROM, strength, and special tests.[26]
- Intra-articular pathologies do not have palpable areas of tenderness, although compensation for longstanding intra-articular problems may result in tenderness of muscles or bursae.
- Motor strength and neurovascular examinations must be performed for the entire lower extremity.
- It is important to rule out other causes of pain referred to the hip.
  - Spinal pain usually is localized at the posterior buttock and sacroiliac region and may radiate to the lower extremity.
  - Injuries to the sacrum and sacroiliac joint are recognized by a positive gapping or transverse anterior stress test.
  - Abdominal injuries are recognized by basic inspection and palpation of the abdomen for a mass or fascial hernia, which can be evaluated by isometric contraction of the rectus abdominis and obliques.
  - Abdominal muscle injury is recognized by pain during contraction of the rectus abdominis and obliques.
  - Herniography may be used to rule out hernias.
    - Particularly difficult to diagnose is the sports hernia (Gilmore's groin).
  - Genitourinary tract
    - Injuries to the pelvic area, such as pubic symphysis and intrapelvic problems, are recognized by the gapping/transverse anterior stress test.
- Specific tests for the hip include the following:
  - McCarthy test: distinction of internal hip pathology such as torn acetabular labrum or lateral rim impingement
  - Stinchfield and Fulcrum test: diagnosis of internal derangements, primarily of the anterior portion of the acetabulum
  - Scour test: associated with micro-instability or combined anterior anteversion; acetabular anteversion summation; hyperlaxity; or strain of the iliofemoral ligament
  - Thomas test: tests for flexion contracture. Extension to 0 degrees (in line with the body) without low back motion is normal. Less than full extension without rotating the pelvis or lifting the lower back is consistent with a flexion contracture.
  - Ober test: used to evaluate iliotibial band tightness. The test is positive when the upper knee remains in the abducted position after the hip is passively extended and abducted, then adducted, with the knee flexed. If, when the hip and knee are allowed to adduct while the hip is held in neutral rotation, the knee adducts past midline, the hip abductors are not tight; whereas if the knee does not reach to midline, then the hip abductors are tight.
  - Ely's test: if on flexion of the knee the ipsilateral hip also flexes, then the rectus femoris is tight.
  - Trendelenburg test: indicative of hip abductor weakness, and may indicate labrum pathology that affects neuroproprioceptive function. If the pelvis (iliac crest or posterior superior iliac spine) of the ipsilateral hip of the leg that is lifted elevates from the neutral standing position, this is normal. If the pelvis drops below the contralateral pelvis or from the starting position (ie, iliac crest/posterior superior iliac spine) this is considered a positive Trendelenburg sign and indicative of hip abductor weakness of the muscles on the extremity standing on the ground. If the pelvis stays level, then this is indicative of mild weakness and recorded as level.
  - Patrick's test (FABER test): indicative of sacroiliac abnormalities or iliopsoas spasm. Pain may be felt with downward stress on the flexed knee. Pain in the posterior pelvis may be considered a positive finding that indicates the pain is coming from the sacroiliac joint.
  - Labral stress test: indicative of labral tear. The patient will note groin pain or a click in a consistent position as the hip is being rotated.
  - Piriformis test: pain in the lateral hip or buttock reproduced by this maneuver is consistent with pain from the piriformis.
  - Impingement test: pain in the groin is a positive test and is consistent with femoroacetabular impingement.

IMAGING AND OTHER DIAGNOSTIC STUDIES

- Routine anteroposterior (AP) and lateral (usually cross-table lateral) radiographs should be obtained in all patients with hip pain to evaluate variations in bony architecture and visualization of areas that may present with hip pain such as the pubic symphysis, sacrum, sacroiliac joints, ilium, and ischium.
  - Radiographs help exclude degenerative joint changes, osteonecrosis, loose bodies, stress fractures, or other osseous pathology, and help assess for acetabular dysplasia and femoral neck abnormalities (bump or cam lesion) and femoroacetabular impingement (**FIG 2A,B**).
- Bone scan or radionuclide imaging is sensitive in detecting fractures, arthritis, neoplasm, infections, and vascular abnormalities, but has low specificity and poor anatomic resolution.
- MRI is used to detect stress fractures of the femoral neck and to identify sources of hip pain such as osteonecrosis, pigmented villonodular synovitis, synovial chondromatosis, osteochondromas, and other intra-articular pathology.
  - MRI arthrography can increase the ability to diagnose and describe labral pathology and articular cartilage loss (**FIG 2C**).

- MRI combined with the use of intra-articular local anesthetic with gadolinium is used to assess pain relief and provide evidence that intra-articular pathology may be causing pain.
- CT, MRI, and occasionally radioisotope imaging typically are required to help diagnose labral tears, hip instability, iliopsoas tendinitis, inflammatory arthritis, early avascular necrosis, occult fractures, psoas abscess, tumor, upper lumbar radiculopathy, or vascular abnormalities.
  - CT scan can be useful to measure ante- and retroversion of the femoral neck and acetabulum, to show the size and shape of the acetabulum and femoral head and neck, to elucidate bony architecture, to confirm concentric reduction after hip dislocation, and to rule out loose bodies.
- Ultrasound is a nonirradiating way of evaluating intra-articular effusions and soft tissue swelling.
- Iliopsoas bursography is the choice imaging modality to detect iliopsoas bursitis and internal snapping hip.
  - Iliopsoas bursitis and internal snapping hip may be evaluated with real-time dynamic ultrasound.
  - Three-dimensional CT is used to assess bony deformities, including oseophytes of the acetabulum and femoral neck bony lesions, which may cause impingement (**FIG 2D**).

DIFFERENTIAL DIAGNOSIS

- Labral tear
- Chondral delamination or degeneration
- Dysplasia
- Femoroacetabular impingement
- Synovitis
- Synovial chondromatosis
- Synovial osteochondromatosis
- Loose bodies
- Ligamentum teres tear
- Ligamentum teres hypertrophy
- Sepsis of the hip
- Arthritis of the hip
- Hip dislocation or subluxation
- Avascular necrosis of the femoral head
- Sacroiliac joint pathology, including ankylosing spondylitis
- Trochanteric bursitis
- Athletic pubalgia
- Femur, pelvic, or acetabular fractures or stress fractures
- Myotendinous strains
- Piriformis syndrome
- Myositis ossification
- Neurologic irritation
- Hamstring syndrome
- Iliotibial band syndrome
- Iliopsoas tendon problems (eg, snapping and tendinitis)
- Tendinitis
- Tendon injuries (iliopsoas, piriformis, rectus, hamstring, or adductor)
- Benign tumors (eg, osteoid osteoma, osteochondroma)
- Occult hernia
- Lumbar spine (mechanical pain and herniated discs)
- Abdomen
- Osteitis pubis

A
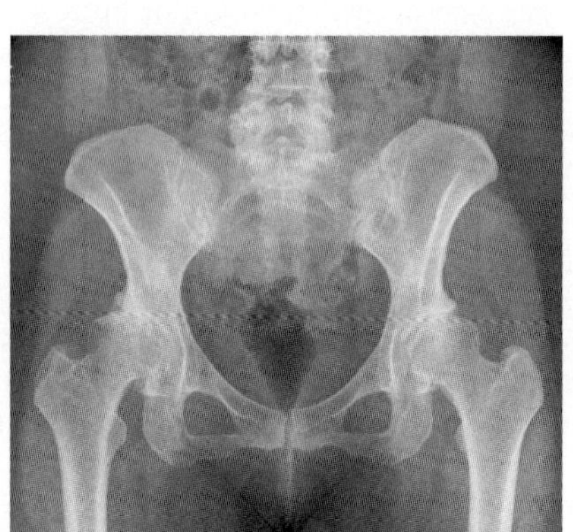
B
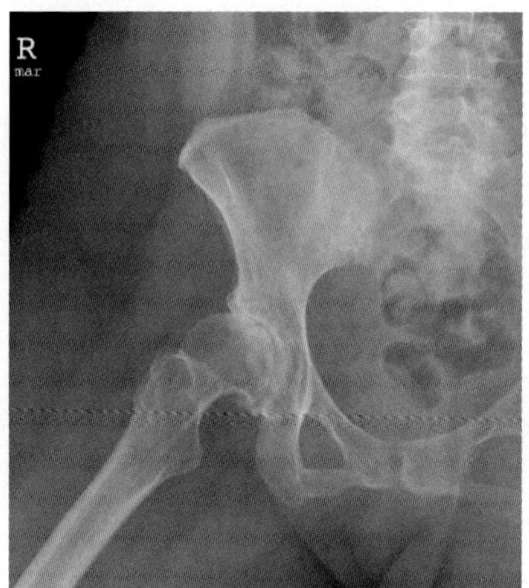

C
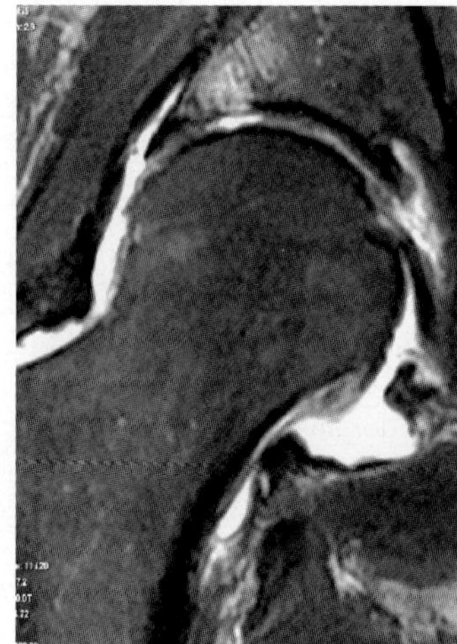
D
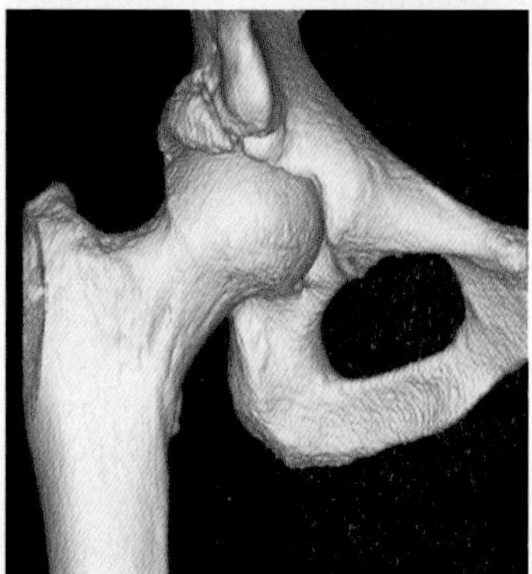

FIG 2 • AP radiographs of the pelvis (**A**) and lateral hip (**B**) of a patient with concomitant developmental dysplasia of the hip and degenerative joint disease. **C.** MRI arthrogram of patient with femoroacetabular impingement. Note the subchondral edema and chondral lesion. **D.** Three-dimensional CT scan showing cam impingement with non-union of a superior acetabular stress fracture in a 32-year-old athletic man.

NONOPERATIVE MANAGEMENT

- Conservative therapy includes rest, ambulatory support, nonsteroidal anti-inflammatory drugs, and physical therapy.
- Most pathologies about the hip usually are treated initially with conservative management, including relative rest, NSAIDs, and rehabilitation. Occasionally, use of ambulatory assist devices may be needed.
- However, several intra-articular pathologies do not resolve or heal with nonoperative management, including labral tears, loose bodies, articular cartilage lesions, and femoroacetabular impingement.

SURGICAL MANAGEMENT

- Proper patient selection is essential for a successful surgical outcome.
- Arthroscopy is most successful for patients with recent, symptomatic intra-articular hip joint pathology, particularly those with mechanical symptoms, and minimal arthritic changes.
- Arthroscopy should be considered if hip pain is persistent, is reproducible on physical examination, and does not respond to conservative treatment.
- Pain relief with intra-articular injection of local anesthetic also is a good predictive sign for success.
- Indications for arthroscopy include loose bodies, foreign objects, labral tears, chondral injuries, synovial disease, femoroacetabular impingement, mild degenerative disease with mechanical symptoms, osteonecrosis of femoral head, osteochondritis dissecans, ruptured ligamentum teres, snapping hip syndrome, impinging osteophytes, adhesive capuslitis, iliopsoas tendon release, iliopsoas bursitis, trochanteric bursectomy, iliotibial band resection, crystalline hip arthropathy, hip instability, joint sepsis, osteoid osteoma, osteochondroma, and unresolved hip pain.
- ROM should be evaluated before arthroscopy to determine the presence of contractures.
- Arthroscopy can be a means to delay total arthroplasty for DJD.
- Contraindications include systemic illness, open wounds, soft tissue disorders, poor bone quality (ie, unable to withstand traction), non-progressing avascular necrosis of the femoral head, arthrofibrosis or capsular constriction, and ankylosis of the hip.
- Severe obesity is a relative contraindication that may be circumvented with extra-length instruments.
- Indications for labrectomy include relief of pain with intra-articular injection of anesthesia, no pain relief with physical therapy or nonsteriodal anti-inflammatory drugs, missed time due to delayed diagnosis, and symptoms for longer than 4 weeks.
- Arthroscopy for DJD should be considered for younger patients with mild–moderate disease who present with mechanical sympotoms and no deformity.
- Microfracture is indicated for grade IV chondral lesions with healthy surrounding articular surface and intact subchondral bone.
- Treatment of sepsis involves drainage, lavage, débridement, and postoperative antibiotics, and requires early diagnosis.
  - Sepsis in the setting of joint arthroplasty requires prompt arthroscopic débridement, well-fixed components, a sensitive microorganism, and patient tolerance to and compliance with antibiotic therapy.[15]

Preoperative Planning

- A physical examination should be completed and radiographs and other imaging reviewed before arthroscopy.
- A three-dimensional CT scan may be obtained to further assess bony abnormalities (see Fig 2D).
- Arthroscopy usually is performed under general anesthesia.
- If epidural anesthesia is used, it also requires adequate motor block to relax muscle tone.
- Typical instrumentation includes a marking pen; no. 11 blade scalpel; 6-inch 17-gauge spinal needles; 60-mL syringe of saline with extension tubing; a Nitanol guidewire; 4.5-, 5.0-, and 5.5-mm cannulas with cannulated and solid obturators; a switching stick; a separate inflow adaptor; and a modified probe.
- Fluid used can be introduced by gravity or a pump.
- Specialized arthroscopy equipment for the hip is available that is extra-long and extra-strong to withstand the lever arm due to the extra length. These instruments include shavers, burrs, biters, probes, curettes, and loose body retrievers.

Positioning

- The patient may be placed in either the supine or lateral decubitus position on a fracture table or attachment that allows for distraction of the hip joint.
  - The lateral decubitus position offers the benefit of directing fat away from the operative site.
- The involved hip joint is in neutral rotation, abducted at 10 to 25 degrees, and in neutral flexion–extension (**FIG 3A**).
- Flexion of the involved hip during distraction and portal placement increases the risk of injury to the sciatic nerve.
- The nonoperative hip also is abducted and is placed under slight traction to stabilize the patient and allow placement of the image intensifier between the legs and directed over the operative hip.
- A heavily padded perineal post is placed against the pubic ramus and ischial tuberosity, but lateralized against the medial thigh of the operative hip, with care taken to protect perineal structures (**FIG 3B**).
- It is important to lateralize the traction vector such that it is parallel to the femoral neck to minimize risk of pressure neuropraxia to the pudendal nerve, and to optimize distraction of the joint.
- The surgeon, assistant, and scrub nurse stand on the operative side, facing the arthroscopic monitor on the opposite side of the patient (**FIG 3C,D**).
- The fluoroscopy monitor is placed at the foot of the fracture table.

Approach

- Portal placement and arthroscopic technique do not differ between the supine and lateral decubitus postions.
- Hip arthroscopy usually is performed through three portals: anterolateral, anterior, and posterolateral.
- A shortened bridge can accommodate the use of 4.5-, 5.0-, and 5.5-mm cannulas.
  - Although a 5.0-mm cannula is used for initial entry of the arthroscope, a 4.5-mm cannula permits interchange of the inflow, arthroscope, and instruments, and a 5.5-mm cannula allows entry of larger instruments (eg, shaver blades).

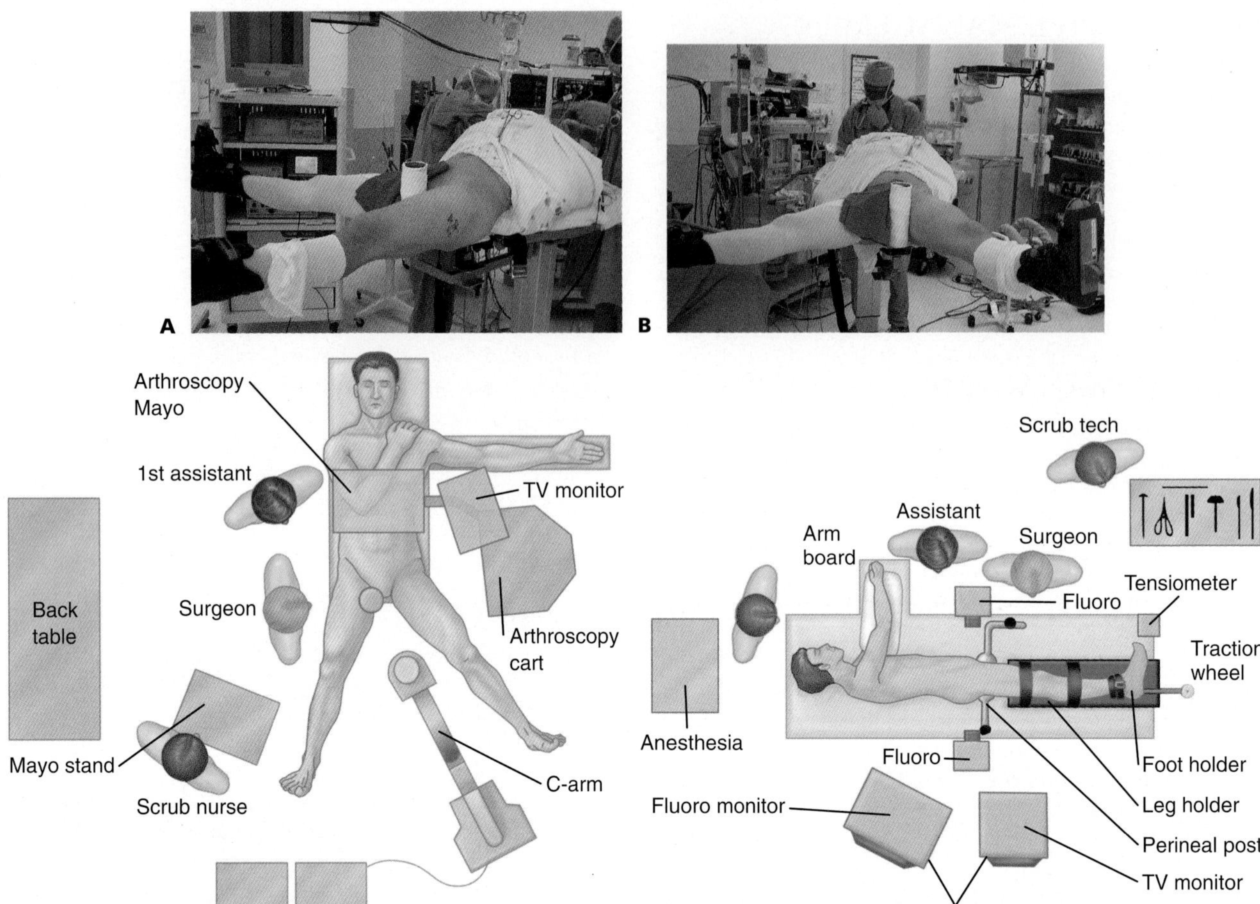

FIG 3 • **A.** Operating room setup for hip arthroscopy. The patient is supine on a fracture table, with the unaffected leg abducted approximately 60 degrees, and the hip to be operated on in neutral flexion–extension, neutral internal–external rotation, and 15 degrees of abduction. **B.** A well-padded peroneal post allows lateralization of the surgical hip in addition to distal displacement of the femoral head with distraction. **C,D.** Schematic representation of hip arthroscopy in the supine and lateral positions. The arthroscopic monitor is on the opposite side of the patient for hip arthroscopy. The fluoroscopic monitor is at the foot of the table; the fluoroscope is brought either between the legs or from the contralateral side of the patient for supine hip arthroscopy. For lateral hip arthroscopy, the fluoroscopic monitor is on the opposite side of the patient from the surgeon and the fluoroscope is next to the surgeon.

- A 30-degree videoarticulated arthroscope provides best visualization of the central portion of the acetabulum, the femoral head, and the superior aspect of the acetabular fossa.
  - A 70-degree videoarthroscope provides optimal visualization of the periphery of the joint, the acetabular labrum, and the inferior aspect of the acetabular fossa.
- The holmium YAG laser and radiofrequency device are used to ablate tissue and can offer increased manueverability over shavers.
- Extra-length convex and concave curved shaver blades are used to remove tissue around the femoral head.
- Fragile, extra-length instruments designed for other arthroscopic procedures should be avoided, because these have a greater tendency to break.

TECHNIQUES

HIP DISTRACTION

- The patient is prepared with chlorhexidine (Hibiclens) or povidone-iodine (Betadine).
- Traction is applied to distract the joint 7 to 10 mm.
- A tensiometer may be used to monitor traction force (typically 25 to 50 pounds).
- Traction time should be monitored. It is important to limit the time to less than 2 hours to prevent complications such as compression of the pudendal nerve or injury to other nerves.
- The spinal needle is introduced under fluoroscopy at the anterolateral position into the joint capsule to equilibrate the space with the ambient pressure (**TECH FIG 1A,B**).
- Pressure in the joint may be equilibrated with air or saline (**TECH FIG 1C**).
- Care should be taken to avoid penetrating the labrum and articular surfaces with the spinal needle.

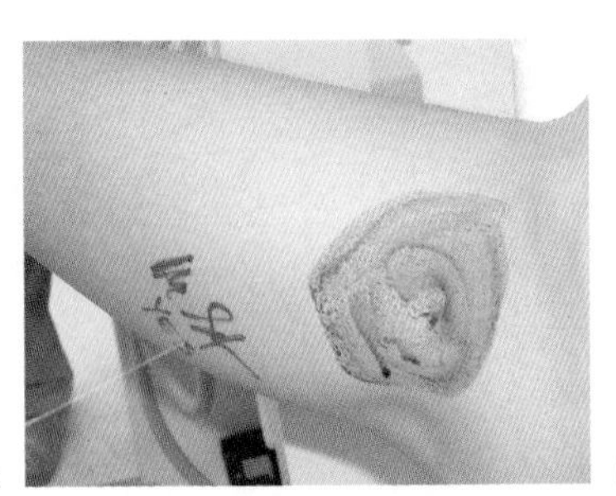

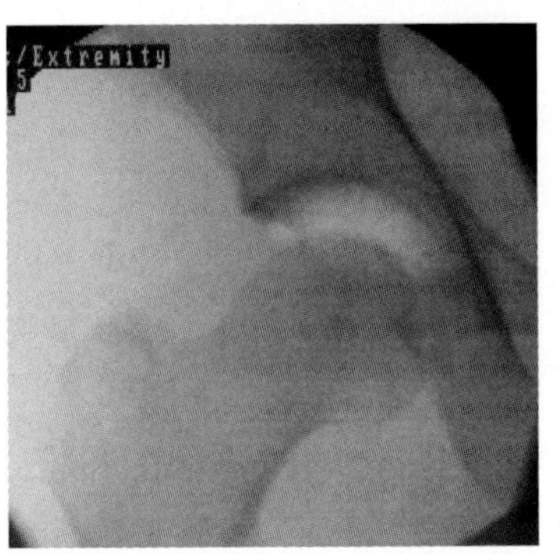

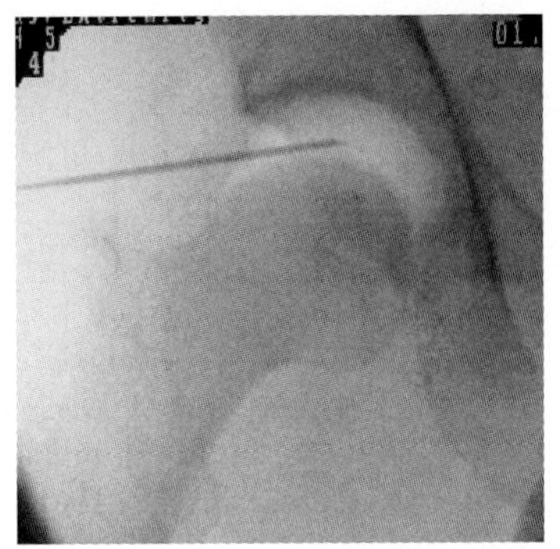

A B C

TECH FIG 1 • **A.** Equilibration of intra-articular pressure with ambient pressure. A spinal needle is introduced under fluoroscopic guidance in a prepped patient to relieve the suction cup effect of the negative intra-articular pressure to confirm adequate distraction prior to starting the hip arthroscopy. **B,C.** Fluoroscopic images taken during the initial stages of hip arthroscopy. **B.** The joint is distracted prior to introducing the spinal needle. **C.** Once the spinal needle has been introduced and the trocar removed, an air arthrogram is made, as evidenced by the air seen laterally in the joint, and the increase in joint distraction without adding more traction force.

MAKING THE PORTALS

- Portals are established by penetrating the skin with a 6-inch 17-gauge spinal needle and positioning the needle into the respective joint space.
- The trocar of the spinal needle is removed and a Nitanol guidewire (Smith & Nephew Endoscopy, Andover, MA) is run through the needle into the joint space (TECH FIG 2A,B).
- The needle is removed.
- A skin incision is made at the entry site, large enough to faciliate entry of a 5.0-mm cannula.
- A long cannula sheath with cannulated trocar is advanced over the guidewire into the joint space (TECH FIG 2C–E).
- The cannulated obturator should be kept off the femoral head to avoid articular damage.
- It is important to avoid cannula removal and reintroduction, because this may damage cartilage.
- It may be necessary to release the capsule with an arthroscopic knife.
- The weight-bearing portion of the femoral head is visualized by using the arthroscope in all three central compartment portals with the 70- and 30-degree lenses or by internally and externally rotating the hip intraoperatively.
- The fossa and ligamentum teres typically are visualized from all three portals, particularly using the 30-degree lens.

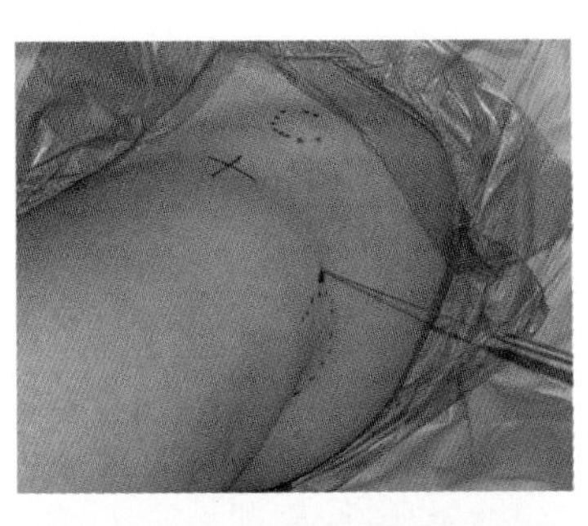

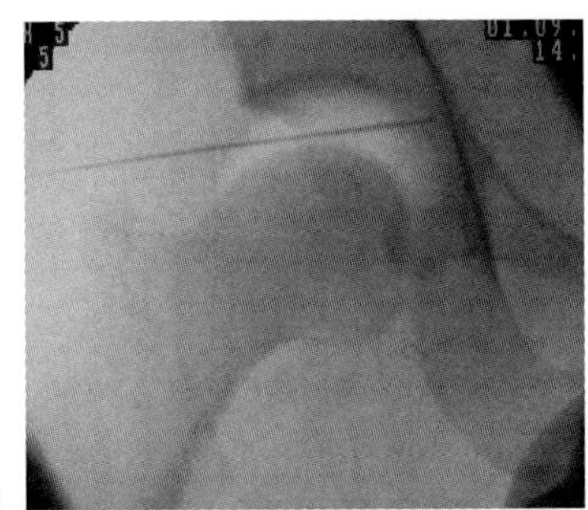

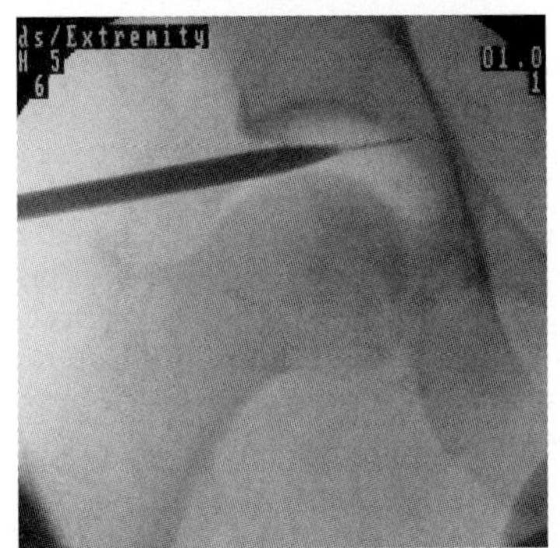

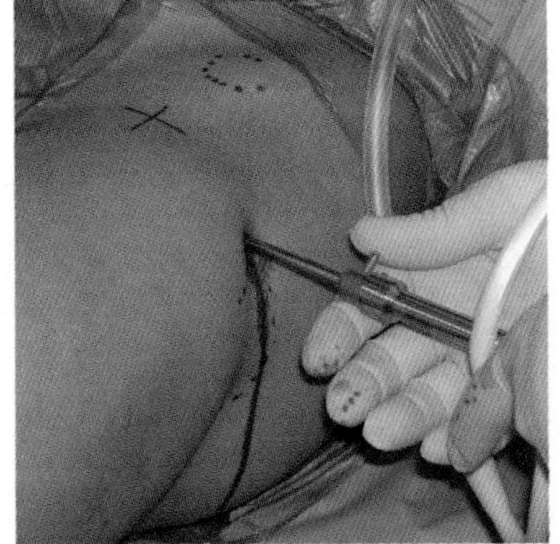

A B C D

TECH FIG 2 • **A.** Guidewire in the anterolateral portal. The spinal needle has been exchanged for a guidewire which, in turn, is being used to guide the trocar and sheathed cannula. **B.** Fluoroscopic view of the guidewire in the distracted joint, after removing the spinal needle. **C.** Fluoroscopic view of the trocar with sheathed cannula within the joint over the guidewire. **D.** The arthroscope placed in the anterolateral portal.

ANTEROLATERAL PORTAL

- The anterolateral portal is created first because it is the safest, being the most distant from and posing least risk of injury to the femoral and sciatic neurovascular structures.
- The portal penetrates the gluteus medius muscle and is positioned directly over the superior aspect of the greater trochanter at its anterior margin to enter the lateral capsule at its anterior margin (**TECH FIG 3**).
- When creating the anterolateral portal, it is important to introduce the spinal needle in the coronal plane by keeping it parallel to the floor (see Tech Fig 2A).
- As the cannula is positioned into the intra-articular space, care should be taken to avoid damage to the labrum or articular surfaces.
- The portal provides visualization of most of the acetabular cartilage, labrum, and weight-bearing femoral head within the central compartment, as well as visualization of the peripheral compartment, such as the non-weight-bearing femoral head, the anterior neck, the anterior intrinsic capsular folds, and the synovial tissues beneath the zona orbicularis and the anterior labrum.
- The superior gluteal nerve is the closest neurovascular structure and runs 4.4 cm posterior to the portal.

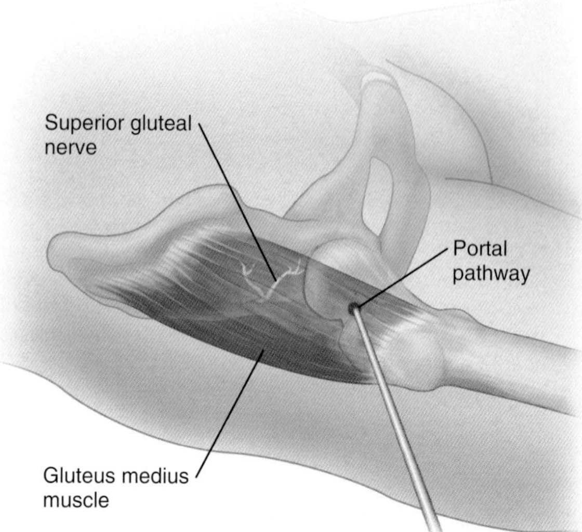

TECH FIG 3 • The anterolateral portal starts just anterior to the superior aspect of the greater trochanter and pierces the gluteus medius muscle.

ANTERIOR PORTAL

- I prefer to establish the anterior portal after the anterolateral portal, although some prefer to establish the anterior portal first.
- Arthroscopic visualization from the anterolateral portal and fluoroscopy facilitate correct portal placement, helping to avoid damage to the labrum or articular surfaces.
- The anterior portal enters at the junction of a line drawn distally from the anterosuperior iliac spine and a transverse line across the superior margin of the greater trochanter (**TECH FIG 4A**).
- The portal penetrates the sartorius and rectus femoris muscles as it is directed 45 degrees cephalad and 30 degrees medially to enter the anterior capsule (**TECH FIG 4B,C**).
- As the cannulated obturator enters the joint space, it should be kept off the articular surface and directed underneath the acetabular labrum.
- The portal allows visualization of the anterior femoral neck, the anterior aspect of the joint, the superior retinacular fold, the ligamentum teres, and the lateral labrum.

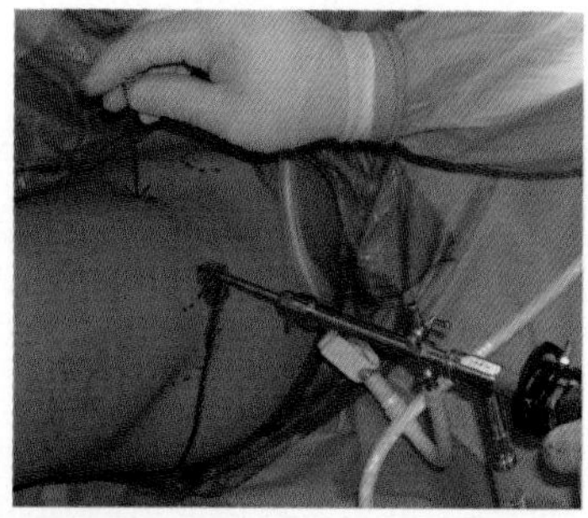
A

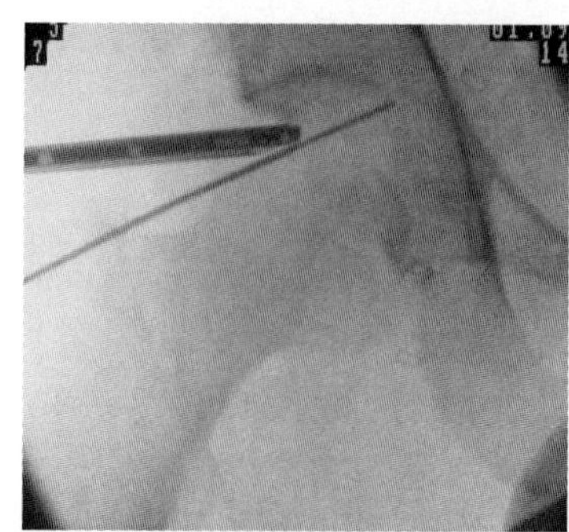
B

TECH FIG 4 • The anterior portal usually is the second portal made and is created under arthroscopic visualization with a 70-degree arthroscopic lens from the anterolateral portal and fluoroscopic visualization. **A.** Introduction of the spinal needle using the junction of the superior aspect of the greater trochanter and a line drawn inferiorly from the anterior superior iliac spine (ASIS) as the starting point. **B.** Fluoroscopic view of the arthroscope in the anterolateral portal and spinal needle being introduced from the anterior portal. *(continued)*

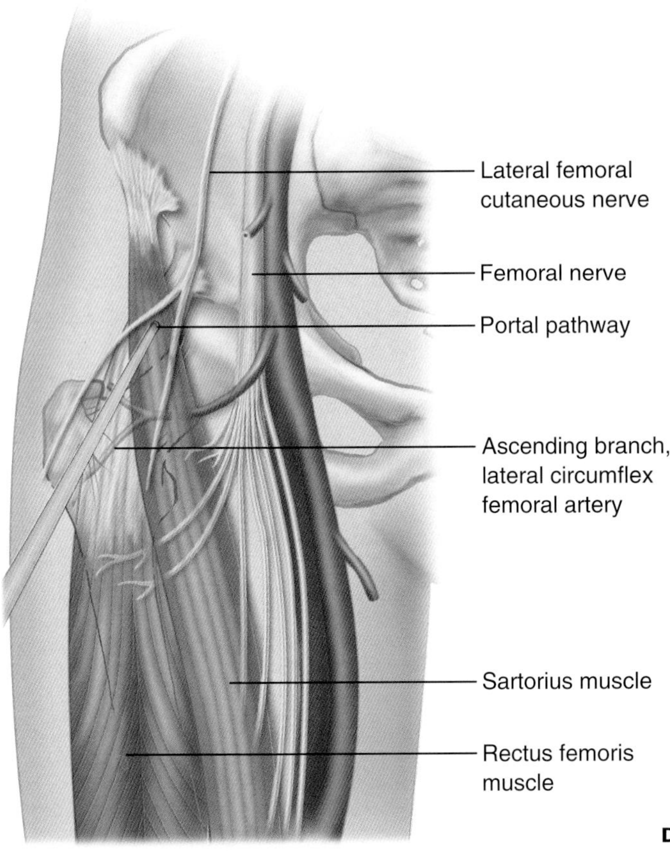

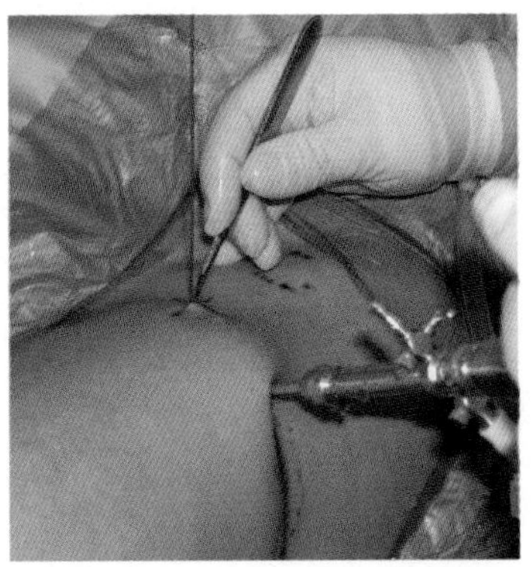

TECH FIG 4 • *(continued)* **C.** Schematic depiction of the location of the portal adjacent to the branches of the lateral femoral cutaneous nerve, penetrating the sartorius and rectus femoris muscles. **D.** Care is taken only to cut the skin when making the anterior portal, to help reduce the risk of laceration of the lateral femoral cutaneous nerve.

- Care should be taken to minimize injury to branches of the lateral femoral cutaneous nerve by directing movement medially, avoiding deep cuts at the entry site, not using vigorous instrumentation, and using a 70-degree arthroscope at the anterolateral portal to guide entry (TECH FIG 4D).
- The femoral nerve is 3.2 cm medial and runs tangential to the portal.
- The ascending branch of the lateral femoral circumflex artery is 3.7 cm inferior to the portal, but terminal branches may be within millimeters of the portal at the capsular level.

POSTEROLATERAL PORTAL

- The posterolateral portal is established after the anterior portal (TECH FIG 5A).
- Arthroscopic visualization and fluoroscopy are used to guide portal placement.
- The portal penetrates the gluteus medius and minimus muscles and is directed over the superior aspect of the greater trochanter at its posterior border to enter the lateral capsule at its posterior margin (TECH FIG 5B).
- The portal is superior and anterior to the piriformis.
- The portal allows visualization of the posterior aspect of the femoral head, the posterior labrum, the posterior capsule, and the inferior edge of the ischiofemoral ligament (TECH FIG 5C).
- The sciatic nerve is 2.9 cm posterior to the portal at the level of the capsule.
  - It is important to maintain the leg in neutral rotation and extension, and to introduce the spinal needle horizontally to avoid injury to the sciatic nerve.

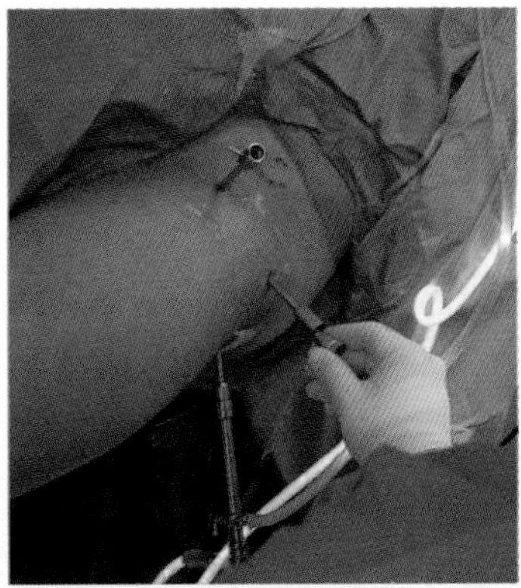

TECH FIG 5 • Posterolateral portal. The posterolateral portal usually is the last central portal made, although it can be made before the anterior portal. **A.** How the posterolateral portal is made, relative to the other portals. *(continued)*

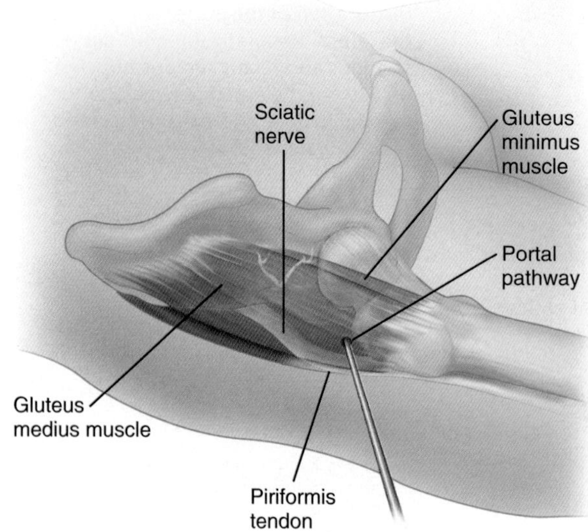

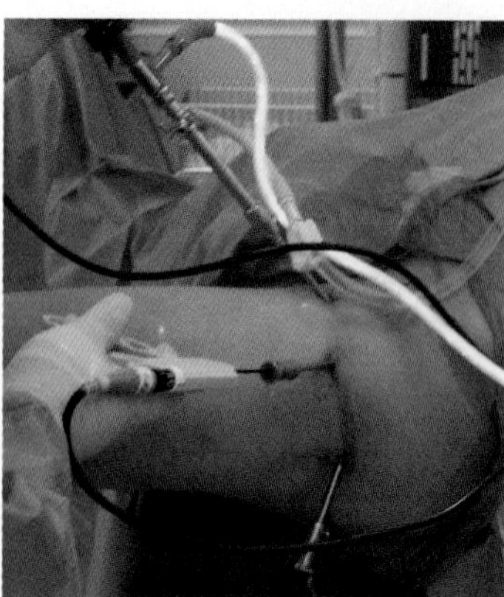

TECH FIG 5 • *(continued)* **B.** The posterolateral portal proceeds through the gluteus medius and minimus muscles. Note its relation to the superior gluteal nerve. **C.** View of obturators in all three central compartment portals to allow for complete central compartment hip arthroscopy. Both a 30- and a 70-degree lens are used in all the portals to allow for full visualization of the femoroacetabular joint to perform a complete hip arthroscopy of the central compartment.

DISTAL ANTEROLATERAL PORTAL

- To access the peripheral compartment–femoral neck region, two portals are used after traction is removed from the extremity.
- Peripheral compartment arthroscopy can be done in hip flexion to relax the anterior capsule or in neutral flexion extension.
- The anterolateral portal is used as one portal.
- A distal anterolateral portal is established 3 to 5 cm distal to the anterolateral portal, just anterior to the lateral aspect of the proximal femoral shaft and neck (TECH FIG 6).
- Fluoroscopy is used to guide portal placement.
- The portal penetrates the gluteus medius muscle and upper vastus lateralis.
- The spinal needle should enter the peripheral compartment laterally. The guidewire is brought through the spinal needle and can be gently advanced to the medial capsule—the easy passage until the medial capsule is reached helps confirm that one is in the peripheral compartment.
- The skin incision is made, and the trocar and the sheath are passed over the guidewire.
- The sheath and guidewire are exchanged for the arthroscope or instrumentation.
- Arthroscopy and fluoroscopy can be used together to perform surgery in the peripheral compartment.

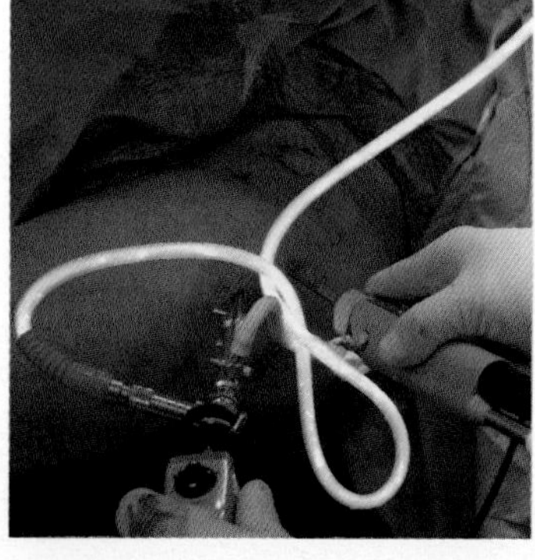

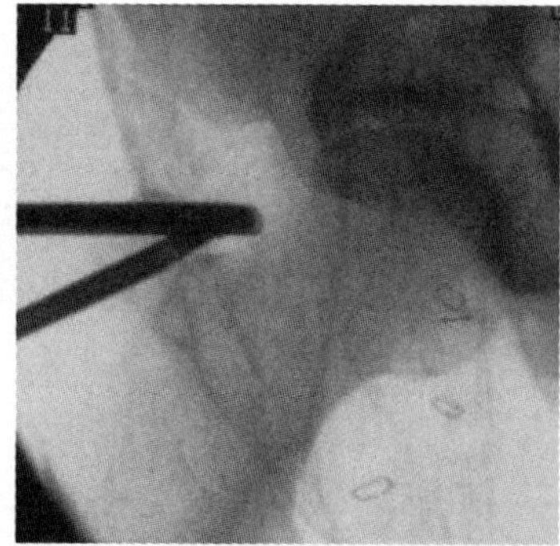

TECH FIG 6 • Distal anterolateral portal. The distal anterolateral portal allows a second portal for peripheral compartment arthroscopy. This portal is 2.5 to 5 cm distal to the anterolateral portal (**A**). This example shows the hip in neutral flexion–extension, which makes it easier to perform a chielectomy or osteoplasty for cam-type femoroacetabular impingement to maintain orientation while using fluoroscopy to assist with the procedure (**B**). Alternatively, the hip can be flexed, relaxing the anterior capsule, making entry into the joint easier.

PEARLS AND PITFALLS

Patient selection	■ A careful patient history, physical examination, and appropriate imaging should be performed. ■ Distinguish intra-articular conditions that may require surgery from extra-articular problems that may only require conservative treatment. ■ Patients should have clear expectations of outcomes.
Hip distraction	■ Distract the hip with as much force as necessary to safely introduce instruments, typically 8 to 10 mm. ■ Limit traction time to 2 hours or take a traction break if it is necessary to exceed this time. ■ Too little traction may result in injury to the articular surfaces. ■ Too much traction can result in nerve injury or injury to the perineum, knee, foot, or ankle.
Patient positioning	■ Obtain the correct vector of joint distraction with minimal force necessary to distract the joint. ■ The perineal post should be adequately padded and lateralized against the involved hip.
Portal placement	■ Proper placement of the anterolateral portal is key to successful placement of other portals. ■ It is important to avoid damaging the labrum or articular surfaces with either the spinal needle or cannula introduction. ■ Use inflow from the secondary portal to improve fluid dynamics or use a pump. ■ Use both 30- and 70-degree cannulas in each portal. ■ Use specialized hip arthroscopy instruments and metal cannulas to reduce risk of instrument breakage and allow proper technique. ■ Avoid inserting the cannula multiple times to reduce fluid extravasation and the risk of damage to labrum, cartilage, and neurovascular structures. ■ Maintain systolic blood pressure below 100 mm Hg and use a radiofrequency device to minimize bleeding.

POSTOPERATIVE CARE

- Traction is released.
- Long-acting local anesthetic is injected into the joint.
- The portals are sutured, and a sterile dressing is applied to the wounds.
- Arthroscopy is an outpatient procedure, and the patient typically leaves recovery after 1 to 3 hours.
- If arthroscopy does not involve bony recontouring of the femoral neck, labral repair, or microfracture of the articular surfaces, then the patient is allowed to walk immediately, although weight bearing should be limited by crutches for 3 to 7 days or until gait pattern is normalized.
- Rehabiliation should take into consideration soft tissue healing constraints, control of swelling and pain, early ROM, limitations on weight bearing, early initiation of muscle activity and neuromuscular control, progressive lower extremity strengthening and proprioceptive retraining, cardiovascular training, and sport-specific training.
- Swelling and pain are controlled by ice and non-aspirin nonsteroidal anti-inflammatory drugs.
- The dressing is removed on the first or second postoperative day, and the wound is covered with adhesive bandages.
- Portal sutures are removed a few days after surgery.
- Patients who undergo labrum repairs on the anterior superior region and capsulorraphy should follow specific ROM and weight bearing guidelines.
- Patients who undergo osteoplasty should limit impact activities that increase the risk of femoral neck fracture during the initial several weeks.
- Patients who undergo microfracture should adhere to 8 to 10 weeks of protected weight bearing on crutches.

OUTCOMES

- Record functional and prosthetic survivorship data, as applicable.
- Loose bodies are the clearest indication for arthroscopy, resulting in less morbidity and faster recovery than open surgery.[8]
- Labral débridement has been shown to result in successful outcomes in 68% to 82% of cases, with positive outcomes associated with isolated tears and poorer prognosis associated with arthritis.[2,10,27]
- Débridement of ligamentum teres, like labral débridement, has shown best results when lesions are isolated and without associated acetabular fracture or significant osteochondral defect of either the acetabulum or femoral head.
- Treatment of hip DJD by arthroscopy has shown unpredictable results, with a range of 34% to 60% of patients reporting improvement of symptoms after arthroscopic débridement for DJD.[11,31]
- One study reported that 86% of patients treated for chondral lesions by microfracture showed a successful response at 2-year follow-up.[1]
- Arthroscopic synovectomy is palliative, and success is based on the integrity of the articular cartilage.
- Treatment of femoroacetabular impingement has shown better outcomes when there is less DJD.
- Treatment of AVN is controversial—the results are better when the articular surface is not disrupted or when treating mechanical symptoms.
  - O'Leary[23] reported 40% of patients improved at 30-month follow-up.
- More specifics are provided in the chapters describing specific techniques for the different processes treated about the hip.

COMPLICATIONS

- Traction neurapraxia
- Direct trauma to pudendal, lateral femoral cutaneous, femoral, and sciatic nerves
- Iatrogenic labral and chondral damage
- Fluid extravasation
- Vaginal tear
- Pressure necrosis to scrotum, labia and perineum, and foot
- Labia and perineum hematoma

- Knee ligament injury
- Ankle fracture
- Femoral head avascular necrosis
- Fracture of femoral neck
- Instrument breakage
- Portal hematoma and bleeding

REFERENCES

1. Byrd JWT, Jones KS. Microfracture for grade IV chondral lesions of the hip. Arthroscopy 2004;20:89.
2. Byrd JWT, Jones KS. Prospective analysis of hip arthroscopy with two year follow up. Arthroscopy 2000;16:578–587.
3. Carreira D, Bush-Joseph CA. Hip arthroscopy. Orthopedics 2006;29: 517–523.
4. Clarke MT, Arora A, Villar RN. Hip arthroscopy: complications in 1054 cases. Clin Orthop Relat Res 2003;406:84–88.
5. Czerny C, Hofmann S, Neuhold A, et al. Lesions of the acetabular labrum: accuracy of MR imaging and MR arthrography in detection and staging. Radiology 1996;200:225–230.
6. Czerny C, Kramer J, Neuhold A, et al. Magnetic resonance imaging and magnetic resonance arthroscopy of the acetabular labrum: comparison with surgical findings. Rofo Fortschr Geb Rontgenstr Neuen Blidgeb Verfahr 2001;173:702–707.
7. Dvorak M, Duncan CP, Day B. Arthroscopic anatomy of the hip. Arthroscopy 1990;6:264–273.
8. Epstein H. Posterior fracture-dislocations of the hip: comparison of open and closed methods of treatment in certain types. J Bone Joint Surg Am 1961;43A:1079–1098.
9. Eriksson E, Sebik A. Arthroscopy and arthroscopic surgery in a gas versus a fluid medium. Orthop Clin North Am 1982;13:293–298.
10. Farjo LA, Glick JM, Sampson TG. Hip arthroscopy for acetabular labrum tears. Arthroscopy 1999;15:132–137.
11. Farjo LA, Glick JM, Sampson TG. Hip arthroscopy for degenerative joint disease. Arthroscopy 1998;14:435.
12. Fitzgerald RH. Anterior labrum tears—diagnosis and treatment. Clin Orthop Relat Res 1995;311:60–68.
13. Glick JM, Sampson TG, Gordon RB, et al. Hip arthroscopy by the lateral approach. Arthroscopy 1987;3:4–12.
14. Glick JM. Hip arthroscopy. The lateral approach. Clin Sports Med 2001;20:733–747.
15. Hyman JL, Salvati EA, Laurencin CT, et al. The arthroscopic drainage, irrigation, and debridement of late, acute total hip arthroplasty infections: average 6 year follow up. J Arthroplasty 1999;14: 903–910.
16. Jacobson T, Allen WC. Surgical correction of the snapping iliopsoas tendon. Am J Sports Med 1990;18:470–474.
17. Johnson L. Arthroscopic Surgery Principles and Practice. St. Louis: Mosby, 1986.
18. Kelly BT, Williams RJ III, Philippon MJ. Hip arthroscopy: current indications, treatment options, and management issues. Am J Sports Med 2003;31(6):1020–1037.
19. Lee D. The Pelvic Girdle, ed 2. Edinburgh: Churchill Livingstone, 1999.
20. McCarthy JC, Noble PC, Schuck MR, et al. The role of labral lesions to development of early degenerative hip disease. Clin Orthop Relat Res 2001;393:25–37.
21. McCarthy JC, Noble PC, Schuck MR, et al. The Otto E. Aufranc Award: The role of labral lesions to develepment of early degenerative hip disease. Clinical Orthop Relat Res 2001 Dec;(393):25–37.
22. Mullis BH, Dahners LE. Hip arthroscopy to remove loose bodies after traumatic dislocation. J Orthop Trauma 2006;20:22–26.
23. O'Leary JA, Berend K, Vail TP. The relationship between diagnosis and outcome in arthroscopy of the hip. Arthroscopy 2001;17: 181–188.
24. Philippon MJ. Arthroscopy of the hip in the management of the athlete. In McGinty HJ, ed. Operative Arthroscopy, ed 3. Philadelphia: Lippincott Williams & Wilkins, 2003:879–883.
25. Philippon MJ. Debridement of acetabular labral tears with associated thermal capsulorrhaphy. Oper Tech Sports Med 2002;10: 215–218.
26. Safran MR. Evaluation of the hip: history, physical examination, and imaging. Oper Tech Sports Med 2005;13:2–12.
27. Santori N, Villar RN. Acetabular labral tears: results of arthroscopic partial limbectomy. Arthroscopy 2000;16:11–15.
28. Schaberg JE, Harper MC, Allen WC. The snapping hip syndrome. Am J Sports Med 1984;12:361–365.
29. Stalzer S, Wahoff M, Scanlan M. Rehabilitation following hip arthroscopy. Clin Sports Med 2006;25:337–357.
30. Villar RN. Hip arthroscopy. J Bone Joint Surg Br 1995;77B:517–518.
31. Villar RN. Arthroscopic debridement of the hip: a minimally invasive approach to osteoarthritis. J Bone Joint Surg Br 1991;73B: 170–171.

Chapter 25 Arthroscopy for Soft Tissue Pathology of the Hip

J. W. Thomas Byrd and MaCalus V. Hogan

DEFINITION

- Soft tissue pathology of the hip includes labral tears, articular damage, and lesions of the ligamentum teres, all of which share several common features.
- The clinical presentations may be indistinguishable, and these lesions often coexist. They represent significant causes of disabling hip pain that can be elusive to clinical detection.
- The diagnosis sometimes is based just on maintaining an index of suspicion. Often these lesions have gone undiagnosed and untreated, with the patient simply resigned to living within the constraints of their symptoms.

ANATOMY

- The horseshoe or lunate articular surface of the acetabulum surrounds the acetabular fossa (**FIG 1**).
- The articular surface of the femoral head forms about two thirds of the sphere, with an indentation medially where the ligamentum teres attaches at the fovea capitis.
- The diameter of the femoral neck normally is 65% of the diameter of the femoral head, allowing clearance of the acetabulum during range of motion (ROM).
- The fibrocartilaginous labrum is triangular in cross section, forming a rim around the articular surface of the acetabulum.
  - Inferiorly, it is contiguous with the transverse acetabular ligament, which traverses the inferior aspect of the fossa. Its morphology and size can be quite variable, especially anterior and superior.
  - The shape of the posterior labrum is the most consistent and least often damaged landmark, representing a useful reference in the arthroscopic assessment of labral pathology.
  - Unlike the shoulder, there is no capsulolabral complex; the capsule attaches directly to the acetabulum separate from the labrum. Thus, acetabular labral pathology is not as synonymous with instability as that of the glenoid.
  - Konrath et al[17] have shown that the labrum has minimal mechanical properties for distributing forces across the acetabular surface. Similarly, Ferguson[13] has demonstrated that the labrum has minimal mechanical properties for stabilizing the joint, but its hydraulic seal is important.
- The ligamentum teres has a serpentine course from its acetabular attachment in the posterior fossa to the fovea capitis of the femoral head. Its precise function remains an enigma.

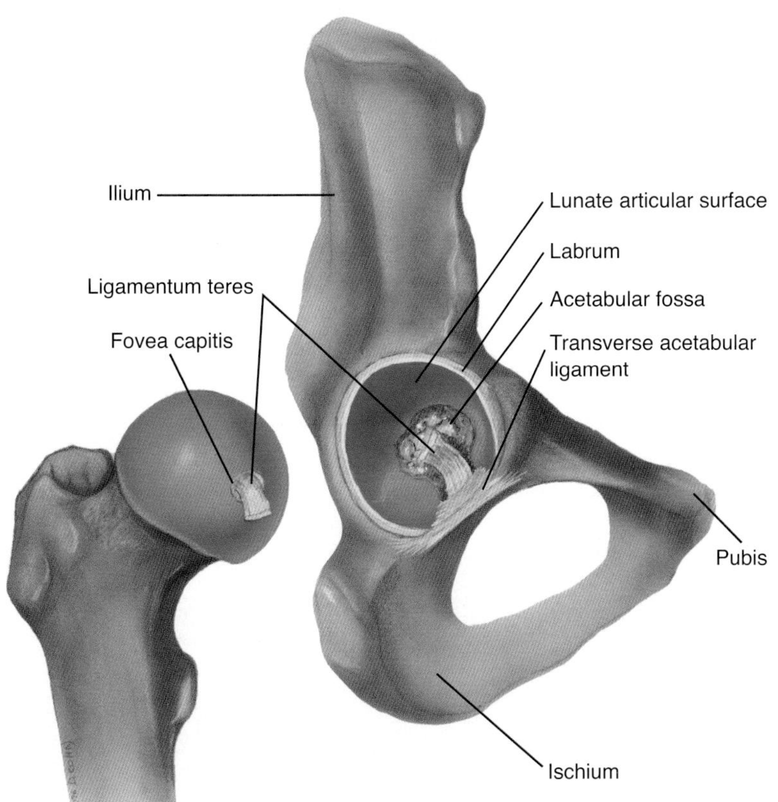

FIG 1 • Macroscopic anatomy of the hip joint. (Courtesy of Delilah Cohn.)

- In childhood, its vessel contributes to the blood supply of the femoral head. Its redundant nature implies that it contributes little to joint stability, but it may have nociceptive and proprioceptive functions.
- Gray and Villar[15] have postulated that its windshield wiper effect during ROM may facilitate joint lubrication. Its dimensions are variable, and sometimes it is absent in adulthood.

PATHOGENESIS

- The etiologies of soft tissue lesions in the hip are numerous and variable. Breakdown may result from supraphysiologic loads on normal tissue, physiologic loads on abnormal tissue, or, commonly, mildly supraphysiologic loads on mildly abnormal tissue.
- Supraphysiologic loads may be the result of macrotrauma or repetitive microtrauma.
- Athletes are especially prone to pushing their bodies beyond the physiologic limits where breakdown occurs.
- Once this point has been passed, reversal of the damage often is incomplete, even with surgical intervention. Variable joint morphology often is a contributing factor.
- Labral tears can occur from compression, commonly associated with impingement; traction associated with excessive translation of the femoral head; and shear forces, typically associated with acetabular dysplasia.
  - Articular damage can be caused by acute trauma or degenerative disease. A propensity for acute articular fracture has been identified in physically fit young men, resulting from a direct lateral blow to the trochanter.[2]
  - There is little adipose tissue over the trochanter to cushion the blow; and with high bone density fracture does not occur, so the force is delivered directly to the joint surface.
- Lesions of the ligamentum teres can occur from acute trauma or degeneration.
  - The ligament is most taut with adduction and external rotation, but acute rupture has been identified with a variety of mechanisms.
  - Deterioration of the ligament occurs with degenerative disease, and the ligament is sometimes hypertrophied, making it more susceptible to degenerate rupture.
- Femoroacetabular impingement (both pincer and cam type) has been recognized as a causative factor in the development of soft tissue joint damage.[14] It is the soft tissue damage that then becomes symptomatic, necessitating treatment.
  - Pincer impingement is associated primarily with labral pathology due to excessive compression and then secondary development of articular breakdown (**FIG 2A**).
  - Cam impingement is associated with selective articular delamination of the anterolateral acetabulum with a variable amount of associated labral pathology (**FIG 2B**).
- Dysplasia is associated with breakdown of the labrum, articular surface, and ligamentum teres.[4]
  - The labrum often is enlarged, with more weight-bearing responsibility, making it susceptible to a breakdown from shear forces. It also can become inverted within the joint and susceptible to deterioration.
  - The reduced surface area of the acetabulum results in increased contact forces, which may exceed the structural integrity of the articular cartilage.
  - Hypertrophy of the ligamentum teres occurs in association with dysplasia, and the hypertrophied ligament is more susceptible to degenerative rupture.

NATURAL HISTORY

- The natural history of these soft tissue lesions is variable. Some conditions deteriorate quickly, whereas others may remain stable for a protracted period of time, and some become asymptomatic.

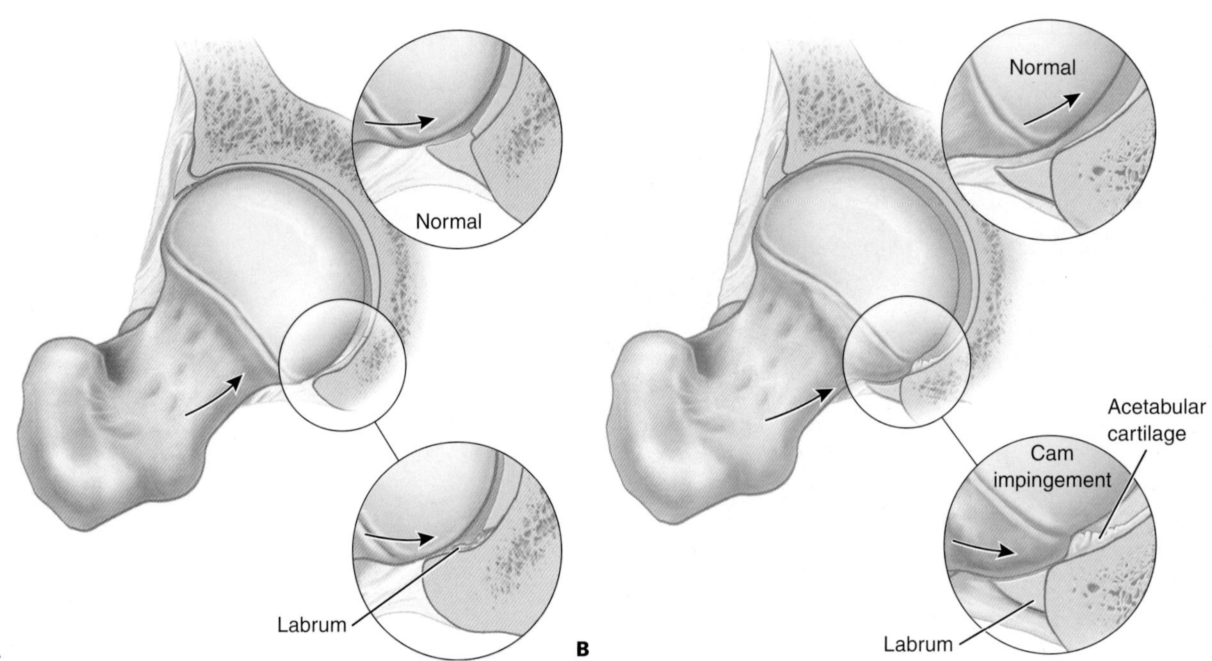

FIG 2 • **A.** Pincer impingement: mechanism of labral breakdown. **B.** Cam impingement: mechanism of articular delamination.

- Labral degeneration has been observed as an unavoidable consequence of age and is found to be uniformly present in persons over 70 years of age.[18]
- Abnormal hip morphology, including impingement and dysplasia, may be found even in absence of joint pathology.
- When symptomatic soft tissue pathology occurs, it is important to assess for predisposing morphology. Some conditions may remain stable for an indefinite period; however, progressive worsening of symptoms usually dictates more proactive intervention.

PATIENT HISTORY AND PHYSICAL FINDINGS

- Examination of the hip joint is fairly straightforward.[3] Much of the assessment revolves around ruling out other problems.
- Patients with chronic hip joint pathology will start to develop other conditions secondarily as they compensate for the joint.
  - The secondary conditions, such as gluteal pain or trochanteric bursitis, may be more evident, obscuring the underlying diagnosis. In addition, other conditions such as lumbar spine disease may coexist with hip joint disease.
  - There is a significant correlation between hip joint pathology and athletic pubalgia in athletes.
    - Increased pelvic motion compensates for restricted hip motion, placing more stress on the pelvic stabilizers and resulting in the soft tissue breakdown characterized by athletic pubalgia.
- The history of injury is variable, with some patients describing a major traumatic event. Others may recount an acute episode such as twisting. In these circumstances, however, the clinician should look closely for predisposing factors, because a healthy joint should be able to withstand these forces.
- Some patients simply describe the insidious or gradual onset of symptoms, further indicative of underlying disease.
- A history of a significant traumatic event indicates a more favorable prognosis of a potentially correctable problem.
  - Similarly, mechanical symptoms such as sharp stabbing pain, catching, or locking are favorable indicators for surgical intervention.
- Simply having pain, with or without activity, is a poorer prognostic indicator for the success of arthroscopy.
- Numerous characteristic features of hip joint symptoms have been identified.[3]
  - Straight plane activities, including running, often are well tolerated.
  - Pivoting and twisting maneuvers usually are more troublesome.
  - Squatting and prolonged hip flexion such as sitting often will exacerbate hip symptoms.
  - Patients may experience a catching sensation when rising from a seated position.
  - Ascending and descending stairs or inclines is more troublesome than walking on level surfaces.
  - Entering and exiting an automobile is very characteristic for recreating symptoms, because it loads the hip in a flexed position while introducing a torsional component.
  - Dyspareunia due to hip pain is uniformly present in sexually active individuals.
  - Difficulty getting shoes and socks on and off usually indicates restricted motion and more advanced disease.
- Localization of the symptoms starts with an understanding that the L3 nerve root serves as the principal innervation of the hip.
- Symptoms, therefore, are sometimes referred to the L3 dermatome, explaining the presence of medial-sided thigh and knee pain.
  - The C-sign is very characteristic of hip joint pathology.
    - Describing their symptoms, patients will cup their hand in the shape of a C above the greater trochanter, gripping their fingers into the groin.
    - Most patients describe groin or anterolateral pain.
- Posterior pain rarely is indicative of hip joint pathology, but may occasionally be a presenting feature.
- It is important to record ROM in a consistent fashion for comparing sides as well as for comparison on subsequent examination.
- Recording flexion and extension must take into account the contributing components of pelvic and lumbar motion. Rotational motion is different when measured in extension versus flexion.
- The log roll test is the most specific test for hip joint pathology:
  - The leg is rolled back and forth, rotating only the femoral head in relation to the acetabulum and capsule, without tensioning any of the surrounding soft tissue structures.
- The impingement test generally has been found positive for virtually any irritable hip joint, regardless of the nature of the pathology.
  - The leg is placed in maximal flexion, adduction, and internal rotation.
  - This maneuver is more sensitive for hip joint pathology, but may be uncomfortable even in a healthy hip. Thus, it is important to compare the symptomatic to the asymptomatic side.
  - It also is important to distinguish whether this test recreates the type of symptoms that the patient experiences with activity, more than simply whether or not it is uncomfortable.
- Abduction with external rotation also can be sensitive for eliciting hip joint symptoms.
  - It may impinge upon posterior lesions or exacerbate anterior symptoms from translation of the femoral head and, thus, is not especially specific for the location or type of intra-articular pathology.

IMAGING AND OTHER DIAGNOSTIC STUDIES

- Radiographs are important for assessing hip morphology.
- A properly centered anteroposterior pelvis radiograph is essential for assessing the morphology of the hip and comparing the affected to the unaffected side (**FIG 3**).
- The optimal lateral view has yet to be determined, but a standardized reproducible lateral radiograph of the affected hip should be obtained in every case.
- Radiographs usually are normal with regard to specific findings indicative of soft tissue pathology in the hip.
- The soft tissue disease usually is far advanced before any radiographic indices emerge.
- Thus, it is important to scrutinize the radiographs carefully, assessing for subtle indicators of change.
  - For example, slight joint space narrowing usually indicates advanced intra-articular disease, and should be viewed

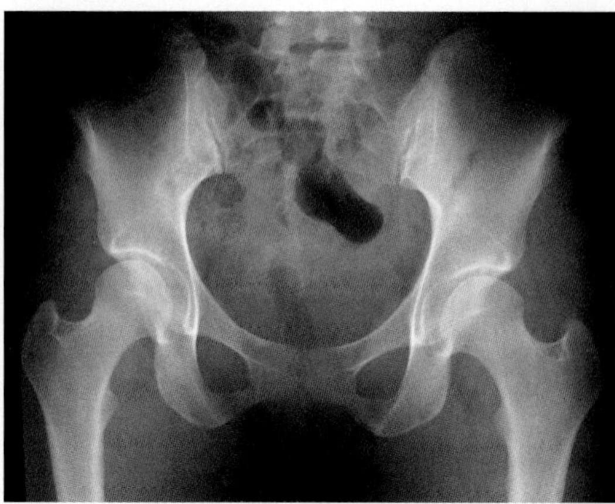

FIG 3 • An AP radiograph allows comparison of the affected and unaffected hips as well as an assessment of the surrounding bony architecture. It must be properly centered without rotation to assess the radiographic indices of hip morphology accurately. (Courtesy of J. W. Thomas Byrd, MD.)

as a cautious indicator in counseling patients on the role of arthoscopy.

- MRI can be useful for the evaluation of hip pathology.
  - Low-resolution studies (eg, open magnets and small scanners) are unreliable at detecting hip joint pathology.
  - High-resolution scans (eg, 1.5-Tesla magnet, surface coils) are superior but still present limitations.[5]
    - They are best at detecting labral pathology but generally poor at assessing the articular surface or the status of the ligamentum teres.
    - Caution is necessary in assessing labral lesions, because these have been identified in studies of asymptomatic volunteers and occur uniformly as a consequence of age.
    - Indirect findings often are the most reliable.
    - Evidence of an effusion in a symptomatic hip is highly indicative of joint pathology.
    - Paralabral cysts are pathognomonic of labral damage and subchondral cysts are indicative of associated articular damage.
- Gadolinium arthrography with MRI (MRA) has a greater sensitivity than MRI, but introduces some risk of overinterpreting pathology.[5]
  - A particular challenge is differentiating a labral tear from a normal labral cleft.
  - Assessment of the patient's symptomatic response to the anesthetic effect of an intra-articular injection is the most reliable diagnostic feature.
    - The intra-articular injection always should include a long-acting anesthetic (eg, bupivacaine).
    - However, this evaluation depends on the patient being able to perform activities that recreate pain prior to injection so that the same activities can be recreated post-injection to assess the amount of pain relief.
- CT can be superior to MRI for assessing bony architecture.
  - Three-dimensional reconstructions are especially useful in assessing cam impingement.
- Bone scans are relatively inexpensive, provide a good skeletal survey tool, and can be helpful in assessing osseous homeostasis around the hip.

DIFFERENTIAL DIAGNOSIS

- Hip flexor or adductor strain
- Hernia
- Athletic pubalgia
- Nerve entrapment
- Upper lumbar disc
- Referred from visceral origin (eg, gastrointestinal, genitourinary, gynecologic)

NONOPERATIVE MANAGEMENT

- Nonoperative management begins with informing the patient on the nature of the disorder; and education regarding warning signs of progressive damage, especially worsening symptoms.
- Activity modification often is necessary to modulate associated discomfort. This may be temporary while managing the acute phase of an injury, or may be long-term for patients coping with a chronic process.
- Distraction mobilization techniques may reduce discomfort and improve function while optimizing ROM.
- Closed-chain stabilization exercises usually are well tolerated and help to protect the joint.
- Trunk and core strengthening are integral to functional recovery.

SURGICAL MANAGEMENT

- Surgical intervention is indicated for mechanical symptoms in the presence of clinically suspected joint pathology.
- Conservative treatment may be appropriate for stable, manageable symptoms. A more proactive approach may be indicated if the symptoms are not manageable or demonstrate progressive worsening with time.
- In selecting patients for surgical management, the most important assessment tools are the history and physical examination.[5]
- Imaging studies are helpful only when interpreted in the context of the overall clinical evaluation.
- The surgeon should not be lured by false-positive interpretations or dissuaded by false-negative results.

Preoperative Planning

- Numerous intra-articular hip lesions may have similar clinical presentations.
- Imaging studies may only partly reflect the extent of pathology.
- Recent radiographs should be available for review in addition to any other tests that have been performed.
  - Radiographic evidence of joint deterioration can occur within a few months; thus, old radiographs are not useful.
- Findings of progressive joint space loss may contraindicate a planned arthroscopic procedure.
- The patient must be properly informed regarding the suspected nature of the joint pathology and also any comorbid conditions that will not be addressed by the procedure.
- The patient should have reasonable expectations of what can be accomplished and the uncertainty regarding what associated pathology may be encountered.

Positioning

- Arthroscopy of the intra-articular ("central") compartment of the hip requires distraction.

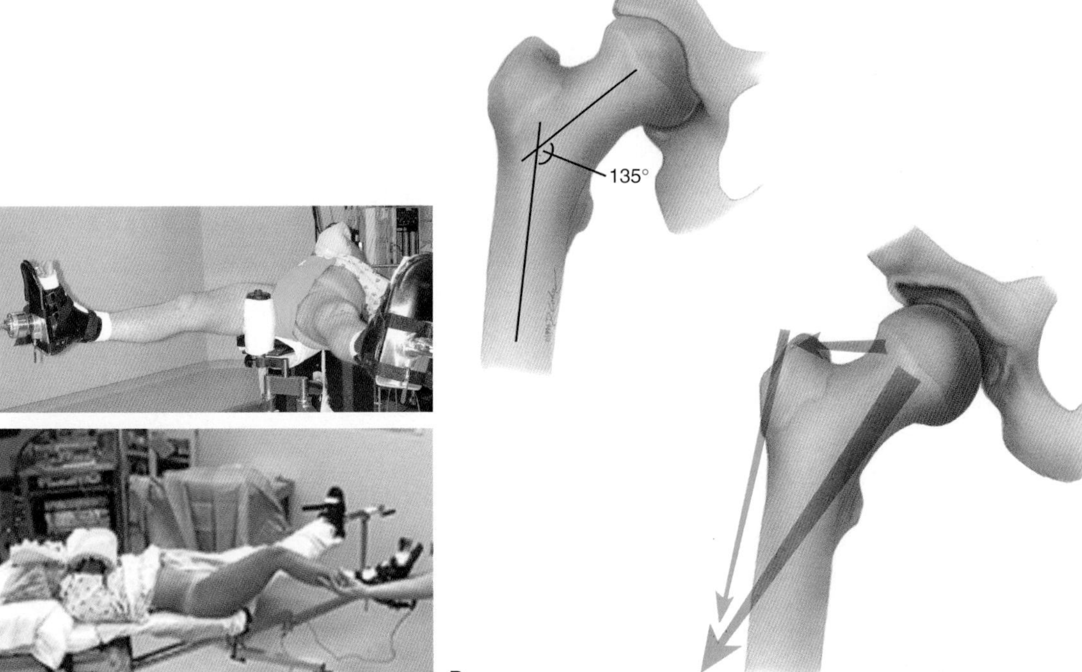

FIG 4 • **A.** The patient is positioned on the fracture table so that the perineal post is placed as far laterally as possible toward the surgical hip resting against the medial thigh. **B.** The optimal vector for distraction is oblique relative to the axis of the body and coincides more closely with the axis of the femoral neck than the femoral shaft. This oblique vector is created partially by abduction of the hip and accentuated by a small transverse component to the vector created by lateralizing the perineal post. **C.** The surgical area remains covered in sterile drapes while the traction is then released and the hip flexed 45 degrees. The figure shows the position of the hip without the overlying drape. (**A:** Reprinted with permission from The supine approach. In: Byrd JWT, ed. Operative Hip Arthroscopy, ed 2. New York: Springer, 2005:145–169; **B:** Courtesy of Delilah Cohn; **C:** Courtesy of J. W. Thomas Byrd, MD.)

- Proper positioning is essential to the safety and efficacy of the procedure.
  - A well-padded perineal post should be secured against the ischium but lateralized against the medial thigh (**FIG 4A**).
    - This keeps the post away from the pudendal nerve and aids in achieving the optimal vector for distraction.
  - Applying slight counter-traction to the nonoperative leg stabilizes the pelvis and keeps the post from shifting as traction is then applied to the operative leg.
  - The amount of abduction of the operative leg can be variable.
    - Less abduction may be necessary with a varus hip to make it possible to introduce the cannulas above the trochanter but enter the joint underneath the lateral lip of the acetabulum.
  - Neutral rotation during portal placement maintains a consistent relationship between the greater trochanter and the joint.
  - Slight flexion (10 degrees) relaxes the capsule and may facilitate distraction (**FIG 4B**).
    - Excessive flexion should be avoided, because it can place tension on the sciatic nerve and reduce anterior access to the joint.
- Most standard fracture tables can accomplish the positioning necessary for hip arthroscopy.
- Specialized positioning devices are more practical for ambulatory surgery centers. These are more affordable and transportable, adapting to standard OR tables.
- Arthroscopy of the peripheral compartment is performed with traction released and hip flexed (**FIG 4C**).
  - Traction is released only after the instruments have been removed from the central compartment.
  - Flexion relaxes the capsule, opening the space within the periphery.

Approach

- For the intra-articular ("central") compartment, three standard portals (anterior, anterolateral, and posterolateral) allow access for virtually all procedures (**FIG 5A,B**).[10]
  - The lateral two portals usually are the easiest to position, but the anterior portal provides the greatest versatility and access to the medial joint space.
  - Eighty percent of the intra-articular pathology resides in the anterior half of the hip and is accessible from the two anteriormost portals.
  - However, the posterolateral portal is important for routine inspection of the posterior recesses as well as access for posteriorly based lesions and the acetabular fossa.
- Two portals usually are sufficient for the peripheral compartment, but the positioning is widely variable, depending on the nature and location of the pathology to be addressed (**FIG 5C,D**).

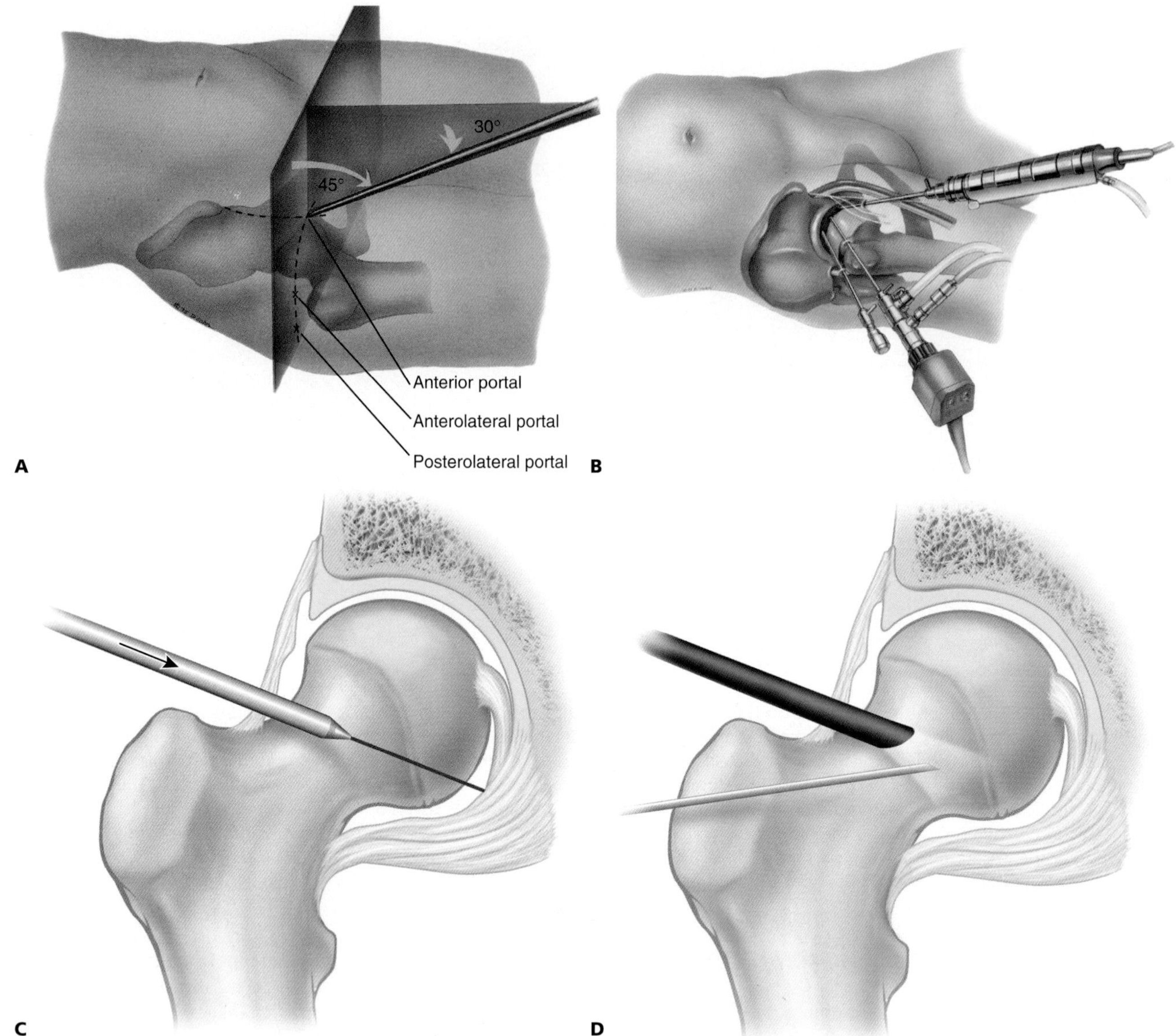

FIG 5 • **A.** The site of the anterior portal coincides with the intersection of a sagittal line drawn distally from the anterior superior iliac spine and a transverse line across the superior margin of the greater trochanter. The direction of this portal courses approximately 45 degrees cephalad and 30 degrees toward the midline. The antero- and posterolateral portals are positioned directly over the superior aspect of the trochanter at its anterior and posterior borders. **B.** The relation of the major neurovascular structures to the three standard portals is demonstrated. The femoral artery and nerve lie well medial to the anterior portal. The sciatic nerve lies posterior to the posterolateral portal. Small branches of the lateral femoral cutaneous nerve lie close to the anterior portal. Injury to these is avoided by using proper technique in portal placement. The anterolateral portal is established first, because it lies most centrally in the safe zone for arthroscopy. **C.** From the anterolateral entry site, the arthroscope cannula is redirected over the guidewire through the anterior capsule, onto the neck of the femur. **D.** With the arthroscope in place, prepositioning is performed with a spinal needle for placement of an ancillary portal distally. (**A,B:** Courtesy of Delilah Cohn.)

TECHNIQUES

LABRAL DÉBRIDEMENT

- Most symptomatic labral tears are managed with selective débridement of the damaged portion (**TECH FIG 1**).
- Emphasis is given to preserving healthy tissue, because removal of normal labrum can lead to poorer results.
- A complete joint survey is performed with thorough inspection and palpation of the labrum, identifying its damaged portion.
- Most labral resection is carried out with a power shaver, debulking the damaged tissue.
  - Hand instruments and an arthroscopic knife may aid in this resection.
- It is important to preserve the healthy tissue but create a stable transition zone when completing the débridement.
  - A radiofrequency device is especially useful for this because of the limited maneuverability imposed by the architecture of the joint.
  - Diseased tissue has an increased water content and responds selectively to the thermal device.

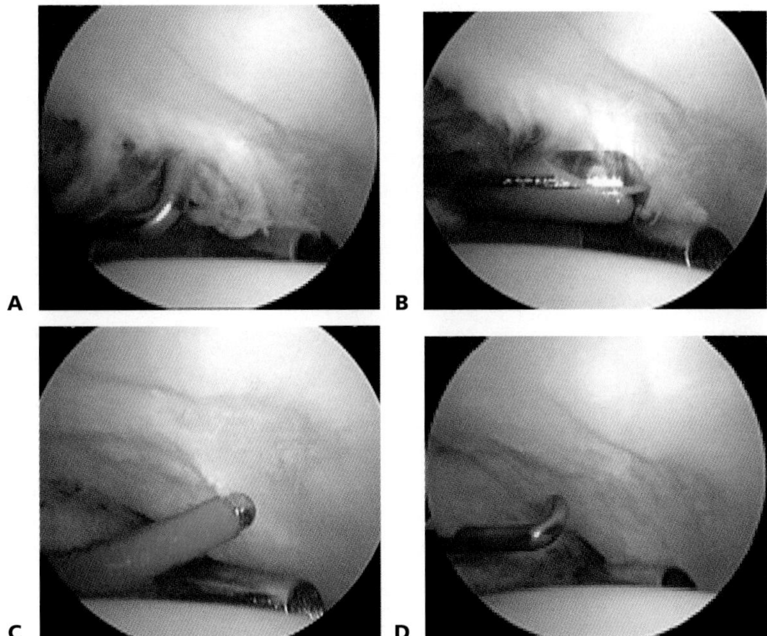

TECH FIG 1 • Arthroscopic view of a right hip from the anterior portal. **A.** A fragmented labral tear with degeneration within its substance is identified. **B.** Débridement is initiated with the power shaver. **C.** A portion of the comminuted labral tear is conservatively stabilized with a radiofrequency probe. **D.** The damaged portion has been removed, preserving the healthy substance of the labrum.

LABRAL REPAIR

- Labral repair is best suited for young patients when it is believed that simple débridement may result in inordinate sacrifice of healthy tissue (TECH FIG 2).
  - An optimal pattern is a tear at the articulolabral junction where a large segment of otherwise healthy tissue has been detached.
- Labral function is most dependent on its fluid seal.[2] Thus, the goal of repair is to reapproximate the labrum to the adjacent acetabulum.
- The mechanical properties of the labrum are minimal; therefore, the recreation of a bolster effect such as that in the shoulder is not necessary.

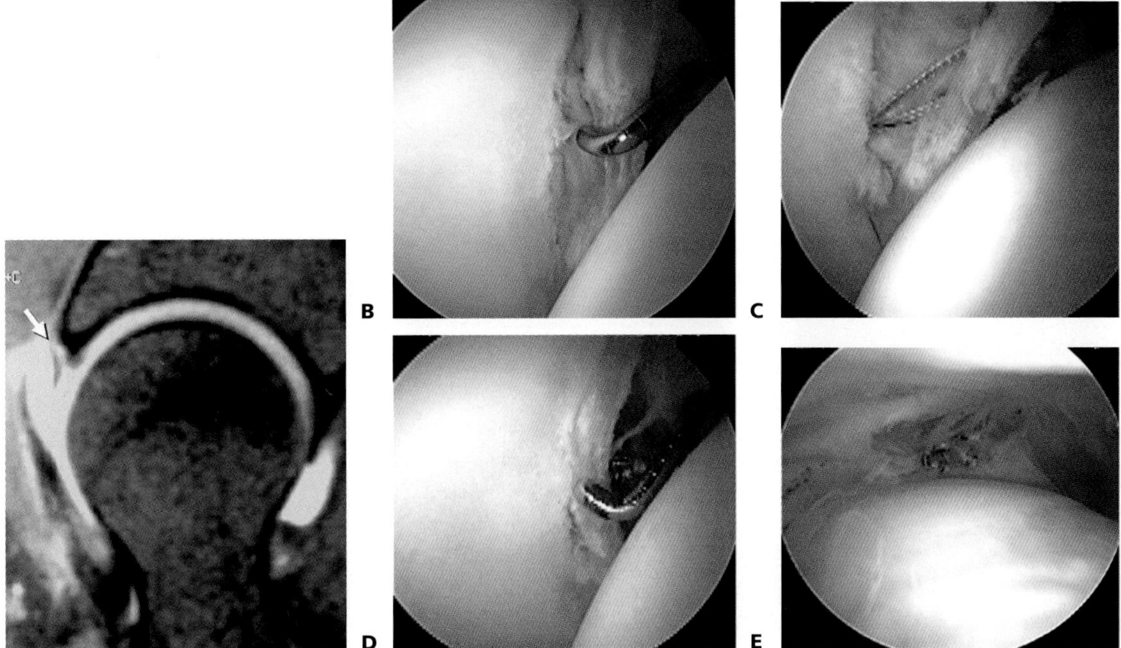

TECH FIG 2 • **A.** Sagittal MRA image demonstrates an anterior labral tear (*arrow*). **B.** Arthroscopy reveals a traumatic detachment of the anterior labrum (indicated by the probe). **C.** An anchor has been placed with suture limbs passed in a mattress fashion through the detached labrum. **D.** The labrum has been reapproximated to the articular edge. **E.** Viewing the peripheral aspect of the labrum, the suture is seen on its capsular surface, avoiding contact with the articular surface of the femoral head. (Courtesy of J. W. Thomas Byrd, MD.)

- An anchor should be placed adjacent to the articular edge; it is not necessary for it to be placed on its surface.
- The angle created by the articular surface and the bony edge of the acetabulum is more acute than its counterpart in the shoulder, which is created by the articular surface and bony face of the glenoid.
- Thus, the direction of anchor entry is more critical, especially to avoid perforation of the articular cartilage. This direction is dictated by the position of the cannula.
- The standard portal placements lend themselves well to anchor placement, but if the direction of entry does not seem appropriate, it is best to simply establish another portal with the proper angle for anchor entry.
- The anchor is seated adjacent to the articular surface, between it and the detached labrum.
- Passage of the suture limbs through the detached labrum can then be accomplished with various suture-passing devices.
  - It is important that the sutures not be left interposed between the labrum and the articular surface of the femoral head, because this can result in third-body wear on the articular cartilage.
  - Passing the sutures in a mattress fashion accomplishes reapproximation of the labrum, recreating the seal and avoiding interposed suture in the joint.

CHONDROPLASTY

- Chondroplasty of unstable articular fragments is performed in the hip, just as in other joints.
- Technical challenges are imposed by the limited instrument maneuverability.
- Curved shaver blades aid in navigating the constrained joint architecture (**TECH FIG 3A–C**).
- Radiofrequency devices can further assist in ablating damaged tissue, even within the constraints of the joint. Judicious use is imperative to avoid thermal injury.
- Like other joints, microfracture of select grade IV lesions can be performed (**TECH FIG 3D–G**).
  - Microfracture is indicated primarily for discrete lesions with healthy surrounding articular surface.

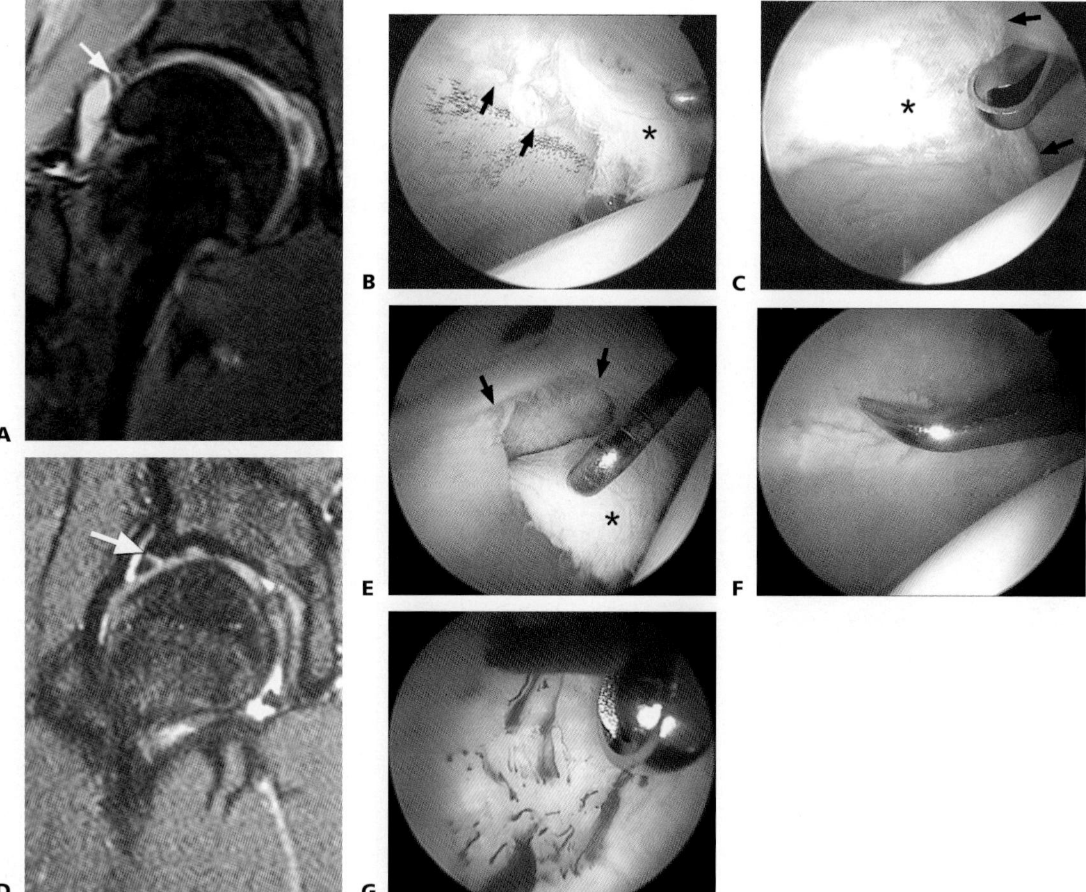

TECH FIG 3 • **A.** Coronal MRI demonstrates evidence of labral pathology (*arrow*). **B.** Arthroscopy reveals extensive tearing of the anterior labrum (*) as well as an adjoining area of grade III articular fragmentation (*arrows*). **C.** The labral tear has been resected to a stable rim (*arrows*), and chondroplasty of the grade III articular damage (*) is being performed. **D.** Coronal MRI demonstrates evidence of labral pathology (*arrow*). **E.** Arthroscopy reveals the labral tear (*arrows*), but also an area of adjoining grade IV articular loss (*). **F.** Microfracture of the exposed subchondral bone is performed. **G.** Occluding the inflow of fluid confirms vascular access through the areas of perforation. (Courtesy of J. W. Thomas Byrd, MD.)

ARTHROSCOPIC REPAIR OF LESIONS OF THE LIGAMENTUM TERES AND PULVINAR

- Disrupted fibers of the ligamentum teres, whether from trauma or degeneration, can be quite painful, creating soft tissue impingement within the joint.
- Associated with this soft tissue impingement, the pulvinar tissue often is hyperplastic or fibrosed and also can create painful symptoms.
- Indiscriminate débridement of the ligamentum teres should be avoided and intact fibers preserved; however, débridement of the disrupted portion can be quite beneficial (TECH FIG 4).
- Most of the contents of the acetabular fossa are best accessed from the anterior portal.
- However, a portion of the posterior contents often is best accessed with instrumentation introduced from the posterolateral portal.
- Between these two sites most pathologic processes can be accessed with combinations of straight, curved, and flexible instruments.

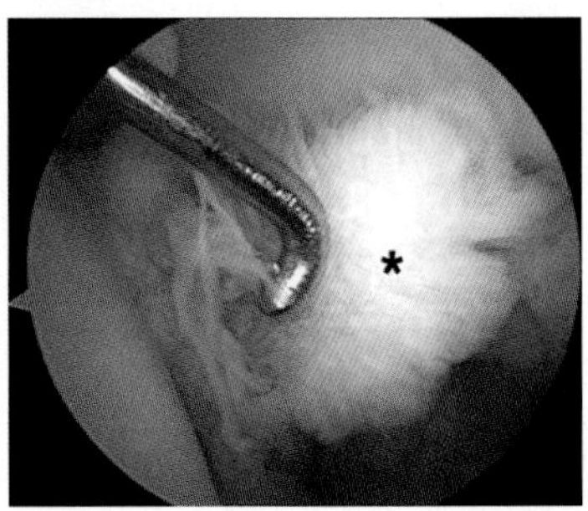

A

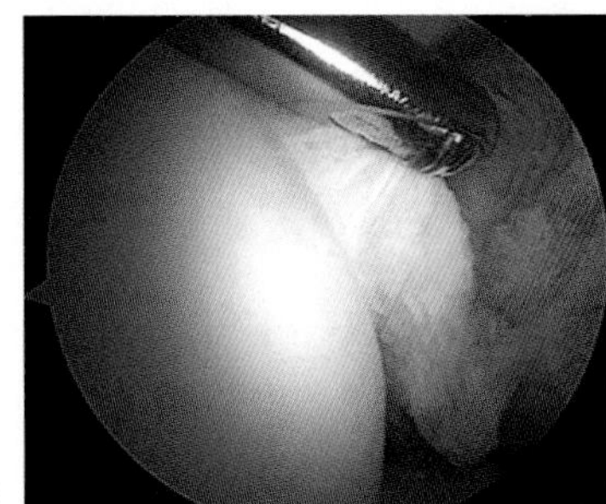
B

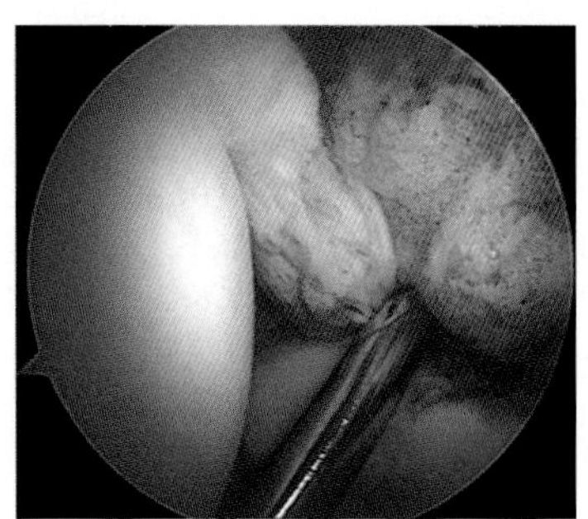
C

TECH FIG 4 • **A.** Arthroscopic view from the anterolateral portal reveals disruption of the ligamentum teres (*). **B.** Débridement is begun with a synovial resector introduced from the anterior portal. **C.** The acetabular attachment of the ligamentum teres in the posterior aspect of the fossa is addressed from the posterolateral portal. (Reprinted with permission from Byrd JWT, Jones KS. Traumatic rupture of the ligamentum teres as a source of hip pain. Arthroscopy 2004;20:385–391.)

PEARLS AND PITFALLS

Patient selection	■ Select patients whose clinical circumstances suggest that they could benefit from arthroscopic intervention. Make sure the patient has reasonable expectations of what can be accomplished. Lastly, surgeons should select cases that match their level of experience, which will, of course, evolve over time.
Patient positioning	■ Proper positioning is essential to the safety and efficacy of the procedure.
Portal placement	■ Proper portal positioning and placement is essential for a well-performed procedure. Proper orientation within the joint optimizes visualization, access, and instrumentation, despite limitations on maneuverability imposed by the constrained architecture.
Avoid iatrogenic damage	■ Every entry of an instrument into the hip should be performed as carefully as possible. With careful attention to technique, the likelihood of "scope trauma" can be diminished.
Avoid excessive labral resection	■ The damaged tissue must be removed, but avoid resection of healthy labrum, which can lead to poorer results.[11]
Avoid advanced disease states	■ Chondroplasty and débridement in the presence of advanced degenerative disease is unlikely to be successful, despite the appeal of a joint-preserving procedure.

POSTOPERATIVE CARE

- For most soft tissue procedures, weight bearing is allowed as tolerated, with crutches needed only until the patient's gait has been normalized, typically 5 or 6 days.
- Home exercises and supervised physical therapy are begun within the first few days.
- Gentle ROM, closed-chain exercises, stabilization, and subsequent functional activities are allowed to progress as dictated by the pathology encountered, the procedure performed, the resources available to the patient, and the patient's goals for returning to activities.
- For labral repairs, patients are kept on a protective weight-bearing status for 6 weeks, with avoidance of external rotation and maximal hip flexion.
- For microfracture, a strict protective weight-bearing status is maintained for 2 months during early maturation of the fibrocartilaginous healing response.

OUTCOMES

- Successful outcomes from labral débridement range from 68% to 82%.[1,12,20]
- Diminished results are observed with associated articular damage, which is present in most cases.

- The poorest results are reported in patients with radiographic evidence of arthritis.
- These observations are supported by a recent study reporting 82% continued successful outcomes at 10-year follow-up for patients undergoing labral débridement in absence of arthritis.[9] Among those with associated arthritis, 79% had been converted to total hip arthroplasty.
- Considerable experience has been gained in labral repair, but few outcome data have been published, with preliminary studies reporting success in two thirds of cases.[16,19]
- These results will improve with a better understanding of patient selection.
- Microfracture of grade IV articular lesions has demonstrated successful outcomes in 86% of properly selected cases.[6]
- Successful results also have been reported with excision of painful unstable fragments caused by macrotrauma.
- Soft tissue impingement due to disrupted fibers of the ligamentum teres tends to be quite painful and responds remarkably well to arthroscopic débridement, with success comparable to loose body removal.[7]
- The results of many of these procedures will continue to improve with better understanding of underlying causative factors such as femoroacetabular impingement.

COMPLICATIONS

- The reported complication rate for hip arthroscopy among large cohorts ranges from 1.3% to 6.4%.[8] Most complications are minor or transient, but a few major problems have been reported.
- Iatrogenic intra-articular damage may be the most common complication. Occasional joint scuffing may not be avoidable, but the concerns can be minimized by use of meticulous technique.
- Traction neuropraxia can be associated with prolonged or excessive traction, but also can occur even when surgery is performed within established guidelines.
- Direct trauma to major neurovascular structures should be avoidable, but, rarely, a partial neuropraxia of the lateral femoral cutaneous nerve can occur in association with the anterior portal.
- Life-threatening intra-abdominal fluid extravasation has been reported, emphasizing the importance of maintaining an awareness of fluid use during surgery.

REFERENCES

1. Byrd JWT, Jones KS. Prospective analysis of hip arthroscopy with two year follow up. Arthroscopy 2000;16:578–587.
2. Byrd JWT. Lateral impact injury: a source of occult hip pathology. Clin Sports Med 2001;20:801–816.
3. Byrd JWT. Hip arthroscopy: patient assessment and indications. Instr Course Lect 2003;52:711–719.
4. Byrd JWT, Jones KS. Results of hip arthroscopy in the presence of dysplasia. Arthroscopy 2003;19:1055–1060.
5. Byrd JWT, Jones KS. Diagnostic accuracy of clinical assessment, MRI, gadolinium MRI, and intraarticular injection in hip arthroscopy patients. Am J Sports 2004;32:1668–1674.
6. Byrd JWT, Jones KS. Microfracture for grade IV chondral lesions of the hip. Arthroscopy 2004;20:89.
7. Byrd JWT, Jones KS. Traumatic rupture of the ligamentum teres as a source of hip pain. Arthroscopy 2004;20:385–391.
8. Byrd JWT. Complications associated with hip arthroscopy. In: Byrd JWT, ed. Operative Hip Arthroscopy, ed 2. New York: Springer, 2005:229–235.
9. Byrd JWT, Jones KS. Prospecive analysis of hip arthroscopy with ten year follow up [abstract]. AAOS Annual Meeting, San Diego, February 14–16, 2007:641.
10. Byrd JWT, Pappas JN, Pedley MJ. Hip arthroscopy: an anatomic study of portal placement and relationship to the extraarticular structures. Arthroscopy 1995;11:418–423.
11. Espinosa N, Rothenfluh DA, Beck M, et al. Treatment of femoroacetabular impingement: preliminary results of labral refixation. J Bone Joint Surg Am 2006;88A;925–935.
12. Farjo LA, Glick JM, Sampson TG. Hip arthroscopy for acetabular labrum tears. Arthroscopy 1999;15:132–137.
13. Ferguson SJ, Bryant JT, Ganz R, et al. The acetabular labrum seal: a poroeleastic finite element model. Clin Biomech 2000;15:463–468.
14. Ganz R, Parvizi J, Beck M, et al. Femoroacetabular impingement: a cause for osteoarthritis of the hip. Clin Orthop Relat Res 2003:417; 112–120.
15. Gray AJR, Villar RN. The ligamentum teres of the hip: an arthroscopic classification of its pathology. Arthroscopy 1997;13: 575–578.
16. Kelly BT, Weiland DE, Schenker ML, Philippon MJ. Arthroscopic labral repair in the hip: surgical technique and review of the literature. Arthroscopy 2005;12:1496–1504.
17. Konrath GA, Hamel AJ, Olson SA, et al. The role of the acetabular labrum and the transverse acetabular ligament in load transmission in the hip. J Bone Joint Surg Am 1998;80A:1781–1788.
18. McCarthy JC, Noble PC, Schuck MR, et al. The watershed labral lesion: its relationship to early arthritis of the hip. J Arthroplasty 2001;16(8 Suppl 1):81–87.
19. Murphy KP, Ross AE, Javernick MA, et al. Repair of the adult acetabular labrum. Arthroscopy 2006;5:567.el-3.
20. Santori N, Villar RN. Acetabular labral tears: results of arthroscopic partial limbectomy. Arthroscopy 2000;16:11–15.

Chapter 26 Arthroscopic Management of Femoroacetabular Impingement

Christopher M. Larson and Rebecca M. Stone

DEFINITION

- Femoroacetabular impingement (FAI) is the result of abnormal contact between the proximal femur and the acetabular rim.
- Abnormalities can be identified on either the femoral or acetabular side, but are more commonly seen on both sides.
- This abnormal contact can lead to acetabular chondral lesions and or labral lesions, leading to hip pain and the development of diffuse osteoarthritis of the affected hip if left untreated.[1,2,3]

ANATOMY

- The proximal femur and acetabulum normally articulate without abutment through a physiologic range of motion (ROM).
- The acetabulum normally is anteverted 12 to 16.5 degrees.
- The acetabulum covers the femoral head to a depth that avoids impingement (ie, overcoverage) and instablility (ie, dysplasia or undercoverage) with a horizontal, thin, sourcil (ie, the weight-bearing zone).
- The proximal femur has a spherical head-neck contour that allows for impingement-free ROM.
- The normal femoral neck shaft angle is 120 to 135 degrees; the femoral neck typically is anteverted and is 12 to 15 degrees.
- It is important to recognize and respect the location of the retinacular vessels that have been shown to enter the antero- and posterolateral portions of the femoral neck and supply the majority of the femoral head's blood supply.

PATHOGENESIS

- There are two primary mechanisms of FAI: pincer and cam impingement.[1–3]
- Pincer impingement is the result of contact between an abnormal acetabular rim and normal femoral head–neck junction (**FIG 1A**).
  - Pincer impingement typically is the result of a deep acetabulum (coxa profunda), local anterior overcoverage (acetabular retroversion), or, less commonly, posterior overcoverage.
  - It leads to labral bruising and tearing, and eventually may result in ossification of the labrum and contrecoup posterior acetabular chondral injury.
- Cam impingement is the result of contact between an abnormal femoral head–neck junction and the acetabulum (**FIG 1B**).
  - The abnormal femoral head neck junction usually is secondary to an aspherical anterolateral head neck junction, but also can be secondary to a slipped capital femoral epiphysis, femoral retroversion, coxa vara, malreduced femoral neck fracture, and, occasionally, posterior femoral head neck abnormalities.
  - Cam impingement results in a shearing stress to the anterosuperior acetabulum, with predictable chondral delamination and labral detachment or tearing in some cases.

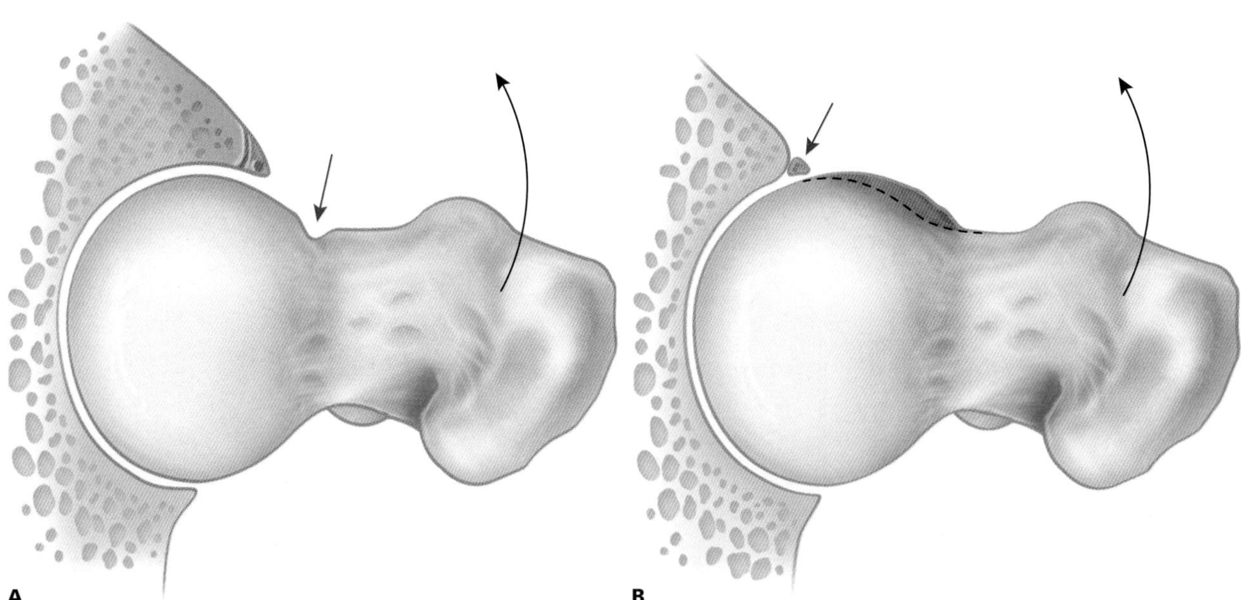

FIG 1 • **A.** Pincer impingement is the result of contact between an abnormal acetabular rim and a normal femoral head–neck junction. **B.** Cam impingement is the result of contact between an abnormal femoral head–neck junction and the acetabulum.

- Although cam impingement is reported to predominate in young athletic males and pincer impingement in middle-aged women, most patients with FAI have a combination of both cam and pincer impingement.

NATURAL HISTORY

- The likelihood of an individual with untreated FAI developing hip osteoarthritis is unknown, because there have been no longitudinal studies prospectively following these patients before the development of symptoms.
- Clinical experience with over 600 surgical dislocations of the hip in patients with FAI has revealed a strong association of this disorder with progressive acetabular chondral degeneration, labral tears, and progressive osteoarthritis.[1–3]
- It is now well accepted that many patients with FAI will develop progressive chondral and labral injury that can ultimately lead to end-stage hip osteoarthritis.

PATIENT HISTORY AND PHYSICAL FINDINGS

- Patients typically are young to middle aged (2nd through 4th decade) with complaints of groin pain exacerbated by physical activity.
- Prolonged sitting, arising from a chair, putting on shoes and socks, getting in and out of a car, and sitting with their legs crossed often exacerbate the symptoms.
- We have found that patients may have a history of siblings, parents, and grandparents with hip pain or osteoarthritis of the hip, and patients may have milder or similar symptoms in the contralateral hip.
- Patients often have had pain for months to years with the diagnosis of chronic low back pathology, hip flexor strains, and sports hernias, and not infrequently have had other surgeries without relief of their pain.
- Physical examinations should include:
- Evaluation of hip ROM: global ROM restriction indicates advanced osteoarthritis.
- Anterior impingement test: groin pain indicates anterolateral rim pathology.
- Posterior impingement test: groin pain or posterolateral pain indicates posterolateral rim pathology.
  - FABER test: FABER means flexion, abduction, and external rotation of the hip. Increased distance from the lateral knee to the examination table can indicate femoroacetabular impingement.

IMAGING AND OTHER DIAGNOSTIC STUDIES

- Plain radiographs including an anteroposterior (AP) pelvis, frog lateral, and ideally a cross-table lateral and false profile view are obtained.
- The AP radiograph should have a coccyx to symphyseal distance of 0 to 2 cm with the coccyx centered over the symphysis to properly evaluate acetabular version.
- The following are measured on the AP radiograph (**FIG 2A**):
  - A lateral center edge angle of 25 to 40 degrees distinguishes deep acetabulum from dysplasia.
  - The presence of a crossover sign indicates local anterior overcoverage (retroversion).
  - The posterior wall sign indicates posterior undercoverage (retroversion).
  - Cam impingement indicates decreased head-neck offset.
  - A femoral neck shaft angle indicates that coxa vara may contribute to impingement.
- The frog-leg lateral and cross-table lateral views with 15 degrees internal rotation ideally evaluate:
  - *Alpha angle:* normally less than 50 to 55 degrees (anterolateral prominence/aspherical femoral head neck junction; **FIG 2B**)
  - Femoral head neck cystic changes and sclerosis
  - *Femoral neck version:* retroversion may contribute to impingement.
- The false profile is used to evaluate:
  - *Anterior center edge angle:* anterior over- and undercoverage
- An MRI arthrogram is useful to evaluate for labral and chondral pathology, acetabular retroversion, or a prominence of the femoral head neck junction which is best seen on the axial cuts (**FIG 2C**).
- Synovial herniation pits at the femoral head neck junction are also indicative of FAI.
- An anesthetic agent should be included with the gadolinium to verify the hip joint as the source of pain, which is indicated by temporary pain relief with provocative maneuvers in the first couple of hours after the injection.
- Occasionally it is helpful to obtain a three-dimensional CT study to appropriately map the area of impingement.

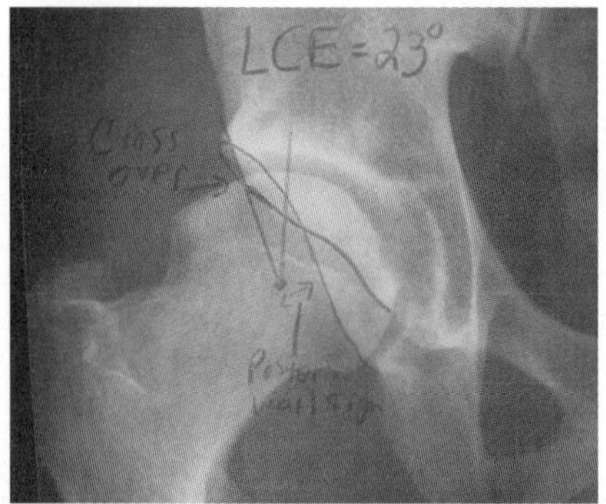

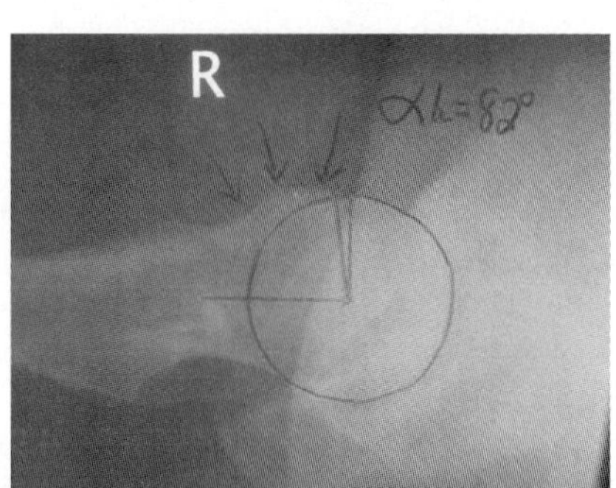

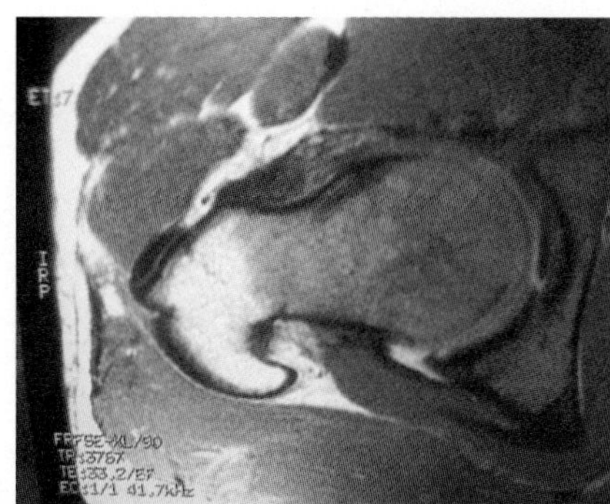

FIG 2 • **A.** Lateral center edge angle, posterior wall sign, and crossover sign are depicted. **B.** Alpha (α) angle is elevated in cam impingement. **C.** Prominence of the anterolateral femoral head–neck junction is seen on axial MRI images.

- This may be done routinely or in cases of subtle FAI or suspected unusual locations of FAI (eg, posterior femoral head / neck prominences).

DIFFERENTIAL DIAGNOSIS

- Sports hernia or athletic pubalgia
- Lumbar spine pathology
- Gynecologic or urologic pathology
- Intra-abdominal pathology
- Hip flexor pathology or iliopsoas snapping
- Iliotibial band pathology or snapping
- Pelvic stress fracture
- Intra-articular pathology not related to FAI

NONOPERATIVE MANAGEMENT

- Nonoperative management of FAI consists of avoiding painful activities such as deep hip flexion, aggressive hip flexion–based weight training, and athletic activities that aggravate symptoms.
- Intra-articular pathology often progresses without symptoms early in the disease, and there is concern that without surgical treatment arthritis eventually will develop.
- Nonoperative management may be best employed in the already degenerative hip with joint space narrowing prior to total hip arthroplasty, and consists of activity modification, core trunk strengthening exercises, and occasional intra-articular corticosteroid or hyaluronic acid injections.

SURGICAL MANAGEMENT

- Physical examination and imaging studies consistent with FAI
- Pain despite activity modification
- Pain in patient who is unable or unwilling to modify activity
- Minimal to no degenerative changes
- Arthroscopic versus open procedure for FAI (Table 1)
  - There are no strict indications for open versus arthroscopic management of FAI.

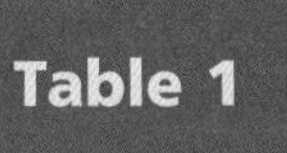

Table 1 Guidelines for Arthroscopic Versus Open Repair of Femoroacetabular Impingement

Pincer impingement

Lateral center edge angle

>25 degrees: arthroscopic acetabular rim trimming

20–25 degrees: avoid excessive rim trimming laterally

>16 to 20 degrees: consider osteotomy

Cam impingement

If resection of >30% of the width of the neck is required to restore the alpha angle to normal, consider concomitant osteotomy (severe pistol grip deformity)

If significant femoral neck retroversion or coxa vara is present, a concomitant or staged osteotomy is considered when impingement is still present after arthroscopic proximal femoral osteoplasty.

Posterior areas of femoral head–neck impingement can be more challenging, and, depending on the surgeon's experience, may be better addressed through an open approach.

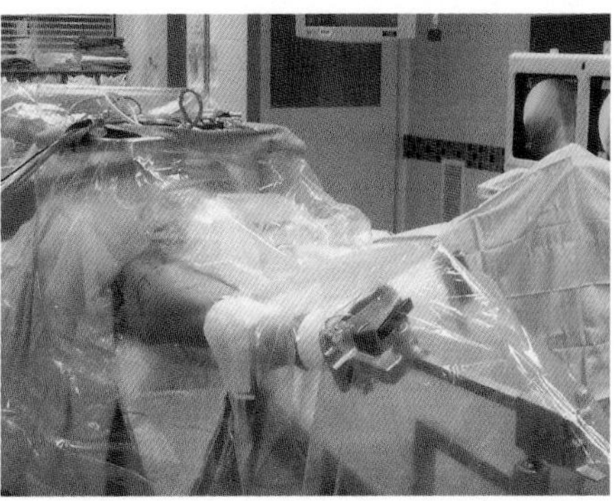

FIG 3 • The operative leg is placed in neutral abduction, slight flexion, and internal rotation. The nonoperative leg is abducted with slight traction with a well-padded post in the peroneal region.

- The goal of arthroscopy is to reproduce the open approach for managing FAI.
- Although controversial, some higher-level athletes may prefer a less invasive arthroscopic approach with a more predictable return to sports.[10]

Preoperative Planning

- Initially, a fluoroscopic evaluation is done, including anteroposterior, frog lateral, and cross-table lateral evaluation of the acetabulum and proximal femur.
- Dynamic fluoroscopic evaluation by abduction of the hip in flexion, external rotation, and extension with internal and external rotation occasionally reveals impingement of the acetabulum on the proximal femur and results in a vacuum effect in the joint as the proximal femur is levered out of the acetabulum.

Positioning

- Arthroscopic management of FAI begins with standard hip positioning in either the supine or lateral position.
- We prefer the supine position with the hip in slight flexion, neutral abduction, and internal rotation (**FIG 3**).

Approach

- Most cases can be performed using the standard anterior paratrochanteric and anterior portals, with occasional use of the posterior paratrochanteric or accessory distal portal (**FIG 4**).

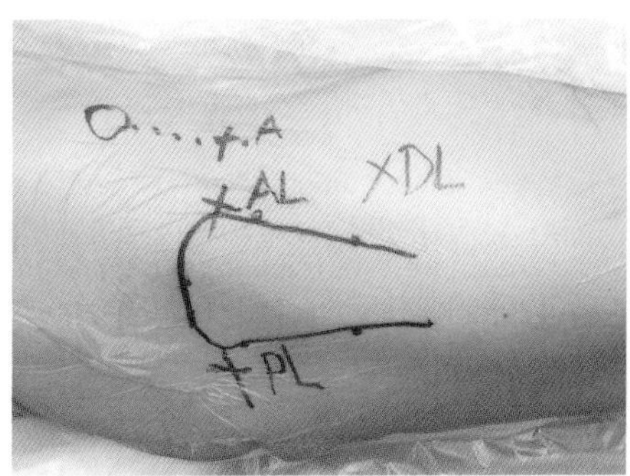

FIG 4 • The standard approach involves use of the anterior (*A*) and anterior paratrochanteric portals (*AL*), with occasional use of the posterior paratrochanteric (*PL*) and distal lateral (*DL*) accessory portal.

DIAGNOSTIC ARTHROSCOPY

- Initially the intra-articular portions of the hip are evaluated, including the acetabular labrum, acetabulum, and femoral head articular cartilage; fovea; ligamentum teres; transverse acetabular ligament; and capsular structures (**TECH FIG 1A,B**).
- The peripheral compartment is evaluated, including the femoral head, labrum, zona orbicularis, medial synovial fold, femoral neck, and peripheral capsular attachments (**TECH FIG 1C**).
- The pathology present helps to define the pathologic mechanisms present, with chondral delamination in the anterior superior acetabulum indicating cam impingement (**TECH FIG 1D**), and labral ecchymosis, tearing, and linear posterior acetabular chondral wear indicating pincer impingement (**TECH FIG 1E**).

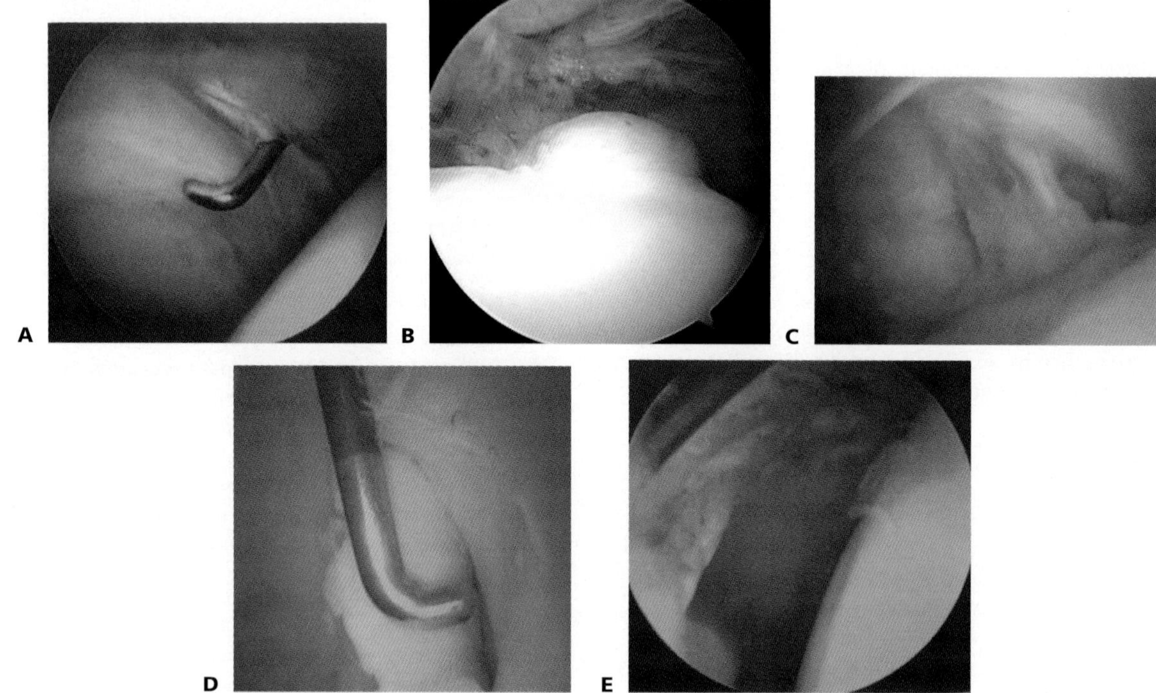

TECH FIG 1 • **A.** View from the anterior paratrochanteric portal reveals the anterolateral labrum, acetabulum (*left*), and femoral head (*right*). **B.** View of the fovea (*top*), ligamentum teres (*center*), and medial femoral head (*bottom*). **C.** View of the peripheral compartment through the anterior portal reveals the zona orbicularis (*top*), femoral neck and medial synovial fold (*center*), and femoral head–neck junction (*bottom*). **D.** Chondral delamination of the anterior superior acetabulum consistent with cam impingement. **E.** Diffuse labral ecchymosis (*left*) consistent with pincer impingement.

PINCER IMPINGEMENT

- When pincer impingment is present, the labrum is evaluated, and any tearing is carefully débrided, taking care to preserve the peripheral labrum when possible.
- If complex tearing of the labrum is present, the labrum is generously débrided; however, the periphery of the labrum often remains intact and is amenable to repair or refixation (**TECH FIG 2A**).
- If the labrum is amenable to repair or refixation, it is carefully detached from the acetabulum using a Beaver blade and shaver, beginning at the periphery and extending to the articular side of the labrum (**TECH FIG 2B**).
- Care must be taken to detach as much of the labrum as possible without cutting too deep on the articular side, which could result in inadvertent delamination of the acetabular articular cartilage.
- The labral detachment usually extends from the anterior portal to the 12:00 position. More or less may be detached further, superiorly and posteriorly, depending on the extent of acetabular overcoverage anterolaterally or posteriorly, and should include detachment of all of the torn or ecchymotic labrum.

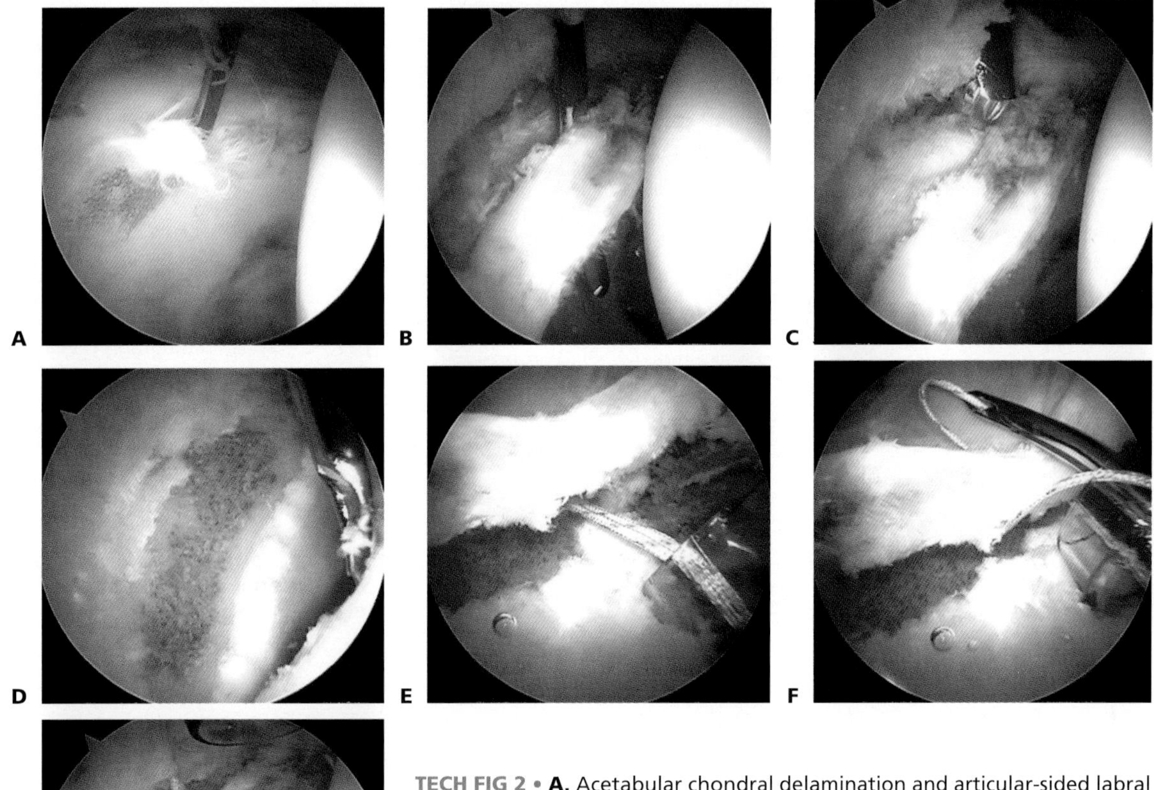

TECH FIG 2 • **A.** Acetabular chondral delamination and articular-sided labral tear (*left*) with preserved peripheral labral tissue. **B.** A Beaver blade is used to detach the labrum from the acetabulum (*left*), creating a bucket handle labral tear. **C.** A burr is used to begin the acetabular rim trimming, starting at the level of the anterior portal site. **D.** Completion of the rim trimming to the anterolateral acetabulum. The labrum is retracted into the joint (*right*). **E.** A suture anchor is placed just below the subchondral bone of the acetabulum, taking care not to enter the acetabular chondral surface. **F.** One limb of the suture is passed under the labrum and then pulled over or through the labrum. **G.** Completion of the acetabular rim trimming and labral refixation with two suture anchors. *Left:* labral repair; *right:* femoral head.

- The labrum then falls into the joint, creating a bucket handle tear, and a 5.5-mm burr is used to trim the acetabular rim to a depth of 5 to 10 mm (TECH FIG 2C,D).
- An attempt is made to trim all of the acetabulum with abnormal articular cartilage to a residual lateral center edge angle of 25 to 30 degrees, taking more or less according to the preoperative center edge angles.
- If areas of grade 4 chondromalacia remain after acetabular rim trimming, microfracture is performed on the exposed bone.
- Suture anchors (usually two to four anchors) are then placed just under the acetabular subchondral bone, and the sutures are first passed under the labrum and then pulled over or through the labrum, securing the labrum to the rim with standard knot-tying techniques (TECH FIG 2E–G).
- Care is taken to place the knot on the capsular or medial side of the labrum to avoid damaging the femoral articular cartilage with prominent suture during weight bearing and ROM.

OS ACETABULI/PINCER IMPINGEMENT

- Occasionally an os acetabuli is responsible for local anterior overcoverage and typically is attached to the acetabulum just peripheral to the labrum.
- The os is exposed and excised using a burr beyond the fibrocartilage attachment of the native acetabulum with or without labral débridement or detachment and refixation (TECH FIG 3).

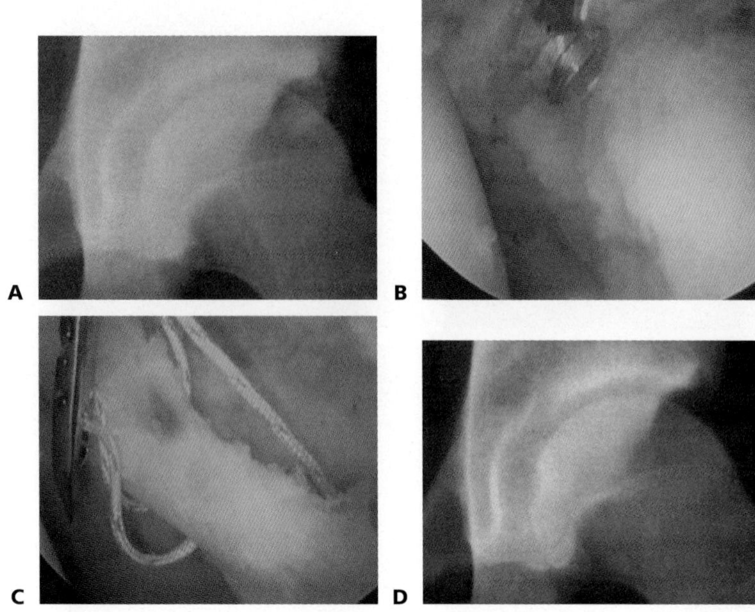

TECH FIG 3 • **A.** AP radiograph revealing a 2-cm × 1-cm os acetabuli involving the anterosuperior acetabulum. **B.** A burr is used to excise the os acetabuli (*right*); the femoral head also is seen (*left*). **C.** The labrum is reattached to the acetabular rim with two suture anchors. **D.** AP radiograph confirms complete excision of the os acetabuli—a proximal femoral osteoplasty also was performed because of associated cam impingement.

CAM IMPINGEMENT

- Exposure of the femoral head–neck junction can be performed using a generous capsulotomy, capsulectomy, or small capsular window.
- We prefer a generous capsulotomy beginning anterior to the anterior portal and extending to the posterolateral portal site (TECH FIG 4A).
- Traction is then released, and the hip is flexed to varying degrees, allowing for visualization of the peripheral head–neck junction and the cam lesion.
- The normal head–neck junction is spherical (TECH FIG 4B), whereas in cam impingement it appears egg-shaped, flat, or with a prominence at the head–neck junction (TECH FIG 4C).
- The cam lesion is covered with healthy-appearing articular cartilage with varying mild degrees of eburnation, progressing very early in the process to a more degenerative peripheral head–neck junction with clefts and intraosseous cysts in more advanced cases (TECH FIG 4D).
- A 5.5-mm burr is used to reshape the anterolateral prominence, typically removing 5 to 10 mm and occasionally more, depending on the size of the lesion and thickness of the neck (TECH FIG 4E,F).
- A recent cadaveric study recommended resecting no more than 30% of the thickness of the femoral neck to avoid pathologic fractures postoperatively.[6]
- A frog lateral and cross-table lateral view with internal rotation are used to verify restoration of a normal alpha angle (TECH FIG 4G,H).
- For more superior and posterior lesions, the hip is slowly extended and internally rotated, and the working and

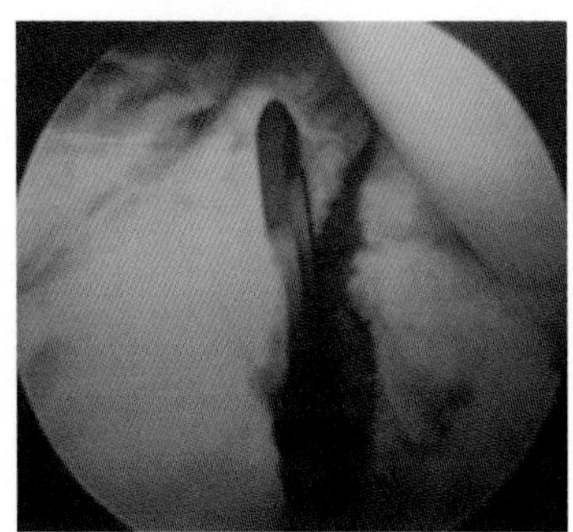

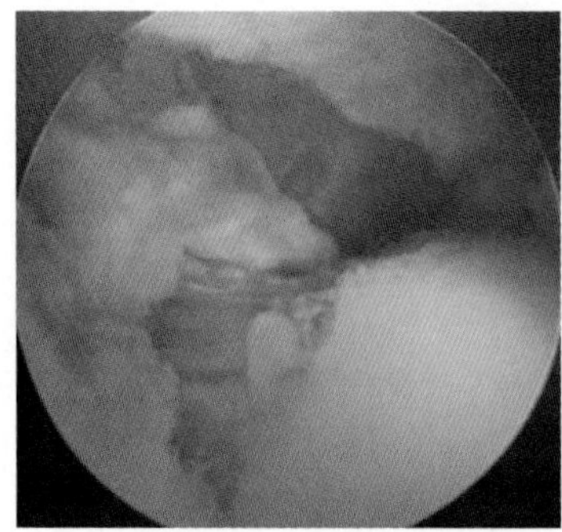

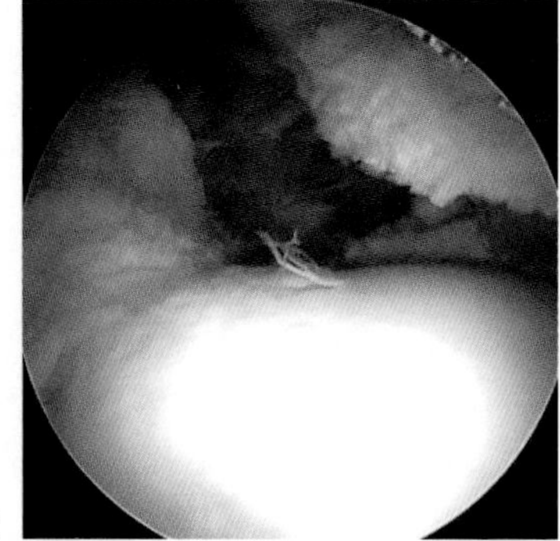

TECH FIG 4 • **A.** A generous capsulotomy is performed to allow exposure of the peripheral head–neck junction. The labrum (*left*) and femoral head (*right*) are seen. **B.** Arthroscopic view of the normal, spherical, femoral head–neck junction in the right hip. **C.** Cam impingement as indicated by a nonspherical, egg-shaped femoral head–neck junction in the right hip. *(continued)*

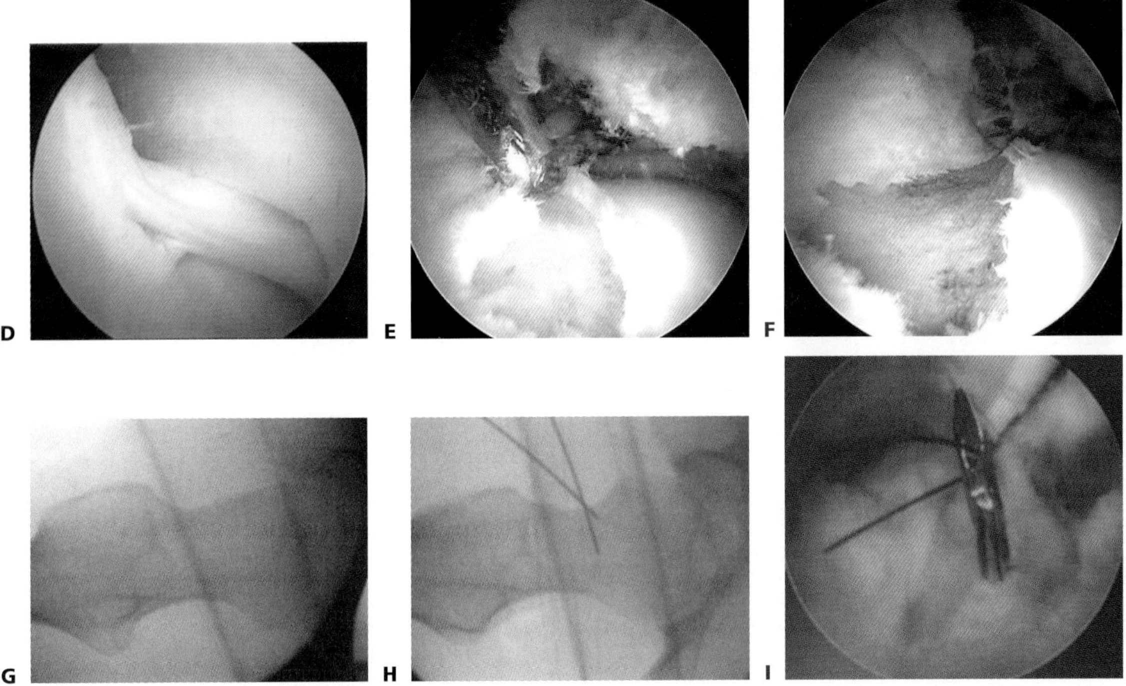

TECH FIG 4 • (*continued*) **D.** Arthroscopic image of the lateral synovial fold (site of the retinacular vessels) in the left hip. **E.** A burr is used to excise and recontour the femoral head–neck junction, seen here in the right hip. **F.** Completion of the osteoplasty restores normal femoral head–neck sphericity, seen here in the right hip. **G.** Intraoperative cross-table lateral fluoroscopic image showing prominence of the anterolateral femoral head–neck junction consistent with cam impingement. **H.** Intraoperative cross-table lateral fluoroscopic image after proximal femoral osteoplasty confirming appropriate resection of the femoral head–neck junction. **I.** Arthroscopic closure of the capsulotomy after proximal femoral osteoplasty and acetabular rim trimming, seen here in the left hip.

arthroscopic portals can be exchanged from the anterior and anterior paratrochanteric portals to the anterior and posterior paratrochanteric portals for better visualization.

- Care is taken to avoid aggressive resection down the anterolateral and posterolateral regions of the femoral neck to avoid damage to the retinacular vessels which should be visualized and protected throughout the case.
- The typical pattern of cam impingement extends down the neck on the anterolateral femoral head–neck junction and closer to the articular cartilage margin of the femoral head, more superiorly in the region of the retinacular vessels.
- Final confirmation of adequate resection is then verified arthroscopically by flexing the hip more than 90 degrees with maximal internal rotation, external rotation, and abduction.
- Capsular closure is then performed with one or two absorbable sutures passed through one side of the capsule with a looped suture passer and grasped through the other side of the capsule (TECH FIG 4I).
- A knot is then tied blindly at the periphery of the capsule using standard arthroscopic knot-tying techniques.
- The hip is then infiltrated with an anesthetic, and the portals are closed in the usual fashion.

PEARLS AND PITFALLS

Indications	■ History, physical examination, and imaging studies should be consistent with femoroacetabular impingement. ■ Intra-articular anesthetic injection should confirm the hip as the source of pain.
Exposure	■ Care should be taken to excise the labrum peripherally and detach on the articular surface without undermining the acetabular chondral surface to allow for adequate tissue for refixation. ■ Adequate capsulotomy or capsulectomy should be performed to allow for exposure of the femoral head–neck junction. ■ Flexion, extension, and rotation allow for complete visualization of the femoral head neck prominence in cam impingement.
Pincer	■ Generally 5 mm of acetabulum is trimmed with more removed based on the extent of chondral damage taking care not to create a dysplastic acetabulum based on preoperative center edge angles.

Cam	■ Adequate (usually 5 to 10 mm) but not overly aggressive femoral osteoplasty is confirmed by repeated arthroscopic ROM evaluation and fluoroscopic frog lateral, cross-table lateral, and anteroposterior images.
Complications	■ More complex cases of FAI managed arthroscopically can be lengthy procedures, and alternating between traction and flexion or release of traction can help prevent traction-based neuropraxias. ■ Meticulous irrigation of all bony debris and postoperative use of nonsteroidal anti-inflammatories can help to minimize the incidence of heterotopic bone formation.

POSTOPERATIVE CARE

- Pre- and postoperative radiographs confirm adequate osteoplasty and rim trimming (**FIG 5**).
- Postoperative restrictions are not consistent from one surgeon to the next and are based on the procedures done.
- We impose the following restrictions:
  - Proximal femoral osteoplasty is treated with protected weight bearing with crutches for 2 weeks and no high-impact or running activities for 2.5 to 3 months.
  - Acetabular rim trimming with labral débridement requires no specific restrictions.

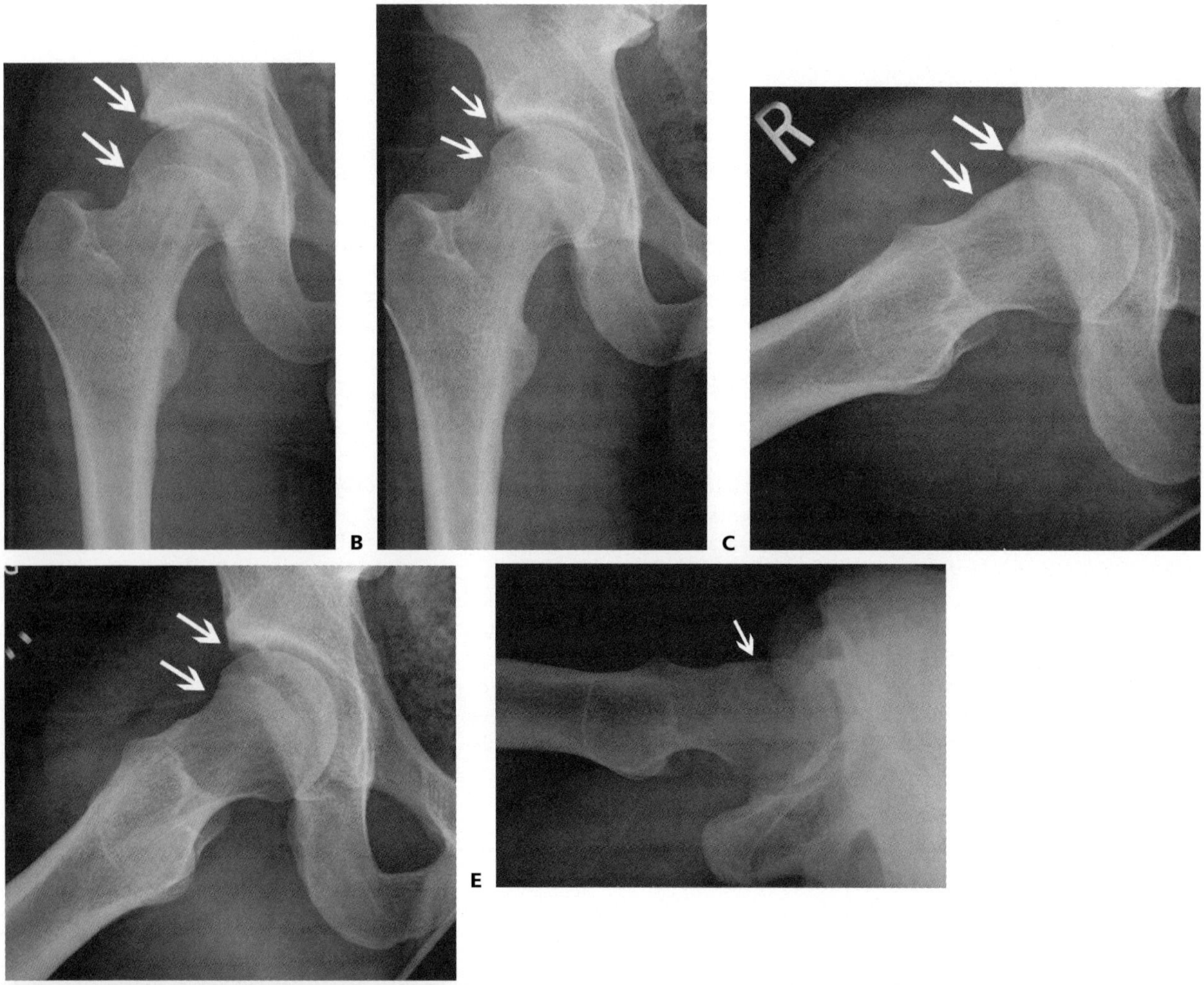

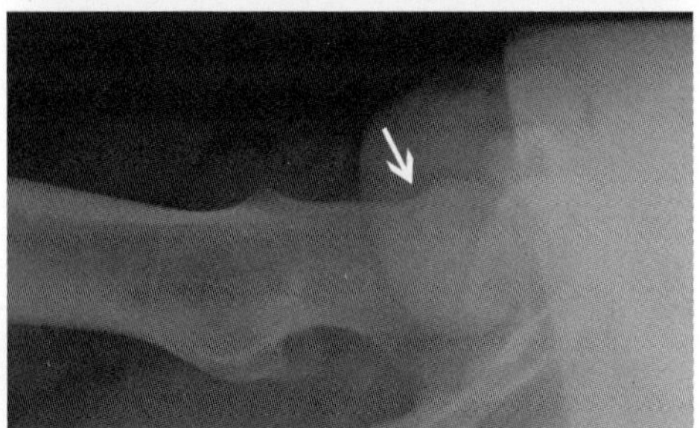

FIG 5 • **A.** Preoperative AP radiograph with a positive crossover sign, indicating cephalad anterior overcoverage of the acetabulum and cam impingement. **B.** Post–acetabular rim trimming and labral refixation radiograph confirming adequate removal of the anterior acetabular overcoverage (*arrows*). **C.** Preoperative frog-leg lateral radiograph showing prominence of the anterolateral head–neck junction (*arrows*). **D.** Post–proximal femoral osteoplasty radiograph confirming restoration of normal anterolateral head–neck sphericity (*arrows*). **E.** Preoperative cross-table lateral radiograph showing flattening of the anterolateral femoral head–neck junction (*arrow*). **F.** Post-proximal femoral osteoplasty radiograph confirming restoration of the normal anterolateral femoral head–neck sphericity (*arrow*).

- Acetabular labral repair and refixation is treated with toe-touch weight bearing for 2 weeks and avoidance of the extremes of external rotation for 2 weeks.
- Microfracture procedures are treated with 6 to 8 weeks of toe-touch weight bearing.
- The first 2 months focus on restoration of ROM, gait and pelvic alignment, and gentle core strengthening.

- At 2 months, more aggressive core strengthening is instituted, with resumption of full sporting activities at 3 to 6 months based on functional improvement.
- Further research is required to develop the optimal rehabilitation programs after the various procedures that have been discussed.

OUTCOMES

- Early and midterm results of open procedures for FAI indicate that reduction in pain and functional improvement directly correlate with the degree of osteoarthritic changes found at the time of surgery.[1,2,7,9]
    - Some evidence indicates that repair or refixation of the labrum results in improved outcomes when compared to labral débridement or excision in a consecutive series.[2,4]
    - It is unclear, however, whether the improvement is the result of labral preservation or of improved technical skills, because the study was performed in a consecutive series of patients.[2,4]
- Little has been published in the literature with respect to outcomes after arthroscopic management of FAI.
    - In a review of 45 professional and Olympic level athletes with FAI treated arthroscopically, all had symptomatic improvement and returned to play.[10]
    - In another series of 320 patients with FAI treated arthroscopically, 90% had elimination of the impingement sign and were reportedly satisfied with their results.[12]
    - Larson and Giveans[5] prospectively followed 100 patients with FAI treated arthroscopically for up to 3 years, with a statistically significant improvement in Harris hip, SF-12, and visual analogue pain scoring consistent with that seen after open management of FAI.
- No well-designed, long-term, or randomized studies have been done to evaluate outcomes of management of FAI to determine whether osteoarthritis has been delayed or prevented in this patient population. Longer-term follow-up and studies of open versus arthroscopic treatment should better define the optimal indications and procedure for patients with FAI.

COMPLICATIONS

- Anterolateral femoral cutaneous nerve neuropraxia
- Heterotopic bone or myositis ossificans formation
- Iatrogenic acetabular and femoral chondral damage
- Rarely postoperative femoral neck fracture
- Potential for sciatic or pudendal nerve neuropraxia
- Potential for avascular necrosis

REFERENCES

1. Beck M, Leunig M, Parvizi J, et al. Anterior femoroacetabular impingement: part II. Midterm results of surgical treatment. Clin Orthop Relat Res 2004;418:67–73.
2. Espinosa N, Rothenfluh DA, Beck M, et al. Treatment of femoroacetabular impingement: preliminary results of labral refixation. J Bone Joint Surg Am 2006;88A:925–935.
3. Ganz R, Parvizi J, Beck M, et al. Femoroacetabular impingement: a cause for osteoarthritis of the hip. Clin Orthop Relat Res 2003;417: 112–120.
4. Larson CM, Giveans M. Arthroscopic debridement versus refixation of the acetabular labrum associated with femoroacetabular impingement. Arthroscopy 2009;25(4):369–376.
5. Larson CM, Giveans M. Arthroscopic management of femoroacetabular impingement: early outcomes measures. Arthroscopy 2008;5(24): 540–546.
6. Mardones RM, Gonzalez C, Chen Q, et al. Surgical treatment of femoroacetabular impingement: evaluation of the effect of the size of the resection: surgical technique. J Bone Joint Surg Am 2006;88A (suppl 1):84–91.
7. Murphy S, Tannast M, Kim YJ, et al. Debridement of the adult hip for femoroacetabular impingement. Clin Orthop Relat Res 2004;429: 178–181.
8. Notzli HP, Wyss TF, Stoecklin CH, et al. The contour of the femoral head-neck junction as a predictor for the risk of anterior impingement. J Bone Joint Surg Br 2002;84B:556–560.
9. Peters CL, Erickson JA. Treatment of femoro-acetabular impingement with surgical dislocation and debridement in young adults. J Bone Joint Surg Am 2006;88A:1735–1741.
10. Philippon MJ, Schenker ML. Arthroscopy for the treatment of femoroacetabular impingement in the athlete. Clin Sports Med 2006; 25:299–308.
11. Philippon MJ, Schenker ML, Briggs KK, et al. Clinical presentation of femoroacetabular impingement. American Orthopaedic Society for Sports Medicine Annual Meeting, 2006.
12. Sampson TG, Glick JM. Hip arthroscopy by the lateral approach. Instr Course Lect 2006;55:317–323. Abstract presented June 29, 2006. Hershey, PA.

Chapter 27 Snapping Hip

J. W. Thomas Byrd and MaCalus V. Hogan

DEFINITION

- *Coxa saltans* is a term popularized by Allen and various coauthors.[1]
  - Initially they described an internal type (iliopsoas tendon) and an external type (iliotibial band).
  - More recently, they proposed an intra-articular type, which is simply a catch-all for numerous intra-articular lesions.
- Snapping hip syndrome most clearly represents an extra-articular dynamic tendinous phenomenon of either the iliopsoas tendon or iliotibial band.

ANATOMY

- The iliopsoas complex, a powerful hip flexor, is formed from the psoas major and iliacus muscles (**FIG 1A**).
  - The psoas major originates from the lumbar transverse processes and the sides of the vertebral bodies and intervertebral discs from T12 to L5; the iliacus originates from the superior two thirds of the iliac fossa, the sacral ala, and the anterior sacroiliac ligaments.
  - The tendon forms first from the psoas proximal to the inguinal ligament and then rotates such that its anterior surface comes to lie medial and its posterior surface lateral.
  - The tendon then spreads out to insert over the lesser trochanter.
  - It is joined by an accessory tendon from the iliacus, and the tendons then fuse together before forming the enthesis of the iliopsoas. Some muscle fibers of the iliacus remain separate, attaching directly to bone.
  - In the sagittal plane, as the iliopsoas exits the pelvis, it is redirected 40 to 45 degrees over the pectineal eminence toward its insertion site.
- Iliotibial band (**FIG 1B**): The fascia lata covers the entire hip region, encasing its three superficial muscles, ie, the tensor fascia lata, sartorius, and gluteus maximus.
  - A confluence of the tensor fascia lata and gluteus maximus forms the iliotibial band.
  - The gluteus maximus also partly inserts into the proximal femur at the gluteal tuberosity.
  - This fibromuscular sheath was described by Henry[7] as the "pelvic deltoid," reflecting on the fashion in which it covers the hip, much as the deltoid muscle covers the shoulder.

PATHOGENESIS

- The snapping occurs as the iliopsoas tendon subluxes from lateral to medial while the hip is brought from a flexed abducted, externally rotated position into extension with internal rotation (**FIG 2A,B**).
  - It is variously proposed that the anterior aspect of the femoral head and capsule, or pectineal eminence, is

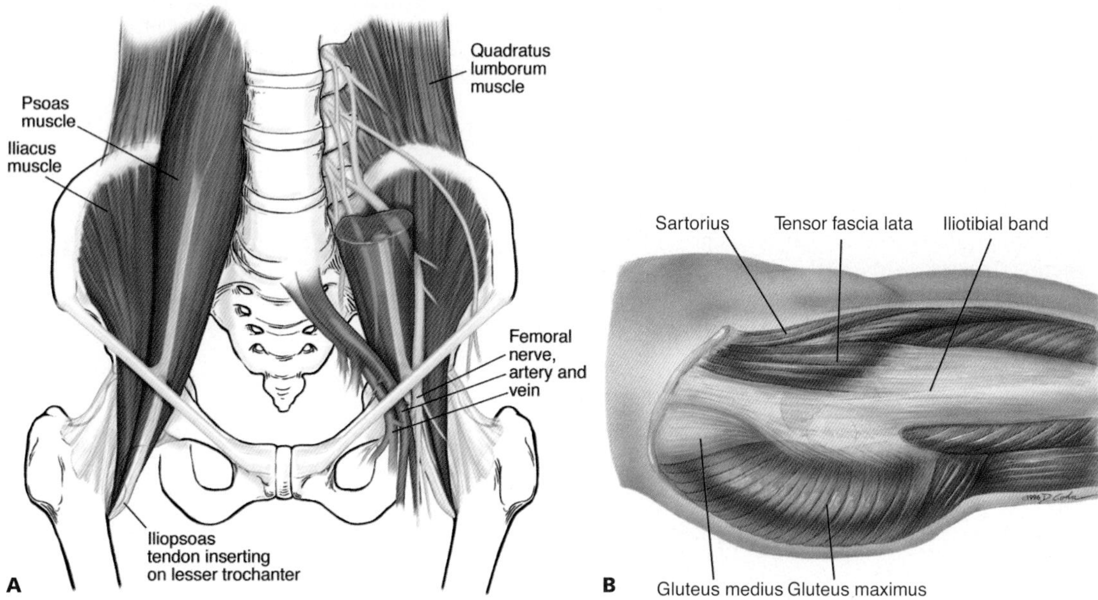

FIG 1 • **A.** Depicted on the right, the proximal portion of the iliospoas has been cut away, revealing the lumbar plexus, embedded in its posterior portion. Distally, the femoral neurovascular structures are noted coursing over the iliospoas, which forms the lateral floor of the femoral triangle. On the left, the tendon is formed first from the psoas, which is then joined by the iliacus prior to its insertion on to the lesser trochanter. **B.** Superficial muscle layer of the hip. (**A:** Courtesy of J. W. Thomas Byrd, MD; **B:** Courtesy of Delilah Cohn.)

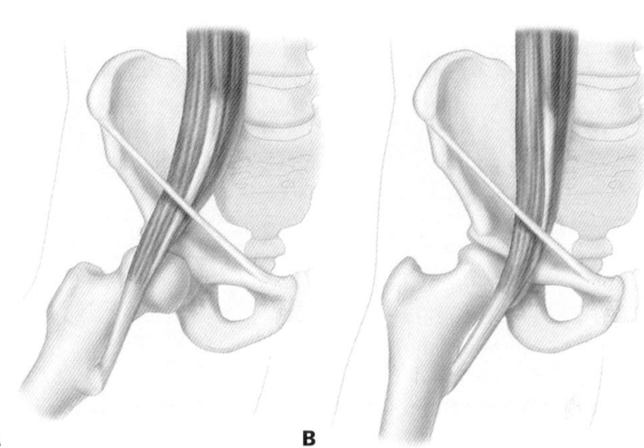

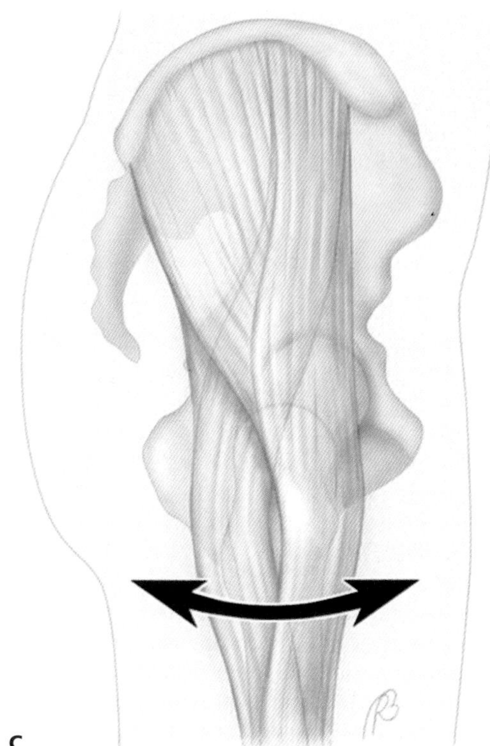

FIG 2 • The iliopsoas tendon flipping back and forth across the anterior hip and pectineal eminence. **A.** With flexion of the hip, the iliospoas tendon lies lateral to the center of the femoral head. **B.** With extension of the hip, the iliospoas shifts medial to the center of the femoral head. **C.** As the iliotibial band snaps back and forth across the greater trochanter, the tendinous portion may flip across the trochanter with flexion and extension, or the trochanter may move back and forth underneath the stationary tendon with internal and external rotation. (Courtesy of J. W. Thomas Byrd, MD.)

responsible for transiently impeding the tendon and creating the snapping.
- Incidental asymptomatic snapping of the iliopsoas tendon is estimated to be present in at least 10% of a normal, active population.
- Painful snapping may be precipitated by macrotrauma or repetitive microtrauma in patients with a predilection for certain activities such as ballet.
- The exact structural alteration that occurs when symptomatic snapping develops has not been defined.

- The snapping occurs as the iliotibial band flips back and forth across the greater trochanter, and often is attributed to a thickening of the posterior part of the iliotibial tract or anterior border of the gluteus medius (**FIG 2C**).
  - The thickened portion lies posterior to the trochanter in extension and flips forward as the hip begins to flex.
  - Coxa vara and reduced bi-iliac width have been proposed as predisposing anatomic factors.
  - Tightness of the iliotibial band also may be an exacerbating factor.
  - Like snapping of the iliopsoas tendon, snapping of the iliotibial band may be an incidental finding without precipitating cause or symptoms.
  - Painful snapping may occur following trauma, but is more commonly associated with repetitive activities, classically being described in the downhill leg of runners training on a sloped roadside surface.
  - It also has been reported as an iatrogenic process following surgical procedures that leave the greater trochanter more prominent, or reconstructive procedures around the knee that alter the iliotibial band.

NATURAL HISTORY

- For most people, the snapping hip remains asymptomatic, never requiring treatment.
- In patients in whom the snapping hip is symptomatic, the course is variable, but there are no apparent long-term consequences of a chronic snapping hip.
- Spontaneous resolution may occur but is uncommon.

PATIENT HISTORY AND PHYSICAL FINDINGS

Iliopsoas Tendon

- The history of onset of symptoms is variable and may be insidious, owing to specific repetitive maneuvers or an acute injury.
  - The patient typically describes a clicking sensation emanating from deep within the anterior groin, which often is audible enough to be characterized as a "clunk."
  - Although the symptoms typically are referred to the anterior groin, some patients may describe flank or sacroiliac discomfort, reflecting irritation around the origin of the psoas and iliacus muscles.
  - The characteristic examination maneuver is performed with the patient lying supine, bringing the hip from a flexed, abducted, externally rotated position down into extension with internal rotation, creating the snap.
  - Sometimes this is a dynamic process that the patient can demonstrate actively better than the examiner can produce passively. Although often prominent, it may be subtle, and may occur more as a sensation experienced by the patient rather than one that the examiner can observe objectively.

- Applying pressure over the anterior joint can block the tendon from snapping and assist in confirming the diagnosis.
- Variously, patients may be able to demonstrate this best lying, sitting, or standing, or with walking. However, regardless of the position, the snapping uniformly occurs as the hip goes from a flexed toward an extended position.

Iliotibial Band

- As with the iliopsoas tendon, patients may describe the onset of symptoms as being insidious, due to specific repetitive activities, or in response to acute trauma.
  - Whereas snapping of the iliopsoas tendon often can be heard from across the room, snapping of the iliotibial band can be seen from across the room.
  - Patients describe a sense that the hip is subluxing or dislocating. This is termed "pseudosubluxation," because the visual appearance may suggest that the hip is subluxing but radiographs uniformly demonstrate that the hip remains concentrically reduced.
  - The patient always relates a snapping or subluxation-type sensation. The symptoms are located laterally, and patients typically can illustrate this while standing.
  - As with the iliopsoas, this often is a dynamic process, better demonstrated by the patient than produced by passive examination. It may be detected with the patient lying on the side and then passively flexing and extending the hip.
  - The snap can be palpated over the greater trochanter, and its origin is confirmed by applying pressure, which can block the snap from occurring.
  - The Ober test evaluates for tightness of the iliotibial band, which may accompany symptomatic snapping.

IMAGING AND OTHER DIAGNOSTIC STUDIES

- The diagnosis of a snapping iliopsoas tendon is based primarily on the history and physical examination.
- Iliopsoas bursography and ultrasonography may be helpful to rule in, but not rule out, the diagnosis (**FIG 3**).
  - These imaging modalities are technically limited because of a significant rate of false-negative interpretation.
- Similarly, snapping of the iliotibial band is based on the clinical assessment, and investigative studies offer little aid in substantiating or discounting the diagnosis.
- Nonetheless, plain radiographs remain an essential tool in the assessment of any hip problem, and other investigative studies such as MRI and magnetic resonance arthrography may be important to evaluate for associated conditions such as intra-articular pathology.

DIFFERENTIAL DIAGNOSIS

- Snapping iliotibial band
- Hip instability
- Snapping iliopsoas tendon
- Intra-articular pathology
- Pelvic instability (eg, sacroiliac joint or symphysis pubis)
- Osteochondroma

NONOPERATIVE MANAGEMENT

- Treatment often involves little more than establishing the diagnosis and assuring the patient that the snapping is not harmful or indicative of future problems.
- Oral anti-inflammatory medications may be helpful in addition to a flexibility and stabilization exercise program.
- For recalcitrant cases:
  - A period of activity modification to diminish symptoms may be necessary.
  - Judicious use of corticosteroid injections may be appropriate, with the goal of providing transient improvement to supplement the effect of other therapeutic modalities.

SURGICAL MANAGEMENT

Iliopsoas Tendon

- Various open procedures have been described for releasing the tendinous portion of the iliopsoas, with generally favorable results.[1,5,6,12]
- However, superior results have been reported with endoscopic methods.[4,9] These superior results are due only partly to the less invasive nature of the technique.
- Most cases with a painful snapping iliopsoas tendon also were found to have associated intra-articular pathology, which also was addressed.

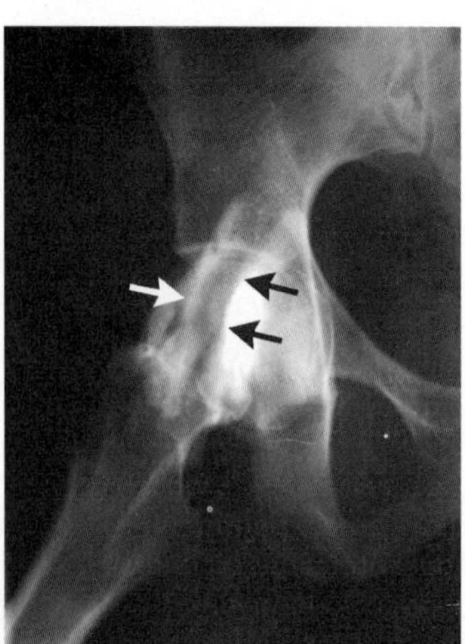

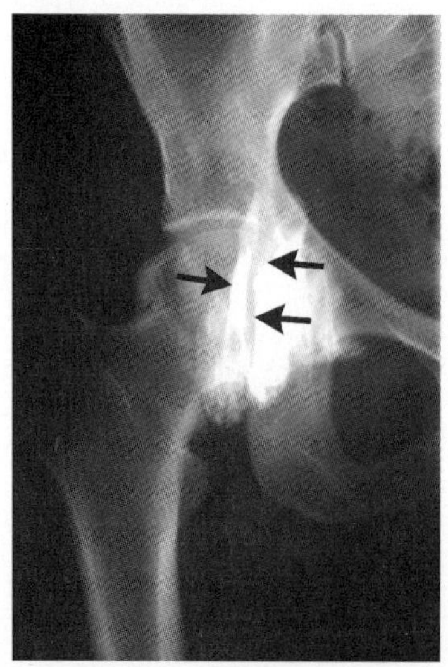

FIG 3 • Iliopsoas bursography silhouettes the iliopsoas tendon (*arrows*) with contrast. **A.** In flexion, the iliopsoas tendon lies lateral to the femoral head. **B.** In extension, the iliopsoas tendon moves medial. (Courtesy of J. W. Thomas Byrd, MD.)

- Failure to inspect the interior of the hip joint and address associated pathology may be a significant contributing factor to less optimal results with traditional open techniques.

Iliotibial Band

- Various techniques have been described for correcting snapping of the iliotibial band.
- One complex procedure is a Z-plasty lengthening, the results of which have ranged from poor to good.[2,10,11]
- Several techniques have employed a simpler approach, creating a relaxing incision in the portion of the iliotibial band over the greater trochanter, and these have shown to be effective at eliminating the snapping in most cases.[3,15] Violation of the tendon structure is minimized, which diminishes the morbidity of the procedure and facilitates the postoperative recovery.
- Endoscopic methods have been developed that may accomplish this same goal.[8]

Preoperative Planning

- Clinical assessment of the snapping iliopsoas tendon and iliotibial band is relatively straightforward.
- However, careful assessment is necessary to ensure that the snapping is clearly the source of the patient's symptoms and also to evaluate other associated conditions, especially concomitant intra-articular pathology.
- Perhaps most important is a careful assessment of the patient's motivation, understanding, and goals of recovery.
- It is important to bear in mind that coxa saltans often is encountered in asymptomatic individuals.
- Surgery is considered only if the patient has exhausted efforts at conservative treatment and demonstrates sufficient motivation for the postoperative recovery.

Positioning

- Iliopsoas tendon
  - Endoscopic release of the iliopsoas tendon is performed in conjunction with routine arthroscopy of the joint.
  - Arthroscopy can be performed with the patient in either the supine or lateral position.
  - The supine position may provide better access to these structures, and is the method described.
- Iliotibial band
  - Open procedures employ the lateral decubitus position, and this also has been the preferred orientation for endoscopic methods.

Approach

- Iliopsoas tendon
  - Most endoscopic reports have described releasing the tendon from its insertion on the lesser trochanter within the iliopsoas bursa.[4,9]
  - This is the endoscopic counterpart to the open method described by Taylor and Clarke.[12] For the occasional case of a snapping iliopsoas tendon associated with a total hip arthroplasty, it clearly is the preferred approach.
  - Another endoscopic technique, in which the iliopsoas tendon is approached from the peripheral compartment, seems to provide a comparable effect of releasing the tendon.[14] The method is analogous to the open method described by Allen et al.[1] Theoretically, it may have an advantage of reduced morbidity.
- Iliotibial band
  - The various open approaches use a common, lateral, longitudinal incision over the greater trochanter.
  - Endoscopic methods employ laterally based portals, approaching the tendon from its superficial subcutaneous surface.

TECHNIQUES

ENDOSCOPIC ILIOPSOAS RELEASE

Lesser Trochanter (Iliopsoas Bursa)

- After completing routine hip arthroscopy, including intra-articular and peripheral compartments, the leg is repositioned in 20 degrees of flexion and full external rotation.
- Slight flexion partially relaxes the tendon but maintains some tension.
- External rotation brings the lesser trochanter more anterior for access from the laterally based portals (**TECH FIG 1A**).
- A portal is established distal to the standard anterolateral hip portal at the level of the lesser trochanter, using fluoroscopic guidance (**TECH FIG 1B**).
  - This exposes the tendon within the iliopsoas bursa, which is the largest bursa in the body.
- Another portal is then placed distally, converging toward the lesser trochanter (**TECH FIG 1C**).
- The arthroscope and instruments are switched between these two portals for thorough visualization and instrumentation of the iliopsoas tendon (**TECH FIG 1D**).
- Adhesions within the bursa can be cleared, providing excellent visualization of the iliopsoas tendon.
- The tendinous portion of the iliopsoas is transected adjacent to its insertion on the lesser trochanter.
  - This is facilitated with the use of a flexible radiofrequency device.
- For safest technique, the medial side of the tendon is fully visualized, and the tendon is then released from medial to lateral. Its fibers will separate 1 to 2 cm.
- Muscular attachments of the iliacus muscle are preserved.

Peripheral Compartment

- After completing arthroscopy of the intra-articular compartment with a standard supine technique, the traction is released, the hip is flexed 45 degrees, and standard portals are established in the peripheral compartment (**TECH FIG 2**).
- The iliopsoas tendon can be exposed in line with the medial synovial fold, proximal to the zona orbicularis.
  - Occasionally, a communication is present at this location between the joint and the iliopsoas bursa.
  - If no communication is present, a capsular window can be created with a shaver.
- The capsule in this location is thin, and often the tendon is visible or palpable through the thin capsule.

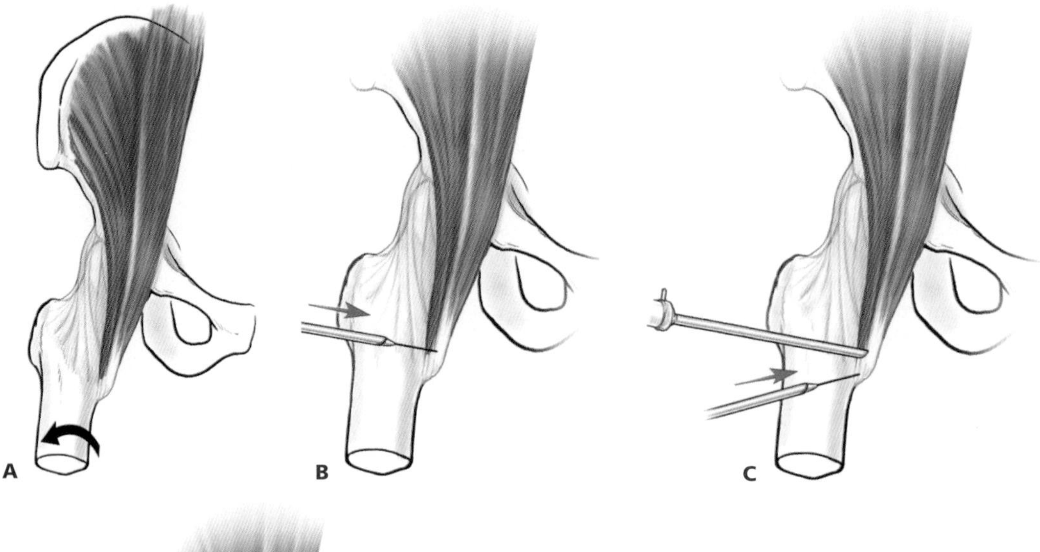

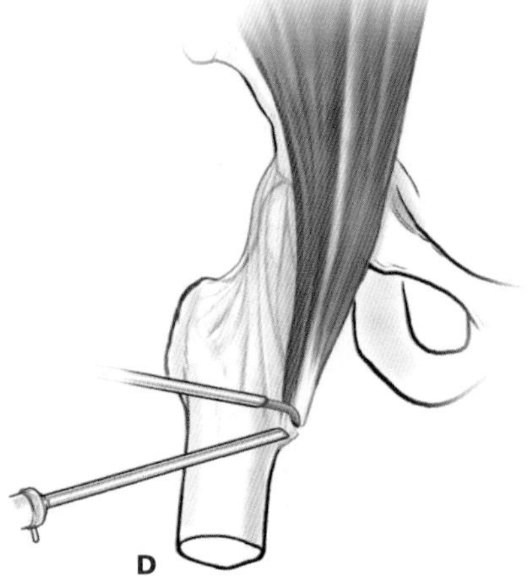

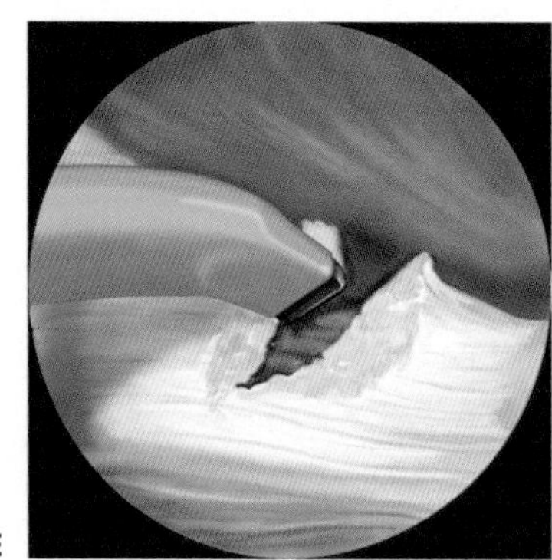

TECH FIG 1 • Release of right iliopsoas tendon from lesser trochanter. **A.** The hip is flexed approximately 20 degrees and externally rotated. **B.** Initial portal established at level of lesser trochanter. **C.** Ancillary portal is established distally under direct arthroscopic visualization. **D.** The arthroscope has been switched to the more distal portal with a flexible radiofrequency (RF) device introduced proximally. **E.** Arthroscopic illustration shows release of the tendinous portion of the iliopsoas. (Courtesy of J. W. Thomas Byrd, MD.)

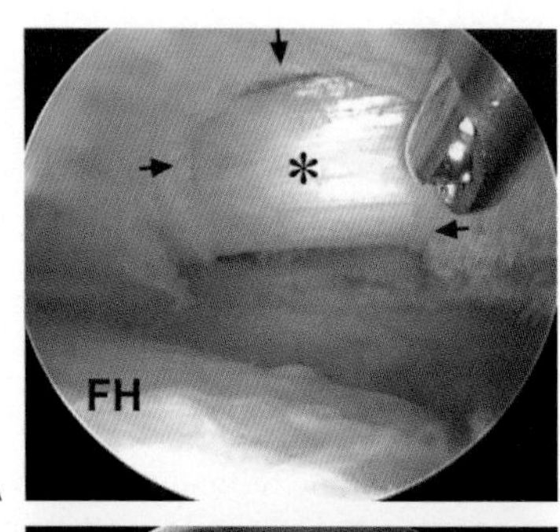

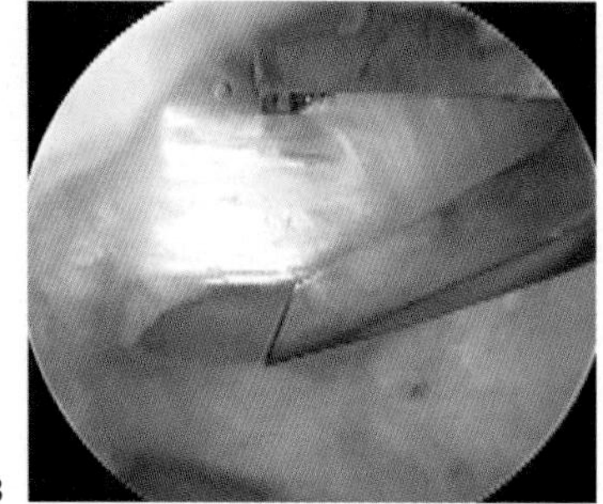

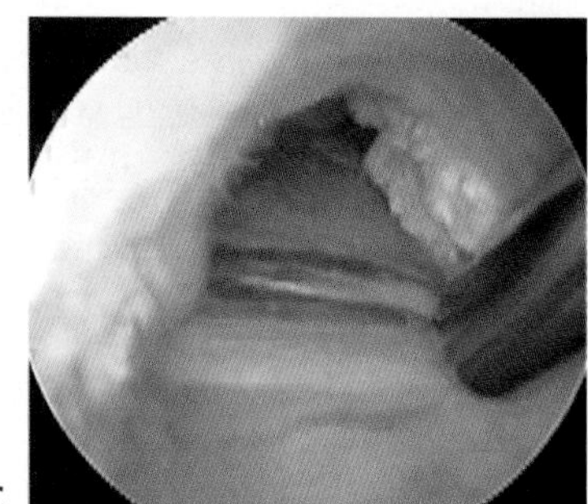

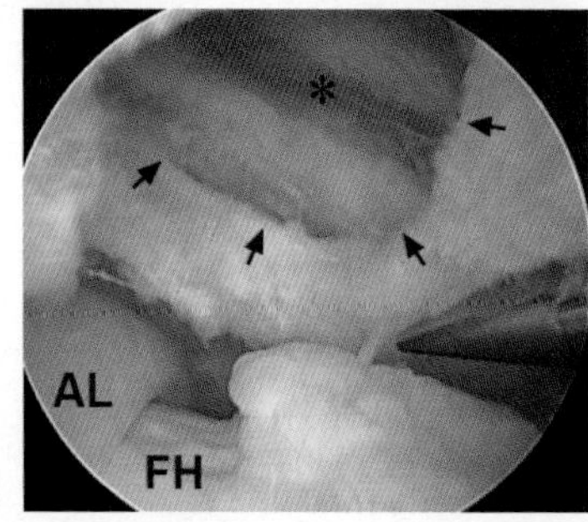

TECH FIG 2 • Arthroscopic view from the peripheral compartment of a right hip. **A.** A window (*arrows*) has been created through the thin medial capsule, exposing the iliopsoas tendon (*) anterior to the femoral head (*FH*). **B.** The tendinous portion is released with a basket. **C.** The final fibers are débrided with a power shaver. **D.** Through the capsular window (*arrows*) the tendon has been completely released, preserving the muscular fibers (*). The relation between the capsular window and the acetabular labrum (*AL*) and femoral head (*FH*) is identified. (Courtesy of J. W. Thomas Byrd, MD.)

- If the glistening tendon is not immediately visible, it should come into view after the capsular window is extended laterally.
- At the level of the joint, the tendon fibers of the iliopsoas lie on the posterior surface of its muscular portion.
- The muscular portion separates the tendon from the femoral nerve, which is the most lateral of the femoral neurovascular structures.
- The tendon can be transected with a combination of hand biter instruments, power shaver, and thermal device.

TENDOPLASTY OF THE ILIOTIBIAL BAND

Open Technique

- A straight, lateral longitudinal incision is centered over the greater trochanter (TECH FIG 3).
  - The length is dictated by the amount of exposure needed to precisely accomplish the tendoplasty.
  - A smaller incision is more cosmetic and can be accomplished with dissection of the subcutaneous tissues and selective retraction but should not compromise visualization for the procedure.
  - Several authors have described variations of a similar method for relaxing the tendon. These are based on an 8- to 10-cm longitudinal incision just posterior to the mid part of the greater trochanter in the thickest portion of the iliotibial band.
- Relaxation of the tendon is completed with paired or staggered 1- to 1.5-cm transverse incisions.
- The field is relatively bloodless, but meticulous hemostasis should be maintained and the subcutaneous tissues closed in layers to avoid formation of a hematoma.

Endoscopic Technique

- Two portals are used: one 3 cm proximal to the tip of the greater trochanter and one 3 cm distal.
- The arthroscope is placed from the distal portal site down to the subcutaneous surface of the iliotibial band.
- Then, with arthroscopic visualization, the proximal portal is established for dissection to release the subcutaneous tissue from the superficial surface of the tendon (TECH FIG 4).
- A 4- to 5-cm longitudinal incision within the tendon is created using a shaver and a radiofrequency (RF) probe.
- An anteriorly based transverse incision is then made and the flaps resected, creating a long, obtuse triangle.
  - This provides better visualization to determine the relation of the iliotibial band and the underlying greater trochanter.
- Portions of the trochanteric bursa can be resected as necessary for treatment and clearing the field of view.
- Lastly, a posterior transverse incision is made and the flaps excised, creating a diamond-shaped pattern of resection.
- Hemostasis should be meticulously maintained and a compressive dressing applied to minimize the formation of a hematoma.

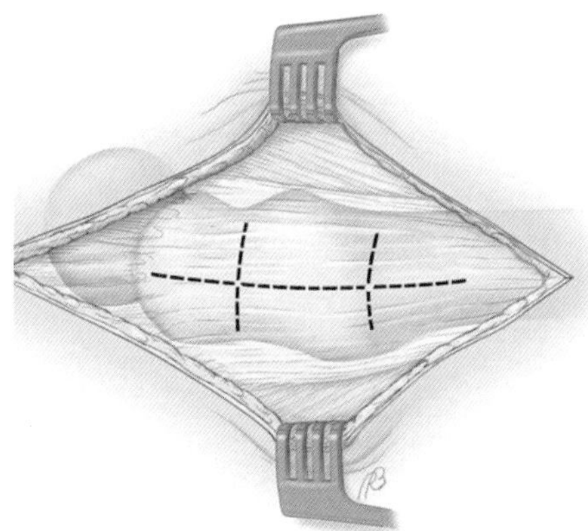

A

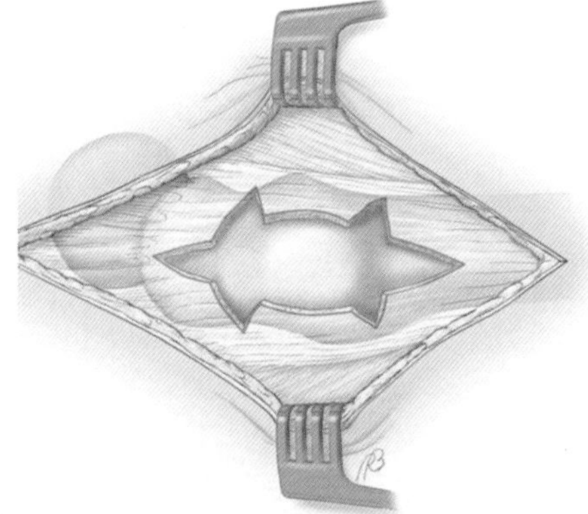

B

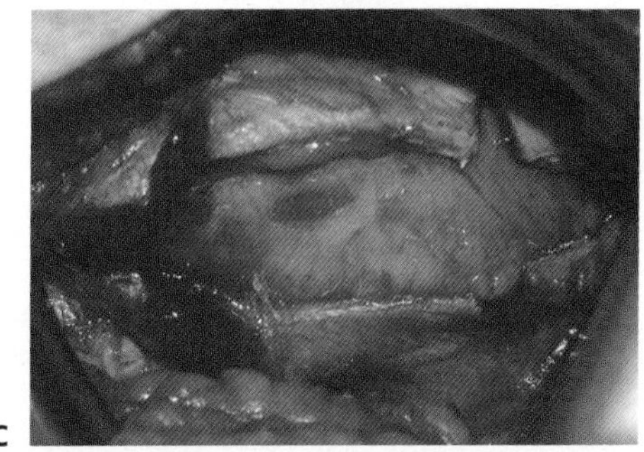

C

TECH FIG 3 • Our preferred approach includes an 8- to 10-cm longitudinal incision, posterior to the midpoint of the greater trochanter, with two pairs of 1- to 1.5-cm transverse incisions. This relaxes the iliotibial band, eliminating the snapping, without creating any suture repair lines that would necessitate prolonged convalescence. **A.** Incision pattern. **B.** Relaxing response to incision. **C.** Appearance at surgery. (Courtesy of J. W. Thomas Byrd, MD.)

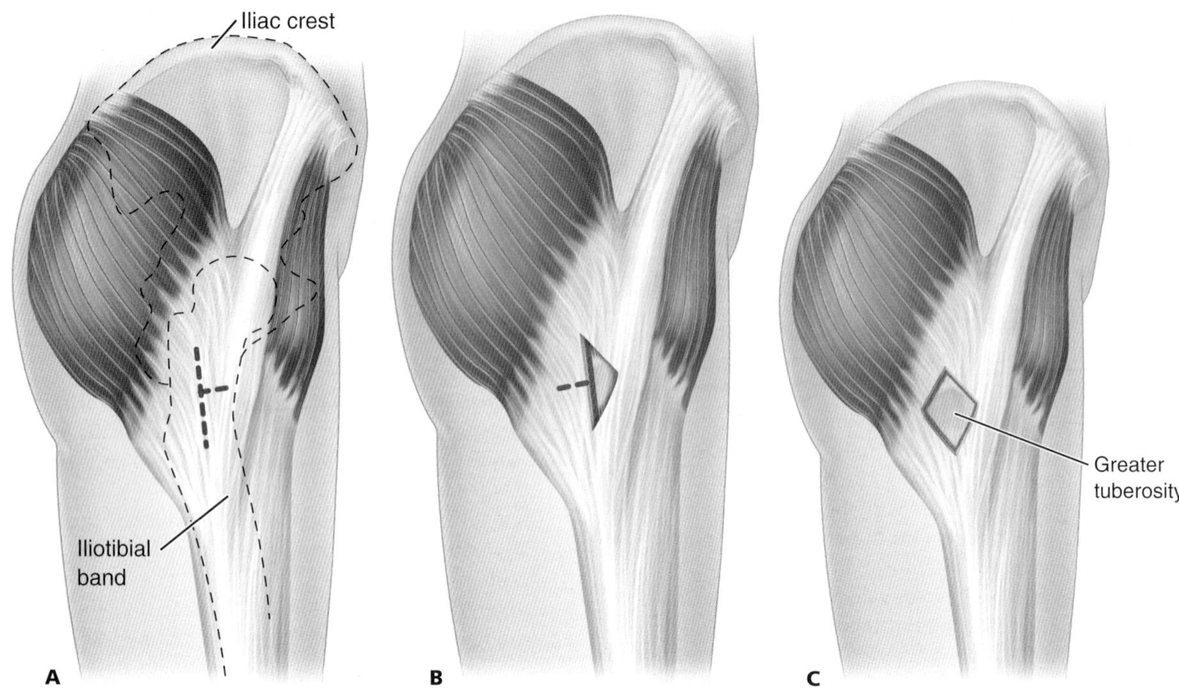

TECH FIG 4 • Endoscopic method of iliotibial band tendoplasty, shown in the right hip. **A.** After creating the longitudinal incision, the anterior limb is created by a perpendicular incision. **B.** Resecting the edges creates a triangle that aids in visualization of the underlying structures. **C.** The posterior limb is then created, and resection completes the diamond pattern of the tendoplasty. (Adapted from Ilizaliturri VM Jr, Martinez-Escalante FA, Chaidez PA, et al. Endoscopic iliotibial band release for external snapping hip syndrome. Arthroscopy 2006;22:505–510.)

PEARLS AND PITFALLS

Visualization	■ With any endoscopic technique, good visualization is essential. Poor visualization will result in a poorly performed procedure. Visualization is facilitated by use of a high-flow fluid management system and control of hemostasis by keeping the systolic blood pressure below 100 mm Hg, adding diluted epinephrine to the fluid, and judicious use of cauterization.
Violation of iliopsoas tendon	■ Surgical violation of the iliopsoas tendon carries the risk of heterotopic ossification, in either an open or arthroscopic procedure. It is prudent to use pharmacologic prophylaxis for this condition.
Failure to fully release tendon	■ The iliopsoas tendon forms from the psoas and iliacus muscles. The tendon sometimes may remain bifid all the way to its insertion on the lesser trochanter. Whether addressing the tendon from the peripheral compartment (**FIG 4A–G**) or from its insertion within the iliopsoas bursa (**FIG 4H,I**), if the tendon looks inordinately small, search for a separate portion of the tendon. Failure to fully release the tendon fibers may result in incomplete resolution of the snapping.
Inadequate tendoplasty	■ Inadequate tendoplasty of the iliotibial band can result in incomplete resolution of symptoms; but excessive release can compromise the functional integrity of the abductor mechanism, rendering it virtually unsalvageable.
Proper diagnosis	■ With proper diagnosis, the surgical results for snapping of the iliopsoas tendon and the iliotibial band are highly predictable and finite in terms of resolution of the snapping. ■ However, the subjective response to surgery is highly dependent on the patient's expectations and motivations, which are equally essential in the evaluation process.

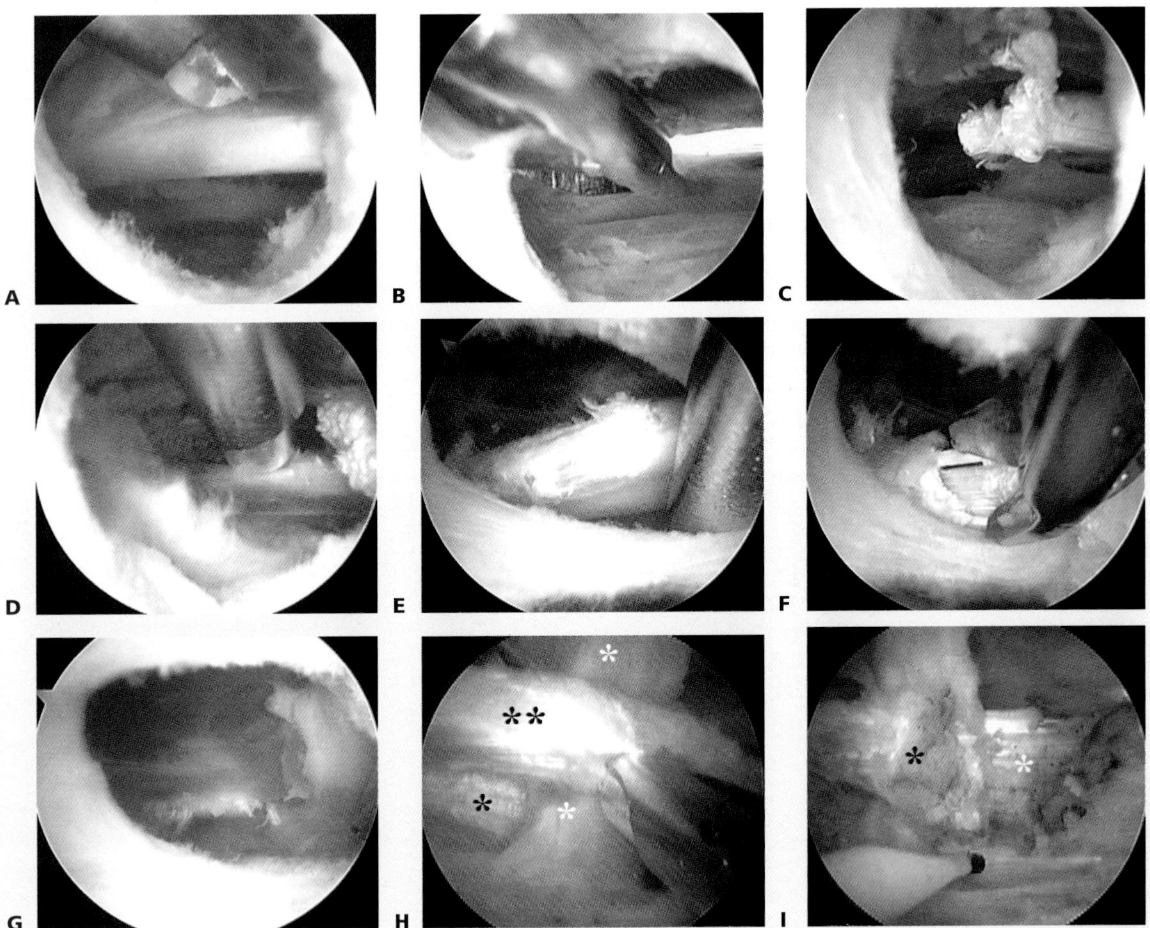

FIG 4 • **A–G.** The iliopsoas tendon of the right hip is exposed from the peripheral compartment. **A.** The initial tendon viewed through a capsular window is fully identified, but is abnormally small. **B.** This tendon is released with a basket. **C.** A stump remains. **D.** This is resected with a shaver. **E.** Further dissection exposes a more substantial portion of the iliopsoas tendon. **F.** This is released as well. **G.** Complete release of the bifid tendon is documented. **H,I.** Viewing the iliopsoas tendon of a right hip at its insertion on the lesser trochanter within the iliopsoas bursa. **H.** A bifid iliopsoas tendon is identified with medial (*) and lateral (**) bands separated by a vessel (*two white asterisks*) coursing perpendicular. **I.** The lateral band (*black asterisks*) has been released with a flexible RF device, revealing the medial band (*white asterisk*) which subsequently is released. (Courtesy of J. W. Thomas Byrd, MD.)

POSTOPERATIVE CARE

- After these procedures, the patient is capable of full weight bearing, but crutches are used for about 2 weeks until the gait pattern is normalized.
- Gentle range-of-motion, closed-chain, and stabilization exercises are introduced as symptoms allow.
- For iliopsoas release, aggressive hip flexion strengthening is avoided for the first 6 weeks; for the iliotibial band, aggressive stretching generally is not necessary.
- The patient should not anticipate returning to vigorous activities for at least 3 months.

OUTCOMES

- For endoscopic release of the iliopsoas tendon, several studies have reported highly predictable results in terms of eliminating the snapping and patient satisfaction.[4,9]
- However, we have observed two cases of heterotopic ossification that occurred following release of the iliopsoas tendon from the lesser trochanter.
- These observations are consistent with reports in the literature on open techniques of the iliopsoas tendon that have noted a propensity for heterotopic bone formation.[13]
- For snapping of the iliotibial band, tendon-relaxing procedures that maintain the structural integrity of the abductor mechanism, whether performed open or endoscopically, have predictably corrected the snapping with minimal morbidity.[3,8,15]

COMPLICATIONS

- No reports have been published of complications with endoscopic release of the iliopsoas tendon.
- We have observed two cases of heterotopic ossification, for which the use of pharmacologic prophylaxis is recommended.[13]
- Potential complication due to damage to surrounding structures (eg, femoral neurovascular bundle)
- No complications have been reported in conjunction with the less extensive tendon-relaxing procedures for a snapping iliotibial band. Careful attention to the precision of the release

can help avoid inadequate or excessive tendoplasty. Inadequate release could result in residual symptoms, whereas excessive release could result in a virtually unsalvageable compromise of the abductor mechanism.

REFERENCES

1. Allen WC, Cope R. Coxa saltans: the snapping hip revisited. J Am Acad Orthop Surg 1995;3:303–308.
2. Brignall CG, Stainsby GD. The snapping hip, treatment by Z-plasty. J Bone Joint Surg Br 1991;73B:253–254.
3. Byrd JWT. Snapping hip. Oper Tech Sports Med 2005:13:46–54.
4. Byrd JWT. Evaluation and management of the snapping iliopsoas tendon. Instr Course Lect 2006;55:347–355.
5. Dobbs MB, Gordon JE, Luhmann SJ, et al. Surgical correction of the snapping iliopsoas tendon in adolescents. J Bone Joint Surg Am 2002;84A:420–424.
6. Gruen GS, Scioscia TN, Lowenstein JE. The surgical treatment of internal snapping hip. Am J Sports Med 2002;30:607–613.
7. Henry AK. Extensile Exposure, ed 2. New York: Churchill Livingstone, 1973.
8. Ilizaliturri VM Jr, Martinez-Escalante FA, Chaidez PA, et al. Endoscopic iliotibial band release for external snapping hip syndrome. Arthroscopy 2006;22:505–510.
9. Ilizaliturri VM Jr, Villalobos FE Jr, Chaidez PA, et al. Internal snapping hip syndrome: treatment by endoscopic release of the iliopsoas tendon. Arthroscopy 2005;21:1375–1380.
10. Kim DH, Baechler MF, Berkowitz MJ, et al. Coxa saltans externa treated with Z-plasty of the iliotibial tract in a military population. Military Medicine 2002;167:172–173.
11. Provencher MT, Hofmeister EP, Muldoon MP. The surgical treatment of external coxa saltans (the snapping hip) by Z-plasty of the iliotibial band. Am J Sports Med 2004;32:470–476.
12. Taylor GR, Clarke NMP. Surgical release of the "snapping iliopsoas tendon." J Bone Joint Surg Br 1995;77B:881–883.
13. Velasco AD, Allan DB, Wroblewski BM. Psoas tenotomy and heterotopic ossification after Charnley low-friction arthroplasty. Clin Orthop Relat Res 1993;291:93–95.
14. Wettstein M, Jung J, Dienst M. Arthroscopic psoas tenotomy. Arthroscopy 2006;22:907.e1–4.
15. White RA, Hughes MS, Burd T, et al. A new operative approach in the correction of external coxa saltans: the snapping hip. Am J Sports Med 2004:32:1504–1508.

Chapter 28 Athletic Pubalgia

Jesse C. Botker, Robert F. LaPrade, and David R. Joesting

DEFINITION

- *Athletic pubalgia* refers to a range of groin injuries in athletes. The terms *athletic pubalgia* and *sports hernia* sometimes are used interchangeably.
- Diagnosis of the cause of groin pain is difficult, because the anatomy is complex and two or more injuries may coexist.
  - Intra-abdominal pathology, genitourinary abnormalities, referred lumbosacral pain, and hip joint disorders must first be excluded.
- Adductor strains are the most common cause of groin pain in athletes.
  - The adductors usually are strained in an eccentric contraction, often one that occurs at the myotendinous junction, but the strain also can occur in the tendon itself or its bony insertion.
  - Other muscles in and around the groin region also can be strained, including the rectus femoris, the sartorius, and the abdominal muscles, as can the conjoint tendon.
- *Sports hernia* is a condition of chronic groin pain that is caused by a tear in the inguinal floor without a clinically obvious hernia.[8,12]
  - It results in an occult injury that usually is not identified by most examiners. However, with increasing experience, the examiner can feel an abnormal inguinal floor and appreciate abnormal tenderness inside the external ring.
  - In contrast, indirect and direct hernias involve easily palpable defects in the inguinal canal or through the anterior abdominal musculature, respectively.
  - Duration of symptoms typically is months, and pain is resistant to conservative measures.
- *Osteitis pubis* is characterized by symphysis pain and joint disruption and occurs commonly in distance runners and soccer players.
  - It may be difficult to distinguish from adductor strains, and the two conditions may coincide.
- Stress fractures are rare injuries that result from repetitive cyclic loading of the bone.
  - The pubic rami are the most common location for stress fractures in the pelvis. These fractures are most common in long distance runners.

ANATOMY

- The anatomy in and around the groin is complex (**FIG 1**), and a thorough understanding of it is crucial in diagnosing the various groin injuries.
  - Thorough knowledge of the origins and insertions is very helpful during examination and palpation of the area.
- The posterior inguinal wall consists primarily of the transversalis fascia, along with the conjoint tendon, made up of the internal abdominal oblique and transversus abdominis aponeuroses.[8]

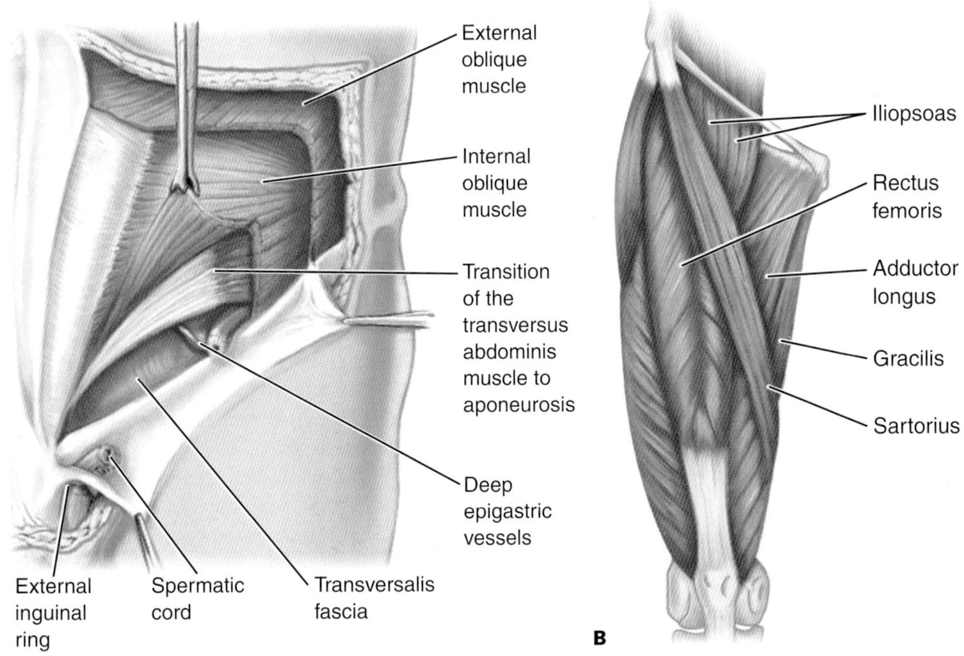

FIG 1 • Anatomy of the abdominal (**A**) and groin (**B**) musculature.

- The conjoint tendon inserts onto the pubic tubercle and along the iliopubic track.
- The pubic symphysis is a rigid, nonsynovial, amphiarthrodial joint consisting of layers of hyaline cartilage encasing a fibrocartilaginous disc.[6]

PATHOGENESIS

- Adductor strains are most commonly seen in soccer or ice hockey players.
  - Most happen acutely, and the patient recalls a sudden intense pain in the groin.
  - Eventually the medial thigh swells and ecchymosis is noted over the next 2 to 3 days.
  - The pain improves when the muscle warms up.
- Sports hernia is seen in competitive athletes and occasional work injuries and may involve a particular traumatic episode, but most times is insidious and worsens over time with overuse.
  - Patients describe a deep, disabling groin pain.
  - Kicking and endurance running tend to increase the symptoms.
  - Coughing or Valsalva maneuver increases intra-abdominal pressure and can increase tenderness, as can a resisted sit-up.
- The most likely mechanism for osteitis pubis is that of increased forces placed on the symphysis pubis from the pull of the pelvic musculature or repetitive stress from increased shearing forces.[4]
  - Some cases of osteitis pubis probably are secondary to or coexist with a sports hernia.
- Stress fractures of the pubic rami present as an insidious onset of deep pelvic and groin pain that is worsened after high-impact exercises.
  - The pain is worse immediately during and after the activity and improves with rest.
  - These injuries usually occur in conjunction with an acute increase in the intensity of training.

NATURAL HISTORY

- Acute adductor strains, if not properly rehabilitated, may progress to chronic strains or tendinopathy.
- Most patients with sports hernia have had a prolonged course of conservative treatment with continued pain and do not get better.[17] A hallmark of sports hernias is that patients have less pain when they are inactive and more pain when active.
- Osteitis pubis is self-limited but may take, on average, about 9 months to heal.[5]
- If the stress fracture is not addressed, pain will continue to increase and can be debilitating.

PATIENT HISTORY AND PHYSICAL FINDINGS

- Patient history is the most important aspect of the evaluation of athletic pubalgia.
- The patient must be asked for duration of symptoms, any inciting events, relieving and exacerbating factors, and timing of pain.
- To directly assess for hernia:
  - In men: insert the finger into inguinal ring at level of external opening. Invaginate the loose scrotal skin and gently insert the finger into the external ring (**FIG 2**). Gently feel the inguinal floor and ask the patient to perform the Valsalva maneuver. One can occasionally feel the tear tighten on one's fingertip. Apply gentle pressure medially and laterally looking for abnormal asymmetric tenderness.

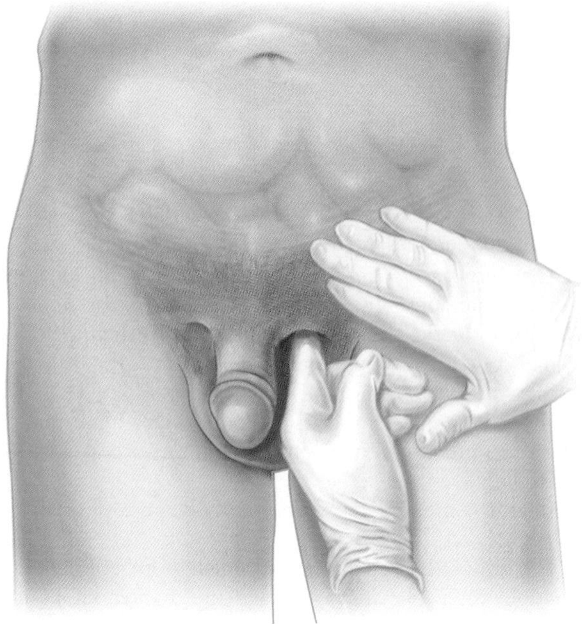

FIG 2 • Assessment for inguinal hernia. The finger is inserted into the inguinal ring at the level of the external opening. The loose scrotal skin is invaginated and the finger is gently inserted into the external ring.

  - In women: palpate the superior aspect of the labia majora and upward to lateral to the pubic tubercle.
- The groin is examined using these methods:
  - Straight leg raise: In patients with radicular low back pain, this will reproduce the pain they are having.
  - Palpation of insertion of conjoint tendon: tenderness may increase, and a bulge may be felt by having the patient perform a Valsalva maneuver.
  - Palpation of the adductor tendon: helps to diagnose an adductor strain or tear
  - Groin adduction resistance: helps to diagnose an adductor strain or tear
  - Palpation of the pubic symphysis: characteristic of osteitis pubis
  - Hip range of motion (ROM) may isolate a source of pain arising from the hip.
  - Thomas test: tightness in extension is a sign of a tight iliopsoas muscle.
  - Hip extension against resistance tests the strength of the hip extensors.
  - Hip flexion against resistance: tests the strength of the iliopsoas and may detect a strain or tear of this muscle.
  - Ober's test: patient inability to lower the upper leg completely to the examination table is pathognomonic of a tight iliotibial band.

IMAGING AND OTHER DIAGNOSTIC STUDIES

- Radiographs can be helpful in excluding fractures or avulsions.[9]
- Stress fractures usually are not evident on radiographs.

  - Bone scanning or MRI is most sensitive, especially in the early stages.
- MRI can be used to confirm muscle strain or tears, and partial or complete tendon tears (**FIG 3A**).
  - MRI has been used to detect sports hernias, although it is not always successful.[3]
- Dynamic ultrasound has been found, in certain cases, to detect posterior wall defects but is highly operator dependent.[16]
- Radiographs, CT scans, and bone scans can rule out other diagnoses; none are reliable in detecting sports hernias.
- Herniography, which involves an intraperitoneal injection of contrast dye followed by fluoroscopy or radiography, has been shown to identify sports hernias but has limited sensitivity and a substantial risk of perforation in up to 5% of patients.[2]
- Osteitis pubis has characteristic radiologic findings, including bone resorption, widening of the pubic symphysis, and irregular contour of articular surfaces or periarticular sclerosis (**FIG 3B**).
  - A bone scan may show increased uptake in the area of the pubic symphysis in osteitis pubis; however, not all patients who have symptoms show an abnormality.[13]
  - MRI has become increasingly useful in the diagnosis of osteitis pubis. Findings can include bone marrow edema or symphyseal disc extrusion.[15]

DIFFERENTIAL DIAGNOSIS

- Groin disruption or strain
- Osteitis pubis
- Pelvic stress fractures
- Indirect and direct hernia
- Avascular necrosis of the hip
- Labral tear of the hip
- Hip osteoarthritis
- Abdominal muscle tear
- Lumbar radiculopathy
- Nerve entrapment
- Tumors
- Genitourinary problems
- Inflammatory bowel disease
- Endometriosis
- Pelvic inflammatory disease

NONOPERATIVE MANAGEMENT

- Acute treatment of adductor strain includes rest, ice, compression, and elevation.
- The next goal is restoration of ROM and prevention of atrophy. Once the patient can tolerate this, the focus should be to regain strength, flexibility, and endurance.[9]
- Nonoperative management of sports hernia includes physical therapy,[10] anti-inflammatory drugs, and corticosteroid injections at the site of pain.[1]
- Osteitis pubis is a self-limiting condition; therapy should focus on hip ROM, as well as adductor stretching and strengthening.
- Corticosteroid injection in osteitis pubis is controversial but may be helpful in select populations of athletic patients.[11,15]
- Treatment in pelvic stress fractures is straightforward and involves 4 to 6 weeks of rest from the activities aggravating the area.

SURGICAL MANAGEMENT

- Many approaches have been tried in the surgical management of sports hernias.
- Tissue repairs require longer rehabilitation and pose a greater risk for recurrence, primarily because of collegenases which are currently being described.
- Laparoscopic repairs fail too often because they do not deal with the anterior mechanisms of groin pain.
- Purely anterior repairs fail occasionally because they do not provide adequate posterior support.
- Mesh repairs are standard.
  - Some mesh repairs fail because the mesh chosen is too heavy and tightly woven.
  - Other mesh repairs fail because of surgical technique (eg, metal tackers, permanent sutures in the periosteum, tight sutures involving nerves and causing necrotic tissue).
  - The most logical and successful repair is the use of two-layered lightweight mesh, which provides both posterior and anterior support and allows normalization of the torn anatomy.

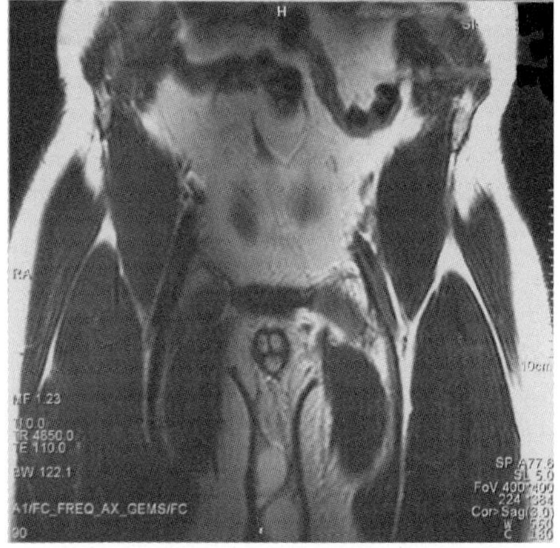

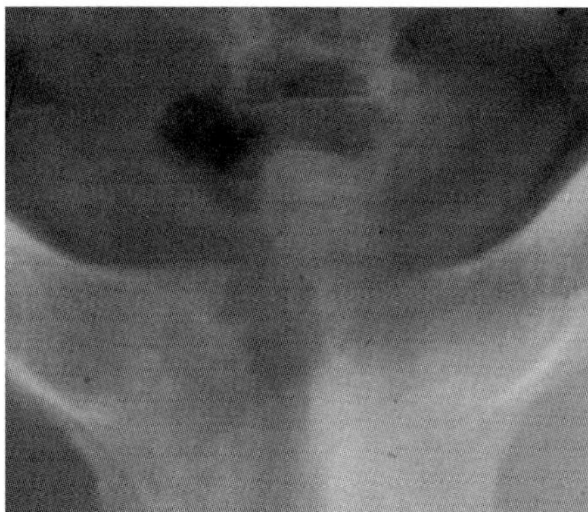

FIG 3 • **A.** MRI of an adductor tear in a hockey player. There is increased signal at the origin of the adductor tendon near the pubis. **B.** Characteristic radiograph of osteitis pubis. Notice the bone resorption, widening of the pubic symphysis, and irregular contour of articular surfaces.

Preoperative Planning

- Preoperative planning involves extreme care to ascertain that the patient really does have the injury for which surgery is being planned. This requires a complete history and physical examination performed by an examiner who understands the pathophysiology of this injury.
- Imaging is valuable to rule out alternative pathology.
- Preemptive analgesia is important to reduce postoperative pain and to make the anesthetic experience smoother. Also, local anesthesia is bactericidal, reducing the risk of infection.
  - We suggest ½% lidocaine with epinephrine and sodium bicarbonate.

Positioning

- The patient is positioned supine and draped.

ULTRAPRO HERNIA SYSTEM (JOHNSON & JOHNSON GATEWAY)

Incision, Dissection, and Site Evaluation

- The incision is made along the path of the inguinal ligament, perhaps 1 cm medial and superior to the ligament. A length of 5 to 6 cm is adequate.
- Dissection is performed down to the external oblique tying veins. Too much cautery increases the risk of a subcutaneous infection.
- The external oblique is incised to the external ring, and the fascia is mobilized both medially and laterally.
- The spermatic cord is carefully evaluated and mobilized, looking for an indirect sac.
- The inguinal floor is carefully evaluated, looking for a torn transversalis fascia or a torn transversus abdominis.
  - Occasionally, the yellow preperitoneal fat can be seen outlining a tear.
- The inguinal floor is palpated. The disruption often can be felt.

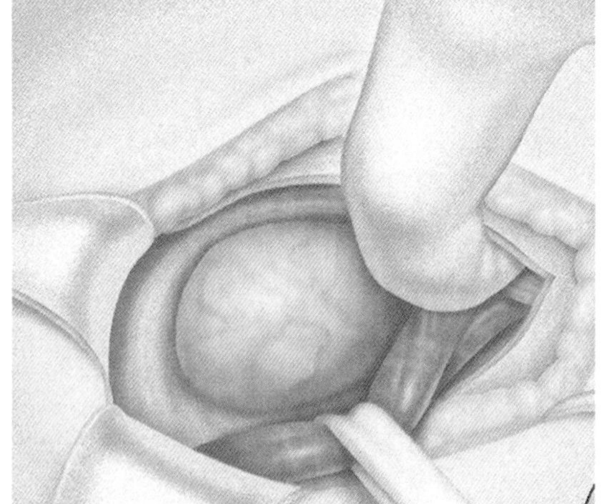
A

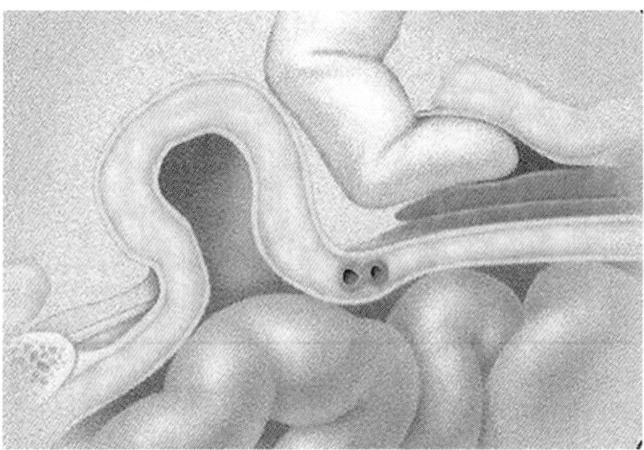
B

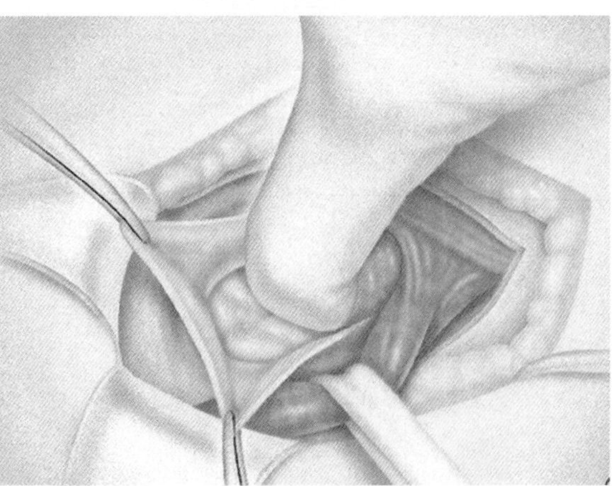
C

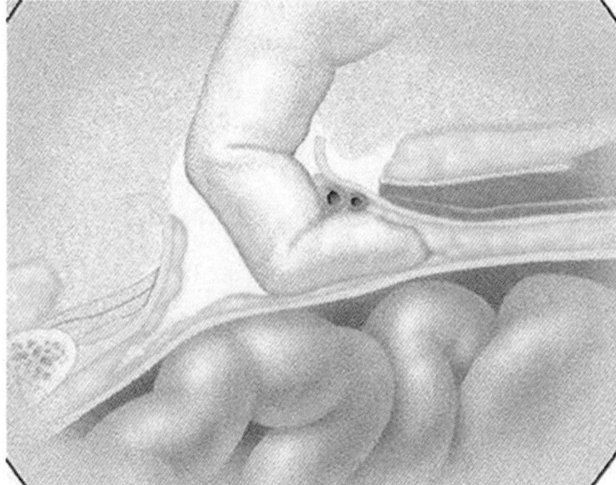
D

TECH FIG 1 • A,B. The anterior pocket is developed under the external oblique to optimize placement of the onlay patch and dissected out laterally to ensure the onlay patch will lie flat. **C.** After the posterior wall has been opened, visual confirmation is made of location in the preperitoneal space by identifying the yellow preperitoneal fat and by visualizing Cooper's ligament. **D.** Then, using the forefinger, sweep circumferentially medial, then lateral to actualize the preperitoneal space. *(continued)*

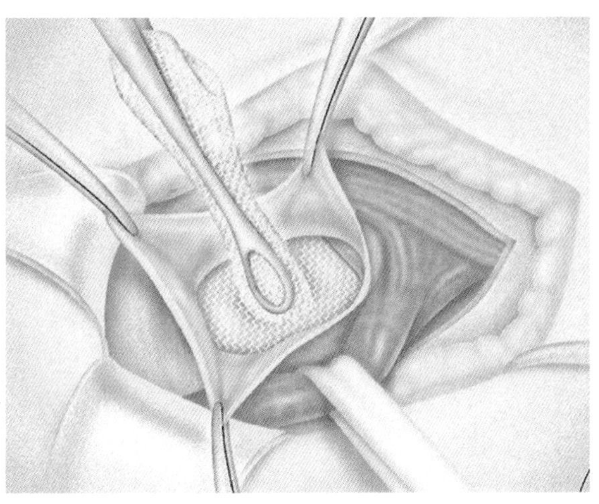

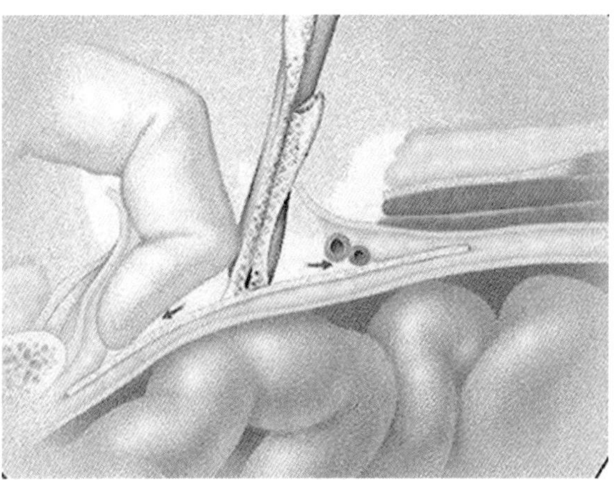

TECH FIG 1 • *(continued)* **E,F.** With the onlay patch grasped down to the connector with sponge forceps, insert the device completely into the defect and deploy the underlay with forceps or finger. (Courtesy of Ethicon Surgery, a Johnson & Johnson company.)

Positioning the Patches

- The preperitoneal space is opened and prepared. Dissection is extended out laterally so the onlay patch will lie flat (**TECH FIG 1A,B**).
  - It should be possible to clearly feel under the rectus, the pubis, Cooper's ligament, and up along the iliofemoral vessels (**TECH FIG 1C,D**).
- The posterior (round) patch of the UHSL is positioned in the space that has been prepared (**TECH FIG 1E,F**).
- The transversalis and transversus abdominis are closed around the connector with an absorbable suture tied loosely (an air knot). The technique is evolving, and in the near future, the mesh probably will be attached with tissue glue.

Affixing the Patches

- The onlay patch is attached to the fascia overlying the pubic tubercle, to the internal oblique fascia medially and to the iliopubic track laterally.
  - A lateral slit is made in the mesh for the spermatic cord, attaching the mesh to the shelving edge of the inguinal ligament. Excess mesh is trimmed away.
  - The mesh should never be tight, and fewer sutures are better than many, as long as the mesh is anatomically placed (**TECH FIG 2A–C**).
- Marcaine is injected thoroughly, and the external oblique, Scarpa's fascia, and skin are clsoed with an absorbable suture (**TECH FIG 2D,E**).

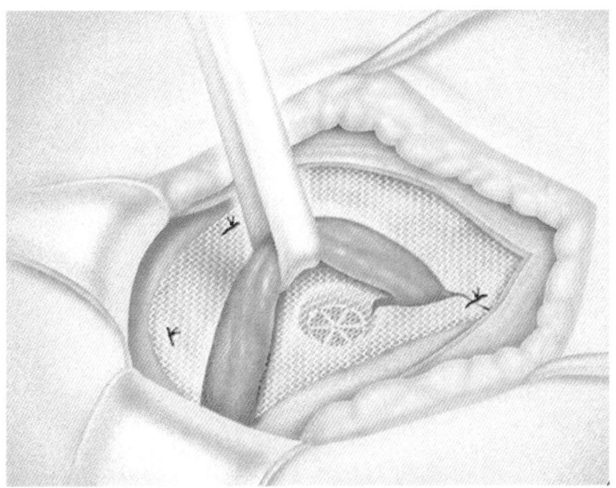

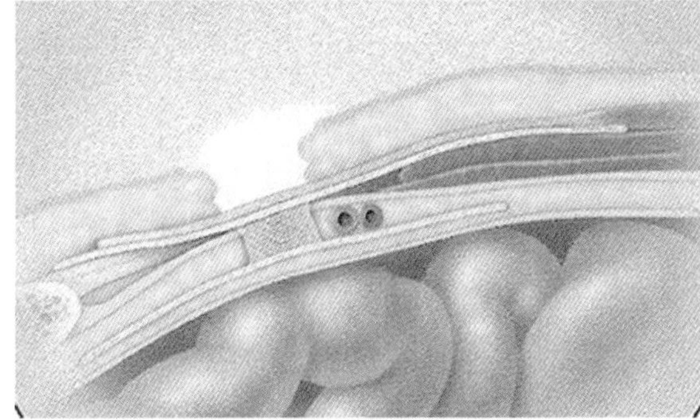

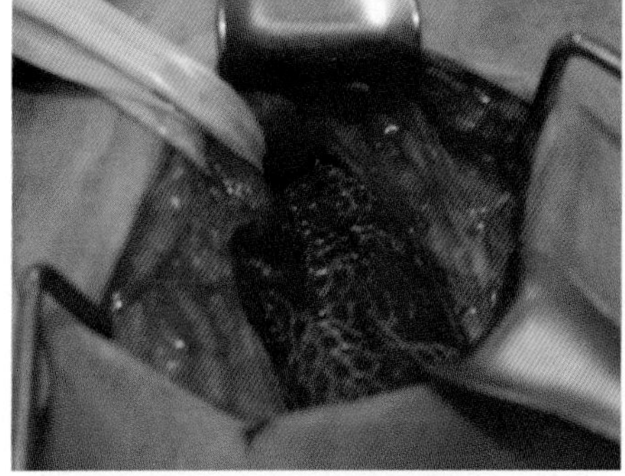

TECH FIG 2 • A,B. Sutures are used to fixate the onlay patch over the pubic tubercle (essential) and to the mid-portion of the transverse aponeurotic arch (optional). A slit is created in the onlay patch to accommodate the spermatic cord, and the mesh is sutured to close the slit. **C.** The spermatic cord comes through the onlay patch. *(continued)*

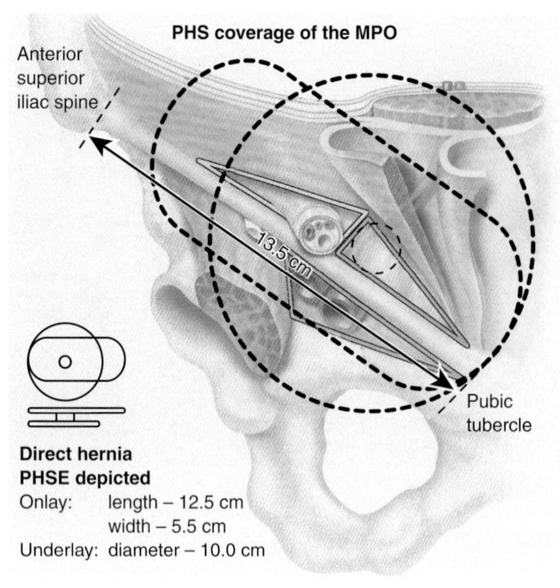

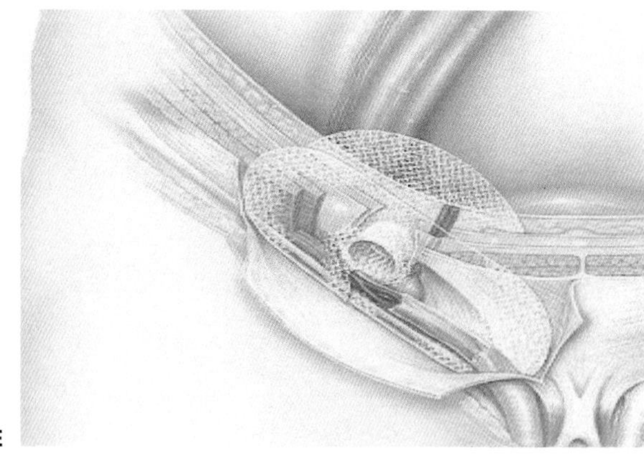

TECH FIG 2 • *(continued)* **D.** Schematic drawing of where the patch will lie. **E.** Finished position of the mesh. (Courtesy of Ethicon Surgery, a Johnson & Johnson company.)

PEARLS AND PITFALLS

Operate only if the patient has a good mechanism of injury, a good history, and clear indications on physical examination.	■ If the patient's pain does not improve with rest, he or she probably does not have a sports hernia.
Tight sutures, tacks, or tight mesh may cause chronic postoperative pain.	■ For the best results, both the anterior and posterior mechanisms of pain must be addressed.
The principle of this surgery (and all abdominal wall hernia surgery) is to normalize the tissue and reinforce the normalized tissue with lightweight, flexible mesh.	

POSTOPERATIVE CARE

- Standard post–inguinal hernia surgery care is advised.
- It is important to emphasize a rapid return to normal non-physical activity (starting the day after surgery) and a progressive incremental return to sports and working out in preparation for sports. This is best accomplished with the help of a trainer.
- The goal of rehabilitation is to establish a full and normal ROM and flexibility followed by incremental increases in resistence for strength training.
- Contact athletes should be able to return to competition in 3 to 4 weeks.
- Runners should be running in 2 weeks and golfers golfing in 1 week.

OUTCOMES

- With appropriate indications and surgical technique, success rates in sports hernia repair have been as high as 97% to 100% in high-performance athletes, with success measured as a return to previous levels of performance and freedom from pain.[7,14]

COMPLICATIONS

- Recurrence
- Thigh pain in the early postoperative period
- Infection
- Hematoma
- Continued pain

REFERENCES

1. Ashby EC. Chronic obscure groin pain is commonly caused by enthesopathy: "tennis elbow" of the groin. Br J Surg 1994;81:1632–1634.
2. Calder F, Evans R, Neilson D. Value of herniography in the management of occult hernia and groin pain in adults. Br J Surg 2000;87:824–825.
3. Ekberg O, Sjoberg S, Westlin N. Sports-related groin pain: evaluation with MR imaging. Eur Radiology 1996;6:52–55.
4. Fricker P. Osteitis pubis. Sports Med Arthroscopy Rev 1997;5:305–312.
5. Fricker P, Taunton J, Ammann W. Osteitis pubis in athletes. Infection, inflammation or injury? Sports Med 1991;12:266–279.
6. Gamble J, Simmons S, Freedman M. The symphysis pubis: anatomic and pathologic considerations. Clin Orthop Relat Res 1986;203:261–272.
7. Genitsaris M, Goulimaris I, Sikas N. Laparoscopic repair of groin pain in athletes. Am J Sports Med 2004;32:1238–1242.
8. Hackney RG. The sports hernia: a cause of chronic groin pain. Br J Sports Med 1993;27:58–62.
9. Holmich P. Adductor related groin pain in athletes. Sports Med Arthroscopy Rev 1997;5:285–291.
10. Holmich P, Uhrskou P, Ulnits L, et al. Effectiveness of active physical training as treatment for longstanding adductor-related groin pain in athletes. The Lancet 1999;353:439–443.
11. Holt M, Keene J, Graf B, et al. Treatment of osteitis pubis in athletes. Results of corticosteroid injections. Am J Sports Med 1995;23:601–606.

12. Joesting DR. Diagnosis and treatment of sportsman's hernia. Curr Sports Med Rep 2002;1:121–124.
13. Karlsson J, Jerre R. The use of radiography, magnetic resonance, and ultrasound in the diagnosis of hip, pelvis, and groin injuries. Sports Med Arthroscopy Rev 1997;5:268–273.
14. Meyers WC, Foley DP, Garrett WE, et al. Management of severe lower abdominal or inguinal pain in high-performance athletes. Am J Sports Med 2000;28:2–8.
15. O'Connell M, Powell T, McCaffrey N. Symphyseal cleft injection in the diagnosis and treatment of osteitis pubis in athletes. Am J Roentgenol 2002;179:955–959.
16. Orchard JW, Read JW, Neophyton J. Groin pain associated with ultrasound finding of inguinal canal posterior wall deficiency in Australian Rules footballers. Br J Sports Med 1998;32:134–139.
17. Taylor DC, Meyers WC, Moylan JA. Abdominal musculature abnormalities as a cause of groin pain in athletes. Inguinal hernias and pubalgia. Am J Sports Med 1991;19:239–242.

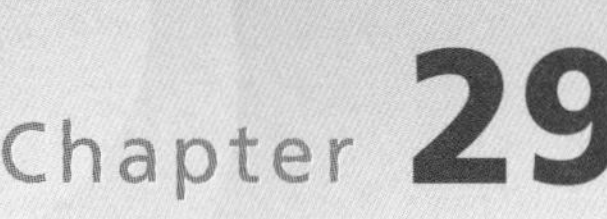

Chapter 29

Adductor Longus–Related Groin Pain

Robert T. Sullivan and William E. Garrett

DEFINITION

- Groin injuries are common among athletes, accounting for 2% to 5% of all athletic injuries.[12]
- A broad spectrum of pathology can cause groin pain in the athlete, and the differential diagnosis is critical.
- Adductor longus–related pain is the most common entity, particularly in athletes participating in kicking sports, such as soccer, and in sports requiring rapid directional changes such as ice hockey and American football.[6,7,12,13]
- Most acute adductor-related groin pain represents strain at the muscle–tendon junction. Although rare, complete avulsions of the adductor longus origin from the pubis can occur.
- Chronic adductor pain typically occurs as an isolated enthesopathy or in concert with athletic pubalgia or pre-hernia complex.

ANATOMY

- The adductor longus is a large, fan-shaped muscle that originates from the anteromedial aspect of the superior pubic ramus just inferior to the pubic tubercle and inserts on the linea aspera of the femur.
- Innervated by the anterior division of the obturator nerve, the origin of the adductor longus consists of direct attachment of both muscle fibers and tendon to the pubis. The proximal tendon has a narrow cross-sectional area.[12]
- The proximal tendon is readily identified on the anterior surface of the muscle with an oblique muscle–tendon junction. The proximal posterior surface usually is entirely muscular in origin.[13]
- A common anomaly is muscle fibers forming the lateral 5 to 11 mm of the anterior origin (**FIG 1**).[13]
- In maturity, the fibrocartilage of the symphysis pubis develops a small, central fluid-filled cavity or cleft.This cleft manifests as a central focus of high signal intensity at T2-weighted and fat-suppressed short T1 inversion recovery (STIR) imaging.[3]

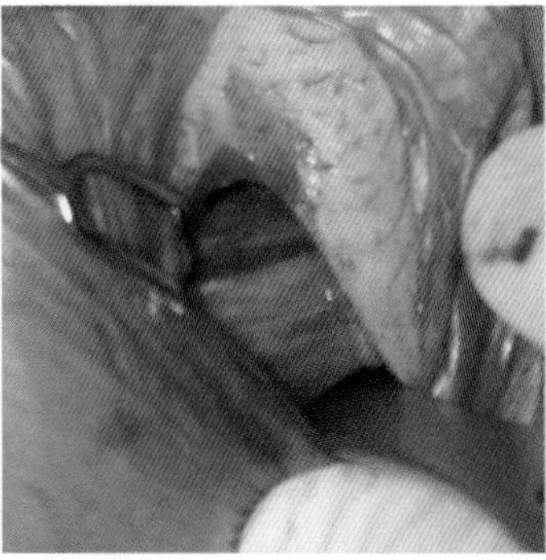

FIG 1 • Muscle fibers forming the most lateral aspect of the adductor longus origin.

PATHOGENESIS

- The pathogenesis of chronic adductor strains and frequently associated sports hernias or athletic pubalgia is poorly understood.
- The problem usually is seen in athletes using powerful and ballistic muscle action involving a rapid change from a trunk rotated posteriorly to the plant foot with simultaneous hip extension and abduction followed by a sudden anterior trunk rotation with hip flexion and adduction.
- Examples are an in-step kick in soccer or a fast gait in hockey when the trailing leg is pulled forward, where these actions create strong muscle activity around the lower abdominal muscles and hip adductors and flexors.
- Many of these conditions are chronic or acute on chronic.
- The possibility of a subtle degree of pelvic instability has been considered, but it is difficult to prove.[2–4]
- Hip adductor involvement is more likely an abnormality at the insertion than a chronic tendinitis or tendinosis.[2–4]

NATURAL HISTORY

- Acute adductor strains at the musculotendinous junction, like other muscle strain injuries, vary considerably in time to recovery based on the severity of the injury. These are almost always managed without surgery.
- Prior adductor strain has been shown to be a significant risk factor for injury.[14]
- An adductor-to-abductor muscle strength ratio of less than 80% is predictive for a future adductor strain as well. Preseason hip strengthening regimens can lower the incidence of adductor strains.[14,15]
- In the rare instance of a complete adductor longus avulsion, nonoperative management is preferred.[11]
- Chronic adductor pain presenting as an enthesopathy may occur simultaneously with athletic pubalgia or may follow an acute strain. Enthesopathy can lead to resistant, chronic groin pain, warranting operative intervention.

PATIENT HISTORY AND PHYSICAL FINDINGS

- The diagnosis of an acute adductor strain is relatively straightforward, because the athlete typically presents with a sudden injury to the groin incurred during athletic competition.
- There is tenderness to palpation at the muscle tendon junction. This pain is exacerbated with resisted adduction and passive abduction. Imaging rarely is required for acute strains, but is more commonly obtained for professional athletes.
- In the setting of a more severe acute injury or avulsion, edema and ecchymosis are present and a defect may be palpated.
- The diagnosis of chronic groin pain is not as straightforward because of the broad spectrum of clinical entities that can cause pain in this region and their similar presentations.
- There is no current diagnostic gold standard for chronic groin pain.

- The differential diagnosis is critical owing to the possibility of other serious disorders; thus, a comprehensive history and physical is warranted in the patient with chronic groin pain.
- The physical findings of chronic adductor pain are similar findings to those of an acute strain, but the examiner is more likely to elicit pain with palpation of the pubic symphysis and is more reliant on imaging, coupled with the examination, for a definitive diagnosis.
- Involvement of the symphysis pubis detected by physical and even radiographic examination is common.
- Chronic adductor-related pain often occurs in conjunction with athletic pubalgia. Sports hernias can present with complaints of vague and migratory lower abdominal pain radiating to the medial thigh.
- Sports hernia findings are pain with a sit-up maneuver or resisted internal rotation of a flexed hip. Tenderness to palpation is found above the inguinal ligament and superior to the pubic tubercle. Tenderness may be more focal, involving the external inguinal ring without a palpable hernia or in the vicinity of the conjoint tendon.
- Physical examination should include:
  - Palpation of the adductor longus. Focal tenderness suggests adductor-realated groin pain. A palpable defect implies adductor avulsion.
  - Squeeze test. The presence or absence of pain is noted. Strength is graded as follows: mild—minimal loss of strength; moderate—clear loss of strength; severe—complete loss of strength. Pain with or without a strength deficit implies adductor-related groin pain.
  - Passive stretch of adductors. Pain localized to the adductor implies adductor-related groin pain.
  - Palpation of external inguinal ring. Pain in the absence of a palpable hernia implies a sports hernia.
  - Sit-up against resistance. Adductor pain implies a concomitant or isolated sports hernia.

IMAGING AND OTHER DIAGNOSTIC STUDIES

- Imaging studies are most effective when selected on the basis of a thorough history and physical examination.
- MRI is the imaging modality of choice to evaluate chronic adductor-related pain.
- Muscle strains have high T2 signal at the muscle–tendon junction, which can extend along the epimysium.
- Enthesopathy, an overuse inury, reveals signal change within the adductor origin and, often, the pubic marrow.
- We believe that osteitis pubis, ie, marrow changes within the pubis, is a radiologic sign rather than a diagnosis, because these changes are most often present in the setting of adductor-related symptoms.
  - Robinson demonstrated that patient symptoms and MRI abnormalities within the pubis correlated significantly and reproducibly with symptomatic adductor enthesopathy or chronic myotendinous strain.[2,10] Thus, pubic marrow changes should alert the clinician to consider an adductor or lower abdominal wall injury.[9,10]
- Additionally, Cunningham[4] demonstrated pubic marrow changes are frequently associated with adductor injury, but adductor enthesopathy is also commonly identified in the absence of pubic marrow changes. This suggests adductor dysfunction most likely precedes pubic marrrow changes.

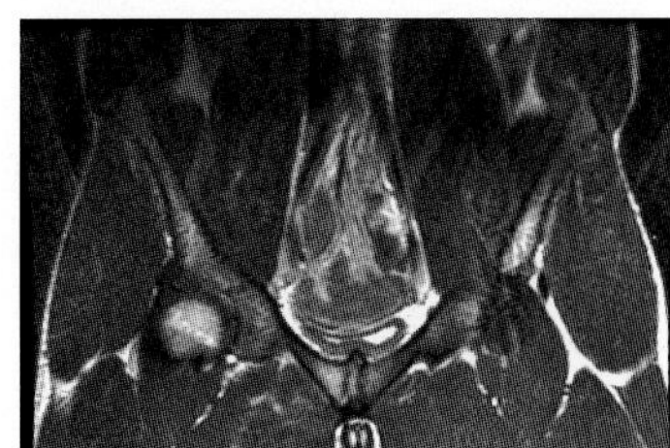

FIG 2 • Secondary cleft sign seen on T2-weighted coronal MRI, suggesting a partial avulsion of the adductor longus on the right.

- In addition to signal changes within the adductor origin, muscle tendon junction, or pubis, a secondary cleft sign may be present.
  - Brennan et al[3] defined the abnormal secondary cleft as an extension of the normal hyperintense signal seen within the central symphyseal cleft to a location lateral to the midline or inferior to the joint.
  - The secondary cleft is best visualized on a coronal STIR image (**FIG 2**). This secondary cleft, like pubic marrow changes, is thought to be a consequence of prolonged traction on the pubic rami and common aponeurosis anterior to the symphysis.
  - Chronic injury leads to a communication between the central and secondary clefts owing to a microtear or partial avulsion of the adductor longus from the pubis.[3,4]

DIFFERENTIAL DIAGNOSIS

- Athletic pubalgia (sports hernia)
- Inguinal hernia
- Acetabular labral tear
- Hip arthritis
- Femoral neck stress fracture
- Hip synovitis
- Referred testicular pain
- Gynecologic pathology
- Coxa saltans
- Iliopsoas strain
- Intra-abdominal disorders

NONOPERATIVE MANAGEMENT

- Adductor-related acute strains and overuse injuries are all initially managed with rest, ice, compression, and elevation (the RICE method) and a brief period of nonsteroidal anti-inflammatory drugs (NSAIDs). Differentiation between a strain and an enthesopathy is critical, because musculotendinous strains are managed much more aggressively with early, active therapy.
- Early on, active and passive range of motion without pain is initiated.
  - Once full, painless range of motion has been achieved, a progressive strengthening regimen is started. Increased emphasis is placed on core stabilzation and strengthening of the pelvic musculature.
- Resistance training consists predominantly of eccentric exercise for the hip and pelvic musculature.

- Holmich et al[5] demonstrated that an active strengthening and coordination program for the pelvic musculature was significantly better than conventional physical therapy in treating chronic athletic-related groin pain.

- Nonoperative therapy is completed with sport-specific training and eventual return to play.
- Early return to play is not advised because of the high risk of recurrent injury. Tyler et al[14,15] showed the best predictor of a future groin strain was an adductor-to-abductor muscle strength ratio of less than 80%.
- Acute adductor avulsions are best managed with nonoperative means, despite reports of successful repair.[8,11]
  - Schlegel et al[11] reported on 19 acute avulsions in NFL players, where those managed nonoperatively had good outcomes and a markedly shorter recovery time.
- Verall[16] reported on a specific nonoperative regimen for sports-related groin pain with MRI-documented pubic stress changes. Twenty-seven athletes were rested for 12 weeks, followed by an active therapy regimen. When evaluated by return to sport criteria, outcomes were excellent.
  - However, results were satisfcatory only if the criterion of ongoing symptoms was used, because nearly a third of individuals remained symptomatic during their second season post–nonoperative treatment.
  - Additionally, 26% of these athletes were participating at a lower level of competition.
- Holmich et al[5] reported on 23 of 29 athletes with chronic adductor-related groin pain returning to symptom-free play at 19 weeks as a result of an active therapy program. Long-term follow-up was not obtained, and these injuries were not stratified regarding strain versus enthesopathy versus avulsion.

SURGICAL MANAGEMENT

- Chronic adductor-related groin pain that has failed nonoperative measures, including an active therapy program focused on strengthening of the pelvic musculature and core stabilization, can be successfully treated with tenotomy of the adductor longus.[1] Although adductor tenotomy previously was reserved for patients with spasticity, it clearly has a role in the management of chronic and disabling groin pain in the athlete. Tenotomy is performed as an isolated procedure or in conjunction with a sports hernia repair.
- Individuals suspected of having a concomitant sports hernia are referred to a general surgeon for definitive management.

Preoperative Planning

- Surgical planning consists primarily of an extensive history and physical examination to confirm that the pain is isolated to the adductor and that all appropriate nonoperative measures have been exhausted.
- Additionally, a confirmatory MRI revealing enthesopathy or chronic strain with associated pubic marrow changes or cleft sign is warranted.

Positioning

- The patient is placed in the supine position with the operative extremity in an abducted and externally rotated position (**FIG 3**). The adductor origin is easily palpated in this position. Only the ipsilateral groin is prepped and draped.

Approach

- The adductor longus is superficial and proximal to the adductor brevis and adductor magnus origins.
- A 3-cm incision is marked about 1 cm inferior and parallel to the inguinal crease. This incision is centered over the palpable tendinous mass.

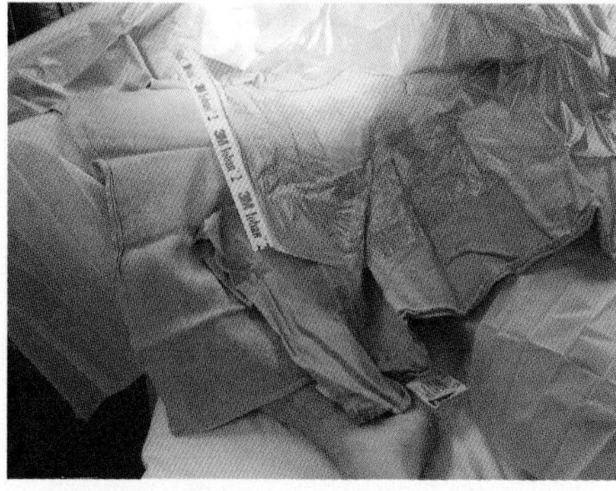

FIG 3 • The operative thigh is flexed, abducted, and externally rotated to provide excellent exposure and easy palpation of the adductor origin.

TECHNIQUES

OPEN ADDUCTOR LONGUS TENOTOMY

- The skin is incised in line with the previous mark down to the underlying fascia (**TECH FIG 1A**). The fascia is incised in a similar fashion, parallel to the skin incision, revealing the underlying adductor longus proximal tendon.
- The tendon is readily identified, and care is taken to identify the medial and lateral borders, noting that the lateral aspect often is composed of muscle fibers without a true tendinous component.
- Once the borders are defined, the tendon is elevated from the underlying adductor brevis and divided with cautery about 1 cm from its pubic origin while protecting the underlying adductor brevis (**TECH FIG 1B**). Note that the undersurface of the adductor longus is entirely muscular.
- Remaining proximal also protects the anterior division of the obturator nerve as it runs its course along the anterior aspect of the adductor brevis.
- Although some have reported suturing the distal stump of the cut tendon to the overlying fascia, this is not necessary; no distal retraction or deformity has been encountered in our experience.
- The fascia is repaired with an absorbable suture, and the overlying skin is approximated.

TECHNIQUES

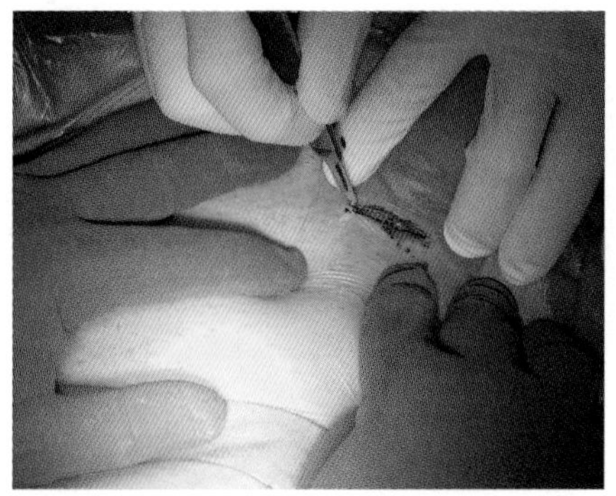

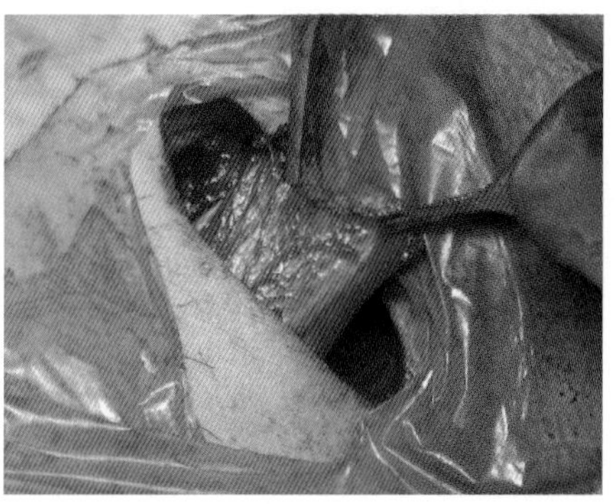

TECH FIG 1 • **A.** The skin incision is 3 to 4 cm long, just inferior and parallel to the inguinal crease, centered over the adductor origin. **B.** The distal free edge of the transected adductor longus tendon.

PEARLS AND PITFALLS

Indications	▪ Surgical release or tenotomy of the addcutor longus has a role in sports medicine for chronic and recalcitrant adductor-related groin pain.
Concomitant pathology	▪ Adductor-related groin pain often is associated with athletic pubalgia. A general surgery evaluation is warranted before considering an isiolated adductor tenotomy.
Anatomy	▪ Muscle fibers often make up the lateral 5 to 11 mm of the adductor longus origin. The presence or absence of these fibers must be confirmed to ensure a complete tenotomy is accomplished.

POSTOPERATIVE CARE

- Immediate ambulation is permitted without assistive devices. Stretching is avoided until the incision has healed.
- Once the incision has healed, a progresive strengthening and stretching routine is initiated, with an emphasis on core stabilization.

OUTCOMES

- Akermark[1] performed isolated adductor tenotomy in 16 athletes with chronic adductor-related groin pain. All patients reported significant improvement. Fifteen of 16 returned to sporting activities within 6 to 8 weeks, and 12 of 16 returned to competitive sports by 14 weeks. Only 10 athletes returned to full athletic competition; five returned to a reduced level of competition.
- As one might expect, patients had decreasesd isokinetic testing relative to the nonoperative side. However, these patients were reported to maintain functional sports activity despite the measured deficit.[1]
- A definitive recommendation to proceed with adductor tenotomy is difficult, particularly in the high-performance athlete. Therefore, adductor tenotomy is reserved as a last-ditch effort to return the chronicaly disabled athlete to competitive sports with the possibility of participation at a reduced level of performance.
- Additional study investigating nonoperative and surgical intervention of adductor-related groin pain clearly is warranted.

COMPLICATIONS

- There are no reported complications for adductor tenotomy, because few series have been reported.
- We suspect that persistent groin pain attributed to an incorrect diagnosis or an untreated concomitant sports hernia is the most prevalent complication from adductor-related surgery.

REFERENCES

1. Akermark C, Johansson C. Tenotomy of the adductor longus tendon in the treatment of chronic groin pain in athletes. Am J Sports Med 1992;20:640–643.
2. Albers S, Spritzer C, Garrett WE, et al. MR findings in athletes with pubalgia. Skeletal Radiol 2001;30:270–277.
3. Brennan D, O'Connel M, Ryan M, et al. Secondary cleft sign as a marker of injury in athletes with groin pain: MR image, appearance and interpretation. Radiology 2005;235:162–167.
4. Cunningham P, Brennan D, O'Connel M, et al. Patterns of bone and soft-tissue injury at the symphysis pubis in soccer players: observations at MRI. AJR Am J Roentgenol 2007;188:W291–W296.
5. Holmich P, Uhrskou P, Ulnits L, et al. Effectiveness of active physical training as treatment for long-standing adductor-related groin pain in athletes: randomised trial. Lancet 1999;353:1444–1445.
6. Holmich P. Long-standing groin pain in sportspeople falls into three primary patterns, a "clinical entity" approach: a prospective study of 207 patients. Br J Sports Med 2007;41:247–252.
7. Meyers W, Foley D, Garrett W, et al. Management of severe lower abdominal or inguinal pain in high-performance athletes. Am J Sports Med 2000;28:2–8.
8. Rizzio L, Salvo J, Schürhoff M, et al. Adductor longus rupture in professional football players: acute repair with suture anchors: a report of two cases. Am J Sports Med 2004;32:243–245.
9. Robinson P, Salehi F, Grainger A, et al. Cadaveric and MRI study of the musculotendinous contributions to the capsule of the symphysis pubis. AJR Am J Roentgenol 2007;188:W440–W445.
10. Robinson P, Barron D, Parsons W, et al. Adductor-related groin pain in athletes: correlation of MR imaging with clinical findings. Skeletal Radiol 2004;33:451–457.

11. Schlegel T, Boublik M, Godfrey J. Complete proximal adductor longus ruptures in professional football players. Presented at American Orthopaedic Society for Sports Medicine Specialty Day, Chicago, March 25, 2006.
12. Strauss E, Campbell K, Bosco J. Analysis of the cross-sectional area of the adductor longus tendon. Am J Sports Med 2007;35:996–999. Epub 2007 Feb 16.
13. Tuite D, Finegan P, Siliaris A, et al. Anatomy of the proximal musculotendinous junction of the adductor longus muscle. Knee Surg Sports Traumatol Arthrosc 1998;6:134–137.
14. Tyler T, Nicholas S, Campbell R, et al. The association of hip strength and flexibility with the incidence of adductor muscle strains in professional ice hockey players. Am J Sports Med 2001;29: 124–128.
15. Tyler T, Nicholas S, Campbell R, et al. The effectiveness of a preseason exercise program to prevent adductor muscle strains in professional ice hockey players. Am J Sports Med 2002;30:680–683.
16. Verall G, Slavotinek J, Fon G, et al. Outcome of conservative management of athletic chronic groin injury diagnosed as pubic bone stress injury. Am J Sports Med 2007;35:467–474.

Chapter 30 Proximal Hamstring Injury

Robert T. Sullivan and William E. Garrett

DEFINITION

- Stretch-induced proximal hamstring injury is common among athletes.
- These injuries represent a continuum including strain at the musculotendinous junction (MTJ), partial tear of the tendon, or complete avulsion of the hamstring muscle complex from the ischial tuberosity.[1,9]

ANATOMY

- The hamstring muscle group consists of three muscles: the biceps femoris (long and short heads); the semitendinosus; and the semimembranosus. All three muscles, except for the short head of the biceps femoris, originate from the ischial tuberosity of the pelvis.
- The biceps femoris and semitendinosus have a common origin.
- The hamstrings are biarticular muscles bridging the hip and knee.
- The proximal tendons of the biceps femoris and semimembranosus have been shown to extend for about 62% and 73%, respectively, of their muscle bellies.[9,11]
- The sciatic nerve lies immediately lateral to the hamstring origin.

PATHOGENESIS

- Eccentric activation while under stretch, as seen in a flexed hip and extended knee when the hamstrings attempt to decelerate the leg during knee extension in high-speed sports-related activity, is thought to be the principal mechanism of injury.[2,21]
- An additional, but rare, mechanism for hamstring injury is extreme stretch with an uncertain amount of muscle activation. This may occur in situations such as waterskiing or when the knee is extended and there is sudden hip flexion.[1,9,11,18]

NATURAL HISTORY

- The natural history of these injuries varies considerably, with a more proximal injury resulting in a longer time for recovery to pre-injury status and a greater likelihood of surgical intervention due to the persistent and significant disability associated with hamstring avulsion.[1]
- Partial or complete hamstring avulsions should not be confused with strain at the musculotendinous junction. Avulsions can be extremely disabling and, unlike strain at the musculotendinous junction, may warrant surgical intervention. Avulsions cause symptoms of weakness and loss of muscle control, especially during fast-paced running.
- Fortunately, most proximal hamstring injuries are strains at the musculotendinous junction that are best managed nonoperatively. Strains most often occur in the biceps femoris, and the most common location is near the muscle–tendon junction. Recovery time has been correlated directly with the percentage of muscle involved by measuring the cross-sectional area or the longitudinal length of abnormal muscle signal on MRI.[1,5,13,20]
- Injuries involving over 50% of the cross-sectional area result in a recovery period longer than 6 weeks, whereas normal imaging findings result in a recovery period of approximately 1 week.[13]
- The greatest risk factor for injury to the hamstring muscle complex is a history of previous injury to the same place.[16,21] Peterson[17] reported the recurrence rate for hamstring injury to be 12% to 31%. Whether the reinjury is attributed to insufficient rehabilitation and early return to sport or the persistence of pre-existing risk factors, the treating physician must have the ability to assess the degree of injury, a knowledge of the reparative process of healing muscle, and an understanding of the rehabilitative and preventive measures for hamstring injury.

PATIENT HISTORY AND PHYSICAL FINDINGS

- Proximal hamstring injury typically results in sudden onset of pain in the posterior proximal thigh during athletic competition or training.
- Severe injury, such as an avulsion, may present with a visible deformity, swelling, ecchymosis, and a palpable defect. Focal tenderness to palpation and pain on provocation with resisted knee flexion are consistent findings.
- With the patient lying prone and the hamstrings activated, palpation of proximal hamstring origin is undertaken.
  - A palpable defect implies proximal avulsion.
  - Pain without a defect suggests partial avulsion.
- Obvious increase in apparent hamstring flexibility of the injured extremity implies proximal avulsion.
- The current classification of muscle injuries identifies mild, moderate, and severe injuries, based on the degree of clinical impairment.
  - *Mild muscle injury* is minimal to no loss of strength, whereas *moderate injury* is a clear loss of strength.
  - *Severe injury* is the complete absence of muscle function. In severe injury, neurogenic symptoms may be present secondary to direct compression or a traction neuritis on the adjacent sciatic nerve.

IMAGING AND OTHER DIAGNOSTIC STUDIES

- Plain radiographs are useful in evaluating for a bony avulsion.
- MRI is the imaging of choice to confirm the existence of a muscle injury or avulson, particularly when a discrepancy exists between the examiner's findings and the patient's symptoms.

- In separate investigations Connell, Kouloris, Askling, and Slavotinek correlated rehabilitation time to the percentage of muscle involved by measuring the cross-sectional area or the longitudinal length of abnormal muscle signal on MRI.
  - Kouloris stated injuries involving greater than 50% of the cross-sectional area resulted in a greater than 6 week recovery period, whereas normal imaging resulted in a recovery period of approximately 1 week.[1,5,13,20]
  - Schneider-Kolsky et al[19] questioned the ability of MRI to predict rehabilitation time for minor and moderate injury. Despite a limitation of variable methods of rehabilitation, they concluded MRI to be useful in predicting the duration of convalescence for moderate and severe injury. Conversely, they determined clinical assessment to be slightly better than MRI for minor injury.
  - Verall reported on a subset of patients with a clear clinical diagnosis of hamstring strain, but an MRI negative for muscle injury. Like Schneider-Kolsky's findings, Verall reported patients with hamstring muscle strain injuries demonstrable by MRI had a poorer prognosis than those whose posterior thigh injury was not MRI-positive. Askling also demonstrated a correlation between the location of injury by MRI and time to recovery. He found longer recovery times for injuries in close proximity to the hamstring origin. In other words, the more cranial the injury the longer the recovery time. Interestingly, the prediction of recovery time was equally good using the point of highest pain on palpation, established within 3 weeks of the injury.
- MRI is most useful in the setting of moderate or severe injury to predict recovery time based on injury location or percentage of involved muscle or to detect an avulsion imperceptible on physical exam due to a massive hematoma or swelling (**FIG 1**).

DIFFERENTIAL DIAGNOSIS

- Referred lower back pain (discogenic, arthropathy, etc.)
- Radiculopathy (HNP, spinal stenosis)
- Sciatica
- Tumor
- Piriformis syndrome
- Apophysitis
- Pelvic stress fracture

NONOPERATIVE MANAGEMENT

- The vast majority of proximal hamstring injuries involve strain at the musculotendinous junction and are managed with nonoperative measures focusing on restoration of flexibility and muscle strength.[8,10]
- Treatment of a proximal hamstring injury is predicated on the grade or severity of the injury and an understanding of the balanced progression of muscle regeneration and scar formation.[10]
- Proximal hamstring strains are typically treated with a few days of rest based on the grade of injury followed by early active and passive mobilization within the limits of pain.
  - Ice and compression are useful adjuncts to diminish bleeding and inflammation as large hematomas may adversely influence scar formation.
  - Sport specific training usually starts approximately 2 weeks post injury.
  - If there is no improvement by 3 to 4 weeks, an MRI should be obtained.
  - Once athletes return to their sports, they should continue an in-season strengthening and stretching program, as prevention of reinjury is critical due to the high rate of recurrence.[2,6,17,21,22]

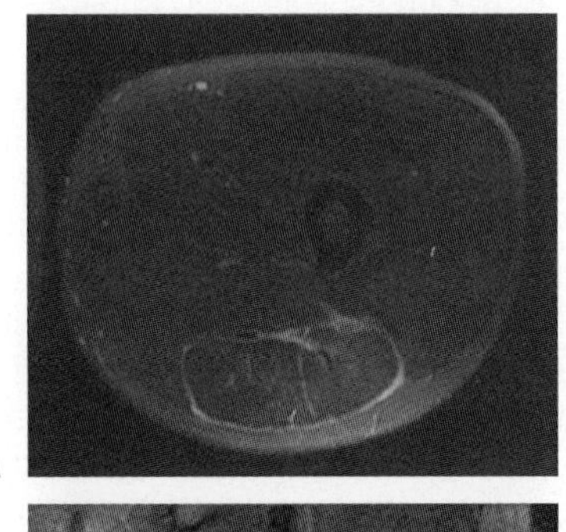

A

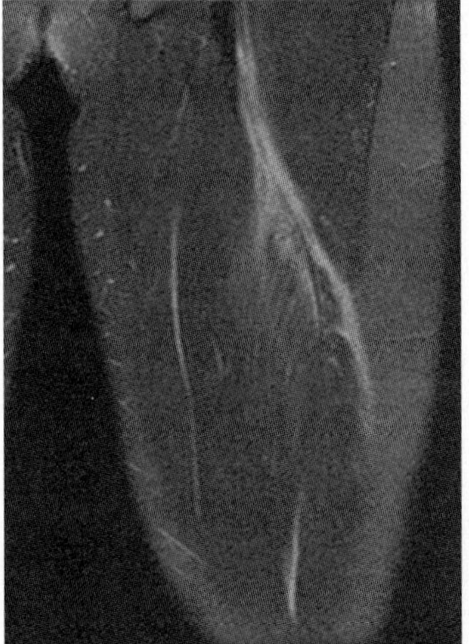

B

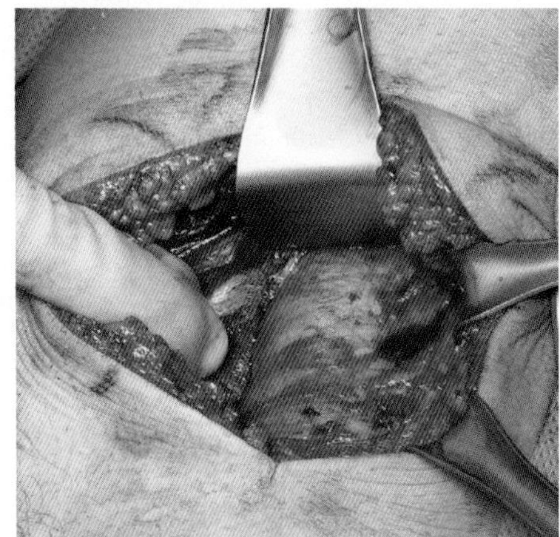

C

FIG 1 • **A,B.** Hamstring strain reveals increased T2 signal along the entire length of the left hamstrings, particularly along the musculotendinous junction, involving the biceps femoris and to a lesser degree the semitendinosus and semimembranosus. **C.** Surgical exposure reveals complete avulsion of the proximal tendon from the ischial tuberosity. (**C:** Courtesy of Gary Fetzer, MD, and Brad Nelson, MD, Minneapolis.)

SURGICAL MANAGEMENT

- Unlike proximal hamstring strains, treatment of hamstring avulsion may necessitate surgical repair, particularly in the high demand athlete or in individuals with complete rupture of the proximal hamstring complex. Complete avulsion has been rarely reported, as most avulsion injuries are partial and involve the biceps femoris.
- Several authors have reported on acute and delayed surgical intervention for partial and complete proximal hamstring avulsions with satisfactory outcomes.[3,4,7,12,14,15] Late diagnosis and delayed intervention are believed to lead to an inferior result. Most arguments for surgical intervention are derived from Sallay's initial report on the poor outcome from nonoperative management in five waterskiers with complete avulsions who were unable to run or return to sporting activity. Sallay also reported on a prolonged recovery time and diminished function in seven individuals with partial avulsions.
- There is some interest in the surgical treatment of partial avulsions, but there are few studies proving poor results in nonoperatively managed partial avulsions.[14]

Preoperative Planning

- Plain radiographs of the pelvis are obtained to evaluate for a bony avulsion.
- MRI is obtained to confirm a partial or complete avulsion and to assess the degeree of hamstring retraction.
- A neurovascular exam of the affected extremity is documented.
- EMG may be considered to evaluate a persistent, perceived neurologic deficit.

Positioning

- The patient is placed in the prone position over chest rolls.
- The operative extremity is draped free to allow for hip and knee flexion and extension.

Approach

- In acute cases with minimal hamstring retraction, we use a tranverse incison within the gluteal crease.
- A longitudinal incision starting from the ischial tuberosity, over the posterior thigh, is used in chronic cases requiring significant mobilization or fractional lengthening of the hamstrings or sciatic neurolysis. A longitudinal incision is also employed in acute cases with significant retraction (**FIG 2**).

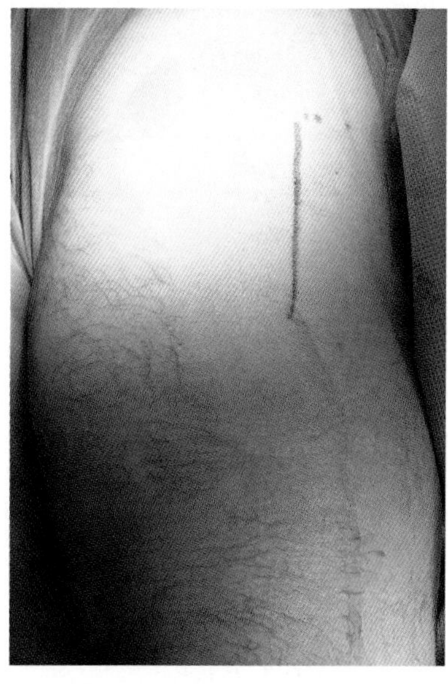

FIG 2 • A longitudinal incision starting from the ischial tuberosity, over the posterior thigh, is used in chronic cases requiring significant mobilization or fractional lengthening of the hamstrings or sciatic neurolysis. A longitudinal incision is also employed in acute cases with significant retraction. (Courtesy of Gary Fetzer, MD, and Brad Nelson, MD, Minneapolis, MN.)

REPAIR OF HAMSTRING COMPLETE AVULSION

TECHNIQUES

- The posterior femoral cutaneous nerve and its proximal branches are identified running deep to fascia down the back of the thigh obliquely crossing the long head of the biceps femoris.
  - Branches of the posterior femoral cutaneous nerve are the inferior cluneals and perineals.
  - The inferior clunial nerves, three or four in number, turn upward around the lower border of the gluteus maximus.
  - The perineal branches are distributed to the skin at the upper and medial side of the thigh.
- The inferior border of the gluteus maximus muscle is mobilized by dividing the posterior fascia and retracting the muscle superiorly in order to expose the ischial tuberosity and avulsed tendon stumps.
- Starting distally from normal anatomy, the sciatic nerve is identified lateral to the ischium.
  - If required, a careful sciatic neurolysis is performed in chronic cases.
  - Care is taken to identify and protect the branches to the semimembranosus.
- The avulsed tendon stumps are identified and tagged with a grasping suture using a no. 2 high strength suture (**TECH FIG 1A**).
- Mobilization of the tendon stumps and proximal musculature is carefully performed in order to minimize tension on the repair and limit the amount of knee flexion, if any, required to aproximate the tendons to their origin on the lateral aspect of the ischial tuberosity. In chronic cases, a distal hamstring lengthening may be necessary.
- If there is an adequate residual, proximal tendon stump, a direct repair is performed. Otherwise the repair is performed using suture anchors after clearing the soft tissue from the the anatomic footprint on the ischial tuberosity (**TECH FIG 1B**).
- If a tendon cannot be mobilized to its anatomic origin on the ischium other authors have reported tenodesing the tendon to the adjacent myotendinous complex.
- The fascia and overlying skin are then approximated in separate layers.

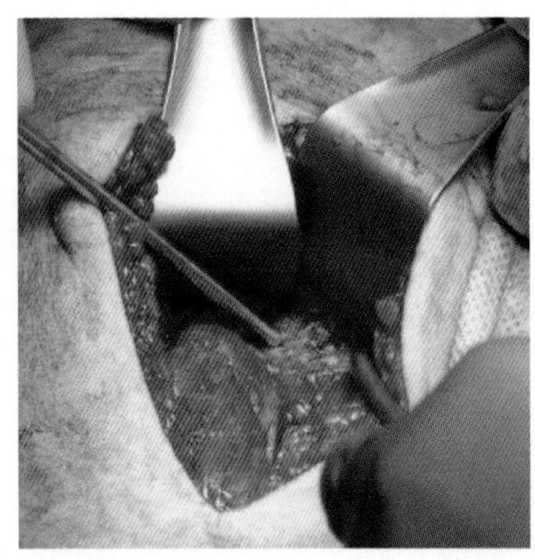

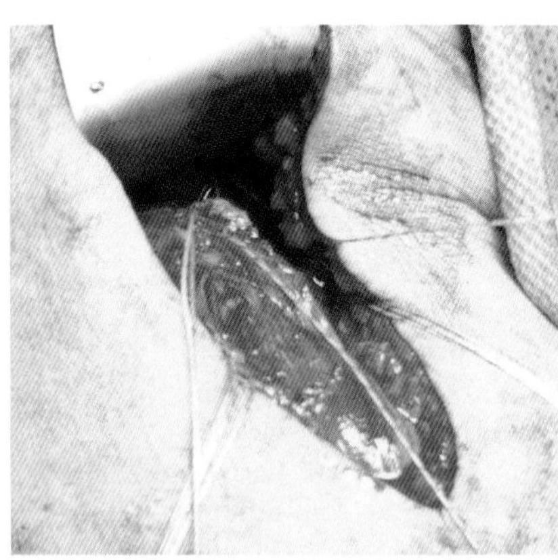

TECH FIG 1 • **A.** The repair is performed using suture anchors after clearing the soft tissue from the anatomic footprint. **B.** Final suture passage is completed, demonstrating reapproximation of the avulsed tendon to the ischial tuberosity. (Courtesy of Gary Fetzer, MD, and Brad Nelson, MD, Minneapolis.)

PEARLS AND PITFALLS

Indications	■ Complete, proximal hamstring avulsions confirmed by exam and imaging are best managed with acute repair, especially in the high performance athlete.
Anatomy	■ The biceps femoris and semitendinosus share a common origin on the lateral aspect of the ischial tuberosity.
Surgical exposure	■ The cluneal and sciatic nerves lie in close proximity to the hamstring origin and must be identified and protected from direct injury or stretch due to overzealous retraction.

POSTOPERATIVE CARE

■ The knee is held in the minimal amount of flexion to limit tension on the repair for approximatley 3 to 4 weeks.

■ Range of motion is initiated thereafter in order to obtain a normal gait by 6 weeks post surgery.

■ A progressive strengthening regimen is initiated after 6 weeks with a return to sports related activity no earlier than 3 months after surgery.

OUTCOMES

■ Klingele[13] reported on suture anchor fixation in 11 individuals (average age 41.5 years) with complete proximal avulsion injuries. There were 7 acute and 4 chronic (>4 weeks) injuries treated with a 78% return to sport by 6 months and a 91% satisfaction after a minimum 2 year follow-up. Varying degrees of hamstring mobilization and fractional lengthening were performed in the chronic cases. However, for patients who underwent repair of chronic injuries the average hamstring muscle strength was 89% of the uninjured extremity by cybex testing at an average 34-month follow-up.

■ Chakravarthy performed either direct or suture anchor repair in 4 patients, 1 acute and 3 chronic, with all patients obtaining normal strength and near-normal flexibility at an average 15 months of follow-up.[4] Three of these four patients returned to their preinjury level of sport.

■ Cross performed repairs on 9 patients (average age 34 years) with chronic, complete avulsions at an average of 36 months post injury.[7] These patients were held at 90 degrees of knee flexion for 8 weeks after surgery with full knee range of motion obtained by 14 weeks in all cases. At an average 4 year follow-up, hamstring strength was 60% of the unaffected side with 7 of 9 patients having returned to a lower level of sports.

■ Brucker performed surgical repair in 8 complete avulsions, 6 acute and 2 chronic, also immobilizing the operative extremity at 90 degrees of knee flexion for 6 weeks post surgery.[3] Full range of motion was obtained in all patients by 16 weeks. At 33 months follow-up all patients were satisfied and 7 had returned to sports. The minimum time to return to sports was 6 to 8 months with 2 individuals delayed more than 24 months. Objective measures revealed no difference in hamstring flexibility relative to the contralateral extremity. Cybex dynanometer testing revealed an average peak torque of the operated hamstring muscles of 88.8% compared to the opposite limb.

■ Orava described surgical intervention in 8 patients, 5 acute and 3 chronic, with complete or incomplete proximal avulsions using suture anchors, drill holes, or tenodesis of the avulsed hamstring to an adjacent and intact hamstring.[15] Hip and knee flexion were avoided for 1 month with full weight bearing initiated at 1 month. All 5 acutes exhibited normal strength and full range of motion at 5.7 year follow-up. However, those patients surgically treated 3 or more months from their injury had inferior outcomes.

■ Lempainen recently described surgical repair of 48 MRI confirmed partial proximal hamstring avulsions or tendon tears in athletes who failed to respond to nonsurgical measures.[14] Forty-three of these injuries were operated on more than 4 weeks from the time of injury with an average delay of 13 months. No immobilization was performed and full weight bearing was initiated at 2 weeks after repair. Eighty-eight percent of these patients reported good or excellent results and 87% returned to their preinjury level of sport at a mean follow-up of 36 months. However, this population predominantly consisted of patients who had failed conservative treatment. There are no reports on the number of patients successfully managed with nonoperative measures for partial avulsions.

- Despite variable technique, degree of chronicity, and heterogeneous patient populations, these reports indicate repair of acute and chronic complete or partial proximal hamstring avulsion can improve patient outcomes. Early surgical intervention for complete tears is preferred in order to limit hamstring retraction and muscle atrophy and to obtain a better functional outcome. Whether or not surgical treatment should be considered in the acute setting for partial injuries remains unclear. The delay in return to sport and the persistent functional impairment associated with partial avulsions as reported by Sallay and Lempainen suggests further study is warranted regarding the indications and timing of surgical intervention in this population.

COMPLICATIONS

- Surgical repair of proximal hamstring avulsions have resulted in satisfactory outcomes; however, several authors have reported on several patients with persistent pain and/or spasm associated with strenuous exercise.
- Brucker reported on a loss of fixation for a single suture anchor from the ischial tuberosity. The anchor was removed in a second surgical procedure due to pain in a sitting position.
- Others have reported on perisitent sciatica mandating a neurolysis to address postoperative scarring.

REFERENCES

1. Askling C, Saartok T, Thorstensson A. Type of acute hamstring strain affects flexibility, strength and time to return to pre-injury level. Br J Sports Med 2006;40:40–44.
2. Brooks J, Fuller C, Kemp S, et al. Incidence, risk, and prevention of hamstring muscle injuries in professional rugby union. Am J Sports Med 2006;34;1297–1304.
3. Brucker P, Imhoff A. Functional assessment after acute and chronic complete ruptures of the proximal hamstring tendons. Knee Surg Sports Traumatol Arthrosc 2005;13:411–418.
4. Chakravarthy J, Ramisetty N, Pimpalnerkar A, et al. Surgical repair of complete proximal hamstring tendon ruptures in water skiers and bull riders: a report of four cases and review of the literature. Br J Sports Med 2005;39:569–572.
5. Connell D, Schneider-Kolsky M, Hoving J, et al. Longitudinal study comparing sonographic and MRI assessments of acute and healing hamstring injuries. Am J Radiol 2004;183:975–984.
6. Crosier J. Factors associated with recurrent hamstring injuries. Sports Med 2004;34:681–695.
7. Cross M, Vandersluis R, Wood D, et al. Surgical repair of chronic complete hamstring tendon rupture in the adult patient. Am J Sports Med 1998;26:785–788.
8. De Smet A, Best T. MR imaging of the distribution and location of acute hamstring injuries in athletes. Am J Radiol 2000;174:393–399.
9. Garrett W Jr. Muscle strain injuries. Am J Sports Med 1996;24(6 Suppl):S2–S8.
10. Jarvinen TA, Jarvinen TL, Kalimo H, et al. Muscle injuries: biology and treatment. Am J Sports Med 2005;33:745–764.
11. Kirkendall D, Garrett W Jr. Clinical perspectives regarding eccentric muscle injury. Clin Orthop Relat Res 2002;430S:S81–S89.
12. Klingele K, Sallay P. Surgical repair of complete proximal hamstring tendon rupture. Am.J Sports Med 2002;30:742–747.
13. Koulouris G, Connell D. Evaluation of the hamstring muscle complex following acute injury. Skeletal Radiol 2003;32:582–589.
14. Lempainen L, Sarimo J, Heikkila J, et al. Surgical treatment of partial tears of the proximal origin of the hamstring muscles. Br J Sports Med 2006;40:688–691.
15. Orava S, Kujala U. Rupture of the ischial origin of the hamstring muscles. Am J Sports Med 1995;23:702–705.
16. Orchard J. Intrinsic and extrinsic risk factors for muscle strains in Australian football. Am J Sports Med 2001;29:300–303.
17. Peterson J, Holmich P.Evidence based prevention of hamstring injuries in sport. Br J Sports Med 2005;39:319–323.
18. Sallay P, Friedman R, Coogan P, et al. Hamstring muscle injuries among water skiers: functional outcome and prevention. Am J Sports Med 1996;24:130–136.
19. Scneider-Kolsky M, Hoving J, Warren P, et al. A comparison between clinical assessment and magnetic resonance imaging of acute hamstring injuries. Am J Sports Med 2006;34:1008–1015.
20. Slavotinek J, Verall G, Fon G. Hamstring injury in athletes: using MR imaging measurements to compare extent of muscle injury with amount of time lost from competition. Am J Radiol 2002;179:1621–1628.
21. Verall G, Slaovotinek P, Barnes P, et al. Clinical risk factors for hamstring muscle strain injury: a prospective study with correlation of injury by magnetic resonance imaging. B J Sports Med 2001;35:435–439.
22. Verall G, Slavotinek P, Barnes P. The effect of sports specific training on reducing the incidence of hamstring injuries in professional Australian Rules football players. Br J Sports Med 2005;39:363–368.

Chapter 31 Knee Arthroscopy: The Basics

Steven A. Aviles and Christina R. Allen

DEFINITION

- Knee arthroscopy is a video-assisted surgical intervention for intra-articular disease of the knee.

ANATOMY

- The knee can be divided into three compartments: the patellofemoral joint, the lateral tibiofemoral joint, and the medial tibiofemoral joint.
- The patellofemoral compartment is composed of the suprapatellar pouch, the patella bone, its femoral articulation (called the trochlea), the medial and lateral femoral condyles, and the medial and lateral patellofemoral ligaments.
- The suprapatellar pouch is a potential space that develops when the knee joint is insufflated with fluid. Within this area, adhesions, plicae, and loose bodies may be found. Adhesions are commonly found with revision surgery.
  - Synovial plicae are bands of synovium that are remnants from fetal development. Their location and size may contribute to snapping sensations and inflammation within the joint. In the suprapatellar pouch, however, they most commonly provide a location for loose bodies to hide.
  - Suprapatellar plicae may partition an entire compartment within the pouch, leaving only a centralized hole by which loose bodies may gain entrance. These holes are called porta.
- The patella is one of the sesamoid bones of the body. It has a medial and a lateral facet that articulate with its respective condyles. Centrally, there is an apex of the bone that sits in the trochlea.
  - The patella has the thickest cartilage in the body, which is used to withstand forces up to five times body weight.
  - With normal articulation of the patella on the femur, the cartilage of the medial facet touches the medial femoral condyle. This can be visualized with arthroscopy.
  - The patella begins to engage the trochlea at approximately 20 degrees and fully engages at 45 degrees. Lack of contact of the medial facet with the medial femoral condyle at these points in the range of motion suggests malalignment.
- The medial and lateral patellofemoral ligaments are thickenings of the medial and lateral retinaculum respectively. They originate centrally on the patella and insert onto the medial and lateral epicondyles of the femur.
  - The medial patellofemoral ligament may become disrupted or attenuated with patellar dislocations. This may predispose to further dislocations, necessitating operative repair.
  - The lateral patellofemoral ligament and retinaculum are often released in efforts to restore patellofemoral alignment.
- The medial tibiofemoral compartment is composed of the medial gutter and the tibiofemoral articulation.
  - The medial gutter is a fold of synovium in the posteromedial aspect of the joint where loose bodies may hide. Ballottement of this space is essentially to ensure that no potential sources of pain exist within this region.
  - The medial tibial plateau is larger in the sagittal plane than the lateral plateau (**FIG 1**). It is a concave surface that articulates with a convex femoral condyle, but the plateau has a much flatter curvature than the femoral condyle. Given the relative incongruence, contact pressures would be focused on a smaller surface area, leading to higher point contact stresses and cartilage degeneration.
  - The medial meniscus exists to alleviate this problem. The medial meniscus is a C-shaped structure on the perimeter of the medial tibiofemoral articulation. On cross section, it is triangular, with the wider area along the periphery.
    - The meniscus provides better congruence between the two surfaces, participates in load sharing, and decreases point contact pressures throughout the articulation.
    - It is connected to the tibial plateau at the posterior and anterior ends at the meniscal roots. The deep medial collateral ligament attaches to the medial meniscus at its body centrally, providing stability. It is also attached to the capsule along its periphery.
    - The undersurface of the meniscus is not adherent to the plateau and can be lifted up, permitting inspection when one is suspicious of undersurface tears of the meniscus.
- In the lateral tibiofemoral compartment, the meniscus is shaped more like an O than a C. It has a similar cross-sectional anatomy as the medial meniscus, except it covers about 75% of the lateral tibiofemoral articulation. This is due to the geometry of the bony structures.
- Although the lateral femoral condyle is quite similar to the medial femoral condyle, the lateral tibial plateau is substantially different.
  - The lateral femoral condyle and the lateral tibial plateau are two convex surfaces. To provide appropriate congruence, a larger meniscus is necessary.

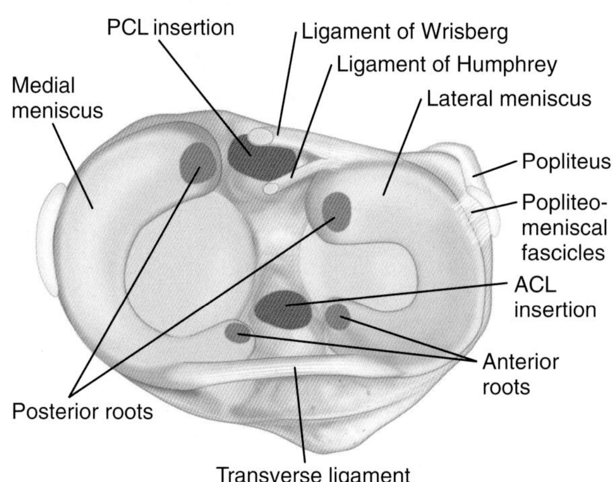

FIG 1 • The tibial plateau.

- The popliteus tendon inserts onto the posterior body of the lateral meniscus and provides stability to the meniscal body. It attaches to the meniscus by means of three popliteomeniscal fascicles: the anteroinferior, posterosuperior, and posteroinferior fascicles. Anterior and posterior to the insertion of the tendon on the lateral meniscus is a recess of the joint capsule that does not insert onto the periphery of the meniscus. This makes the lateral meniscus more mobile than the medial meniscus.
- Along the posterior horn of the meniscus originate two ligaments that insert into the femur. The ligament of Wrisberg travels posterior to the posterior cruciate ligament (PCL) to insert onto the femur; the ligament of Humphrey travels anterior to the PCL and inserts onto the femur.

- Between the medial and lateral articulations is the intercondylar notch. It is a nonarticular portion of the knee that extends distally and posteriorly from the trochlea.
  - In the most anterior aspect of the notch lies the transverse meniscal ligament. This is a ligament that originates at the anterior horn of the medial meniscus away from the anterior root and inserts on the anterior horn of the lateral meniscus anterior to the anterior root of the lateral meniscus.
  - This space between the transverse ligament and the anterior horn of the medial and lateral menisci is often mistaken for a tear of the menisci on magnetic resonance imaging (MRI).
  - There is significant bony variation in terms of the width of the intercondylar notch; this may contribute to the decision to perform a notchplasty or notch widening when performing an anterior cruciate ligament (ACL) reconstruction.
  - The ACL and PCL reside within the intercondylar notch.
    - The ACL originates at the posterolateral position (about 10:30 on a right knee and 1:30 on a left knee) of the inner wall of the notch and inserts centrally and anteriorly on the tibia. In the sagittal plane, it inserts slightly posterior to the anterior horn of the lateral meniscus and about 7 mm anterior to the PCL fibers.
    - The PCL originates from the anterior aspect of the medial wall of the notch and has a broad origination that begins at about 12 o'clock and ends around 3:30 (on a right knee). This ligament travels posterior to the ACL and inserts centrally on the posterior aspect of the tibial plateau about 10 to 15 mm inferior to the joint line. The fibers run quite close to the posterior root of the medial meniscus and one must be careful not to deviate medially when débriding PCL remnants in this region during a PCL reconstruction.

SURGICAL MANAGEMENT

Preoperative Planning

- Each patient is unique and the equipment needed for each surgery will vary. The surgeon must review the case specifics and studies before surgery and ensure that all necessary equipment is available when the surgery begins.
- On the day of surgery, the surgeon should reconfirm with the patient the laterality of the procedure, "sign your site," and verify that there has been no change in the signs and symptoms of the injury since the last office visit.
- The surgeon performs an examination under anesthesia to reconfirm the diagnosis because this is crucial to understanding the nature of the injury. With sedation, the patient is more relaxed and able to give a more sensitive examination.

Positioning

- The patient should be supine and close to the edge of the bed.
  - The surgeon should verify that he or she will be able to get proper flexion of the leg should it be necessary to drop the foot of the bed.
- The contralateral leg can be placed in a well-padded leg holder or secured to the bed with circumferential padding.
- The use of a thigh holder versus a lateral post for arthroscopy is based on surgeon preference.
  - The thigh holder can be used with the foot of the bed dropped to 90 degrees, or the leg may be abducted and brought over the side of the bed (**FIG 2A**).
  - Commercial knee holders may not be capable of holding very large knees or pediatric knees. In these cases, a lateral post is preferred (**FIG 2B**).

Approach

- The approach largely depends on what arthroscopic knee procedure is going to be performed.
- Regardless, portal placement is the key to successful knee arthroscopy.

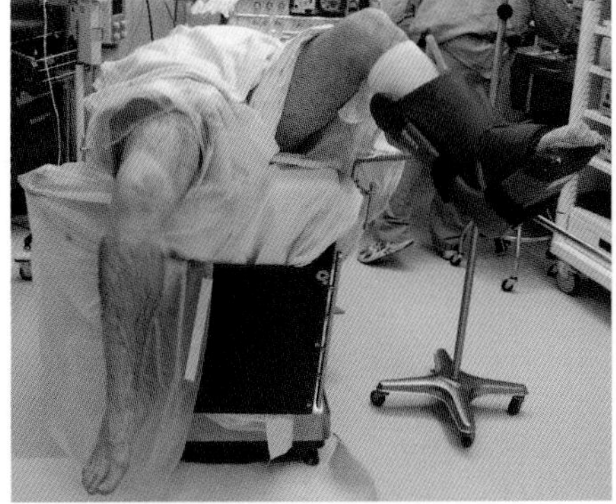
A

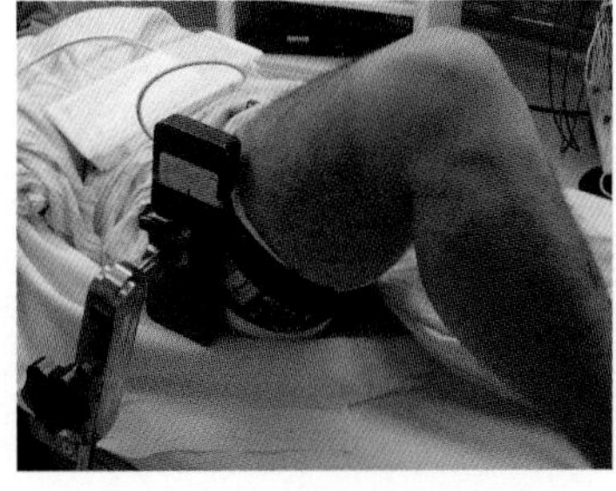
B

FIG 2 • **A.** Use of a thigh holder for the right surgical leg, with left leg elevated and protected in a "well-leg" holder. **B.** Use of a lateral post for right knee positioning during arthroscopy.

TECHNIQUES

PORTAL PLACEMENT

- TECH FIG 1 shows the locations of the far lateral, anterolateral, anteromedial, and far medial portals and their relationships to landmarks of the knee.

Anterolateral Portal

- Most arthroscopic visualization is performed through this portal.
- It is created just lateral to the patella tendon. The incision is usually placed just inferior to the inferior aspect of the patella. Alternatively, the incision can also be referenced from the tibia.
- The incision should measure 1 cm long.
- Typically the incision is made vertically, but some surgeons prefer a horizontal incision, which may aid in preventing inadvertent laceration to the infrapatellar branch of the saphenous nerve.

Anteromedial Portal

- This is the primary working portal.
- Its position is highly dependent on the work that needs to be done.
- Traditionally, it is slightly more inferior than the anterolateral portal and just medial to the patella tendon, but the surgeon should be liberal about moving the location of this portal to optimize the surgical goals of the arthroscopy (ie, meniscal surgery versus mosaicplasty).
- The surgeon can use a spinal needle to localize the optimal portal placement before making the anteromedial portal incision.

Superomedial or Superolateral Portal

- A superior portal can be placed either medial or lateral to the quadriceps tendon.
  - We prefer a superolateral portal because it results in less vastus medialis oblique inhibition.
- This portal can be used as an inflow or outflow portal or to perform procedures in the suprapatellar pouch (ie, loose body removal, medial retinaculum plication, synovectomy, or evaluation of patella tracking).
- This portal is placed about 2.5 cm proximal to the superior pole of the patella at the edge of the quadriceps tendon.

Central (Transpatellar) Portal

- This portal uses a vertical incision through the central third of the patellar tendon at the level of the joint line.
- It is mostly used to facilitate access to the intercondylar notch.

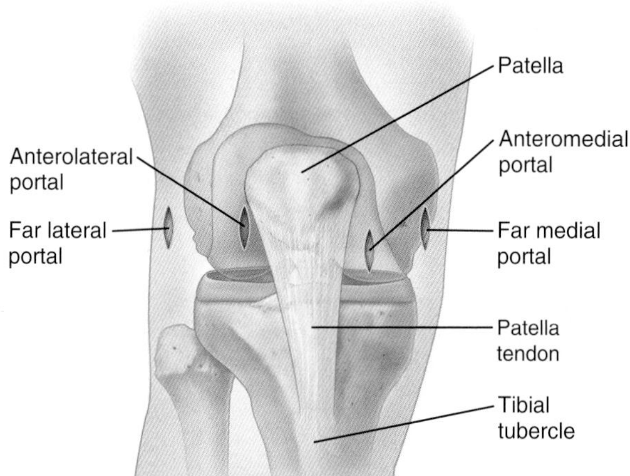

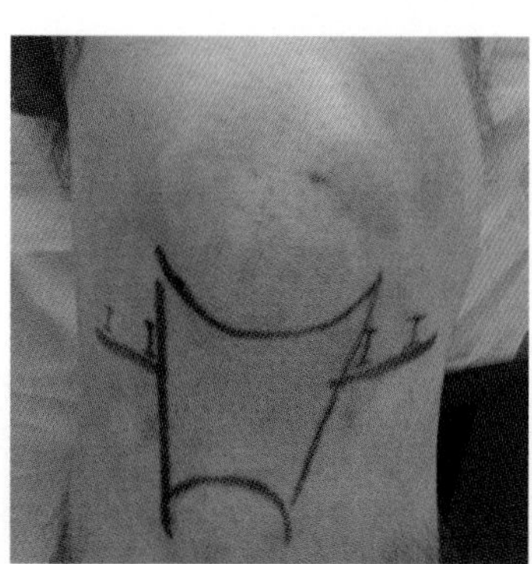

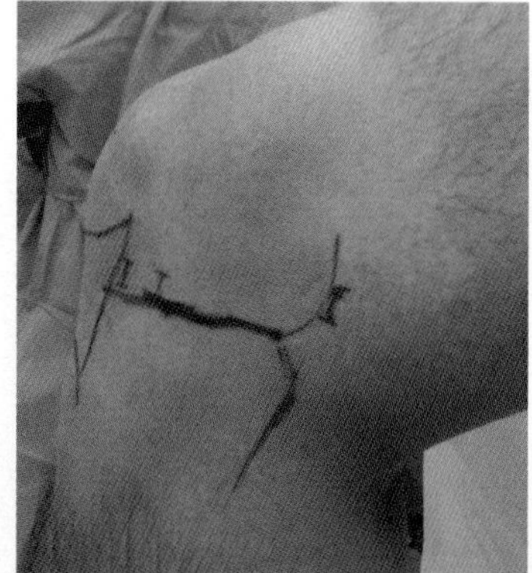

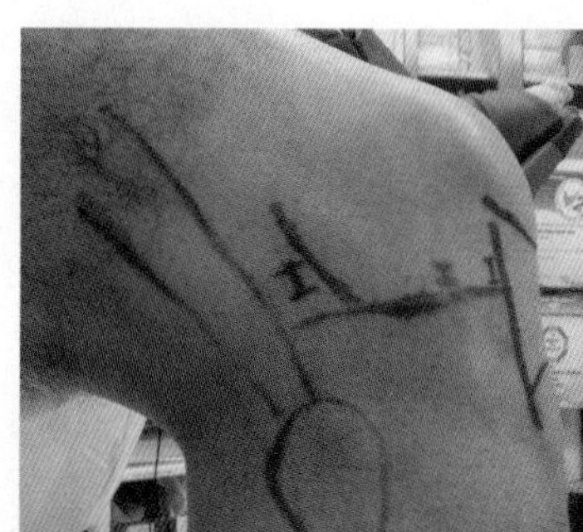

TECH FIG 1 • Artist's rendition (**A**) and anterior view (**B**) of the right knee showing portal placement of far lateral, anterolateral, anteromedial, and far medial portals and their relationships to the inferior pole of the patella, the medial and lateral joint line, and the patellar tendon. **C.** Medial view of right knee showing anteromedial, far medial, and posteromedial portal placement and their relationships to the medial tibial plateau and medial femoral condyle. **D.** Lateral view of right knee far lateral, anterolateral, and posterolateral portal placement and their relationships to the lateral tibial plateau, lateral femoral condyle, fibula, and biceps tendon.

- Occasionally, this portal may be required when performing a modified Gillquist maneuver (examination of the posterior horns of the menisci through the intercondylar notch) in a patient with a stenotic intercondylar notch.

Posteromedial Portal

- When pathology presents in the posteromedial knee, this portal may be used as a working portal.
- To assess the proper placement of this portal, the surgeon performs a modified Gillquist maneuver through the anterolateral portal (technique details are given in the Diagnostic Arthroscopy section) and uses the 70-degree arthroscope to transilluminate the skin overlying the posteromedial capsule.
  - A spinal needle is placed at the center of the transilluminated skin. This position should be about 1 to 2 cm above the joint line.
  - When comfortable with the position of the needle, the surgeon makes a 1-cm skin incision with a no. 11 blade and places a cannula with a blunt obturator to penetrate the capsule. This helps to protect the soft tissues in this area from damage and reduces fluid extravasation into the surrounding soft tissues.
  - The saphenous nerve travels near this area and is at risk of injury with creation of this portal.

Posterolateral Portal

- The indications and technique for this portal are similar to those for the posteromedial portal.
- The surgeon perform the modified Gillquist maneuver through the anteromedial portal and transilluminates the skin overlying the posterolateral capsule of the knee with the 70-degree arthroscope as described above.
- A spinal needle is used to confirm proper portal placement. This portal should be at the lateral aspect of the posterolateral compartment to avoid the large neurovascular structures.
- Before making the skin incision, the surgeon should ensure that the planned incision is anterior to the biceps tendon to avoid the peroneal nerve.

Far Lateral and Far Medial Portals

- These portals are made 2 cm either lateral or medial to their respective anterior portals.
- They can be used to aid in work that needs to be done posterior to the femoral condyles.

DIAGNOSTIC ARTHROSCOPY

Marking Landmarks

- Marking the landmarks of the knee with a sterile surgical marker can be helpful.
- The surgeon can mark the inferior pole of the patella, the patella tendon, and the tibial tubercle.
- The tibial joint line is marked off medially and laterally. This will assist in the accurate placement of the anterolateral and anteromedial portals.

Anterolateral Portal

- Using a no. 11 blade knife, the surgeon places a vertically oriented 1-cm incision just lateral to the patellar tendon and inferior to the patella with the knee at 60 to 90 degrees of flexion.
- The bevel of the knife is buried (blade facing away from the meniscus) to ensure the capsule has been penetrated.
- The knife is angled toward the intercondylar notch to prevent damage to the lateral femoral condyle.

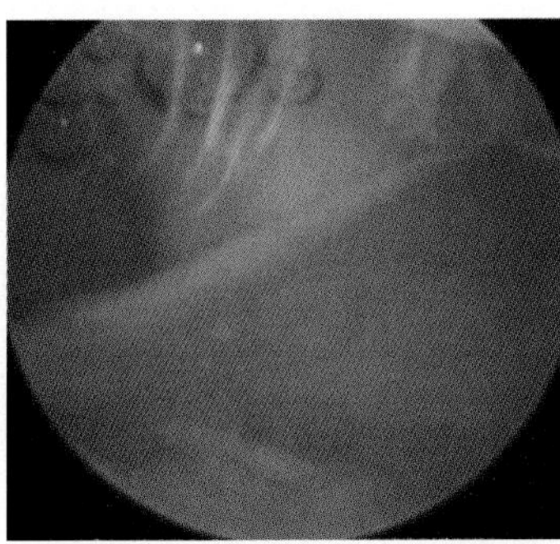

TECH FIG 2 • Arthroscopic view of the suprapatellar pouch showing adhesion running obliquely.

Anteromedial Portal

- Creation of an anteromedial portal is necessary to complete a thorough diagnostic arthroscopy.
- The surgeon may use a probe placed though this portal to palpate the cartilage for injury and perform a complete evaluation of the menisci once the arthroscope has been inserted.
- The position of this portal varies depending on the work being performed. Typically, it is 1 cm medial to the patella tendon and slightly inferior to the anterolateral portal.

Introduction of Obturator and Sheath

- With the knee flexed at 60 to 90 degrees, the arthroscope sheath is placed with a blunt obturator through the anterolateral portal, aiming toward the intercondylar notch.
- Intra-articular position is confirmed by palpating the obturator anterior to the medial compartment.
- By dropping his or her hand, the surgeon pulls the obturator and sheath back slightly.
- As the knee is brought to an extended position, the obturator and sheath is gently advanced in the suprapatellar pouch.

Visualization of Suprapatellar Pouch

- The camera is placed in the suprapatellar pouch (**TECH FIG 2**).
- The size of the pouch is evaluated.
- The surgeon looks for adhesions and loose bodies.

Visualization of the Patella

- The camera is aimed anteriorly (toward the ceiling) to visualize the patella.

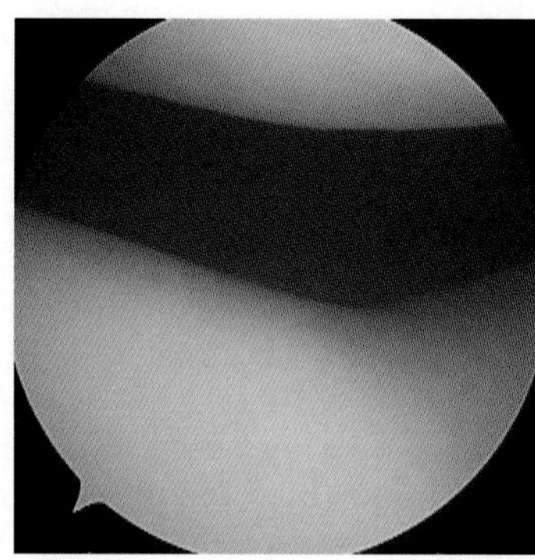

TECH FIG 3 • Arthroscopic view of the apex of the patella and trochlea.

- The arthroscope is retracted until the patella comes into view (TECH FIG 3).
- Pictures of the medial and lateral facets are taken.
- The surgeon's free hand can be used to mobilize the patella for better visualization.
- The cartilage of the patella is probed for evidence for softening, chondral flaps, or fissures.

Visualization of the Trochlea and Condyles

- The arthroscope is aimed toward the femur, and the trochlea and anterior aspects of the medial and lateral femoral condyles are inspected.
- The probe is used to palpate the cartilage for evidence of softening, fissures, and unstable cartilage flaps.

Assessment of Patellar Tracking

- The arthroscope is retracted further and the knee is ranged from flexion to extension to assess patellar tracking.
- The medial facet of the patella should engage the medial aspect of the trochlea at 20 degrees and fully engage in the trochlea at 45 degrees.
- Lateral facet overhang may suggest a tight lateral retinaculum and maltracking.

Lateral Gutter

- The arthroscope is advanced up into the suprapatellar pouch so the tip is proximal to the patella.
- With the patient's knee extended, the surgeon brings the arthroscope over the lateral femoral condyle. The surgeon's hand is raised so that the camera is angling down toward the floor, and the light source is turned so that it is looking distally (TECH FIG 4A).
- The lateral gutter (located between the lateral femoral condyle and the lateral capsule of the knee joint) will be visualized.
- By pushing posteriorly, the insertion of the popliteus tendon and its three popliteomeniscal fascicles of the lateral meniscus may be visualized (TECH FIG 4B,C).

Visualization of the Lateral Meniscocapsular Junction and the Anterior Knee

- The arthroscope is retracted to visualize the attachment of the lateral meniscus to the capsule. This is best performed with the knee in 20 degrees of flexion.

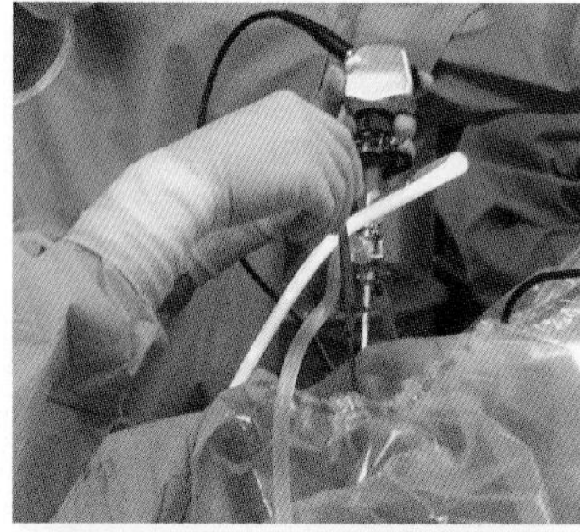

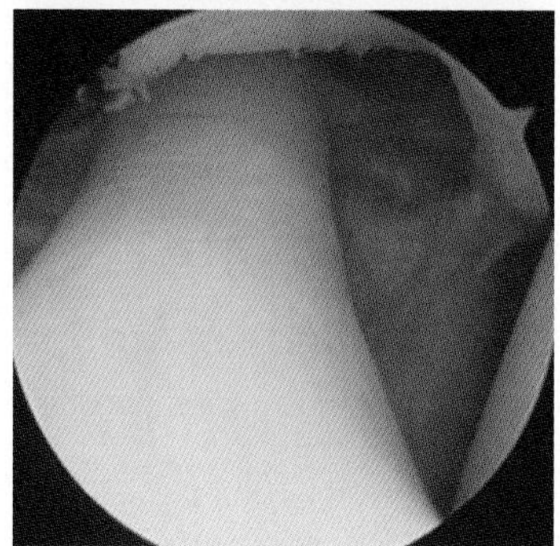

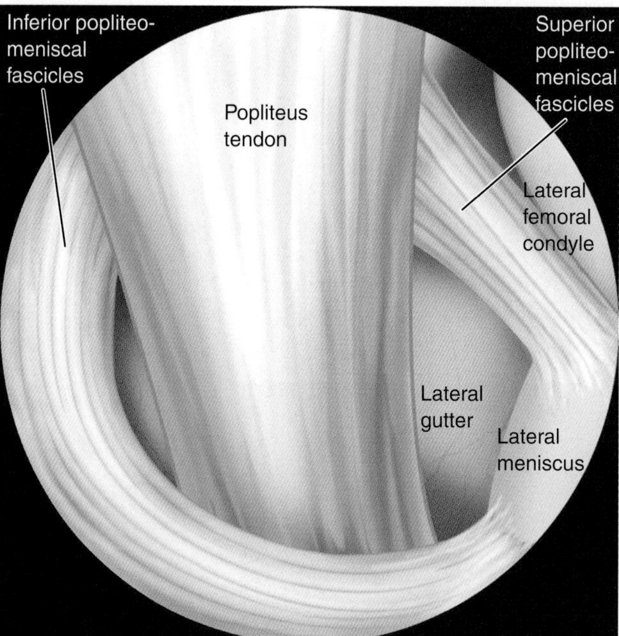

TECH FIG 4 • **A.** Surgeon and arthroscope positioning for performing arthroscopic evaluation of the posterolateral corner of the knee. Arthroscopic view (**B**) and artist's rendition (**C**) of the posterolateral corner of the knee. The popliteus runs superiorly, and the popliteomensical fascicles attach the posterior horn of the lateral meniscus to the popliteus.

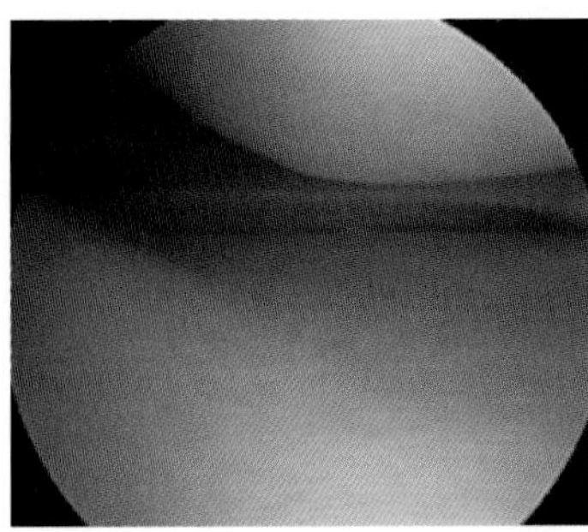

TECH FIG 5 • Arthroscopic view of the medial compartment, including the medial femoral condyle, medial tibial plateau, and medial meniscus.

- A varus stress is applied to the knee at 30 degrees of flexion.
- The lens of the arthroscope is turned medially to visualize the anterior horn of the lateral meniscus.
- The anterior horn of the medial meniscus may also be seen more medially if the view is not blocked by synovium or the anterior fat pad.

Medial Gutter

- The arthroscope is returned to the suprapatellar pouch, and then the surgeon migrates over the medial femoral condyle to the medial gutter.
- By lifting his or her hand and aiming the light source so that the arthroscope is angling toward the floor again, the surgeon can visualize the medial gutter (space between the medial femoral condyle and the medial capsule of the knee joint).
- Ballottement is performed to check for loose bodies.
- A medial meniscal cyst and displaced medial meniscal flap tears may be visualized using this view as well.

Medial Compartment

- From the medial gutter, the medial compartment is entered by bringing the arthroscope toward the midline until the medial femoral condyle is viewed (**TECH FIG 5**).
- The knee is moved through a range of motion from full extension to full flexion. The entire medial femoral condyle is evaluated for cartilage defects.
- The surgeon probes for softening, fissures, and flaps and checks for plica snapping over the condyle as well.
- The posterior portion of the medial compartment is usually best visualized with the leg at 30 degrees, with a valgus stress applied to the knee.
- The medial compartment may widen abnormally with valgus stress so that significant space between the medial tibial plateau and medial femoral condyle exists.
  - The surgeon should suspect a medial collateral ligament injury when this occurs. This is especially true if the meniscus lifts up off the tibial plateau, indicating significant tibial-sided medial collateral ligament laxity.
- The tibial plateau is visualized and probed for chondral abnormalities. The surgeon should visualize the posterior root, posterior horn, body, anterior horn, and anterior root of the meniscus.
- The undersurface of the meniscus is probed and inspected. The meniscus is tested with a hoop stress test.
- The perimeter of the tibial plateau is probed for flipped flap tears of the meniscus.
- In patients who are not ligamentously lax, the posterior horn periphery may be difficult to visualize.
  - In this case a modified Gillquist maneuver may allow better visualization of the posterior horn of the medial meniscus.
- Instruments angled up work best in the medial compartment because the tibial plateau is a convex surface.

Posteromedial Knee

- The surgeon performs the modified Gillquist maneuver.
  - The arthroscope is removed from the sheath and the blunt obturator is placed in the sheath. The knee should not be placed in 70–90 degrees of flexion.
  - The blunt obturator and sheath is placed into the anterolateral portal and advanced into the space between the medial aspect of the intercondylar notch and the posterior cruciate ligament (**TECH FIG 6A**).
  - Gentle pressure is applied until the obturator slides posteriorly.

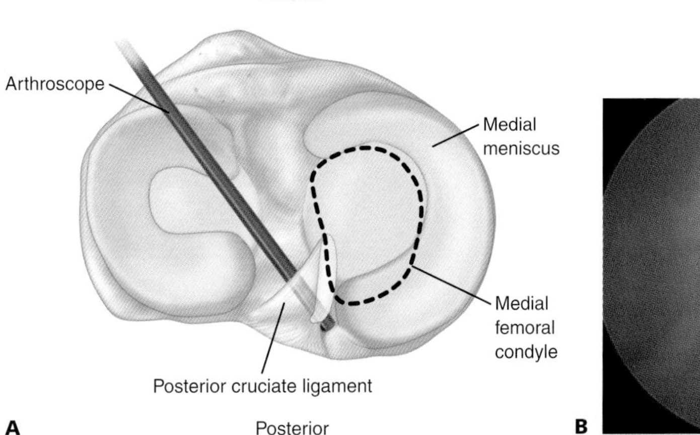

B

TECH FIG 6 • **A.** Artist's rendition of modified Gillquist maneuver, showing arthroscope passing between posterior cruciate ligament and medial femoral condyle. **B.** Arthroscopic view of the posteromedial knee after Gillquist maneuver using a 70-degree arthroscope, including the medial meniscocapsular junction, medial femoral condyle, and medial gutter.

- The blunt obturator is replaced with the 70-degree arthroscope and camera, and the surgeon visualizes the posterior horn of the medial meniscus, the posterior medial femoral condyle, the posterior meniscal root and the capsular attachment, and the insertion of the PCL on the back of the tibial plateau (**TECH FIG 6B**). The surgeon can check for loose bodies as well.

Intercondylar Notch

- The leg is relaxed and allowed to dangle at the side of the bed.
- The cruciate ligaments are inspected in the intercondylar notch and their competency and laxity are tested (**TECH FIG 7**).

Lateral Compartment

- The arthroscope and probe can be situated in the intercondylar notch near the medial aspect of the lateral femoral condyle.
- The leg is placed in a figure 4 position with the knee flexed to 90 degrees while varus stress is applied. Ninety degrees of flexion is the optimal position for visualizing the posterolateral compartment of the knee.
    - When using a leg holder, varus stress can produce similar results.
- When the lateral compartment opens up so there is significant space between the lateral tibial plateau and lateral femoral condyle, the surgeon should suspect a posterolateral corner injury.
- The knee is moved through a range of motion from full extension to full flexion and the entire lateral femoral condyle and lateral tibial plateau are evaluated for cartilage defects (**TECH FIG 8**).

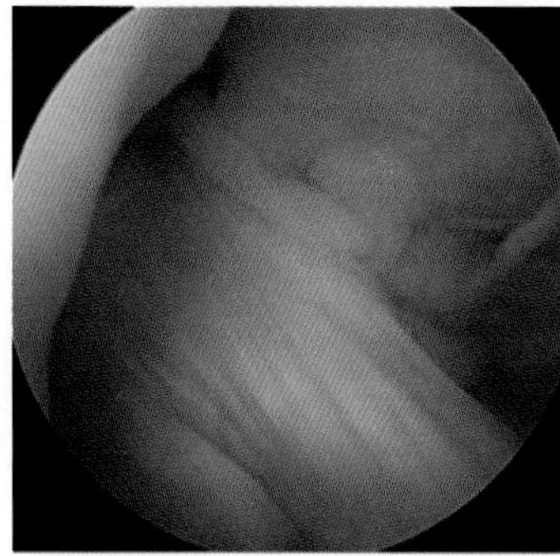

TECH FIG 7 • Arthroscopic view of the intercondylar notch. The anterior cruciate ligament is well visualized on the left, with the posterior cruciate ligament on the right more obscured by fat and synovial tissue.

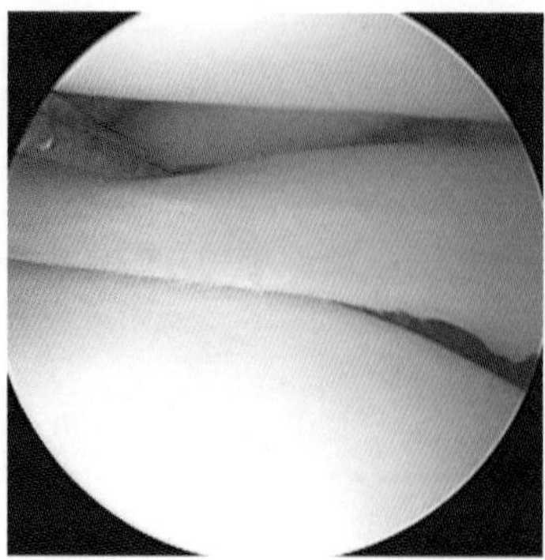

TECH FIG 8 • Arthroscopic view of the lateral compartment, including the lateral femoral condyle, lateral tibial plateau, lateral meniscus, and popliteus tendon.

- The surgeon should probe for softening, fissures, and flaps.
- The meniscus is inspected and probed on its surface and undersurface.
- The popliteus tendon is checked for tears.
- The popliteal hiatus is checked for abnormal instability.
- The surgeon should visualize the posterior root, posterior horn, body, anterior horn, and anterior root of the meniscus.
- The undersurface of the meniscus is probed and inspected, and the meniscus is tested with a hoop stress test.
- The perimeter of the tibial plateau is probed for flipped flap tears of the meniscus.
- The surgeon should inspect the posterior horn of the lateral meniscus. This may require a variation of the modified Gillquist maneuver (mentioned previously).

Modified Gillquist Maneuver for the Posterolateral Compartment

- The arthroscope is removed from the sheath and the blunt obturator is placed in the sheath. The knee should not be placed in 70–90 degrees of flexion.
- The blunt obturator and sheath is placed into the anteromedial portal and advanced into the space between the lateral aspect of the intercondylar notch and the ACL.
- Gentle pressure is applied until the obturator slides under the ACL next to the lateral femoral condyle posteriorly to the posterolateral compartment.
- The blunt obturator is replaced with the 70-degree arthroscope and camera. The posterior horn of the lateral meniscus, the posterior lateral femoral condyle, the posterior meniscal root, and the capsular attachment are visualized. The surgeon can check for loose bodies as well.

PEARLS AND PITFALLS

Preoperative planning	■ The surgeon should be sure to have all instruments and implants available that will be helpful to the surgery. A 70-degree arthroscope can be useful in most cases. Shoulder arthroscopy instrumentation and cannula systems can be helpful with more complex surgeries as well. The surgeon should talk to the patient before the surgery and perform an examination under anesthesia to confirm the pathology necessitating surgery.
Proper portal placement	■ Surgical portal incisions should be tailored to the needs of the case. If a portal is not adequate or optimal, the surgeon should make a new portal. Larger or heavier patients may require larger portals for better maneuvering.

Avoiding the fat pad and synovium	■ These soft tissue structures have a rich vascular supply and nervous innervation. Débridement of these structures will increase postoperative pain and prolong rehabilitation.
Pump pressure	■ High pump pressures can result in fluid extravasation into the soft tissues, leading to the potential for compartment syndrome. This is especially true in trauma patients and older patients. The surgeon may want to consider gravity inflow or lower pump pressures in such situations.
Older patients	■ Older patients are more likely to sustain an injury to the collateral ligaments when varus or valgus stresses are applied to gain compartment visualization. The surgeon should be gentle with their knees.
Tight compartments	■ Some patients have ligamentously tight knees, making it difficult to reach the posterior aspect of the medial and lateral tibiofemoral compartments. The surgeon should use all portals available, including the far medial and lateral as well as the posteromedial and posterolateral portals, to properly address the pathology.

POSTOPERATIVE CARE

- Once the procedure has ended, postoperative care has begun.
- Excess fluid is eliminated from the knee with suction.
- Although there is some variation in portal closure, we prefer a simple skin closure with a nonabsorbable monofilament suture.
  - Regardless of suture type or technique, the surgeon should obtain a tight closure.
- Intra-articular and portal injection of local anesthetic may help with postoperative pain management.
- Deep vein thrombosis prophylaxis may be accomplished with a compression dressing from the toes to the thigh, elevation, mobilization, and ankle pumps.
- Regardless of postoperative weight-bearing status, most patients will require crutches for mobility.
- Cryotherapy has been shown to improve pain scores after knee arthroscopy and is recommended.
- Motion and weight-bearing status are determined by the procedure performed and the patient's needs.
- Pain control with narcotics will likely be necessary for the first few weeks.

COMPLICATIONS

- Infection
- Loss of motion
- Iatrogenic cartilage injury
- Nerve injury: saphenous nerve, peroneal nerve, femoral nerve, sciatic nerve
- Vascular injury
- Deep vein thrombosis
- Compartment syndrome
- Arthrofibrosis
- Reflex sympathetic dystrophy
- Persistent hemarthrosis

REFERENCES

1. DeLee JC. Complications of arthroscopy and arthroscopic surgery: results of a national survey. Arthroscopy 1985;1:214–220.
2. Furie E, Yerys P, Cutcliffe D, et al. Risk factors for arthroscopic popliteal artery laceration. Arthroscopy 1995;11:324–327.
3. Gillquist J, Hagberg G. A new modification of the technique of arthroscopy of the knee joint. Acta Chir Scand 1976;142:123–130.
4. Hungerford DS, Barry M. Biomechanics of the patellofemoral joint. Clin Orthop 1989;241:203.
5. Jaureguito JW, Greenwald AE, Wilcox JF, et al. The incidence of deep venous thrombosis after arthroscopic knee surgery. Am J Sports Med 1999;27:707–710.
6. Kim TK, Savino RM, McFarland EG, et al. Neurovascular complications of knee arthroscopy. Am J Sports Med 2002;30:619–626.
7. Williams JS Jr, Hulstyn MJ, Fadale PD, et al. Incidence of deep vein thrombosis after arthroscopic knee surgery: a prospective study. Arthroscopy 1995;11:701–705.

Chapter 32 Arthroscopic Synovectomy

Anne E. Colton, Charles Bush-Joseph, and Jeffrey S. Earhart

DEFINITION

- Synovitis is inflammation of the synovial membrane. The synovial lining undergoes hyperplasia, most prominent in rheumatoid arthritis. A mononuclear infiltration often makes up the sublining. Redundant synovial folds and villae may be present.
- Synovitis secondary to inflammatory conditions can lead to painful, swollen, and stiff knees.
- After medical management has been exhausted, surgery is indicated if the patient experiences continued pain, swelling, and mechanical symptoms.
- Conditions associated with knee synovitis include rheumatoid arthritis, pigmented villonodular synovitis (PVNS), synovial osteochondromatosis, psoriatic arthritis, osteoarthritis, lupus arthrosis, gout, synovial hemangiomas, plicae, intra-articular adhesions, fat pad fibrosis, posttraumatic synovitis, hemophilic synovitis, and fibrotic ligamentum muscosum.[1–3,5,6,9,14,15]

ANATOMY

- Synovial tissue is a specialized mesenchymal lining of joints.
- Normal synovium supplies nutrients for the articular cartilage and produces lubricants that bathe the joint surfaces to allow smooth gliding. It is a specialized mesenchymal tissue.
- Histologic hallmarks of chronic synovitis include hyperplasia of the intimal lining, lymphocyte infiltration, and blood vessel proliferation.
- Patients with chronic synovitis can have localized or diffuse disease, depending on their underlying condition. When localized, imaging studies such as magnetic resonance imaging (MRI) can help direct arthroscopy. With diffuse disease, it is vital to visualize all aspects of the knee.

PATHOGENESIS

- In chronic synovitis, the synovial lining undergoes hyperplasia, angiogenesis, and increased cellularity (inflammatory cells such as lymphocytes and macrophages).
- Rheumatoid arthritis is one of many immunoinflammatory diseases. It presents as an insidious onset of morning stiffness with multiple joint involvement. The synovitis that ensues is likely an acute autoantibody-mediated inflammatory response.
- PVNS is a proliferation of nodules and villi in the synovium of joints. Typically it is monoarticular, most commonly affecting the knee.
- Hemophilia is an X-linked deficiency of clotting factors, leading to bleeding of varying severity.
  - The knee is the most common site of hemarthrosis. The repeated hemarthroses can lead to a chronic, progressive synovial hyperplasia.

NATURAL HISTORY

- Repeated bouts of acute synovitis or chronically inflamed synovium can lead to chronic pain, limited range of motion, and ultimately joint degeneration and arthrosis.

PATIENT HISTORY AND PHYSICAL FINDINGS

- A full personal and family history of rheumatologic and hematologic disorders should be elicited, including involvement of other joints and episodes of knee or other joint swelling in the past.
- The patient may have a history of recurrent swelling, pain, warmth, stiffness, and mechanical symptoms (**FIG 1**).
  - Patients may have the stigmata of psoriasis or lupus.
- PVNS can cause mechanical symptoms such as locking, not unlike a meniscal tear. A palpable mass may be present.
  - Intermittent symptoms are more common with localized PVNS; diffuse PVNS has more of a chronic presentation.
- In rheumatoid arthritis, the cervical spine is commonly involved and must be evaluated before surgical intervention. Also, the disease is often not limited to the musculoskeletal system: patients can also have vasculitis, subcutaneous nodules, and pericarditis.
- During the physical examination the surgeon should look for effusion, tenderness, warmth, mass, and synovial thickening.
  - Range of motion: Loss of flexion or extension may indicate arthrofibrosis.
  - Lachman test: assesses competence of anterior cruciate ligament
  - Posterior drawer test: assesses competence of posterior cruciate ligament
  - Varus stress test: assesses competence of lateral collateral ligament
  - Valgus stress test: assesses competence of medial collateral ligament
- Malalignment and ligamentous insufficiencies are noted and will likely preclude arthroscopic synovectomy, given their association with joint destruction.
- Joint aspiration can be therapeutic and diagnostic.
  - Synovial fluid analysis should include documentation of fluid color (ie, brownish in PVNS, indicating recurrent

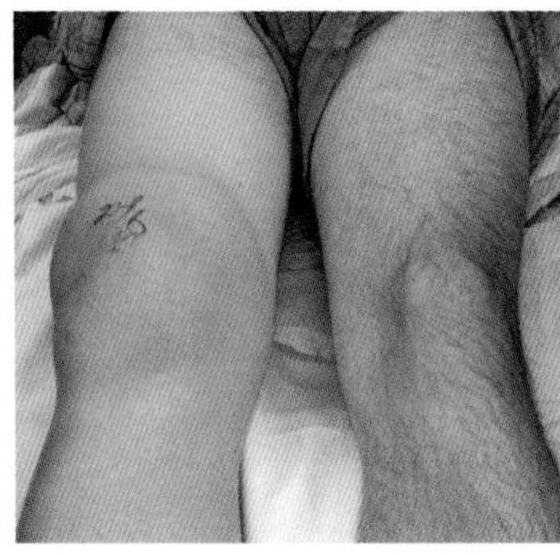

FIG 1 • Patient with a long history of chronic synovitis in his right knee.

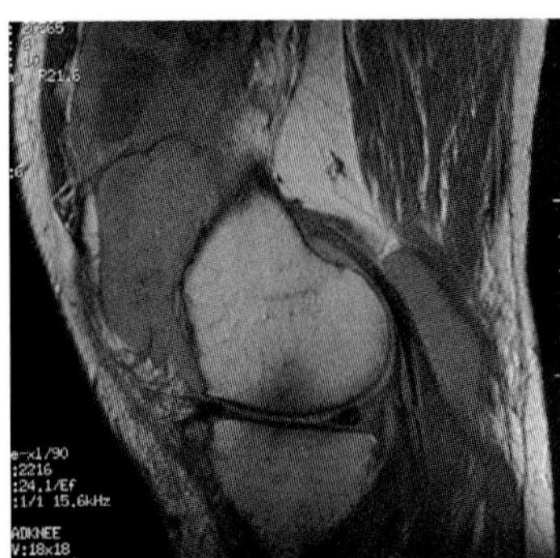

FIG 2 • T2-weighted MRI reveals large effusion in patient's knee, subsequently diagnosed by arthroscopic synovectomy as rheumatoid arthritis.

bleeding), testing for rheumatoid factor, complement levels, cell count, Gram stain, culture, and crystal analysis.

IMAGING AND OTHER DIAGNOSTIC STUDIES

- Radiographs are important to document the extent of joint destruction.
  - The surgeon should look for the characteristic rheumatologic signs of periarticular erosions and osteopenia.
  - Radiologic signs of PVNS and gout include cystic, sclerotic, or erosive lesions.
  - Synovial chondromatosis is often visible.
- Advanced degenerative disease is associated with a poorer prognosis after arthroscopy.[12]
- MRI is helpful to assess the scope of joint involvement before surgery (**FIG 2**).
  - Nodular PVNS can be readily seen as low signal on both T1 and T2 images.

DIFFERENTIAL DIAGNOSIS

- Synovial disorders
- Infection
- Degenerative joint arthrosis

NONOPERATIVE MANAGEMENT

- Conservative treatment includes medical management of the underlying disease.
- Oral anti-inflammatory medications may be used, as well as intra-articular corticosteroid injections.
- Gentle physical therapy can aid in maintenance of range of motion.

SURGICAL MANAGEMENT

- Arthroscopic synovectomy allows the identification and management of synovial lesions that may be missed with open procedures and also allows re-evaluation after the index procedure with a low morbidity.[7,13]
- Arthroscopic synovectomy can provide definitive treatment for the many synovial disorders.
- For more chronic or recurring conditions such as rheumatoid arthritis or hemophilic synovitis, this surgery can reduce the severity of pain and dysfunction commonly associated with these pathologies. It can reduce the number of recurrences and may slow the progression of joint arthrosis.[7]

Preoperative Planning

- Preoperative flexion and extension cervical spine radiographs are necessary to rule out instability in rheumatoid patients.
- Appropriate medical clearance is necessary to keep perioperative complications to a minimum.
- General anesthesia rather than local anesthesia is recommended because the procedure can be lengthy. An epidural may also be used when medically indicated and may aid in postoperative pain relief. A Foley catheter may be used in anticipation of prolonged anesthesia.
- Equipment
  - 4.5-mm 30-degree arthroscope
  - 4.5-mm 70-degree arthroscope (available if visualization is not adequate with 30-degree scope)
  - Small suction shaver
  - Arthroscopic electrocautery
  - Arthroscopic basket
- The examination under anesthesia should document the presence of effusion, range of motion, ligamentous stability, and patellar mobility and tracking. Examination of the contralateral knee should always be performed for comparison.

Positioning

- The patient is placed supine and brought to the edge of the bed to ensure that the leg may be easily hung over the side.
  - An arthroscopic leg holder is not used because it may prohibit the use of the superomedial and superolateral portals.
- A well-padded thigh tourniquet is placed high on the operative leg.
- The contralateral leg is placed in a well-padded leg holder, flexing the hip and knee, with the hip in slight abduction. Compressive wrapping or sequential compression stockings should be used on the contralateral leg owing to the length of the procedure (**FIG 3**).
- The foot of the bed is dropped, allowing the operative leg to hang free. The bed is also flexed to produce slight hip flexion, decreasing the chance of femoral nerve palsy that may be associated with excessive hip extension and leg traction.

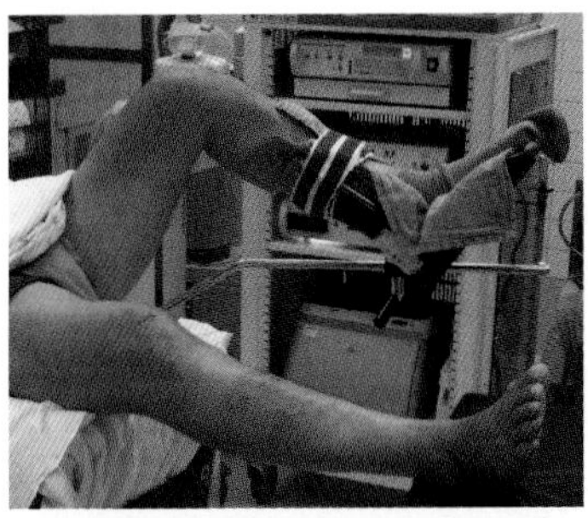

FIG 3 • Patient positioning for arthroscopic synovectomy.

- An arthroscopic lateral post may be placed midthigh on the side of the operative bed.
- A suction canister trap should be set up for biopsy collection.

Approach

- Portals are marked on the skin; five or six are generally needed for a complete synovectomy (**FIG 4**).

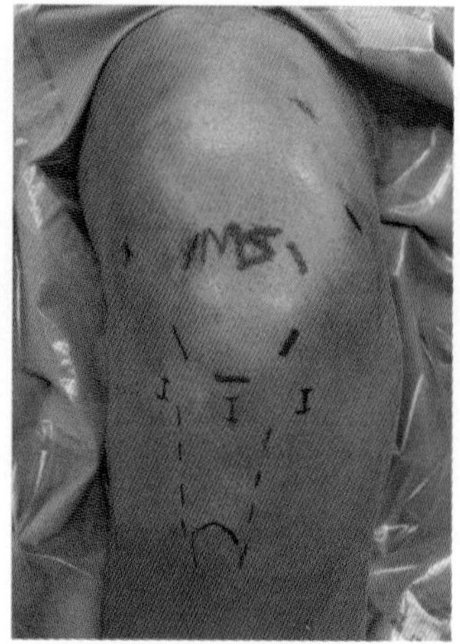

FIG 4 • Arthroscopic portals marked on the right knee.

TECHNIQUES

DIAGNOSTIC ARTHROSCOPY

- The operative limb is exsanguinated and the tourniquet is inflated to 250 to 300 mm Hg (**TECH FIG 1A**).
- The procedure is begun with outflow in the superomedial portal because this is rarely used as a viewing portal (**TECH FIG 1B**).
- An incision is made in the inferolateral portal. The arthroscope is placed into the suprapatellar pouch with the knee in extension. A superolateral working portal is established (**TECH FIG 1C,D**).

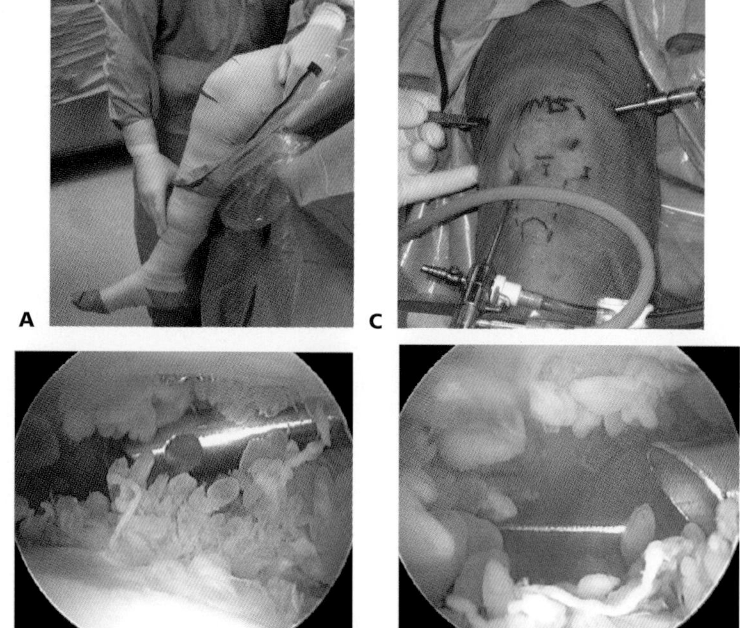

TECH FIG 1 • **A.** The limb is exsanguinated with an Esmarch bandage. **B.** Arthroscopic view reveals the outflow in the superomedial portal. **C.** The superolateral portal is established. **D.** Arthroscopic view shows establishment of the superolateral working portal under direct visualization.

SYNOVECTOMY

Suprapatellar Pouch, Medial and Lateral Gutter, and Intercondylar Notch

- With the arthroscope in the inferolateral portal, the shaver is placed in the superolateral portal. The synovium is resected from the suprapatellar pouch and the lateral gutter (**TECH FIG 2A,B**).
- The shaver is moved to the inferomedial portal. The synovium is excised from the medial gutter and the medial aspect of the suprapatellar pouch (**TECH FIG 2C,D**).

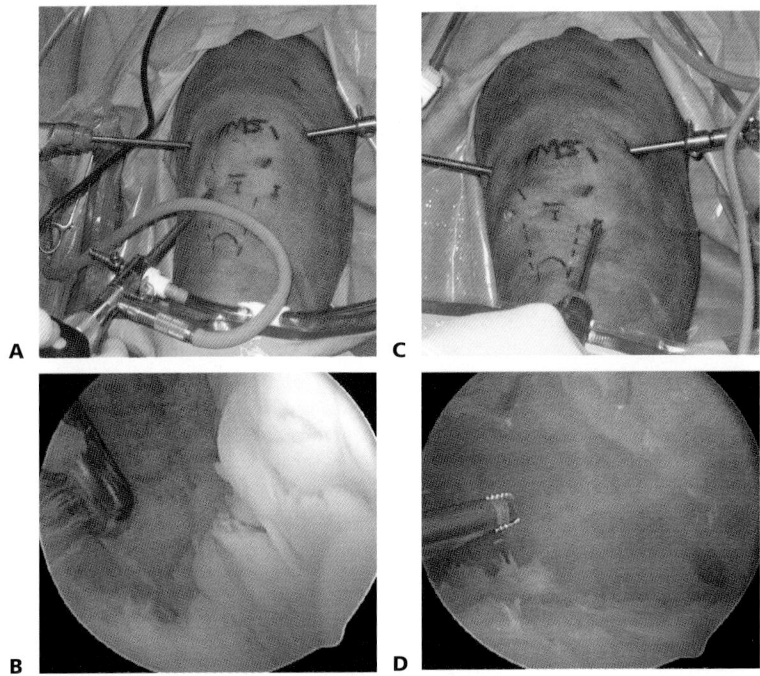

TECH FIG 2 • **A.** The shaver is placed into the superolateral working portal. **B.** Arthroscopic view showing partial resection of the lateral gutter synovium. **C.** The shaver is moved to the inferomedial portal. **D.** Arthroscopic resection of medial synovium.

Retropatellar Pouch, Inferolateral and Inferomedial Gutters

- The arthroscope is moved to the superolateral portal and the shaver is placed in the inferolateral portal. This enables synovial resection from the inferolateral gutter and the retropatellar space (TECH FIG 3A,B).
- The shaver is placed in the inferomedial portal to complete the synovectomy of the retropatellar space and the inferomedial gutter (TECH FIG 3C,D).

Intercondylar Notch

- The arthroscope is returned to the inferolateral portal and the shaver is maintained in the inferomedial portal (TECH FIG 4A,B).
- Resection of synovium in the intercondylar notch and around the cruciate ligaments is carefully performed (TECH FIG 4C).
  - This establishes adequate working space within the notch to allow visualization of the posterior compartments of the knee.
  - Care must be taken to distinguish synovium from ligament.

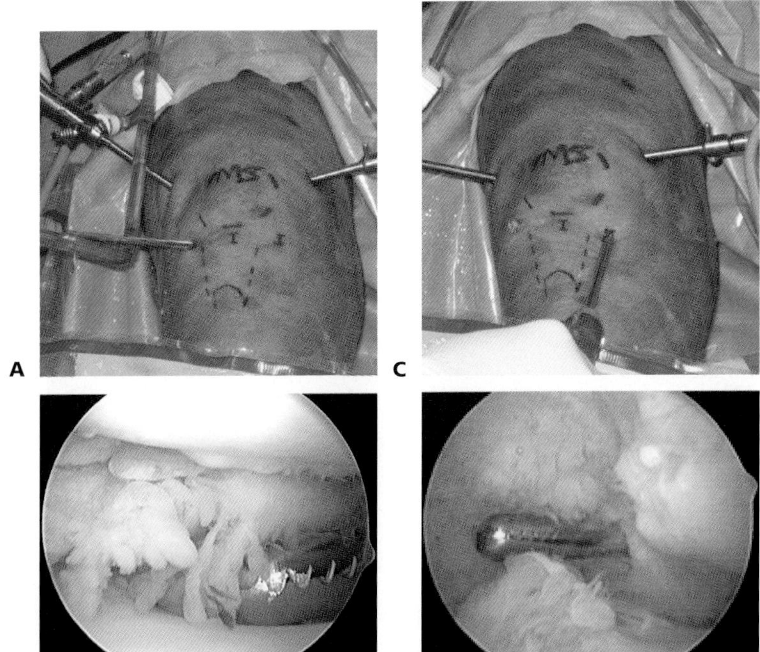

TECH FIG 3 • **A.** The arthroscope is moved to the superolateral portal, and the shaver is placed in the inferolateral portal. **B.** Arthroscopic view of the resection in the retropatellar space and lateral gutter. **C.** The arthroscope is moved to the inferomedial portal, and the shaver is placed in the inferolateral portal. **D.** Arthroscopic view of inferomedial gutter synovial resection.

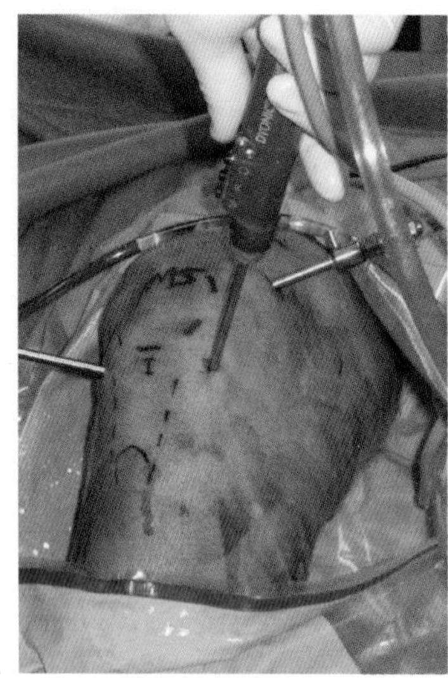

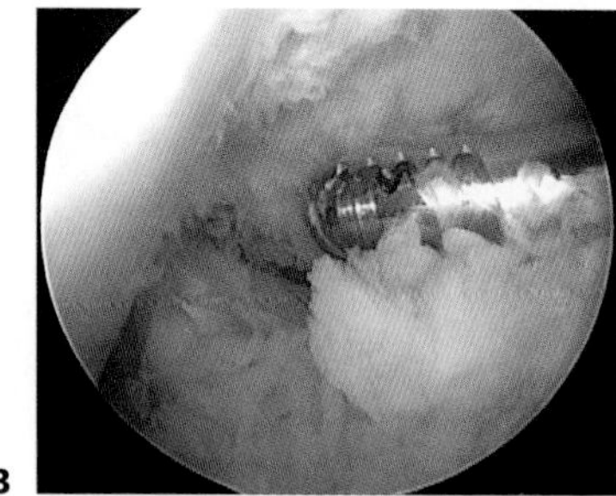

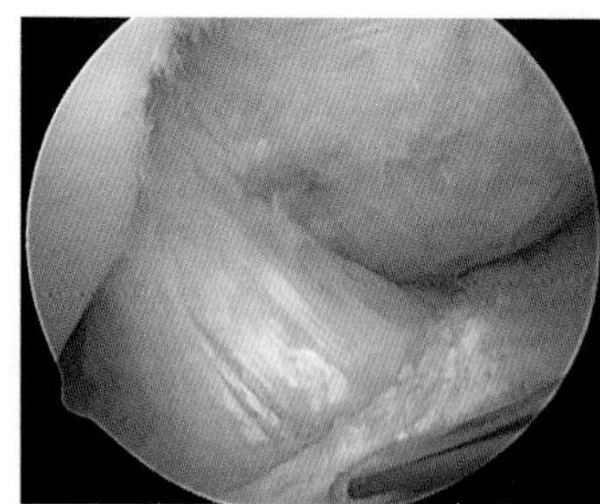

TECH FIG 4 • **A.** The arthroscope is returned to the inferolateral portal, and the shaver is in the inferomedial portal. **B.** Arthroscopic photograph shows the resection of synovectomy in the notch. **C.** Arthroscopic photo shows complete resection of synovium in the notch. The anterior cruciate ligament is now apparent.

Posteromedial Compartment

- For access to the posteromedial compartment, a blunt-tipped trocar is placed in its arthroscopic sheath and inserted through the inferolateral portal.
  - Alternatively, a switching stick can be placed through the inferolateral portal under direct visualization with the arthroscope placed in the inferomedial portal.
- The medial femoral condyle is palpated with the tip and the trocar is pushed posteriorly in the interval between the medial femoral condyle and the posterior cruciate ligament, raising the hand to accommodate the posterior slope of the tibia.
- The trocar should push into the posteromedial compartment without too much force.
  - If this proves difficult to accomplish, a central patellar tendon portal may allow easier access to the posterior compartment.
- The trocar is removed and the arthroscope is inserted. From this position, the posterior aspect of the medial femoral condyle and the posterior horn of the medial meniscus can be visualized.
- While looking medially, a posteromedial working portal is developed under direct visualization.
  - A spinal needle is inserted anterior to the medial head of the gastrocnemius to avoid the neurovascular structures (TECH FIG 5A).
- Once in the appropriate position, a small, longitudinal incision is made through the skin.
- Using a hemostat, the soft tissue is spread until the capsule is reached.
- Using a blunt-tipped trocar and arthroscopic cannula, the hemostat is replaced to establish a working portal.
  - The surgeon inserts the shaver after removing the trocar and proceeds with resection of the synovium in the posteromedial compartment (TECH FIG 5B,C).

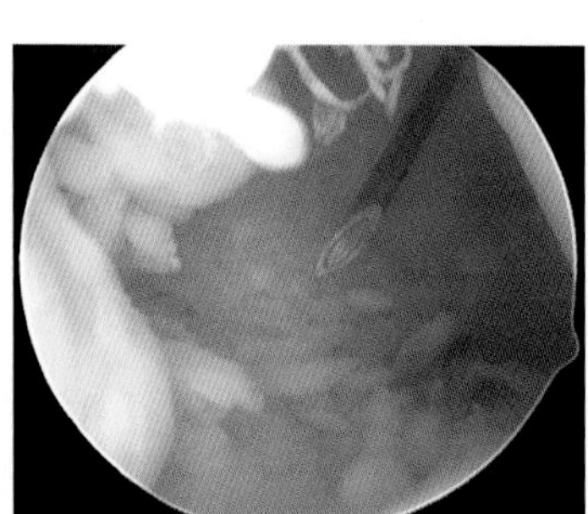

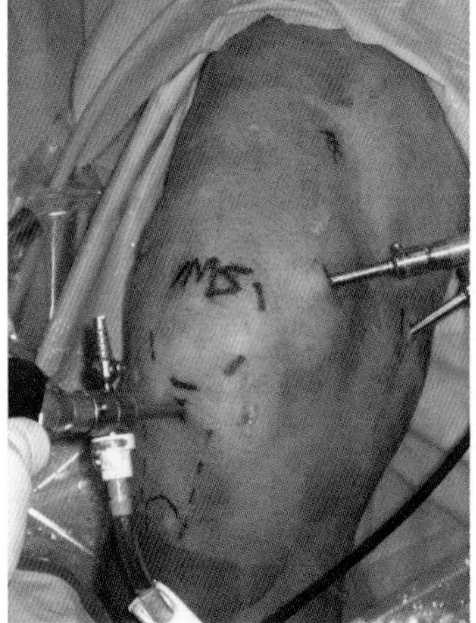

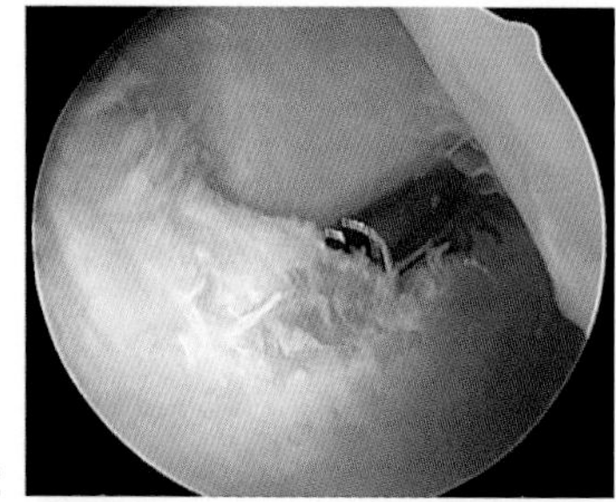

TECH FIG 5 • **A.** Arthroscopic photograph showing establishment of the posteromedial portal. **B.** Arthroscope is placed through the notch into the posteromedial compartment with shaver placed into the posteromedial portal. **C.** Synovial resection in the posteromedial compartment.

Posterolateral Compartment

- With a blunt trocar in the arthroscopic cannula, the trocar is placed in the inferomedial portal.
- The lateral femoral condyle is palpated with the trocar and pushed along the notch between the condyle and the anterior cruciate ligament (TECH FIG 6A).
  - This can also be done with a switching stick, as described in the previous section.
  - Again, the hand is raised to accommodate the posterior slope of the tibial plateau.
- The trocar should give way, indicating passage into the posterolateral compartment. It is important not to push through any great resistance to avoid penetrating the capsule and damaging the neurovascular structures.
- The arthroscope is placed into the cannula. The posterior aspect of the lateral femoral condyle as well as the posterior horn of the lateral meniscus should be seen.
- A posterolateral portal is made by inserting a spinal needle into the compartment under direct visualization (TECH FIG 6B,C).
  - The needle should be inserted posterior to the fibular collateral ligament and anterior to the lateral head of the gastrocnemius.
  - The soft spot anterior to the biceps femoris muscle and posterior to the iliotibial tract will ensure protection of the peroneal nerve.
- When making the posterolateral and posteromedial portals, the surgeon should make sure that the instruments can be directed in the coronal plane behind the corresponding femoral condyle.
- In a manner similar to the posteromedial portal, the skin is incised with a scalpel and the surgeon dissects to and then through the posterior capsule with a hemostat under direct visualization.
- Maintaining the same angle, the surgeon replaces the hemostat with a blunt trocar in an operative cannula.
  - The surgeon inserts the shaver and proceeds with débridement of the posterolateral compartment (TECH FIG 6D,E).
- Hypertrophied synovium on the posterior capsule and posterior septum should be resected.
- The suction must be monitored carefully because the posterior capsule may be penetrated, placing the neurovascular structures at risk.
- After completion of the synovectomy, the tourniquet is released and hemostasis is achieved with electrocautery.
- The entire suction canister should be sent for pathology and microbiology testing (TECH FIG 6F).
- A suction drain is typically used for 24 hours postoperatively to minimize hemarthrosis.
- Light compressive dressing and cryotherapy are used to minimize swelling and encourage early joint motion.

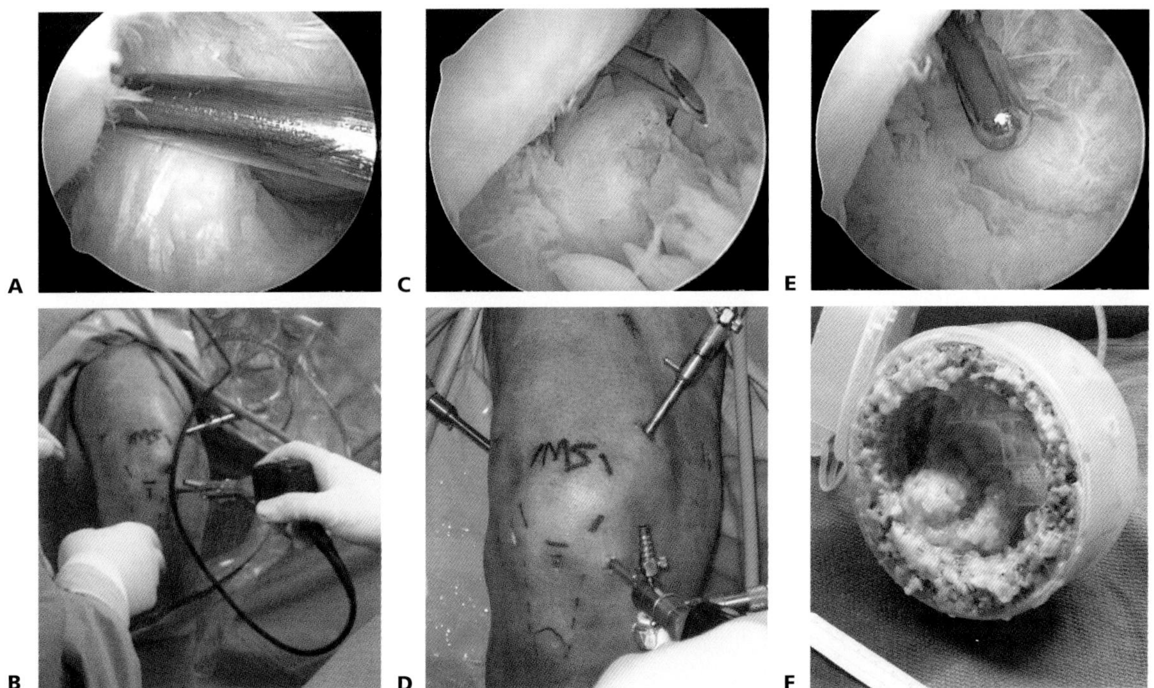

TECH FIG 6 • **A.** A switching stick is placed into the posterolateral compartment under direct visualization. **B.** The posterolateral portal is made using needle localization. **C.** Arthroscopic photograph reveals needle localization for the establishment of the posterolateral portal. **D.** The shaver is placed in the posterolateral portal. **E.** Arthroscopic photograph showing the resection of synovium in the posterolateral compartment. **F.** Suction canister filter traps synovial biopsy specimen.

PEARLS AND PITFALLS

Hemostasis	■ At the end of the procedure, hemostasis must be obtained. Failure to do so may result in hemarthrosis and procedure failure.
Portal placement	■ The surgeon must be prepared to view the knee from multiple portals. ■ Portals must be placed under direct visualization to protect neurovascular structures. ■ Cannulas should be used when possible to ensure atraumatic entry and exit of instruments, avoiding soft tissue injury.
Technique	■ The surgeon must approach the arthroscopic synovectomy with a well-defined stepwise approach to excise the pathologic tissue in its entirety.
Biopsy	■ Enough tissue must be obtained for pathologic evaluation and diagnosis.
Therapy	■ Regaining and maintaining full knee range of motion and quadriceps function is critical.

POSTOPERATIVE CARE

- The patient is weight bearing as tolerated.
- Continuous passive motion is advised in cases of complete synovectomy, advancing as tolerated over 1 to 3 days.
- Physical therapy is initiated after removal of the suction drain. Closed-chain exercises are emphasized.

OUTCOMES

- When comparing arthroscopic synovectomy to open synovectomy, the arthroscopic technique is associated with lower morbidity and more rapid return of function and lower rates of recurrence in rheumatoid, hemophilia, and other inflammatory arthritides.[7,10,13] In addition, synovectomy can be more complete with accurate visualization of the posterior compartments.[15]
- One study of 96 rheumatoid arthritic knees found significant decreases in pain and synovitis at an average of 4 years after arthroscopic synovectomy.[11]
- Along with the use of rheumatoid medications, arthroscopic synovectomy can reduce inflammation and help preserve range of motion.[2]
  - Success rates in the relief of pain and swelling have been as high as 80% in the treatment of rheumatoid arthritis.[10]
- Arthroscopic synovectomy has been used successfully in the treatment of PVNS.
  - In the past, open synovectomies led to stiffness and pain after the procedure. In a series of 18 patients with diffuse PVNS, one third of the patients had a recurrence after open synovectomy, and in most patients the knee was manipulated in an attempt to decrease stiffness.[4]
  - Recurrence rates with arthroscopic synovectomy of PVNS have been as low as 11%, with improved range of motion.[9]
- Localized PVNS has responded best to arthroscopic treatment.
  - Multiple series have reported no recurrences at follow-up after excision of the lesion.[8,9,15]
  - The procedure allows improved visualization of lesions and facilitates the discovery of small, localized forms of PVNS.
- Hemophilic synovitis, also associated with aggressive joint destruction, has responded well symptomatically to arthroscopic synovectomy.
  - Unlike most forms of synovitis, this usually requires a short period of hospitalization because of the underlying systemic disorder.
  - The procedure has been effective in reducing recurrent hemarthrosis and maintaining range of motion.
  - However, joint deterioration continues to occur, although probably at a slower rate.[14]

COMPLICATIONS

- Recurrent hemarthrosis, often requiring repeat aspirations or surgical irrigation and débridement
- Loss of range of motion
  - Joint stiffness and flexion contracture can be challenging to treat.
  - Dynamic bracing can be used.
- Rare complications include infection, either superficial or intra-articular, neurovascular injury, rapid onset of joint arthrosis, or cruciate ligament damage.

REFERENCES

1. Comin JA, Rodriguez-Merchan EC. Arthroscopic synovectomy in the management of painful localized post-traumatic synovitis of the knee joint. Arthroscopy 1997;13:606–608.
2. Fiacco U, Cozzi L, Rigon C, et al. Arthroscopic synovectomy in rheumatoid and psoriatic knee joint synovitis: long-term outcome. Br J Rheumatol 1996;35:463–470.
3. Gilbert MS, Radomisli TE. Therapeutic options in the management of hemophilic synovitis. Clin Orthop Relat Res 1997;343:88–92.
4. Johansson JE, Ajjoub S, Coughlin LP, et al. Pigmented villonodular synovitis of joints. Clin Orthop Relat Res 1982;163:159–166.
5. Klein W, Jensen KU. Arthroscopic synovectomy of the knee joint: indication, technique and follow-up results. Arthroscopy 1988;4: 63–71.
6. Lee BI, Yoo JE, Lee SH, et al. Localized pigmented villonodular synovitis of the knee: arthroscopic treatment. Arthroscopy 1998;14: 764–768.
7. Matsui N, Taneda Y, Ohta H, et al. Arthroscopic versus open synovectomy in the rheumatoid knee. Int Orthop 1989;13:17–20.
8. Moskovich R, Parisien JS. Localized pigmented villonodular synovitis of the knee. Clin Orthop Relat Res 1991;271:218–224.
9. Oglivie-Harris DJ, McLean J, Zarnett ME. Pigmented villonodular synovitis of the knee. J Bone Joint Surg Am 1992;74A:119–123.
10. Ogilvie-Harris DJ, Weisleder L. Arthroscopic synovectomy of the knee: is it helpful? Arthroscopy 1995;11:91–95.
11. Ogilvie-Harris DJ, Basinski A. Arthroscopic synovectomy of the knee for rheumatoid arthritis. Arthroscopy 1991;7:91.
12. Roch-Bras F, Daures JP, Legouffe MC, et al. Treatment of chronic knee synovitis with arthroscopic synovectomy: long-term results. Rheumatology 2002;29:1171–1175.
13. Shibata T, Shiraoka K, Takubo N. Comparison between arthroscopic and open synovectomy for the knee in rheumatoid arthritis. Arch Orthop Trauma Surg 1986;105:257–262.
14. Wiedel JD. Arthroscopic synovectomy of the knee in hemophilia: 10 to 15 year follow-up. Clin Orthop Relat Res 1996;328:46–53.
15. Zvijac JE, Lau AC, Hechtman KS, et al. Arthroscopic treatment of pigmented villonodular synovitis of the knee. Arthroscopy 1999;15: 613–617.

Chapter 33 Arthroscopic Meniscectomy

Frederick M. Azar

DEFINITION

- Irreparable meniscal tears are those for which no healing response is possible.
  - This may include all or part of a meniscus, prompting partial, subtotal, or total meniscectomy.
- Meniscal injuries in the "white zone" (central avascular portion; **FIG 1**) most often require partial meniscectomy.
  - This usually involves the inner two thirds of the meniscus.
- Symptomatic tears of discoid lateral menisci also may require partial or subtotal saucerization of the meniscus.
- Numerous classifications of tears of the menisci have been proposed based on location or type of tear, etiology, and other factors; most of the commonly used classifications are based on the type of tear found at surgery (**FIG 2**).
  - Longitudinal tears
  - Transverse and oblique tears
  - A combination of longitudinal and transverse tears
  - Tears associated with cystic menisci
  - Tears associated with discoid menisci
- The most common type of tear is the longitudinal tear, usually involving the posterior segment of either the medial or lateral meniscus.
- More lateral meniscal tears have been diagnosed than medial tears.
  - Although no definitive study comparing the incidence of medial to lateral tears has been reported, the two types are believed to occur with almost equal frequency.
  - Most partial-thickness tears involve the inferior rather than the superior surface of the meniscus.

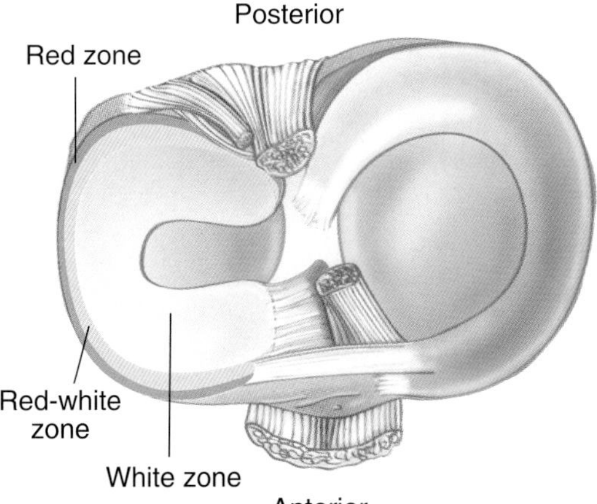

FIG 1 • Tears in the central avascular portion of the meniscus (white zone) usually require partial meniscectomy, those in the vascular red zone have good healing potential, and those in the red-white zone have limited healing potential.

- Certain patterns of meniscal tears are associated with mechanical locking.
  - Small longitudinal tears limited to the posterior horn usually are not capable of producing locking but rather cause pain, recurrent swelling, and subjective instability.
  - Extensive longitudinal tears can cause locking by displacing into the intercondylar notch.
  - A pedunculated fragment may result if either the posterior or anterior attachment of the bucket-handle fragment becomes detached.
- Transverse, radial, or oblique tears can occur in either meniscus but are more common in the lateral, usually at the junction of the anterior and middle thirds.
- Transverse tears also can result from degenerative changes that make the meniscus less mobile.
- Complex transverse and longitudinal tears may occur with degeneration or repeated traumatic episodes.
- Meniscal cysts frequently are associated with tears and are nine times more common on the lateral than on the medial side.
- Discoid menisci are abnormal in terms of both mobility and tissue bulk, making them vulnerable to compression and rotary stress.

ANATOMY

- The menisci are crescents that are roughly triangular in cross section.
- They cover one half to two thirds of the articular surface of the corresponding tibial plateau.
- They are composed of dense, tightly woven collagen fibers arranged in a pattern providing great elasticity and ability to withstand compression.
  - The major orientation of collagen fibers in the meniscus is circumferential.
  - Radial fibers and perforating fibers also are present (**FIG 3A**).
  - The arrangement of these collagen fibers determines to some extent the characteristic patterns of meniscal tears (**FIG 3B,C**).
  - When meniscal samples are tested by applying a force perpendicular to the fiber direction, the strength is decreased to less than 10% because collagen fibers function primarily to resist tensile forces along the direction of the fibers.[4]
  - The circumferential fibers act in a similar manner as metal hoops placed around a pressurized wooden barrel: the tension in the hoops keeps the wooden staves in place (**FIG 3D,E**).
  - Hoop tension is lost when a single radial cut or tear extends to the capsular margin.
- The peripheral edges of the menisci are convex, fixed, and attached to the inner surface of the knee joint capsule, except where the popliteus is interposed laterally; the peripheral edges also are attached loosely via coronary ligament to the borders of the tibial plateaus.
- The inner edges are concave, thin, and unattached.

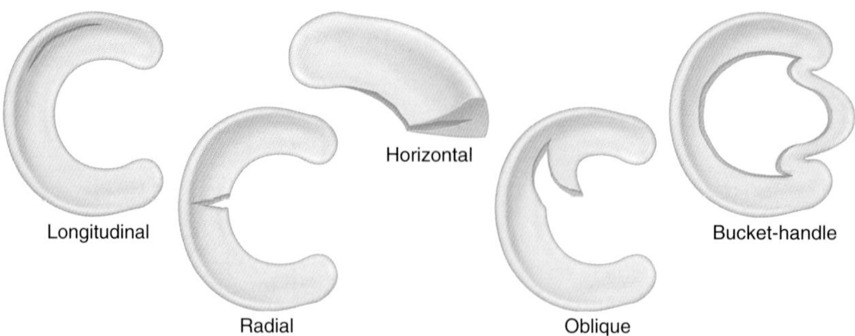

FIG 2 • Patterns of meniscal tears.

- The menisci are largely avascular except near their peripheral attachment.
- The inferior surface of each meniscus is flat, whereas the superior surface is concave, corresponding to the contour of the associated bony anatomy.
- The medial meniscus is a C-shaped structure larger in radius than the lateral meniscus, with the posterior horn being wider than the anterior (**FIG 4**).[6]
- The anterior horn is attached firmly to the tibia anterior to the intercondylar eminence and to the anterior cruciate ligament (ACL).
- Most of the weight is borne on the posterior portion of the meniscus.
- The posterior horn is anchored immediately in front of the attachments of the posterior cruciate ligament posterior to the intercondylar eminence.

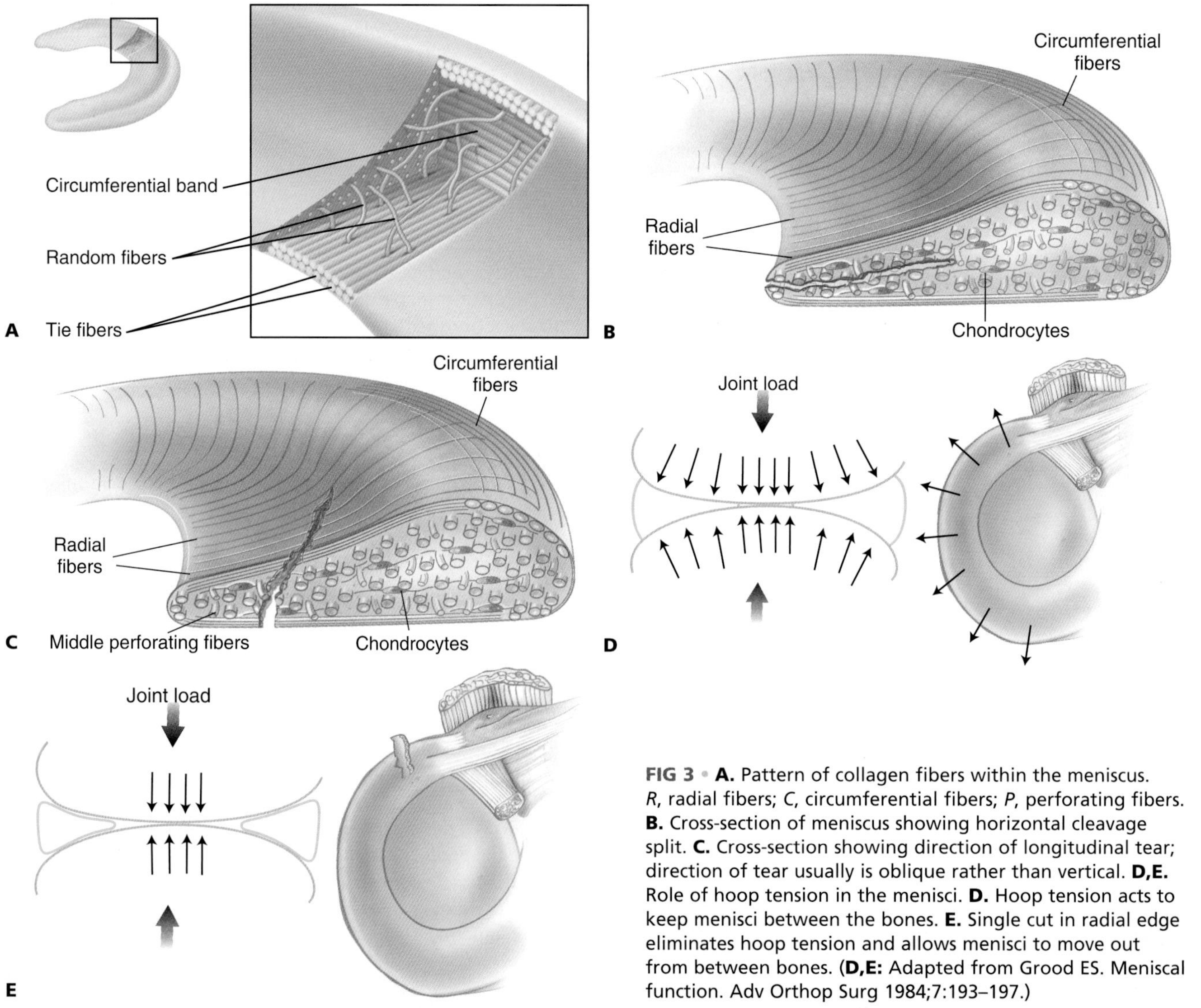

FIG 3 • **A.** Pattern of collagen fibers within the meniscus. *R*, radial fibers; *C*, circumferential fibers; *P*, perforating fibers. **B.** Cross-section of meniscus showing horizontal cleavage split. **C.** Cross-section showing direction of longitudinal tear; direction of tear usually is oblique rather than vertical. **D,E.** Role of hoop tension in the menisci. **D.** Hoop tension acts to keep menisci between the bones. **E.** Single cut in radial edge eliminates hoop tension and allows menisci to move out from between bones. (**D,E:** Adapted from Grood ES. Meniscal function. Adv Orthop Surg 1984;7:193–197.)

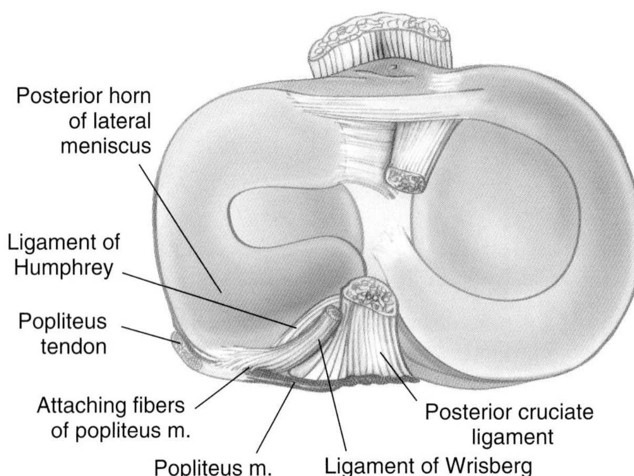

FIG 4 • Superior view of tibial condyles. Lateral meniscus is smaller in diameter, thicker about its periphery, wider in body, and more mobile than the medial meniscus; posteriorly it is attached to the medial femoral condyle by either the anterior or posterior meniscofemoral ligament, depending on which is present, and to the popliteus muscle.

- Its entire peripheral border is firmly attached to the medial capsule and through the coronary ligament to the upper border of the tibia.
- The lateral meniscus is more circular in form, covering up to two thirds of the articular surface of the underlying tibial plateau.
  - The anterior horn is attached to the tibia medially in front of the intercondylar eminence.
  - The posterior horn inserts into the posterior aspect of the intercondylar eminence and in front of the posterior attachment of the medial meniscus.
  - The posterior horn often receives anchorage also to the femur via the ligament of Wrisberg and the ligament of Humphrey and from fascia covering the popliteus muscle and the arcuate complex at the posterolateral corner of the knee.
  - The inner border, like that of the medial meniscus, is thin, concave, and free.
  - The tendon of the popliteus muscle separates the posterolateral periphery of the lateral meniscus from the joint capsule and the lateral collateral ligament. This tendon is enveloped in a synovial membrane and forms an oblique groove on the lateral border of the meniscus.
  - The lateral meniscus is smaller in diameter, thicker in periphery, wider in body, and more mobile than the medial meniscus.
- The menisci follow the tibial condyles during flexion and extension, but during rotation they follow the femur and move on the tibia (**FIG 5**).
  - Consequently, the medial meniscus becomes distorted.
  - Its anterior and posterior attachments follow the tibia, but its intervening part follows the femur; thus, it is likely to be injured during rotation.
  - However, the lateral meniscus, because it is firmly attached to the popliteus muscle and to the ligament of Wrisberg or of Humphrey, follows the lateral femoral condyle during rotation and therefore is less likely to be injured.
  - In addition, when the tibia is rotated internally and the knee flexed, the popliteus muscle, by way of the arcuate ligament complex, draws the posterior segment of the lateral meniscus backward, thereby preventing the meniscus from being caught between the condyle of the femur and the plateau of the tibia.
- The vascular supply to the medial and lateral menisci originates predominately from the lateral and medial geniculate vessels (both inferior and superior).
  - Branches from these vessels give rise to a perimeniscal capillary plexus within the synovial and capsular tissue, which supplies the peripheral border of the meniscus throughout its attachment to the joint capsule.
  - These vessels are oriented in a predominantly circumferential pattern, with radial branches directed toward the center of the joint.
  - Arnoczky and Warren[3,4] used microinjection techniques to show that the depth of peripheral vascular penetration is 10% to 30% of the width of the medial meniscus and 10% to 25% of the width of the lateral meniscus.
  - The medial geniculate artery, along with a few terminal branches of the medial and lateral geniculate artery, also supplies vessels to the menisci through the vascular synovial covering.
- The menisci have several proposed functions in the knee joint.
  - They act as a joint filler, compensating for gross incongruity between the femoral and tibial articulating surfaces.
  - They are believed to have a joint lubrication function, distributing synovial fluid and aiding the nutrition of the articular cartilage.

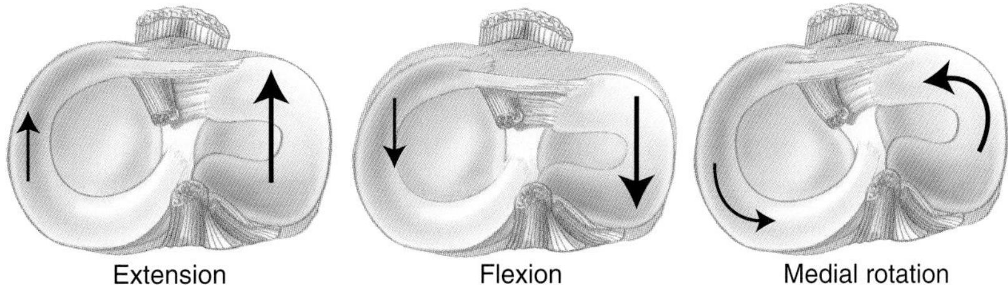

FIG 5 • Kinematics of the menisci with knee flexion, extension, and rotation. Although the lateral meniscus and lateral tibial plateau have a smaller AP width, the lateral meniscus moves more than the medial meniscus through each range of motion. (Adapted from Tria AJ Jr, Klein KS. An Illustrated Guide to the Knee. New York: Churchill Livingstone, 1992.)

- They serve as important secondary stabilizers in all planes, especially providing rotary stability to the joint, and allowing for smooth gliding or rotary motion as the knee extends.

PATHOGENESIS

- Meniscal injuries generally have either a traumatic or degenerative cause.
  - Traumatic injuries in young, active individuals are often associated with tears of the anterior and posterior cruciate ligaments.
  - The most common traumatic tears are vertical longitudinal tears, followed by vertical transverse tears.
  - Degenerative meniscal tears occur most often in patients older than 40 years of age, typically with no history of a specific traumatic event and often in association with other degenerative changes in the knee joint.
  - Degenerative tears of the menisci have minimal or no healing potential.
  - The most common degenerative tear patterns are horizontal cleavage tears, flap tears, and complex tears (see Fig 2).
- Miller, Warner, and Harner[17] classified meniscal tears based on their location in three zones of vascularity and use this classification to determine the potential for healing after repair (see Fig 1):
  - Red: fully within the vascular area
  - Red-white: at the border of the vascular area
  - White: within the avascular area
- After injury within the peripheral vascular zone, a fibrin clot forms that is rich in inflammatory cells.
  - Vessels from the perimeniscal capillary plexus proliferate throughout this fibrin scaffold and are accompanied by the proliferations of differentiated mesenchymal cells.
  - Eventually the lesion is filled with cellular fibrovascular scar tissue that glues the wound edges together and appears continuous with the adjacent normal meniscal fibrocartilage.
  - Experimental studies in animals have shown that complete radial lesions of the meniscus are completely healed with a young fibrocartilaginous scar by 10 weeks, although several months are required for maturation to fibrocartilage that appears normal.
- Controversy exists about the ability of a meniscus or a meniscus-like tissue to regenerate after meniscectomy.
  - It is now generally accepted that to have any regeneration, the entire meniscus must be resected to expose the vascular synovial tissue, or, in subtotal meniscectomy, the excision must extend to the peripheral vasculature of the meniscus.
  - The frequency and degree of regeneration of the meniscus have not been determined precisely.
- Traumatic lesions of the menisci are produced most commonly by rotation as the flexed knee moves toward an extended position.
- The most common location for injury is the posterior horn of the meniscus, and longitudinal tears are the most common type of injury.
- The length, depth, and position of the tear depend on the position of the posterior horn in relation to the femoral and tibial condyles at the time of injury.
- Less significant trauma is needed to injure a meniscus that is degenerated or made less mobile from prior injury, previous surgery, disease, or congenital anomaly (ie, discoid meniscus).

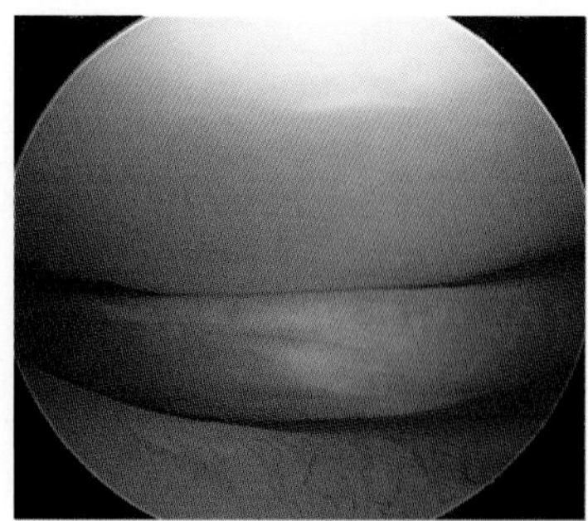

FIG 6 • Classic bucket-handle meniscal tear.

- The menisci are also at increased risk in the presence of joint incongruities, ligamentous instability, profound muscle weakness, or congenitally relaxed joints.
- As the knee is internally rotated during flexion, the medial meniscus is forced posteriorly. If the peripheral attachment stretches or tears, the posterior part of the meniscus is forced centrally, caught between the femur and tibia, and torn longitudinally as the knee extends.
- If this longitudinal tear extends anteriorly beyond the medial collateral ligament, the inner segment of the meniscus is caught in the intercondylar notch and cannot return to its former position; thus, a classic bucket-handle tear with locking of the joint is produced (**FIG 6**).
- The same mechanism can produce a posterior peripheral or a longitudinal tear of the lateral meniscus.
- Because of its mobility and structure, the lateral meniscus is not as susceptible to bucket-handle tears, but incomplete transverse tears are more common here than in the medial meniscus.

NATURAL HISTORY

- The effects of meniscectomy on joint laxity have been studied for anteroposterior and varus–valgus motions and rotation.
  - These studies indicated that the effect on joint laxity depends on whether the ligaments of the knee are intact and whether the joint is bearing weight.
  - In the presence of intact ligamentous structures, excision of the menisci produces small increases in joint laxity.
  - When combined with ligamentous insufficiency, these increased instabilities caused by meniscectomy are greatly exaggerated.
- In an ACL-deficient knee, medial meniscectomy has been shown to increase tibial translation by 58% at 90 degrees, whereas primary anterior and posterior translations were not affected by lateral meniscectomy.
- Anatomically, the capsular components that attach the lateral meniscus to the tibia do not affix the lateral meniscus as firmly as they do the medial meniscus.
  - These results indicate that in contrast to the medial meniscus, the lateral meniscus does not act as an efficient posterior wedge to resist anterior translation of the tibia on the femur.
  - Therefore, in knees that lack an ACL, the lateral meniscus is subjected to different forces than those that occur on the medial side.
- Allen et al,[2] in a biomechanical study, determined that force in the medial meniscus increased significantly in response to an anterior tibial load after ACL transection, which may

account for some of the differences in injury patterns between the medial and lateral menisci in the anterior cruciate-deficient knee.

- Walker and Erkman[27] noted that under loads of up to 150 kg, the lateral meniscus appeared to carry 70% of the load on that side of the joint, whereas on the medial side the load was shared about equally by the meniscus and the exposed articular cartilage.
  - Medial meniscectomy decreases contact area by 50% to 70% and increases contact stress by 100%.
  - Lateral meniscectomy decreases contact area by 40% to 50% but dramatically increases contact stress by 200% to 300% because of the relative convex surface of the lateral tibial plateau.
  - Presumably the menisci provide mediolateral stability where the load is supported by the entire width of the tibial articular surface. Without the menisci the load is supported centrally on each plateau, diminishing the lever arm of load support.
- Radiographic changes apparent after meniscectomy include narrowing of the joint space, flattening of the femoral condyle, and formation of osteophytes.

PATIENT HISTORY AND PHYSICAL FINDINGS

- Mechanical symptoms, such as catching, popping, and locking, usually occur only with longitudinal tears and are much more common with bucket-handle tears, usually of the medial meniscus.
- Locking of the knee is not pathognomonic of a bucket-handle tear of a meniscus: other conditions such as loose body, patellar maltracking, and intra-articular tumor can cause similar findings.
- The following clues can be important in the differential diagnosis:
  - Sensation of giving way
  - Effusion
  - Atrophy of the quadriceps
  - Tenderness over the joint line (or the meniscus)
  - Reproduction of a click by manipulative maneuvers during the physical examination
- Probably the most important physical finding is localized tenderness along the posteromedial or posterolateral joint line, which is most commonly caused by reactive synovitis.
- A history of specific injury may not be obtained, especially when tears of abnormal or degenerative menisci have occurred.
- A patient without locking typically gives a history of several episodes of trouble referable to the knee, often resulting in effusion and a brief period of disability but no definite locking.
- A sensation of giving way or snaps, clicks, catches, or jerks in the knee may be described, or the history may be even more indefinite, with recurrent episodes of pain and mild effusion in the knee and tenderness in the anterior joint space after excessive activity.
- The injured knee should be compared with the opposite knee, which can exhibit 5 to 10 degrees of physiologic recurvatum. In this case, the injured knee can be locked and still extend to neutral position.
- Regardless of its cause, locking that is unrelieved after aspiration of the hemarthrosis and a period of conservative treatment may require surgical treatment.
  - A serious error would be failure to distinguish locking from false locking.
  - False locking occurs most often soon after an injury in which hemorrhage about the posterior part of the capsule or a collateral ligament with associated hamstring spasm prevents complete extension of the knee.
  - Aspiration and a short period of rest until the reaction has partially subsided usually will differentiate locking from false locking of the joint, and magnetic resonance imaging (MRI) can confirm the diagnosis.
- A sensation of giving way is often present but is not specific to meniscal tear.
- Effusion indicates that something is irritating the synovium; therefore, it has limited specific diagnostic value.
  - The sudden onset of effusion after an injury usually denotes a hemarthrosis, and it can occur when the vascularized periphery of a meniscus is torn.
  - Tears occurring within the body of a meniscus or in degenerative areas may not produce a hemarthrosis.
  - Repeated displacement of a pedunculated or torn portion of a meniscus can produce sufficient synovial irritation to produce a chronic synovitis with an effusion of a nonbloody nature.
  - The absence of an effusion or hemarthrosis does not rule out a tear of the meniscus.
- Atrophy of the musculature about the knee suggests a recurring disability of the knee but does not indicate its cause.
- Clicks, snaps, or catches, either audible or detected by palpation during flexion, extension, and rotary motions of the joint, can be valuable diagnostically, and efforts should be made to reproduce and accurately locate them.
- Numerous manipulative tests have been described, but the McMurray test is most commonly used. Although other tests cannot be considered diagnostic, they are useful enough to be included in the routine examination of the knee.
  - For the McMurray test, with the knee completely flexed, the examiner palpates the joint line with one hand and uses the other hand to rotate the foot internally while extending the knee. The maneuver is repeated with the foot externally rotated. If a meniscal tear is present, a click may be heard or felt in the joint line of the affected side during this maneuver.
  - The grinding test, as described by Apley, is another test for isolating meniscal pathology. With the patient prone, the knee is flexed to 90 degrees and the anterior thigh is fixed against the examining table. Traction on the foot is used to distract the joint and the foot is rotated. Next, with the knee in the same position, the foot and leg are pressed downward and rotated as the joint is slowly flexed and extended.
  - Another useful test, the squat test, consists of several repetitions of a full squat with the feet and legs alternately fully internally and externally rotated as the squat is performed. Reproduction of pain on the medial or lateral side of the knee is suggestive although not diagnostic of meniscal tear.
- The diagnosis of internal derangement of the knee caused by a meniscal tear can be difficult to make even for an experienced orthopedic surgeon, but a careful history and physical examination combined with appropriate imaging studies help to limit errors in diagnosis and unnecessary arthroscopy.

- During an injury, damage to other structures of the knee such as the ligaments and articular cartilage is common. For simplicity, tears of the menisci are discussed here as though they were isolated injuries, but evidence of other injuries always must be sought.

IMAGING AND OTHER DIAGNOSTIC STUDIES

- Imaging includes standing anteroposterior, 45-degree posteroanterior, and patellofemoral views to exclude other causes of knee pain such as joint degeneration, loose bodies, and osteochondritis dissecans.
- Other noninvasive diagnostic studies, such as ultrasonography, scintigraphy, computed tomography (CT), and MRI, have been shown to improve diagnostic accuracy in many knee disorders.
- Compared with arthroscopy, MRI has been shown to have 98% accuracy for medial meniscal tears and 90% for lateral meniscal tears.
- Others have reported that MRI had a positive predictive value of 75%, a negative predictive value of 90%, a sensitivity of 83%, and a specificity of 84% for pathologic changes in the menisci.
- MR arthrography may be useful in evaluating knees with prior meniscectomy or meniscal repair.
- High-resolution CT has been reported to have a sensitivity of 96.5%, specificity of 81.3%, and accuracy of 91%, but we usually use this study to evaluate the patellofemoral joint.

DIFFERENTIAL DIAGNOSIS

- Ligament injury
- Chondral injury
- Osteochondral loose body
- Pathologic plica
- Patellar maltracking
- Intra-articular tumor

NONOPERATIVE MANAGEMENT

- An incomplete meniscal tear or a small (5-mm) stable peripheral tear with no other pathologic condition, such as a torn ACL, can be treated nonoperatively with predictably good results. Many incomplete tears will not progress to complete tears if the knee is stable.
- Small stable peripheral tears have been observed to heal after 6 to 8 weeks of protection.
- Stable vertical longitudinal tears, which tend to occur in the peripheral vascular portions of the menisci, have been reported to heal with nonoperative treatment.
- Meniscal tears that cause infrequent and minimal symptoms can be treated with rehabilitation and restricted activity.
- Tears associated with ligamentous instabilities can be treated nonoperatively if the patient defers ligament reconstruction or if reconstruction is contraindicated.
- Nonsurgical management consists of activity modification, nonsteroidal anti-inflammatories, and physical therapy.
- If symptoms recur after a period of nonoperative treatment, surgical repair or removal of the damaged meniscus may be necessary.
- The most important aspect of nonoperative treatment, once the acute pain and effusion have subsided, is restoration of the normal knee range of motion and muscle strength. This can be accomplished through a regular program of progressive exercises to include the quadriceps, hamstrings, hip flexors, and hip abductors.

SURGICAL MANAGEMENT

- Indications for surgical treatment of meniscal tears include:
  - Symptoms that affect sports participation or activities of daily living or work (locking, giving way, frequent effusions)
  - Failure of nonoperative treatment
  - Absence of other causes of knee pain (based on complete clinical and imaging evaluations)
- Meniscectomy is categorized into three types depending on the amount of meniscus removed:
  - Partial meniscectomy, in which only loose, unstable meniscal fragments are excised and a stable and balanced peripheral rim of healthy meniscal tissue is preserved (**FIG 7**)
  - Subtotal meniscectomy, in which the type and extent of the tear require excision of a portion of the peripheral rim, usually leaving most of the anterior horn and a portion of the middle third intact
  - Total meniscectomy
- Historically, the indications and surgical techniques for excision of torn menisci have been controversial.
  - Some have advocated total excision of torn menisci, whereas others have proposed subtotal excision.
  - Justification for total excision often was based on short-term, functional recovery criteria; however, longer follow-up showed associated degenerative changes.
  - Removal of even one third of the meniscus has been shown to increase joint contact forces by up to 350%.
  - The amount of degenerative change in the articular cartilage appears to be directly proportional to the amount of meniscus removed.
- If meniscal pathology produces almost daily symptoms, frequent locking, or repeated or chronic effusions, the pathologic portion of the meniscus should be removed because the problems caused by the present disability far outweigh the probability or significance of future degenerative arthritis.
- If a significant portion of the peripheral rim can be retained by subtotal meniscal excision, the long-term result is improved.
- Partial meniscectomy by arthroscopic technique has sufficient support and clinical results to indicate its routine use.
- Subtotal meniscectomy is justified only when it is irreparably torn, and the meniscal rim should be preserved if at all possible.
- Total meniscectomy is no longer considered the treatment of choice in young athletes or other people whose daily activities require vigorous use of the knee.

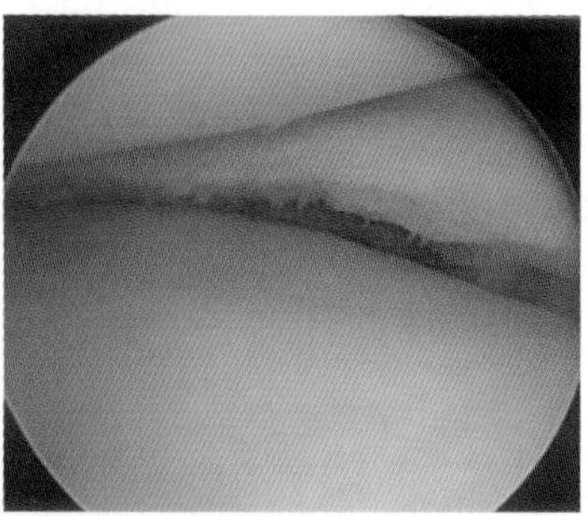

FIG 7 • Partial meniscectomy: loose unstable fragments are excised and a stable and balanced peripheral rim of healthy meniscal tissue is preserved.

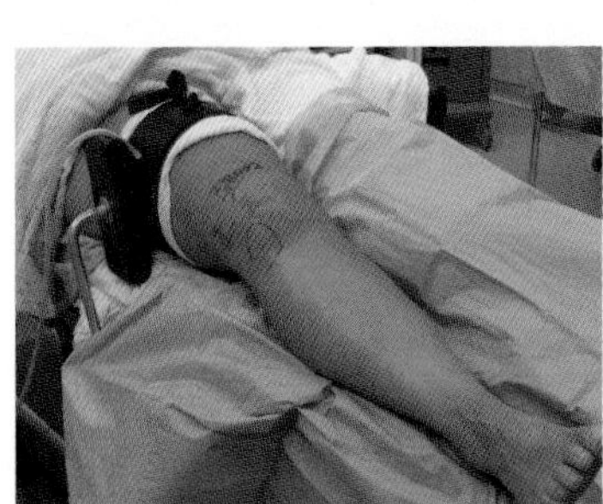

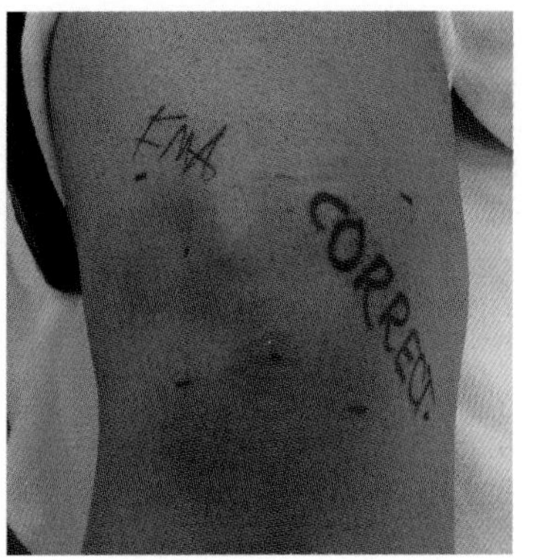

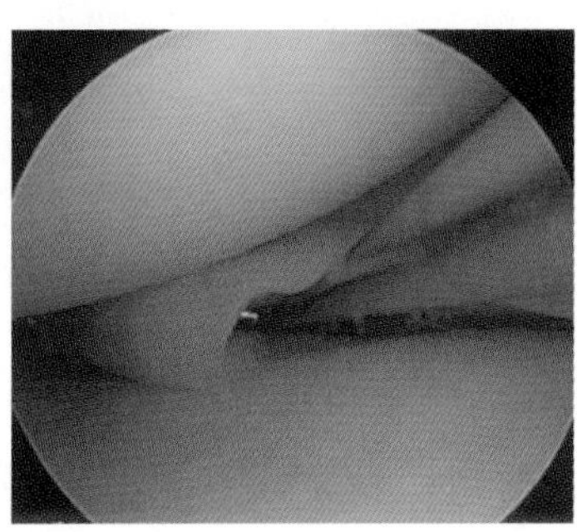

A B C

FIG 8 • **A.** Patient positioning for meniscectomy. **B.** Surgical landmarks are outlined; operative extremity is clearly identified and surgeon has "signed the site." **C.** Arthroscopic probe used to determine extent of meniscal tear.

Preoperative Planning

- A discussion regarding meniscal repair versus removal should be conducted preoperatively. The patient should understand the risks, benefits, alternatives, and potential complications of both, as well as the variations in postoperative recovery time and rehabilitation.
- The patient also should understand the potential for recurrent meniscal tear and long-term consequences of meniscectomy.
- A discussion also should be held about the treatment of additional pathology, such as chondral lesions, that may be a source of continued symptoms postoperatively.
- The necessary equipment should be present to treat whatever meniscal or chondral pathology might be encountered.

Positioning

- The patient is placed supine with the nonoperative leg in a leg holder that brings the extremity into flexion at the hip and knee (**FIG 8A**).
- The use of a proximal leg holder for the operative knee places the patient's foot on the surgeon's iliac crest, eliminating the need for an assistant to hold the leg.

Approach

- After an examination under anesthesia, joint lines and soft tissue and bony landmarks are drawn on the skin before joint distention (**FIG 8B**).
  - Typically, these are the outlines of the patella and patellar tendon, the medial and lateral joint lines, and the posterior contours of the medial and lateral femoral condyles.
- Standard and optional arthroscopic portals are marked (see Chap. SM-31).
  - A small outflow, needle-type cannula can be placed superomedially or superolaterally, with inflow through the arthroscope, but this often is not needed for meniscectomy.
- A two-portal or three-portal technique can be used (see Chap. SM-31).
  - The anterolateral and anteromedial portals are most commonly used with the two-portal technique.
- Occasionally, a posteromedial, accessory medial, or central portal is used to assist in removal of displaced meniscal fragments.
- Thorough, systematic arthroscopic examination of the knee joint must be done before the decision is made for partial or subtotal meniscectomy (see Chap. SM-31).
  - An arthroscopic probe should be used to examine the meniscal tear to determine its anterior and posterior extents (**FIG 8C**). The probe should be used to palpate the superior and inferior extents of the meniscus.
- When an irreparable meniscal tear is identified, all mobile fragments that can be pulled past the inner margin of the meniscus into the joint should be removed and the remaining meniscus contoured to reduce the risk of leaving a defect that can propagate into a larger tear.
- The meniscal rim does not need to be perfectly smooth, and the amount of meniscus removed and contouring of the rim must be weighed against the risk of degenerative changes (the risk of degenerative changes is directly proportional to the amount of meniscus removed).
- The goal is to remove the tear entirely while removing as little meniscus as possible.

ARTHROSCOPIC PARTIAL MENISCECTOMY FOR CONVENTIONAL TEARS

- The goals of surgery are to remove the mobile segment at the meniscal base and to contour the remaining meniscus to leave as wide a rim as possible.
- Any tags or pieces of meniscus that may catch in the joint or can be displaced into the center of the joint are resected with meniscal forceps, baskets, scissors, or graspers (**TECH FIG 1**).
- Full-radius resectors and motorized suction shavers are used to remove damaged cartilage, smooth the meniscal rim, and remove loose pieces of meniscus and cartilage.
- Various ablation devices can be used to contour tears; however, care must be taken not to damage adjacent articular cartilage.
- For horizontal cleavage tears, one or both "leaves" can be resected, depending on surgeon preference. No definitive study has shown that preserving either the superior or inferior leaf improves results.

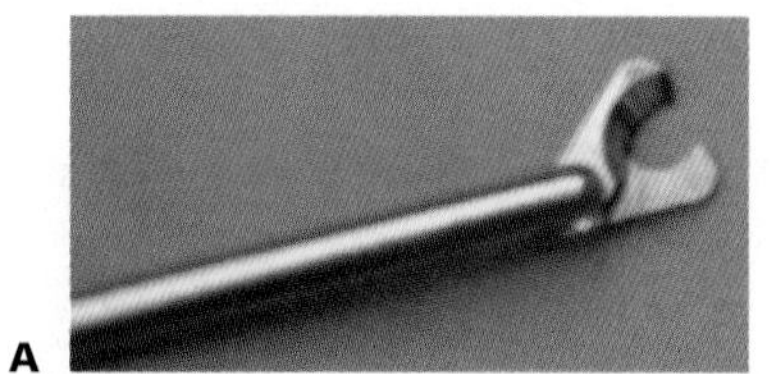

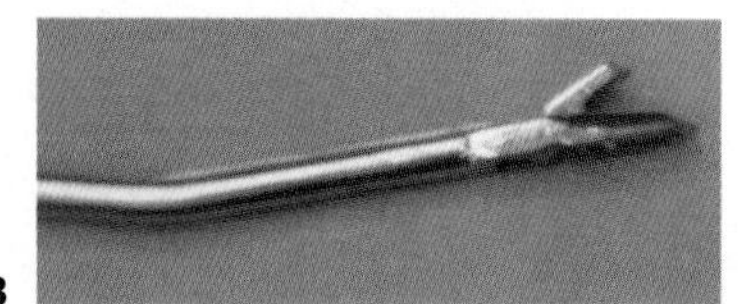

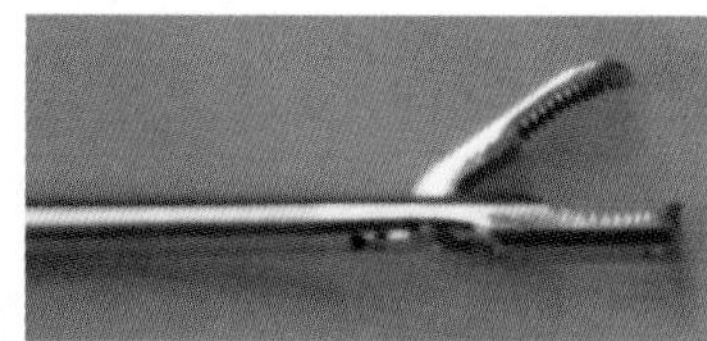

TECH FIG 1 • **A.** Meniscal scissors. **B.** Meniscal basket. **C.** Meniscal grasper.

ARTHROSCOPIC PARTIAL MENISCECTOMY FOR BUCKET-HANDLE TEARS

- A probe or blunt trocar is used to reduce the fragment to its normal position (TECH FIG 2A).
- Partial division of the posterior attachment of the meniscal fragment is done with basket forceps, scissors, or an arthroscopic knife. The cut should go almost completely through the posterior attachment of the mobile fragment at its junction with the remaining normal meniscal rim (TECH FIG 2B).
- To avoid damage to the normal meniscus or articular cartilage, this cut should not be made blindly. Exposure can be aided by passing the arthroscope through the intercondylar notch to view the posterior horn of the meniscus while cutting. Alternatively, a posteromedial portal can be made for direct observation.
- A small tag of meniscal tissue is left intact posteriorly to prevent the meniscus from becoming a loose body in the joint after anterior release.
- The anterior horn attachment is divided with angled scissors, basket forceps, or an arthroscopic knife. The release should be made flush with the intact anterior rim so that no stump or dog-ear remains (TECH FIG 2C).
- If access to the anterior horn attachment is difficult through the ipsilateral portal, changing portal sites and approaching from the contralateral portal with the

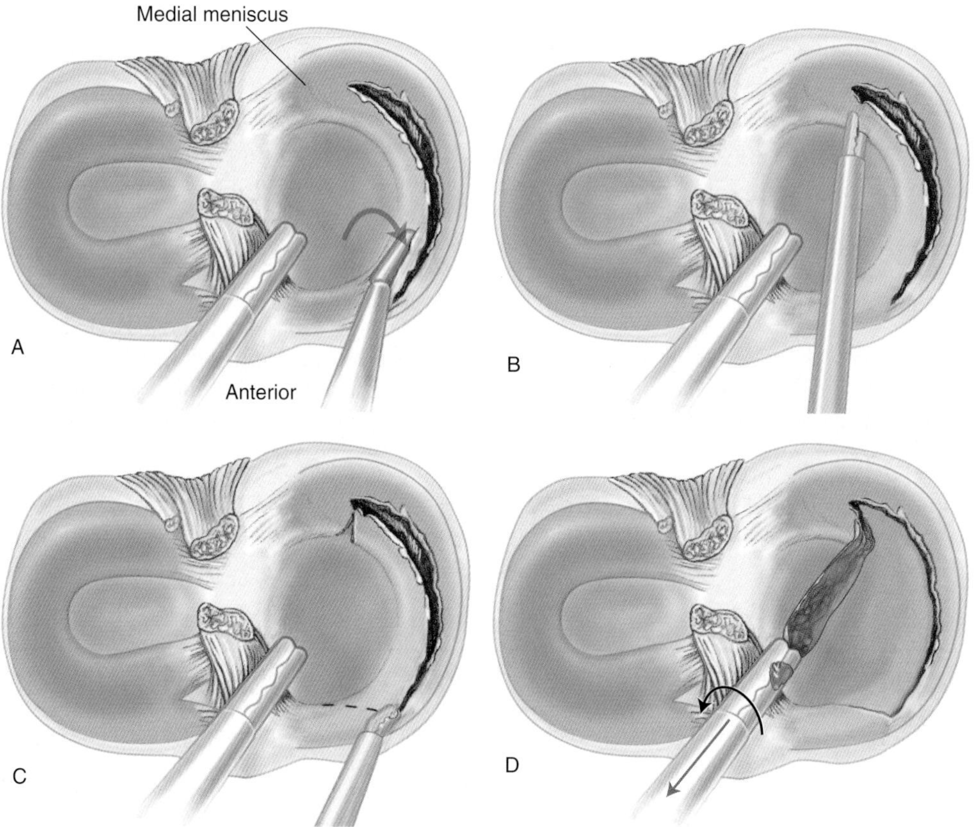

TECH FIG 2 • Meniscectomy for a bucket-handle tear. **A.** Displaced fragment is reduced into normal position with a probe. **B.** Posterior attachment is almost transected with a meniscal biter. **C.** Anterior attachment is transected with a meniscal biter or knife. **D.** Fragment is grasped and rotated to avulse the few remaining strands of meniscal tissue. (Adapted from Scott N. The Knee. St. Louis: Mosby, 1994.)

instrument often makes this easier. Rarely, a midpatellar portal is necessary so that both anterior portals can be used for instruments.

- A hemostat is used to enlarge the capsular incision before attempting meniscal removal.
- A grasping clamp is inserted through the ipsilateral portal to grasp the meniscal fragment as close to its remaining posterior attachment as possible. With the fragment in view, the grasping forceps are twisted and rotated while applying traction to avulse the few remaining strands of meniscus, and the fragment is removed from the joint (TECH FIG 2D).
- Occasionally, the meniscal fragment cannot be detached with the grasping forceps alone. With a grasper through the lateral portal for traction on the meniscus, an arthroscopic scissor can be passed through the same portal to complete the resection. If necessary, an accessory portal can be made for the scope so that the two anterior portals can be used for instruments.
- A motorized meniscal shaver is used to smooth the remaining rim.

ARTHROSCOPIC PARTIAL MENISCECTOMY AND MENISCAL CYST DECOMPRESSION

- The meniscus is carefully probed to identify the extent of the meniscal tear. Radial tears are trimmed to a stable peripheral rim. For stable horizontal tears, only the inferior leaf is resected and the superior leaf is gently trimmed.
- The cyst is palpated externally, which may push the cyst material into the joint and decompress the cyst, allowing identification of the cyst communication.
- If this is not successful, a spinal needle can be inserted percutaneously through the cystic mass to help locate the track between the cyst and the meniscus. Punch forceps passed through the tear and tracked into the cyst may widen the track enough for the contents of the cyst to be evacuated into the joint.
- If necessary, a small, motorized shaver is inserted into the cyst to break up loculations, assist in cyst decompression, and stimulate inflammation and scarring of the cyst.

ARTHROSCOPIC PARTIAL EXCISION OF DISCOID LATERAL MENISCUS

- The following principles can be applied to all three types of discoid lateral menisci, including incomplete, complete, and Wrisberg types.
- In young patients with small knees, a 2.7-mm arthroscope and small-joint instruments should be used.
- In older individuals, the standard 4-mm arthroscope is used. In addition to standard technique, anteromedial and lateral portals can be used for instrumentation while viewing through a medial midpatellar portal.
- With the knee in a figure 4 position, basket forceps are used to begin the central resection of the discoid tissue (TECH FIG 3A).
- With the discoid meniscus under direct observation, resection is planned so that a healthy peripheral meniscus about 8 mm wide remains.
- When the desired amount of meniscal tissue has been removed and the rim is balanced, the thickness of the inner edge is much greater than that after routine partial meniscectomy (TECH FIG 3B).
- For a Wrisberg-type discoid meniscus, a repair with saucerization is recommended; however, if an inadequate posterior tibial attachment is present, total meniscectomy may be indicated.

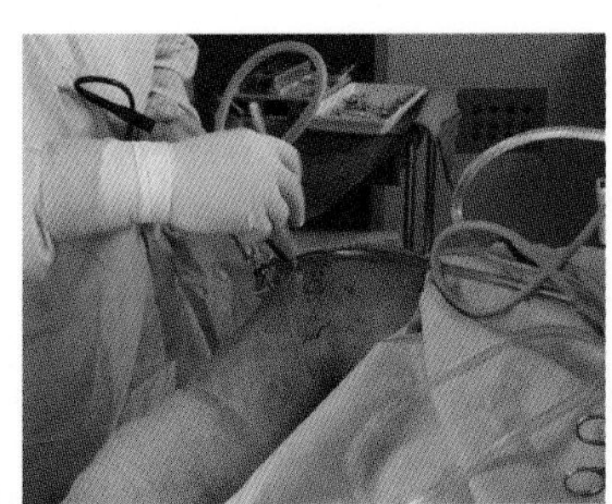

A

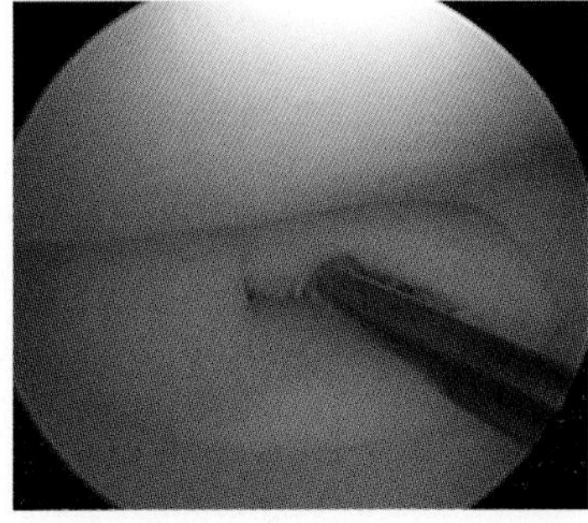

B

TECH FIG 3 • **A.** Knee is placed in figure 4 position for resection of discoid meniscus. **B.** Discoid meniscus with radial tear.

PEARLS AND PITFALLS

The number of portals should be minimized.	■ With multiple portals, the surgeon must watch for fluid extravasation.
The knife blade is directed medially or laterally away from the patellar tendon for horizontal portals and superiorly away from the anterior of the menisci for vertical portals.	
The leg holder or post is placed about 10 cm above the superior pole of the patella.	■ If too proximal or distal, the surgeon cannot obtain sufficient valgus stress to open the medial joint for inspection.
A systematic approach is used so that any pathology present can be identified.	1. The surgeon inspects the following: a. Anterior compartment (suprapatellar region, patellofemoral joint [including tracking], lower trochlea). b. Medial and lateral gutters c. Medial and lateral compartments d. Posterior compartment (by directing arthroscope medial to posterior cruciate ligament) 2. The surgeon probes the menisci superiorly and inferiorly: can have up to 5 mm physiologic excursion of posterior horn of medial meniscus; can have up to 10 mm physiologic excursion posterior horn of lateral meniscus. 3. The surgeon inspects for pathologic plicae that may mimic meniscal tear. 4. The surgeon inspects and probes for displaced meniscal fragments, which may be submeniscal or in the posterior compartment (**FIG 9**).

A 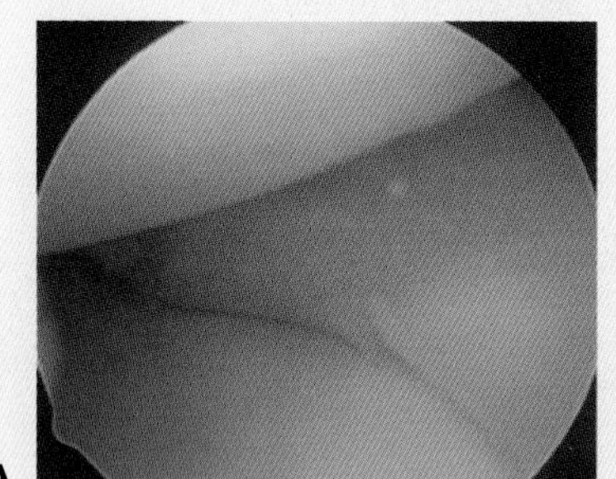

B 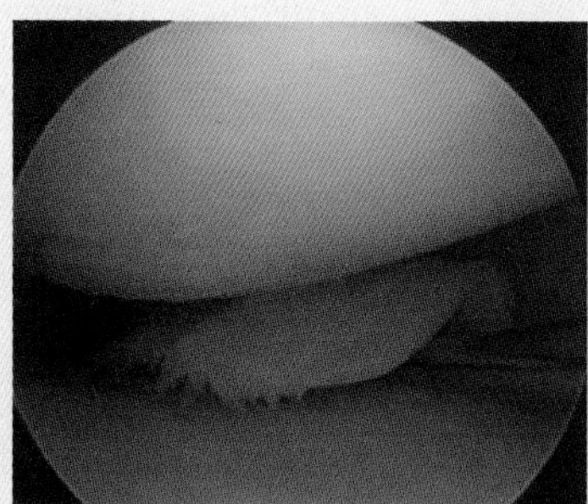

FIG 9 • Displaced meniscal fragment (**A**), which must be located and removed (**B**).

POSTOPERATIVE CARE

- No brace or range-of-motion restrictions
- Immediate full weight bearing with crutches as needed
- Cold therapy
- Nonsteroidal anti-inflammatories at 2 weeks if not contraindicated
- Active, passive, and active-assisted range of motion immediately postoperatively
- Straight-leg-raise exercises immediately
- Return to sports when full range of motion is regained, no effusion is present, and strength is 80% of uninjured side (usually 4 to 6 weeks minimum)

OUTCOMES

- The knee can function well without the meniscus, sometimes for the rest of a patient's life, but late degenerative changes within the joint sometimes occur, and the loss of the meniscus undoubtedly plays some part in producing these changes.
- In addition to the condition of the meniscus, numerous other factors can influence long-term function, such as joint alignment, laxity of the capsular or ligamentous structures, and incomplete rehabilitation of the musculature about the knee.
- Fairbank[10] described three changes he had observed in the knee, alone or in combination, in patients who had had a meniscectomy, at intervals ranging from 3 months to 14 years after the surgery:
  - The development of an anteroposterior ridge that projected distally from the margin of the femoral condyle
  - Flattening of the peripheral half of the articular surface of the condyle
  - Narrowing of the joint space
  - These changes have been reported in 40% to 90% of patients with meniscectomy in ACL-deficient knees. Considerable evidence indicates that meniscectomy often is followed by degenerative changes within the joint, but whether the injury, the damaged meniscus itself, or its excision led to the degenerative changes cannot be determined with certainty in most of these studies. Probably all these factors, and others as well, have an influence.
- Partial meniscectomy has been proven to have significantly better outcomes than total meniscectomy (90% and 68% good results, respectively, reported in comparison study).

- Generally, outcomes after medial partial meniscectomy (80% to 100% good to excellent results) have been better than after lateral partial meniscectomy (54% to 92% good to excellent results). A recent review of the literature, however, reported that there were consistently no significant differences in radiographic or functional outcome between medial and lateral meniscal injury in the studies included in their analysis.
- Reported results of partial meniscectomy for discoid meniscus in children are generally good (87% to 100% good to excellent results).
- Results tend to deteriorate with time because of degenerative changes in the knee joint; however, continued good to excellent results have been reported with follow-up as long as 20 years.
- Two primary factors associated with worse results of partial meniscectomy are preexisting osteoarthritis and ACL deficiency. Other factors suggested to predispose to poor outcomes are age more than 35 years, female gender, presence of medial cartilage degeneration, resection of the posterior third of the meniscus, and meniscal rim resection.
- Preoperative participation in sports has been shown to be a predictor of a better outcome.

COMPLICATIONS

- Possible complications after partial or total meniscectomy are the same as those after any arthroscopic procedure on the knee (see Chap. SM-31).
- Patients should be informed of the risks of infection, deep vein thrombosis (with or without pulmonary embolism), recurrent effusions, incomplete tear removal, synovial–cutaneous fistula, arteriovenous fistula, popliteal pseudoaneurysm, and compartment syndrome.

REFERENCES

1. Alford JW, Lewis P, Kang RW, et al. Rapid progression of chondral disease in the lateral compartment of the knee following meniscectomy. Arthroscopy 2005;21:1505–1509.
2. Allen CR, Wong EK, Livesay GA, et al. Importance of the medial meniscus in the anterior cruciate ligament-deficient knee. J Orthop Res 2000;18:109–115.
3. Anderson-Molina H, Karlsson H, Rockborn P. Arthroscopic partial and total meniscectomy: a long-term follow-up study with matched controls. Arthroscopy 2002;18:183–189.
4. Arnoczky SP, Warren RF. Microvasculature of the human meniscus. Am J Sports Med 1982;10:90–95.
5. Arnoczky SP, Warren RF, Kaplan N. Meniscal remodeling following partial meniscectomy: an experimental study in the dog. Arthroscopy 1985;1:247–252.
6. Bowen TR, Feldmann DD, Miller MD. Return to play following surgical treatment of meniscal and chondral injuries to the knee. Clin Sports Med 2004;23:381–393.
7. Charalambous CP, Tryfonidis M, Alvi F, et al. Purely intra-articular versus general anesthesia for proposed arthroscopic partial meniscectomy of the knee: a randomized controlled trial. Arthroscopy 2006; 22:972–977.
8. Chastain F, Robinson SH, Adeleine P, et al. The natural history of the knee following arthroscopic medial meniscectomy. Knee Surg Sports Traumatol Arthrosc 2001;9:15–18.
9. Ericsson YB, Roos EM, Dahlberg L. Muscle strength, functional performance, and self-reported outcomes four years after arthroscopic partial meniscectomy in middle-aged patients. Arthritis Rheum 2006; 55:946–952.
10. Fairbank TJ. Knee joint changes after meniscectomy. J Bone Joint Surg Br 1948;30:664-670.
11. Good CR, Green DW, Griffith MH, et al. Arthroscopic treatment of symptomatic discoid meniscus in children: classification, technique, and results. Arthroscopy 2007;23:157–163.
12. Haemer JM, Wang MJ, Carter DR, et al. Benefit of single-leaf resection for horizontal meniscus tear. Clin Orthop Relat Res 2007;457: 194–202.
13. Herrlin S, Hallander M, Wange P, et al. Arthroscopic or conservative treatment of degenerative medial meniscal tears: a prospective randomised trial. Knee Surg Sports Traumatol Arthrosc 2007;15: 393–401.
14. Higuchi H, Kimura M, Shirakura K, et al. Factors affecting long-term results after arthroscopic partial meniscectomy. Clin Orthop Relat Res 2000;377:161–168.
15. Kuraishi J, Akizuki S, Takizawa T, et al. Arthroscopic lateral meniscectomy in knees with lateral compartment osteoarthritis: a case series study. Arthroscopy 2006;22:878–883.
16. Lee SJ, Aadalen KJ, Malaviya P, et al. Tibiofemoral contact mechanics after serial medial meniscectomies in the human cadaveric knee. Am J Sports Med 2006;34:1334–1344.
17. McDermott ID, Amis AA. The consequences of meniscectomy. J Bone Joint Surg Br 2006;88B:1549–1556.
18. Meredith DS, Losian E, Mahomed NN, et al. Factors predicting functional and radiographic outcomes after arthroscopic partial meniscectomy: a review of the literature. Arthroscopy 2005;21:211–223.
19. Miller MD, Warner JJP, Harner CD. Meniscal repair. In: Fu HH, Harner CD, Vince KG, eds. Knee Surgery. Baltimore: Williams & Wilkins, 1994.
20. Okazaki K, Miura H, Matsuda S, et al. Arthroscopic resection of the discoid lateral meniscus: long-term follow-up for 16 years. Arthroscopy 2006;22:967–971.
21. Pena E, Calvo B, Martinez MA, et al. Why lateral meniscectomy is more dangerous than medial meniscectomy: a finite element study. J Orthop Res 2006;24:1001–1010.
22. Phillips BB: Arthroscopy of the lower extremity. In: Canale ST, Beaty JH, eds. Campbell's Operative Orthopaedics, ed 11. Philadelphia: Elsevier, 2008.
23. Scheller G, Sobau C, Bulow JU. Arthroscopic partial lateral meniscectomy in an otherwise normal knee: clinical, functional, and radiographic results of a long-term follow-up study. Arthroscopy 2001; 17:946–952.
24. Shelbourne KD, Carr DR. Meniscal repair compared with meniscectomy for bucket-handle medial meniscal tears in anterior cruciate ligament-reconstructed knees. Am J Sports Med 2003;31:718–723.
25. Shelbourne KD, Dickens JF. Digital radiographic evaluation of medial joint space narrowing after partial meniscectomy of bucket-handle medial meniscus tears in anterior cruciate ligament-intact knees. Am J Sports Med 2006;34:1648–1655.
26. Soto G, Safran MR. Arthroscopic meniscectomy. In: Miller MD, Cole BJ, eds. Textbook of Arthroscopy. Philadelphia: WB Saunders, 2004.
27. Walker PS, Erkman MJ. The role of the menisci in force transmission across the knee. Clin Orthop Rel Res 1975;109:184–192.
28. Wojtys EM, Chan DB. Meniscus structure and function. AAOS Instr Course Lect 2005;54:323–330.

Chapter 34 Meniscal Repair

Nicholas A. Sgaglione and Michael J. Angel

DEFINITION

- A meniscus tear results in mechanical disruption of the gross structure of the medial or lateral meniscus or both.
- The goals of meniscus repair are to preserve and optimize meniscus function and to restore joint biomechanics.

ANATOMY

- The medial meniscus and the lateral meniscus are crescent-shaped and triangular in cross section.
- The medial meniscus is C-shaped. It covers about 64% of the tibial plateau. Its width varies from anterior to posterior, with an average of 10 mm (**FIG 1**).
- The lateral meniscus is more circular. It covers about 84% of the tibial plateau, with an average width of 12 to 13 mm.
- The menisci are fibrocartilaginous structures made up of collagen (90% type I and the remainder made up of types II, III, V, and VI), fibrochondrocytes, and water.
- The collagen fibers are arranged in a circumferential pattern in the peripheral third, whereas the inner two thirds is organized with a combination of radial and circumferential fibers (see Fig 3A in Chap. SM-33).
- The menisci function to deepen the articular surface of the tibial plateau, providing shock absorption and compensating for gross incongruity between the articulating surfaces, acting as joint stabilizers. They provide joint lubrication and maintenance of synovial fluid and assist in providing nutrition of articular cartilage.[16]
- The vascular supply comes from the perimeniscal capillary plexus supplied by the medial and lateral inferior and superior geniculate arteries. The plexus penetrates the meniscus peripherally and its abundance decreases as it crosses centrally.
  - This difference in vascularity creates the red-red, red-white, and white-white zones.[2]
- The meniscus contains free nerve endings and corpuscular mechanoreceptors, providing pain and proprioception in the knee joint.[16]

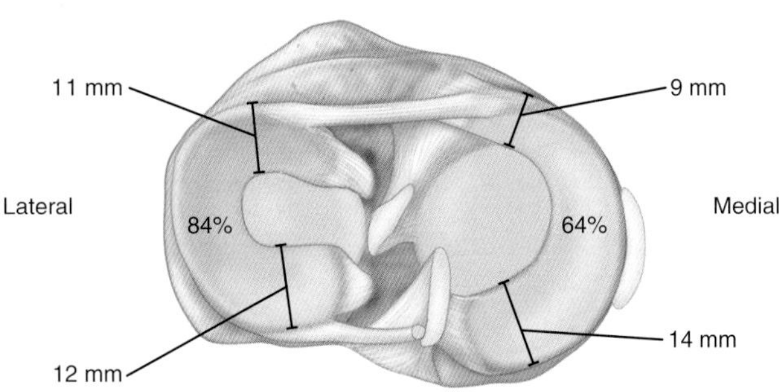

FIG 1 • Anatomy of the meniscus, showing the average sizes of the components of the medial and lateral meniscus with the average amount of tibial plateau coverage.

PATHOGENESIS

- Acute tears typically occur in younger patients from compression and rotational injury of the knee joint as it moves from a flexed to an extended position.
- Degenerative tears are typically chronic in nature, are found in older patients, are complex, and are usually irreparable.
- Medial meniscus tears most often occur in the stable knee or chronic anterior cruciate ligament (ACL)-deficient knee, whereas lateral tears occur more often in younger patients with acute ACL tears.
  - Associated injuries are often found. The "terrible triad" consists of tears of the lateral meniscus, ACL, and medial collateral ligament. It is often sustained from a hyperextension with a valgus stress, such as during a "clipping" injury in football.
- Tears may be classified according to anatomic zone (as described by Cooper et al[7]), vascularity (red-red, red-white, white-white), or by tear pattern.
- Tear patterns are described as horizontal, radial, longitudinal, bucket-handle, oblique, or complex (see Fig 2 in Chap. SM-33).[7]

NATURAL HISTORY

- Walker and Erkman[24] in 1975 found that with loads up to 150 kg, the lateral meniscus bore most of the weight bearing in that compartment, whereas the medial meniscus shared about 50% of the load with the articulating surfaces of the tibiofemoral joint.
  - Partial and total meniscectomy has been shown to increase the contact stresses exerted on the articular cartilage, resulting in its degeneration and ultimately osteoarthritis.
  - After partial meniscectomy, femoral–tibial contact areas decrease by about 10%, with peak local contact stresses (PLCS) increasing by about 65%. After total meniscectomy, contact areas decrease about 75% and PLCS increases about 235%.[3]
  - PLCSs and contact areas were found to be the same with meniscus repair.[3]
- Partial meniscectomy has been shown to improve prognosis and decrease chondral wear compared to total meniscectomy.

PATIENT HISTORY AND PHYSICAL FINDINGS

- The history should include location of pain (joint line tenderness), recent traumas, prior injuries and surgery, as well as evidence of effusions, locking, catching, or instability (which may indicate associated ligamentous pathology).
- In addition, questions should be asked about the patient's age, function, activity level, occupation, goals, expectations, and other pertinent medical problems. These will help the surgeon decide on nonsurgical versus surgical treatment and resection versus repair.

- A complete examination of the knee should be performed, including evaluation for:
  - Anterior and posterior ligament injury: Lachman, anterior and posterior drawer, pivot shift, along with a history of hearing a "pop" with injury and acute swelling
  - Posterolateral corner injury: injury of the popliteus tendon, iliotibial band, popliteofibular ligament, biceps, and posterior capsule. Asymmetry on the dial (external rotation) test is the most sensitive examination.
  - Collateral ligament injury: Medial and lateral collateral ligament injuries may be assessed by palpation and widening with varus–valgus stresses at 30 degrees and at full extension.
- The examiner should also:
- Inspect for effusion. The presence of diffuse joint effusion is not specific enough. A localized swelling at the joint line may indicate a parameniscal cyst.
- Palpate all ligament and tendon insertions, as well as the patellofemoral joint; this may indicate associated pathology.
- Evaluate range of motion. Loss of extension or locking may relate to a displaced or bucket-handle tear. Pain with squatting may indicate a posterior horn tear.
- Perform the McMurray test to evaluate varus–valgus stress. Positive valgus stress indicates a medial meniscus tear. Positive varus stress indicates a lateral meniscus tear.
- Perform the Apley test to look for a meniscus tear. Relief on distraction is found if a meniscus tear is the only pathology, but no relief will be found if a concomitant collateral ligament injury is present.
- Perform the Childress test, which is positive if the patient has pain or mechanical blocking; this may indicate a meniscus tear.
- While assessing for the Merkel sign, pain with internal rotation of tibia is consistent with a medial meniscus tear; pain with external rotation is consistent with a lateral meniscus tear.

IMAGING AND OTHER DIAGNOSTIC STUDIES

- Plain radiographs should be taken to evaluate for bony pathology, extremity alignment, arthritis, chondrocalcinosis, or findings consistent with associated injuries such as a Segond sign (ACL injury), osteochondritis dissecans lesion, or osteochondral fracture.
  - Typically four views are obtained: a 30- or 45-degree posteroanterior flexion weight-bearing view, a true lateral view, a notch view, and a patella skyline view.
- Magnetic resonance imaging (MRI) is not always indicated to evaluate for meniscal pathology, but it is typically used and helpful in evaluation of associated injuries when a meniscus tear is suspected. The sensitivity of MRI for meniscus tears is reported as high as 96%, with a specificity of 97%.[13]
- MRI classification is as follows:
  - Grade 1: small focal area of increased signal, not extending to the joint surface
  - Grade 2: linear area of increased signal, not extending to the joint surface
  - Grade 3: linear area of increased signal extending to the joint surface
- A linear abnormality is identified as extension to the articular surface on two consecutive images and is considered to have a high likelihood of being a true tear (**FIG 2A**).
- A bucket-handle tear may be identified by the "double PCL" (posterior cruciate ligament) sign (**FIG 2B,C**).

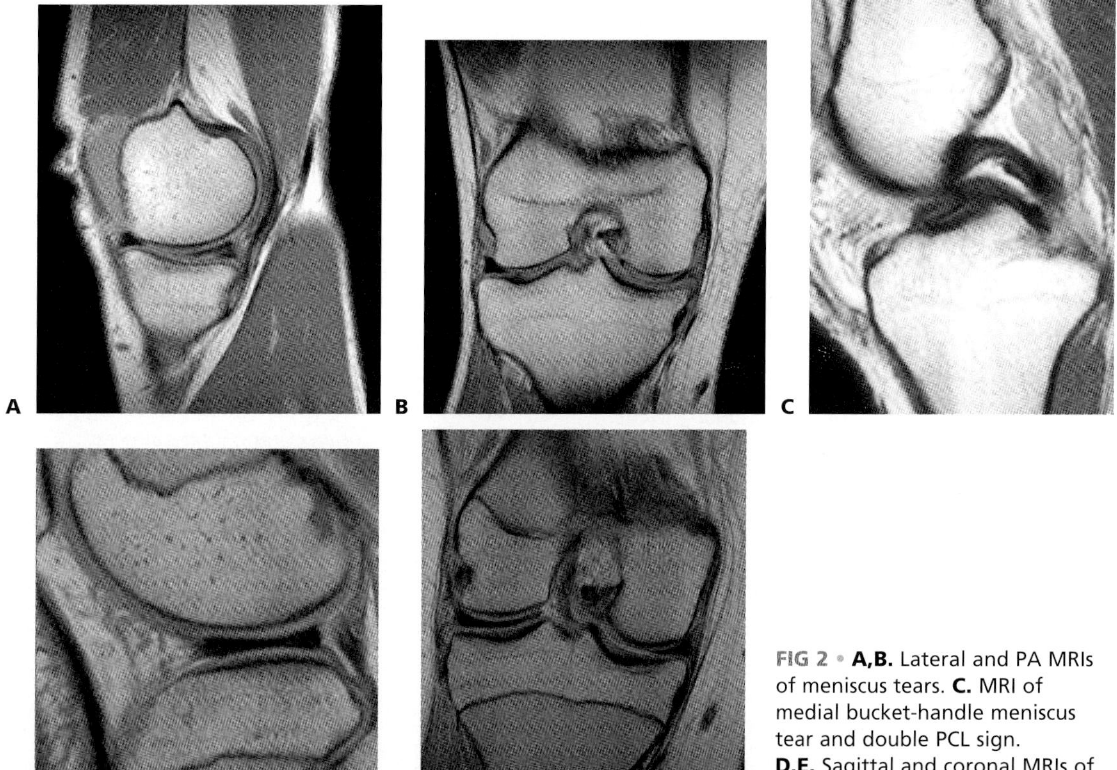

FIG 2 • **A,B.** Lateral and PA MRIs of meniscus tears. **C.** MRI of medial bucket-handle meniscus tear and double PCL sign. **D,E.** Sagittal and coronal MRIs of discoid lateral meniscus tears.

- Evaluation of the meniscus postoperatively presents a challenge because the repair site becomes filled with fibrous scar and may continue to produce abnormal MR signal on postoperative imaging. Currently the best method of evaluation is with a gadolinium-enhanced MRI.
- A discoid meniscus may be evident on MRI as a rectangular meniscus on all slices as opposed to the wedge shape typically seen. It is more commonly found in the lateral meniscus (**FIG 2D,E**).

DIFFERENTIAL DIAGNOSIS

- ACL or PCL tear
- Medial or lateral collateral ligament tear
- Osteochondritis dissecans lesion
- Patellofemoral syndrome
- Osteoarthritis
- Chondrocalcinosis

NONOPERATIVE MANAGEMENT

- Conservative treatment options include physical therapy, nonsteroidal anti-inflammatory medications, steroid injections, and activity modification.
- Typically, a stable longitudinal tear in the periphery less than 10 mm is likely to heal on its own.
- Bracing usually is not indicated in the treatment of meniscus tears.
- The expected result of nonoperative treatment is improved symptoms in 6 weeks, with return to full activities by 3 months.

SURGICAL MANAGEMENT

- Intervention may proceed after failure of conservative treatment or more urgently if the patient shows mechanical symptoms such as locking or catching. These may represent loose bodies or an unstable torn meniscus (ie, bucket-handle tear), which can cause significant articular damage if left untreated.
- With all meniscus pathology, the goal is to preserve as much meniscus as possible.
- Repair versus resection
  - The potential long-term benefit of repairing the meniscus is chondroprotection.
  - The surgeon should consider tear location, pattern, vascularity, and associated pathology when determining whether to repair or resect the meniscus.
  - The surgeon should consider the patient's age, activity level, overall health, and compliance with a limited postoperative activity regimen.
  - When resection is performed, all efforts should be made to preserve as much viable meniscus as possible. Mobile, unstable meniscus fragments should be resected, leaving a smooth contour.
  - The meniscosynovial junction should be preserved because this is where the circumferential collagen fibers form the predominant amount of "hoop stresses."
  - The surgeon should consider leaving a stable tear alone. An unstable tear will be easily mobilized, displaced at least 7 mm, and/or will have the ability to "roll" (**FIG 3**).

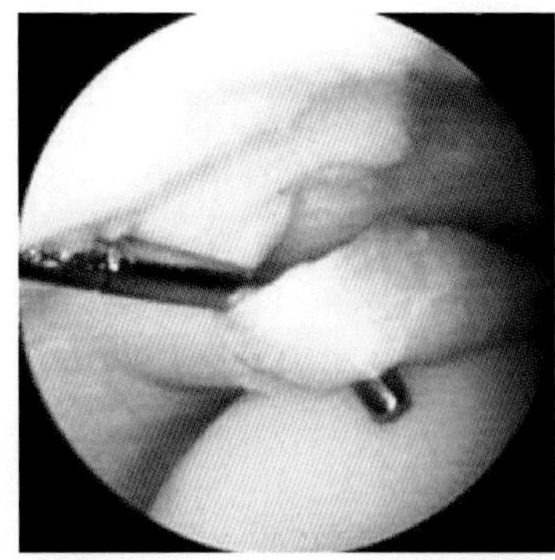

FIG 3 • Intraoperative evaluation of the ability to "roll" the meniscus.

  - The healing potential for a meniscus repair in conjunction with an anterior cruciate ligament reconstruction is far superior to that of a repair alone.

Preoperative Planning

- Before the surgery, all radiologic studies should be reviewed.
- The knee should be examined under anesthesia before beginning the surgery in an attempt to detect associated pathology.
- The surgeon should discuss with the patient the risks and benefits of the surgery as well as the principle of informed consent.
- All patients should be apprised of the possibility of meniscus resection versus repair.
  - They should understand the implications of each in terms of short- and long-term consequences and postoperative rehabilitation protocols.
  - The surgeon may discuss the potential for associated pathology and may obtain a better understanding of the patient's treatment preferences before entering the operating room.
  - This may be a particularly crucial conversation with an elite athlete who would prefer to undergo a resection in an attempt to return to competitive sport faster.
- The anesthesia used is typically decided on by the anesthesiologist and orthopedist before entering the operating room. General anesthesia or a laryngeal mask airway (LMA) may be used.
  - We prefer to have the anesthesiologist provide sedation in conjunction with a local anesthetic administered by the surgeon.
  - We typically use a mixture of 0.5% bupivacaine and 1% lidocaine with epinephrine in equal proportions. About 30 to 40 cc is injected intra-articularly, and about 5 cc is injected into each portal site.

Positioning

- Typically the patient is lying supine.
- The two most popular methods of leg support are a knee holder (thigh immobilizer) and a lateral post.
  - The knee holder should be placed perpendicular to the position of the femur at a level above the patella and portals that allows for a valgus force on the knee. The end of the table is dropped down below 90 degrees from horizontal to allow both legs to hang freely from the knees.
  - The lateral post should be placed above the patella and angled outwardly to allow for a valgus force on the operative knee. This technique is performed without dropping the end of the table. The surgeon should check that the knee may be taken through a range of motion by abducting the leg against the lateral post with flexion of the knee off the side of the table.

- A tourniquet may be placed on the upper thigh if bleeding is suspected, such as in débridement of a hypertrophic fat pad.
- Padding of the contralateral leg is used to prevent pressure-related injury to the bony prominences or superficial nerves.

Approach

- The typical portal sites are a superomedial, anteromedial, and anterolateral portal (**FIG 4**).
    - The superomedial portal is typically made proximal to the superior pole of the patella in line with the medial border of the patella (medial to the quadriceps) and is directed in an oblique manner into the joint. This portal is typically used for outflow or inflow.
    - The anterolateral portal is created by making a small (about 6 mm) stab incision 1 cm proximal to the joint line and 1 cm lateral to the patella tendon. This area can be identified as the "soft spot." This portal is used for insertion of the arthroscope.
- The anteromedial portal is considered the working portal for insertion of instruments. It is typically made under direct visualization by inserting a spinal needle into the medial "soft spot" 1 cm medial to the patella tendon and 1 cm proximal to the joint line.
- Accessory portals may include superolateral, posteromedial, posterolateral, midpatella, central, far medial, or lateral (Fig 4).
- The tears may be stimulated to heal with either rasping or trephination.
    - Rasping may be performed with either an arthroscopic shaver or a meniscal rasp that lightly abrades both the tibial and femoral edges of the tear site, as well as the meniscosynovial junction, to stimulate vascularity.

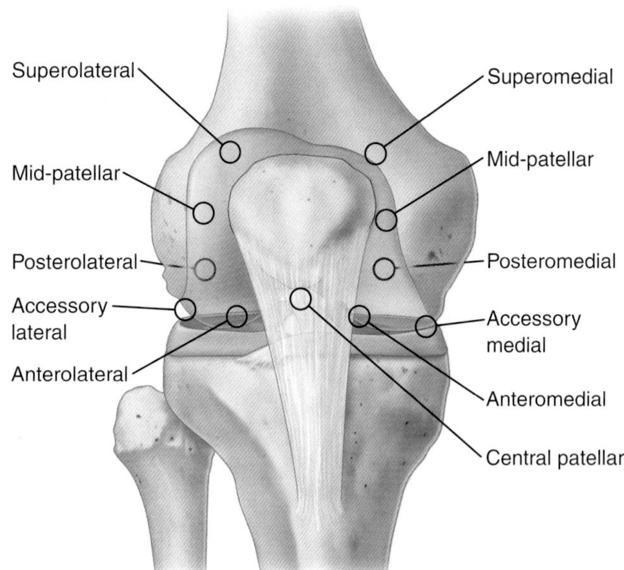

FIG 4 • Placement of the standard (superolateral, anteromedial, and anterolateral) and accessory arthroscopic portals in the knee.

- Trephination is performed by inserting a long 18-gauge needle either percutaneously or through the arthroscopic portals across the meniscus tear to create vascular channels. The surgeon should avoid perforation of the meniscus surface, causing further injury.

INSIDE-OUT TECHNIQUE

- This technique requires passage of double-loaded 2-0 or 0 nonabsorbable sutures with long flexible needles passed arthroscopically through thin cannulas (**TECH FIG 1**).
- It is best used for posterior horn, middle third, peripheral capsule, and bucket-handle tears.
- Before passage of the sutures, an incision is made posteromedial or posterolaterally to capture the needles as they exit through the capsule. In this manner, all neurovascular structures are protected.
- For passage of a needle through the medial compartment, the knee is placed in 20 to 30 degrees of flexion to avoid tethering the capsule.
    - A 4- to 6-cm posteromedial incision is made just posterior to the medial collateral ligament, extending about one-third above and two-thirds below the joint line.
    - Dissection is continued anterior to the sartorius and semimembranosus musculature, deep to the medial head of the gastrocnemius.
- The posterolateral incision is made with the knee in 90 degrees of flexion to allow the peroneal nerve, popliteus, and lateral inferior geniculate artery to fall posteriorly.
    - A 4- to 6-cm incision is made just posterior to the lateral collateral ligament, anterior to the biceps femoris tendon, extending one-third above and two-thirds below the joint line.
    - Dissection is continued between the iliotibial band and the biceps tendon and then proceeds deep and anterior to the lateral head of the gastrocnemius.
- On exposure of the capsule, a "spoon" or popliteal retractor is placed against the capsule to visualize the exiting needles.
- A single- or double-lumen cannula is passed through the arthroscopic portals to the site of the tear.
- Long flexible needles are then passed through the cannula, piercing the meniscus above and below the tear site and creating vertical mattress sutures.
- The needles are captured one at a time by an assistant who is retracting on the capsule. Care is taken not to pull either suture all the way through until both needles are passed.
- The sutures are then tensioned and tied to the capsule while viewing the repair arthroscopically.

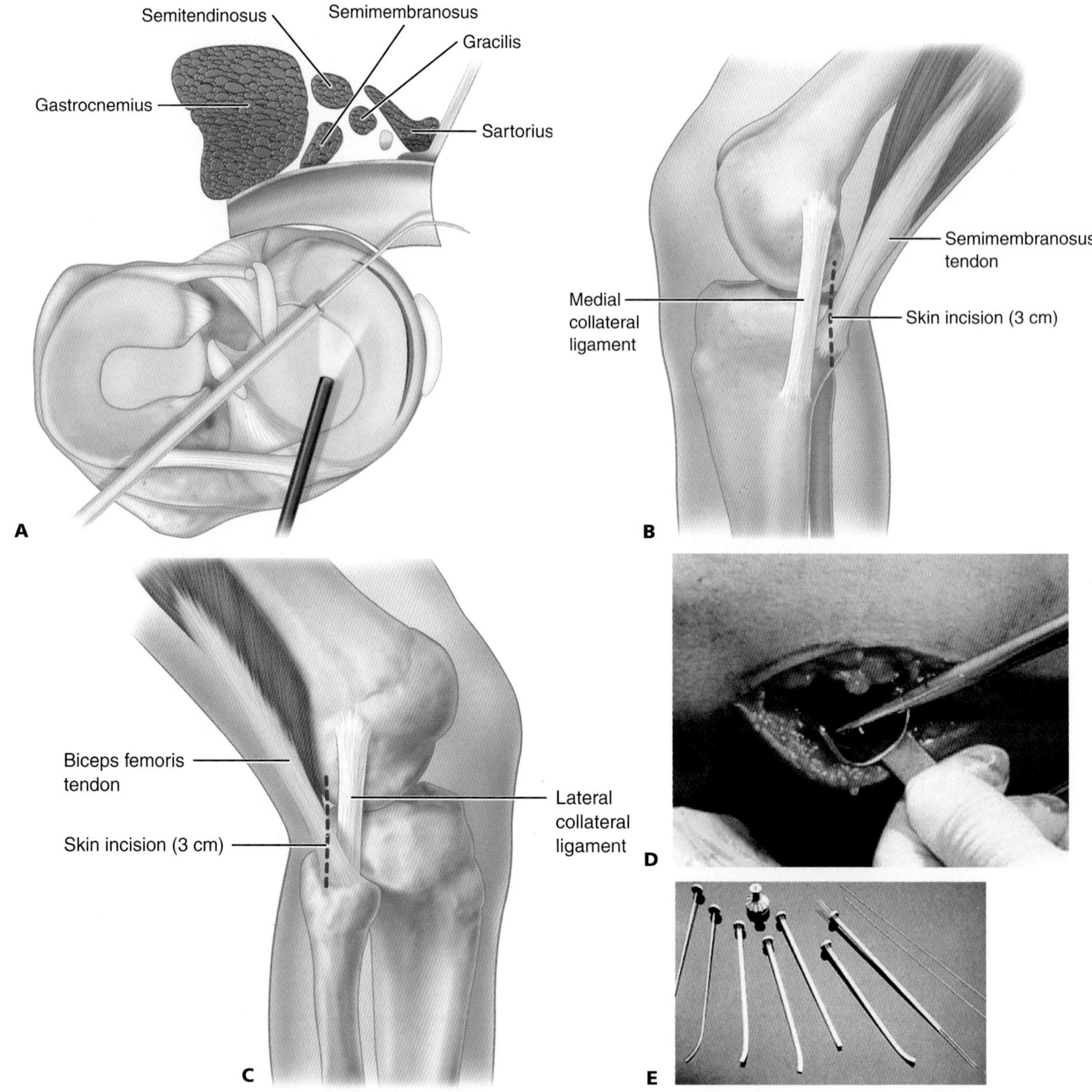

TECH FIG 1 • Inside-out repair technique. **A.** Diagram of technique. **B.** Skin incision on medial side. **C.** Skin incision on lateral side. **D.** Intraoperative image and popliteal retractor in place. **E.** The cannulas used to pass the needles.

OUTSIDE-IN TECHNIQUE

- This technique is performed by passing multiple long 18-gauge spinal needles percutaneously from outside of the knee to inside the knee joint (TECH FIG 2).
- This technique is best performed on tears of the anterior and middle third, as well as radial tears.
- Needles should be spaced about 3 to 5 mm apart.
- The needle should enter the joint through the periphery to achieve a vertical or horizontal mattress suture configuration.
- An absorbable monofilament suture is passed into the joint.
- A second needle with a wire retriever trocar is passed through the tear to retrieve the suture.
- After tensioning of the mattress suture, a 3- to 5-mm skin incision is made near the suture strands and blunt dissection carried down to the capsule with a hemostat.
- A probe may be used to retrieve the sutures and tie them down to the capsule under direct visualization, taking care to avoid incarceration of any neurovascular structures.

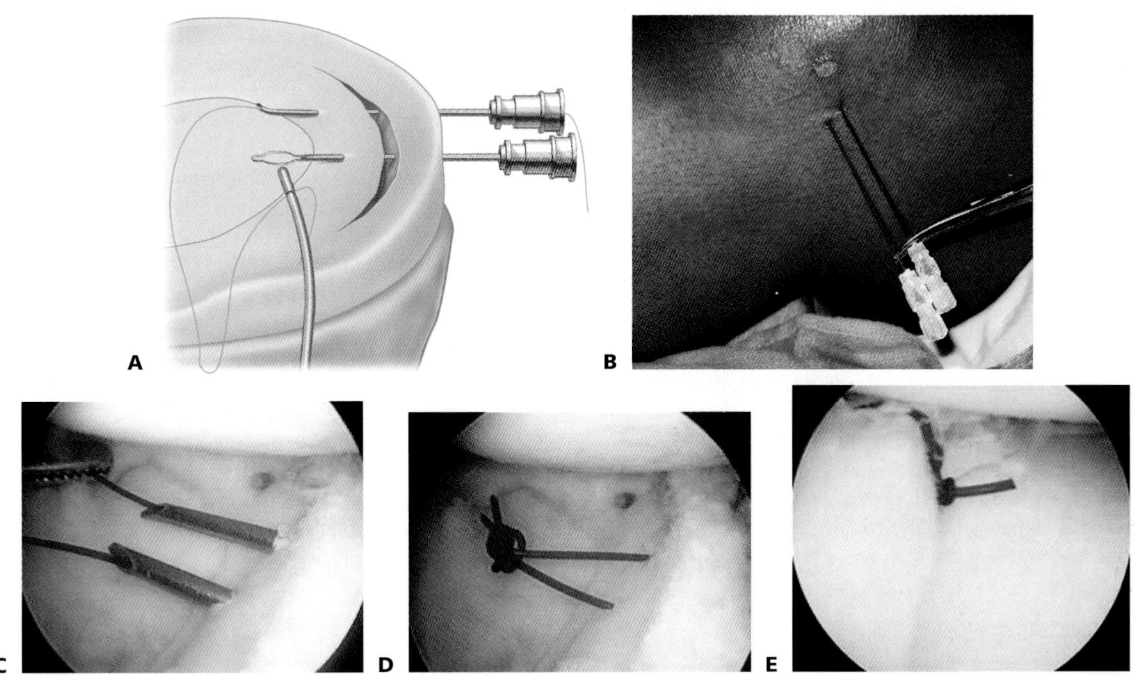

TECH FIG 2 • Outside-in repair technique. **A.** Illustration of horizontal mattress technique without intra-articular knots. **B.** Placement of needles. **C,D.** Arthroscopic views of passage of knots. **E.** Arthroscopic view of mattress suture with outside-in technique.

ALL-INSIDE FIXATION TECHNIQUE

- Multiple proprietary fixation devices are available with variations on the popular reverse-barbed fishhook design (eg, Meniscus Arrow, Bionx, Blue Bell, PA; Biostinger, and ConMed Linvatec, Largo, FL; Dart, Arthrex, Naples, FL) (TECH FIG 3).
  - They are also referred to as first-generation fixators.
- These devices are best used in vertical longitudinal tears in the red-white zone of the posterior horn.
- They are typically made of bioabsorbable copolymers such as poly-L-lactic acid and poly-D-lactic acid.
- After identification of the tear site, accurate measurement of the size of the meniscus is performed with an arthroscopic measuring device.
- Insertion of the fixator must be performed perpendicular to the tear and parallel to the tibial surface.
- Fixators can be placed at 3- to 5-mm intervals.
- Care must be taken to implant the fixator so that it is seated flush or countersunk to the meniscus surface while spanning the tear equally on both sides to appropriately compress the tear.

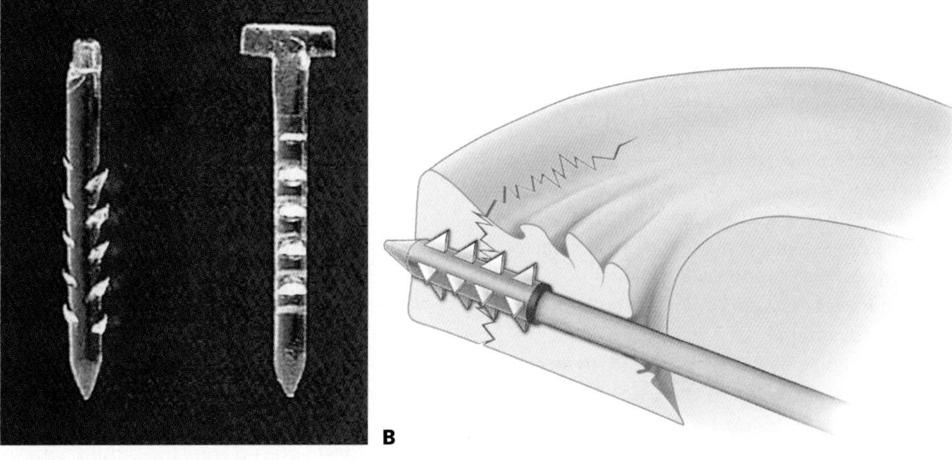

TECH FIG 3 • Use of arthroscopic fixator. **A.** Meniscal fixators. **B.** Placement of meniscal arrow.

ALL-INSIDE SUTURE FIXATION TECHNIQUE

- Multiple proprietary designs are available (eg, FasT-Fix, Smith and Nephew, Andover, MA; RapidLoc, Mitek, Westwood, MA) (TECH FIG 4).
  - They are also referred to as second-generation fixators.
- The suture fixators are designed to allow repair of the meniscus with mattress sutures without creating an incision through the skin.
- The devices deploy two absorbable or nonabsorbable suture anchors with attached nonabsorbable sutures between them.
- The sutures can then be arthroscopically tied or they may come pretied, depending on proprietary design.
- After preparing the tear in the standard manner, the fixator should be inserted from the contralateral portal.
- Use of a curved needle provides the surgeon with more options compared to the straight needle with regard to position and reduction and insertion angles.
- Insertion of the needle through a sheath or insertion cannula prevents the delivery system from getting caught on loose tissue.
- The surgeon starts the repair from the center and works outward. This avoids gapping, ruffling, and dog-ears.
- The use of an outside-in stay suture may aid in holding the reduction until the mattress sutures can be placed.
- The devices are placed perpendicular to the tear.
- The first anchor should be placed superiorly and posteriorly and the second should be placed inferiorly and anteriorly across the tear to create a vertical mattress.
- The knot pusher is used to slide and manually assist in cinching down the knot; however, the surgeon should avoid overtightening and puckering the repair.
- The devices are placed about 4 to 5 mm apart.

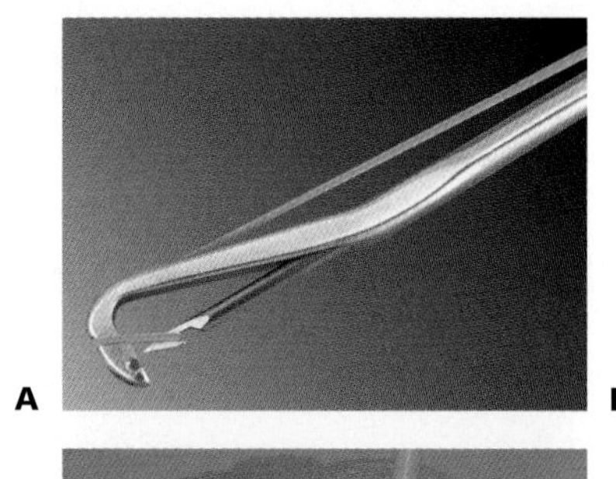
A

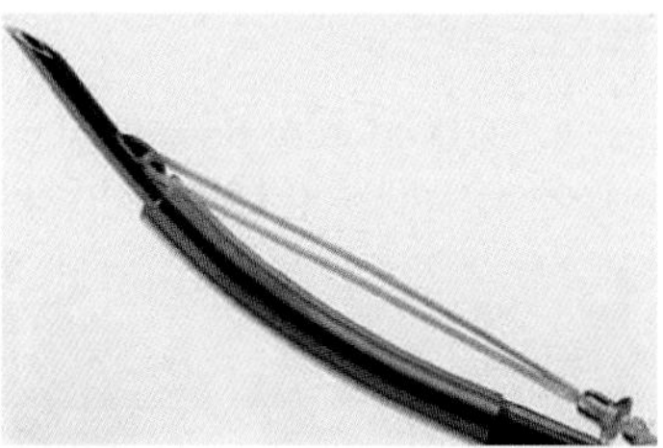
B

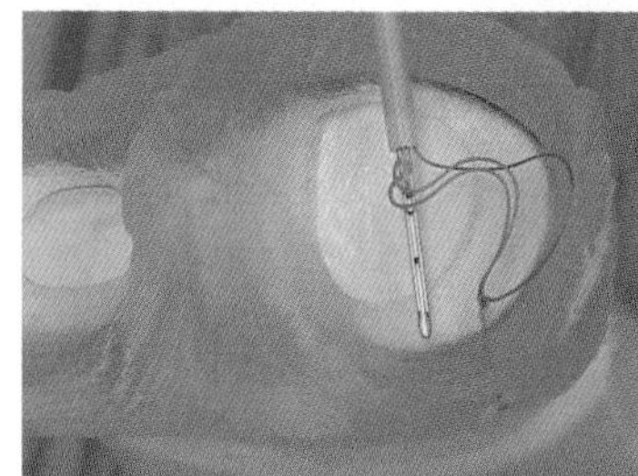
C

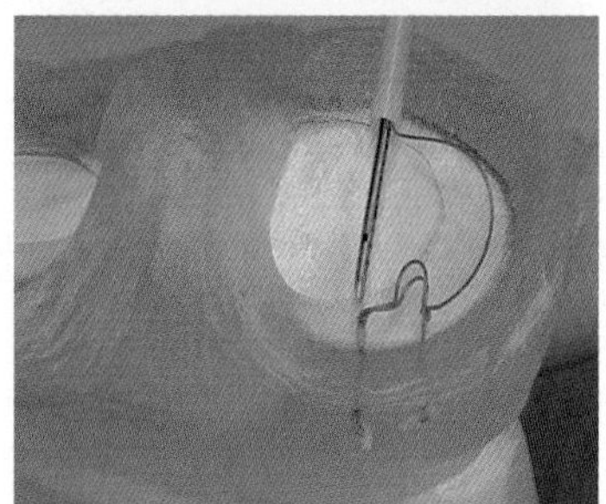
D

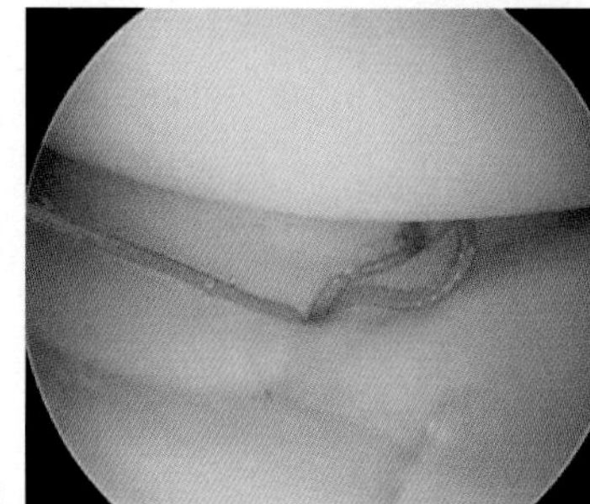
E

TECH FIG 4 • Use of arthroscopic suture fixators. **A,B.** Design of two commercially available suture fixators. **C,D.** Placement of arthroscopic sutures in mattress configuration. **E.** The "self-tying" arthroscopic knot thrown with a suture fixator.

REPAIR BIOLOGIC AUGMENTATION METHODS

- These techniques are indicated in cases of isolated meniscus repair (no concomitant ACL reconstruction) in which there is concern for healing.
- It is generally accepted that results of meniscus repair are improved when performed in conjunction with ACL reconstruction. The reason for the success is theoretically secondary to the release of intraosseous growth factors and cytokines when bone tunnels are drilled.
- Several methods have been used in an attempt to recreate that biologic advantage.
- Trephination or rasping may be performed in an attempt to increase vascularity delivered to the tear site.
- The use of fibrin clot or platelet-rich fibrin matrix attempts to deliver biologically active factors directly to the repair site.
  - The fibrin clot technique introduces a concentrated autologous platelet-rich matrix to the repair site. The platelet-rich matrix technique is a refinement of the fibrin clot technique designed to deliver a more concentrated and volume-stable matrix to the repair site.
  - The fibrin clot is performed by first obtaining 30 to 50 mL of blood from the patient intraoperatively and transferring it to a glass container. The blood is stirred with a sintered glass rod. A clot will form, which is blotted dry and then inserted using an arthroscopic grasper to the repair site. The clot is best placed with the fluid flow turned down and is best placed on the tibial site of the repair (TECH FIG 5A,B).

- The platelet-rich fibrin matrix technique is performed by obtaining a smaller sample of autologous blood intraoperatively (about 10 mL) and placing it in a centrifuge for about 20 minutes. After centrifugation is completed, the fibrin matrix is retrieved and placed arthroscopically into the repair site in similar fashion to the fibrin clot. Proprietary technology is available (Cascade Autologous Platelet System, MTF, Edison, NJ) to perform this method (**TECH FIG 5C,D**).

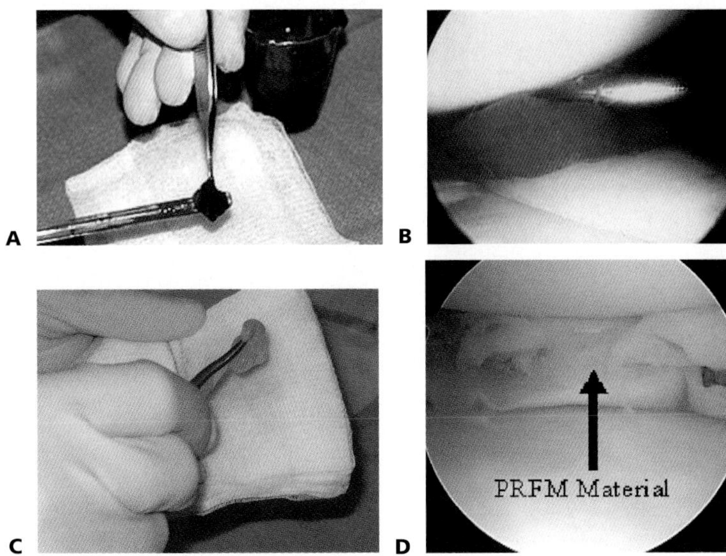

TECH FIG 5 • Preparation and placement of a fibrin clot (**A,B**) and of platelet-rich fibrin matrix (**C,D**).

PEARLS AND PITFALLS

Indications	■ Repair of red-white and red-red tears only optimally. ■ If concurrent pathology is present, meniscus tears should always be repaired in conjunction with anterior cruciate ligament reconstruction.
Tear site management	■ The tear should be approached from the contralateral portal. ■ Preparation of the tear site with abrasion, débridement, or trephination is essential. ■ The tear should be reduced accurately and reduction should be maintained during fixator placement. ■ Tears should be bisected with reduction to avoid a dog-ear result. ■ An anchoring stitch may assist with tear reduction. ■ Hybrid techniques are very effective. ■ Accessory portals improve access and fixation configuration.
Fixation placement	■ Implants should be separated by about 5 mm. ■ Implants should be placed perpendicular to the tibia. ■ Implants should not be left proud.
Suture techniques	■ Vertical mattress sutures are used when possible. ■ Skin incisions are made in 90 degrees of flexion for posteromedial and posterolateral approaches. ■ Sutures are passed in 20 degrees of flexion for medial tears and 90 degrees of flexion for lateral tears.
Rehabilitation	■ Programs should be individualized for each patient in terms of protection, weight bearing, range of motion, and return to activities.

POSTOPERATIVE CARE

- Postoperative care must be individualized based on tear geometry, repair construct strength, associated surgical procedures, and surgeon preference.
- In the operating room, our patients are placed in a knee immobilizer or hinged brace locked in extension.
- A patient with an isolated meniscus repair will remain partially weight bearing with crutches for about 1 month.
- Early range of motion is performed passively from postoperative day 1.
- Typically, range of motion is limited to 90 degrees for the first 3 weeks for nondisplaced meniscus tears and 4 to 6 weeks for displaced bucket-handle tears.
- Crutches are discontinued when the patient shows good quadriceps function and no antalgia.

- Return to pivoting sports ranges from 4 to 6 months, or when the patient has no point tenderness or effusion and can show full extension and painless terminal flexion.

OUTCOMES

- The success rate of meniscus repair has been estimated at 50% to 90%, with a higher likelihood of success when repair is performed in conjunction with an ACL reconstruction.
  - Early studies by Cannon and Vittori[6] reported on inside-out repairs of 90 knees. Overall clinical success was found to be 82%. Those repaired in conjunction with ACL reconstruction had a 93% success rate while isolated repairs were successful in only 50% of cases.
  - Henning et al[19] reported on 260 repairs in 240 patients with follow-up of about 2 years. On arthroscopic second-look or arthrogram evaluation, inside-out repairs had a 62% success rate, with 17% incompletely healed and 21% not healed. Ninety-two percent of the knees were stable and ACL reconstruction was performed on 80% of them.
  - Rodeo et al[17] found an overall success rate of 87% with use of the outside-in technique in 90 patients. He noted failure in 38% of the unstable knees, 15% in stable knees, and 5% in ACL-reconstructed knees.
- Studies have shown inside-out vertical mattress suture placement to be the strongest fixation technique, whereas the all-inside suture fixators provide excellent repair strength. The all-inside first-generation fixators have shown inferior results compared to the newer fixators.
  - Biomechanical testing of longitudinal tears in adult porcine meniscus showed mean load to failure of inside-out vertical mattress sutures to be 80.4 N, FasT-Fix 70.9 to 72.1 N (vertical and horizontal configuration), the Dart 61.7 N, horizontal sutures 55.9 N, Rapidloc 43.3 N, and Meniscus Screw (Arthrotek, Biomet, Warsaw, IN) 28.1 N.[4]
  - Two recent studies showed early and intermediate success of Rapidloc.
    - One study found a 90.7% success rate with the use of Rapidloc to repair 54 menisci in 49 patients with an average follow-up of 34.8 months.[15]
    - Another prospective analysis of 32 meniscus repairs performed with Rapidloc, at an average of 32 months of follow-up, found clinical success in 87.5% of patients.[5]
  - A recent study of 61 menisci repaired with the FasT-Fix found, at an average follow-up of 18 months, a 90% success rate. ACL reconstruction was performed in 62% of them. Excellent or good clinical results were found on Lysholm knee scoring in 88%.[10]
  - Spindler et al[22] compared 47 inside-out suture repairs to 98 all-inside meniscal arrow repairs, with clinical failure as defined as reoperation. They found seven failures in each group, but the mean time to follow-up was 68 months for the inside-out repairs and only 27 months for the all-inside group.
  - One study of 60 meniscus repairs using the meniscal arrow showed a failure rate of 28% on MRI and repeat arthroscopy at a mean follow-up of 54 months. They found an increasing rate of significant complications in addition to meniscus repair failure, including chondral scoring, fixator breakage, and joint-line irritation.[11]
  - Lee and Diduch[12] also showed deteriorating results with first-generation fixators. They studied 32 meniscus repairs, all performed exclusively with arrows in conjunction with an ACL reconstruction. They reported a success rate of 90.6% at a mean follow-up of 2.3 years; subsequent reports of those same patients found a 71.4% success rate at a mean follow-up of 6.6 years.

COMPLICATIONS

- The overall incidence of complications from arthroscopic meniscus surgery is 0.56% to 8.2%.[21]
- Meniscus repair surgery has a higher complication rate than meniscus resection, with reports as high as 18%.[20]
- Commonly discussed complications include infection, deep vein thrombosis, vascular injury, and neurologic complications.
- The rate of infection is 0.23% to 0.42%, with an increasing incidence associated with extended operating time, extended tourniquet time, performance of multiple concurrent procedures, and a history of prior surgeries.[1]
  - There is no clear consensus on the use of prophylactic perioperative antibiotics.
  - There are published reports of an increased incidence of infection associated with intra-articular corticosteroid injections given intraoperatively.[14]
  - When an infection has been diagnosed after a repair, it is appropriate to leave the implant or sutures in place; however, there is a higher failure rate associated with it.
- The incidence of deep vein thrombosis ranges from 1.2% to 4.9% after arthroscopic knee surgery.[8] No clear consensus exists with regard to perioperative anticoagulation.
- The overall incidence of vascular complications is 0.54% to 1.0%, with complications including popliteal artery injury, pseudoaneurysm, and arteriovenous fistulas.[9]
- Neurologic complications include direct or indirect nerve injury or complex regional pain syndrome. The overall incidence is 0.06% to 2.0%.[18]
  - Medial meniscus repairs using an inside-out or outside-in technique can result in saphenous neuropathy or neuropraxia, with reports of up to 43% of cases.[23]
- More recent reports of neuropathy with all-inside techniques have yet to be published.
- The most common complications associated with the inside-out and outside-in techniques are traumatic neuropathy to the saphenous or peroneal nerves.
- The all-arthroscopic implant fixators can be associated with complications such as retained fragments that fail to resorb, broken implants, fixator migration, and inflammatory responses to the implant. A retained implant may cause further chondral damage secondary to implant abrasion.[11]

REFERENCES

1. Armstrong R, Bolding F, Joseph R. Septic arthritis following arthroscopy, clinical syndromes and analysis of risk factors. Arthroscopy 1992;8:213–223.
2. Arnoczky SP, Warren RF. The microvasculature of the meniscus and its response to injury: an experimental study in the dog. Am J Sports Med 1983;11:131–141.
3. Baratz M, Fu F, Mengato R. Meniscal tears: the effect of meniscectomy and of repair on intraarticular contact areas and stress in the human knee: a preliminary report. Am J Sports Med 1986;14:270–275.
4. Barber FA, Berber MA, Richards D. Load to failure testing of new meniscal repair devices. Arthroscopy 2004;40:45–50.
5. Barber FA, Coons DA, Ruiz-Suarez M. Meniscal repair with the Rapidloc meniscal repair device. Arthroscopy 2006;22:962–966.

6. Cannon W, Vittori J. The incidence of healing in arthroscopic meniscal repairs in ACL-reconstructed knees versus stable knees. Am J Sports Med 1992;20:176–181.
7. Cooper DE, Arnoczky SP, Warren RF. Arthroscopic meniscal repair. Clin Sports Med 1990;9:589–607.
8. Jauregito J, Geenwald A, Wilcox J, et al. The incidence of deep vein thrombosis after arthroscopic knee surgery. Am J Sports Med 1999; 27:707–710.
9. Kim T, Savino R, McFarland E, et al. Neurovascular complications of knee arthroscopy. Am J Sports Med 2002;30:619–629.
10. Kotsovolos E, Hantes M, Mastrokalos D, et al. Results of all-inside meniscal repair with the FasT-fix meniscal repair system. Arthroscopy 2006;22:3–9.
11. Kurzweil P, Tifford C, Ignacio E. Unsatisfactory clinical results of meniscal repair using the Meniscus Arrow. Arthroscopy 2005;21: 905:e1–e7.
12. Lee G, Diduch D. Deteriorating outcomes after meniscal repair using the Meniscus Arrow in knees undergoing concurrent anterior cruciate ligament reconstruction: increased failure with long-term follow-up. Am J Sports Med 2005;33:1138–1141.
13. Magee T, Williams W. 3.0 T MRI of meniscal tears. Am J Radiol 2006;187:371–375.
14. Montgomery S, Campbell J. Septic arthritis following arthroscopy and intraarticular steroids. J Bone Joint Surg Am 1989;71A:540–544.
15. Quinby JS, Golish, SR, Hart J, et al. All-inside meniscal repair using a new flexible, tensionable device. Am J Sports Med 2006;34:1281–1286.
16. Renstrom P, Johnson RJ. Anatomy and biomechanics of the menisci. Clin Sports Med 1990;9:523–538.
17. Rodeo S. Arthroscopic meniscal repairs with use of the outside-to-inside technique. J Bone Joint Surg Am 2000;82A:127–141.
18. Rodeo S, Forster R, Weiland A. Neurological complications due to arthroscopy. J Bone Joint Surg Am 1993;75:917–926.
19. Scott GA, Jolly B, Henning CE. Combined posterior incision and arthroscopic intraarticular repair of the meniscus: an examination of factors affecting healing, J Bone Joint Surg Am 1986;68:847–861.
20. Sherman O, Fox J, Snyder S, et al. Arthroscopy: "no problem surgery"—analysis of complications in 2640 cases. J Bone Joint Surg Am 1986;68A:256–265.
21. Small N. Complications in arthroscopic surgery performed by experienced arthroscopists. Arthroscopy 1988;4:215–221.
22. Spindler KP, McCarty EC, Warren TA, et al. Prospective comparison of arthroscopic medial meniscal repair technique: inside-out suture versus entirely arthroscopic arrows. Am J Sports Med 2003; 31:929–934.
23. Stone R, Miller G. A technique of arthroscopic suture of a torn meniscus. Arthroscopy 1985;1:226–232.
24. Walker PS, Erkman MJ. The role of the menisci in force transmission across the knee. Clin Orthop 1975;109:184 192.

Chapter 35 Meniscal Transplant

Roland S. Kent, Christopher A. Kurtz, and Kevin F. Bonner

DEFINITION

- An estimated 850,000 meniscal procedures are performed yearly in the United States.
- Although meniscus preservation is always preferable, large irreparable tears often require partial or subtotal meniscal excision.
- Many patients will become symptomatic in the meniscal-deficient compartment as the result of increased articular cartilage contact stresses and progressive cartilage deterioration.
- Meniscal allograft transplantation is an option in the carefully selected patient with symptomatic meniscal deficiency.

ANATOMY

- The menisci are semilunar fibrocartilaginous discs made of predominantly type I collagen. Water, which accounts for 70% of meniscal composition, is trapped within the matrix by negatively charged glycosaminoglycans (**FIG 1**).
- Only the peripheral third of the meniscus is vascularized (10% adjacent to popliteal hiatus). Blood is supplied via the perimeniscal capillary plexus with contributions from the superior and inferior medial and lateral geniculate arteries.
- Medial meniscus
  - The medial meniscus covers a smaller percentage of medial compartment surface than the lateral meniscus.
  - A portion of the anterior cruciate ligament (ACL) tibial insertion footprint lies between the anterior and posterior horn attachment sites.
- Lateral meniscus
  - The lateral meniscus covers a relatively larger percentage of the articular surface in its respective compartment than the medial meniscus.
  - The anterior horn attaches adjacent to the ACL and the posterior horn attachment is behind the intercondylar eminence.
  - The anterior and posterior horn attachments are closer to each other than the medial meniscus without a ligament insertion footprint interposed between the two sites. This makes the lateral meniscus more amenable to a bone bridge transplantation technique.
  - A discoid variant is found in 3.5% to 5% of patients.

The views expressed in this article are those of the authors and do not reflect the official policy or position of the Department of the Navy, Department of Defense, or the United States Government.

PATHOGENESIS

- Meniscal pathology is generally of two types:
  - Acute traumatic tears
    - These injuries typically occur in a previously relatively "healthy" meniscus in patients younger than 35.
    - They may also occur in older individuals, but typically in the setting of an acute ACL tear.
    - Traumatic tears often include unstable longitudinal tears in the vascular zone, which are optimal candidates for meniscal repair.
    - They often occur in association with combined knee injuries (ACL, medial collateral ligament).
  - Degenerative tears
    - This is a more complex tear pattern that typically occurs in patients older than 35.
    - Often a relatively minor trauma or event "breaks the camel's back" and a tear propagates through degenerative meniscal tissue.
  - These are not repairable.
- Risk factors for meniscal tears include sports participation (especially jumping and cutting sports at risk for concurrent ACL injury), age, higher body mass index, occupational kneeling and squatting (associated with degenerative rather than acute traumatic meniscal lesions), level of activity, and ACL instability.
- The association of meniscal tears with ACL tears is well documented. Lateral meniscal injuries occur more frequently with acute ACL disruption, while medial meniscal injuries occur more often in the setting of chronic ACL insufficiency.
- Irreparable tear patterns or failed previous meniscal repairs often necessitate arthroscopic meniscal excision of the tear component. The degree of tear propagation typically dictates the resection required.

NATURAL HISTORY

- Meniscectomy can decrease contact area by 75% and increase joint contact stresses by over 200%.[1]
- Contact stresses increase as a function of the amount of meniscus resected.
- These increases in joint contact stress often lead to premature cartilage deterioration and the development of osteoarthritis. Although patients often remain relatively asymptomatic until they have advanced degenerative changes, many patients (who tend to be younger and more active) develop pain earlier in the degenerative process.
- Lateral meniscectomy is considered to have a poorer prognosis than medial meniscectomy.
- The medial meniscus is the secondary stabilizer to anterior tibial translation. Medial meniscectomy (posterior horn) in the ACL-deficient knee often increases tibial translation and instability.

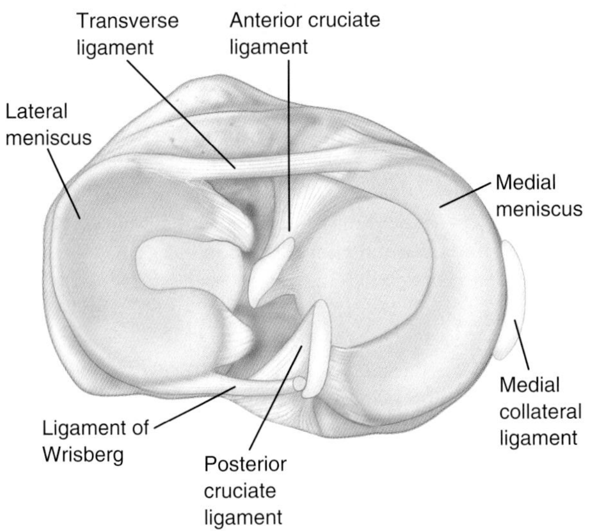

FIG 1 • Meniscal anatomy.

- Meniscus implantation decreases peak stresses and improves contact mechanics but does not restore perfect knee mechanics.[5,9]

PATIENT HISTORY AND PHYSICAL FINDINGS

- Potential transplant patients are typically younger than 40 years of age, with an absent or nonfunctioning meniscus, who are symptomatic from their meniscal insufficiency. The upper limit is generally age 50 (not absolute) for highly active patients who are not good candidates for arthroplasty.
- A detailed history includes specific symptoms, prior injuries, and subsequent surgery. Arthroscopy pictures are helpful in determining the degree of meniscal resection and the condition of the articular cartilage.
- Symptomatic postmeniscectomy patients typically present with joint line pain (sometimes subtle), swelling, and pain associated with barometric pressure changes. Symptoms are usually activity-related.
- The physical examination should focus on determining pain location, ligament stability, and alignment, assessing the cartilage, and ruling out elements of the differential diagnosis.
  - Palpating the joint line for tenderness will localize the source of pain.
  - Sharp pain on the McMurray test may indicate recurrent meniscal injury or chondral lesion versus meniscal insufficiency (dull ache).
  - The Lachman test assesses for concomitant ACL pathology, which should be addressed at the time of surgery.
  - Concerns about malalignment and gait problems necessitate long-leg alignment films.
  - Symmetric range of motion is needed before the transplant.

IMAGING AND OTHER DIAGNOSTIC STUDIES

- Plain radiographs
  - Anteroposterior (AP) view of both knees in full extension (**FIG 2A**): Look for subtle joint space narrowing.

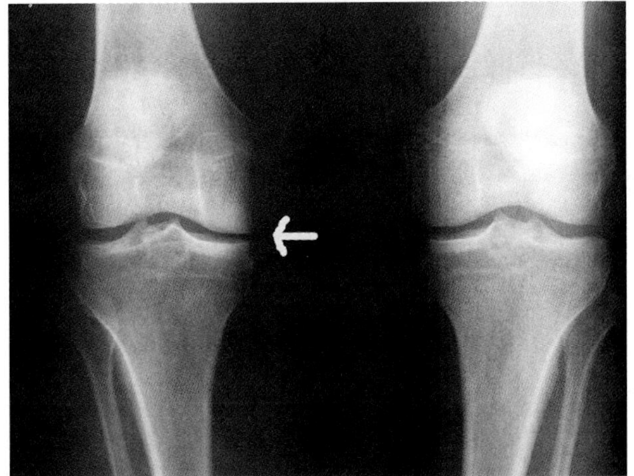

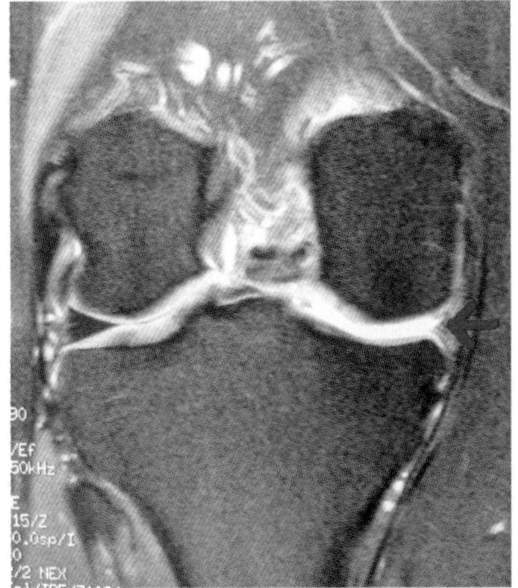

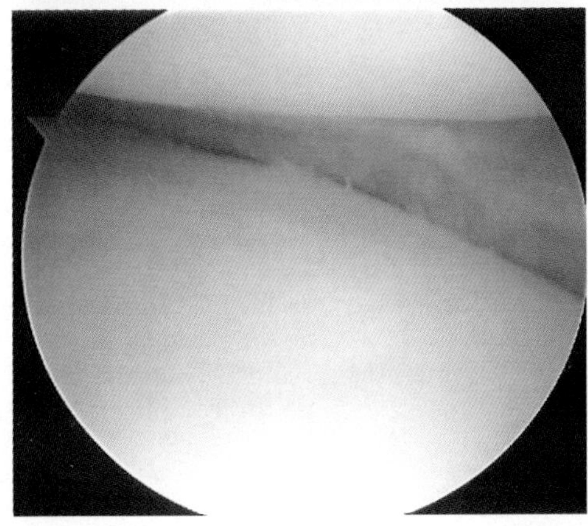

FIG 2 • **A.** AP weight-bearing bilateral knee views showing subtle medial compartment joint space narrowing of the right knee (*arrow*). **B.** MRI showing deficient medial meniscus. **C.** Arthroscopic image of right knee showing deficient medial meniscus.

Table 1 Meniscal Allograft Sizing Methods

Sizing Method	Strengths and Weaknesses
Direct measurement	Contralateral knee may be used for sizing, though some variability exists in menisci of opposite knees.
Plain radiographs	The consistent relationship between meniscal size and landmarks in plain radiographs often is used by tissue banks for allograft sizing. By using measurements of the length and width of the medial and lateral tibial plateaus, McDermott et al determined that meniscal size can be predicted with a mean error rate of 5%.[8]
MRI	Although compared to plain radiographs MRI is historically considered to be slightly more accurate at sizing allografts, Shaffer et al found that only 35% of menisci measured with MRI were found to be within 2 mm of the actual size needed.[13]
CT	Carpenter et al reported that MRI consistently underestimated the anteroposterior and mediolateral sizes of both the medial and lateral menisci but was more accurate in estimating meniscal height. They concluded that CT and plain radiographs were more useful in allograft sizing.[2]

- Weight-bearing 45-degree flexion posteroanterior view: Look for subtle joint space narrowing.
- Merchant view
- Non-weight-bearing lateral views
- Long-leg alignment films (if malalignment is suspected)

- MRI: to assess menisci, articular cartilage, and subchondral bone) (**FIG 2B**)
- Bone scan can be considered and may reveal increased activity in the involved compartment. However, it is not typically used and its sensitivity in this setting is unknown.
- Diagnostic arthroscopy is often recommended.
  - It will accurately define the extent of meniscectomy and the degree of arthrosis if previous arthroscopic images are unavailable or unclear, or if more than 1 year has elapsed since the last arthroscopy (**FIG 2C**).
- Outerbridge grade III or less articular cartilage damage is acceptable (grade I or II is preferable) unless a focal grade IV lesion is addressed concurrently with a cartilage resurfacing procedure.

DIFFERENTIAL DIAGNOSIS

- Recurrent meniscal tear
- Chondral or osteochondral lesion (may be the primary cause of pain but may require chondroprotection of meniscus transplant)
- Advanced bipolar degenerative arthritis
- Synovitis
- Patellofemoral pain (radiating medial)
- Extra-articular sources (ie, hamstring or pes tendinitis)

NONOPERATIVE MANAGEMENT

- Activity modification (nonimpact activities and exercises)
- Appropriate pharmacologic therapy
- Injection therapy (may be helpful for diagnostic purposes as well)
- Unloader braces
- A potential exception to nonsurgical management may be in the setting of the chronically ACL-insufficient knee or failed ACL-reconstructed knee with medial meniscal deficiency.
  - A concomitant reconstruction of the ACL with meniscal allograft replacement may improve joint stability, ACL graft survival, and eventual clinical outcome.
  - This is a new relative indication.

SURGICAL MANAGEMENT

- Indications are patient younger than 40 years with an absent or nonfunctioning meniscus and with pain due to meniscal insufficiency or progressive joint space narrowing.
  - Upper limit is generally age 50 for highly active patients who are not good candidates for arthroplasty.
- Contraindications to surgery include immunodeficiency, inflammatory arthritis, prior deep knee infection, osteophytes indicating bony architectural changes, marked obesity, Outerbridge grade IV articular changes (focal chondral defects can be addressed concurrently), knee instability, or marked malalignment (unless these issues are corrected).

Preoperative Planning

- Graft sizing: Although size matching of meniscal allografts to recipient knees is thought to be critical, the tolerance of size mismatch is unknown. While various sizing methods have been proposed, measurements based on plain radiographs and MRI are most commonly used (Table 1).
- Meniscal allografts are procured under strict aseptic conditions within 12 hours of cold ischemic time in accordance with standards established by the American Association of Tissue Banks for donor suitability and testing (Table 2).

Table 2 Meniscal Allograft Preservation Methods

Preservation Method	Strengths and Weaknesses
Fresh grafts	Can be stored for only up to 7 days, making graft sizing and serologic testing difficult. These grafts have not been shown to improve efficacy in vivo.
Fresh-frozen allograft	Preparation is easier and less expensive than cryopreservation. Despite lack of donor cell viability, allograft survival and outcome of meniscal transplant have not been affected. Use is increasing. Recommended graft material.
Cryopreserved allografts	Technically difficult to prepare and expensive, thus limiting their use. They maintain a cell viability of 10% to 40% and are invaded by host cells as early as 4 weeks after transplantation.
Freeze-drying (lyophilization)	Allows indefinite storage but produces alterations in the biomechanical properties and the size of the allografts. Currently not recommended.
Secondary sterilization via ethylene oxide or gamma irradiation	Ethylene oxide may cause soft tissue synovitis and gamma irradiation negatively affects the mechanical properties of collagen-containing tissues.

- All equipment should be ordered and readily available (ie, commercially available meniscal workstations).
- An experienced assistant is very valuable for this procedure.

Positioning

- The patient is placed in the supine position with the knee at the table break (**FIG 3**).
- For a lateral meniscal transplant, there is the option of a figure 4 position versus the leg over the table break for femoral distractor application (see Approach).
- On occasion it may be helpful to use a femoral distractor to optimize and maintain distraction of the involved compartment with the knee in flexion (currently not used by the senior author [KFB]).[7]

Approach

- For the lateral meniscus, a lateral parapatellar arthrotomy with posterolateral meniscus repair approach is used.
- For the medial meniscus, a medial parapatellar arthrotomy with posteromedial meniscus repair approach is used.

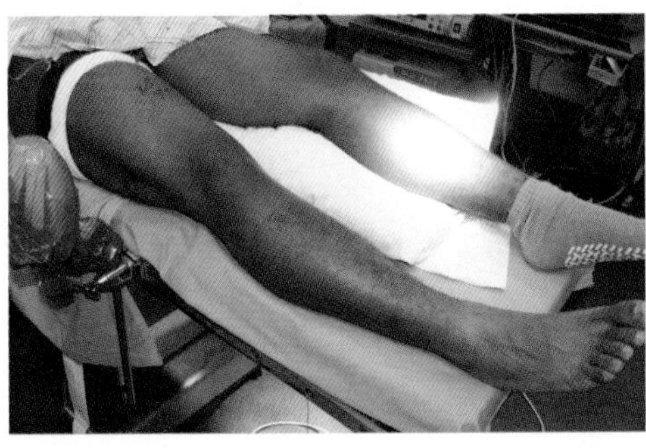

FIG 3 • Patient positioned with the knee at the table break. Femoral distractor optimizes compartment distraction with the knee flexed.

LATERAL MENISCUS GRAFT PREPARATION

- A previously size-matched lateral meniscus with the attached tibial plateau is thawed in a saline and antibiotic solution.
- Remove soft tissue from the meniscus (capsular tissue) (**TECH FIG 1A**).
- Always use the bone bridge-in-slot technique; it maintains the bridge of bone between the anterior and posterior insertion sites.
- Commercially available meniscus workstations can facilitate bone bridge preparation into various shapes that will match tibial recipient sites (Arthrex, Naples, FL) (**TECH FIG 1B,C**).
- The most common bone preparation techniques include keyhole, dovetail, and slot configurations (**TECH FIG 1D**).
- Prepare the bone bridge shape between the meniscus insertion sites using the appropriate workstation (**TECH FIG 1E**).
- During bone preparation, be careful not to injure the meniscus insertion sites.
- Mark the superior surface of the meniscus and the popliteal hiatus with a surgical marker.
- Using 10-inch flexible meniscus repair needles (Ethibond, Somerville, NJ), place one or two vertical mattress sutures (may place up to four if desired) through the posterior horn of the meniscus (**TECH FIG 1F,G**). Do not cut off the needles. These will serve as passage sutures and are used for fixation as well.

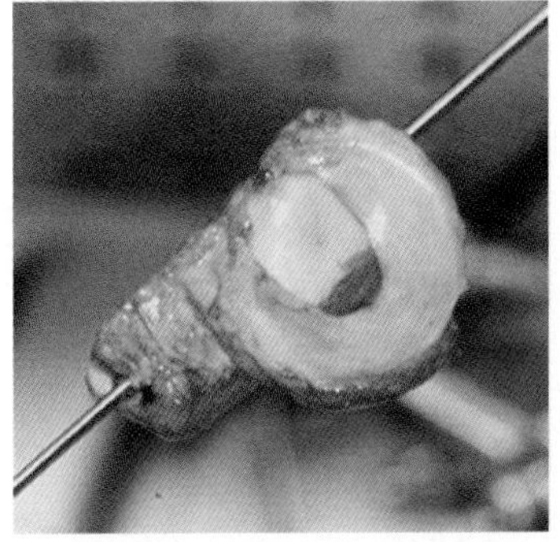

A

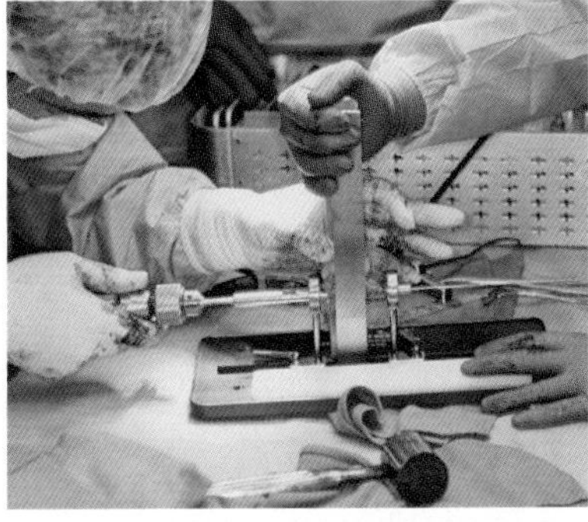

B

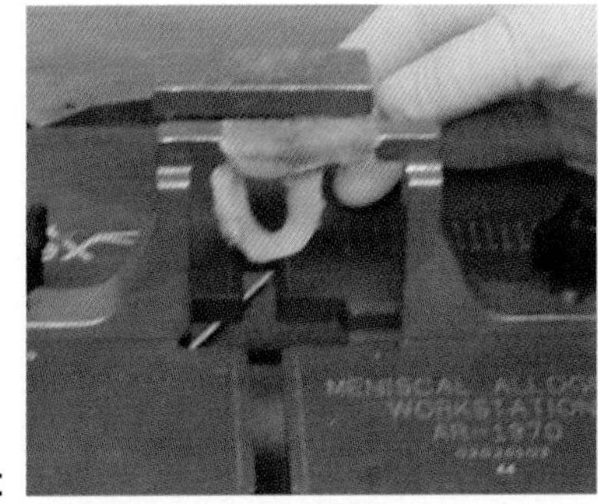

C

TECH FIG 1 • Lateral meniscus graft preparation. **A.** Prepreparation lateral meniscus graft (after capsular soft tissue has been removed). **B.** Preparing a keyhole graft with the workstation. **C.** Dovetail workstation. *(continued)*

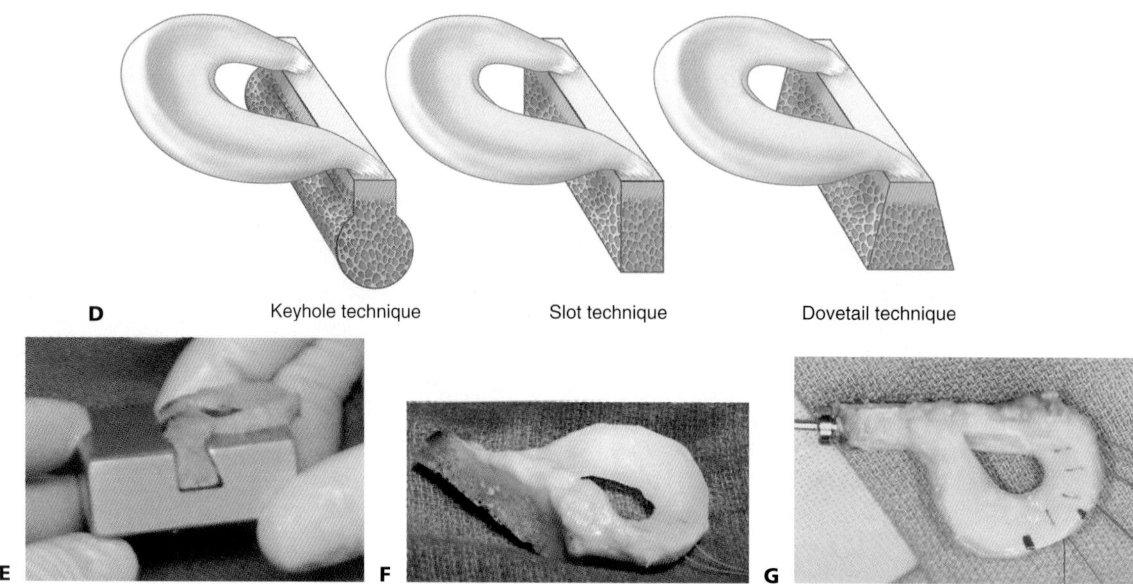

TECH FIG 1 • *(continued)* **D.** Common bone bridge shapes. **E.** Dovetail preparation. **F.** Dovetail graft with single passage suture. **G.** Keyhole graft with four passage sutures.

LATERAL MENISCUS APPROACH AND TIBIAL PREPARATION

- A combined arthroscopic and lateral parapatellar arthrotomy approach is performed.
- Perform an arthroscopic débridement and excoriation to the far peripheral meniscal rim or joint capsule with a shaver or meniscal rasp.
- A no. 15 blade may be used to excise the anterior horn and any remnant of the body.
- Use an arthroscopic burr to create a small trough in line with the anterior and posterior horn attachments (guide for recipient site) (**TECH FIG 2A**).
- Expose the proximal tibia through a small lateral parapatellar arthrotomy in line with the trough (**TECH FIG 2B**).
- Commercially available instrumentation will facilitate creation of the tibial recipient site in line with the anterior and posterior horn attachments (Arthrex, Naples, FL) (**TECH FIG 2C–E**).
- Take care to avoid penetration through the posterior cortex.
- Perform posterolateral exposure to receive inside-out sutures (meniscus repair approach) (**TECH FIG 2F**).

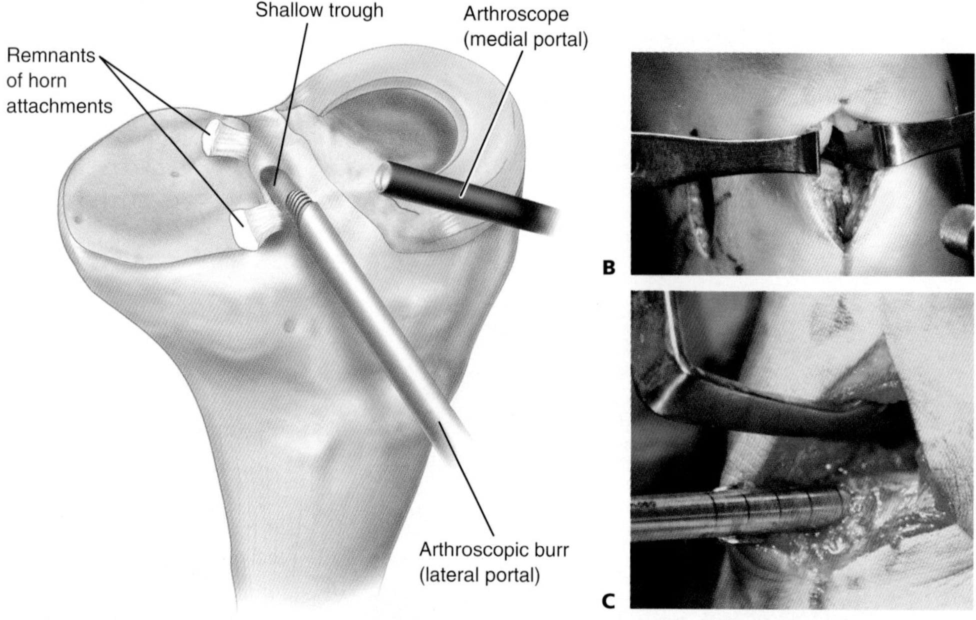

TECH FIG 2 • Lateral meniscal approach and tibial preparation. **A.** Creation of a small trough between the anterior and posterior horn attachments. **B.** Lateral parapatellar approach. **C.** Preparation of keyhole recipient site. *(continued)*

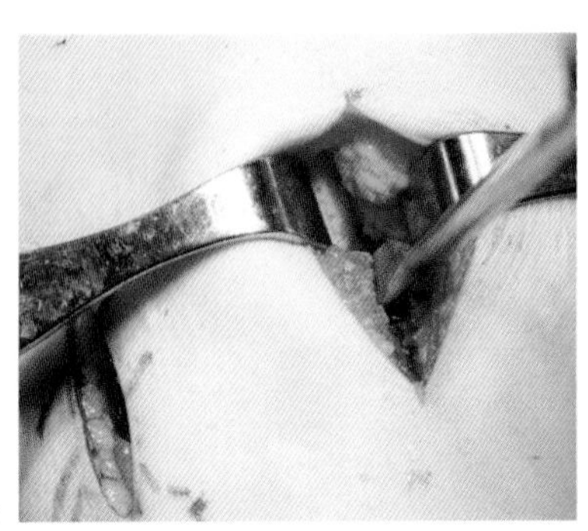
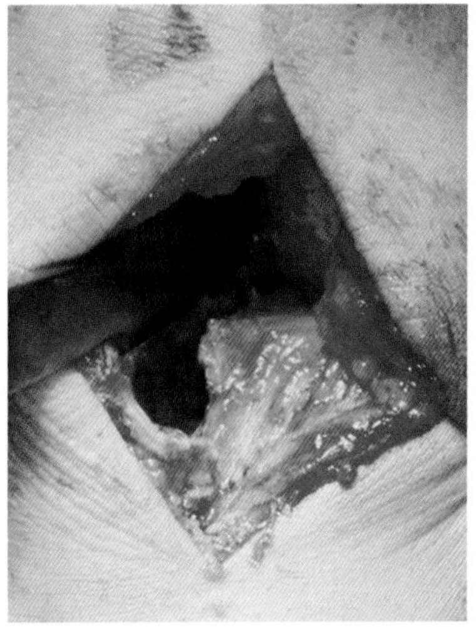
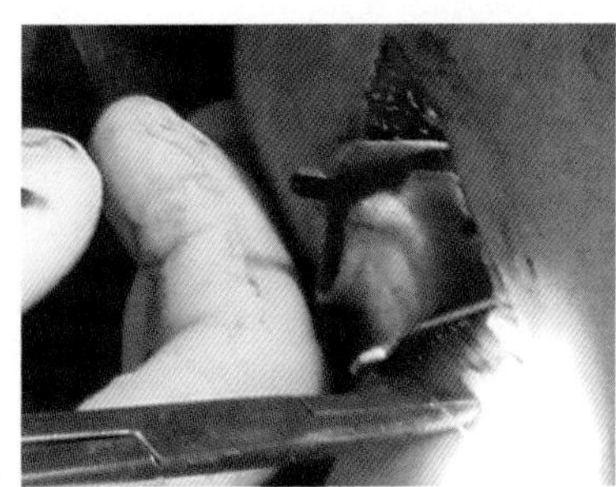

TECH FIG 2 • *(continued)* **D.** Preparation of dovetail recipient site. **E.** Completed keyhole recipient site. **F.** Posterolateral exposure.

DELIVERY AND FIXATION OF LATERAL MENISCUS

- Before delivery of the graft into the recipient site, place the 10-inch needles from the passage sutures through the miniarthrotomy and posterolateral capsule to assist in delivery of the graft (TECH FIG 3A).
- Exposure, retraction, and needle retrieval are identical to an inside-out repair technique.
- Plan optimal placement of sutures through the capsule relative to their position in the meniscus (TECH FIG 3B). Use the popliteus tendon and the popliteal hiatus in the graft as a guide for suture placement.
- By simultaneously inserting the shape-matched donor graft into the tibial recipient site and pulling on the posterior inside-out passage suture, the graft is delivered to re-establish the normal insertion site (TECH FIG 3C).
- A varus stress to the knee, combined with pulling on the posterior passage sutures, will help reduce the posterior horn under the femoral condyle (TECH FIG 3D).
- Matching the anterior cortices (graft and recipient) and bringing the knee through a range of motion will assist in final anteroposterior positioning.
- Place additional inside-out meniscus sutures with the suture cannula placed in the medial portal. The scope is placed into the miniarthrotomy.

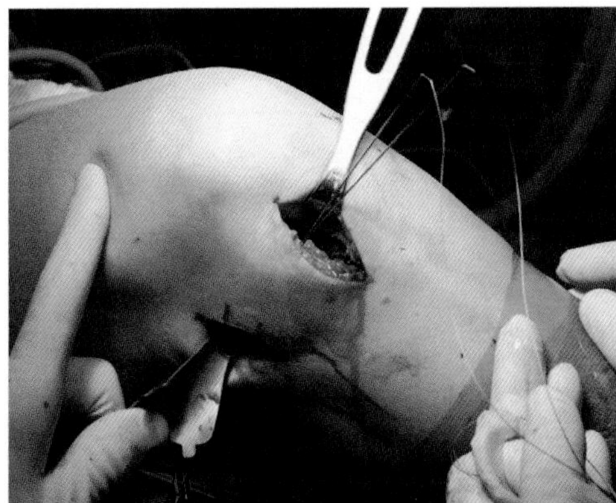

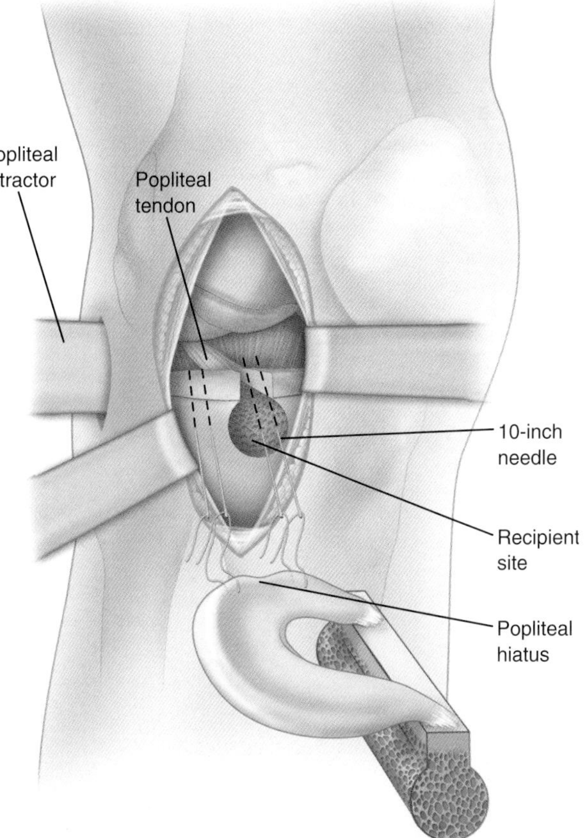

TECH FIG 3 • Delivery of lateral meniscus. **A.** Ten-inch needles from the passage suture are placed through the posterolateral capsule and retrieved by the assistant. **B.** Inside-out vertical sutures are placed through the appropriate location within the posterolateral capsule. *(continued)*

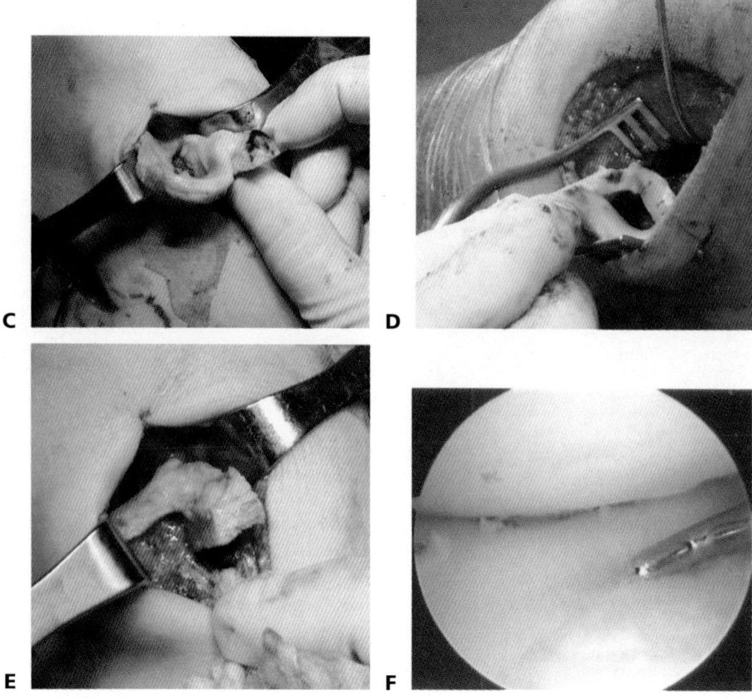

TECH FIG 3 • *(continued)* **C,D.** The dovetail graft is delivered into the recipient site. **E.** Posterior horn is reduced by pulling on the posterior passage suture combined with varus stress to the knee. **F.** Completed lateral meniscus transplant.

- Additional anterior sutures can be placed through the anterior arthrotomy using standard open suturing techniques.
- Tie sutures with the knee in flexion (TECH FIG 3E,F).
- An interference screw or transosseous suture fixation may be placed with the slot technique, but this is typically unnecessary with the dovetail and keyhole technique.

MEDIAL MENISCUS GRAFT PREPARATION

- A previously size-matched medial meniscus with the attached tibial plateau is thawed in a saline and antibiotic solution. Remove soft tissue as described for the lateral meniscus.
- Medial meniscal allografts may be fashioned with or without bone plugs at the anterior and posterior horn insertion sites (TECH FIG 4A,B).
- For preparation without bone plugs, detach the anterior and posterior horns from the bone block and whipstitch each horn with heavy nonabsorbable suture. We do not typically use this technique unless a plug fractures.
- For preparation with bone plugs (recommended), place a 2.4-mm Beath guide pin through the bone block into the posterior insertion site at about a 60-degree angle. Place

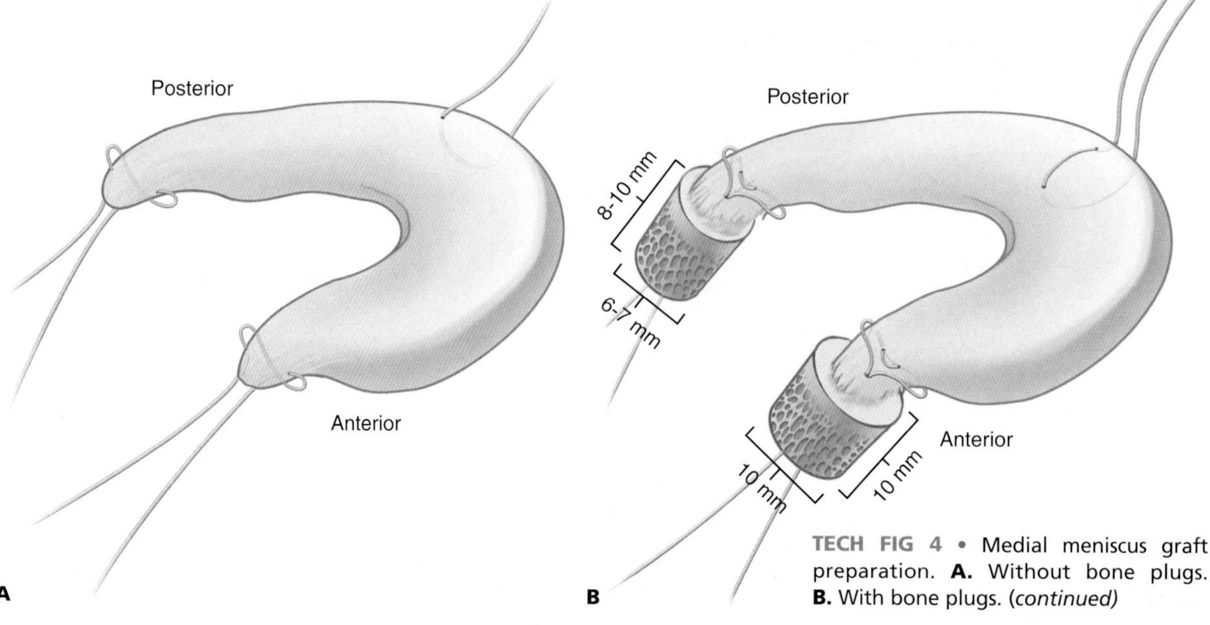

TECH FIG 4 • Medial meniscus graft preparation. **A.** Without bone plugs. **B.** With bone plugs. *(continued)*

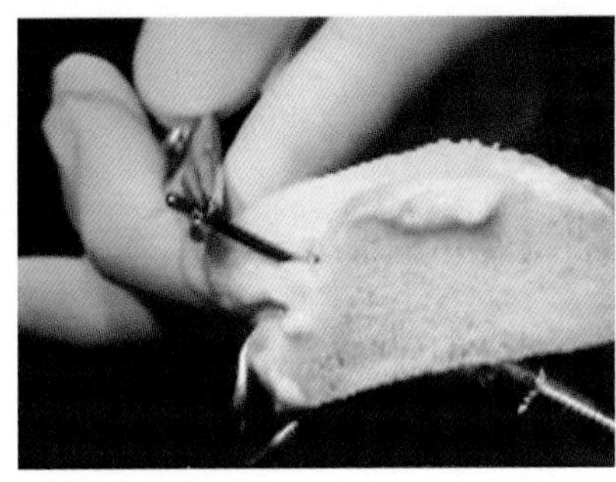

TECH FIG 4 • *(continued)* **C.** Coring reamer over collared pin.

a commercially available collared pin into the 2.4-mm hole. Ream over the collared pin using an 7- or 8-mm coring reamer (creates a plug 6 or 7 mm in diameter) (TECH FIG 4C). Trim and taper the end to create a 10-mm-long plug.

- Repeat these steps for the anterior horn insertion, but angle the guide pin approximately 20 degrees and create a bone plug 10 mm in diameter. Place a heavy nonabsorbable suture (no. 2 FiberWire) up the guide pin hole, through the meniscal tissue, then back down the guide pin hole for each bone plug.
- Place a vertical passing stitch of nonabsorbable suture at the junction of the posterior and middle thirds of the meniscus.
- Mark the anterior and posterior horns on the superior meniscal surface.

MEDIAL MENISCUS APPROACH AND TIBIAL PREPARATION

- The case is performed via arthroscopic, medial parapatellar, and posteromedial meniscal repair approaches (TECH FIG 5A).
- The remaining meniscus is débrided, leaving 1 mm of meniscal rim. The surrounding capsule and meniscal bed is abraded with the shaver and rasps.
- To visualize and access the posterior horn insertion site, perform a small notchplasty of the medial wall of the notch inferior to the posterior cruciate ligament (PCL) insertion. Likewise, débride back the medial tibial spine until easy access is obtained (TECH FIG 5B).
- Perform a medial parapatellar incision, extending distally to allow access to the anteromedial proximal tibia. Do not perform the arthrotomy portion until the posterior tunnel is complete.

TECH FIG 5 • Medial meniscus technique. **A.** Medial approach. **B.** Notchplasty performed under posterior cruciate ligament. **C,D.** Guide pin placement into the posterior horn insertion. **E.** Shuttle suture through the posterior tunnel exiting the medial portal. **F.** Anterior arthrotomy incorporating medial portal.

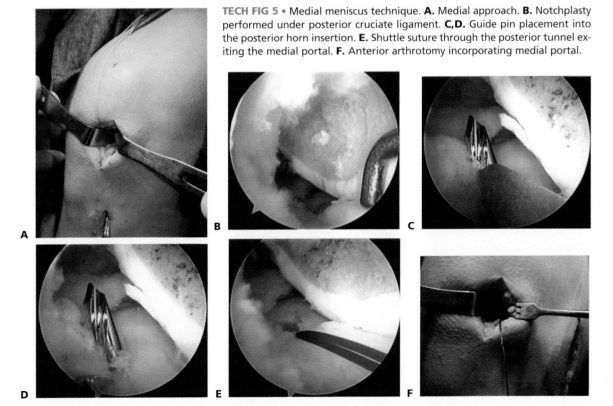

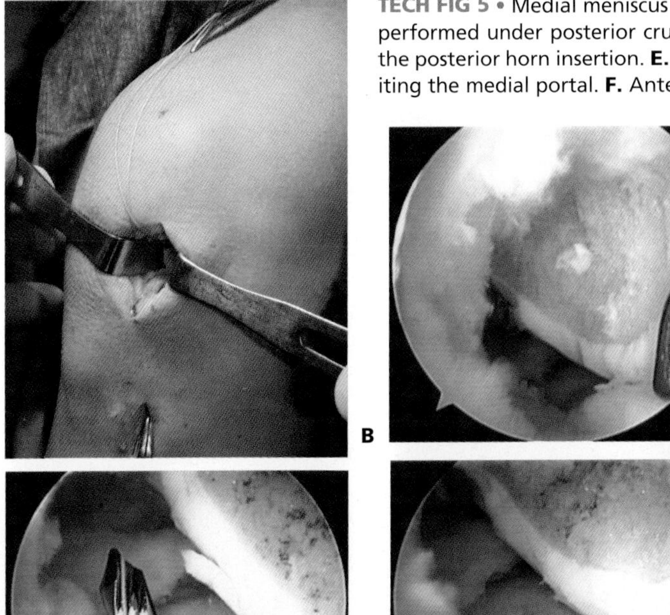

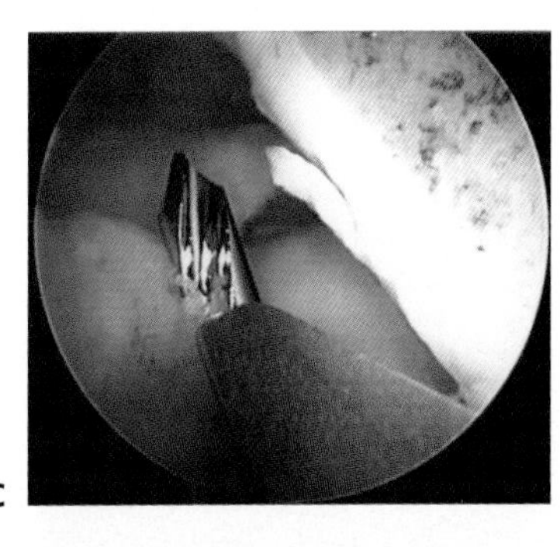

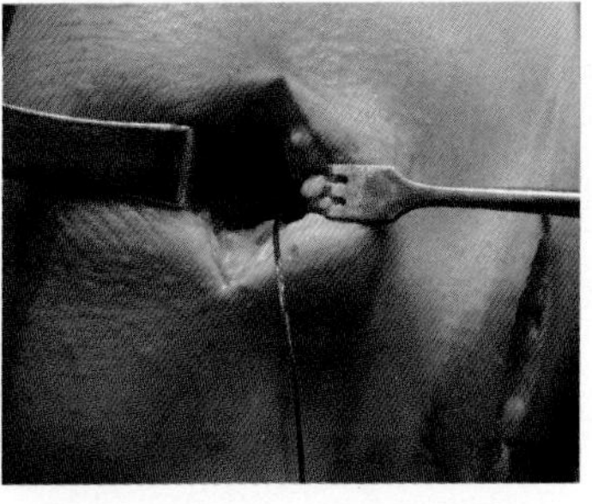

- Under direct visualization, position a variable-angle ACL-PCL tibial drill guide such that the guide pin will exit in the center of the native posterior horn insertion site footprint (TECH FIG 5C,D).
- Drill a 9-mm tibial tunnel. Débride and chamfer the intra-articular portion of the tunnel. Pass a shuttle suture up the tunnel and out the medial portal (TECH FIG 5E).
- Complete the medial parapatellar arthrotomy, incorporating the medial portal (do not cut the shuttle suture) (TECH FIG 5F).
- Perform posteromedial exposure to receive inside-out sutures (meniscus repair approach).

DELIVERY AND FIXATION OF MEDIAL MENISCUS

- Shuttle-exchange the shuttle sutures with the posterior bone plug suture and allograft passing suture. Via the parapatellar arthrotomy, deliver the meniscal allograft into the knee and fully seat the posterior bone plug into the posterior tunnel (TECH FIG 6A,B). Apply a valgus stress to the knee while pulling on the posterior bone plug sutures and the posterior passing sutures.
- Using zone-specific cannulas (Linvatec, Largo, FL), suture the allograft to the periphery approximately two thirds of the way posterior to anterior with multiple vertical mattress sutures.
- Through the parapatellar arthrotomy, determine the anterior horn insertion site and place a Beath guide pin in its center.
- Drill a blind 10-mm tunnel vertically to a depth sufficient to accept the anterior allograft bone plug (TECH FIG 6C).
  - Drill a 2-mm hole perpendicular to the tunnel from the anterior tibial cortex entering the tunnel base.

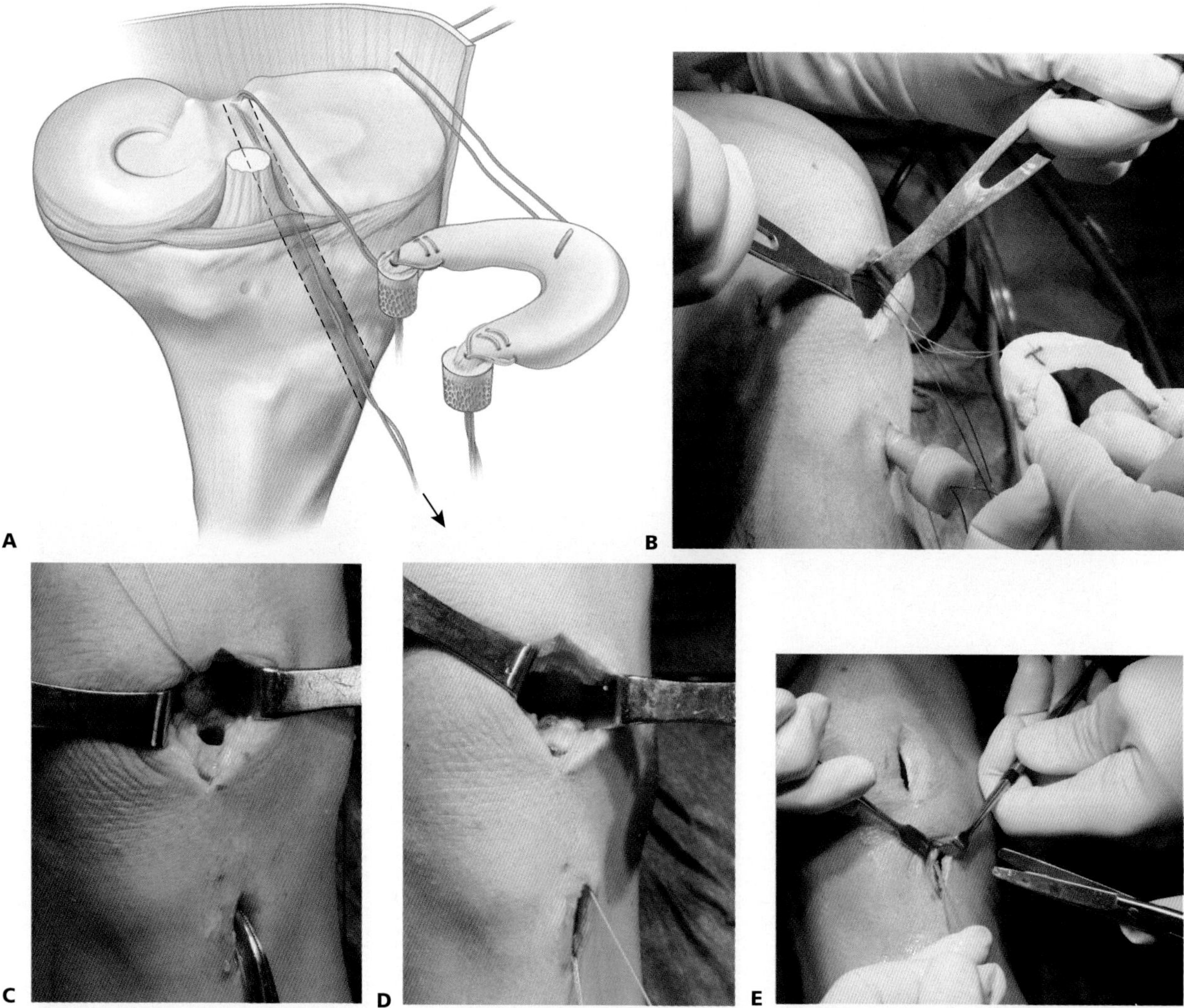

TECH FIG 6 • **A,B.** Meniscus delivery. Shuttle suture and delivery of the posterior bone plug and meniscus. **C.** Anterior recipient tunnel created by reaming over guide pin. **D.** Anterior bone plug seated into tunnel. **E.** Bone plug sutures tied over anterior bone bridge. *(continued)*

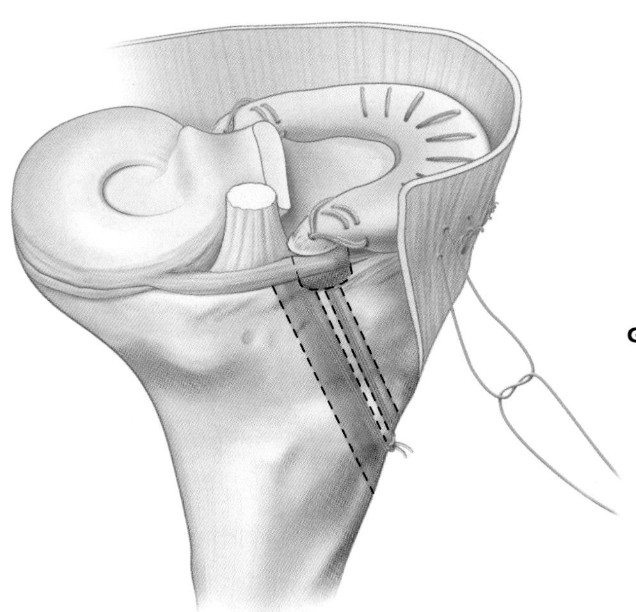

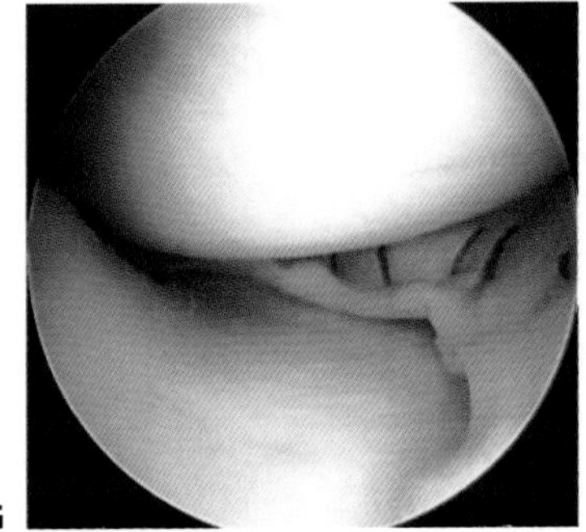

TECH FIG 6 • *(continued)* **F.** Schematic of bone plug and meniscus fixation. **G.** Arthroscopic view of final graft in position.

- Place a shuttle stitch through the 2-mm hole and exit up the anterior tunnel.
- Shuttle-exchange the shuttle stitch and the anterior bone plug suture. Deliver and fully seat the anterior bone plug in the tunnel (TECH FIG 6D).
- Tie the bone plug sutures over the bone bridge rather than tying the sutures over a plastic ligament button. (TECH FIG 6E).
- Complete the meniscal repair to the anterior capsule using an open repair technique (TECH FIG 6F,G).

PEARLS AND PITFALLS

Indications	■ The surgeon must ensure that meniscal deficiency is the symptom generator. ■ The procedure should be performed in the window of opportunity between the onset of symptoms and the development of advanced degenerative change.
Graft management	■ Bone plugs should be 1 mm smaller than tunnels. The surgeon should avoid "press fit" to facilitate passage. ■ For lateral transplants, the surgeon should strongly consider commercially available graft preparation instrumentation. ■ For medial transplants, if the bone plug detaches or fractures, it should be reattached with suture or converted to plugless technique.
Graft passage	■ Valgus stress is applied while pulling on passage sutures. ■ The surgeon may need to "pie-crust" the medial collateral ligament in a tight medial compartment. ■ If the medial graft cannot be passed from front to back, it may be delivered via a posteromedial arthrotomy.

POSTOPERATIVE CARE

- Postoperative rehabilitation may need to be altered based on concomitant procedures.
- A hinged knee brace locked in extension is used for 6 weeks.
- Weight bearing as tolerated is typically permitted with the knee braced in full extension (this may be limited by other procedures).
- Range of motion is limited between 0 and 90 degrees for the first 6 weeks. Flexion is increased between 6 and 12 weeks.
- Closed-chain exercises, cycling, and swimming are started at 6 weeks.
- Running may begin at 4 to 6 months.
- Squatting and pivoting sports are not allowed for 6 to 9 months.

OUTCOMES

- With appropriate indications, current success rates for allograft meniscus transplantation are about 75% to 85%.[3,4,6,10]
- Bone plug fixation may improve outcomes, although this is controversial.
- Poor results are typically associated with more advanced articular cartilage degeneration.

- Meniscus transplants that are combined with articular cartilage resurfacing or realignment procedures can yield favorable outcomes.
- One study reported that 86% of patients with a combined ACL reconstruction and meniscus transplant had normal or near-normal International Knee Documentation Committee (IKDC) scores, with an average maximum KT arthrometer side-to-side difference of 1.5 mm.[12]

COMPLICATIONS

- Nonhealing or incomplete healing
- Infection
- Neurovascular injury
- Loss of motion
- Meniscus tear or extrusion (late)
- Persistent or progressive symptoms (typically related to articular cartilage)

REFERENCES

1. Baratz ME, Fu FH, Mengato R. Meniscal tears: the effect of meniscectomy and of repair on intraarticular contact areas and stress in the human knee: a preliminary report. Am J Sports Med 1986;14:270–275.
2. Carpenter JE, Wojtys EM, Huston LJ, et al. Abstract: preoperative sizing of meniscal allografts. Arthrosocopy 1993;9:344.
3. Cole BJ, Carter TR, Rodeo SA. Allograft meniscal transplantation: background, techniques, and results. J Bone Joint Surg Am 2002;84A:1236–1250.
4. Cole BJ, Dennis MG, Lee S, et al. Prospective evaluation of allograft meniscus transplantation: minimum 2-year follow-up. Am J Sports Med 2006;13:1–9.
5. Huang A, Hull ML, Howell SM. The level of compressive load affects conclusions from statistical analyses to determine whether a lateral meniscal autograft restores tibial contact pressure to normal: a study in human cadaveric knees. J Orthop Res 2003;21:459–464.
6. Kang RW, Lattermann C, Cole BJ. Allograft meniscus transplantation: background, indications, techniques, and outcomes. J Knee Surg 2006;19:220–230.
7. Kurtz CA, Bonner KG, Sekiya JK. Technical note: meniscus transplantation utilizing the femoral distractor. Arthroscopy 2006;22:568e1–3.
8. McDermott ID, Sharifi F, Full AM, et al. An anatomical study of meniscal allograft sizing. Knee Surg Sports Traumatol Arthrosc 2004;12:130–135.
9. Paletta GA Jr, Manning T, Snell E, et al. The effect of allograft meniscal replacement on intraarticular contact area and pressures in the human knee: a biomechanical study. Am J Sports Med 1997;25:692–698.
10. Rodeo SA. Meniscal allografts: where do we stand? Am J Sports Med 2001;29:246–261.
11. Sekiya JK, Ellingson CI. Meniscal allograft transplantation. J Am Acad Orthop Surg 2006;14:164–174.
12. Sekiya JK, Giffin JR, Irrgang JJ, et al. Clinical outcomes after combined meniscal allograft transplantation and anterior cruciate ligament reconstruction. Am J Sports Med 2003;31:896–906.
13. Shaffer B, Kennedy S, Klimkiewicz J, et al. Preoperative sizing of meniscal allografts in meniscal transplantation. Am J Sports Med 2000;28:524–533.

Chapter 36 Microfracture Chondroplasty

J. Richard Steadman and William G. Rodkey

DEFINITION

- Chondral defects in the knee are common.
- The lesions may be partial- or full-thickness (**FIG 1**), through all layers of the articular cartilage down to the level of the subchondral bone.
- Chondral defects may be acute or chronic.
- These articular cartilage lesions may present in a variety of clinical settings and at different ages.[5–10]

ANATOMY

- The articular cartilage of the knee is 2 to 4 mm thick, depending on the location within the joint.
- The articular cartilage is avascular tissue that is devoid of nerves and lymphatics.
- Relatively few cells (chondrocytes) are present in the abundant extracellular matrix.
- These factors are critical in the lack of a spontaneous or naturally occurring repair response after injury to articular cartilage.

PATHOGENESIS

- The shearing forces of the femur on the tibia as a single event may result in trauma to the articular cartilage (**FIG 2**), causing the cartilage to fracture, lacerate, and separate from the underlying subchondral bone or separate with a piece of the subchondral bone.
- Chronic repetitive loading in excess of normal physiologic levels also may result in fatigue and failure of the chondral surface.
- Single events usually occur in younger patients, whereas chronic degenerative lesions are seen more commonly in persons of middle age and older.[5–10]
- Repetitive impacts can cause cartilage swelling, an increase in collagen fiber diameter, and an alteration in the relation between collagen and proteoglycans.

NATURAL HISTORY

- Articular cartilage defects that extend for the full thickness to subchondral bone rarely heal without intervention.[5–10]
- Some patients may not develop clinically significant problems from acute full-thickness chondral defects, but most eventually suffer from degenerative changes that can be debilitating.

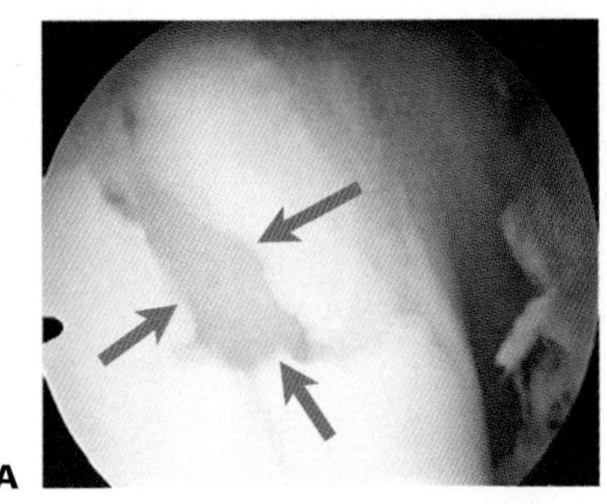

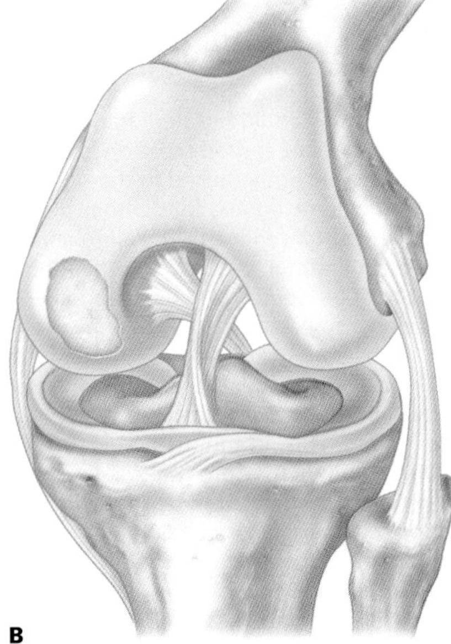

FIG 1 • **A.** A full-thickness chondral defect through all layers of the articular cartilage is outlined (*arrows*). **B.** A full-thickness chondral lesion.

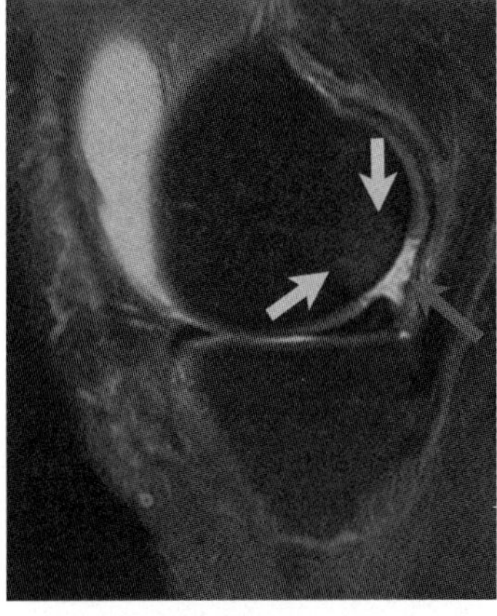

FIG 2 • A shearing injury has resulted in a full-thickness chondral defect, as seen on this MRI scan. The dark arrow denotes the cartilage defect, and the light arrows show the limits of the subchondral bone edema secondary to the shearing injury. (Courtesy of Dr. Charles Ho, Vail, CO.)

- Acute events may not result in full-thickness cartilage loss but, rather, may start a degenerative cascade that can lead to chronic full-thickness loss.
- The degenerative cascade typically includes early softening and fibrillation (grade I); fissures and cracks in the surface of the cartilage (grade II); severe fissures and cracks with a "crab meat" appearance (grade III); and, finally, exposure of the subchondral bone (grade IV).

PATIENT HISTORY AND PHYSICAL FINDINGS

- The physical diagnosis can be difficult to establish, especially if the chondral defect is isolated.
- Chondral lesions can be located on the joint surfaces of the femur, tibia, or patella.
- Point tenderness over a femoral condyle or tibial plateau is a useful finding, but is not diagnostic.
- If compression of the patella elicits pain, a patellar or trochlear lesion may be indicated.
- Joint effusion may be present, but it is not a consistent finding.
- Catching or clicking may be present, especially if there is an elevated flap of cartilage.
- Restricted range of motion (ROM) can be associated with many pathologic conditions of the knee, but the ROM should be documented as a baseline prior to any treatment.
- Physical examinations should be performed, as follows:
  - The patella is palpated in superior-inferior and medial-lateral directions for evidence of effusion. About 50% of patients with chondral defects have an effusion.
  - The Lachman test is used to rule out ligamentous instability by applying anterior force to the tibia with the knee in 20 to 30 degrees of flexion.
  - The thumb and index finger are used to place digital pressure over all geographic areas of the knee to detect point tenderness; this finding is useful but is not in itself diagnostic.
  - A palpable or audible pop in combination with pain is considered a positive result to the McMurray's test, indicating a meniscus lesion rather than a chondral lesion.

IMAGING AND OTHER DIAGNOSTIC STUDIES

- For diagnostic imaging, angular deformity and joint space narrowing are assessed using long standing radiographs.
- Two methods for radiographic measurement of the biomechanical alignment of the weight-bearing axis of the knee are used in our facility:
  - The angle between the femur and tibia on anterorposterior (AP) views obtained with the patient standing
  - The weight-bearing mechanical axis drawn from the center of the femoral head to the center of the tibiotarsal joint on long (~51 inches/130 cm) standing radiographs (**FIG 3A**).
- If the angle drawn between the tibia and femur shows more than 5 degrees of varus or valgus compared with the normal knee, this amount of axial malalignment would be a relative contraindication for microfracture.
- We rely most often on the mechanical axis. It is preferable for the mechanical axis weight-bearing line to be in the central quarter of the tibial plateau of either the medial or lateral compartment.

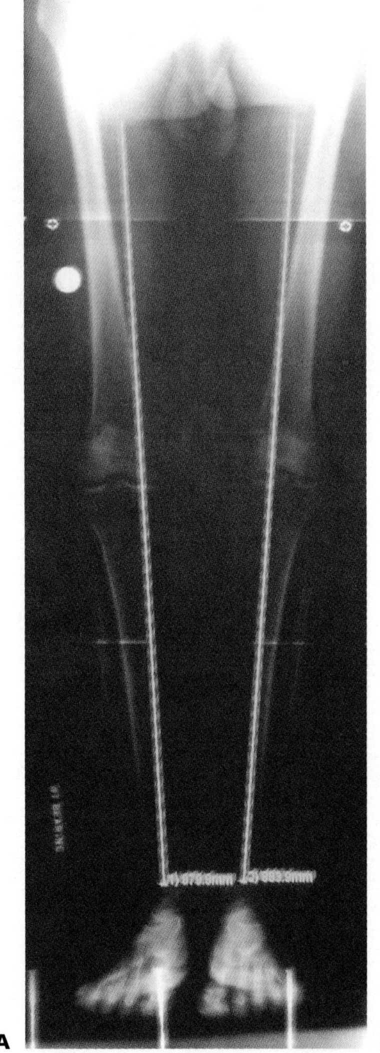

A

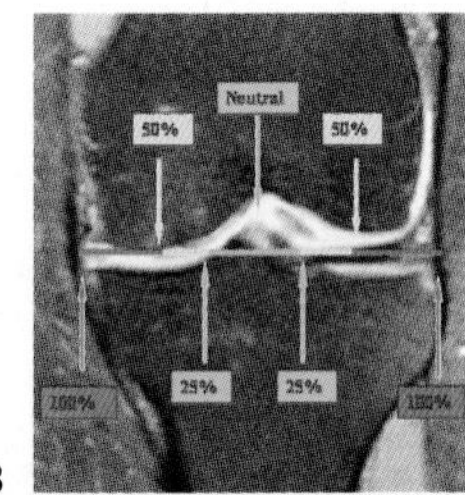

B

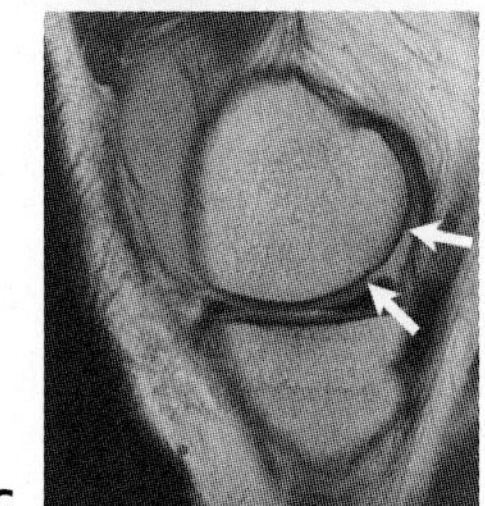

C

FIG 3 • **A.** On this long standing radiographic view, the weight-bearing axis is seen to have shifted somewhat medially in the left knee, but it is significantly shifted in the right knee (*green line*). **B.** If the weight-bearing axis falls within the neutral 25% of either compartment (*green area*), the alignment of the knee would be considered normal. If the weight-bearing axis is between 25% and 50% (*yellow area*), a realignment procedure should be considered in conjunction with a microfracture chondroplasty. If the weight-bearing axis is greater than 50% (*red area*) in either compartment, then this would be an absolute contraindication to microfracture unless a realignment procedure was done first or in conjunction with the microfracture. **C.** MRI clearly shows an acute full-thickness chondral defect, the extent of which is noted by the white arrows. (**C:** Courtesy of Dr. Charles Ho, Vail, CO.)

- If the mechanical axis weight-bearing line falls outside the quarter of the plateaus closest to the center (**FIG 3B**), either medial or lateral, this weight-bearing shift also would be a relative contraindication if left uncorrected. In such cases, a realignment procedure should be included as a part of the overall treatment regimen.

- Standard AP, lateral, and weight-bearing radiographic views with knees flexed to 30 to 45 degrees also are obtained.
- MRI that uses newer diagnostic sequences specific for articular cartilage is crucial to our diagnostic workup of patients with suspected chondral lesions (**FIG 3C**).

DIFFERENTIAL DIAGNOSIS

- Meniscus tear
- Loose bodies
- Attached chondral flap
- Symptomatic plica
- Synovitis
- Chondral bruising, with or without subchondral edema

NONOPERATIVE MANAGEMENT

- Patients with acute chondral injuries are treated as soon as practical after the diagnosis is made, especially if the knee is being treated concurrently for meniscus or anterior cruciate ligament pathology.
- Patients with chronic or degenerative chondral lesions often are treated nonoperatively (conservatively) for at least 12 weeks after a suspected chondral lesion is diagnosed clinically.
- This treatment regimen includes activity modification, physical therapy, nonsteroidal anti-inflammatory drugs, viscosupplement injections, and possibly dietary supplements that may have cartilage-stimulating properties.
- If nonoperative treatment is not successful, then surgical treatment is considered.

SURGICAL MANAGEMENT

- Microfracture initially was designed for patients with posttraumatic articular cartilage lesions of the knee that had progressed to full-thickness chondral defects.
- The microfracture technique still is most commonly indicated for full-thickness loss of articular cartilage in either a weight-bearing area between the femur and tibia or an area of contact between the patella and the trochlear groove.
- Unstable cartilage that overlies the subchondral bone also is an indication for microfracture (**FIG 4**).
- If a partial-thickness lesion is probed and the cartilage simply scrapes off down to bone, we consider this a full-thickness lesion.

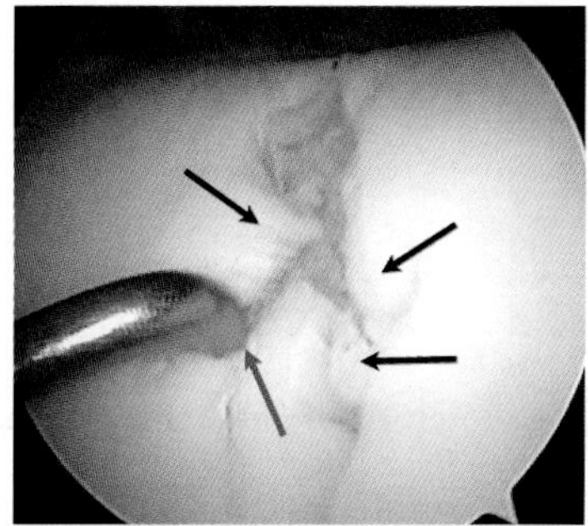

FIG 4 • The probe (*red arrow*) shows that this chondral defect has areas of unstable cartilage (*black arrows*) that are fissured fully to subchondral bone. These unstable cartilage segments must be removed until a stable margin is achieved.

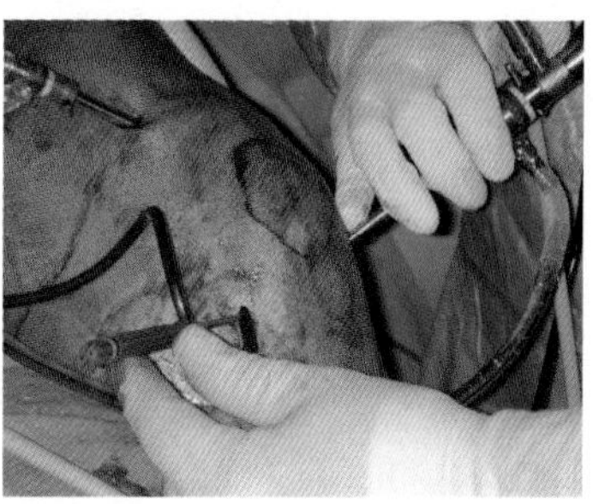

FIG 5 • For the definitive procedure, the distal portion of the table is lowered so that the foot is off the table and the knee is flexed 90 degrees.

- Degenerative joint disease in a knee that has proper axial alignment is another common indication for microfracture.
- These lesions all involve loss of articular cartilage at the bone–cartilage interface.

Preoperative Planning

- All imaging studies are reviewed.
- MRI scans are re-reviewed for presence of concomitant pathology.
- Radiographs are carefully studied for fractures, loose bodies, axial alignment, and joint space narrowing.
- The surgical plan should include addressing concomitant pathology concurrently, as appropriate.
- Examination under anesthesia should be accomplished before skin preparation and draping.

Positioning

- The patient is positioned supine.
- Initially, for the diagnostic portion of the arthroscopy, the foot is on the table.
- For the definitive procedure, the distal portion of the table is lowered so that the foot is off the table and the knee is flexed 90 degrees (**FIG 5**).
- A lateral post is raised so that a varus force can be placed on the joint to increase visualization as necessary.

Approach

- Our primary approach to chondral lesions is arthroscopic microfracture chondroplasty (Table 1).[5–10]

Table 1 Indications and Contraindications for Microfracture

Indications	Contraindications
Full-thickness defect (grade IV), acute or chronic	Partial-thickness defects
Unstable full-thickness lesion	Uncorrected axial malalignment
Degenerative joint disease lesion (requires proper knee alignment)	Inability to commit to rehabilitation protocol
Patient capable of rehabilitation protocol	Global degenerative osteoarthrosis

DIAGNOSTIC ARTHROSCOPY

- Three portals routinely are made about the knee for use of the inflow cannula, the arthroscope, and the working instruments (**TECH FIG 1**).
- Typically, a tourniquet is not used during the microfracture procedure; rather, the arthroscopic fluid pump pressure is varied to control bleeding.
- An initial, thorough diagnostic examination of the knee should be done.
- All geographic areas of the knee must be inspected carefully, including the suprapatellar pouch, the medial and lateral gutters, the patellofemoral joint, the intercondylar notch and its contents, and the medial and lateral compartments, including the posterior horns of both menisci.
- All other intra-articular procedures are done before microfracture.
  - This technique helps prevent loss of visualization when fat droplets and blood enter the knee from the microfracture holes.
- Importantly, particular attention must be paid to soft tissues such as plicae and the lateral retinaculum that potentially could produce increased compression between cartilage surfaces.

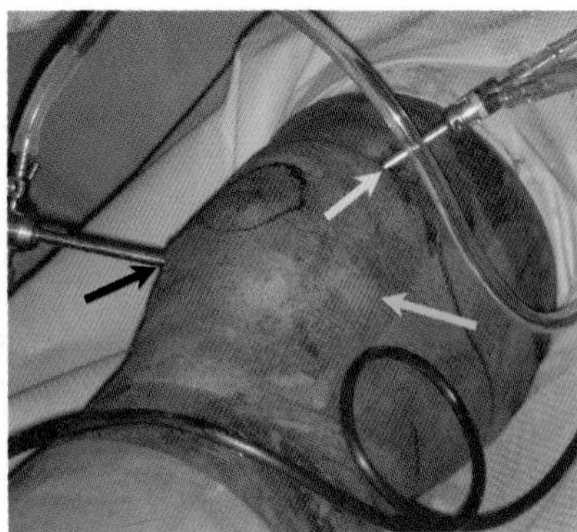

TECH FIG 1 • Three portals routinely are made about the knee for use of the inflow cannula (*yellow arrow*), the arthroscope (*black arrow*), and the working instruments (*green arrow* indicates the approximate location where this portal will be made).

INITIAL PREPARATION

- After careful assessment of the full-thickness articular cartilage lesion, the exposed bone is débrided of all remaining unstable cartilage.
- A hand-held curved curette (**TECH FIG 2A**) and a full radius resector (**TECH FIG 2B**) are used to débride the cartilage.
  - It is critical to débride all loose or marginally attached cartilage from the surrounding rim of the lesion.
  - The calcified cartilage layer that remains as a cap to many lesions must be removed, preferably with a curette (**TECH FIG 2C**).
  - Thorough and complete removal of the calcified cartilage layer is extremely important, based on animal studies we have completed.[1,2]
  - Care should be taken to maintain the integrity of the subchondral plate by not débriding too deeply.
- This prepared lesion, with a stable perpendicular edge of healthy, well-attached viable cartilage surrounding the defect (**TECH FIG 2D**), provides a pool that helps hold the marrow clot—"super clot"—as it forms.

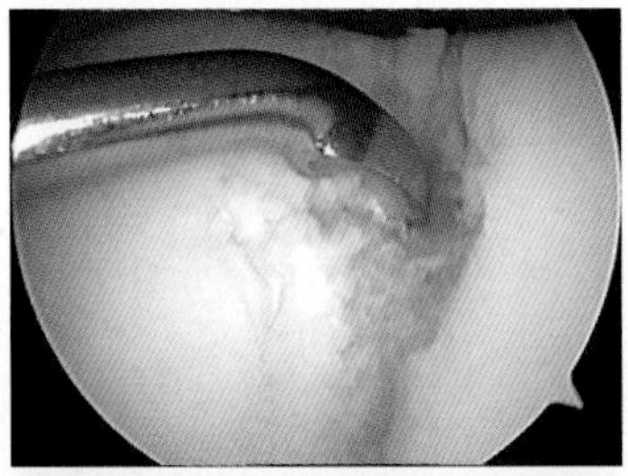

A

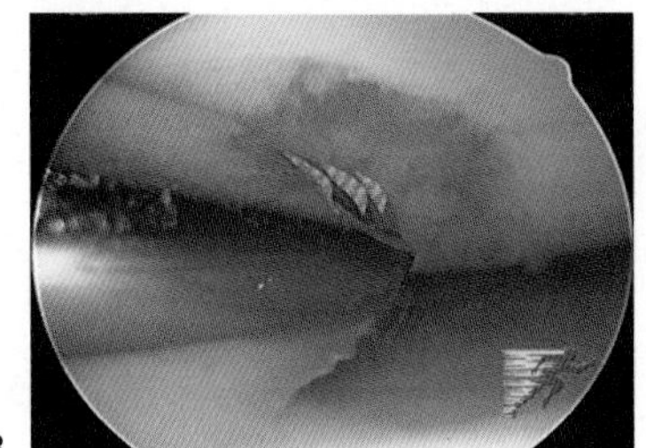

B

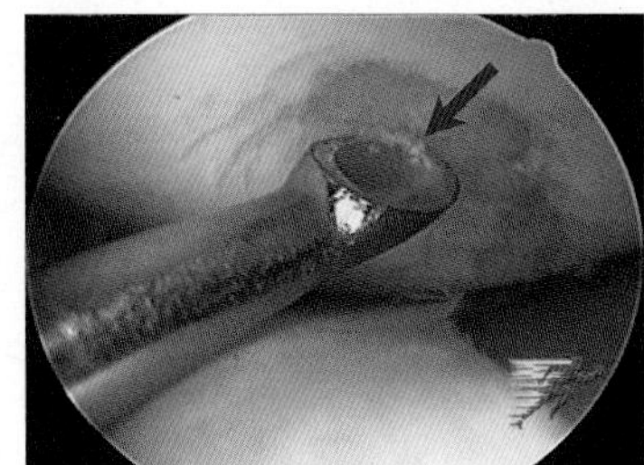

C

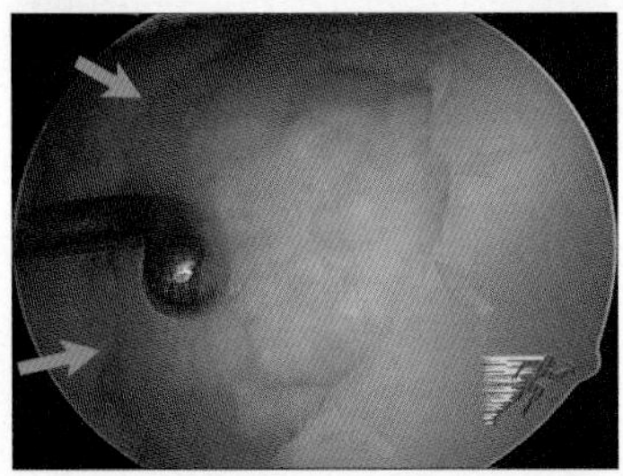

D

TECH FIG 2 • **A.** A handheld, curved curette is used to remove unstable and damaged cartilage segments. **B.** A full-radius resector also may be used to remove unstable or damaged cartilage from the lesion in preparation for the microfracture procedure. **C.** The calcified cartilage layer that remains as a cap to many lesions must be removed, preferably by using a curette as noted by the blue arrow. **D.** This prepared lesion has a stable perpendicular edge of healthy, well-attached viable cartilage surrounding the defect, as noted by the green arrows. A properly prepared lesion provides a pool that helps hold the marrow clot—"super clot"—as it forms.

MICROFRACTURE

- After preparation of the lesion, an arthroscopic awl is used to make multiple holes, or "microfractures," in the exposed subchondral bone plate.
- An awl with an angle that permits the tip to be perpendicular to the bone as it is advanced, typically 30 or 45 degrees, is used.
- A 90-degree awl is available that should be used only on the patella or other soft bone. The 90-degree awl should be advanced only manually, not with a mallet.
- The holes are made as close together as possible but not so close that one breaks into another, thus damaging the subchondral plate between them.
  - This technique usually results in microfracture holes that are approximately 3 to 4 mm apart.
- When fat droplets can be seen coming from the marrow cavity, the appropriate depth (approximately 2–4 mm) has been reached.
- Arthroscopic awls produce essentially no thermal necrosis of the bone compared with hand-driven or motorized drills.
- Microfracture holes around the periphery of the defect should be made first, immediately adjacent to the healthy stable cartilage rim (TECH FIG 3A,B).
- The process is completed by making the microfracture holes toward the center of the defect (TECH FIG 3C).

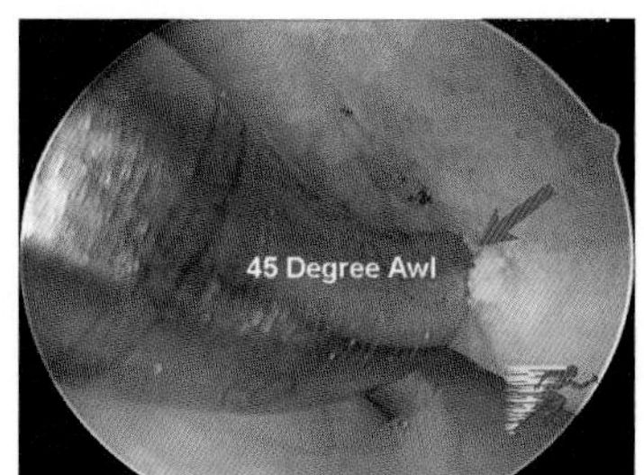

A

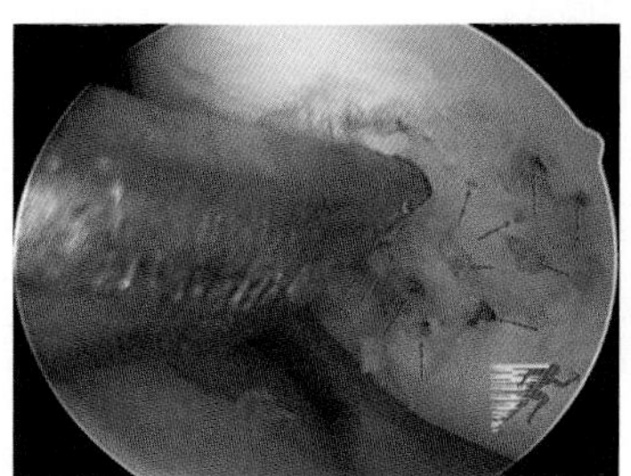

C

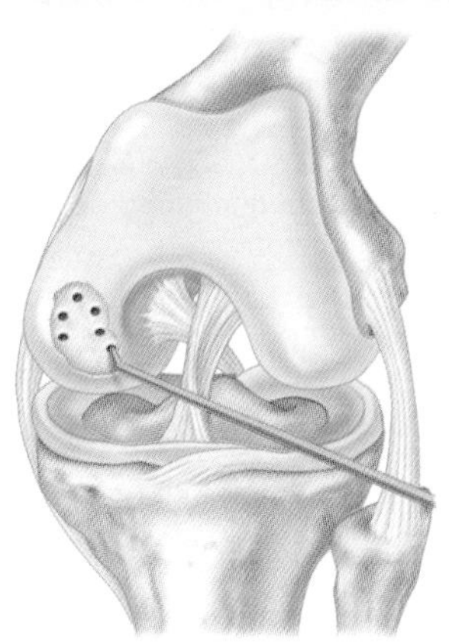

B

TECH FIG 3 • **A.** An awl is used with an angle that permits the tip to be perpendicular to the bone as it is advanced, typically 30 or 45 degrees. Microfracture holes are made around the periphery of the defect first, immediately adjacent to the healthy stable cartilage rim (*purple arrow*). **B.** The microfracture holes are made starting at the periphery of the prepared lesion, keeping the awl perpendicular to the bone. **C.** The microfracture process is completed by making the microfracture holes (*red arrows*) toward the center of the defect. The holes are as close together as possible, 3 to 4 mm apart, but without any hole breaking into another and disrupting the integrity of the subchondral bone plate.

ASSESSMENT

- The treated lesion is assessed at the conclusion of the microfracture to ensure a sufficient number of holes have been made before reducing the arthroscopic irrigation fluid flow.
- After the arthroscopic irrigation fluid pump pressure is reduced, the release of marrow fat droplets and blood from the microfracture holes into the subchondral bone is observed under direct visualization (TECH FIG 4).
- The quantity of marrow contents flowing into the joint is judged to be adequate when marrow is observed emanating from all microfracture holes.
- Finally, all instruments are removed from the knee and the joint is cleared of fluid.

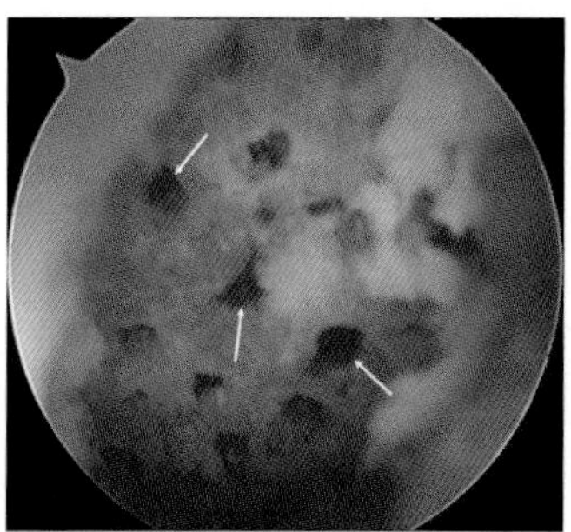

TECH FIG 4 • Marrow elements, including blood and fat droplets, accessed by the subchondral bone microfracture can be seen coming from essentially all of the microfracture holes (*white arrows*) after the arthroscopic irrigation fluid pressure has been reduced.

TECHNIQUES

ADDITIONAL CONSIDERATIONS

- Intra-articular drains should not be used, because the goal is for the surgically induced marrow clot, rich in marrow elements, to form and to stabilize while covering the lesion.
- Chronic degenerative chondral lesions commonly have extensive eburnated bone and bony sclerosis with thickening of the subchondral plate, thus making it difficult to do an adequate microfracture procedure (TECH FIG 5).
- In these instances, and when the axial alignment and other indications for microfracture are met, first a few microfracture holes are made with the awls in various locations of the lesion to assess the thickness of the eburnated bone, and then a motorized burr is used to remove the sclerotic bone until punctate bleeding is seen.
- After the bleeding appears uniformly over the surface of the lesion, a microfracture procedure can be performed as described.
- We have observed noticeably improved results for these patients with chronic chondral lesions since we began using this technique. However, if the surrounding cartilage is too thin to establish a perpendicular rim to hold the marrow clot, we probably would not do a microfracture procedure in patients with degenerative lesions that have advanced to that degree.

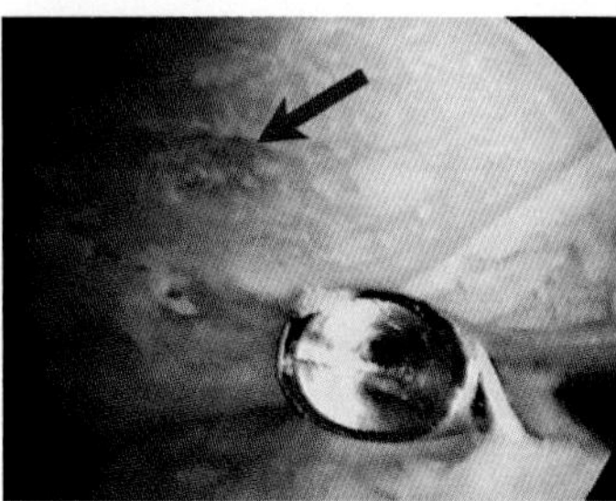

TECH FIG 5 • Chronic degenerative chondral lesions commonly have extensive eburnated bone and bony sclerosis with thickening of the subchondral plate, making it difficult to do an adequate microfracture procedure. The black arrow points to a single microfracture hole that has been made to help assess the depth of eburnated or sclerotic bone that must be removed before performing the microfracture procedure.

PEARLS AND PITFALLS

Initial procedures	■ Complete a thorough arthroscopic diagnostic examination, inspecting all geographic areas of the knee. Perform all other intra-articular procedures before completing microfracture.
Chondroplasty	■ Assess the chondral lesion. Remove all loose or marginally attached cartilage down to exposed bone. ■ Thoroughly and completely remove the calcified cartilage layer with a hand-held curette, but do not penetrate the subchondral bone. ■ Use a microfracture awl to make microfracture holes in the subchondral bone, first working all the way around the periphery and then into the center of the lesion. ■ Remove all instruments and evacuate the joint. Do *not* use a drain in the joint.
Postoperative management	■ Follow the rehabilitation protocol carefully to improve the likelihood of success.

POSTOPERATIVE CARE

- We prescribe cold therapy for all patients postoperatively, and it is continued for 1 to 7 days.[5–10]
- The specific post-microfracture rehabilitation protocol recommended depends on both the anatomic location and the size of the defect.[3,4]
- If other intra-articular procedures are done concurrently with microfracture, such as anterior cruciate ligament reconstruction, we do not hesitate to alter the rehabilitation program as necessary.[3]
- After microfracture of lesions on the weight-bearing surfaces of the femoral condyles or tibial plateaus, we initiate immediate motion with a continuous passive motion (CPM) machine in the recovery room.[5–10]
  - The initial ROM typically is 30 to 70 degrees, which is increased as tolerated in 10- to 20-degree increments until full passive ROM is achieved.
  - The machine usually is set at 1 cycle per minute, but the rate can be varied based on patient preference and comfort.
- The goal is to have the patient in the CPM machine for 6 to 8 hours every 24 hours.
  - If the patient is unable to use the CPM machine, instructions are given for passive flexion and extension of the knee with 500 repetitions three times per day and encouragement to gain full passive ROM of the injured knee as soon as possible after surgery.
- Crutch-assisted touchdown weight-bearing ambulation (10% of body weight) is prescribed for 6 to 8 weeks, depending on the size of the lesion.
- Patients with lesions on the femoral condyles or tibial plateaus rarely use a brace during the initial postoperative period.
- Patients begin therapy immediately after surgery with an emphasis on patellar mobility and ROM, with instructions to perform medial to lateral and superior to inferior movement

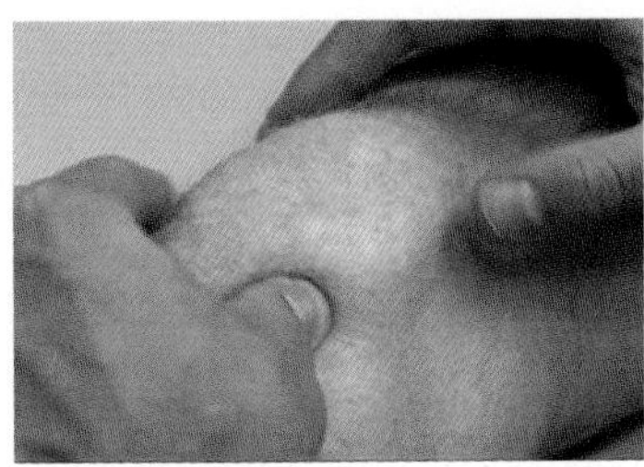

FIG 6 • We place great emphasis on patellar mobility and range of motion with instructions to perform medial to lateral and superior to inferior movement of the patella as well as medial to lateral movement of the quadriceps and patellar tendons as shown here.

of the patella as well as medial to lateral movement of the quadriceps and patellar tendons (**FIG 6**).

- This mobilization is crucial in preventing patellar tendon adhesions and associated increases in patellofemoral joint reaction forces.

- ROM exercises (without ROM limitations), quadriceps sets, straight leg raises, hamstring stretching, and ankle pumps also are initiated the day of surgery.
- Stationary biking without resistance and a deep water exercise program are initiated at 1 to 2 weeks postoperatively.
- After 8 weeks of touchdown weight bearing, the patient is progressed to weight bearing as tolerated, typically weaning off crutches within 1 week.
- Restoration of normal muscular function through the use of low-impact exercices is emphasized during weeks 9 through 16.
- Depending on the clinical examination, the patient's size, the sport, and the size of the lesion, we usually recommend that patients not return to sports that involve pivoting, cutting, and jumping until at least 4 to 9 months after microfracture.
- All patients treated by microfracture for patellofemoral lesions must use a brace set at 0 to 20 degrees for the first 8 weeks postoperatively to limit compression of the regenerating surfaces of the trochlea or patella, or both.
- We allow passive motion with the brace removed, but otherwise the brace must be worn at all times.
- Patients with patellofemoral lesions are placed into a continuous passive motion machine set at 0 to 50 degrees immediately postoperatively.
- Apart from the ROM setting, parameters for the CPM are the same as for tibiofemoral lesions.
- With this regimen, patients typically obtain a pain-free and full passive ROM soon after surgery.
- Patients with lesions of the patellofemoral joint treated by microfracture are allowed to bear weight as tolerated in their brace 2 weeks after surgery.
- After 8 weeks, we open the knee brace gradually before it is discontinued, and then patients are allowed to advance their training progressively.
- Stationary biking without resistance is allowed 2 weeks postoperatively; resistance is added at 8 weeks after microfracture.
- Starting 12 weeks after microfracture, the exercise program is the same as that used for femorotibial lesions.

OUTCOMES

- With appropriate indications, surgical technique, and especially use of our prescribed rehabilitation program, the success rate of microfracture chondroplasty is approximately 90%.[3–10]
- In a study that followed 72 patients (95% follow-up rate) for an average of 11 years (range, 7–17 years) following microfracture, results showed improvement in symptoms and function in all patients.[5]
  - Patient-reported pain and swelling decreased at postoperative year 1 and continued to decrease at year 2, and clinical improvements were maintained over the study period.
  - Age was the only independent predictor of functional (Lysholm) improvement, with patients over 35 years of age improving less than patients under 35; however, both groups showed improvement.
- In National Football League (NFL) players treated with microfracture (**FIG 7**) between 1986 and 1997, 76% of players returned to play in the NFL the next football season.[6]

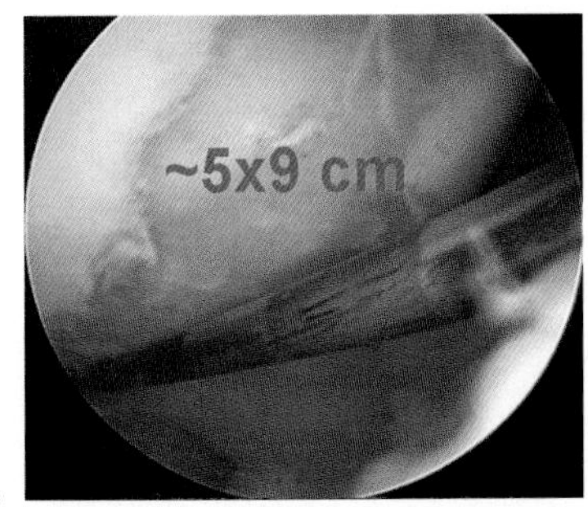

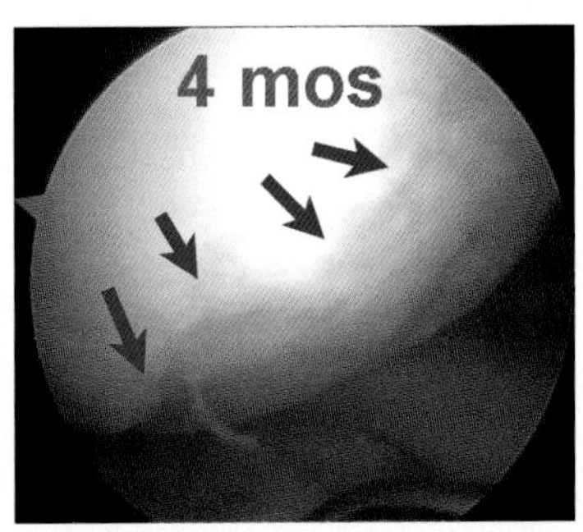

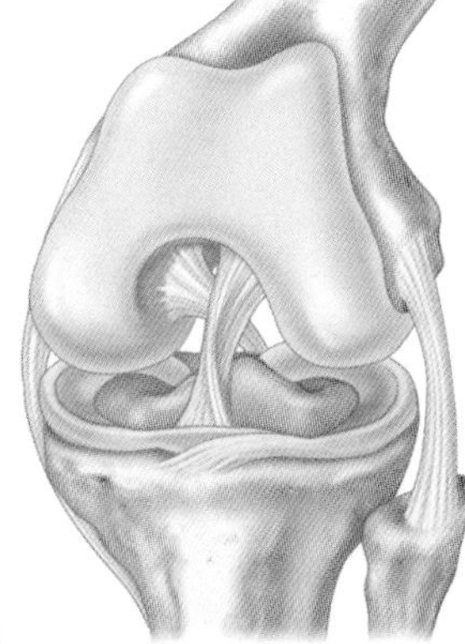

FIG 7 • **A.** A National Football League player presented with a severe defect of the femoral condyle that measured about 5 × 9 cm. This lesion was treated with the microfracture procedure as described here, and the patient was fully compliant with the rehabilitation protocol. **B.** Four months after the microfracture procedure a relook arthroscopy was carried out. The blue arrows show the margins of the lesion, which has been completely filled with repair tissue. **C.** Illustration of how new "repair" cartilage formed over the damaged area.

- Those players played an average of 4.6 additional seasons in the NFL.
- All players showed decreased symptoms and improvement in function.
- Of those players who did not return to play, most had preexisting degenerative changes of the knee.

COMPLICATIONS

- Mild transient pain, most often after microfracture in the patellofemoral joint
- A grating or "gritty" sensation of the joint, especially when a patient discontinues use of the knee brace and begins normal weight bearing through a full ROM
- "Catching" or "locking" as the apex of the patella rides over this lesion during joint motion
- Recurrent effusion between 6 and 8 weeks after microfracture, most commonly when beginning to bear weight on the injured leg after microfracture of a defect on the femoral condyle
- Decreased ROM due to secondary scarring

REFERENCES

1. Frisbie DD, Morisset S, Ho CP, et al. Effects of calcified cartilage on healing of chondral defects treated with microfracture in horses. Am J Sports Med 2006;34:1824–1831.
2. Frisbie DD, Oxford JT, Southwood L, et al. Early events in cartilage repair after subchondral bone microfracture. Clin Orthop 2003;407: 215–227.
3. Hagerman GR, Atkins JA, Dillman C. Rehabilitation of chondral injuries and chronic degenerative arthritis of the knee in the athlete. Oper Tech Sports Med 1995;3:127–135.
4. Irrgang JJ, Pezzullo D. Rehabilitation following surgical procedures to address articular cartilage lesions of the knee. J Orthop Sports Phys Ther 1998;28:232–240.
5. Steadman JR, Briggs KK, Rodrigo JJ, et al. Outcomes of microfracture for traumatic chondral defects of the knee: average 11-year follow-up. Arthroscopy 2003;19:477–484.
6. Steadman JR, Miller BS, Karas SG, et al. The microfracture technique in the treatment of full-thickness chondral lesions of the knee in National Football League players. J Knee Surg 2003;16:83–86.
7. Steadman JR, Rodkey WG, Briggs KK. Microfracture chondroplasty: indications, techniques, and outcomes. Sports Med Arthrosc 2003; 11:236–244.
8. Steadman JR, Rodkey WG, Briggs KK. Microfracture to treat full-thickness chondral defects. J Knee Surg 2002;15:170–176.
9. Steadman JR, Rodkey WG, Briggs KK, et al. Débridement and microfracture for full-thickness articular cartilage defects. In: Scott WN, ed. Insall & Scott Surgery of the Knee. Philadelphia: Churchill Livingstone Elsevier, 2006:359–366.
10. Steadman JR, Rodkey WG, Rodrigo JJ. "Microfracture": surgical technique and rehabilitation to treat chondral defects. Clin Orthop 2001;391S:S362–S369.

Chapter 37

Osteochondral Autograft "Plug" Transfer

F. Alan Barber and David A. Coons

DEFINITION

- Osteochondral autograft "plug" transfer is a technique for treating full-thickness, localized articular cartilage lesions with or without subchondral bone loss in a nonarthritic joint.
- Cylinders or "plugs" of healthy cartilage, with their associated tidemark and subchondral bone, are harvested from one location in the joint and press-fit into same-length recipient holes prepared in the lesion to restore bone contour and the articular surface.
- Multiple plugs may be tranferred to the same region, depending on the defect size.

ANATOMY

- Articular cartilage has a complex structure and plays a vital role in normal and athletic activity. It transmits loads uniformly across the joint and provides a smooth, low-friction, gliding surface.
- Articular cartilage is a smooth, viscoelastic, hypocellular structure with a low coefficient of friction (estimated to be 20% of the friction seen with ice on ice) and the ability to withstand significant recurring compressive loads.
- The articular surfaces of diarthroidal joints are covered with hyaline cartilage.
  - Hyaline cartilage is composed of sparsely distributed chondrocytes in a large extracellular matrix made of about 80% water and 20% collagen.
  - Collagen fibers provide form and tensile strength; water gives it substance.
  - Type II collagen accounts for 95% of the total collagen present. The cellular component (chondrocytes) synthesizes and degrades proteoglycans and is the metabolically active portion of this structure.
- Articular cartilage has four distinct zones: a superficial (tangential) zone; a middle (transitional) zone; a deep (radial) zone; and the calcified zone (**FIG 1**).
- The superficial zone collagen fibers are oriented parallel to the joint surface and resist both compressive and shear forces. This zone is the thinnest and sometimes is called the *gliding zone*.
  - The surface layer, known as the *lamina splendens*, is cell free, and consists mainly of randomly oriented flat bundles of fine collagen fibrils.
  - Under that layer are more densely packed collagen fibers interspersed with elongated, oval chondrocytes oriented parallel to the articular surface.
  - This superficial zone acts as a barrier, limiting the penetration of large molecules into the deeper zone and preventing the loss of molecules from the cartilage into the synovial fluid.
- The middle (transitional) zone collagen fibers are parallel to the plane of joint motion and resist compressive forces.
  - This zone has more proteoglycans and less water and collagen than the superficial zone.
  - The chondrocytes are more spherical with more cellular structures, suggesting a matrix synthesis function.
- The deep (radial) zone fibers are perpendicular to the surface and resist both compressive and shear forces.
  - The collagen bundles are arranged in a formation known as the *arcades of Benninghoff*, in which the round chondrocytes are arranged in columns perpendicular to the joint surface.
- The tidemark is located at the base of the deep zone and resists shear stress. It represents a zone of transition from the deep zone to the zone of calcified cartilage.
- The calcified zone acts as an anchor between the articular cartilage and the subchondral bone.
  - It is the deepest zone and is a thin layer of calcified cartilage creating a boundary with the underlying subchondral bone.
  - The cells in this zone usually are smaller and are surrounded by a cartilaginous matrix.

PATHOGENESIS

- Chondral damage can result from a variety of mechanisms, including a pivoting twisting fall, significant direct impacts on the knee, anterior cruciate ligament (ACL) tears, or a patellar dislocation (**FIG 2**).

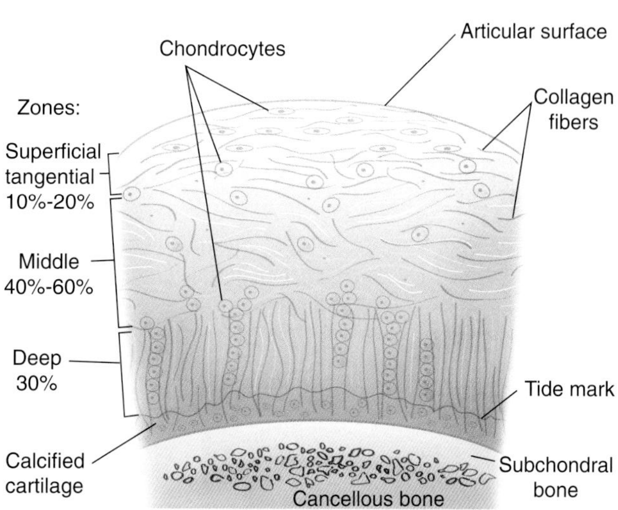

FIG 1 • Articular cartilage has four distinct zones: superficial (tangential); middle (transitional); deep (radial); and calcified. (Modified from Browne JE, Branch TP. Surgical alternative for treatment of articular cartilage lesions. J Am Acad Orthop Surg 2000;8:180–189.)

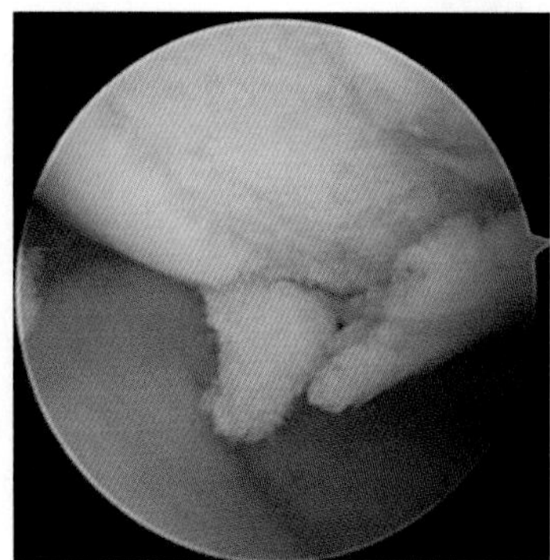

FIG 2 • Chondral damage can result from a variety of mechanisms, including a pivoting twisting fall or significant direct impacts on the knee.

- ACL injuries cause direct contusions to the articular surfaces and may lead to instability and localized, full-thickness articular cartilage defects.
- Osteochondritis dissecans involves the separation of subchondral bone and cartilage from surrounding healthy tissues.
  - It most commonly occurs in the lateral aspect of the medial femoral condyle.
- Traumatic osteochondral lesions include acute bone and cartilage loss due to fracture, crush, or shear injuries.
- Sometimes, even without a clearly remembered traumatic event, the patient develops pain with weight bearing.

NATURAL HISTORY

- Cartilage biopsy samples overlying bone bruises have shown degeneration, necrosis of the chondrocytes, and a loss of proteoglycan.
  - An experimental model suggests that a severe bone bruise and its associated chondral necrosis are precursors to degenerative changes.[20]
- Instability secondary to ACL loss has been shown to contribute to the onset of osteoarthritis after ACL tears.[21]
- Articular cartilage has limited regeneration potential.

PATIENT HISTORY AND PHYSICAL FINDINGS

- Various mechanisms of injury are associated with full-thickness articular cartilage lesions, inncluding pivoting twisting falls, direct impacts, and patellar instability.
- Full-thickness chondral lesions often are clinically silent and should be suspected in the setting of any traumatic hemarthrosis, especially with a ligament disruption.
- Reports of pain localized to one compartment, a persistent dull aching pain worsening after activity, and pain most noticeable when falling asleep are common.
  - Running, stair climbing, rising from a chair, and squatting may aggravate the symptoms, as does sitting for a prolonged period.
- Physical findings include joint line tenderness, effusion, crepitus, grinding, or catching.
- Effusion is nonspecific but suggests intra-articular pathology.
  - Pain on direct palpation of the femoral condyles may indicate cartilage damage.
- Decreased range of motion is nonspecific but often indicates pathology.
- The Lachman test detects ACL instability that may lead to cartilage injury.
- Malalignment of the tibia to the femur when standing may lead to abnormal chondral wear.
- A positive patellar apprehension test signals damage to the medial patellofemoral ligament.

IMAGING AND OTHER DIAGNOSTIC STUDIES

- A standard radiographic knee evaluation should be performed.
  - This includes standing anteroposterior (AP) views in full extension to identify angular changes and to compare joint space height.
  - A 45-degree flexion posteroanterior (PA) weight-bearing view may identify subtle joint space narrowing.
  - A non–weight-bearing lateral view obtained in 45-degree flexion in which the posterior femoral condyles overlap, an axial view of both patellae to help evaluate the patellar alignment, and an AP knee flexion view to outline the femoral intercondylar notch also should be obtained.
- Osteochondritis dissecans lesions most commonly are found in the lateral aspect of the medial femoral condyle (**FIG 3A**) and are best demonstrated on an AP knee flexion view.
- Long-leg hip-to-ankle films accurately determine varus or valgus alignment.
- Proper MRI protocols have high sensitivity and specificity.
  - MRI has evolved into a proven tool to evaluate chondral surfaces and detect full- and partial-thickness lesions that may be clinically silent (**FIG 3B,C**).

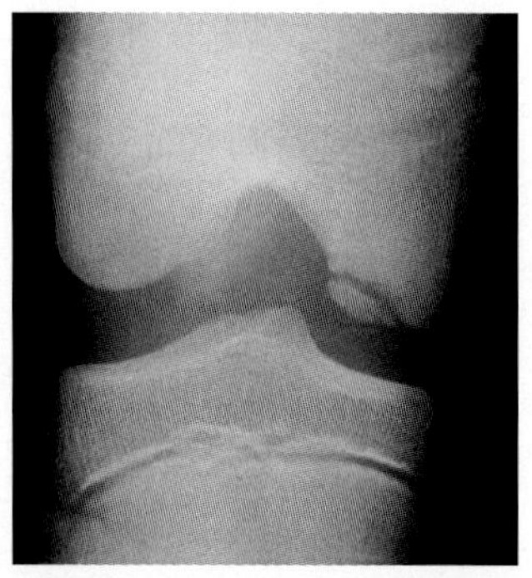

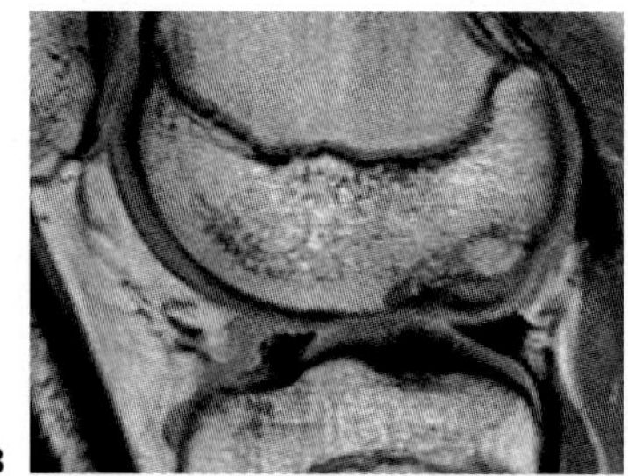

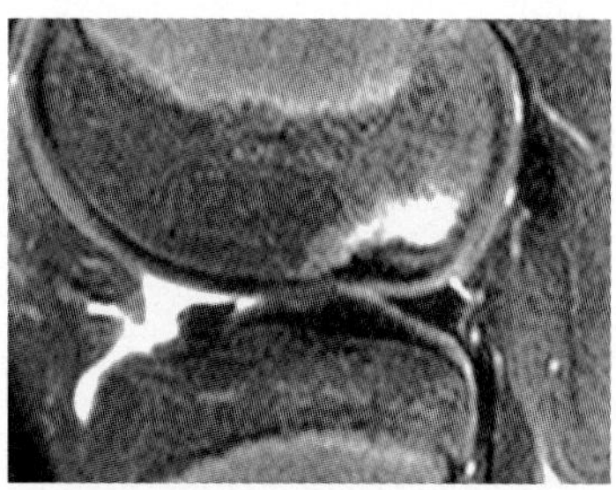

FIG 3 • **A.** Osteochondritis dissecans involves subchondral bone and cartilage separation from the adjacent condyle and is found most commonly in the lateral aspect of the medial femoral condyle. **B,C.** MRI evaluation can detect full- or partial-thickness articular lesions and osteochondritis dissecans that may be clinically silent.

- Clinically proven cartilage-sensitive sequences include T1-weighted gradient echo with fat suppression and fast spin-echo sequences with and without fat suppression.
- Many newer sequences offer promise but have not yet been validated.[22]

DIFFERENTIAL DIAGNOSIS

- Partial- or full-thickness cartilage lesion
- Osteonecrosis
- Osteochondritis dissecans
- Meniscal tear
- Ligament injuries

NONOPERATIVE MANAGEMENT

- Nonoperative treatment for full-thickness, discrete chondral lesions consists of physical therapy, anti-inflamatory medication, and activity modification to avoid high-impact or patella-destabilizing activities.
- Bracing options include patellar stabilizing braces for patellofemoral instability and load-shifting braces that unload the injured compartment.
  - Unloading the compartment also can be accomplished by shoe inserts that provide an appropriate heel and sole wedge.
  - These efforts are more effective for medial femoral condyle lesions than lateral ones.
- It is important to ensure that the patient understands that full-thickness lesions have little spontaneous healing capacity and that further degeneration is likely.

SURGICAL MANAGEMENT

- The indications for osteochondral autograft transplantation include discrete, isolated, full-thickness articular cartilage lesions between 1.0 and 2.5 cm in diameter (**FIG 4**).
  - Acceptable results with larger defects have been reported, but not consistently.
- If the depth of subchondral bone loss exceeds 6 mm, it will be necessary to adjust the harvested graft accordingly.
- Contraindications include opposing full-thickness articular cartilage damage ("kissing" lesions), multiple-compartment full-thickness lesions, significant angular changes, history of joint infection, intra-articular fracture, and rheumatoid arthritis.
- This technique is most commonly performed on the femoral condyle; however, osteochondral autograft transplantation of the trochlea, patella, tibial plateau, humerus, and talus has been reported.
- The COR osteochondral repair system (Depuy Mitek, Raynham, MA) allows for the harvesting of a precisely sized osteochondral plug and transplantation into a precisely drilled defect. The technique illustrated here uses this system.
  - Other systems have been developed, including the osteochondral autologous transfer system (OATS; Arthrex, Naples, FL), and MosaicPlasty (Smith & Nephew Endoscopy, Andover, MA).

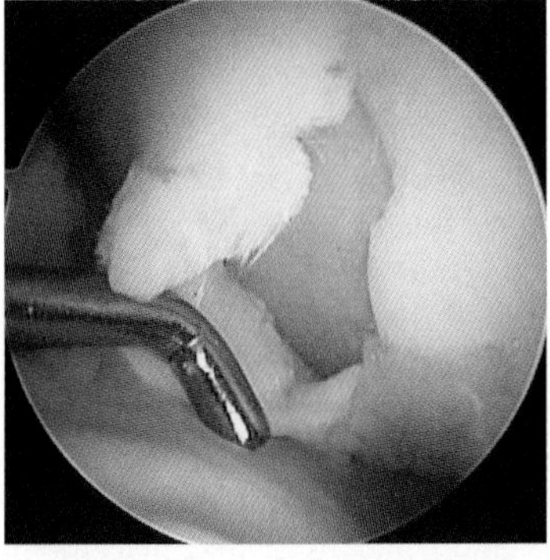

FIG 4 • The indications for osteochondral autograft transplantation include discrete, isolated, full-thickness articular cartilage lesions between 1.0 and 2.5 cm in diameter.

Preoperative Planning

- The success of this procedure depends upon maintaining viable chondrocytes. Confocal microscopy studies demonstrate that greater pressure on the articular cartilage cells leads to cell death. Several technical issues are related to greater transplanted cell death. These include high impact pressure during insertion, proud grafts which are not advanced to the level of the adjacent native articular cartilage, and sunken grafts depressed 2 mm or more compared to the adjacent articular cartilage.
- The ideal technique optimizes graft position and stability, provides for consistent graft length harvesting, and minimizes the forces required to insert the grafts.
- Multiple procedures can be performed at the same time, including meniscal repair and ligament reconstruction.
  - Improved results occur with concomitant ACL reconstruction.[18]
  - Any ligament instability or malalignment should be corrected at the time of autografting to avoid increased failure rates.
- All radiographs and MRI images should be reviewed before surgery to confirm whether the lesion can be treated arthroscopically or whether an arthrotomy is needed.
- Perpendicular placement of the harvester and drill to the articular surface is required.
- The COR transfer system has a unique "perpendicularity" guide which enhances the perpendicular harvest of the donor graft as well as the perpendicular orientation of the drilled recipient site.
- Any allograft or synthetic materials that may be needed should be available in the operating room.
  - Although allograft tissue avoids concerns about harvest site morbidity, it is offset by the risks of transmitted disease and decreased chondrocyte viability[17] as well as significant costs.

Positioning

- Osteochondral autograft transfer in the knee is performed with the patient supine and the operative knee in an arthroscopic leg holder flexed off the table.
  - It is crucial to confirm that the knee can be flexed adequately to access the lesion before operative preparation and draping.
- The contralateral leg should be well padded and positioned out of the operative field.
- It may be necessary to drape the operative leg free of a leg holder to obtain enough knee flexion to access the lesion.

Approach

- Arthroscopic osteochondral autograft transplantation can be techinically difficult, because of the need to achieve perpendicular access to the articular cartilage and adequate knee flexion.

- The use of the intercondylar notch as a donor site allows for ready arthroscopic access and avoids the need for an arthrotomy such as is required when obtaining grafts from either the superior medial or lateral femoral condyles above the linea terminalis.
- A thorough arthroscopic diagnostic knee evaluation should be performed first.
- An arthrotomy can be performed for lesions that cannot be addressed adequately arthroscopically. A spinal needle can be used to determine the best angle for portal creation, ensuring a perpendicular approach to the harvest and defect sites.
- Arthroscopic osteochondral autografting includes five steps: lesion evaluation and preparation, determination of the number of grafts needed, defect preparation, graft harvest, and graft delivery.
- The other plug transfer systems have technique differences including the order in which the donor plugs are harvested and the relative length of the donor plug to the recipient hole.
- The Mosaicplasty system required overdrilling of the recipient site by 2 mm creating room for debris and allowing the graft to "float" into place. The donor plug is harvested first before creating the recipient hole to avoid donor-recipient site mismatch.
- The OATS system requires underdrilling of the recipient sites by 2 mm and requires a final "impaction" designed to improve graft stability but at the same time placing additional impact pressure on the graft articular cartilage. Here too the donor plug is harvested first before creating the recipient hole to avoid donor-recipient site mismatch.

TECHNIQUES

DIAGNOSTIC ARTHROSCOPY

- During the diagnostic evaluation, a complete examination must be performed to rule out other pathology and confirm that no contraindications to the procedure exist.
- It is necessary to look in the posterior recesses and underneath the menisci for chondral pieces.
- Concomitant ligament surgery should be addressed after the transplantation.
- An adequate synovectomy, especially of the fat pad, is needed to facilitate complete visualization of both the defect and harvest sites.
- A spinal needle should be used to identify the correct portal placement for a perpendicular approach.

LESION EVALUATION AND PREPARATION

- A 16-gauge needle can be used to plan the best (perpendicular) approach to both the defect and donor sites.
- The defect is prepared by removing loose debris and freshening the edges with a curette or an arthroscopic knife to create perpendicular chondral walls (**TECH FIG 1**).
- The subchondral bone should be cleared of any residual articular cartilage, but generalized bone bleeding should be avoided.

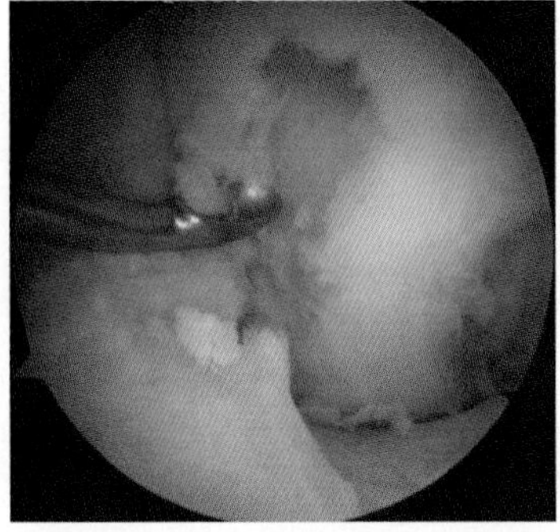

TECH FIG 1 • The defect is prepared by removing loose debris and freshening the edges with a curette or an arthroscopic knife to create perpendicular chondral walls.

DETERMINING NUMBER OF GRAFTS

- The number of grafts required is planned using the probe to obtain a preliminary measurement of the defect's shape and dimensions (**TECH FIG 2A**).
- When using more than 1 graft, a 2–3-mm bone bridge should be maintained between the recipient sites to ensure a good press fit.
- The depth of the lesion should be estimated using the 2-mm marks on the harvester.
  - A series of grafts 6 mm in diameter fills the defect best.
- Larger-plug harvesters are available but may require an arthrotomy and are more likely to encroach on weight-bearing areas at harvest sites.
  - Specifically, given that a 10-mm diameter lesion is an indication for grafting, harvesting a 10-mm graft defeats the purpose of using this grafting technique.
  - The plan should be to place the grafts starting at the periphery of the defect so that the articular cartilage matches the adjacent chondral edge after transplantation (**TECH FIG 2B**).
- The depth of the defect also should be analyzed.
  - In most cases, the standard 10½–12-mm harvester depth is sufficient to fill the defect.
  - Osteochondritis dissecans lesions or those with significant bone loss may require the use of the variable depth harvester and placement of grafts that have cancellous sections standing above the crater base.

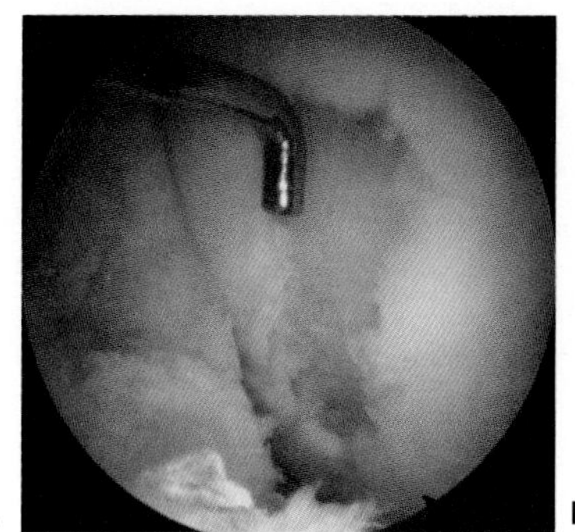

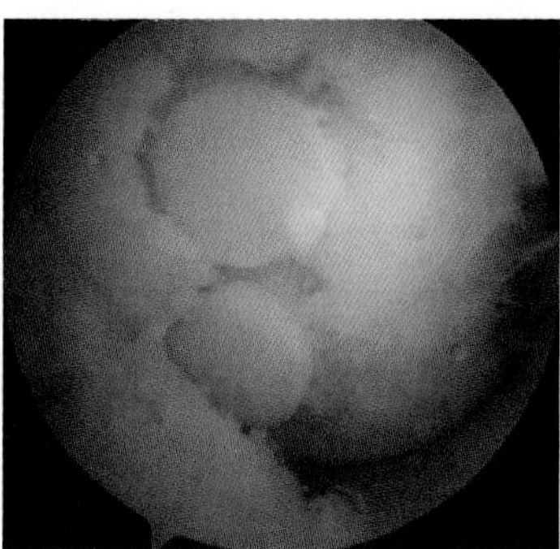

TECH FIG 2 • **A.** The number of grafts required is planned using the probe to obtain a preliminary measurerment of the defect shape and dimensions. **B.** Plugs of healthy cartilage and subchondral bone are harvested from one location and press-fit into the defect, restoring the articular surface. (**B:** Reprinted with permission from Barber FA. Chondral injuries in the knee. In: Johnson DH, Pedowitz RA, eds. Practical Orthopaedic Sports Medicine and Arthroscopy. Philadelphia: Lippincott Williams & Wilkins, 2007:752.)

DEFECT PREPARATION

- Any residual articular cartilage is removed from the subchondral bone, but generalized bone bleeding should be avoided.
- Drilling the recipient site before harvesting the donor autograft plugs allows the selection of the best match on the femoral surface between the donor grafts and the articular cartilage adjacent to the recipient sites.
- Using the COR perpendicularity system reproducibly identifies the best orientation for drilling the recipient site and makes it feasible to drill the recipient site before harvesting the grafts.
- Insert the drill guide with the perpendicularity rod through the portal and into position at the recipient site. With the drill guide positioned in a perpendicular orientation, turn the perpendicularity rod counterclockwise until it disengages and remove the rod.
- The recipient sites in the defect are drilled with the corresponding size COR drill bit under direct arthroscopic visualization, keeping the drill perpendicular to the articular surface.
  - The projecting tooth at the drill tip keeps the drill from "walking" and allows for precise recipient site placement by creating a starter hole (TECH FIG 3).
- The drill is advanced to the appropriate depth using the markings of 5 mm, 8 mm, 10 mm, 12 mm, 15 mm, and 20 mm found on the side of the drill. This line is compared to the adjacent articular cartilage. The fluted drill's concave sides remove bone during drilling and reduce both friction and heat.
- In cases of subchondral bone loss, the depth should be used and the depth underdrilled to restore the contour and height of the articular surface.
  - This is accomplished by aligning the laser mark with the desired articular cartilage height.
- The recipient holes can be drilled at the same time or sequentially after autograft insertion.
- Care should be taken to maintain a bone bridge between recipient sites of 2 to 3 mm and to avoid recipient site convergence.

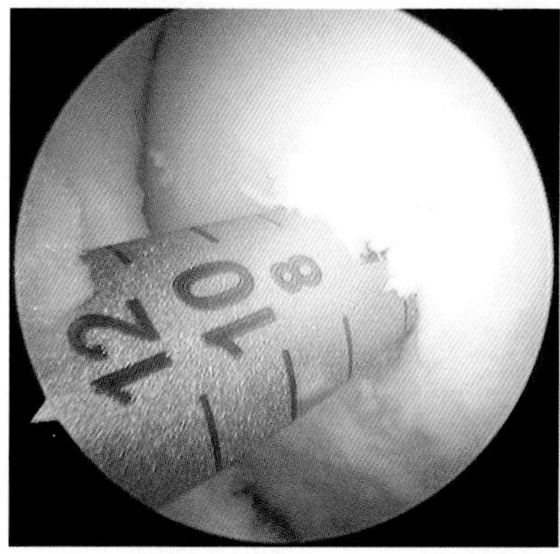

TECH FIG 3 • The recipient sites in the defect are drilled with the corresponding size COR (DePuy Mitek, Inc, Raynham, MA) drill bit under direct arthroscopic visualization, keeping the drill perpendicular to the articular surface.

GRAFT HARVEST

- Potential harvest sites include the lateral and medial trochlea above the linea terminalis and the intercondylar notch.
  - In general, contact pressures are lower in the intercondylar notch and medial trochlea, but available harvest material is limited.[1]
  - Higher contact pressures are found in the lateral trochlea, but these decrease more posteriorly.
  - Harvesting 5-mm plugs from the lateral trochlea did not result in significant increases in stress concentration and loading in one study.[7]
  - We prefer to harvest from the superior and lateral intercondylar notch, because it commonly is obliterated in ACL reconstruction without subsequent morbidity and allows for an entirely arthroscopic procedure (TECH FIG 4A).

- Once the number of plugs to be obtained is determined and the sites prepared, the harvester is inserted into the disposable cutter.
- The retropatellar fat pad is completely débrided to improve visualization and avoid soft tissue entrapment.
- The COR Harvester Delivery Guide comes with the cutting tool pre-assembled as a single unit. The perpendicularity rod should be inserted into this Harvester/Cutter assembly before insertion into the joint. The perpendicularity rod will function as an obturator and minimize both soft tissue capture and fluid loss as the assembly is inserted into the knee.
- The Harvester Delivery Guide/Cutter/perpendicularity rod assembly is positioned on the donor site in preparation for the graft harvest. The perpendicularity rod is used to confirm the perpendicular position of the cutter and then removed.
- The arthroscope is rotated to confirm this alignment from several angles.
  - Perpendicular grafts can be obtained readily with both arthroscopic and open approaches.[4]
- Using a mallet and continuing to hold the harvester perpendicular to the articular cartilage in all planes, use a mallet to tap the Harvester Delivery Guide/Cutter to the desired depth based upon the 5-mm, 8-mm, 10-mm, 12-mm, 15-mm, and 20-mm markings on the side of the harvester (**TECH FIG 4B**).
  - A unique feature of the COR system is the cutter tooth on the harvester which underscores the cancellous bone at the distal end of the harvester tube allowing for a precise and consistent depth cut (**TECH FIG 4C**).
  - The T-handle of the harvester is rotated clockwise at least two full rotations, undercutting the distal bone and creating a precise harvest depth.
- The plug is removed by gently twisting the T-handle while withdrawing the plug. Care should be taken to avoid toggling the donor hole.
- On a firm surface, insert the Harvester Delivery Guide/Cutter into the graft loader and push down firmly until it makes contact with the bottom of the loader. The harvested graft will be pushed from the cancellous bone side

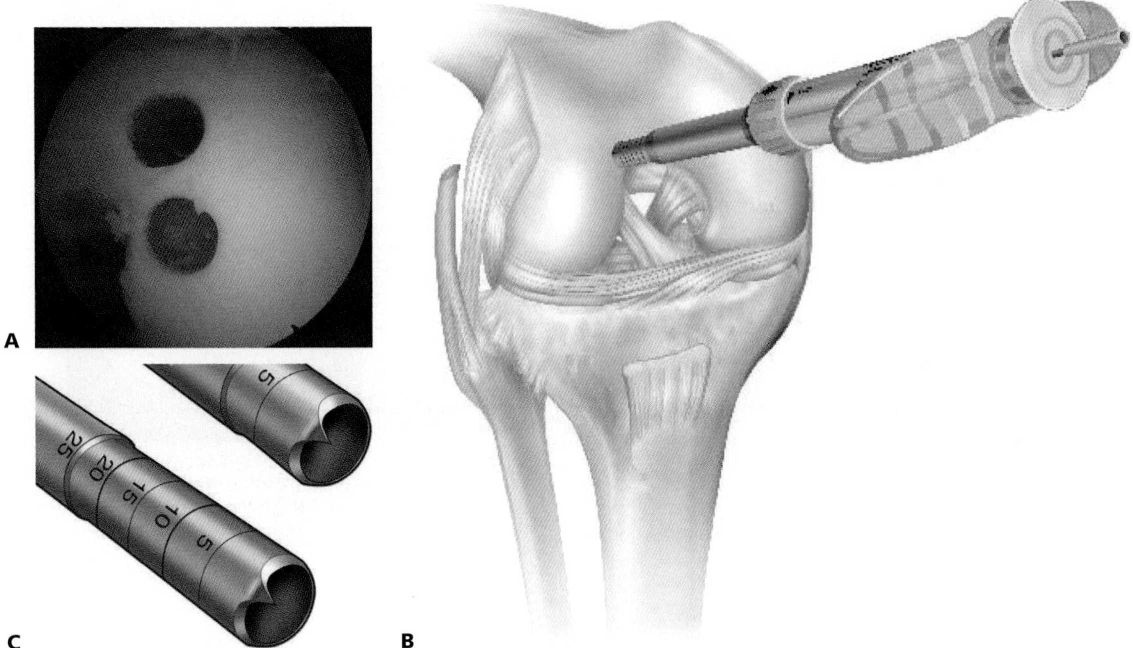

TECH FIG 4 • A. Harvest sites include the superior and lateral intercondylar notch, an area that is commonly removed in anterior cruciate ligament reconstruction notchplasty. **B.** Position the Harvester/Delivery Guide/Cutter with the perpendicularity guide on the selected donor site. After verifying the perpendicularity, remove the guide and then tap the harvester until the desired laser line depth has been reached. **C.** A unique feature of the COR system is the cutting tooth which underscores the cancellous bone at the distal end of the harvester tube and allows for a precise depth cut. (**B,C:** Courtesy of Depuy Mitek, Inc, Raynham, MA.)

of the graft plug upwards into the Harvester/Delivery Guide and out of the cutter section (TECH FIG 5). A loud noise usually accompanies this transfer.

- The harvester is removed from the cutter. The graft plug remains inside the harvester until it is transplanted.
- This transfer system eliminates any loads to the articular surface of the graft and eliminates the danger of chondrocyte damage in this step.

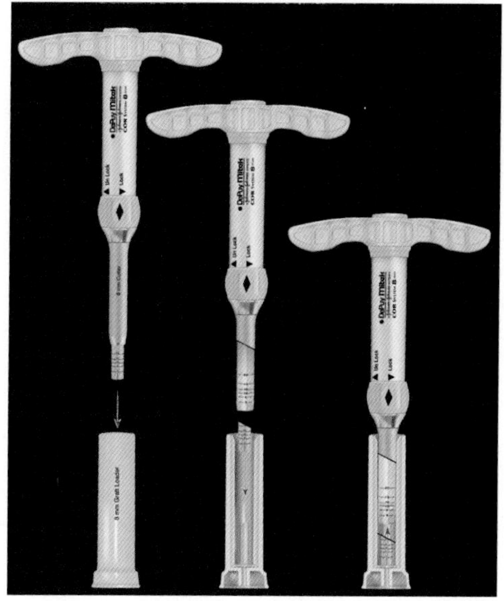

TECH FIG 5 • On a firm surface, insert the Harvester Delivery Guide/Cutter into the graft loader and push down firmly until it makes contact with the bottom of the loader. The harvested graft will be pushed from the cancellous bone side of the graft plug upwards into the Harvester/Delivery Guide and out of the cutter section.

GRAFT INSERTION

- Once the harvester tube is disassembled from the cutter, it is placed in the clear plastic insertion tube with depth markings.
- The plastic plunger is placed in the harvester delivery system before insertion of the delivery system into the joint.
- The loaded harvester–clear plastic delivery guide system is then inserted into the knee. It may be necessary to enlarge the portal slightly to permit this passage.
- The clear end of the delivery system, with the graft tip slightly projecting, is held perpendicularly at the recipient site outlet, and, aligning the articular cartilage of the autograft with the adjacent articular cartilage, implanted with gentle tapping until it is flush with the articular cartilage (TECH FIG 6).
  - The Universal tamp may be used to fine-tune the graft placement.
  - The 8 mm side is recommended for 4 mm and 6 mm grafts and the 12 mm side is recommended for 8 mm and 10 mm grafts.

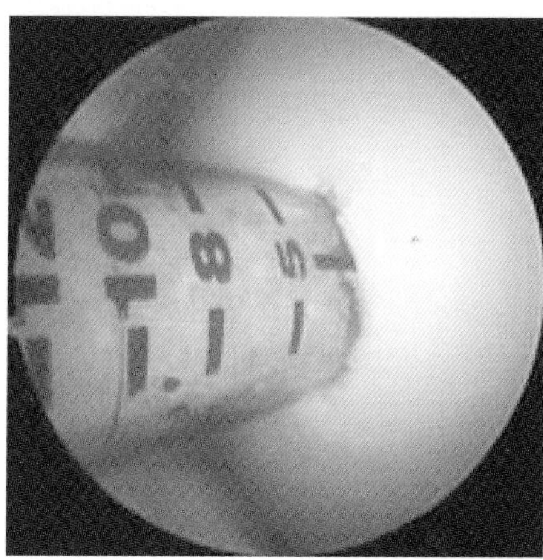

TECH FIG 6 • The loaded harvester–clear plastic delivery guide system is held perpendicular to the articular cartilage and implanted with gentle tapping.

MULTIPLE GRAFT REPAIR

If more than one graft is needed to repair an articular cartilage defect, the Harvester/Delivery Guide and Cutter is reassembled and the process repeated until the defect is completely filled. A 2-mm to 3-mm bone bridge should be maintained between the drilled holes to allow for a secure graft press fit.

TECHNIQUES

BACKFILLING

- Filling the donor sites is recommended, especially for harvested plugs greater than 6 mm in diameter or if multiple plugs have been harvested from a single area.
  - Large-diameter and deep defects can cause excessive stress on the surrounding cartilage and lead to degeneration.[13]
- Allograft or commercially available biodegradable material can be used as backfill material plugs (TECH FIG 7).

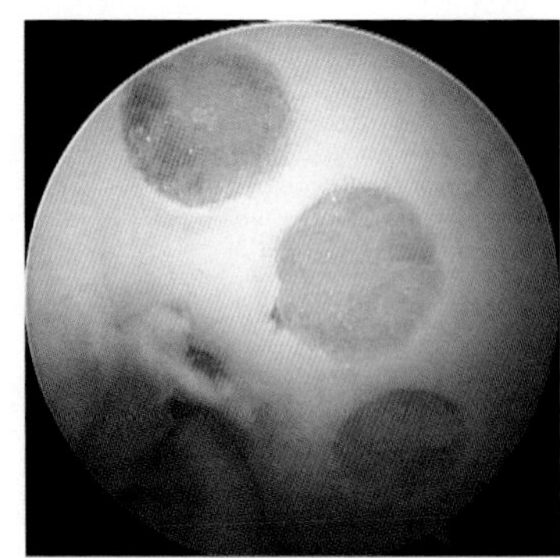

TECH FIG 7 • Grafting (back-filling) the donor sites is recommended, especially for harvested plugs greater than 6 mm in diameter or if multiple plugs are harvested from a single area.

PEARLS AND PITFALLS

Indications	■ Associated instability and malalignment must be addressed. ■ Proper patient selection is the key to good results.
Lesion preparation	■ Maintain perpendicular orientation of the walls during recipient site preparation to avoid loose plugs. ■ Ensure that the recipient site is an appropriate depth to avoid leaving a "proud" plug.
Graft harvesting Implantation	■ Make sure the harvester is rotated and not toggled when removing plugs. ■ Plugs should not be left proud under any circumstances. In circumstances where a plug is "angled" with reference to the surrounding cartilage, the plug should be sunk so that the upper edge of the graft is flush with the surrounding surfaces.[15] ■ Minimize the force used during graft transfer and insert to decrease articular cartilage cell depth.
Graft–recipient site mismatch	■ If the graft diameter is too large, the recipient site may be "upsized" to the proper width. ■ If the graft is too small or unstable, an adjacent 4-mm tunnel may be prepared to wedge in the original graft.
"Proud" graft	■ If the graft is more than 0.5-mm proud, gentle attempts to make it flush should be undertaken. Removing and replacing a graft greatly diminishes graft stability.[5] If the graft is markedly proud and cannot be salvaged, consider replacing with another graft or allograft.[16]

POSTOPERATIVE CARE

- Immediate range-of-motion exercises without a brace are begun.
- Non–weight bearing is observed for 3 weeks, followed by progressive weight bearing during weeks 3 to 6 after surgery and then full weight bearing beginning at 6 weeks after surgery.
- A progressive quadriceps strengthening program is then started.
- Full athletic activity is permitted at 4 months.

OUTCOMES

- Condylar lesions typically have excellent clnical results.
  - Multiple authors report excellent and good results ranging from 78% to 96% at a minimum of 2 years follow-up.[2,6,8,18,19]
- Patellar or patellar and trochlear mosaicplasties have been reported to have good to excellent results in 79% of patients.[9,23]
  - Allograft has been shown to be an effective treatment for patellofemoral disease.[14,23]
- Comparisons of osteochondral transplantation with microfracture, Pridie drilling, and abrasion arthroplasty have shown better results with osteochondral transplantation.[6,10]
- Osteochondral transplantation consistently results in restoration of hyaline cartilage versus "hyaline-like" or fibrocartilage.[2,3,6,12]
- Patients younger than 40 years of age have better results.[6,11,18]

COMPLICATIONS

- Infection
- Loose body if graft loosens
- Graft reabsorption
- Cartilage degeneration due to excessive pressure when seating the graft
- Proud graft leading to excessive contact pressures, graft destruction, and possible "catching" sensation.

REFERENCES

1. Ahmad CS, Cohen ZA, Levine WN, et al. Biomechanical and topographic considerations for autologous osteochondral grafting in the knee. Am J Sports Med 2001;29:201–206.
2. Barber FA, Chow JC. Arthroscopic chondral osseous autograft transplantation (COR procedure) for femoral defects. Arthroscopy 2006;22:10–16.
3. Barber FA, Chow JC. Arthroscopic osteochondral transplantation: histologic results. Arthroscopy 2001;17:832–835.

4. Diduch DR, Chhabra A, Blessey P, et al. Osteochondral autograft plug transfer: achieving perpendicularity. J Knee Surg 2003;16:17–20.
5. Duchow J, Hess T, Kohn D. Primary stability of press-fit-implanted osteochondral grafts. Influence of graft size, repeated insertion, and harvesting technique. Am J Sports Med 2000;28:24–27.
6. Gudas R, Kalesinskas RJ, Kimtys V, et al. A prospective randomized clinical study of mosaic osteochondral autologous transplantation versus microfracture for the treatment of chteochondral defects in the knee joint in young athletes. Arthroscopy 2005; 21:1066–1075.
7. Guettler JH, Demetropoulos CK, Yang KH, Jurist KA. Dynamic evaluation of contact pressure and the effects of graft harvest with subsequent lateral release at osteochondral donor sites in the knee. Arthroscopy 2005;21:715–720.
8. Hangody L, Fules P. Autologous osteochondral mosaicplasty for the treatment of full-thickness defects of weight-bearing joints: ten years of experimental and clinical experience. J Bone Joint Surg Am 2003; 85(Suppl 2):25–32.
9. Hangody L, Rathonyi GK, Duska Z, et al. Autologous osteochondral mosaicplasty. Surgical technique. J Bone Joint Surg Am 2004; 86A(Suppl 1):65–72.
10. Hangody L, Kish G, Karpati Z, et al. Mosaicplasty for the treatment of articular cartilage defects: application in clinical practice. Orthopedics 1998;21:751–756.
11. Hangody L, Kish G, Kárpáti Z. Arthroscopic autogenous osteochondral mosaicplasty—a multicentric, comparative, prospective study. Index Traumat Sport 1998;5:3–9.
12. Horas U, Pelinkovic D, Herr G, et al. Autologous chondrocyte implantation and osteochondral cylinder transplantation in cartilage repair of the knee joint. A prospective, comparative trial. J Bone Joint Surg Am 2003;85A:185–192.
13. Jackson DW, Lalor PA, Aberman HM, et al. Spontaneous repair of full-thickness defects of articular cartilage in a goat model. A preliminary study. J Bone Joint Surg Am 2001;83A:53–64.
14. Jamali AA, Emmerson BC, Chung C, et al. Fresh osteochondral allografts. Clin Orthop Rel Res 2005;437:176–185.
15. Koh JL, Kowalski A, Lautenschlager E. The effect of angled osteochondral grafting on contact pressure: a biomechanical study. Am J Sports Med 2006;34:116–119.
16. Koh JL, Wirsing K, Lautenschlager E, et al. The effect of graft height mismatch on contact pressure following osteochondral grafting: a biomechanical study. Am J Sports Med 2004;32:317–320.
17. Malinin T, Temple T, Buck BE. Transplantation of osteochondral allografts after cold storage. J Bone Joint Surg Am 2006;88A: 762–770.
18. Marcacci M, Kon E, Zaffagnini S, et al. Multiple osteochondral arthroscopic (mosaicplasty) for cartilage defects of the knee: prospective study results at 2-year follow-up. Arthroscopy 2005;21: 462–470.
19. Matsusue Y, Kotake T, Nakagawa Y, et al. Arthroscopic osteochondral autograft transplantation for chondral lesion of the tibial plateau of the knee. Arthroscopy 2001;17:653–659.
20. Nakamae A, Engebretsen L, Bahr R, et al. Natural history of bone bruises after acute knee injury: clinical outcome and histopathological findings. Knee Surg Sports Traumatol Arthrosc 2006;14:1252–1258. Epub 2006 Jun 20.
21. Nelson F, Billinghurst RC, Pidoux I, et al. Early post-traumatic osteoarthritis-like changes in human articular cartilage following rupture of the anterior cruciate ligament. Osteoarthritis Cartilage 2006;14:114–119.
22. Potter HG, Foo LF. Magnetic resonance imaging of articular cartilage: trauma, degeneration and repair. Am J Sports Med 2006;34: 661–677.
23. Torga Spak R, Teitge RA. Fresh osteochondral allografts for patellofemoral arthritis: long term follow-up. Clin Orthop Rel Research 2006;444:193–200.

Chapter 38 Autogenous Cartilage Implantation

Sean M. Jones-Quaidoo and Eric W. Carson

DEFINITION

- Articular cartilage of joints such as the knee is essential to the joint's normal function, in which it acts as a load-bearing structure and provides a nearly friction-free surface. Unfortunately, articular cartilage is particularly suspectible to traumatic injury or pathologic conditions such as osteochondritis dissecans, which can, over time, be significantly disabling in the young athlete and have the potential of degenerating over time.
  - The natural history of articular cartilage injuries currently is poorly understood.
  - The treatment of focal chondral lesions remains a significant challenge for the sports medicine orthopedic surgeon.
- A retrospective review of 31,516 knee arthroscopies examined the prevalence of chondral injuries. This review reported 41% Outerbridge III chondral injuries and 19.2% Outerbridge IV chondral injuries, with an estimated 3% to 4% isolated chondral lesions that were larger than 2 cm^2.[13]
  - The orthopedic surgeon is armed with a variety of surgical treatments for pathologic problems in articular cartilage. Numerous surgical techniques have been proposed to address this difficult and often disabling condition in a young patient population.
- Current articular cartilage resurfacing procedures can be divided into three categories:
  - Bone marrow stimulation
  - Implantation of autologous articular cartilage
  - Transplantation of osteochondral allograft
- The clinical results of all of these surgical procedures have generally good short- and long-term clinical results.[2–5,14,19] All have specific drawbacks: for example, marrow stimulation produces fibrocartilage; the autogenous osteochondral autograft transfer system (OATS) has an issue with donor site morbidity; and allograft OATS has a significant risk of disease transmission along with a possible immune response to the allograft tissue.
- In 1994, Brittberg et al[7] proposed an innovative surgical treatment for articular cartilage injuries, autologous cartilage implantation (ACI).
- ACI is performed in two stages.
  - The initial procedure is a comprehensive arthroscopic evaluation of the articular cartilage defect covering size, location, and depth of lesion (**FIG 1**).
  - At the same time, if the surgical indications are favorable, the orthopedic surgeon can harvest autologous articular cartilage cells. These articular cartilage cells are then digested enzymatically, with the ultimate isolation of mature chondrocytes.
  - The second stage involves implantation of these autologous chondrocyte cells into the defect through a small knee arthrotomy with a periosteal graft sutured over the defect. The cultured chondrocytes are then injected into the defect beneath the periosteal graft.
- This once-experimental procedure, initially directed toward articular cartilage and used for broad-based indications, has become an important procedure for a specific subset of patients. More than 5000 ACI procedures have been performed in the United States by more than 600 orthopedic surgeons.
- Second-look arthroscopy and biopsy of surgically implanted chondrocytes have documented a reconstitution of the articular surface with similar mechanical properties to the surrounding "hyaline-like articular cartilage," with documented durability of clinical results.

ANATOMY

- Articular cartilage consists of four distinct histologic zones: superficial, middle, deep, and calcified (**FIG 2A**).
- The chondrocyte is the cell responsible for the growth of cartilage.
- The metabolic balance of the protein macromolecular complex of articular cartilage is maintained by chondrocytes, which constitute about 5% of the weight of cartilage.
- Water makes up about 75% of the weight of articular cartilage. Water's role as a cation makes it one of the most important elements.
- Glycosaminoglycans provide the compressive strength of articular cartilage and account for about 10% of cartilage weight. These function to trap and hold water with the articular cartilage.
- Collagen, predominantly type II, provides the form and tensile strength of articular cartilage. It makes up about 10% of the weight of cartilage.

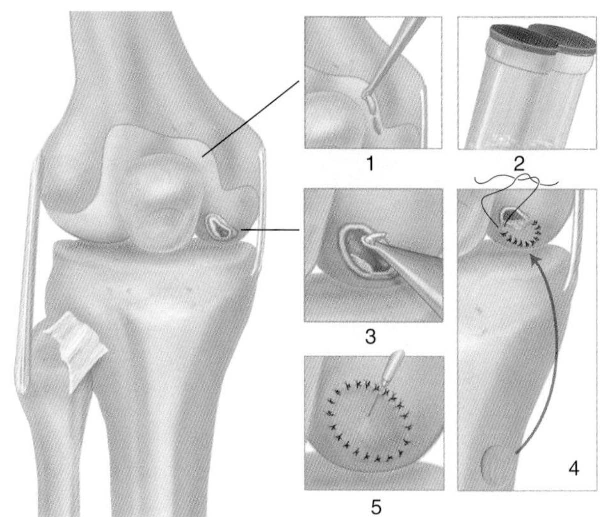

FIG 1 • Overview of the autogenous cartilage implantation (ACI) technique. Step 1: articular cells are harvested. Step 2: cells are grown in culture for 4 to 6 weeks. Step 3: the lesion is débrided. Step 4: harvested periosteum is sutured onto the defect. Step 5: cultured chondrocyte cells are implanted.

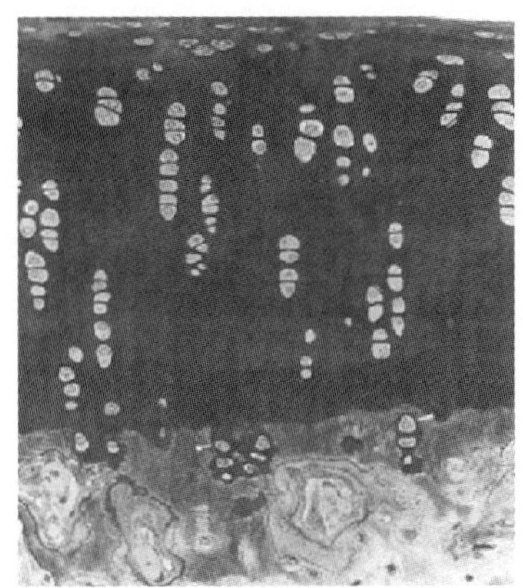

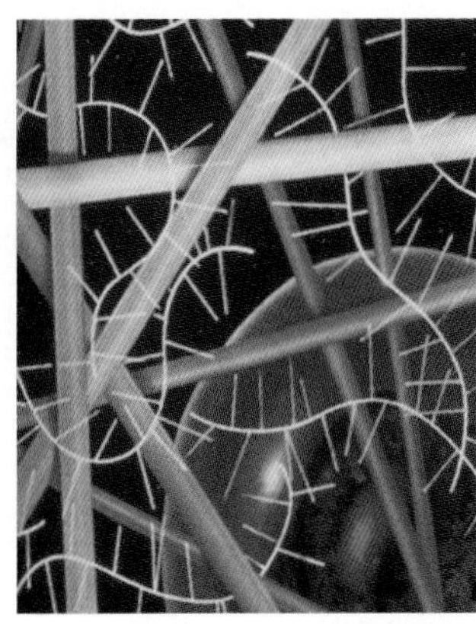

FIG 2 • **A.** Histology of articular cartilage. **B.** Chondrocyte and matrix with labels.

- The chondrocyte is the major producer of collagen, proteoglycans, and noncollagenous proteoglycans, as well as enzymes (**FIG 2B**).
- Articular cartilage receives its nutritional supply from the synovial fluid in which it is bathed; it does not have a true blood supply.[9]

PATHOGENESIS

- Injuries of the articular cartilage can result from either trauma, as in the case of a partial- or full-thickness chondral or osteochondral injury, or a pathologic process such as osteochondritis dissecans or local osteonecrosis.
- Shallow or partial articular cartilage lesions have limited ability to heal, related primarily to the lack of a blood supply.
  - An inflammatory response cannot occur, leading to a defect within the articular cartilage.[11]
- In full-thickness chondral lesions, in contrast, there is penetration of the subchondral plate, leading to the migration of progenitor cells from the vasculature in the subchondral bone marrow meschencymal cells to the surface, an inflammatory response, and an attempted healing response.
  - The mescenchymal progenitor cells differentiate into fibrocartilage.
  - This tissue is a weak substitute for hyaline articular cartilage and lacks its resilient mechanical properties.[11,20]

NATURAL HISTORY

- The natural history of articular cartilage injury is poorly understood. It is well recognized, however, that the human body has a limited capacity—or no capacity—to repair articular cartilage injuries.[11,20]
- Limited studies have demostrated progressive and variable degenerative changes equivalent to those of osteoarthritis.
- The repair tissue often succumbs to mechanical stresses with premature degeneration, delamination, interarticular osteophyte formation, and eventual breakdown and joint destruction over time.
- Some limited studies have been published with long-term follow-up of untreated osteochondritis dissecans that progressed on to osteoarthritis in adulthood.[13]

PATIENT HISTORY AND PHYSICAL FINDINGS

- Articular cartilage injury can present after a trauma sustained during an athletic event or as a slow progression of symptoms, as in osteochondritis dissecans.
  - Patients may present with what intially is believed to be meniscal pathology, with swelling, pain, palpable tenderness, and locking of the knee.
- Articular cartilage chondral flap or more significant osteochondral injury must be part of the differential diagnosis in evaluating the young patient with knee pain.
- Those patients with a more insidious onset and no trauma tend to fit more into the category of osteochondritis dissecans. The findings are more consistent with chronic or recurrent effusion, pain, and mechanical symptoms similar to those of meniscus pathology.

IMAGING AND OTHER DIAGNOSTIC STUDIES

- The following plain radiographs are obtained in weight-bearing knee flexion: anteroposterior view; notch view; sunrise view of the patella and trochlea; and lateral views (**FIG 3A,B**). Although the articular cartilage itself cannot be appreciated, joint space narrowing and other bony defects will be apparent.
  - Full-length lower-extremity radiographs are indicated for most patients to assess overall alignment and in consideration of the possibility of performing a realignment procedure concomitantly at the time of the ACI procedure in those patients with malalignment problems.
- MRI can more clearly demonstrate articular lesions. As the technology advances, better imaging quality is becoming available.
  - MRI can assess the size of the lesion, location, involvement of subchondral bone, and number of lesions (**FIG 3C**).
  - After ACI, MRI also is being used to assess the degree of defect fill, the integration of the repair cartilage to the subchondral bone plate, and the status of the subchondral bone plate and bone marrow.
  - Recently, the development of MRI cartilage sequencing has better defined articular cartilage injuries and postoperative osteochondral fill.
  - T2-weighted MRI mapping techniques give remarkable detail at the proteoglycan level (**FIG 3D,E**).
  - Optical coherence tomography (OCT)[12] involves cross-sectional imaging technology using near-infrared light technology. The high-resolution images provide a noninvasive look at the microstructural level of articular cartilage.

DIFFERENTIAL DIAGNOSIS

- Osteoarthritis
- Osteochondritis dissecans

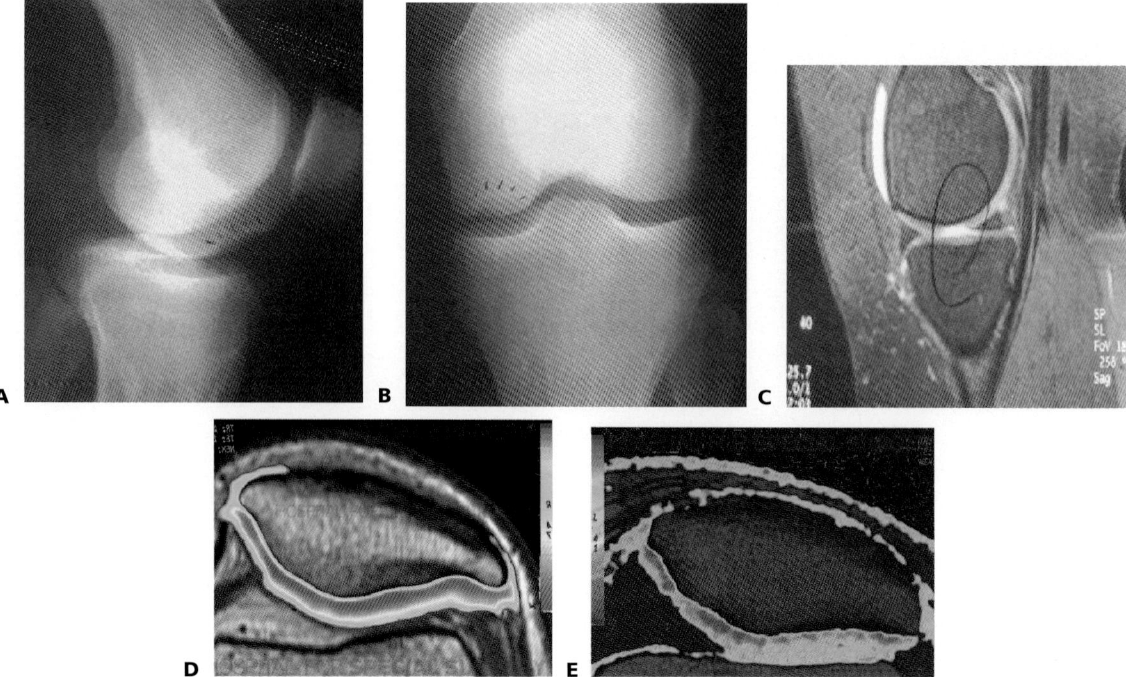

FIG 3 • Lateral (**A**) and AP (**B**) radiographs of osteochondritis dissecans. **C.** MRI of articular cartilage lesion (*circled*) of the medial femoral condyle. **D,E.** T2-weighted MRI mapping of articular cartilage, showing normal articular cartilage and degenerated articular cartilage. (**D,E**: Courtesy of Hollis Potter and Riley Williams, Hospital for Special Surgery, New York, NY.)

- Osteonecrosis
- Meniscus injury
- Loose body
- Chondral flap
- Osteochondral injury

NONOPERATIVE MANAGEMENT

- Nonoperative treament is controversial. Patients without symptoms can be treated nonoperatively, with modification of activity level. This may be effective for a period of time; however, with age there is the potential of developing degenerative arthritis, particularly in those younger patients with large lesions. The true natural history of articular cartilage injuries is not known.
- Some surgeons have proposed aggressive surgical treatment in the hope of preventing degenerative arthritis. Few clinical data are available to support such a treatment algorithim, however.

SURGICAL MANAGEMENT

- Patients who fail conservative treatment for chondral injury must be evaluated for surgical treatment.
- The patient must have a full understanding of the surgical procedure and the extensive rehabilitation it requires.
- The indications for ACI are as follows:
  - Symptomatic weight bearing, unipolar, focal full-thickness chondral injury
  - Cartilage lesions of grade III or IV in the Outerbridge classification[16]
  - Unstable osteochondritis dissecans fragment
  - There is no size restriction on the lesion treated, although lesions typically are larger than 1.5 to 2.0 cm^2.
  - Physiologic young, active patients who will be compliant with the rehabilitation protocol
- Contraindications
  - Osteoarthritis or bipolar lesions with characteristic radiographic Fairbanks changes:
    - Joint space narrowing
    - Osteophyte formation
    - Subchondral bony sclerosis or cyst formation
  - Comorbidities such as ligamentous instability or meniscal pathology, unless they are addressed either concomitantly with the ACI or in a staged fashion
  - Coexisting inflammatory arthritis or active infections

Preoperative Planning

- The size of the lesion and the availability of adequate cartilage cells for ACI are assessed.
- Any bony deficit is assessed for possible bone grafting at the same time as the ACI. This is especially important for those patients with traumatic osteochondral fractures and large osteochondritis dissecans lesions. These lesions are best evaluated with MRI or at the time of the intial knee arthroscopy and direct examination of the lesion.
  - Staged bone grafting can be done at the time of arthroscopic evaluation. In general, 6 months are required between bone grafting and ACI, to allow time for the bone graft to consolidate and recreate a new subchondral plate.
- Alignment of the entire extremity and the status of ligaments and meniscus must be taken into consideration. Biomechanical malalignment, maltracking of the patella, lack of meniscus, and ligament insufficiency are examples of an altered intra-articular environment that can lead to shear stresses, excessive friction, and abnormal compressive loads across the autogenous chondrocyte implantation and thence potentially to failure.

- Improvement in ACI results is directly related to recognizing coexisting knee pathology and addressing it, either in a staged procedure or concomitantly at the time of the ACI.
  - For patients with limb malalignment, the surgeon must consider either proximal tibia osteotomies (opening or closing) for varus alignment or, for those with valgus alignment, a distal femoral osteotomy.
  - Most lesions of the patellofemoral joint require distal patella realignment procedures.
  - Ligamentous insufficiency, whether of the ACL, which is most common, or medial or lateral collateral laxity, even the most subtle, may produce excessive shear forces in the knee, which may irreversibly damage the maturing repair tissue produced by ACI. These ligament injuries must be addressed at the time of the ACI.
  - Patients with significant loss of meniscus tissue, through either subtotal or total menisectomy, must be considered candidates for allograft meniscus transplantation.

Positioning

- The patient is placed on the operating table in the supine position, and the entire lower extremity is sterily prepared and draped so that the knee may be placed in extreme flexion if necessary.
- A tourniquet is applied to the upper thigh.

Approach

- The first stage of a standard arthroscopy is performed for the harvest of articular cartilage followed by implantation of cells into the chondral defect.
- A midline incision usually is recommended, followed by a medial or lateral parapatellar arthrotomy to expose the corresponding site of the chondral defect.
  - A separate incision is made or the proximal incision is continued along its distal extent to harvest the periosteal patch on the proximal medial tibia.

TECHNIQUES

ARTHROSCOPIC ASSESSMENT

- Prior to the arthroscopic evaluation,[15] a comprehensive knee examination is performed, with close detail to the ligament stability of the knee and overall alignment.
  - Any ligament instability or malalignment must be addressed either concomitantly or in a staged procedure.
- Taking into account all factors, including the preoperative evaluation, the arthroscopic evaluation of the osteochondral lesion or defect provides the ultimate determination as to whether a patient is a candidate for ACI. Strict attention is paid to the condition of the intra-articular structures, such as integrity of the ligaments and meniscus.
  - Undiagnosed pathology may be critical to the outcome of ACI surgery.

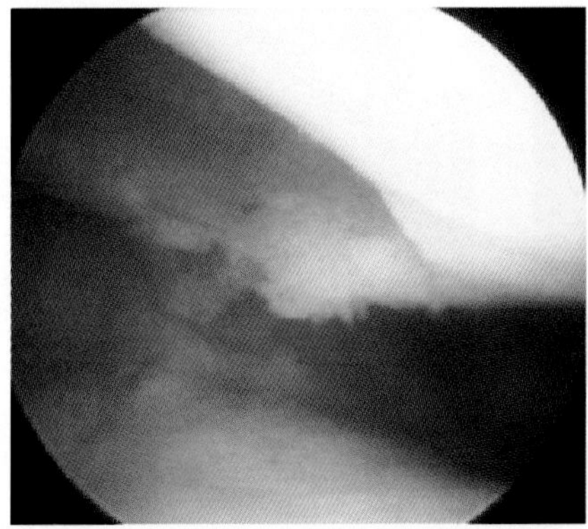

TECH FIG 1 • Arthroscopic view of a full-thickness medial femoral condyle lesion.

- Complete arthroscopic evaluation of the articular surfaces, both visual and probing (TECH FIG 1), is undertaken.
  - Accurate assessment of the osteochondral lesion, including size (anteroposterior and medial–lateral dimensions), is best obtained with a graduated probe. The estimation of size is of the utmost importance with regard to the number of chondrocytes that must be grown in culture to provide optimal fill for the defects.
- The cartilage injury area is probed for depth, size, number, and location of lesions. Additional assessment determines whether the lesion is a contained or uncontained defect, referring to the borders of the lesion.
- The Outerbridge system (Table 1) is a practical working approach to arthroscopic grading of articular cartilage defects.[16]
- A newer, more functional classification has been proposed by the International Cartilage Repair Society (Table 2).[6]

Table 1 Outerbridge Classification of Cartilage Lesions

Grade	Description
I	Articular surface is swollen and soft and may be blistered.
II	Characterized by the presence of fissures and clefts measuring <1 cm in diameter
III	Characterized by the presence of deep fissures extending to the subchondral bone, measuring >1 cm in diameter; loose flaps and joint debris also may be noted.
IV	Subchondral bone exposed

CARTILAGE BIOPSY FOR AUTOLOGOUS CARTILAGE IMPLANTATION

- A biopsy specimen of cartilage can be obtained at the time of the diagnostic arthroscopy.
- Articular cartilage biopsy sites include the superior medial and lateral femoral condyle, as well as the intercondylar notch.
- The best instrument for harvesting is either a ring curette or a curved notchplasty gauge (**TECH FIG 2A**).
- The two biopsies should be full-thickness cartilage measuring 5 × 8 mm, with a total weight of 200 to 300 mg (**TECH FIG 2B**).
- The biopsy specimens are placed in a vial of media in the prepackaged biopsy transport kit from Carticel. This articular cartilage biopsy contains about 200,000 to 300,000 cells, which will be enzymatically digested and grown to approximately 12 million cells per 0.4 mL of culture medium per implanted vial after 4 to 6 weeks, to be used for the implantation procedure.

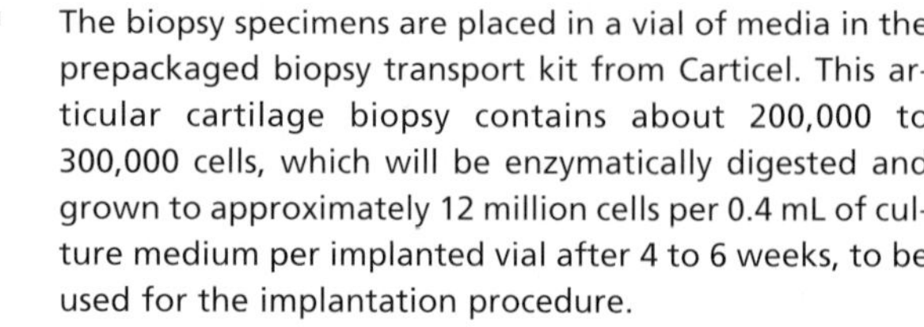

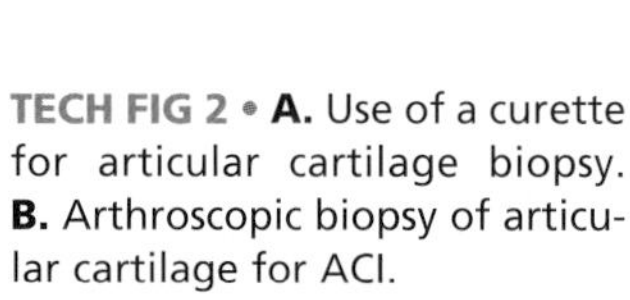

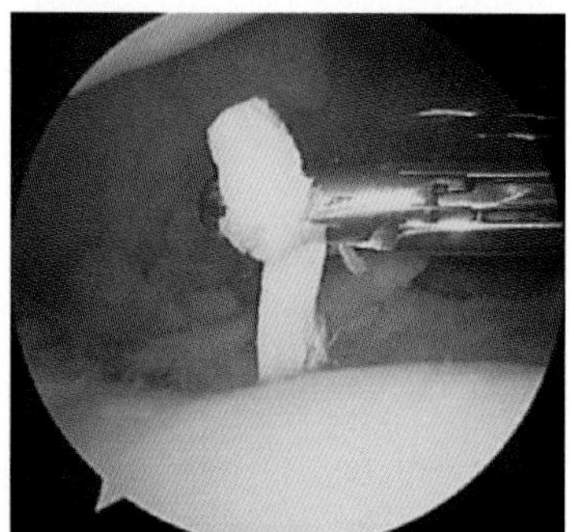

TECH FIG 2 • **A.** Use of a curette for articular cartilage biopsy. **B.** Arthroscopic biopsy of articular cartilage for ACI.

DEFECT PREPARATION

- After the diagnostic arthroscopy, a medial or lateral parapatellar mini-arthrotomy is performed to provide adequate exposure to the osteochondral defect. If a lesion of the patella or trochlea is present, a formal medial parapatellar arthrotomy with eversion of the patella is done for complete exposure.
- Defect preparation is crucial to the outcome of ACI. All of the unhealthy cartilage surrounding and remaining in the lesion must be débrided completely using a curette and a no. 15 scalpel blade.
  - Healthy vertical cartilage borders are necessary for optimal suturing of the periosteum graft (**TECH FIG 3A–E**).
  - The bed of the defect is débrided of fibrous tissue and calcified cartilage, but the subchondral plate must not be violated in the débridement process.

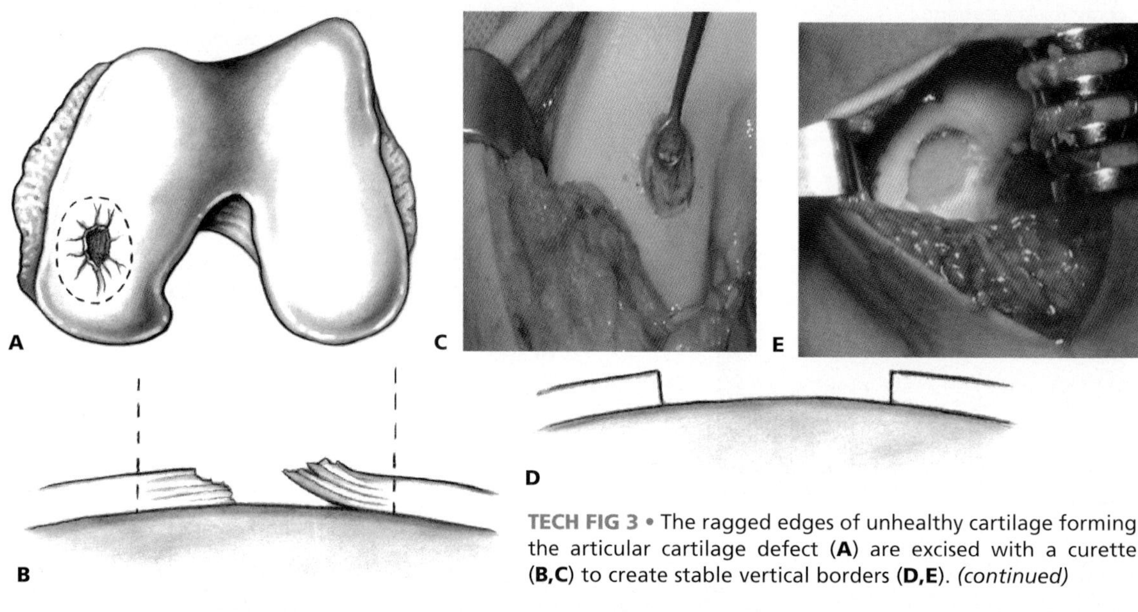

TECH FIG 3 • The ragged edges of unhealthy cartilage forming the articular cartilage defect (**A**) are excised with a curette (**B,C**) to create stable vertical borders (**D,E**). *(continued)*

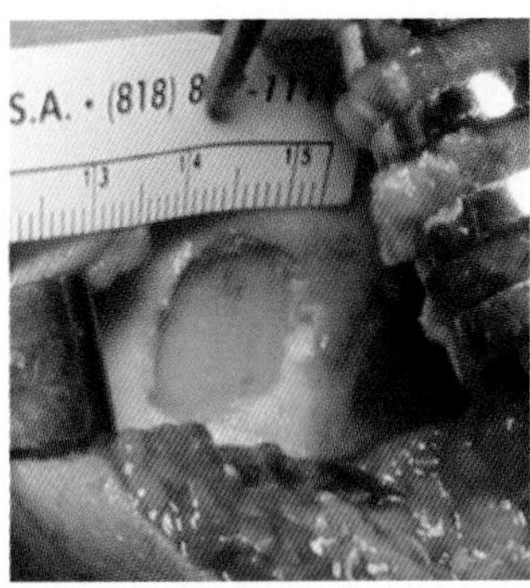

TECH FIG 3 • *(continued)* **F.** Measuring the medial femoral condyle lesion. (**A,B,D,F:** Courtesy of Genzyme, Inc.)

- Bleeding at the cartilage defect must be controlled.
  - Three means of controlling bleeding from the subchondral plate are available:
    - Application of sponges soaked in a 1:1000 solution of epinephrine and saline
    - Application of fibrin glue on sites of bleeding on the subchondral bone
    - Use of a needle-point electrocautery with a needletip Bovie set on low.
- Defect dimensions can be measured with a sterile ruler to determine the size of the periosteal patch.
  - The longest anterior to posterior and medial to lateral dimensions should be measured, after which 2 to 3 mm are added to each dimension to obtain the appropriate dimensions for the periosteal graft (TECH FIG 3F).
  - Another method is to make a template from sterile paper from the surgical gloves. A template is placed on the lesion and the defect is outlined with a permanent marking pen, oversizing by 1 to 2 mm. This template is then placed on the proximal tibia as a guide for the periosteal graft.

PERIOSTEAL GRAFT HARVEST

- The osteochondral defect is measured with a disposable ruler at its widest mediolateral and superoinferior dimensions.
  - An alternative method is to create a template of the lesion with sterile paper, as just described above. The lesion is traced on the paper.
- The proximal medial tibia provides the best site for harvesting periosteum. An alternative site for periosteal tissue is the distal femur.
  - The incision is placed 2.5 cm below the pes anserinus (TECH FIG 4A).
- The dissection is carried out down to the periosteum with complete removal of the subcutaneous tissue and fascia. A sharp dissection is recommended to remove this fascia layer.
- With a permanent marker, the template of the lesion is used to outline the periosteum with 2 to 3 mm added to the measured dimensions of the defect to take into account shrinkage of the periosteal graft after removal from the bone.
- The cambium layer is marked to avoid confusion when suturing the periosteum onto the graft with the cambium layer closest to the defect.
- With a no. 15 knife blade cutting sharply down to bone circumferentially, a sharp periosteal elevator is used to elevate the periosteum from the proximal tibia (TECH FIG 4B). It is lifted off the proximal tibia with a smooth pair of pick-ups so as to not damage the cells of the periosteum.
- The periosteum is kept moist with saline.

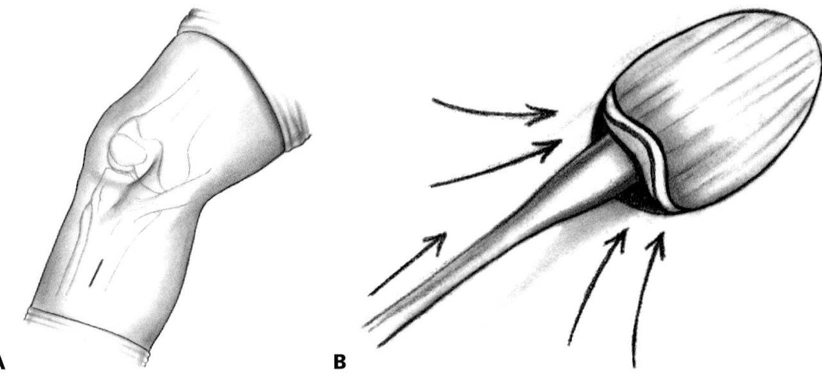

TECH FIG 4 • **A.** The incision for periosteum harvest is located 2.5 cm below the insertion of the pes anserinus. **B.** A small periosteal elevator is used to create an edge around the border of the periosteum graft to be harvested from the proximal tibia. (Courtesy of Genzyme, Inc.)

PERIOSTEUM GRAFT FIXATION

- If a tourniquet has been used, it is deflated at this point, and meticulous hemostatsis of the defect bed is undertaken with the techniques described earlier.
  - Any bleeding can affect the viability of the implanted chondrocytes. Use of thrombin-soaked pledgets in diluted epinephrine along with the use of a needle-point Bovie can help control any bleeding.

- The orientation of moist periosteal graft on the defect is determined, with the cambium layer closet to the defect. Keeping the periosteum moist is of the utmost importance to preserve the viability of the cambium layer.
  - Any excess periosteum overlying the borders of the defect must be trimmed to provide an exact fit of the defect.
- Once the appropriate orientation and size of the graft are established, the periosteum graft is secured in place with a 6.0 Vicryl suture on a P1 cutting needle using simple interrupted suture technique.
  - To facilitate easy passage of the suture through the cartilage and thin periosteum, mineral oil or glycerin is applied to the suture.
- The four corners of the periosteal graft are first secured and tensioned, followed by sequential sutures about 3 to 4 mm apart from each other (**TECH FIG 5A**).
  - This will ensure a watertight seal for the implanted chondrocytes beneath the periosteum graft.
- It is critical for the knots of the suture to be placed on the periosteum side to prevent shearing off of the knot and failure of the periosteal graft as the graft is maturing during early rehabilitation.
  - The suture needle should be passed through the periosteum from outside to inside, approximaely 2 mm from the edge of the periosteum.
  - The needle then is passed though the cartilage using the curvature of the needle, from inside to the outside of the cartilage with the needle entering the cartilage perpendicular to the inside wall of the defect and exiting the articular surface 2 to 3 mm from the débrided defect (**TECH FIG 5B,C**).
- The sutures are placed alternately around the defect, spaced about 3 mm apart, leaving a 5- to 6-mm opening to accommodate an angiocatheter for injection of the chondrocyte cells.
- A watertight integrity test is performed with the placement of the 18-gauge catheter into the superior aspect, and saline is slowly infused to assess the graft suturing (**TECH FIG 5D**).
  - Areas with of saline leakage are reinforced with additional sutures. The area then is retested until the graft is watertight.
  - Once a watertight seal is obtained, the excess saline is aspirated from the defect.
- Commercially prepared fibrin glue, available in most operating rooms, is then passed circumferentially over the periosteum graft–cartilage interface suture line as an additional sealant to prevent leakage of the injected chondrocytes (**TECH FIG 5E,F**).

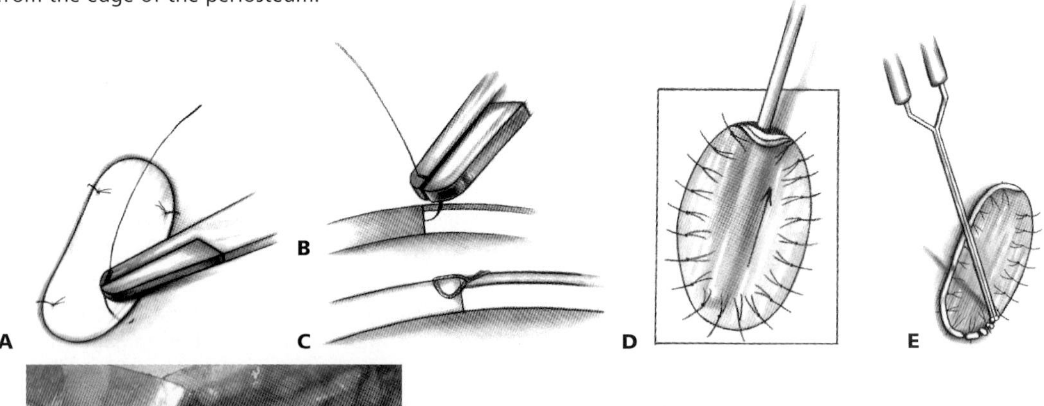

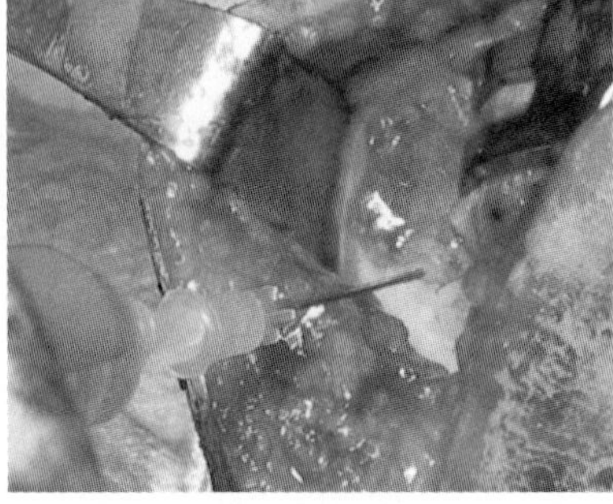

TECH FIG 5 • **A.** The four corners of the periosteum graft are secured first. **B.** The suture needle is angled toward the surface to obtain a bite in the cartilage. **C.** The knot is placed on the periosteum side, not the cartilage rim, to prevent shearing. **D.** Final suturing of the periosteum graft leaves an opening at the most superior point for insertion of an 18-gauge catheter for saline injection to test for a watertight seal. **E,F.** Fibrin glue is applied one drop at a time around the periphery of the defect. (Courtesy of Genzyme, Inc.)

SPECIAL SITUATIONS

- Uncontained defects without vertical cartilage borders on the periphery or encroaching on the intercondylar notch require the use of mini-anchors or suturing into the synovial layer to secure the periosteal graft.
- Those osteochondral defects may require bone grafts. Bone graft can be obtained from the proximal tibia or iliac crest in the standard fashion.
- This can be done either in a staged fashion or concomitantly at the time of the ACI. Those procedures that are staged can have the bone graft packed into the defect with the plan of returning in 3 months after consolidation. If done concomitantly with ACI, the "periosteal graft sandwich" technique is used. Bone graft is placed in the defect, followed by a periosteal patch. Another periosteal graft is then sutured into place as described previously. The chondrocyte cells are then slowly injected between the two periosteum layers.

IMPLANTATION OF AUTOGENOUS CHONDROCYTES

- The chondrocyte cells are delivered into the culture medium inside a Carticel vial (Genzyme Biosurgery, Cambridge, MA; TECH FIG 6A).
  - The cells require resuspension in the medium.
  - A sterile 18-gauge catheter is then inserted into the Carticel vial to mix and resuspend the chondrocytes, which settle to the bottom during shipping. This is repeated until the cells are completely resuspended in the medium.
- The cells then are slowly injected under the periosteal patch into the defect.
- After injection of the cells is completed, the needle is withdrawn, and the small opening for the angiocatheter is then sutured with 6.0 Vicryl and sealed with fibrin glue (TECH FIG 6B,C).
- The arthrotomy wound is copiously irrigated, and the retractors are removed slowly. The arthrotomy is then closed in the standard, layered fashion.
- A sterile dressing is applied. No drain is placed in the joint, because the ACI graft may be damaged by the suction of the drain.

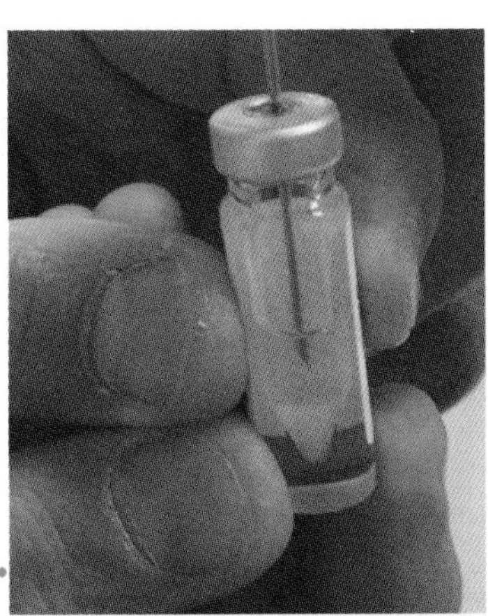
A

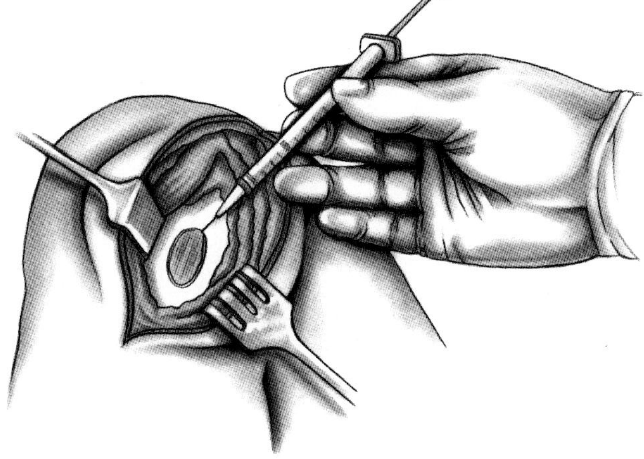
B

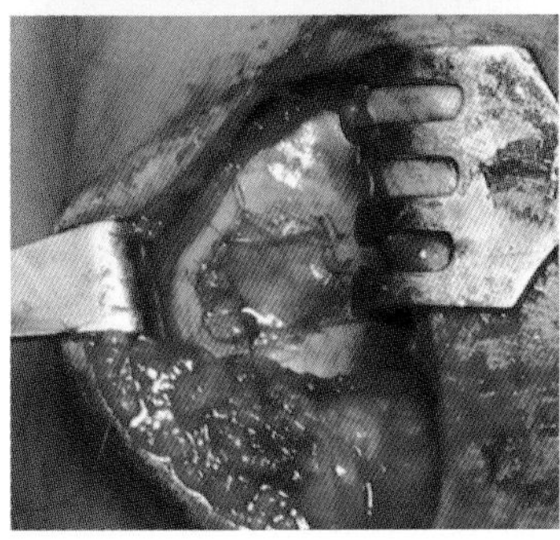
C

TECH FIG 6 • **A.** Vial of chondrocyte for injection. **B.** Injection of cells. **C.** Periosteum graft post injection of cells. (**B:** Courtesy of Genzyme, Inc.)

PEARLS AND PITFALLS

Pitfalls with ACI	■ Leaving unhealthy cartilage: not excising enough cartilage to define true size of lesion ■ Sharp dissection and the taking of bone when harvesting the periosteum ■ Not removing the fascia layer off of the periosteum ■ Injecting cells before obtaining adequate hemostasis or watertight seal in defect bed ■ Attaching the periosteum too low into the lesion ■ Tying knots too loosely or on the cartilage rim, or cutting too close to the knot ■ Violating the subchondral bone, causing bleeding and potential lysis of implanted chondrocyte cells ■ Leaving fibrocartilage in the base of the defect from a previous failed marrow-stimulating procedure ■ Not allowing the fibrin glue to congeal before applying it in a drop fashion ■ Not harvesting a large enough amount of periosteum. Needs to be oversized by 2 to 3 mm to accommodate for shrinkage

Table 2 ICRS Arthroscopic Cartilage Grading System

Grade	Description
0	Normal
1	Nearly normal superficial lesions
1A	Soft indentation
1B	Superficial cracks or fissures
2	Abnormal lesion extending down to <50% of cartilage depth
3	Severely abnormal cartilage defects >50% of cartilage depth
3A	Down to calcified layer
3B	Down to but not through subchondral layer
3C	Blistering
4	Exposed subchondral bone

ICRS, International Cartilage Repair Society.
Reprinted with permission from Brittberg M. ICRS: Clinical Cartilage Injury Evaluation System. Third ICRS Symposium, Gothenburg, Sweden, April 28, 2000.

POSTOPERATIVE CARE

- The concept of a slow, gradual time course for healing is critical to understand in post-ACI rehabilitation. The foundation principles of a successful ACI rehabilitation program center on protection of the graft, mobility and motion exercises, muscle strengthening, progressive weight bearing, and patient education.
- Protection of the repaired tissue from execessive intra-articular joint forces is critical during the early postoperative period, although early motion aids in cell orientation of the repaired tissue and prevents arthrofibrosis.
  - If the graft is overloaded with friction and delamination of the ACI tissue, or potential hypertrophy of the ACI tissue occurs, potential complications must be understood.
  - The intra-articular microenvironment must be protective of this complicated interaction of the implantated chondrocytes and the stimulutory aspects of the rehabilitation, such as early motion to allow for the remodeling and maturation of these chondrocytes into a hyaline-like cartilage phenotype.
- During the early phase (day 1 through week 12), the patient is permitted non–weight bearing during weeks 0 to 2, toe-touch weight bearing until weeks 8 to 9, and full weight bearing at 9 weeks.
  - The patient begins continuous passive motion (CPM) 6 to 24 hours after surgery.
  - CPM is performed 6 to 8 hours a day for 6 weeks.
  - The patient should obtain full range of motion.
  - The patient gradually returns to activities of daily living.
- The transition phase is from week 13 through month 6.
  - The patient has increased activities of daily living and increased standing and walking.
  - The patient should have quadricep and hamstring strength greater than 80%.
- The mid-phase is from month 7 through month 9.
  - The patient advances to strength training involving non-pivoting activities.
- The final phase is month 10 through month 18.
  - The patient can perform low-impact activities, such as skating and cycling, during months 9 through 12; repetitive impact activities such as jogging and aerobic classes during months 13 through 15; and high-level pivoting activities such as tennis and basketball during months 16 through 18.
- Rehabilitation of patellar and trochlear lesions requires special consideration. The contact pressure of the patellofemoral articulation is maximal between 40 and 70 degree of knee flexion; therefore, flexion of this magnitude should be avoided during active knee flexion until the graft is mature and can withstand these shear stresses.
  - Early, gentle patella mobility exercises also are important to prevent adhesions and decreased patella mobility.
  - Avoidance of active knee extension during the first 10 to 12 weeks and the use of continuous passive motion is encouraged to give the best clinical results.
  - The gradual progression of active extension exercises also depends on the size and location of the patellar or trochlear lesion as observed in the operating room.

OUTCOMES

- Brittberg et al[7] published their intial results with ACI in *The New England Journal of Medicine,* a study that revealed impressive intial results. Fouteen of 16 patients (87%) with isolated femoral condyle lesions treated with ACI had good to excellent results with 2-year follow-up. Subsequent follow-up of these patients at 11 years revealed the durability of and patient satisfaction with the ACI procedure.[8,17,18]
- A more recent multicenter study assessed the clinical outcome of lesions of the distal femur treated with ACI in 100 patients.[9] Eighty-seven percent of the patients completed a 5-year follow-up assessment. Patients were, on average, 37 years of age and had a mean total defect size of 4.9 cm^2; and 70% of the patients had underogne at least one previous articular cartilage procedure. Seventy-three percent showed significant improvement, with an increase of 4.1 points on the Cincinnati knee rating system, substantiating ACI as a viable option for the treatment of chondral injuries.
- Even though ACI is highly successful, new treatment modalities continue to be developed, including an arthroscopic approach and possibly a one-stage procedure.
  - Matrix-induced autologous chondrocyte transplantation (MACI) is one such treatment modality that is conducted arthroscopically (**FIG 4**). Similar to ACI, autologous chondrocytes are used but are placed into a collagen scaffold for implantation. This constrution can be used instead of a periosteal graft, with stabilization still provided with fibrin glue.
  - The scaffold has a porous surface that can embody the repairing tissue. Different scaffolds are under development. Each scaffold must fulfill specific requirements in regard to biocompatibility, endurance, and structural stability. The scaffold should induce maturation and differentiation of the cellular structures that it supports.
  - About 3200 surgical procedures using this technique have been performed in Europe, with excellent early clinical results.[1]

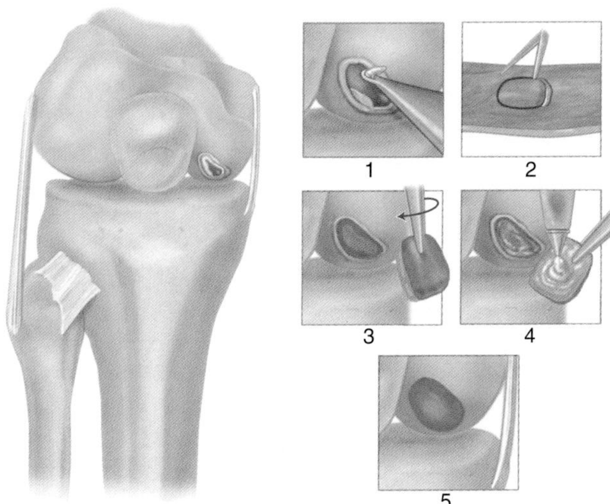

FIG 4 • Overview of the matrix-induced autologous chondrocyte transplantation (MACI) technique. Step 1: the defect is assessed and damaged cartilage débrided. Step 2: MACI membrane is cut according to the template, matching defect size and shape. Step 3: proper membrane orientation, in which cells face the bone bed. Step 4: fibrin sealant is applied to the defect and to the bone bed. Step 5: MACI is held in place with light pressure and fixed by fibrin glue, with no suturing required.

COMPLICATIONS

- Hypertrophy or overgrowth of the periosteum graft
- Delamination of the periosteum graft
- Postoperative stiffness, arthrofibrosis
- Infection
- Donor site morbidity
- Partial or full graft detatchment

REFERENCES

1. Bachmann G, et al. [MRI in the follow-up of matrix-supported autologous chondrocyte transplantation (MACI) and microfracture]. Radiology 2004;44:773–782.
2. Beris AE et al. Advances in articular cartilage repair. Injury 2005;36: Suppl 4:S14–23.
3. Blevins F, Steadman R, Rodrigo J, et al. Treatment of articular cartilage defects in athletes: an analysis of functional outcome and lesion appearance. Orthopedics 1998:21:761–768.
4. Bobic V, Morgan C, Carter T. Osteochondral autologous graft transfer. Oper Tech Sports Med 2000;8:168–178.
5. Borazjani BH et al. Effect of impact on chondrocyte viability during insertion of human osteochondral grafts. J Bone Joint Surg Am 2006;88A:1934–1943.
6. Brittberg M. ICRS: Clinical Cartilage Injury Evaluation System. Third ICRS Symposium, Gothenburg, Sweden, April 28, 2000.
7. Brittberg M, Lindahl A, Ohlsson C, et al. Treatment of deep cartilage defects in the knee with autologous chondrocyte transplantation. N Engl J Med 1994;331:889–895.
8. Brittberg M, Lindahl A, Ohlsson C, et al. Articular cartilage engineering with autologous chondrocyte transplantation: a review of recent developments. J Bone Joint Surg Am 2003:85A:109–115.
9. Browne J, Anderson A, Arciero R, et al. Clinical outcome of autologous chondrocyte implantation at 5 years in US subjects. Clin Orthop 2005;436:237–245.
10. Browne JE, Branchm TP. Surgical alternatives for treatment of articular cartilage lesions. J Am Acad Orthop Surg 2000;8:180–189.
11. Buckwalter JA. Articular cartilage: injuries and potential for healing. J Orthop Sports Phys Ther 1998;28:192–202.
12. Chu C, Lin D, Geisler J, et al. Arthroscopic microscopy of articular cartilage using optical coherence tomography. Am J Sports Med 2004;32:699–709.
13. Curl W, Krome J, Gordan E, et al. Cartilage injuries: a review of 31,516 knee arthroscopies. Arthroscopy 1997;13:456–460.
14. Jackson RW, Marans HJ, Silver RS. Arthroscopic treatment of degenerative arthritis of the knee. J Bone Joint Surg Am 1988;70A: 332–336.
15. Minas T. Surgical manual defect assessment and biopsy procurement and cell implantation procedure. Carticel. Boston: Genzyme Biosurgery, 2004.
16. Outerbridge RE. The etiology of chondromalacia patellae. J Bone Joint Surg Br 1961;43B:752–757.
17. Peterson L, Brittberg M, Kiviranta I, et al. Autologous chondrocyte transplantation: biomechanics and long term durability. Am J Sports Med 2002;30:2–12.
18. Peterson L, Minas T, Brittberg M, et al. Two to 9 year outcome after autologous chondrocyte transplantation of the knee. Clin Orthop 2000;374:212–234.
19. Scopp JM, Mandelbaum BR. A treatment algorithm for the management of articular cartilage defects. Orthop Clin North Am 2005;36: 419–426.
20. Shapiro F, Koide S, Glimcher MJ. Cell origin and differentiation in the repair of full-thickness defects of articular cartilage. J Bone Joint Surg Am 1993;75:532–553.

Chapter 39 Allograft Cartilage Transplantation

Eric C. McCarty, R. David Rabalais, and Kenneth G. Swan, Jr.

DEFINITION

- Articular cartilage lesions are focal, usually isolated, cartilage defects that may be either symptomatic or incidentally found.
- Osteochondritis dissecans is an osteochondral lesion that occurs in adolescents and, therefore, may have different management ramifications from lesions in adults.
- Lesions can be partial- or full-thickness, down to subchondral bone.
- Lesions can be secondary to trauma or atraumatic, as is the case for osteochondritis dissecans.
- Cases with a traumatic etiology may have associated ligamentous or meniscal injury.
- Small full-thickness chondral defects may heal adequately with mechanically inferior fibrocartilage (primarily type I collagen), but larger defects often require cartilage transplant surgery to replace the damaged chondral surface.

ANATOMY

- Articular cartilage is composed primarily of type II collagen.
- Chondrocytes that produce the extracellular matrix are of mesenchymal stem cell origin.
- Osteochondral lesions may occur in all three compartments of the knee.
- Chondral defects after a patellar dislocation may be found on the medial patellar facet or lateral trochlea.
- Classically, osteochondritis dissecans occurs at the lateral aspect of the medial femoral condyle.

PATHOGENESIS

- Osteochondral lesions may be traumatic or may have no known history of trauma.
- Traumatic lesions may be caused by compaction, as with an anterior cruciate ligament tear and lateral-based osteochondral injury, or by a shearing mechanism, as seen with patellar dislocations.
- Atraumatic lesions may be found in young persons, as is the case with osteochondritis dissecans, or in elderly persons, as seen with degenerative lesions.
- The etiology of ostoechondritis dissecans is uncertain. Traumatic, inflammatory, developmental, and ischemic causes have all been proposed but not proven.

NATURAL HISTORY

- Few controlled, prospective outcome studies have been published.
- The natural history for juveniles with nondisplaced osteochondritis dissecans is very favorable.
- Those diagnosed as adults have a less favorable prognosis. In one study, 81% of patients had tricompartmental gonarthrosis at an average of 33 years follow-up.[5]

PATIENT HISTORY AND PHYSICAL FINDINGS

- Patients with focal osteochondral lesions typically are active and young, ranging in age from adolescence to middle age.
- Often, the history does not include a specific traumatic episode. History and physical findings can be subtle.
- Presentation is variable; it may mimic meniscal pathology, with intermittent pain and swelling.
- Condylar defects may present with high-impact loading complaints, whereas patellofemoral defects may produce anterior knee pain–type complaints, with stairs and prolonged sitting causing symptoms.
- Patients with large cartilage lesions who are candidates for osteochondral allograft transplant surgery may have a history of previous knee surgery and previous attempts at cartilage regeneration by other methods (eg, microfracture, autologous chondrocyte implantation, osteochondral autograft transplant).
- Physical findings can be nonspecific and may include joint effusion and painful range of motion.
- Tenderness at the defect, on either the condyle, patellar facets, or trochlea, may be elicited.
- In the case of patellofemoral defects, patellar mobility and apprehension must be assessed.
- Ligament integrity must be determined.
- Mechanical alignment must be assessed, and appropriate imaging studies obtained.
- Failure to identify and address ligamentous deficiency or mechanical malalignment will lead to compromise of restorative cartilage procedures.
- Physical examination of the knee should note the following:
  - Chronic or recurrent effusion associated with, although not predictive of, a chondral lesion
  - Pain at extremes of range of motion (ie, forced flexion or forced extension) may indicate mensical pathology. An extension block may indicate a displaced meniscus tear. Osteochondral defects may cause decreased flexion via effusion, or may have normal range of motion.
  - An isolated lesion may have point tenderness, although it often is difficult to palpate.
  - Increased patellar mobility may indicate generalized ligamentous laxity, increasing suspicion for patellar instabililty.
  - Mechanical axis views are obtained if there is any hint of malalignment based on gait and stance analysis.

IMAGING AND OTHER DIAGNOSTIC STUDIES

- Anteroposterior, lateral, and sunrise views are mandatory to determine overall knee condition, rule out diffuse degenerative arthritis, and assess patellar position within the trochlea.

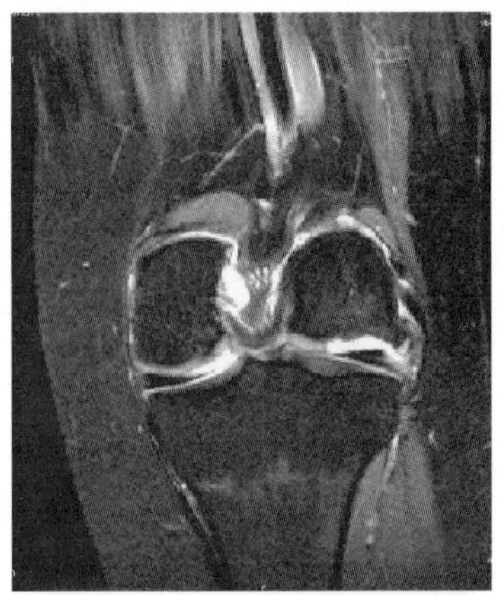
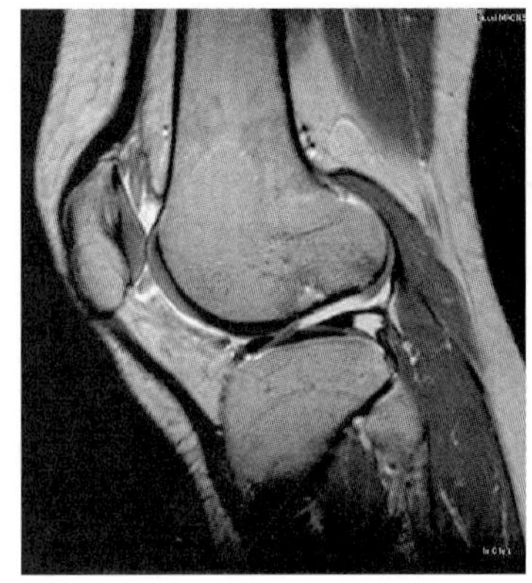
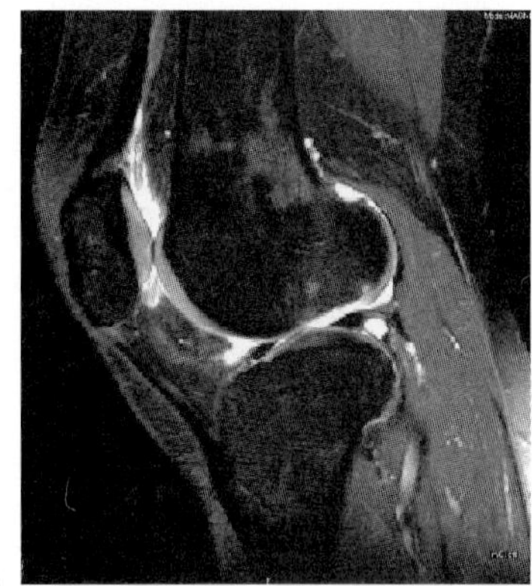
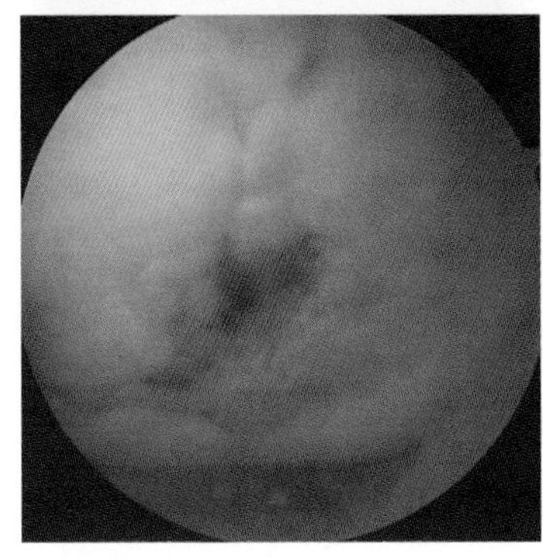

FIG 1 • T2-weighted coronal (**A**), T1-weighted sagittal (**B**), and T2-weighted sagittal (**C**) MRI scans of a right knee with a medial femoral condyle osteochondral defect. **D.** Arthroscopic view of a large osteochondral defect. Full assessment of the lesion was not completed until the defect was débrided to stable rim.

- Large chondral defects may not be visible on plain radiographs, or may have a small radiodense bone fragment attached.
- "Notch views" may better define more central lesions.
- Long-leg mechanical axis views are mandatory in patients with malalignment on physical examination, and should be considered in all candidates for osteochondral autograft transfer.
- MRI is the best modality to determine the presence, size, and location of cartilage lesions, as well as to determine the integrity of menisci and ligaments (**FIG 1A–C**).
- Arthroscopy remains the gold standard for evaluation of articular cartilage lesions (**FIG 1D**).

DIFFERENTIAL DIAGNOSIS

- Meniscal tear
- Degenerative arthritis
- Patellar instability
- Bone contusion
- Avascular necrosis
- Undiagnosed ligamentous injury

NONOPERATIVE MANAGEMENT

- Patients with asymptomatic osteochondral lesions (often found incidentally on standard knee arthroscopy) may be candidates for nonoperative treatment.
- Long-term studies may indicate an increased risk for degenerative arthritis with conservative management,[5] but no randomized controlled studies exist.
- Nonoperative treatment should consist of physical therapy to obtain or maintain painless, full range of motion.
- Aggravating impact activities should be avoided.
- Patients may participate in sports as tolerated.
- Unloader braces or shoe wedges may help alleviate mild symptoms.

SURGICAL MANAGEMENT

- Osteochondral allograft transplantation often is a two-stage procedure.
- The magnitude of the lesion and occasionally the diagnosis itself often are not appreciated until first-look arthroscopy (**FIG 2**).
- Size and location of the cartilage lesion is determined.
- Lesions 1 cm in diameter or larger are considered for allograft transplant. Smaller lesions may be amenable to microfracture or autograft cartilage transplant with single or mutliple plugs.

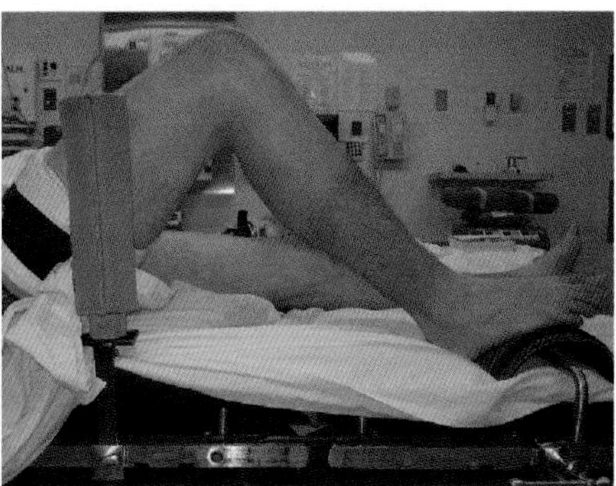

FIG 2 • Patient positioning, with tourniquet, using a lateral post and foot rest.

- The remainder of the knee is inspected to ensure this is not a diffuse cartilage process, and to examine the integrity of the cruciate ligaments and mensici.

Preoperative Planning

- Mechanical alignment must be assessed and, if necessary, osteotomy planned for.
- Templated radiographs are obtained for appropriate allograft sizing, based on the medial–lateral dimension of the lesion.
- The patient must be informed that there is no way to predict when an appropriate-sized donor will become available, and that a moderate waiting period (weeks to months) may be required before surgery can be done.
- Fresh osteochondral allografts are used. Frozen chondral grafts are unacceptable.
- Allografts are harvested within 24 hours of donor death and can be preserved for up to 4 days at 4° C.
- Chondrocyte viability likely declines after 5 days, but prolonged storage—up to 21 days—currently is acceptable.[6]
- After 28 days, chondrocyte viability is unacceptably diminished.[4]
- Tissue matching and immunologic suppression are unnecessary with osteochondral grafts.
- Donors are screened with a multifactorial process promoted by the American Association of Tissue Banks to minimize the risk of disease transmission.

Positioning

- We prefer to have the patient supine, keeping the foot of the table up.
- A lateral post and sliding footrest or taped sandbag allow for 90-degree flexion positioning of the knee.
- The surgeon should be able to flex the knee to 120 degrees if needed.
- A tourniquet is placed but is inflated only if visualization is compromised by intra-articular bleeding.

Approach

- The approach depends on the location of the defect.
- The defect typically is on the medial or lateral femoral condyle, requiring a longitudinal parapatellar tendon arthrotomy.
- Large trochlear or patellar defects amenable to osteochondral allograft transplation (rare) may require a larger parapatellar incision and eversion of the patella.

FEMORAL CONDYLE OSTEOCHONDRAL ALLOGRAFT TRANSPLANT

Diagnostic Arthroscopy

- A brief diagnostic arthroscopy is peformed to fully assess or reassess the condylar defect (TECH FIG 1A) as well as to examine for additional knee pathology and any changes from the original arthroscopy.

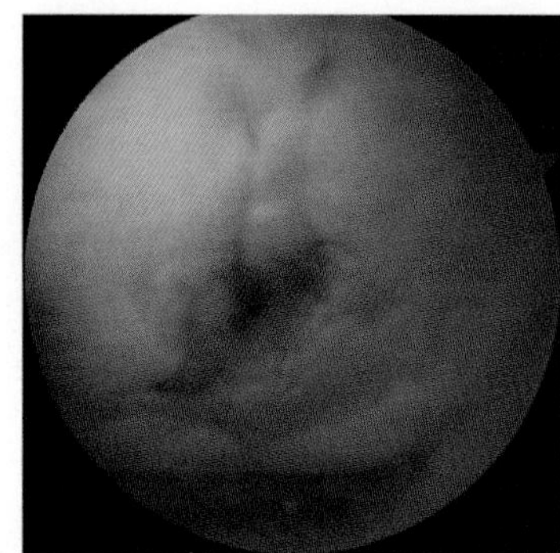

A

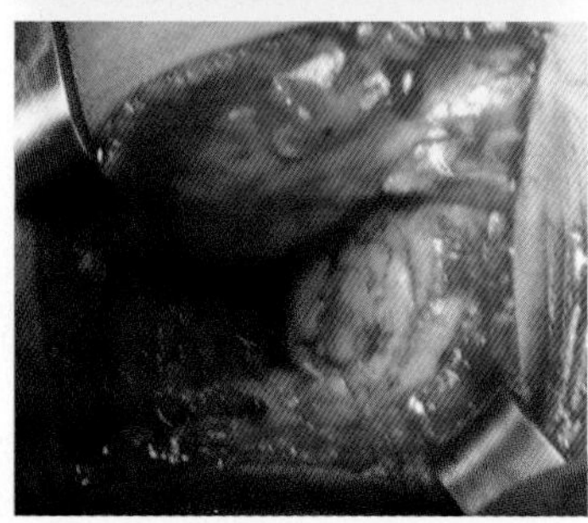

B

TECH FIG 1 • **A.** Arthroscopic view of a large osteochondral defect. **B.** Open view of a large osteochondral defect.

- A standard parapatellar arthrotomy is carried out to expose the defect on the affected side of the knee. It is lateral for a lateral femoral condylar defect and medial for a medial femoral condylar defect (TECH FIG 1B).

Sizing

- The size of the defect is determined using a cannulated cylindrical sizing device.
- A circumferential mark is placed around the sizer to outline the margins of the defect to be grafted (TECH FIG 2A).
- Occasionally, a chondral defect is large or irregularly shaped, and requires more than one allograft. The resultant graft may be in the form of a "snowman," with two or even three differently sized circular grafts stacked on top of one another.
- A central guide pin is placed through the sizer into bone to a depth of 2 to 3 cm. The sizer is then removed (TECH FIG 2B).
- A reference mark is placed at the superior (12 o'clock) position of the recipient site.

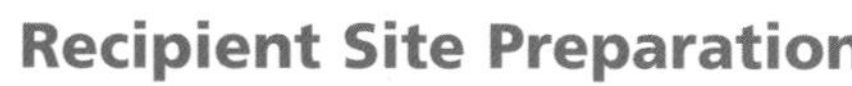

Recipient Site Preparation

- The recipient site is prepared by first scoring the periphery of the lesion (TECH FIG 3A).
- Next, a counterbore or reamer is used to drill the defect to a depth of 8 to 10 mm circumferentially, to bleeding subchondral bone (TECH FIG 3B).
- Following that, the recipient bed should be drilled with a small (1.6 to 2.0 mm) drill bit to stimulate additional vascular response (TECH FIG 3C).
- The recipient site depth is then measured in four positions, as on the face of a clock: 12 o'clock, 3 o'clock,

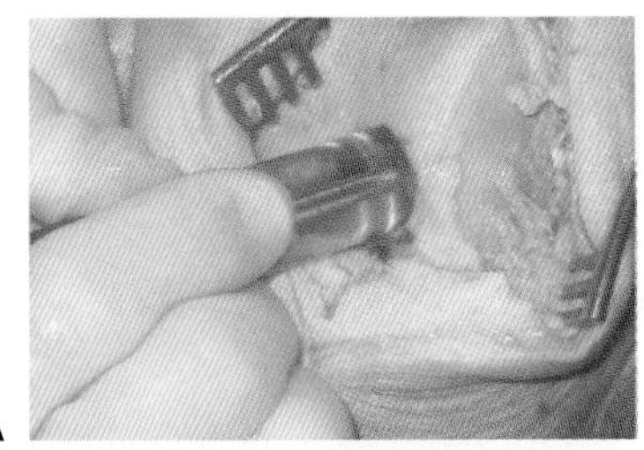

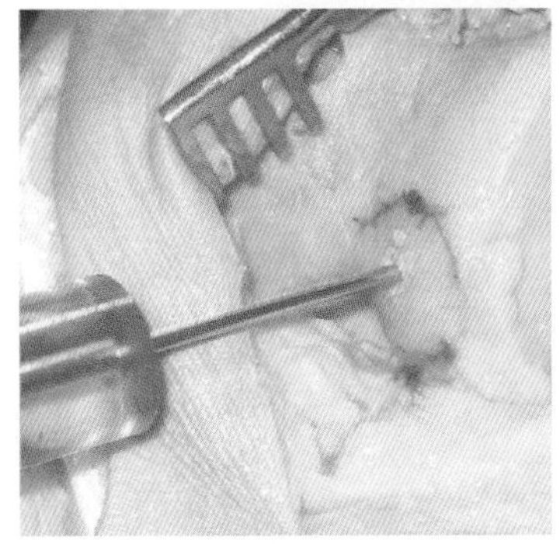

TECH FIG 2 • **A.** Sizing of osteochondral defect. **B.** Placement of a central pin through the center of the sizer into the center of the defect after circumferential marking of the sizer on the condyle.

6 o'clock, and 9 o'clock. This may be done using a standard paper ruler, or by a measuring device supplied by the equipment company (TECH FIG 3D).

- The depth of the recipient site may not be precisely consistent throughout its circumference. Donor modification will allow for fine tuning.

Donor Preparation

- The same sizer used for defect sizing is used to template the allograft hemicondyle on the back table. Careful comparison of defect location (eg, relative to femoral notch) and donor position is imperative to ensure optimal donor–recipient fit (TECH FIG 4A,B).
- We use the Arthrex Osteochondral Allograft Transfer System (OATS) Workstation (Naples, FL) to help secure the donor graft. This instrument allows for multiple degrees of freedom while positioning and contouring the graft (TECH FIG 4C).
- The angle of harvest of the donor tissue must match the angle at which the recipient site was reamed (TECH FIG 4D).
- Next, the donor osteochondral plug(s) is harvested. The Arthrex system makes it possible to completely drill through the donor condyle, which is held in place with the OATS Workstation. The relevant donor graft tissue is then carefully removed from the harvester drill (TECH FIG 4E,F).

Graft Harvest

- The graft depth is now measured and marked to the precise degree that the recipient bed was measured, in the same four quadrants.
- The graft is held using allograft holding forceps, similar to the manner in which the patella is prepared during total knee arthroplasty. The graft cut is made using a power saw, with care taken to match the cut to the previously made depth measurements. The osteochondral portion of the graft should be held within the forceps, so as not to drop the relevant portion of the graft once the cut is completed (TECH FIG 5A–C).

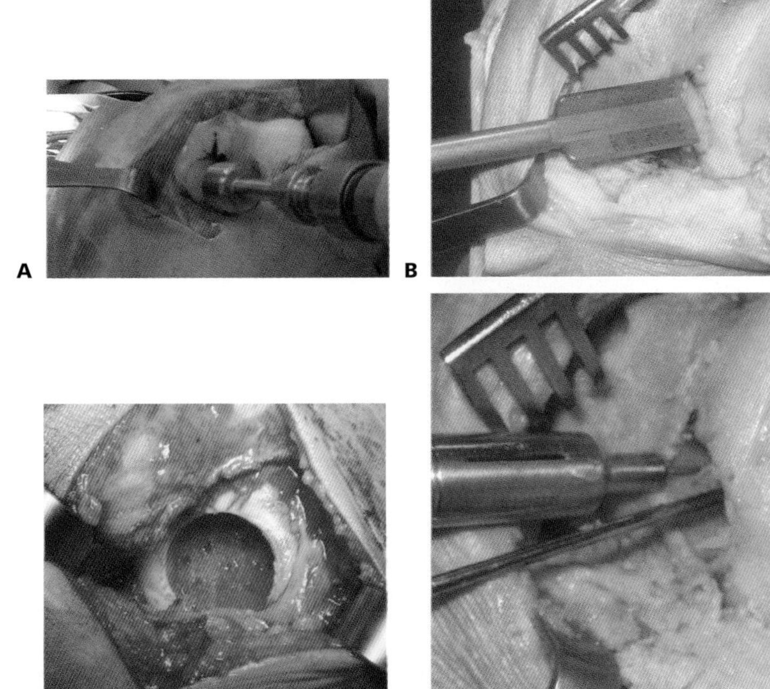

TECH FIG 3 • **A.** Scoring of peripheral cartilage. Note placement of the 12 o'clock reference mark. **B.** Counterbore reaming of a defect, over the central pin, to a depth of 8 to 10 mm. **C.** Recipient site reamed to subchondral bone and drilled with 2.0-mm drill bit to enhance subchondral bleeding. **D.** Measuring of defect depth.

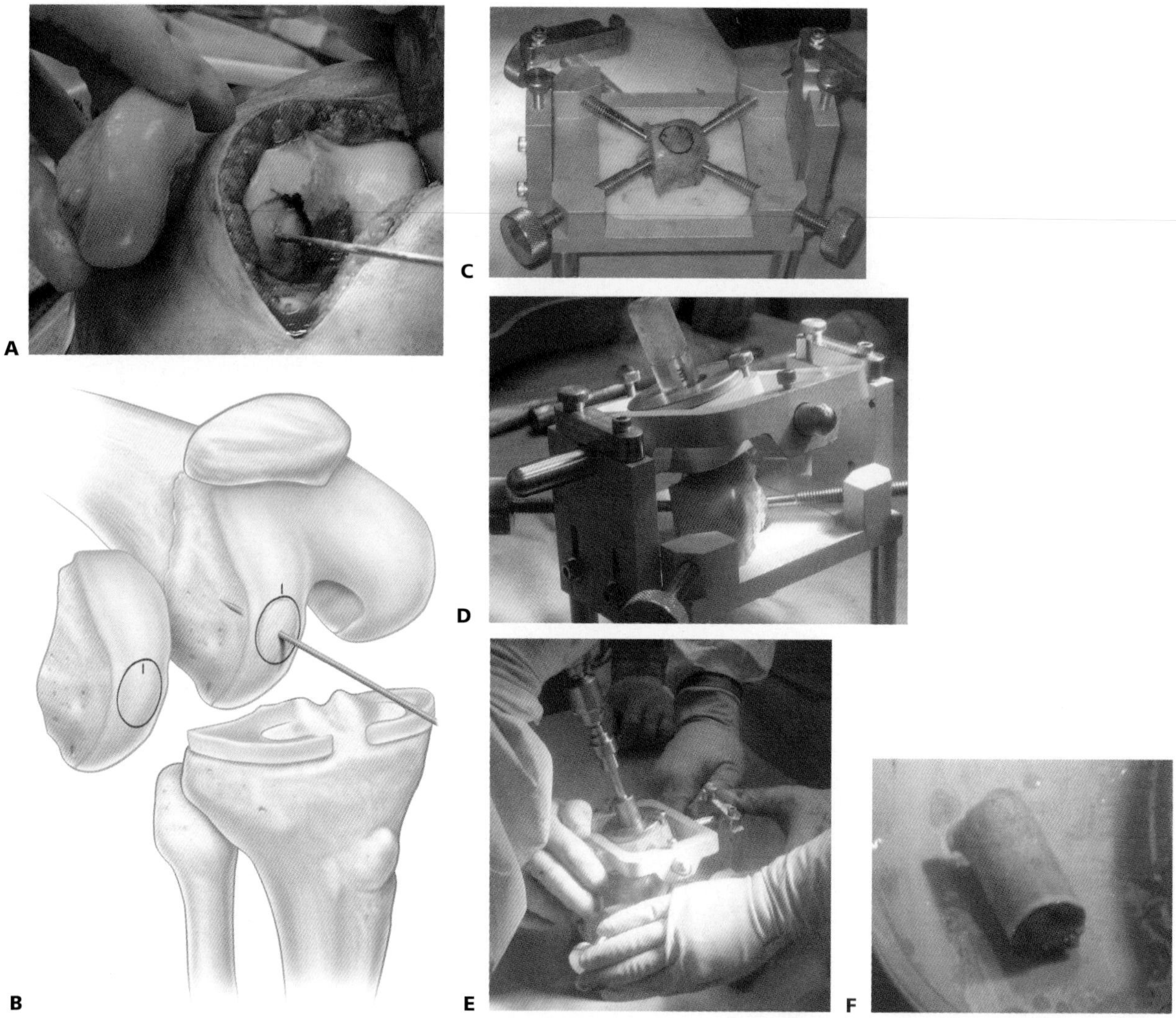

TECH FIG 4 • **A.** Comparing donor hemicondyle to recipient condyle, to specifically localize donor site. **B.** Schematic of intraoperative donor–recipient matching. **C,D.** Donor graft workstation. **E.** Perpendicular drilling of donor condyle. **F.** Precontoured donor plug.

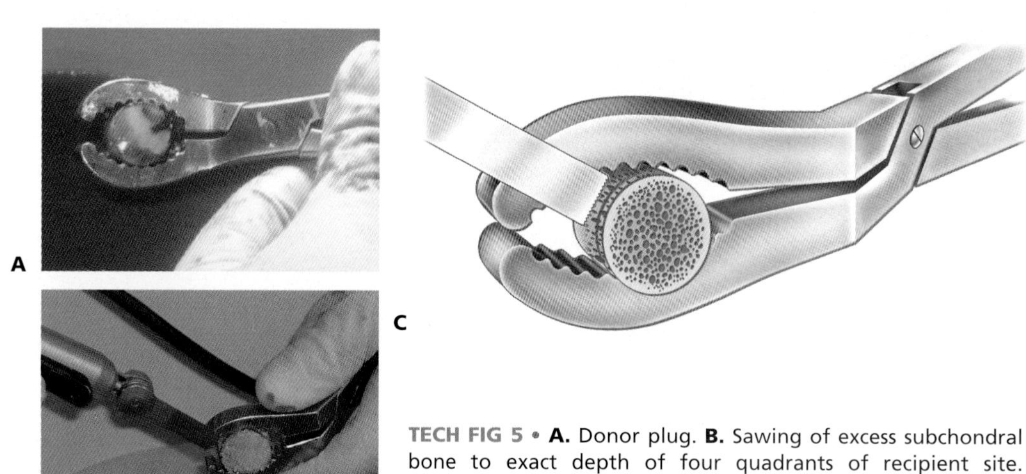

TECH FIG 5 • **A.** Donor plug. **B.** Sawing of excess subchondral bone to exact depth of four quadrants of recipient site. **C.** Diagram of sawing excess bone at precise quadrant levels. *(continued)*

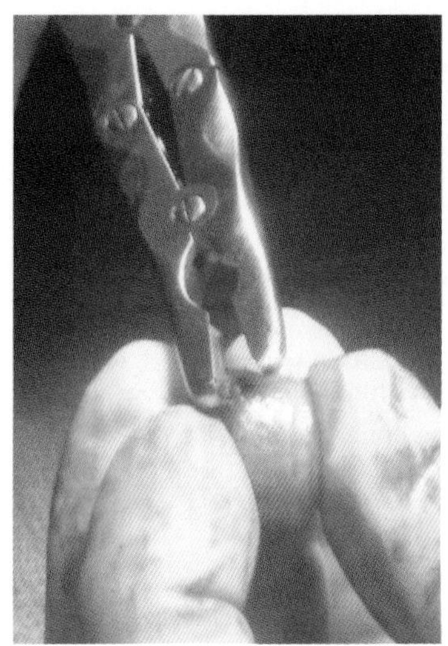

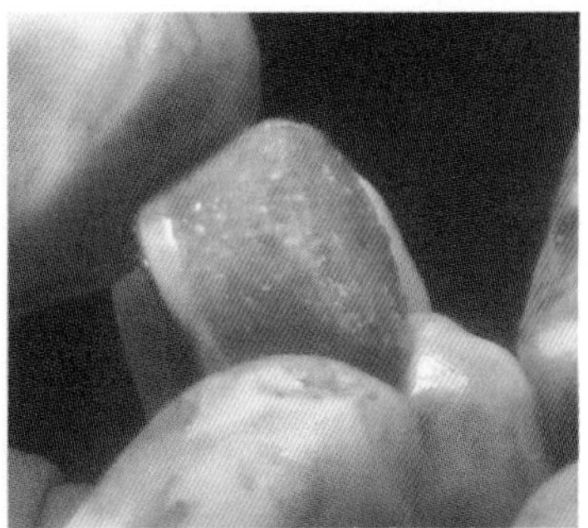

TECH FIG 5 • *(continued)* **D.** Contouring of osteochondral plug. **E.** Fully contoured and "bulletized" osteochondral plug.

- The bony end of the graft's edges should be slightly rounded, or "bulletized," to ease insertion of the graft into the recipient socket (TECH FIG 5D,E).

Delivery

- Before graft insertion, the recipient bed may be further prepared by using a dilator to widen the socket by 0.5 mm and to smooth the socket surfaces. (This step is optional.)
- The graft is then inserted manually, after lining up the 12 o'clock recipient and donor reference marks (TECH FIG 6A). If the press-fit method is inadequate, an appropriately sized tamp is used to gently tap the graft into position (TECH FIG 6B).
- Additional fixation usually is unnecessary (TECH FIG 6C–E).

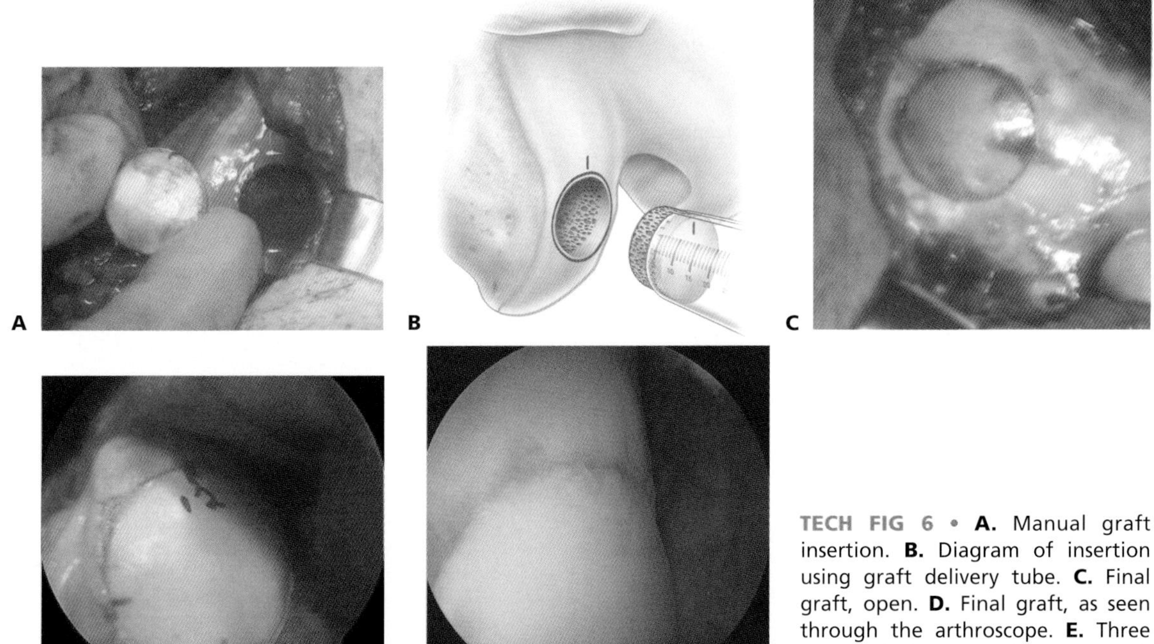

TECH FIG 6 • **A.** Manual graft insertion. **B.** Diagram of insertion using graft delivery tube. **C.** Final graft, open. **D.** Final graft, as seen through the arthroscope. **E.** Three month follow-up, with a second-look arthroscopy.

PEARLS AND PITFALLS

Full-length radiographs to check alignment should be considered in all patients.	■ Malalignment must be corrected before or during the OATS procedure.
Guide pin insertion at the recipient site must be perpendicular and in the center of the lesion. Donor graft must be harvested in same perpendicular plane.	■ Mismatch positioning between recipient and donor will risk early failure of the graft.
Excess donor condyle should be removed with a power saw before it is placed in the workstation.	■ A large condylar block will not fit in the workstation.
Donor graft undergoes pulse lavage before final preparation.	■ Removal of marrow elements from bone will minimize subtle immune response about the allograft plug.
The recipient bed should be drilled with a small, 1.6-mm drill bit to enhance vascular response.	■ Minimal drilling should be done, avoiding fracture of subchondral bone.
Bony edges of the donor plug should be rounded with a rongeur to aid insertion.	■ Sharp edges may make insertion of graft more challenging.

POSTOPERATIVE CARE

- Patients typically are discharged home from same-day surgery.
- An ice cuff about the knee helps alleviate postoperative pain and swelling.
- Bracing is not indicated for isolated OATS.
- Continuous passive motion is begun on day 1 and progressed to full as tolerated; typically 0 to 60 degrees on postoperative day 1, then increased by 5 degrees per day; however, there are no passive range-of-motion restrictions.
- Patients are given strict non–weight-bearing instructions.
- Our preference is strict non–weight bearing for 8 weeks, followed by partial weight bearing for another 4 weeks.
- Patients may be expected to return to full activities by 6 to 8 months.

OUTCOMES

- Gross et al[2] reported on 60 fresh femoral osteochondral allografts at an average of 10 years and 65 fresh tibial plateau osteochondral allografts at 11.8 years (average) with 84% good/excellent results and 86% good/excellent results, respectively, for posttraumatic defects.
  - Kaplan-Meier survivorship analysis determined 95% survival at 5 years, 85% at 10 years, and 74% at 15 years for femoral grafts.
  - Tibial allografts were reported to have 95% survivorship at 5 years, 80% at 10 years, and 65% at 15 years.
  - We determined no negative outcome with meniscal transplant or limb realignment surgery.
- Shasha et al[7] reported the results of 60 fresh femoral allografts for varying etiologies (ie, posttraumatic, osteoarthritis, osteonecrosis, osteochondritis dissecans) with an average follow-up of 10 years.
  - Survivorship data revealed 95% survivorship at 5 years, 85% at 10 years, and 74% at 15 years, with 84% good/excellent results and 12 graft failures.
- Bakay et al[1] reported 22 good/excellent results in 33 patients at 2 years follow-up with cryopreserved or cryoprotected osteochondral allografts in the femur, tibial plateau, and patella.
- Jamali et al[3] reported the results of 20 fresh osteochondral allografts in the patellofemoral joint at 94 months follow-up with 12 good/excellent results and 5 failures.
  - Kaplan-Meier survivorship data determined 67% survivorship at 10 years.

COMPLICATIONS

- Infection
- Stiffness
- Thromboembolic events
- Reflex sympathetic dystrophy
- Graft dislodgment/failure

REFERENCES

1. Bakay A, Csonge L, Papp G, et al. Osteochondral resurfacing of the knee joint with allograft: clinical analysis of 33 cases. Int Orthop 1998;22:277–281.
2. Gross AE, Shasha N, Aubin P. Long-term follow-up of the use of fresh osteochondral allografts for post-traumatic knee defect. Clin Orthop Rel Res 2005;435:79–87.
3. Jamali AA, Emmerson BC, Chung C, et al. Fresh osteochondral allografts. Clin Orthop Rel Res 2005;437:176–185.
4. Kwan MK, Wayne JS, Woo SL, et al. Histological and biomechanical assessment of articular cartilage from stored osteochondral shell allografts. J Orthop Res 1989;7:637–644.
5. Linden B, Malmo S. Osteochondritis dissecans of the femoral condyles. J Bone Joint Surg Am 1977;59:769–776.
6. Shahgaldi BF, Amis A, Heatley FW. Repair of cartilage lesions using biological implants. A comparative histological and biomechanical study in goats. J Bone Joint Surg 1991;73B:57–65.
7. Shasha N, Aubin PP, Cheah HK, et al. Long-term clinical experience with fresh osteochondral allografts for articular knee defects in high demand patients. Cell and Tissue Banking 2002;3:175–182.

Chapter 40 Osteochondritis Dissecans and Avascular Necrosis

Mark J. Billante and David R. Diduch

DEFINITION

- Osteochondritis dissecans (OCD), avascular necrosis (AVN), spontaneous osteonecrosis of the knee, and chondral and osteochondral lesions all occur at or beneath the articular surface of a weight-bearing joint and are easily confused (**FIG 1**).
- OCD lesions occur when a segment of subchondral bone becomes avascular. The wafer of bone plus the overlying articular cartilage may become separated from the underlying bone.
- Chondral lesions on the articular surface do not penetrate subchondral bone; damage is to chondrocytes and extracellular matrix, and there is no inflammatory healing response.
- Osteochondral lesions not only damage articular cartilage but also penetrate subchondral bone, and, therefore, cause an inflammatory healing response.
- AVN occurs when a larger wedge segment of bone loses its blood supply. If the necrosis extends to the subchondral bone, this can lead to subchondral fracture and bone surface collapse.
- In OCD, the avascular fragment separates from a normal, vascular bony bed beneath a sclerotic rim. In AVN the avascular osteochondral surface breaks into multiple fragments and separates from an avascular bed.

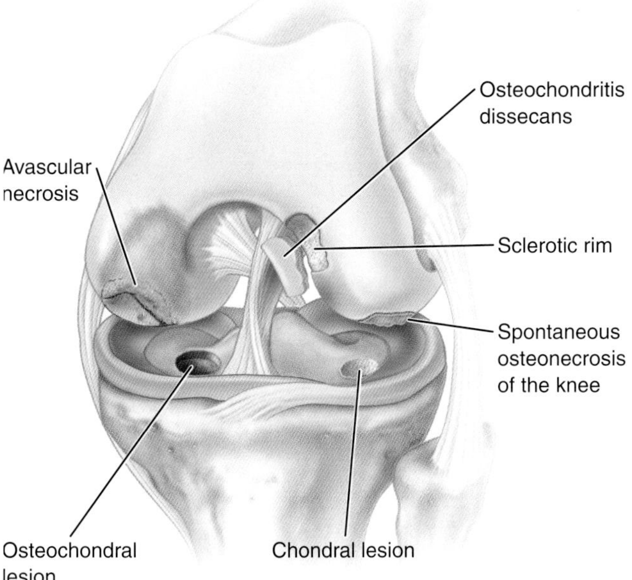

FIG 1 • Avascular necrosis involves a large avascular bony segment, possibly extending to subchondral bone. Osteochondritis dissecans is distinguished by an avascular bony wafer plus overlying cartilage. An osteochondral lesion involves the articular cartilage plus underlying bone, whereas a chondral lesion involves the articular surface only. Spontaneous osteonecrosis of the knee involves focal stress fracture of subchondral bone plate with collapse.

- Spontaneous osteonecrosis of the knee involves a stress fracture of the subchondral bone with secondary collapse. It often is seen in patients post-meniscectomy or with meniscal subluxation.

ANATOMY

Osteochondritis Dissecans

- OCD lesions most often are found in the knee. They also occur commonly in the capitellum and talus.
- In the knee, OCD lesions involve the medial femoral condyle 80% to 85% of the time, the lateral femoral condyle 10% to 15% of the time, and the trochlea less than 1% of the time. Patellar lesions are uncommon, seen in only 5% to 10% of cases, and typically occur in the inferomedial area.[4,7,8]
- Classic lesions occur in the lateral aspect of the medial femoral condyle. Lateral lesions most often are located in the inferocentral region and involve a significant portion of the weight-bearing surface (**FIG 2**).

Avascular Necrosis

- AVN most commonly is seen in the hip. The knee is the second most common location, but accounts for only about 10% as many cases as the hip. AVN can affect the femur, tibia, or both; is bilateral in over 80% of cases; and usually involves multiple condyles (**FIG 3A**).
- AVN involves a larger area of subchondral bone, with extension into the epiphysis and even the metaphysis or diaphysis.

Spontaneous Osteonecrosis of the Knee

- Spontaneous osteonecrosis of the knee is different from AVN. Spontaneous osteonecrosis of the knee occurs in patients older than 55 years, involves only one condyle (most commonly medial), and is unilateral in 99% of cases (**FIG 3B,C**).
- The pathologic lesion in spontaneous osteonecrosis of the knee is a stress fracture of subchondral bone with collapse of the articular surface and secondary joint incongruity and pain.

PATHOGENESIS

Osteochondritis Dissecans

- The definitive cause of OCD lesions remains elusive. Several theories exist, including trauma, ischemia, abnormal ossification involving the physes, genetic predisposition, and combinations of these. Prominent theories are further discussed in the following paragraphs, with most authors suspecting that repetitive stress plays a central role.
- Repetitive microtrauma may create a stress fracture within subchondral bone. If the microtrauma continues and overwhelms the ability of the subchondral bone to heal, necrosis may occur, leading to separation and nonunion of the segment.[4]
- The epiphyseal artery supplies the epiphysis and secondary centers of ossification.
  - Repetitive microtrauma or a trauma in a growing child to one of these small end arteries with a tenuous blood supply

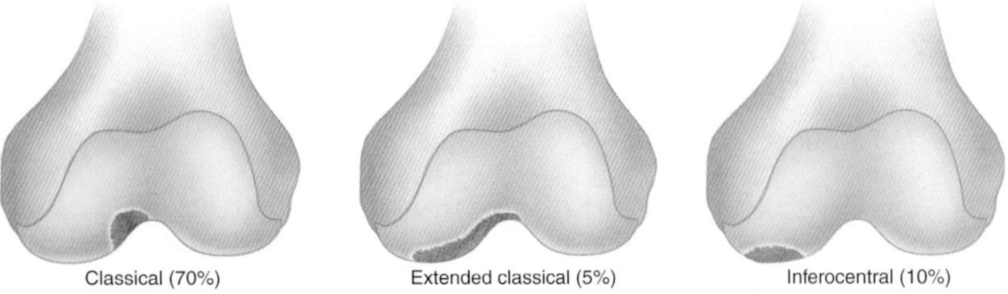

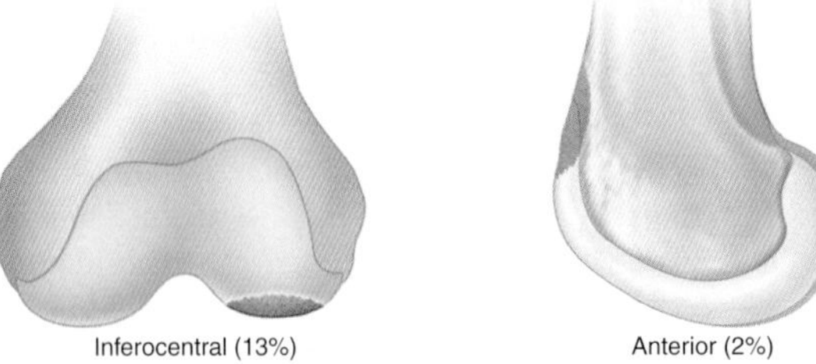

FIG 2 • Locations of OCD in the knee. (Adapted from Williams JS Jr, Bush-Joseph CA, Bach BR. Osteochondritis dissecans of the knee: a review. Am J Knee Surg 1998;11:221–232.)

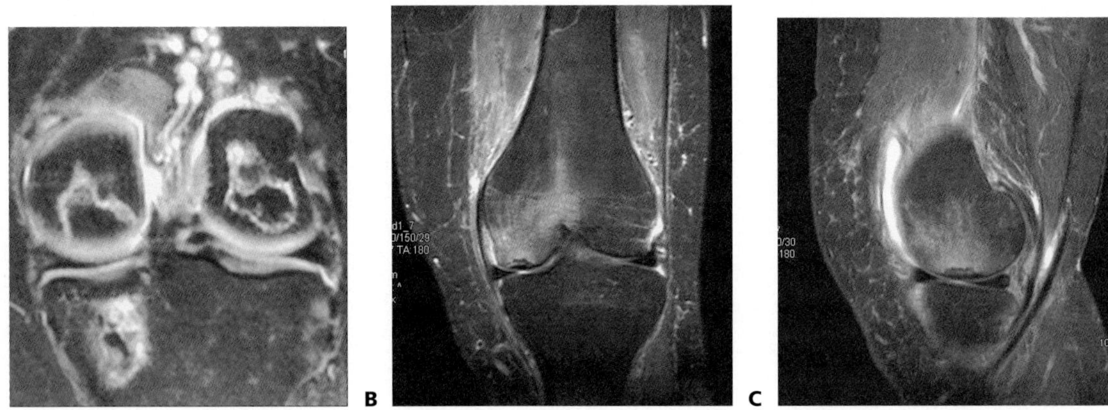

FIG 3 • **A.** MRI scan of AVN involving multiple condyles with extension into the metaphysis. **B,C.** MRI scans of spontaneous osteonecrosis of the knee involving the medial condyle only. Note the edema adjacent to the involved area.

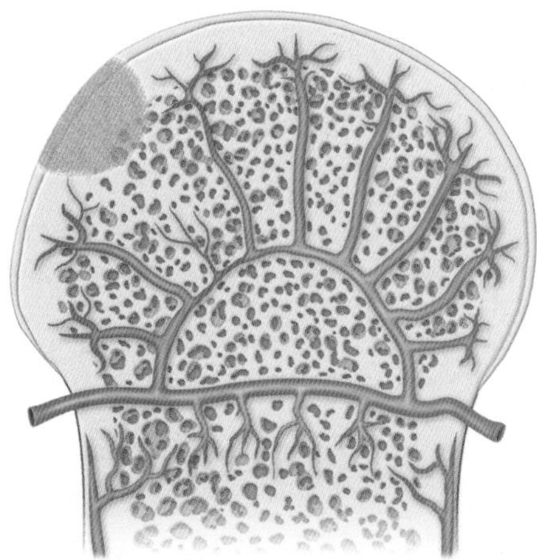

FIG 4 • Osteochondritis lesions can occur from an interruption of the epiphyseal blood supply to a specific area. (Adapted from Williams JS Jr, Bush-Joseph CA, Bach BR. Osteochondritis dissecans of the knee: a review. Am J Knee Surg 1998;11:221–232.)

can result in disruption of the vascular supply to the segment, with resultant development of an OCD lesion[8] (**FIG 4**).

- The alteration of subchondral vascularity is precipitated by insult at a vulnerable point.
  - In juvenile cases, revascularization can occur.
  - In most situations, however, healing is inadequate, and persistent avascularity of the fragment, along with mechanical forces at the subchondral region, leads to articular surface fracture.
- Synovial fluid pumped into the bone around the fragment via knee motion limits healing by preventing fibrin clot formation. The pressurized fluid can even erode bone and create a cystic defect. Loss of fragment stability results in loose body formation.
- Shear stress may be created by the medial tibial spine abutting the medial femoral condyle, possibly coupled with traction from the posterior cruciate ligament origin. However, this theory does not account for the presence of lesions at other locations and the fact that tibial eminence impingement does not occur in connection with normal walking or running.

Avascular Necrosis

- AVN of the knee has been called *ischemic, idiopathic,* or *corticosteroid-associated necrosis.*
  - As with AVN of the hip, necrotic bone leads to subchondral fracture and subsequent joint collapse.[5]
- Similar to OCD lesions, AVN occurs from interruption of blood supply to a segment of bone, but in AVN the interruption is nontraumatic and may involve the epiphysis and also extend into the metaphysis.

NATURAL HISTORY

Osteochondritis Dissecans

- OCD lesions occur in between 15 and 21 per 100,000 population, with a peak between the ages of 10 and 15 years.
- They are more common in males, by a 5:3 ratio.
- A history of previous knee trauma is seen in 40% to 60% of patients.
- Lesions are bilateral in 15% to 30% of patients, usually prompting evaluation of both knees after making the diagnosis.
  - If lesions are bilateral, they typically are in different phases of development.
- Patient maturity aids in prediction of treatment outcome.
  - Juvenile cases with open physes have a high (65% to 75%) potential to heal.
  - Results in adolescent cases are less predictable. About 50% do go on to heal, but the remainder have a progressive, nonhealing course similar to that of adult (ie, patients with closed physes) patients.
  - In skeletally mature patients, healing potential is essentially nonexistent.
- Factors affecting prognosis include size and site of the lesion, fragment stability, joint fluid behind the fragment, status of the articular surface, and duration of the disorder.

Avascular Necrosis

- AVN of the knee occurs most often in patients younger than 55 years of age, involves multiple condyles, and is bilateral more than 80% of the time.
- Patients have AVN in other large joints in 60% to 90% of cases, are predominantly women, and often have a history of systemic lupus erythematosus, sickle cell disease, alcoholism, or systemic corticosteroid use.
- In general, only AVN involving the epiphysis is clinically important. Here, loss of structural support can lead to collapse and fragmentation of the overlying joint surface, resulting in a painful arthritic joint (**FIG 5**).

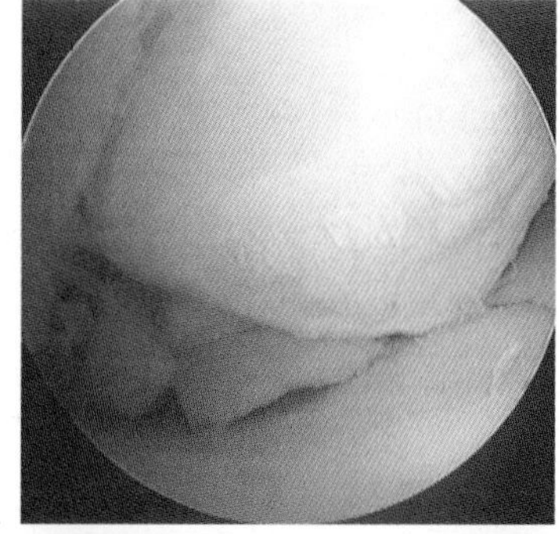
A

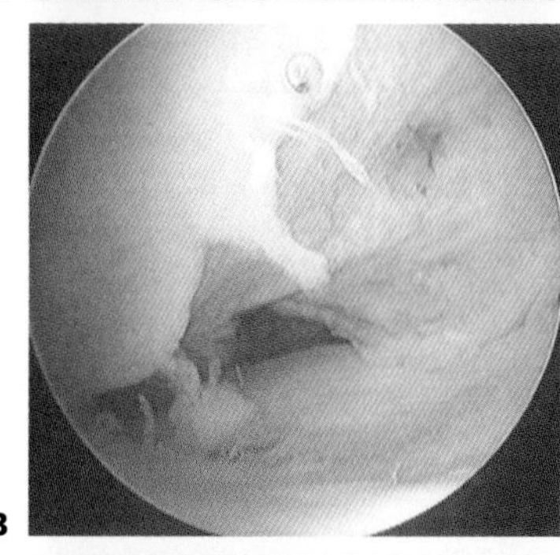
B

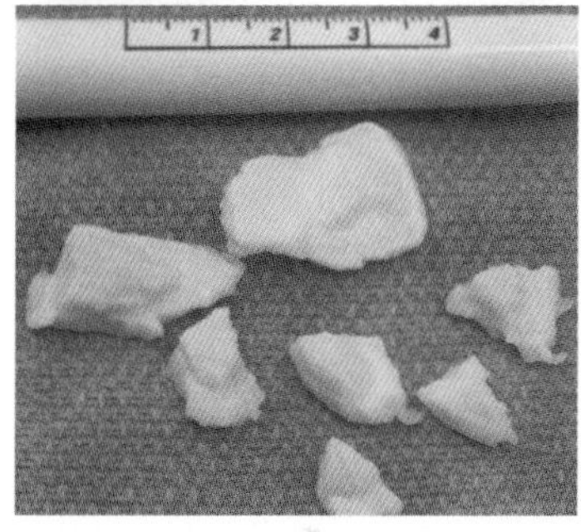
C

FIG 5 • **A.** Fragmentation of the distal femoral condyle with multiple loose bodies. **B.** After débridement of the femoral condyle and removal of loose bodies. **C.** Fragments after arthroscopic removal. (Reprinted with permission from Diduch DR, Hampton BJ. Avascular necrosis drilling in the knee. In: Miller MD, Cole BJ, eds. Textbook of Arthroscopy. Philadelphia: Elsevier, 2004:593–599.)

PATIENT HISTORY AND PHYSICAL FINDINGS

Osteochondritis Dissecans

- Vague, poorly localized complaints of knee pain often are the initial presentation for OCD lesions.
- Swelling is important to note, because an effusion strongly suggests that the fragment is loose to at least some degree.
- Loose or detached lesions may have mechanical symptoms such as crepitus, catching, or locking. These symptoms can mimic meniscal pathology.
  - Symptoms tend to progress with time as continued activity causes a stable lesion to become unstable.

- Quadriceps atrophy may be present as a late finding with chronic lesions.
- Loss of range of motion is uncommon. Pain with range of motion, crepitus, or mechanical symptoms may represent an unstable lesion.
- Wilson's sign is specific for medial femoral condyle lesions and is tested for by flexing the knee to 90 degrees, then internally rotating and slowly extending it.
  - Patients develop pain (positive Wilson's sign) at approximately 30 degrees as the tibial spine abuts against the medial femoral condyle; pain is relieved with external rotation.
  - According to recent studies, this sign may lack sensitivity.[8]
- Patients may walk with an antalgic gait, externally rotating the affected leg to avoid contact of the tibial spine against the medial femoral condyle in the classic lesion.
- Tenderness to direct palpation of the lesion (Axhausen's sign) is found in patients with subchondral instability and is a helpful indicator of progressive healing as the sign abates.

Avascular Necrosis

- Patients with AVN have insidious onset of knee pain.
- The pain may be medial, lateral, or diffuse.
- Mild effusions and joint line tenderness may be present.
- The physical examination often is unremarkable.

IMAGING AND OTHER DIAGNOSTIC STUDIES

Osteochondritis Dissecans

- In OCD, plain films help to localize and characterize the lesion while also providing valuable information regarding skeletal maturity and age of the lesion, and ruling out other bony injuries.
- Radiographic evaluation should include anteroposterior (AP), lateral, tunnel, and sunrise views (**FIG 6A,B**).
  - Tunnel views provide visualization of the femoral condyles in greater profile than can be obtained with AP views (**FIG 6C,D**). The tunnel view often is the most revealing view

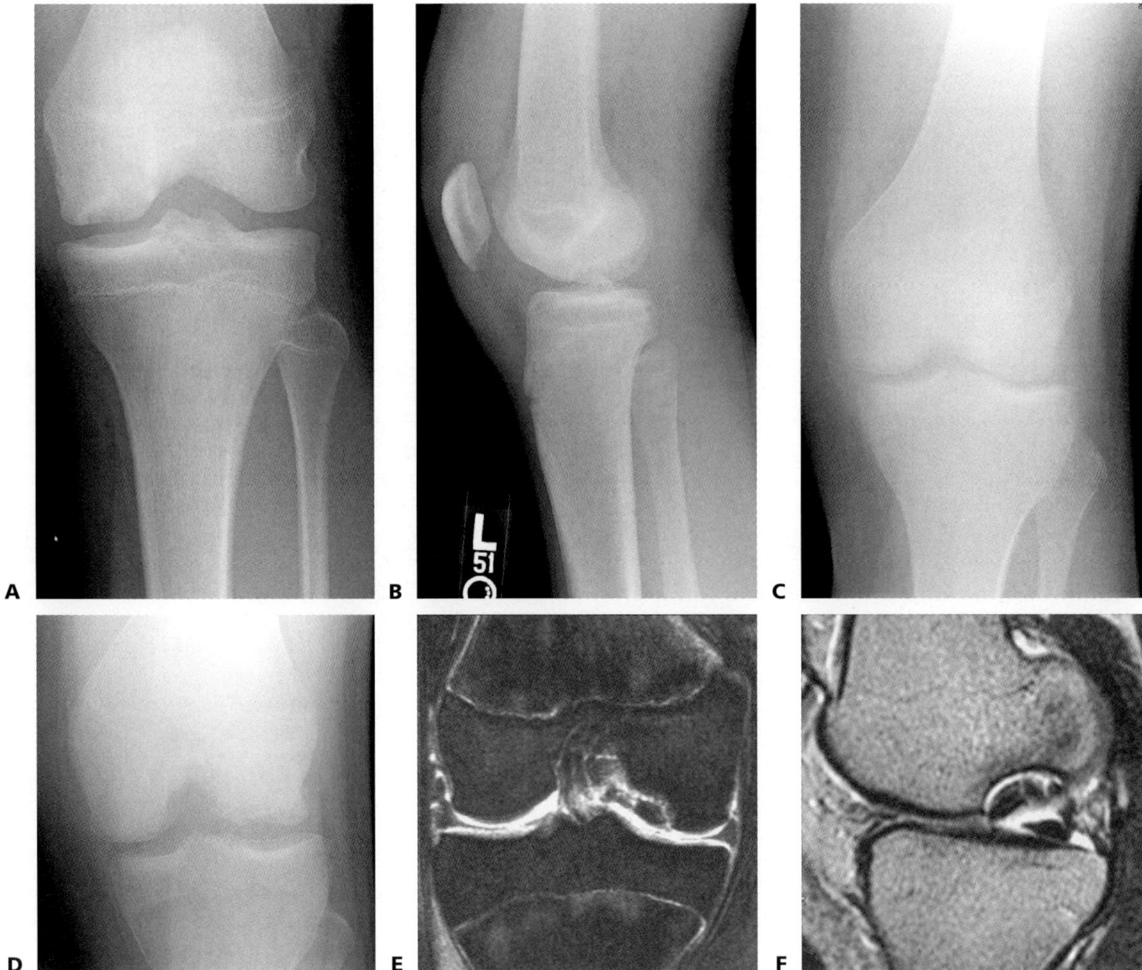

FIG 6 • **A,B.** AP and lateral views demonstrating a lesion in the medial femoral condyle. **C,D.** AP and tunnel views demonstrating an OCD lesion of the lateral femoral condyle. The femoral condyles are in greater profile in the tunnel view, making the lesion easier to appreciate. **E,F.** Coronal and sagittal MRI images of an OCD lesion. Note the joint fluid present beneath the lesion.

because OCD lesions commonly are located on the lateral aspect of the medial femoral condyle.

- Comparison views of the opposite knee should be considered, because 15% to 30% of cases are bilateral.
- Children younger than 7 years of age may have irregularities of the distal femoral ossification centers that simulate OCD lesions. These represent anatomic variants of normal ossification and are asymptomatic.

- MRI is an essential part of the diagnostic evaluation of OCD.
  - It provides critical information regarding the status of cartilage and subchondral bone, size of the lesion, presence of fluid beneath the lesion, extent of bony edema, as well as loose bodies or other knee injuries (**FIG 6E,F**).
  - DeSmet et al[2] found four MRI criteria that are negatively correlated with the ability of OCD lesions to heal after nonoperative treatment: a line of high signal intensity beneath the lesion, indicating synovial fluid, that (1) is at least 5 mm long; (2) is at least 5 mm thick; or (3) communicates with the joint surface; and (4) a focal defect of 5 mm or more in the articular surface.
    - The high-signal line was found in 72% of unstable lesions and was the most common sign in patients who failed nonoperative treatment.[2,6]
- Historically, Cahill and Berg advocated the use of serial technetium 99m bone scans for evaluation of healing.[9] This recommendation was based on the relation between blood flow and osteoblastic activity with scintigraphic activity.
  - Unfortunately, the isotropic tracer remains in the affected area well after healing, making interpretation difficult.
  - The use of serial bone scans for the management of OCD lesions has not been universally accepted, in large part because of the need for intravenous access, time required for the study, and, more importantly, the emergence of MRI.

Avascular Necrosis

- For patients with AVN, plain radiographs and MRI scans should be obtained.
- Once the diagnosis of AVN is established, screening MRI of both hips should be considered.

DIFFERENTIAL DIAGNOSIS

- Normal accessory ossification centers
- Loose bodies
- Meniscus pathology
- Acute osteochondral fracture
- Avascular necrosis
- Epiphyseal dysplasia

NONOPERATIVE MANAGEMENT

Osteochondritis Dissecans

- Initial nonoperative treatment is indicated in children with open physes because of the favorable natural history in this patient population.
  - Cahill reported that 50% of juvenile OCD lesions will heal within 10 to 18 months if the physis remains open and patient compliance is maintained.[10]
- Most authors agree that 6 weeks of protected weight bearing followed by 6 weeks of activity modification and reevaluation with radiographs plus MRI at 3 months constitutes an adequate trial of nonoperative treatment.
- Children present unique challenges with regard to compliance.
  - Some authors advocate use of a knee immobilizer as part of the nonoperative regimen, believing that the combination of a stable lesion, non–weight bearing, knee immobilization, and daily range-of-motion exercises followed by activity modification will result in successful healing by 3 to 6 months in over 90% of cases.
  - Although no randomized prospective data have been released to support use of a knee immobilizer, a brace may be useful to increase compliance with the nonoperative regimen in this difficult patient population.
- Nonoperative management rarely is indicated in the symptomatic adult population because of the unremitting course of the disease.
  - After closure of the physis, healing capacity is greatly reduced, and the possibility of instability, loosening, and subsequent detatchment of the lesion is high.
  - Careful evaluation of adolescent patients nearing skeletal maturity is necessary, because their healing ability also is decreased compared to that of younger patients.
  - Aggressive and early operative intervention usuallly is indicated to preserve the integrity of the joint.

Avascular Necrosis

- In AVN, initial treatment with analgesics, nonsteroidal anti-inflammatory medications, and protected weight bearing for 3 months represents an adequate trial of nonoperative management.
- If symptoms persist, surgical intervention should be considered.

SURGICAL MANAGEMENT

Osteochondritis Dissecans

- In OCD, operative treatment goals are to maintain joint congruity, rigidly fix unstable fragments, and repair osteochondral defects, thereby reducing symptoms and preventing additional cartilage deterioration (**FIG 7**).
- Operative treatment should be performed in skeletally immature patients with unstable or detached lesions, and also in patients who are approaching physeal closure whose lesions have failed nonoperative intervention.
- Surgical intervention in OCD begins with arthroscopy. The stability of the lesion and the intergrity of the overlying cartilage can be assessed directly.
  - Arthroscopic drilling of juvenile OCD lesions is appropriate in patients who have failed nonoperative management in lesions that remain stable with intact articular surfaces. Drilling aims to create channels for possible revascularization and healing.
  - Retrograde drilling across the epiphysis avoids penetration of the articular surface but is technically demanding in terms of drill depth and placement accuracy.
  - Antegrade transarticular drilling is straightforward and creates channels that heal with fibrocartilage on the joint surface.
  - Arthroscopic drilling and fixation in situ can be performed for stable or minimally unstable lesions without evidence of articular cartilage disruption or fluid behind the fragment on MRI.

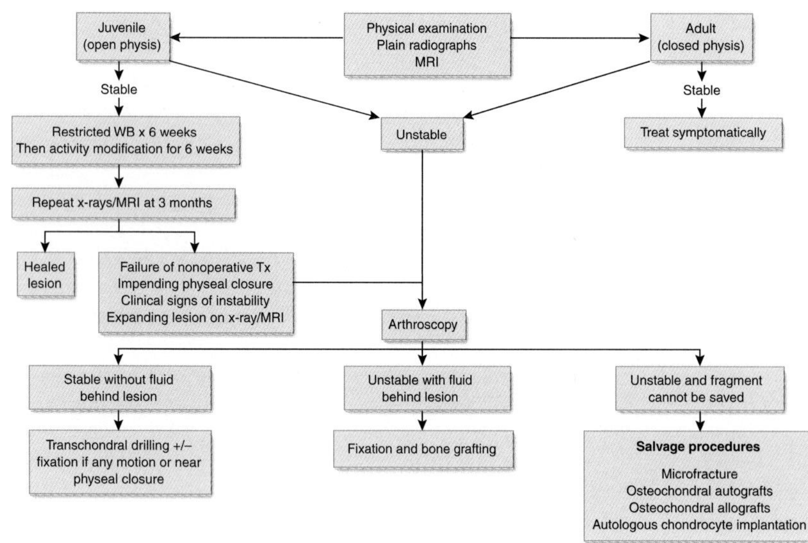

FIG 7 • Treatment algorithm for OCD lesions.

- Fixation can be accomplished by a variety of open or arthroscopic methods, including Kirschner wires, cannulated screws, headless variable pitch compression screws, bone pegs, and bioabsorbable implants. Nonabsorbable fixation requires an additional surgery for hardware removal.
  - Unstable lesions have fibrous tissue and a sclerotic bony rim behind them that is best removed to allow healing to occur (**FIG 8**). Furthermore, any joint fluid beneath a fragment will prevent formation of a fibrin clot, thereby preventing the first step necessary for bony healing.
  - Unstable lesions with subchondral bone loss should be grafted with autogenous bone graft packed into the defect before fragment reduction and subsequent fixation.
    - Bone grafting fills any voids that would prevent the fragment from sitting flush with the surrounding articular cartilage. Local autogenous bone graft sources include the distal femur and proximal tibia.
  - Patients with completely unstable lesions (loose bodies) that have subchondral bone attached can be trimmed to match the defect, bone grafted, and fixed primarily.
- Several salvage options are available for lesions that cannot be repaired primarily.
  - Débridement and lavage are used for incidentally discovered lesions or those not involving a major weight-bearing area in patients with mostly mechanical symptoms. No attempt is made to repair or replace the damaged articular surface.
  - Marrow-stimulating techniques (eg, drilling, abrasion arthroplasty, or microfracture) promote a healing response in the form of fibrocartilage in the area of the lesion.
  - Restorative techniques replace damaged areas with new articular cartilage. These include osteochondral autografting, osteochondral allografting, and autologous chondrocyte implantation.

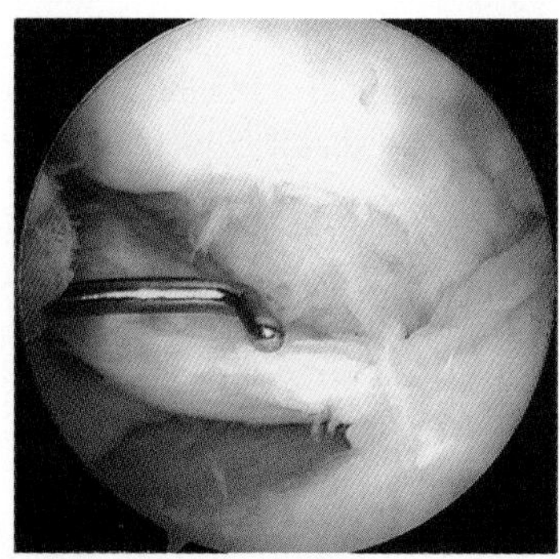

FIG 8 • Arthroscopic image of medial femoral condyle OCD lesion. The probe is used to hinge the lesion open, demonstrating fibrous tissue beneath lesion.

Avascular Necrosis

- Surgical treatment of AVN can include arthroscopic débridement, arthroscopic drilling, core decompression, or high tibial osteotomy.
- Core decompression has been shown to be relatively successful for symptomatic subchondral lesions prior to collapse.
- Resurfacing with osteoarticular allografts or autografts is not generally favored because the bony bed is dead.
- For patients with collapse and secondary arthrosis, unicompartmental arthroplasty and total knee arthroplasty are additional options.

Preoperative Planning

Osteochondritis Dissecans

- Plain radiographs should be reviewed for growth plate status, localization of lesion in both AP and lateral planes, presence or absence of sclerosis, and possible loose bodies.
- MRI scans should be reviewed for accurate estimate of lesion size, status of cartilage and subchondral bone, high-signal zone beneath the fragment, bony edema, presence of loose bodies, or concomitant intra-articular pathology. In particular, the presence of joint fluid or cystic erosions behind the fragment determines the need for bone grafting.

Avascular Necrosis

- In AVN, plain films evaluate for evidence of collapse and secondary arthrosis (**FIG 9**). Once present, core decompression is not indicated.
- MRI aids in determining the location and extent of subchondral bone involvement. Only lesions extending to subchondral

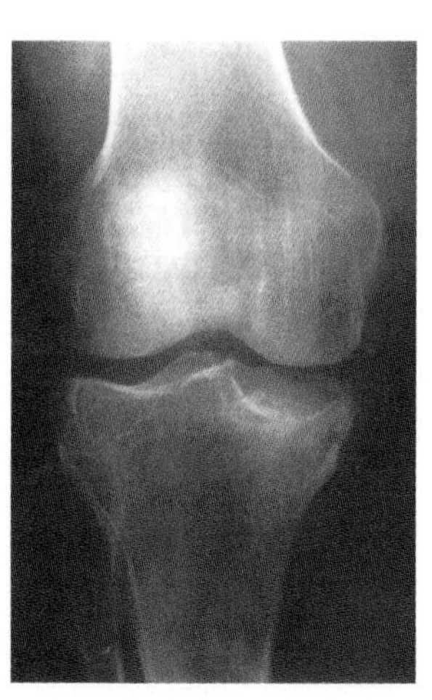

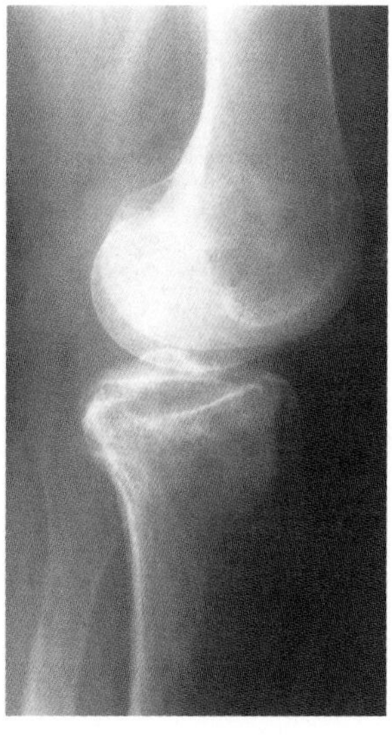

FIG 9 • AP and lateral radiographs demonstrating collapse of the tibial surface in AVN. (Reprinted with permission from Diduch DR, Hampton BJ. Avascular necrosis drilling in the knee. In: Miller MD, Cole BJ, eds. Textbook of Arthroscopy. Philadelphia: Elsevier, 2004:593–599.)

bone are at risk for collapse and, therefore, appropriate for core decompression.

Positioning

- Patients are postitioned supine.
- Retrograde drilling of femoral lesions is aided by placing an image intensifier on the opposite side of a radiolucent table to facilitate intraoperative imaging.
- A tourniquet is placed on the operative thigh, and a lateral post is used to stabilize the extremity for valgus stress. The post also facilitates hip rotation in the figure 4 position, allowing lateral knee access and ease in obtaining lateral imaging.
- The extremity is then prepared and draped, the tourniquet is inflated, and diagnostic arthroscopy is performed.

Approach

- Lesions may be approached using standard arthroscopic techniques.
- The surgeon should have a low threshold for making a limited medial or lateral arthrotomy for direct access to the lesion. It is crucial to be perpendicular to the lesion for placement of hardware or osteochondral grafting.

TECHNIQUES

TRANSCHONDRAL DRILLING OF INTACT OCD LESIONS WITH OR WITHOUT FIXATION

- Drilling can be accomplished using either an antegrade or retrograde technique (TECH FIG 1A).
  - Antegrade techniques are technically easier but violate the articular cartilage.
  - Retrograde techniques avoid violation of the articular surface but involve the technical challenges of maintaining drill depth and placement accuracy, and also require the use of fluoroscopy. A cannulated anterior cruciate ligament (ACL) guide is useful for guiding Kirschner wire placement.
- First, a thorough diagnostic arthroscopy is completed.
  - Careful inspection of the affected condyle is accomplished by varying the degree of knee flexion. Subtle irregularity at the borders of the lesion is looked for; the remaining articular cartilage will appear smooth.
  - The lesion is probed along its borders to ensure that there are no discontinuities in the articular cartilage overlying the subchondral bone (TECH FIG 1B).
- Once the presence of an intact lesion has been verified, several drill holes are made in the lesion using a 0.062-inch Kirschner wire (TECH FIG 1C,D).

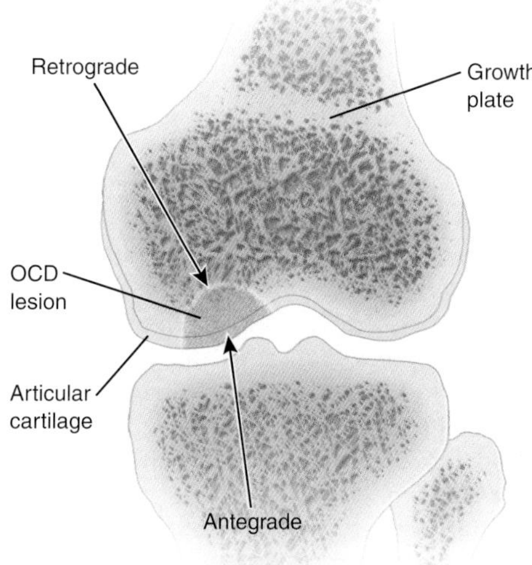

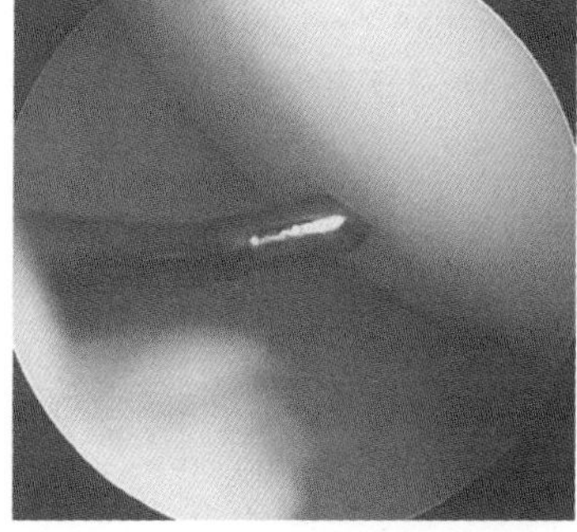

TECH FIG 1 • **A.** Retrograde and antegrade drilling of osteochondritis dissecans (OCD) lesions. **B.** Probe seen indenting the edge of an OCD lesion. *(continued)*

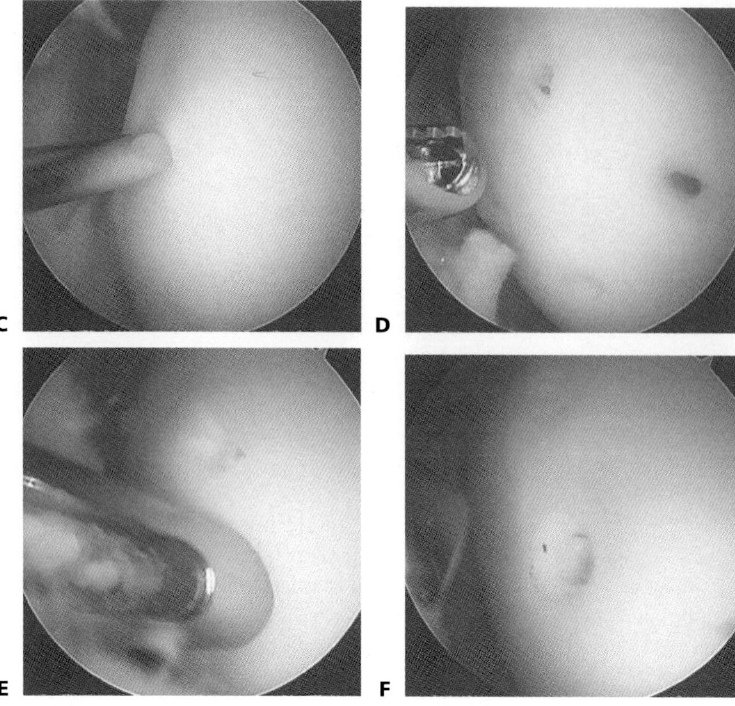

TECH FIG 1 • *(continued)* **C.** Multiple drill holes are made in the lesion. **D.** Wire positioned perpendicular to surface prior to antegrade drilling of lesion. **E.** Absorbable fixation placed perpendicular to the surface of the lesion. **F.** Absorbable fixation countersunk beneath surface of the lesion. (**B–F:** Reprinted with permission from Diduch DR, Hampton BJ. Avascular necrosis drilling in the knee. In: Miller MD, Cole BJ, eds. Textbook of Arthroscopy. Philadelphia: Elsevier, 2004:593–599.)

  - The wire must be positioned perpendicular to the surface.
  - A soft tissue protector or drill sleeve is used over the wire.
- Surgeons should use whichever portal provides perpendicular access to the lesion, whether anteromedial or anterolateral. Large lesions may require use of both portals to access the entire lesion.
- Drilling to a depth of 1.5 to 2 cm is done to encourage vascular access to the lesion. In skeletally immature patients, careful limitation of depth is essential to avoid penetration of the physis.
- If any motion can be created by pressing against the fragment, or if the patient is approaching skeletal maturity, fixation of the fragment also should be performed.
  - Absorbable fixation options include "headed" nails with barbs at the tip to provide compression, our preferred technique (TECH FIG 1E,F); screws, which have more potential to cause joint surface damage; or smooth pins, which require varied angles of insertion to hold the fragment.
  - Metal fixation options include lag screws, variable pitch fully threaded screws, or Kirschner wires (less compression).

PRIMARY FIXATION AND BONE GRAFTING OF OSTEOCHONDRITIS DISSECANS LESIONS

- Primary fixation of OCD lesions of the knee should be attempted whenever possible.
- The presence of subchondral bone on the undersurface of the lesion is a prerequisite for success of primary fixation. A lesion made of cartilage alone will not heal (TECH FIG 2A).
- First, a diagnostic arthroscopy is performed. Once the lesion is identified it is probed and examined for any fibrous tissue in the bed of the lesion.
- The surgeon should have a low threshold for making a mini-arthrotomy for direct access and visualization of the lesion. This facilitates fixation perpendicular to the fragment, thereby maximizing stability and the compression obtained.
  - Mini-arthrotomies can be made by extension of the anteromedial or anterolateral portal, depending on the location of the lesion. Care must be taken to avoid injury to the anterior horn of the meniscus during distal extension of the arthrotomy.
- A limited fat pad excision is helpful to improve visualization.
- Anterior and posterior lesions can be visualized by varying extention or flexion of the knee.
- A curette is used to remove fibrous tissue from both the bed and the undersurface of the lesion until exposed bleeding bone is seen. The arthroscopic burr can help penetrate the dense sclerotic rim.
- Reduction of the fragment is then performed either manually or with Kirschner wires.
  - It is imperative that the reduction sit flush with the articular surface.
  - Any stepoff will result in increased contact stress and shear forces secondary to surface irregularity, with resultant edge loading.

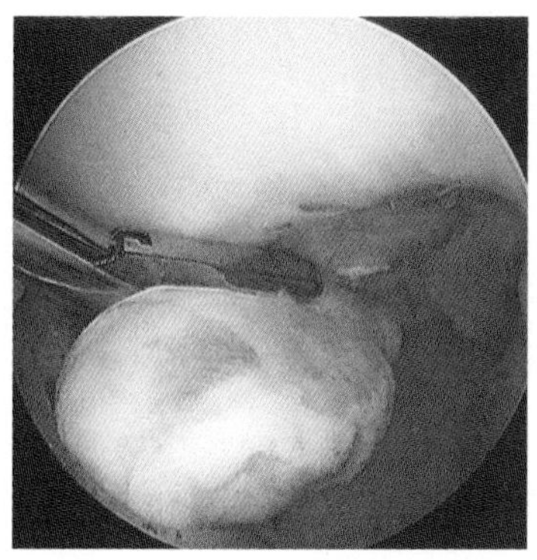

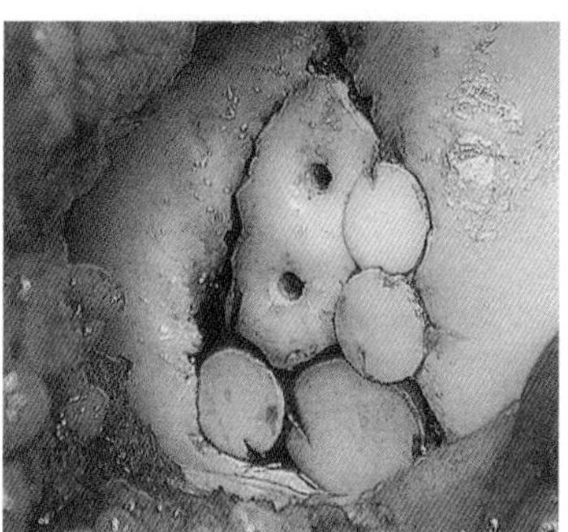

TECH FIG 2 • **A.** Subchondral bone on the undersurface of the OCD fragment appears yellow. **B.** Two absorbable nails used for fixation after bone grafting of large OCD lesion. The remainder of the lesion is filled with four osteochondral autograft plugs, which also provide supplemental fixation. (Reprinted with permission from Diduch DR, Hampton BJ. Avascular necrosis drilling in the knee. In: Miller MD, Cole BJ, eds. Textbook of Arthroscopy. Philadelphia: Elsevier, 2004:593–599.)

- Bone grafting is essential, therefore, to avoid malreduction of the fragment.
- Cancellous autograft can be harvested from local sources such as Gerdy's tubercle on the tibia, or the outer aspect of the distal femur below the physis.
  - In both cases the periosteum is incised, and then a small cortical window is made with an osteotome. A curette is used to harvest the cancellous bone.
  - The cortical window is then replaced, and the periosteum is repaired over the defect.
  - The bone graft is impacted into the bed, followed by repeat reduction and assessment of the chondral surface.
- Fixation is achieved by placing the device perpendicular to the surface.
  - Screw heads should be countersunk beneath the chondral surface to avoid hardware problems.
  - Multiple fixation points may be necessary, depending on the size of the lesion.
  - Combining types or techniques of fixation is acceptable. For instance, a compression screw may be placed centrally in a lesion surrounded by absorbable pins at the periphery of the lesion to enhance fixation. Also, if only a portion of the lesion has subchondral bone attached, it is acceptable to fix that portion of the lesion and use osteochondral plug autografts to fill the remainder of the defect (TECH FIG 2B).
  - Overtightening of screws used for fixation must be avoided. Overly aggressive compression can fracture the fragment.
- Final inspection should demonstrate a congruent reduction with secure fixation of the lesion.

DRILLING OF AVASCULAR NECROSIS IN THE KNEE

- Either an antegrade or a retrograde technique can be used in the femur.

Retrograde Drilling of the Femur

- Retrograde techniques are preferred because they permit creation of a larger channel for a more effective core decompression.
  - Retrograde drilling of femoral lesions requires fluoroscopy plus arthroscopy.
- A 2.4-mm guidewire is used to pierce from skin down to bone.
- The starting point is verified with fluoroscopy in both the AP and lateral planes.
- The guidewire is advanced to within 1–2 mm of the articular surface (TECH FIG 3A).
- Position of the wire is confirmed on the lateral projection by placing a probe against the target condyle's distal articular surface. This technique helps avoid confusion created by overlapping shadows when identifying the target condyle (TECH FIG 3B).

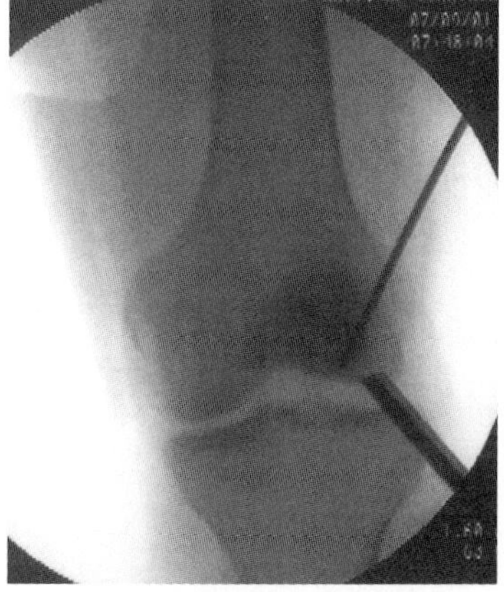

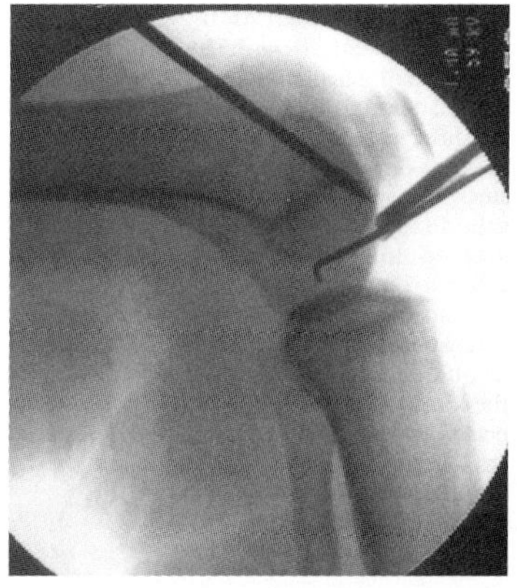

TECH FIG 3 • **A.** Guidewire advanced to articular surface under fluoroscopic guidance using retrograde technique. **B.** Arthroscopic probe placed on the articular surface helps identify target condyle. *(continued)*

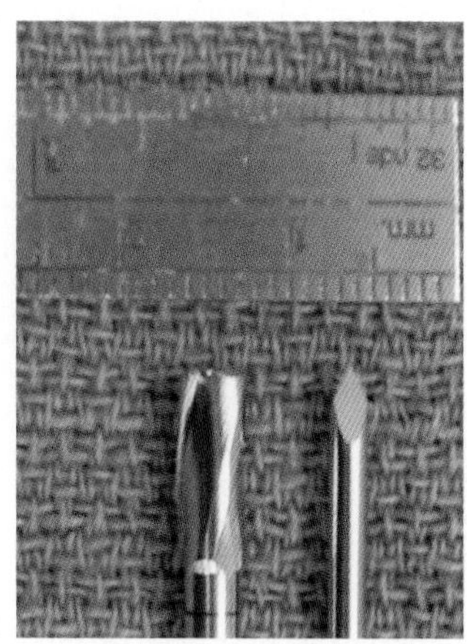
C

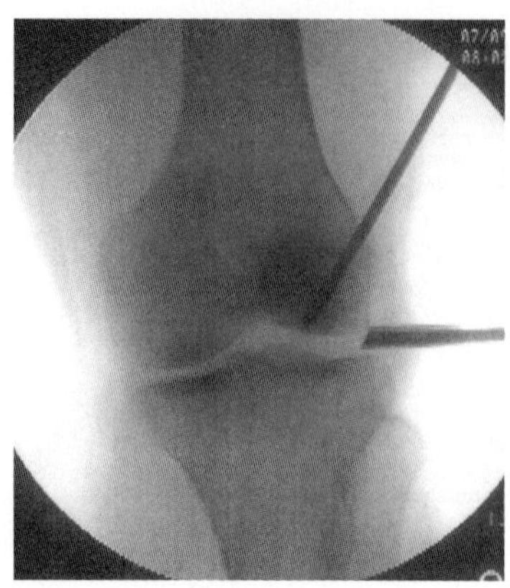
D

TECH FIG 3 • *(continued)* **C.** The cannulated drill is significantly wider in diameter than the guidewire, facilitating core decompression of the AVN lesion. **D.** Fluoroscopic image of the cannulated drill bit over the guidewire using the retrograde technique. (**A,B,D:** Reprinted with permission from Diduch DR, Hampton BJ. Avascular necrosis drilling in the knee. In: Miller MD, Cole BJ, eds. Textbook of Arthroscopy. Philadelphia: Elsevier, 2004:593–599.)

- Arthroscopic visualization is then used to advance the guidewire to barely pierce the articular surface.
- Drilling decompression is performed with a 4.5-mm cannulated drill bit (Endobutton drill bit, Smith & Nephew, Andover, MA) placed over the guidewire.
- As it approaches the articular surface, the drill bit should be advanced by hand for better control.
  - The drill bit is stopped 2 mm short of the articular surface (TECH FIG 3C,D).
  - Two or three passes with the guidewire and cannulated drill bit are required for each lesion.

Antegrade Drilling of the Femur

- Antegrade drilling of femoral lesions involves drilling from the articular surface into the lesion.
- It does not require fluoroscopy.
  - Lesions are localized by correlation of arthroscopic findings with MRI images.
  - Multiple drill holes are made directly into the lesion using a smooth, 1- to 2-mm guidewire to a depth that penetrates through the lesion and into healthy bone.
- The drilled tract is then aspirated for bleeding using the shaver with suction.
  - This bleeding indicates decompression and is evidence that the guidewire passed completely through the necrotic subchondral bone (TECH FIG 4).

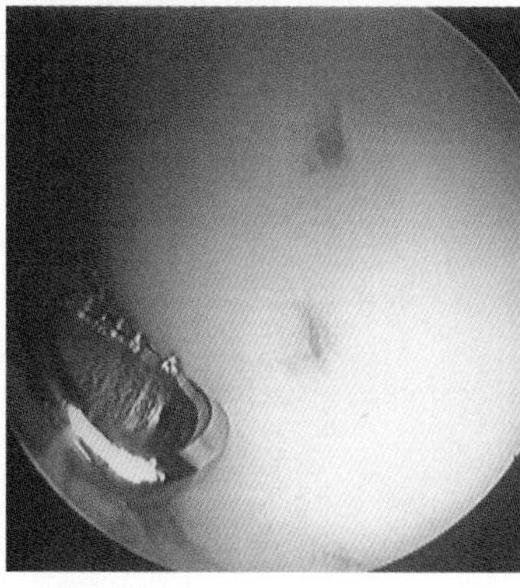

TECH FIG 4 • Motorized shaver with suction can be used to aspirate the drill tract for bleeding using the antegrade technique. (Reprinted with permission from Diduch DR, Hampton BJ. Avascular necrosis drilling in the knee. In: Miller MD, Cole BJ, eds. Textbook of arthroscopy. Philadelphia: Elsevier, 2004:593–599.)

Retrograde Drilling of the Tibia

- Tibial lesions are drilled using a retrograde technique.
- Fluoroscopy is optional.
- An ACL guide is used to target the lesion (TECH FIG 5A).
- Lesions are localized by correlation of arthroscopic findings with MRI images.
- A 2.4-mm guidewire is placed through the ACL guide and allowed to just pierce the articular surface (TECH FIG 5B).
- A 4.5-mm drill bit is then used for drilling decompression, stopping the drill bit just beneath the articular surface.

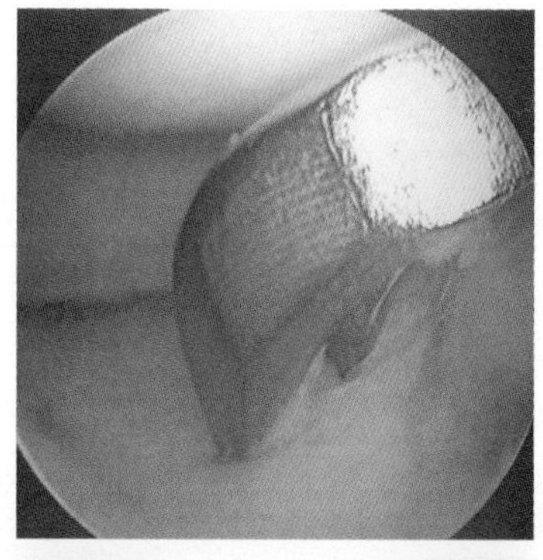
A

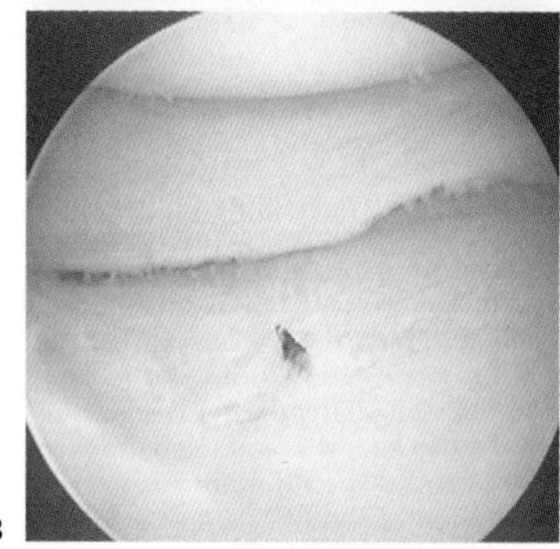
B

TECH FIG 5 • **A.** Tibial lesions can be targeted using an anterior cruciate ligament guide using the retrograde technique. **B.** Guidewire is seen piercing the tibial articular surface using the retrograde technique. (Reprinted with permission from Diduch DR, Hampton BJ. Avascular necrosis drilling in the knee. In: Miller MD, Cole BJ, eds. Textbook of arthroscopy. Philadelphia: Elsevier, 2004:593–599.)

PEARLS AND PITFALLS

Mistakes to avoid when treating OCD	■ Underestimating instability of the lesion and drilling in situ when fixation of the fragment is necessary for healing to occur ■ Underestimating fluid behind the fragment and pinning in situ when fixation and bone grafting are necessary for healing ■ Excision alone of a fragment with subchondral bone on its undersurface when reduction and fixation are necessary ■ Attempting fixation of a fragment that consists of cartilage only. Without subchondral bone, healing will not occur. ■ If in doubt, a mini-arthrotomy should be made for direct access and visualization of the lesion. This facilitates perpendicular fixation, which maximizes healing potential.
Mistakes to avoid when treating AVN	■ Overtreatment of MRI findings. AVN is not always the source of the patient's pain. Look for other pathology in the knee that may account for the patient's symptoms. Only lesions with involvement of subchondral bone with potential for subsequent collapse are clinically relevant. ■ Drilling of AVN lesions should not be abandoned if initial attempts fail. Repeat drilling is effective in 60% of cases.[5]

POSTOPERATIVE CARE

Osteochondritis Dissecans

- After transchondral drilling, with or without fixation of intact OCD lesions, full range-of-motion and closed chain resistance exercises are encouraged.
- Daily range-of-motion exercises are encouraged, because motion is important to provide articular cartilage nutrition via synovial fluid diffusion.
  - Touch-down weight bearing is done for 6 weeks.
  - Advanced weight-bearing and resistance excercises are done from 6 to 12 weeks.
  - Sports or running is avoided until 3 months or radiographic union.
  - Patient compliance is an issue owing to the minimally invasive nature of the surgery.
- After primary fixation and bone grafting of OCD lesions, patients may be placed in a hinged knee brace that is unlocked for self-guided exercises.
  - A continuous passive motion machine may be used for 2 to 3 weeks to help achieve motion.
  - Physical therapy is focused on range of motion for the first 2 weeks, after which gentle, progressive strengthening is initiated.
  - Touch-down weight bearing is permitted during the first 6 weeks, followed by progressive weight bearing.
  - Radiographs are taken 1 to 2 weeks after surgery and on successive visits every 4 weeks thereafter.
  - Once healing is verified radiographically, the patient may be taken back to surgery for hardware removal if necessary. The chondral surface can be inspected and the stability of the lesion can be evaluated at that time.
  - Most authors recommend removal of any metal hardware on the joint surface to minimize secondary wear or possible corrosion from synovial fluid.
  - Return to sports or running usually is not permitted until 6 months after surgery, unless radiographic union is demonstrated before that point.

Avascular Necrosis

- After drilling of AVN, patients are limited to 50% weight bearing for 2 weeks, until repeat radiographs are taken to rule out collapse.
  - Once collapse is ruled out, weight bearing can be advanced as tolerated.
  - Patients may benefit from physical therapy three times a week for 4 weeks. Therapy should focus on quadriceps strengthening and both active and passive range of motion.

OUTCOMES

Osteochondritis Dissecans

- Many authors have found transchondral drilling to be effective in treating OCD lesions in skeletally immature patients. Results are less effective in patients with closed physes.
  - Anderson et al used transchondral drilling to treat 17 patients (20 knees) with open physes and 4 patients with closed physes.[11] The open physes group had a 90% healing rate, whereas the skeletally mature group had a healing rate of 50%.
  - At Children's Hospital of Philadelphia, 51 patients up to 18 years of age were treated with transchondral drilling. Skeletally immature patients had an 83% success rate, as opposed to 75% success in patients with closed physes. Failure to heal was associated with lesions in nonclassic locations, multiple lesions, and other underlying medical conditions.
  - Aglietti et al[12] noted radiographic healing in 16 knees, and all patients were asymptomatic at follow-up of 4 years.
  - Kocher et al[4] reported on 23 patients (30 knees) treated with transchondral drilling with a follow-up of 3.9 years. Radiographic healing was seen in all patients at an average of 4.4 months. Patients also had significant improvement in Lysholm scores.
- Primary fixation of OCD lesions has had positive results.
  - Johnson et al[13] treated 35 patients with an arthroscopically assisted technique that employed cannulated screw fixation of the fragment. Results were good or excellent in 90% of cases.
  - Zuniga et al[14] treated 11 patients with symptomatic OCD lesions of the medial femoral condyle with a combination of Herbert screws and absorbable pins. Radiographic signs of healing correlated with the clinical outcome, which was good or excellent in 81.8% of patients.
  - Cugat et al[15] used cannulated screws for fixation of OCD lesions in 14 patients. All patients returned to their previous sporting activity 3 to 11 months after surgery.

Table 1 Ficat Classification of Avascular Necrosis Modified for the Knee

Stage	Description
I	Normal appearance
II	Cystic or sclerotic lesions, or both
	Normal contour of bone without subchondral collapse or flattening of the articular surface
III	Crescent sign or subchondral collapse
IV	Joint space narrowing with secondary changes on the opposing joint surface

Avascular Necrosis

- Treatment of symptomatic AVN with nonoperative methods such as restricted weight bearing, analgesics, and observation has a clinical failure rate higher than 80%.
  - Core decompression of stage I, II, or III knees (Table 1) provides symptomatic relief, with 79% of patients having good or excellent Knee Society scores at 7 years.
  - For patients who fail initial core decompression, repeat decompression and arthroscopic débridement provides some benefit, with results comparable to those of the initial decompression.
  - Core decompression will not improve symptoms once collapse has occurred, because the joint surface then is irregular and essentially arthritic.

COMPLICATIONS

- Nonunion with loose body formation
- Persistent symptomatic lesions
- Inability to localize the lesion
- Drill bit penetration of the articular surface
- Synovitis or foreign body reactions with absorbable implants
- Postoperative knee stiffness
- Hardware migration or failure
- Damage to adjacent articular surfaces
- Soft tissue irritation or burn from inadequate portal size
- Infection
- Deep venous thrombosis

REFERENCES

1. Crawford DC, Safran MR. Osteochondritis dissecans of the knee. J Am Acad Orthop Surg 2006;14:90–99.
2. De Smet AA, Ilahi OA, Graf BK. Untreated osteochondritis dissecans of the femoral condyles: prediction of patient outcome using radiographic and MR findings. Skeletal Radiol 1997;16:463–467.
3. Diduch DR, Hampton BJ. Avascular necrosis drilling in the knee. In Miller MD, Cole BJ, eds. Textbook of Arthroscopy. Philadelphia: Elsevier Science, 2004:593–599.
4. Kocher MS, Tucker R, Ganley TJ, et al. Management of osteochondritis dissecans of the knee. Am J Sports Med 2006;34:1181–1191.
5. Mont MA, Baumgarten KM, Rifai A, et al. Atraumatic osteonecrosis of the knee. J Bone Joint Surg Am 2000;82A:1279–1290.
6. Pill SG, Ganley TJ, Milam RA, et al. Role of magnetic resonance imaging and clinical criteria in predicting successful nonoperative treatment of osteochondritis dissecans in children. J Pediatr Orthop 2003;23:102–108.
7. Stanitski CL. Articular cartilage lesions and osteochondritis dissecans of the knee in the skeletally immature patient. In: DeLee JC, Drez D Jr, Miller MD, eds. Orthopaedic Sports Medicine: Principles and Practice, vol. 2. Philadelphia: Elsevier Science, 2003:1886–1901.
8. Williams JS Jr, Bush-Joseph CA, Bach BR. Osteochondritis dissecans of the knee: a review. Am J Knee Surg 1998;11:221–232.
9. Cahill BR, Berg BC. 99m-technetium phosphate compound joint scintigraphy in the management of juvenile osteochondritis dissecans of the femoral condyles. Am J Sports Med 1983;11:329–335.
10. Cahill BR. Osteochondritis dissecans of the knee: treatment of juvenile and adult forms. J Am Acad Orthop Surg 1995;3:237–247.
11. Anderson AF, Richards DB, Pagnani MJ, et al. Antegrade drilling for osteochondritis dissecans of the knee. Arthroscopy 1997;13:319–324.
12. Aglietti P, Buzzi R, Bassi PB, et al. Arthroscopic drilling in juvenile osteochondritis dissecans of the medial femoral condyle. Arthroscopy 1994;10:286–291.
13. Johnson LL, Uitvlugt G, Austin MD, et al. Osteochondritis dissecans of the knee: arthroscopic compression screw fixation. Arthroscopy 1990;6:179–188.
14. Zuniga RSJ, Blasco L, Grande M. Arthroscopic use of Herbert screws in osteochondritis dissecans of the knee. Arthroscopy 1993;9:668–670.
15. Cugat R, Garcia M, Cusco X, et al. Osteochondritis dissecans: a historical review and its treatment with cannulated screws. Arthroscopy 1993.9:675–684.

Chapter 41

Single-Bundle Anterior Cruciate Ligament Repair

Mark D. Miller

DEFINITION

- Anterior cruciate ligament (ACL) injuries result in a disruption of the fibers of this ligament and an ACL-deficient knee.
- Although most injuries are complete, partial injuries have been described. In our practice, partial injuries—defined as an asymmetrical Lachman test (or 3 to 4 mm of asymmetry on KT-1000 testing)[1] with a negative pivot shift test during examination under anesthesia, or a one-bundle ACL disruption seen arthroscopically—are rare.
- The key point in determining how to treat partial injuries is to determine whether functional stability of the ACL has been maintained.

ANATOMY

- The ACL is about 33 mm long and 11 mm in diameter.[8]
- The tibial insertion has a broad, irregular diamond shape and is immediately anterior and adjacent to the medial tibial eminence.
- The femoral attachment of the ligament is a semicircular area on the posteromedial aspect of the lateral femoral condyle.
- It extends from the 9 o'clock position to the 11 o'clock position (right knee).
- The ACL is composed of two "bundles"—a more important posterolateral portion, which is tight in extension, and a less critical anteromedial portion, which is tight in flexion.
- It is composed of 90% type I collagen; the remaining collagen is predominantly type III.
- The main blood supply for the ACL is the middle geniculate artery.
- Mechanoreceptor nerve endings have been identified within the ACL and are thought to have a proprioceptive role.

PATHOGENESIS

- ACL injuries usually result from a noncontact pivoting injury, typically involving a change of direction or deceleration maneuver.
- Patients often describe hearing or feeling a "pop" and will develop an acute or subacute effusion (ie, "swells up like a balloon").
- In most cases, the athlete will not be able to return to play and may need assistance to leave the field or slope (we have termed the latter a "positive ski patrol sign").
- Combined ACL, medial collateral ligament (MCL), and meniscal injuries have been referred to as the "unhappy triad."[11]
  - Lateral meniscal tears are more common in acute ACL injuries.

NATURAL HISTORY

- Researchers from Kaiser Permanente in Southern California, including Donald Fithian[7] and the late Dale Daniel,[6] have done much to contribute to our knowledge of the natural history of the ACL-injured knee.
  - From their work, we recognize that patients with a high level of participation in jumping or cutting sports and significant side-to-side differences (>5 mm) on KT-1000 arthrometer measurements are at high risk for recurrent injury without ACL reconstruction.
  - Unfortunately, these same researchers have shown an *increased* incidence of arthritis in the surgically reconstructed ACL group.[6,7]
- The difficulty with these and other studies is that multiple variables are involved, making comparisons difficult and possibly inaccurate.[10]
- It is clear from the literature that the incidence of meniscal tears and chondral injury can be reduced with ACL reconstruction.
- Advocates of double-bundle ACL reconstruction propose that the incidence of arthritis may be reduced with this technique, but that theory has yet to be proved clinically.

PHYSICAL FINDINGS

- Physical examination methods include the following:
  - Effusion: about 70% of acute hemarthrosis cases represent ACL.[6]
  - Range of motion (ROM): loss of extension may be a result of a displaced bucket handle meniscal tear or arthrofibrosis (stiff knee). Loss of flexion may be related to a knee effusion.
  - The Lachman test[13] is highly sensitive for ACL deficiency. The patient must relax for this examination, and effusion or a displaced meniscal tear may give a false endpoint.
  - The anterior drawer test is poorly sensitive and outdated, but is helpful to rule out a posterior cruciate ligament (PCL) injury.
  - The pivot shift test[3] is difficult to perform in the clinic setting, but is an especially helpful and sensitive test during examination under anesthesia.
- A complete examination of the knee also should include evaluation of associated injuries and ruling out differential diagnoses, including (but not limited to) the following:
  - Meniscal tears: joint line tenderness, pain or popping with provocative maneuvers (eg, McMurray, Apley compression, duck walk), and loss of full extension may be present.
  - PCL injury: a "pseudo-Lachman" may be appreciated if the PCL is present, and the unwary examiner may falsely attribute this to an ACL injury. The key is the starting point on the drawer examination. The tibial stepoff in PCL-injured knees will be absent, or the tibia may actually be displaced (or be displaceable) posteriorly, signifying a PCL injury.
  - Posterolateral corner (PLC) injury: Injury to the popliteus, popliteofibular ligament, biceps, iliotibial band, or posterior capsule will result in external rotation asymmetry (dial test), a positive posterolateral drawer test, and external rotation recurvatum.

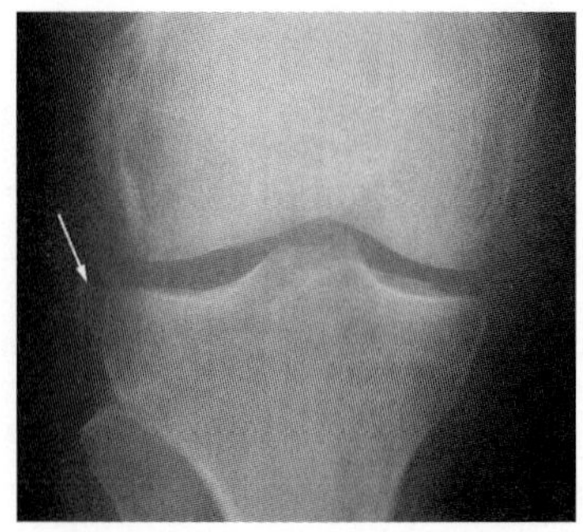

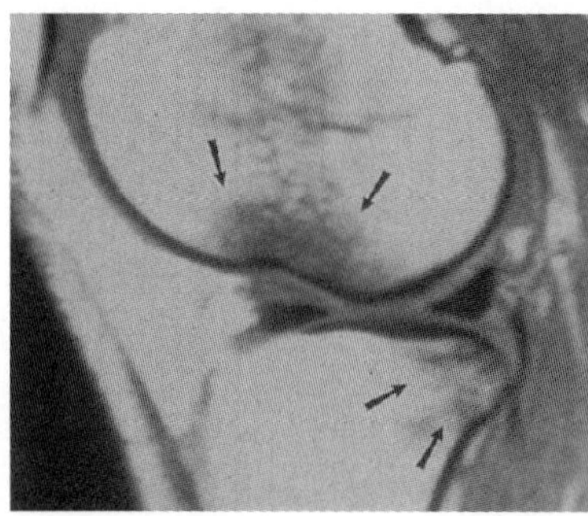

FIG 1 • **A.** Segond (lateral capsular) sign. A small avulsion fracture in this area is highly associated with an ACL injury. **B.** MRI of ACL-injured knee with associated bone bruises. These impaction injuries are in the classic locations—the most lateral aspect of the middle third of the lateral femoral condyle and the posterior aspect of the tibia.

- Collateral ligament injury: MCL injuries are recognized as opening with valgus force, and lateral collateral ligament (LCL) injuries open with varus stress. These examinations are tested in both 30 and 0 degrees of knee flexion. Opening to valgus or varus stress in 0 degrees (ie, full extension) signifies a more severe injury, usually involving one or both cruciate ligaments.
- Patellar instability: localized tenderness or instability with apprehension testing is essential to rule out a patellar dislocation that reduced spontaneously. This type of injury also can cause an acute knee effusion and can be easily confused with an acute ACL injury.

IMAGING AND DIAGNOSTIC STUDIES

- Plain radiographs, including anteroposterior, lateral, and patellar views, should be obtained to rule out bony avulsion fractures or associated injuries.
- A small avulsion fracture off the lateral tibial plateau (**FIG 1A**) represents a lateral capsular avulsion (Segond sign) and is highly associated with an ACL injury. It is very specific, but not sensitive.
- Flexion weight-bearing radiographs are important in older or posttraumatic patients to rule out associated osteoarthritis.
- Long-leg hip-to-ankle radiographs must be obtained in patients with varus or valgus malalignment.
- An osteotomy should be performed before ACL reconstruction in select cases.
- MRI is highly sensitive and specific in diagnosing ACL tears as well as associated injuries.
  - Bone contusions, or bruises, also may be detected in the mid-lateral potion of the lateral femoral condyle (near the sulcus terminalis) and the posterior tibial plateau (**FIG 1B**).

DIFFERENTIAL DIAGNOSIS

- Meniscal tear
- Osteochondral injury
- Contusion
- Patellar dislocation
- Other ligament/capsular injury (eg, MCL, LCL, PLC, multiple ligament injury)

NONOPERATIVE MANAGEMENT

- Although nonoperative management is controversial, patients with less laxity and those who are less involved with high-level pivoting sports may be treated nonoperatively.
- Nonoperative treatment is done in three phases over a period of about 3 months.
  - In the *initial phase,* emphasis is placed on regaining full motion, controlling effusion, and maintaining quadriceps tone. (This is appropriate for patients who are surgical candidates as well.)
  - In the *second phase,* quadriceps and hamstring strengthening is emphasized.
  - In the *third and final phase,* sport-specific rehabilitation is accomplished.
- Patients may attempt to return to sports after their effusion has completely resolved, they have full ROM, their quadriceps tone and strength have been restored (isokinetic testing is

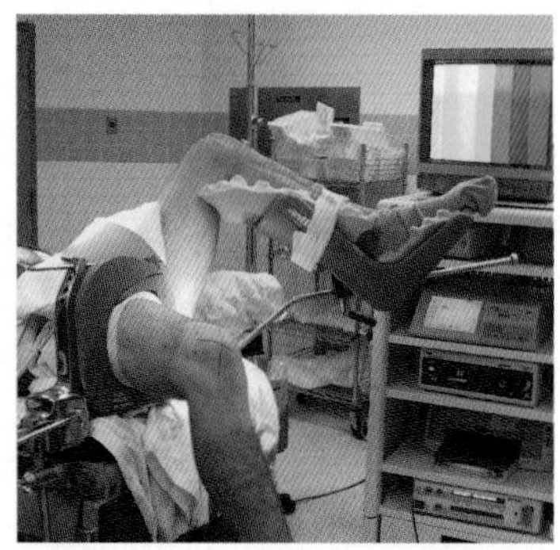

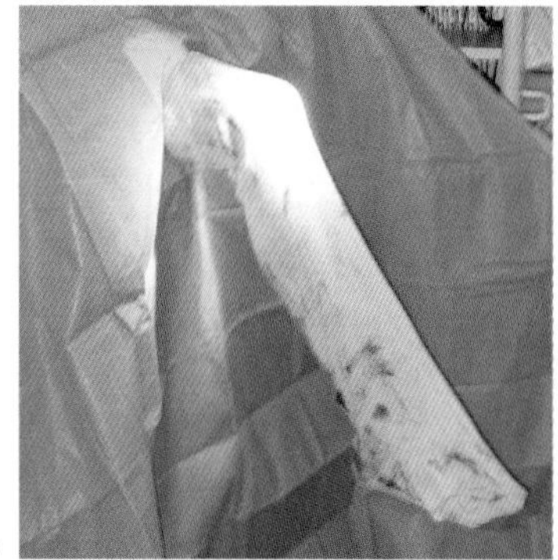

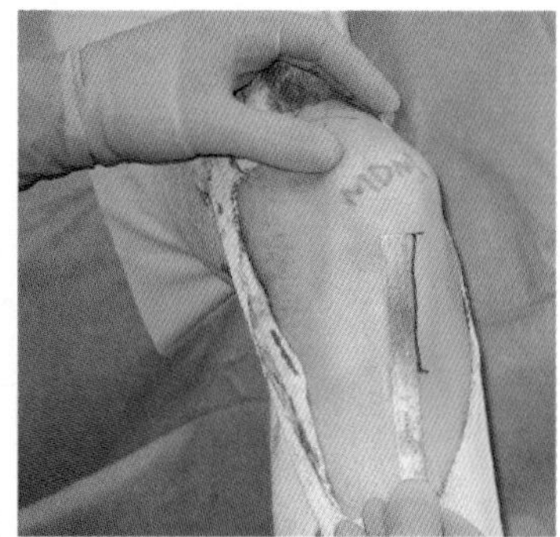

FIG 2 • Positioning for ACL reconstruction. **A.** The foot of the bed is dropped, a leg holder is used for the operative side, and the contralateral leg is cushioned in another holder. **B.** Appropriate draping. The nonoperative leg is not included in the operative field. **C.** The table is dropped to flex the knee. This positioning allows free movement of the operative knee and easy access by the surgeon.

helpful), and they have no residual symptoms of instability (functional testing is helpful).

SURGICAL MANAGEMENT

Preoperative Planning

- All imaging studies are reviewed.
- Plain radiographs should be reviewed for fractures, loose bodies, patellar height and alignment, and the presence of any hardware (from previous procedures) or foreign bodies.
- Associated fractures, meniscal tears, articular cartilage lesions, and multiple ligament injuries should be addressed concurrently.
- Examination under anesthesia should be accomplished prior to positioning.
- Lachman, pivot shift, varus/valgus, and dial testing should be included in the examination under anesthesia.

POSITIONING

- Although some surgeons prefer to perform ACL reconstruction with the patient supine and the foot of the table up, we prefer to drop the foot of the bed and use a commercially available knee holder for the operative knee. We place the contralateral leg in a well-padded holder that is not included in the operative field (**FIG 2**).
- This allows us to freely flex the knee and have global access.

Approach

- The approach depends on graft choice.
- There are two gold standards for ACL grafts—bone–patellar tendon–bone autograft and four-strand semitendinosus gracilis (hamstring) autograft. We use both patellar tendon and hamstring grafts and have found that certain parameters are helpful in determining graft choice (Table 1).
- Other graft choices include quadriceps tendon autograft and a variety of allografts. Although these grafts may be useful in certain cases, they are not popular choices for most surgeons.
- After the graft is selected, the procedure involves arthroscopic diagnosis and repair of pathology, tibial and femoral tunnel placement, graft passage and fixation, and wound closure.

Table 1 ACL Graft Choice Indications

Patellar tendon
Football players
Gymnasts
Sprinters
Ballet dancers
Martial arts participants
Patients with systemic laxity
Revision of prior hamstring grafts
Hamstring
Jumping sport athletes
Clergy, carpenters
Older patients
Those with prior anterior knee pain
Those with patellar chondrosis
Those with narrow patellar tendons
Revision of prior patellar tendon grafts

TECHNIQUES

PATELLAR TENDON GRAFT HARVESTING

- Patellar tendon grafts (TECH FIG 1) are harvested through a 5- to 7-cm paramedian incision.
- Saphenous nerve branches are protected if identified.
- The paratenon is incised vertically and reflected off the underlying tendon.
- The central third of the tendon (typically 10 mm) is harvested, with care taken not to cut across the longitudinal fibers of the tendon.
- Bone blocks (approximately 25 mm long) are obtained using a micro oscillating saw.
- Care is taken to saw no deeper than 10 mm, particularly on the patellar side, to avoid an iatrogenic fracture.
- The tibial bone block can be either more rectangular or more trapezoidal in cross section.
- The patellar bone block should be more triangular in cross section, to avoid injury to the patella.
- The bone blocks are removed using a curved osteotome (again, being careful on the tibial side) and taken to the back table for preparation.
- A rongeur or burr is used to fashion the bone blocks so that they will fit through an appropriately sized tunnel.
- With retraction, the lower portion of the incision can be used to prepare the tibial tunnel.
- If the tendon is harvested at the beginning of the procedure, arthroscopic portals can be made through the incision.

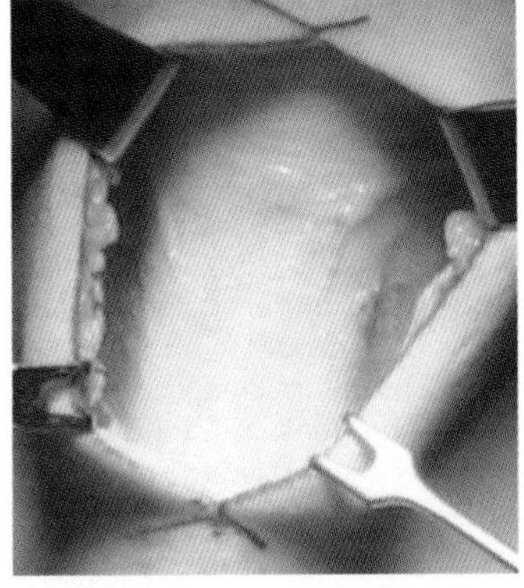
A

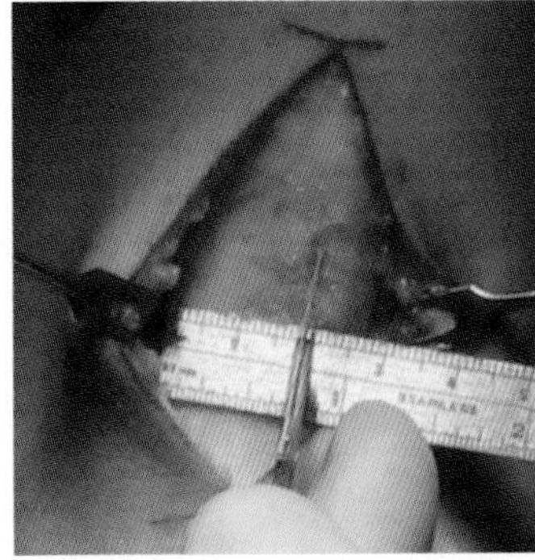
B

TECH FIG 1 • Patellar tendon graft harvesting. **A.** Exposure of the patellar tendon and paratenon. **B.** The middle third (~10 mm) of the patellar tendon is measured. *(continued)*

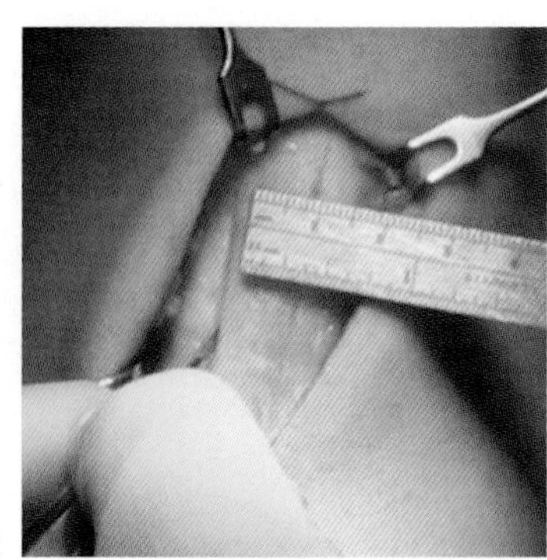

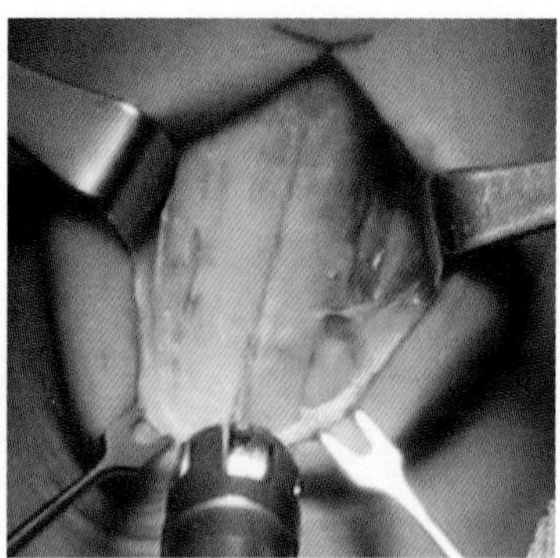

TECH FIG 1 • *(continued)* **C.** Vertical incisions are made, with care taken not to transect any of the longitudinal fibers of the tendon. **D.** After the tendon is excised, bone blocks are made on either end.

HAMSTRING TENDON GRAFT HARVESTING

- Hamstring grafts (TECH FIG 2) are harvested through a 2- to 3-cm paramedian incision centered at the level of the tibial tubercle, approximately 6 cm below the medial joint line.
- The sartorial fascia is exposed, and the tendons are palpated.
- The tendons insert in an oblique fashion and are more horizontal than vertical.
- The gracilis tendon insertion is superior to the semitendinosus tendon insertion, but both tendons converge at the pes anserine.
- It is necessary to reflect the overlying sartorial fascia that covers both tendons.
- Alternatively, the tendons can be exposed from their deep side if their insertions are sharply reflected off the tibia.
- Once the tendons are identified, a whipstitch is placed in them near their insertions so that they can be reflected off their insertions and mobilized.
- Blunt dissection and palpation are essential in mobilizing the tendons.
- Both tendons must be mobilized and all tendinous slips freed.
- The semitendinosus will have one or more large bands that attach to the medial head of the gastrocnemius. These must be incised before a tendon stripper is used, or the tendon will be inadvertently cut at this location.
- After harvesting, the tendons are prepared on the back table.
- Muscle fibers are removed from the tendons using a curette or elevator, a whipstitch is placed in the free end, and the tendons are tensioned using a commercially available graft board.
- The grafts are folded in half and the diameter of the four-strand graft measured before tensioning.
- The harvest incision can easily be used for tibial tunnel placement.
- Standard arthroscopic portals are made through the skin at the level of the joint.

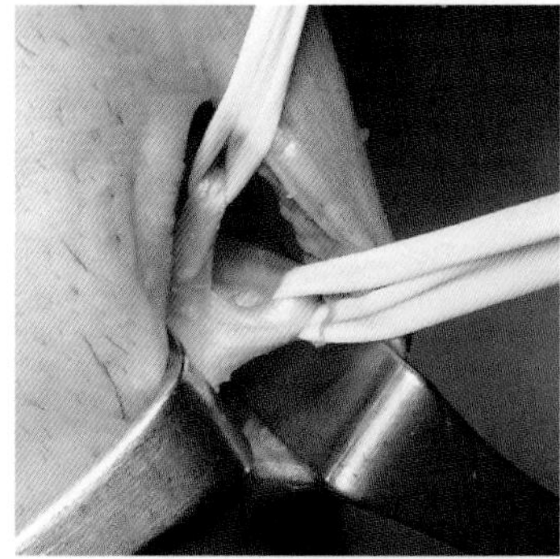

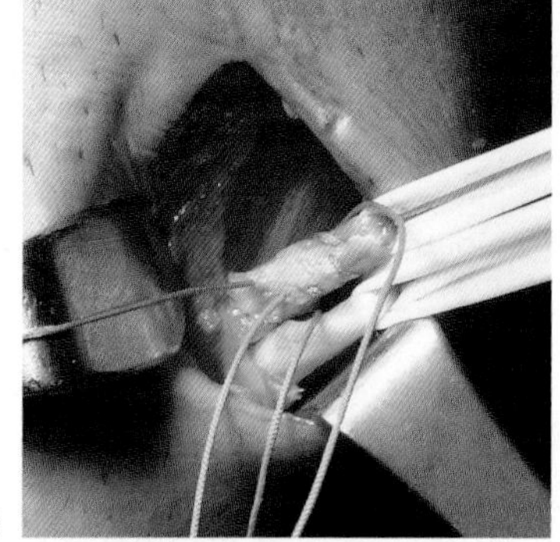

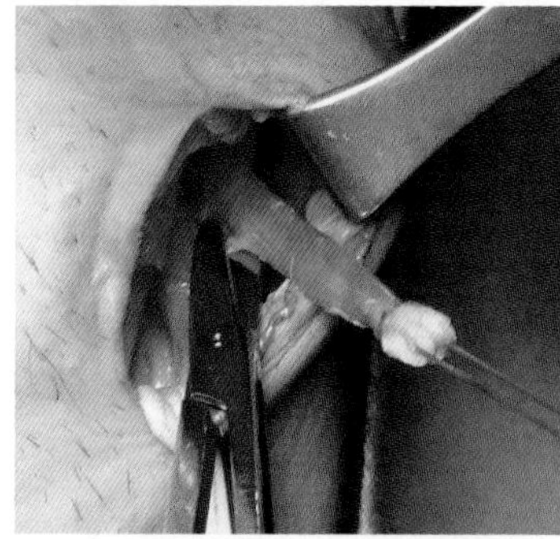

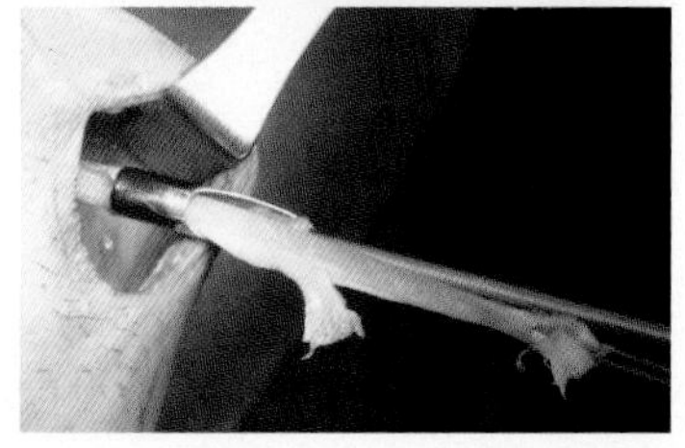

TECH FIG 2 • Hamstring graft harvesting. **A.** The gracilis (*top*) and semitendinosus (*bottom*) tendons are isolated by dissecting under the sartorial fascia. **B.** Whipstitches are placed in the tendons prior to detaching them. **C.** The tendons are freed from any attachments using blunt dissection and scissors. **D.** A tendon stripper is used to harvest the tendons. The tendinous slip that was cut would have prevented the stripper from passing unless it was first released.

ARTHROSCOPY

- Diagnostic arthroscopy is completed, and all pathology is identified.
- Meniscal tears are repaired if possible.
- Articular cartilage lesions are addressed.
- Loose bodies that are identified are removed.
- The ACL is visualized and, if torn, it is débrided with baskets and a shaver.
- The tibial footprint of the ACL and the "over-the-top" position in the back of the notch are cleared of all soft tissue (TECH FIG 3).
- Although most surgeons no longer perform an aggressive notchplasty, it is important to clear enough soft tissue and bone to identify all landmarks and to ensure that the graft will not be impinged upon.
- It also is important to ensure that the roof of the notch will not impinge on the graft. (This is more important in hamstring reconstructions because the anterior portion of the graft may be more easily impinged.)

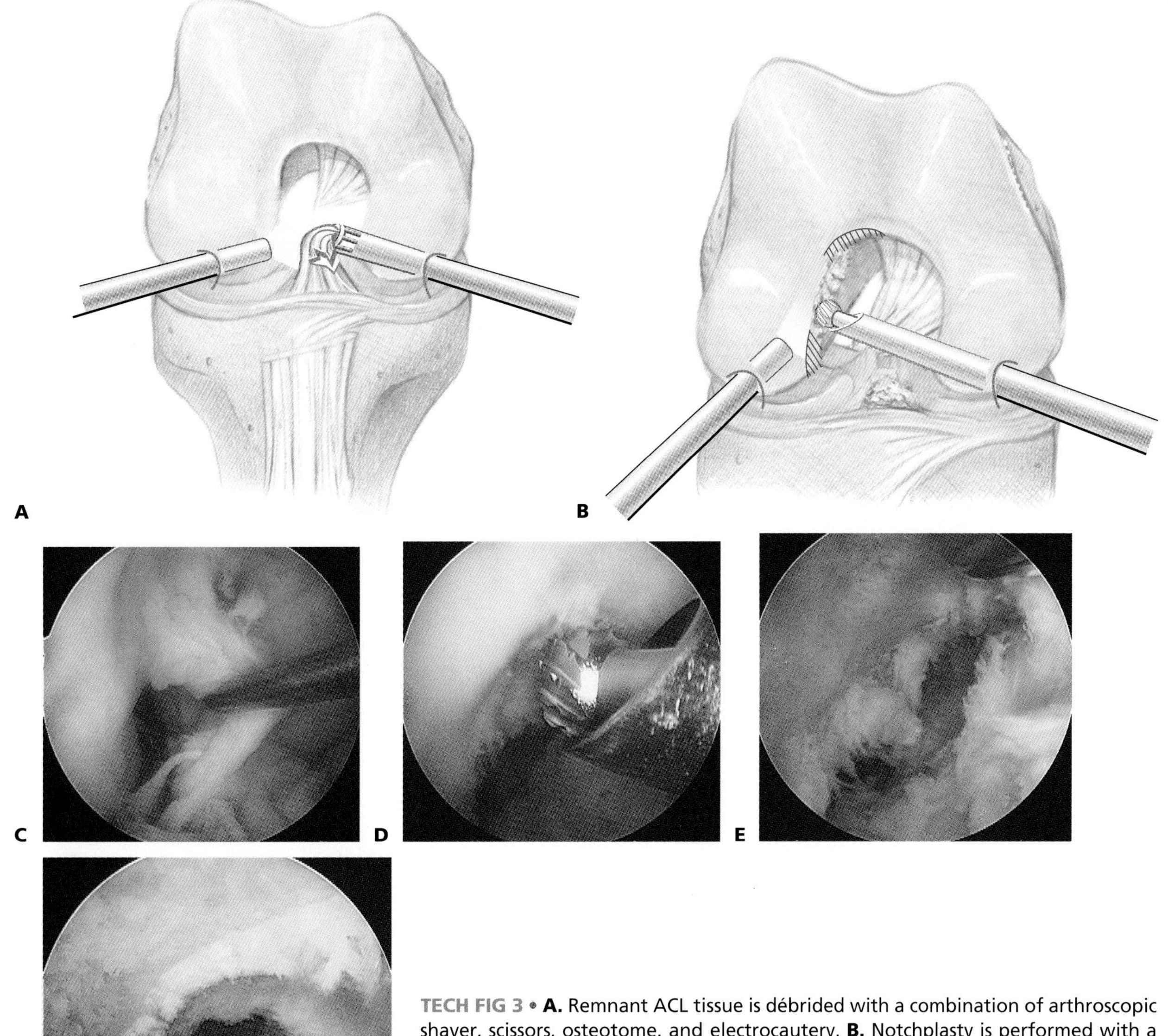

TECH FIG 3 • **A.** Remnant ACL tissue is débrided with a combination of arthroscopic shaver, scissors, osteotome, and electrocautery. **B.** Notchplasty is performed with a combination of a 1/4-inch curved osteotome, mallet, and grasper, or with a spherical motorized burr. Some patients may require minimal or even no notchplasty. The goal is to have enough space for graft placement and visualization purposes. Notchplasty should not extend cephalad to the intercondylar apex. A 3- to 5-mm notchplasty usually is performed, depending on the width of the intercondylar notch. **C.** The torn ACL. **D.** Notchplasty is performed. **E.** Careful débridement of the notch is done before drilling tunnels. **F.** Notchplasty/débridement of the ACL stump.

TIBIAL TUNNEL PLACEMENT

- A commercially available guide is used to place a guidewire for the tibial tunnel.
- The intra-articular landmarks for the tibial tunnel are as follows (TECH FIG 4):
  - Posteromedial aspect of the ACL footprint
  - Adjacent to the slope of the medial eminence
  - Along a line extended from the posterior border of the anterior horn of the lateral meniscus
  - 7 mm in front of the PCL
- The extra-articular portion of the guide should be positioned midway between the tibial tubercle and the posteromedial aspect of the tibia.[5]
- For patellar tendon reconstructions, the angle of the guide should be set based on the "N + 7 rule"[9] and checked based on the "N + 2 rule."[12] That is, the guide is provisionally set at an angle that is 7 degrees more that the tendon length (in mm) between the bone blocks, and the distance is checked on the plunger for the guide—it should be 2 mm longer than the tendon length. The guide is set between 45 and 50 degrees for hamstring grafts.
- Once the guidewire is placed and checked, a cannulated drill is used to complete the tibial tunnel.
- We use a fully threaded drill bit and save the bone graft that collects in the flutes of the drill to fill the patellar defect (it usually is discarded for hamstring graft reconstructions).
- The PCL is protected with a curette during final tunnel drilling.
- The back edge of the tibial tunnel is rasped to keep the graft from being abraded.

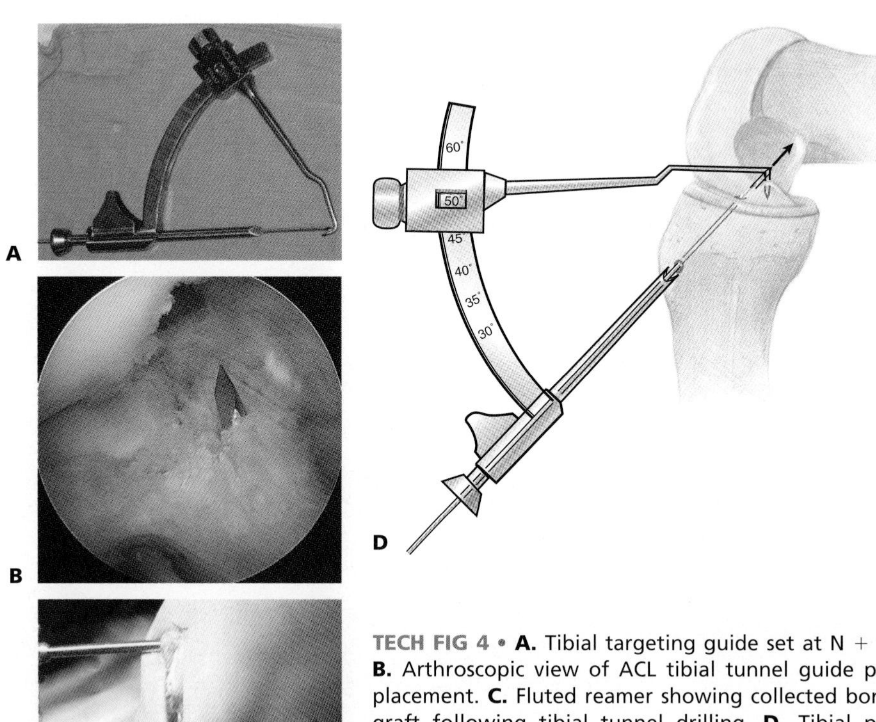

TECH FIG 4 • **A.** Tibial targeting guide set at N + 7. **B.** Arthroscopic view of ACL tibial tunnel guide pin placement. **C.** Fluted reamer showing collected bone graft following tibial tunnel drilling. **D.** Tibial pin placement usually is performed at an angle 10 degrees greater than the graft–soft tissue construct. For example, a 45-mm soft tissue construct usually is drilled at 55 degrees. This illustration demonstrates that if a steeper angle is selected, it may be more difficult to place the femoral tunnel anatomically.

FEMORAL TUNNEL PLACEMENT

- An endoscopic offset guide is placed through the tibial tunnel and off the back of the posterolateral notch (TECH FIG 5). Some surgeons prefer to place this guide through the medial portal with the knee hyperflexed.
- The guide pin should be placed in the 10:30 (right knee) or 1:30 (left knee) position. (While looking arthroscopically, the top of the notch is the 12:00 position.)
- The offset guide should be chosen to retain a 1-mm posterior wall following drilling. A 10-mm tunnel should be

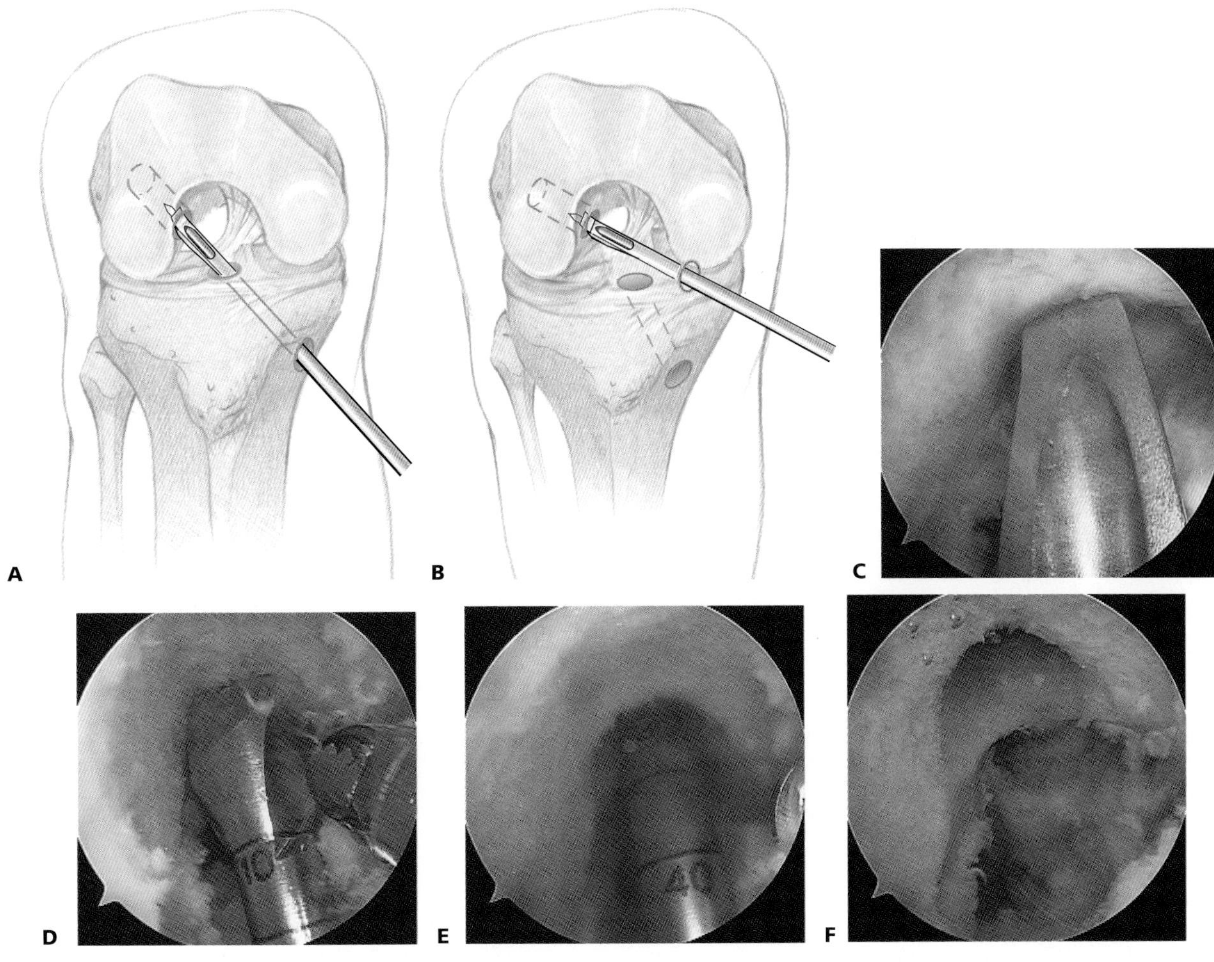

TECH FIG 5 • **A.** Retrograde placement of a 7-mm femoral offset aimer through the tibial tunnel. The knee should be flexed 75 to 90 degrees. **B.** Alternatively, an accessory inferomedial portal can be used to position the aimer. The knee should be flexed at least 110 degrees. **C.** Femoral "over the top" guide in correct position. **D.** Acorn drill bit positioned prior to drilling femoral tunnel. **E.** The femoral tunnel is drilled to a depth of approximately 30 mm for a patellar tendon graft. **F.** View after drilling of tunnel, showing intact posterior wall.

made with a 6-mm offset guide, because the guide is used to place a guidewire for the center of the tunnel and the radius of a 10-mm drill is 5 mm.

- The femoral tunnel is drilled to a depth of approximately 30 mm for a patellar tendon graft and to within 5 to 8 mm of the far cortex for a hamstring graft.
- Depending on the surgeon's choice for femoral graft fixation, additional tunnel preparation may be necessary.
- For Endobutton (Smith & Nephew Arthroscopy, Andover, MA) fixation, a 4.5-mm tunnel is drilled through the far cortex.
- For TransFix (Arthrex, Naples, FL), Bone Mulch (Arthrotek, Warsaw, IN), Rigid Fix (DePuy Mitek, Norwood, MA), and other similar fixation systems, transverse pilot holes are created from lateral to medial.

GRAFT PASSAGE AND FIXATION

- A Beath needle is placed through both tunnels and pierces the quadriceps muscles and skin.
- Sutures from the graft or fixation device are pulled through the tunnels and outside the thigh.
- The graft is pulled into both tunnels and fixed with an interference screw or a fixation device of the surgeon's choice.
- Once the femoral side is fixed, the knee is cycled through the complete ROM, and the graft is tensioned.
- The tibial side is then fixed with an interference screw or secured to the tibia with a screw and washer or staple (TECH FIG 6).
- The graft is probed and inspected before wound closure is performed.

TECHNIQUES

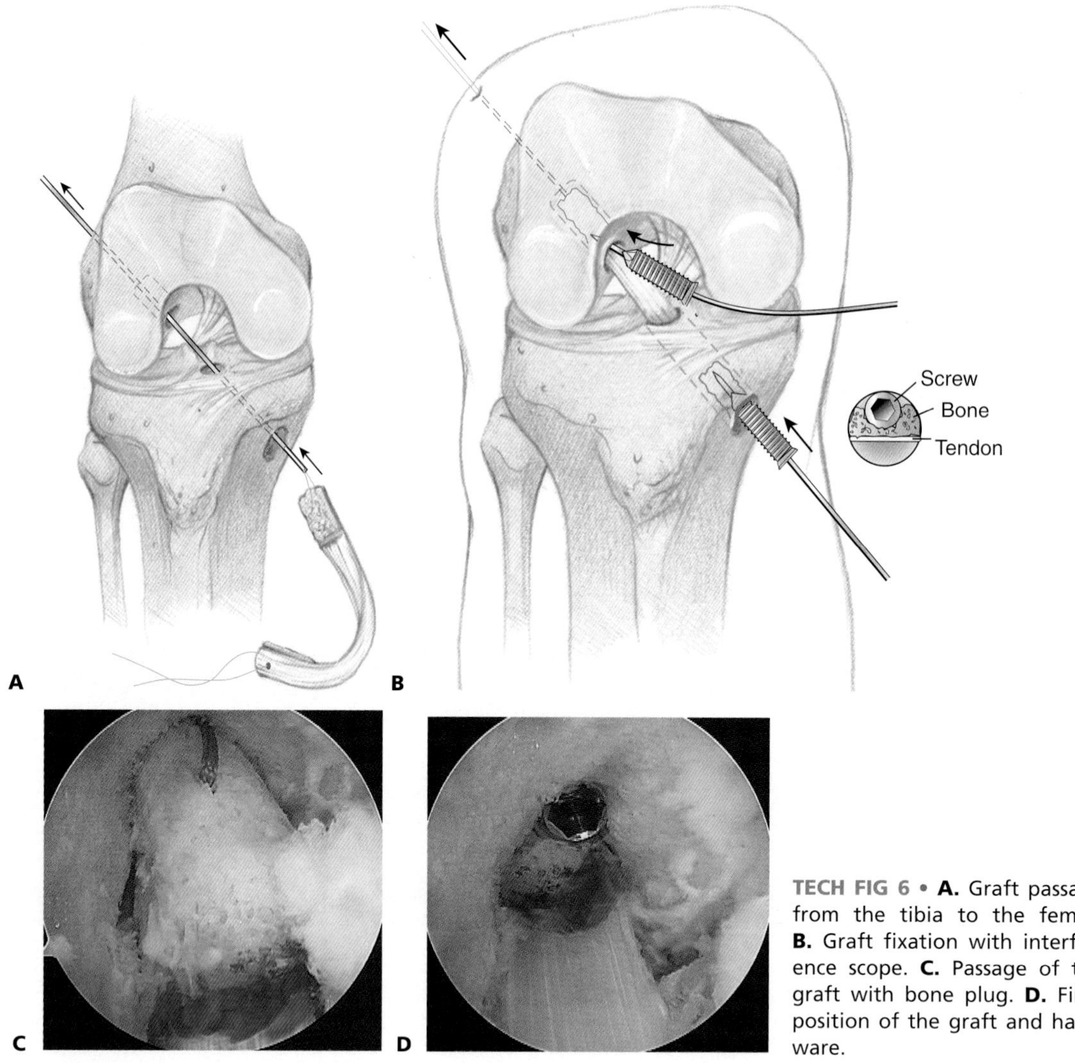

TECH FIG 6 • **A.** Graft passage from the tibia to the femur. **B.** Graft fixation with interference scope. **C.** Passage of the graft with bone plug. **D.** Final position of the graft and hardware.

WOUND CLOSURE

- The wounds are closed in layers.
- Bone graft from the drill bit or bone block preparation is packed into the patellar defect, and the paratenon is closed for patellar tendon graft cases.
- The sartorial fascia is closed for hamstring graft cases.
- Subcutaneous tissue and skin are closed in standard fashion.

PEARLS AND PITFALLS

Indications	■ A complete history and physical examination should be performed. ■ Care must be taken to address associated pathology.
Graft management	■ Extreme care should be taken when harvesting and preparing grafts. ■ Patellar bone blocks should be carefully harvested to avoid fracture. ■ The hamstring must be completely freed prior to harvesting. ■ The graft should be secured at all times and handled carefully.
Tunnel placement	■ Anterior tunnel placement is responsible for most ACL reconstruction failures. ■ Careful tunnel placement should be routine. ■ Intraoperative radiographs can be obtained to check tunnel locations before drilling.

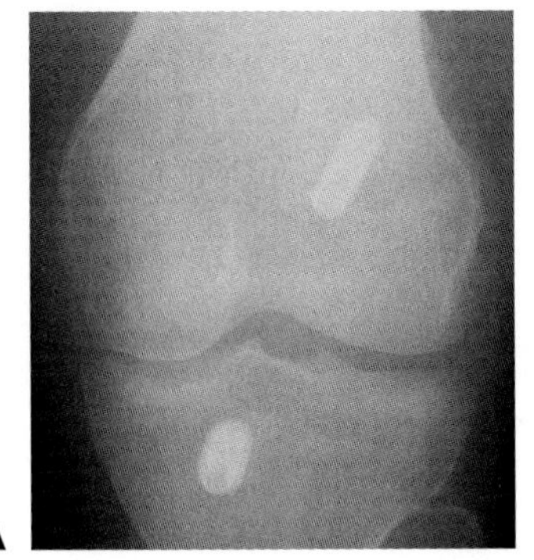
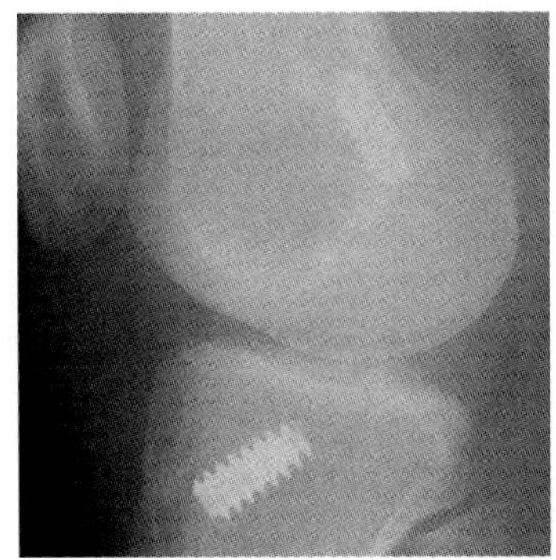
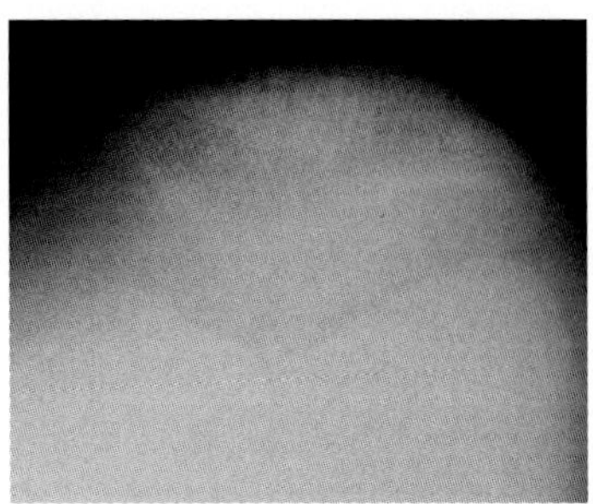

FIG 3 • Postoperative PA (**A**), lateral (**B**), and sunrise (**C**) radiographs of ACL reconstruction with bone–patellar tendon–bone autograft.

Guide pin breakage	■ Knee flexion must not change following guide pin placement. ■ A few degrees of flexion may result in the guidewire bending and shearing by the drill.
Fixation problems	■ Interference screws must be inserted along the path of the tunnel to avoid divergence. ■ For the femoral tunnel, the surgeon should hyperflex the knee and drop his or her hand toward the tibia while inserting the screw. ■ Intraoperative radiographs should be taken so that problems may be recognized and fixed before leaving the operating room.

POSTOPERATIVE CARE

- Radiographs are evaluated to ensure that graft placement and fixation are appropriate (**FIG 3**).
- Some surgeons place the patient in a knee immobilizer or a hinged brace, but we have found that this may restrict their motion and does not provide any benefit.
- Early range of motion (especially extension) is emphasized.
- It is important that a pillow be placed *under the heel* (not under the knee, which is more comfortable), beginning in the recovery room.
- Closed-chain rehabilitation (beginning with a stationary cycle) is emphasized in the early postoperative course.
- Running typically is delayed until 3 or 4 months postoperatively, and most athletes can return to their sport by 6 months.

OUTCOMES

- With appropriate indications and surgical technique, success rates for ACL reconstruction are on the order of 90% to 95%.
- In one study, 96% of patients had KT-1000 side-to-side differences of less than 5 mm.[2]
- Comparisons between patellar tendon and hamstring reconstruction have yielded equivalent results.
- Some studies suggest that hamstring grafts may have slightly increased laxity (1 to 2 mm) compared with patellar grafts.
- Other studies have cited an increased incidence of anterior knee pain following ACL reconstruction with patellar tendon grafts.

COMPLICATIONS

- Intraoperative graft mishandling[4]
- Graft failure or rupture
- Patellar fracture
- Deep venous thrombosis
- Infection
- Loss of motion
- Tunnel enlargement (a later complication)[14]

REFERENCES

1. Bach BR Jr, Nho SJ. Anterior cruciate ligament: diagnosis and decision making. In: Miller MD, Cole BJ, eds. Textbook of Arthroscopy. Philadelphia: Elsevier, 2004:633–643.
2. Bach BR Jr, Tradonsky S, Bojchuk J, et al. Arthroscopically assisted anterior cruciate ligament reconstruction using patellar tendon autograft: Five to nine year follow-up evaluation. Am J Sports Med 1998;26:20–29.
3. Bach BR Jr, Warren RF, Wickiewicz TL. The pivot shift phenomenon: results and a description of a modified clinical test for anterior cruciate ligament insufficiency. Am J Sports Med 1988;16: 571–576.
4. Cain EL Jr, Gillogly SD, Andrews JR. Management of intraoperative complications associated with autogenous patellar tendon graft anterior cruciate ligament reconstruction. Instr Course Lect 2003; 52:359–367.
5. Chhabra A, Diduch DR, Blessey PB, et al. Recreating an acceptable angle of the tibial tunnel in the coronal plane in ACL reconstruction using external landmarks. Arthroscopy 2004;20:328–330.
6. Daniel DM, Stone ML, Dobson BE, et al. Fate of the ACL-injured patient: a prospective outcome study. Am J Sports Med 1994;22: 632–644.
7. Fithian DC, Paxton EW, Stone ML, et al. Prospective trial of a treatment algorithm for the management of the anterior cruciate ligament-injured knee. Am J Sports Med 2005;33:335–346.
8. Girgis FG, Marshall JL, Al Monajem ARS. The cruciate ligaments of the knee joint: anatomical, functional, and experimental analysis. Clin Orthop 1975;106:216–231.
9. Miller MD, Hinkin DT. The N+7 rule for tibial tunnel placement during endoscopic ACL reconstruction. Arthroscopy 1996;12: 124–126.
10. Nedeff D, Bach BR Jr. Arthroscopy assisted ACL reconstruction using patellar tendon autograft: a comprehensive review of contemporary literature. Am J Knee Surg 2001;14:243–258.
11. O'Donoghue DH. Surgical treatment of fresh injuries to the major ligaments of the knee. J Bone Joint Surg Am 1950;32A:721–738.
12. Olszewski AD, Miller MD, Ritchie JR. Ideal tibial tunnel length for endoscopic anterior cruciate ligament injuries. Arthroscopy 1998;14: 9–14.
13. Torg JS, Conrad W, Kalen V. Clinical diagnosis of anterior cruciate ligament instability in athletes. Am J Sports Med 1976;4:84–93.
14. Wilson TC, Kanatara A, Johnson DL. Tunnel enlargement after anterior cruciate ligament surgery. Am J Sports Med 2004;32:543.

Chapter **42**

Anatomic Double-Bundle Anterior Cruciate Ligament Reconstruction

Steven B. Cohen and Freddie H. Fu

DEFINITION

- Anterior cruciate ligament (ACL) tears have been described in detail in Chapter SM-41.
- Any patient with functional instability or pivoting of the knee is considered to have an ACL insufficiency.

ANATOMY

- To fully understand the principles of ACL reconstruction, it is important to understand the complex anatomy of the ACL, which is composed of two major bundles.
  - These bundles are named relative to their relation to the tibial footprint: the posterolateral (PL) bundle is posterior and lateral on the tibial footprint, whereas the anteromedial (AM) bundle is anterior and medial on the tibial footprint.
  - The PL bundle originates more distally and anteriorly relative to the AM bundle on the wall of the intercondylar notch.
- The femoral insertion site of ACL changes based on flexion angle (**FIG 1**).
  - With the knee in full extension, the alignment of the AM and PL bundle insertion sites on the femur is vertical.
  - With the knee in 90 degrees of flexion, the insertion sites are horizontal, with the PL bundle insertion site anterior to that of the AM bundle.
- Measurements of individual bundles have found the AM bundle to be, on average, 38.5 mm long and 7.0 mm wide, whereas the PL bundle is 19.7 mm long and 6.4 mm wide.[4,5,8]
- When the knee is extended, the PL bundle is under tension and the AM bundle is moderately lax.
- With knee flexion, the AM bundle tightens and the PL bundle becomes lax.
- With internal and external rotation of the tibia at 90 degrees of flexion, the PL bundle tightens.

BIOMECHANICAL STUDIES

- ACL single-bundle reconstruction using either patellar tendon or quadrupled hamstring autograft successfully limits anterior tibial translation but provides insufficient control of the combined rotatory load of internal and valgus torque.[9]
- In a single-bundle ACL reconstruction, rotatory stability was improved with the use of the 2 o'clock or 10 o'clock femoral tunnel position compared with the 1 o'clock or 11 o'clock position. Neither the 10 o'clock nor the 11 o'clock tunnel position could restore the kinematics and the in situ forces of the intact knee, however.[6]

PATIENT HISTORY AND PHYSICAL FINDINGS

- The history of a noncontact valgus pivoting injury followed by an effusion of the knee is highly suspicious for an ACL tear.
- The physical examination and methods for examination of the ACL are covered in Chapter SM-41.
- Patients with a partial or single-bundle tear may have either a positive pivot shift or positive Lachman test. For example, an intact AM bundle and torn PL bundle may have a normal Lachman and positive pivot shift, whereas an intact PL bundle and a torn AM bundle may have a normal pivot shift and an increased Lachman test.

IMAGING AND DIAGNOSTIC STUDIES

- Radiographs should include the following views:
  - 30-degree flexion weight-bearing posteroanterior view
  - Lateral
  - Sunrise view of the patella
  - Long-leg alignment view in the case of coronal angular deformity

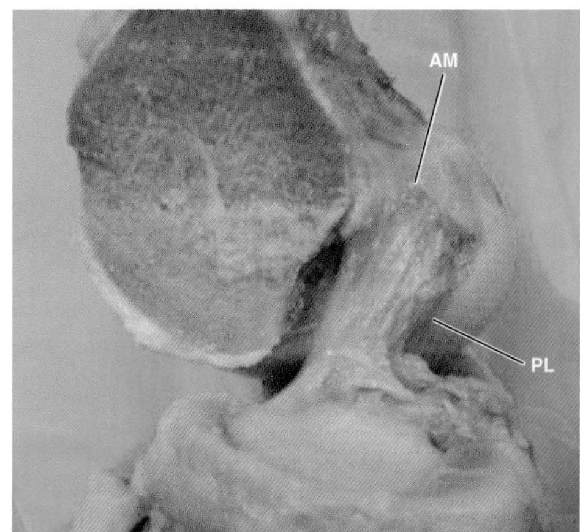

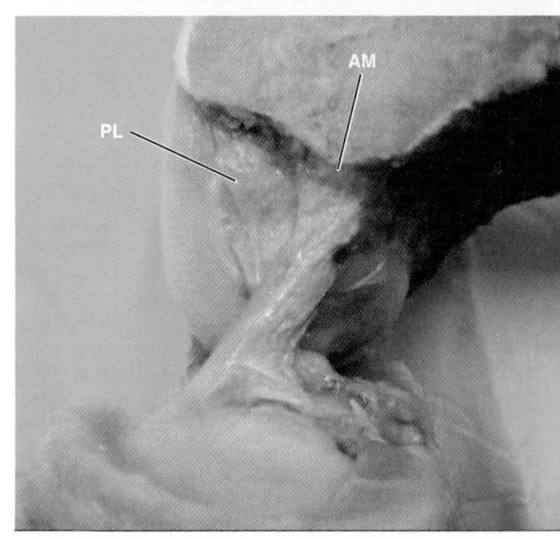

FIG 1 • Anatomy of the anterior cruciate ligament (ACL). The femoral insertion of the anteromedial (AM) and posterolateral (PL) bundles varies based on degree of flexion. At 0 degrees, the femoral insertion is vertical, with the AM bundle superior to the PL bundle (**A**), whereas at 90 degrees, the femoral insertion is horizontal, with the PL bundle anterior to the AM bundle (**B**).

- MRI should be used to confirm the suspicion of an ACL tear and look for associated injuries of the chondral surfaces (including bone bruises), meniscus, patella, and other ligamentous structures.
- A KT-1000 arthrometer test is performed to determine absolute translation and side-to-side translation difference.

DIFFERENTIAL DIAGNOSIS

- Meniscal tear
- Osteochondral injury
- Contusion
- Patellar dislocation
- Other ligament/capsular injury (eg, medial collateral ligament, lateral collateral ligament, posterolateral corner, multiple ligament injury)
- It is important to remember that patella dislocation may mimic the initial presentation of ACL tear.

NONOPERATIVE TREATMENT

- Potential nonoperative candidates and rehabilitation protocol are detailed in Chapter SM-41.

SURGICAL TREATMENT

Indications

- The indications for anatomic double-bundle ACL reconstruction are similar to those for traditional single-bundle reconstruction.
- Patients with recurrent instability or episodes of giving way or those who are unable to return to activities of daily living or sports are appropriate for surgical reconstruction.
- Patients with complaints of instability and a single-bundle or "partial" tear may benefit from single-bundle augmentation, or double-bundle reconstruction in the event the remaining bundle is incompetent.
- Double-bundle reconstruction has been useful in the revision setting, particularly when the previous femoral tunnel placement was in the traditional "over the top" position, which is too high in the femoral notch. This allows anatomic placement of the two femoral tunnels without interfering with the previous tunnel.

Contraindications

- We have not found any contraindication to this procedure in the skeletally mature patient.
- Neither the height of the patient nor the size of the knee has been a factor when performing the surgery.

Evaluation Under Anesthesia

- Range of motion in comparison to the contralateral knee
- Ligamentous examination
  - Lachman
  - Pivot shift
  - Varus and valgus stress
  - Anterior and posterior drawer

Positioning

- The patient is positioned supine on the operating table, and the nonoperative leg is placed in a well-leg holder in the abducted lithotomy position.
- A pneumatic tourniquet is applied around the upper thigh of the operative leg, the operative limb is exsanguinated by elevation for 3 minutes, and the tourniquet is insufflated to 300 to 350 mm Hg, depending on patient size.
- The operative leg is positioned in an arthroscopic leg holder and prepared and draped.

Approach

- The portals used for this procedure[3] are slightly different from standard arthroscopy portals (**FIG 2**).
- The anterolateral portal is placed more superior, at the level of the inferior pole of the patella, just lateral to the patella tendon.
- A central anteromedial portal is placed just below the inferior pole of the patella, approximately 1 cm lateral to the medial edge of the patella tendon (intratendinous central portal).
- An accessory anteromedial portal is established using direct visualization with an 18-gauge spinal needle, which is inserted medially and distally to the inferomedial portal, just above the anterior medial meniscus.
- The accessory medial portal is used for better access to the lateral wall of the intercondylar notch when placing the femoral PL tunnel and femoral AM tunnel if transtibial tunnel location placement is unacceptable.
- The arthroscope is placed in the central anteromedial portal during femoral tunnel placement for better visualization of the intercondylar notch.
- The arthroscope is placed in the anterolateral portal for tibial tunnel placement.

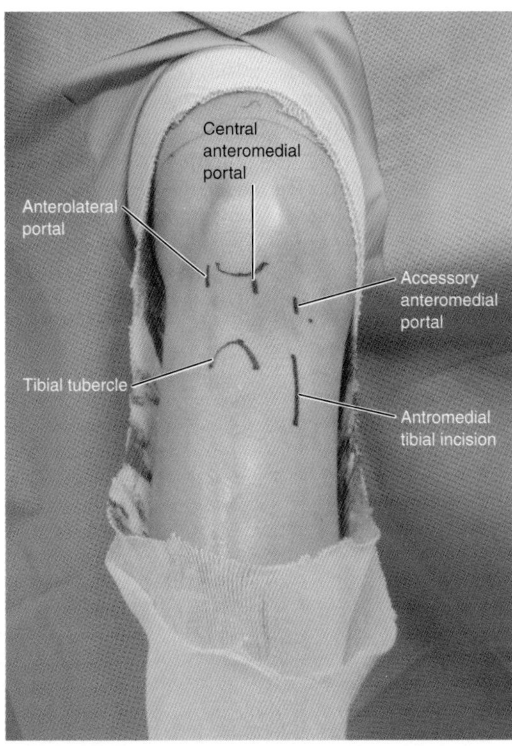

FIG 2 • Portal placement for anatomic double-bundle ACL reconstruction.

DIAGNOSTIC ARTHROSCOPY

- Thorough inspection of the joint, including:
  - Patellofemoral joint compartment
  - Lateral compartment and meniscus
  - Medial compartment and meniscus
  - Posterior cruciate ligament
  - ACL
- Any associated meniscal or chondral lesions are addressed before the ACL reconstruction.
- The torn ACL is dissected carefully using a thermal device to determine the injury pattern and with special attention to the anatomic footprints of the two ACL bundles, on the lateral wall of the intercondylar notch and on the tibial insertion (**TECH FIG 1**).
- Injury patterns may include the following:
  - Tear or stretch of one or both bundles
  - Injury from femoral insertion, tibial insertion, and midsubstance
- There are 25 different injury patterns.
- Anatomic insertion sites of the AM and PL bundles on the tibia and femur are marked.
- The tibial footprints are left intact because of their proprioceptive and vascular contributions.

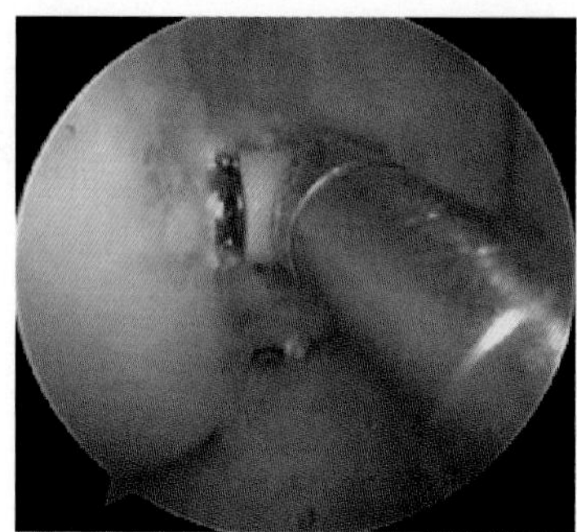

TECH FIG 1 • Dissection and marking of the femoral insertion of the ACL with a thermal device.

POSTEROLATERAL FEMORAL TUNNEL

- The PL femoral tunnel is the first tunnel to be drilled.
- A 3/32 Steinmann pin is inserted through the accessory anteromedial portal.
- The tip of the guidewire is placed on the femoral footprint of the PL bundle on the lateral wall of the intercondylar notch adjacent to the articular surface (**TECH FIG 2A**).
- Once the tip of the guidewire is placed in the correct anatomic position (8 mm from anterior and 5 mm from distal articular cartilage), the knee is flexed to 120 degrees and the guidewire is manually tapped into the femur.
  - Hyperflexion is performed while placing the PL femoral tunnel to avoid injury to the peroneal nerve when passing a Beath pin.
- The guidewire is over-drilled with a 7-mm acorn drill, taking care to avoid injury to the medial femoral condyle articular cartilage.
- The PL tunnel is drilled to a depth of 25 to 30 mm (**TECH FIG 2B**).
- The far cortex is then breached with a 4.5-mm EndoButton drill (Smith & Nephew, Andover, MA), and the depth gauge is used to measure the distance to the far cortex.

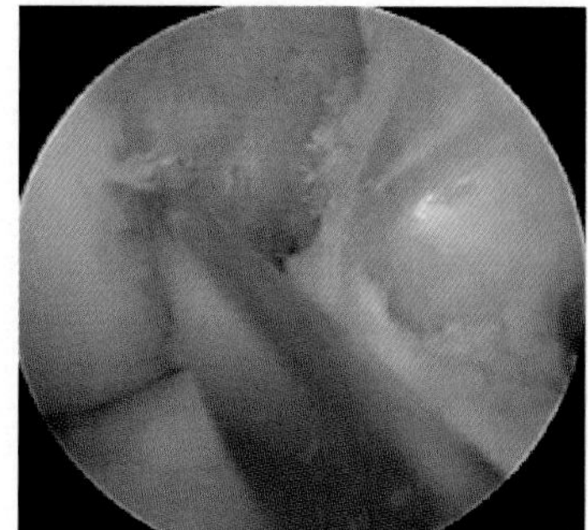

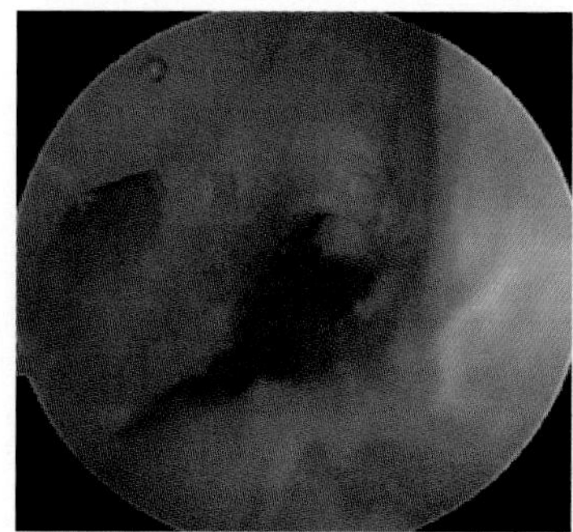

TECH FIG 2 • **A.** Insertion of a guide pin in the femoral insertion of the PL bundle through the accessory anteromedial portal. **B.** PL femoral tunnel drilled to 7 mm diameter.

TIBIAL TUNNELS

- To establish the two tibial tunnels, a 4-cm skin incision is made over the anteromedial surface of the tibia at the level of the tibial tubercle.
- First the PL tunnel is drilled.
- An Accufex (Smith & Nephew, Andover, MA) ACL tibial tunnel tip drill guide set to 55 degrees is placed through the accessory medial portal intra-articularly on the tibial footprint of the PL bundle, which was previously marked using a thermal device (TECH FIG 3A).
- On the tibial cortex, the tibial drill starts just anterior to the superficial medial collateral ligament fibers.
- A 3.2-mm guidewire is then passed into the stump of the PL tibial footprint.
- The AM tibial tunnel is drilled with the tibial drill guide set at 45 degrees and placed through the anteromedial portal, and the tip of the drill guide is placed on the tibial footprint of the AM tunnel (TECH FIG 3B).
- The starting point of the AM tunnel on the tibial cortex is more anterior, central, and proximal than the starting point of the PL tunnel.
- The 3.2-mm guidewire is passed into the stump of the AM tibial footprint, and placement of both guidewires is assessed for satisfactory position (TECH FIG 3C).
- The tibial tunnels are then overdrilled with 7- and 8-mm compaction drill reamers for the PL and AM tunnels, respectively.

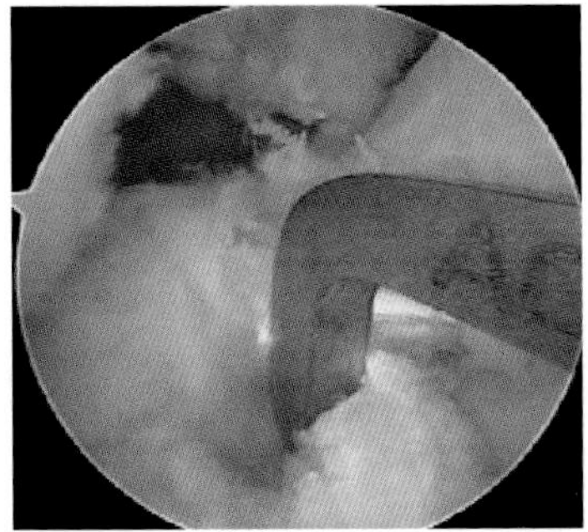

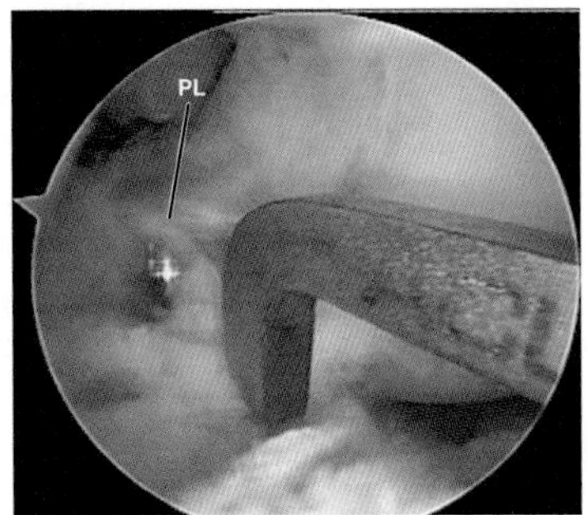

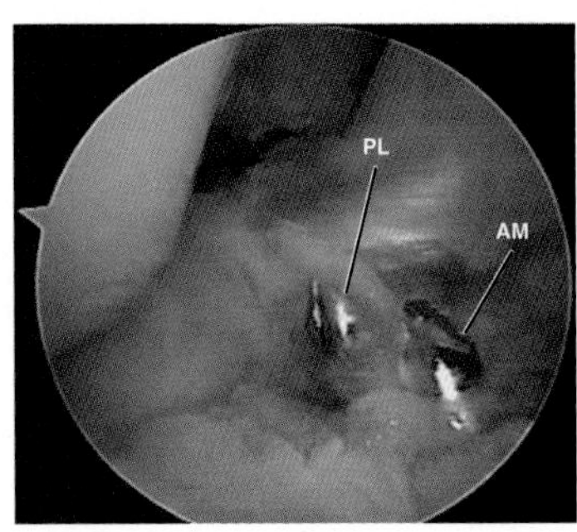

TECH FIG 3 • **A**. Placement of ACL tibial guide (set on 55 degrees) on the tibial PL bundle insertion site through the accessory anteromedial portal. **B.** Placement of ACL tibial guide (set on 45 degrees) placed on the tibial anteromedial (AM) bundle insertion site through the central anteromedial portal. **C**. Appearance of guide pins in the AM and PL tibial insertions of the ACL.

ANTEROMEDIAL FEMORAL TUNNEL

- The femoral AM tunnel is the last tunnel to be drilled.
- A transtibial technique is used most commonly, in a similar fashion to that of a femoral tunnel for ACL single-bundle reconstruction (TECH FIG 4A).
- A guidewire is passed through the AM tibial tunnel, and the tip of the guidewire is placed on the femoral footprint of the AM bundle, which was marked previously with a thermal device.
  - At 90 degrees, the location is directly posterior to the PL femoral tunnel.
- If the location of the guidewire tip is unacceptable, the accessory medial portal is used to insert the guidewire in the proper location.
- After the guidewire is inserted in the desired position, an 8-mm acorn drill is inserted over the guidewire, and the AM femoral tunnel is drilled to a depth of 35 mm to 40 mm (TECH FIG 4B).
- The far cortex of the AM femoral tunnel is breached with a 4.5-mm EndoButton drill, and the depth gauge is used to measure the distance to the far cortex.

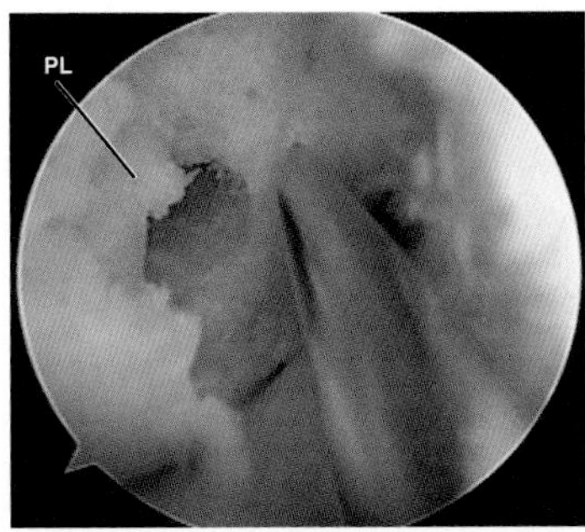

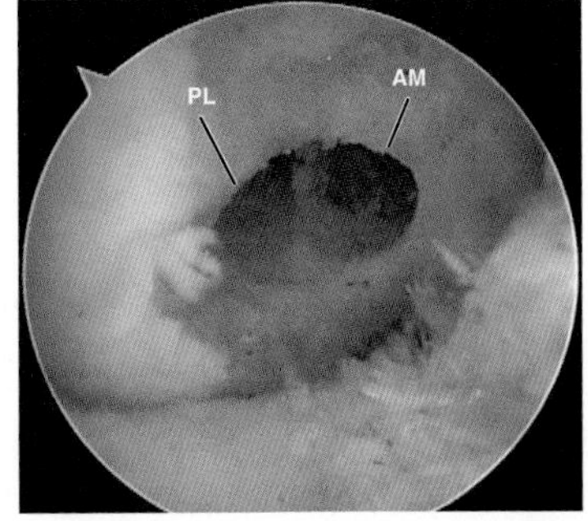

TECH FIG 4 • **A.** Placement of a guide pin into the femoral AM bundle insertion using the transtibial technique. **B.** Appearance of the AM and PL femoral tunnels at 90 degrees after drilling to 8 mm and 7 mm diameter, respectively.

GRAFT CHOICE

- During the arthroscopic procedure, the ACL grafts are prepared on the back table.
- We prefer to use two separate tibialis anterior or tibialis posterior tendon allografts.
- These grafts usually are 24 cm to 30 cm in length, and we fold each tendon graft to obtain 12- to 15-cm double-stranded grafts (TECH FIG 5).
- The AM tendon double-stranded graft typically is 8 mm, and the PL double-stranded graft is 7 mm.
- Alternatively, autogenous semitendinosus and gracilus grafts can be harvested (see Chap. SM-41) and used for the reconstruction.
- The ends of the tendon grafts are sutured using a whipstitch with no. 2 Ticron sutures (Tyco, Waltham, MA).

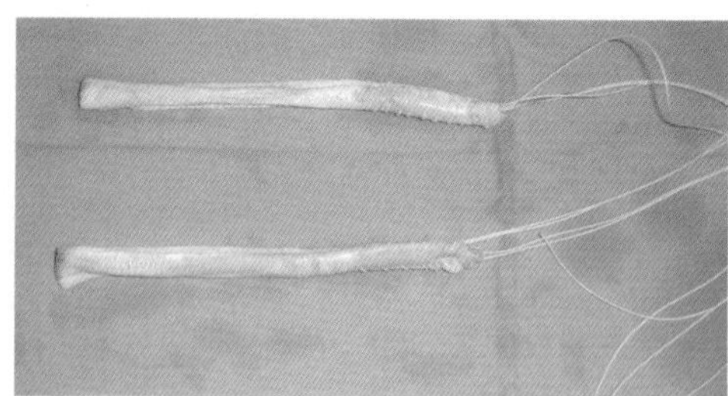

TECH FIG 5 • Double-looped tibialis anterior allografts. An 8-mm graft is used for the AM graft and looped through a 15-mm EndoButton loop. A 7-mm graft is used for the PL graft and is placed through an EndoButton loop.

GRAFT PASSAGE

- The PL bundle graft is passed first. A Beath pin with a long looped suture attached to the eyelet is passed through the accessory anteromedial portal and out the PL femoral tunnel and lateral aspect of the thigh.
- Hyperflexion of the knee is performed to protect the peroneal nerve.
- The looped suture is visualized within the joint and retrieved with an arthroscopic suture grasper through the PL tibial tunnel.
- The graft is passed, and the EndoButton is flipped in standard fashion to establish femoral fixation of the PL bundle graft (TECH FIG 6A).
- Next, the AM bundle graft is passed using the transtibial technique and out the anterolateral thigh with a Beath pin loaded with a looped suture (TECH FIG 6B).
- If the transtibial technique is not used for the AM femoral tunnel, then the graft is passed in a similar fashion to the PL bundle graft.
- The EndoButton is flipped in standard fashion to establish femoral fixation of the AM bundle graft.
- Preconditioning of the grafts is performed by flexing and extending the knee through a range of motion (ROM) from 0 to 120 degrees approximately 20 to 30 times.

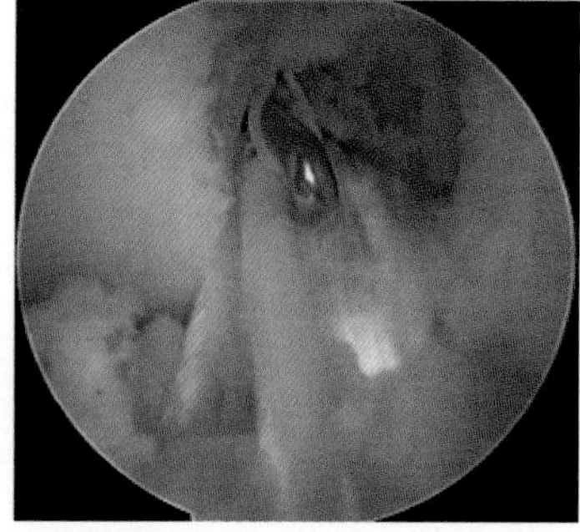

A

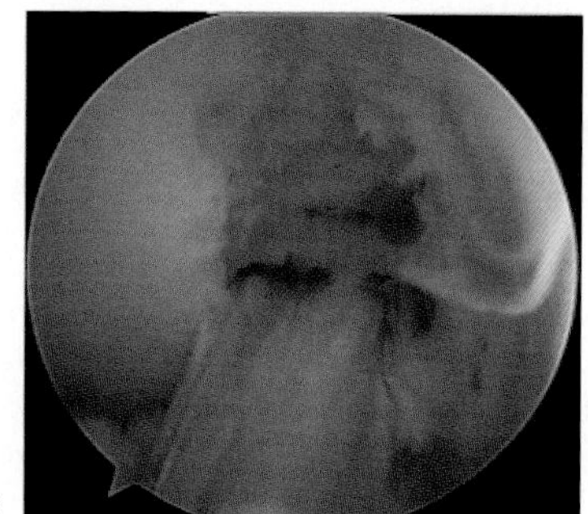

B

TECH FIG 6 • **A.** Arthroscopic view from the anterolateral portal of the passage of the PL bundle graft. The PL graft is passed first, followed by the AM graft. **B.** Arthroscopic view from the central anteromedial portal following passage of the AM and PL grafts, completing the anatomic double-bundle ACL reconstruction.

FIXATION

- Each graft is looped around an EndoButton.
- The length of the EndoButton loop is chosen according to the measured length of the femoral tunnels.
- On the tibial side, we prefer the use of a bioabsorbable interference screw fixation combined with Richards staple fixation (Smith & Nephew Richards, Memphis, TN) for each graft (TECH FIG 7).
- The PL bundle graft is tensioned and fixed at full extension, and the AM bundle graft is tensioned and fixed at 60 degrees of flexion.
- After the fixation is complete, the knee is tested for stability and full ROM. The wounds are closed in standard fashion, and the leg locked in full extension in a hinged knee brace with a Cryocuff (Aircast, Summit, NJ) placed under the brace.

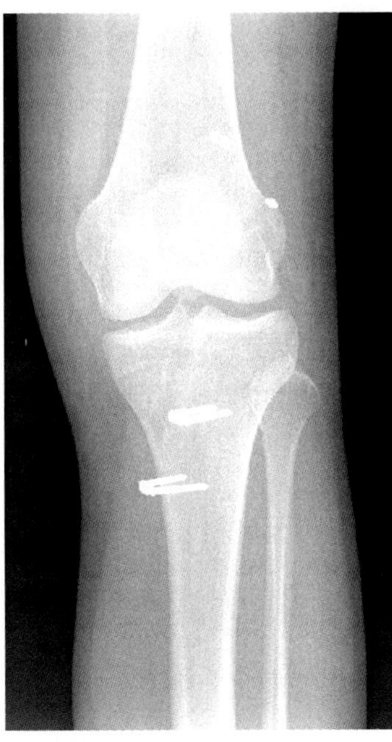

TECH FIG 7 • Postoperative AP radiograph after anatomic double-bundle ACL reconstruction. The femoral fixation uses an EndoButton for each graft, and tibial fixation is obtained using a bioabsorbable interference screw and Richards staple for each graft.

PEARLS AND PITFALLS

Grafts	■ We prefer soft tissue grafts (and prefer allograft over autograft). ■ AM graft: 7 to 8 mm ■ PL graft: 6 to 7 mm
Examination of injury pattern	■ Inspection for tear or stretch of either or both bundles
Portals	■ Three portals are used. ■ The lateral wall is visualized through the central portal.
Tunnel placement	■ Marking anatomic insertion sites ■ PL femoral tunnel placed first ■ AM femoral tunnel based on PL tunnel
Fixation	■ For femur: EndoButton ■ For tibia: biointerference screw plus staple
Postoperatively	■ Early ROM

POSTOPERATIVE CARE

- The authors' postoperative rehabilitation follows the same standard protocol used for patients undergoing ACL single-bundle reconstruction using soft tissue grafts.
- Patients wear a hinged knee brace for 6 weeks.
- For the first week, the brace is locked in extension.
- Continuous passive motion is started immediately after surgery, from 0 to 45 degrees of flexion, and is increased by 10 degrees per day.
- Patients use crutches for 4 weeks postoperatively.
- From the first postoperative day, patients are allowed full weight bearing as tolerated.
- Non-cutting and non-twisting sports such as swimming, biking, and running in a straight line are allowed at 12 weeks after surgery.
- Return to full activity level usually is allowed at 6 months postoperatively.

OUTCOMES

- No current long-term studies on the results of anatomic double-bundle ACL reconstruction have been performed.
- Several short-term studies and multiple prospective studies currently are ongoing in Japan, France, Italy, and the United States.
- Muneta et al[7] reported on 54 patients 2 years after double-bundle ACL reconstruction using autogenous hamstring and found a trend toward improved anterior stability compared with the single-bundle technique.
- Zaricznyj[11] found 86% good or excellent results at 3.6 years follow-up in 14 patients after using doubled hamstring autograft for ACL reconstruction with one femoral and two tibial tunnels. Rotational stability was achieved in each patient, as demonstrated by a negative pivot shift.
- In a case series with 57 consecutive patients, Yasuda et al[10] demonstrated that anatomic ACL double-bundle reconstruction

appears to be a safe technique with satisfactory outcomes. They evaluated functional outcomes at 24 to 36 months follow-up and compared their results with historic data on ACL single-bundle reconstruction. Patients undergoing anatomic ACL double-bundle reconstruction trended toward better AP knee stability, as measured by the KT-2000, compared with the single-bundle group.

- In a prospective, randomized clinical trial including 108 patients, Adachi et al[1] compared the outcomes of anatomic ACL double-bundle reconstruction with the ACL single-bundle technique at an average follow up of 32 months. Their outcome measures included AP knee stability, as measured by the KT-2000, and the joint position sense of the knee. These authors did not find any difference between the ACL double-bundle and the ACL single-bundle group.

COMPLICATIONS

- Traditional complications for single-bundle reconstruction include graft failure, hardware complications, and infection.
- In our series, we have had three graft failures, all occurring after returning to sports.
  - Two failures were sustained during contact injuries while playing collegiate football. The third occurred in a noncompliant patient 3 months after reconstruction when she returned to playing high school basketball without a brace.
  - Four patients have undergone staple removal for symptomatic hardware.
- Specific complications for double-bundle reconstruction include:
  - Risk of femoral condyle fracture
  - Graft impingement
  - Incorrect tunnel placement
  - Tunnel enlargement
  - Difficulty with revision surgery
- We have performed 186 double-bundle ACL reconstructions and have had no fractures and no radiographic signs of femoral condylar avascular necrosis or tunnel widening.
- Bell et al[2] performed biomechanical and computer modeling studies comparing single and double femoral tunnels and the risk of femoral condyle fracture.
  - Results of these studies have shown that fracture risk increased significantly for the single tunnel versus the native condyle procedure, but no significant increase in fracture risk was found for one versus two tunnels.
- ROM studies are in progress. Preliminary results have shown earlier return to full extension and symmetric flexion to the contralateral knee by 3 months after surgery.
- Proper tunnel location is achieved by marking the anatomic sites for each bundle prior to ACL débridement.
- Prospective studies measuring for radiographic tunnel enlargement are ongoing. Thus far, no significant tunnel enlargement has been found; however, follow-up has been short-term only.
- Revision surgery has not been compromised in the two patients in our cohort who have undergone repeat ACL surgery following traumatic re-tear after double-bundle reconstruction.

REFERENCES

1. Adachi N, Ochi M, Uchio Y, et al. Reconstruction of the anterior cruciate ligament. Single- versus double-bundle multistranded hamstring tendons. J Bone Joint Surg Br 2004;86B:515–520.
2. Bell KM, Egan M, Fu FH, et al. Femoral fracture risk analysis of singe- and double-bundle ACL reconstruction. Orthopaedic Research Society Annual Meeting, Chicago, March 19–22, 2006.
3. Cohen SB, Fu FH. The three portal technique for ACL reconstruction: use of a central anteromedial portal—Technical note. Arthroscopy 2007;23:325.
4. Girgis FG, Marshall JL, Monajem A. The cruciate ligaments of the knee joint. Clin Orthop Relat Res 1975;106:216–231.
5. Kummer B, Yamamoto Y. Funktionelle Anatomie der Kreuzbaender. Arthroskopie 1988;1:2–10.
6. Loh JC, Fukuda Y, Tsuda E, et al. Knee stability and graft function following anterior cruciate ligament reconstruction: comparison between 11 o'clock and 10 o'clock femoral tunnel placement. Arthroscopy 2003;19:297–304.
7. Muneta T, Sekiya I, Yagishita K, et al. Two-bundle reconstruction of the anterior cruciate ligament using semitendinosus tendon with endobuttons: operative technique and preliminary results. Arthroscopy 1999;15:618–624.
8. Odensten M, Gillquist J. Functional anatomy of the anterior cruciate ligament and a rationale for reconstruction. J Bone Joint Surg Am 1985;67A:257–262.
9. Woo SL, Kanamori A, Zeminski J, et al. The effectiveness of reconstruction of the anterior cruciate ligament with hamstrings and patellar tendon: a cadaveric study comparing anterior tibial and rotational loads. J Bone Joint Surg Am 2002;84A:907–914.
10. Yasuda K, Kondo E, Ichiyama H, et al. Anatomic reconstruction of the anteromedial and posterolateral bundles of the anterior cruciate ligament using hamstring tendon grafts. Arthroscopy 2004;20:1015–1025.
11. Zaricznyj B. Reconstruction of the anterior cruciate ligament of the knee using a doubled tendon graft. Clin Orthop Relat Res 1987;220: 162–175.

Chapter 43

Revision Anterior Cruciate Ligament Repair

David R. McAllister and David L. Feingold

DEFINITION

- The anterior cruciate ligament (ACL) is the primary stabilizer preventing anterior displacement of the tibia. The ligament is made up of an anteromedial and a posterolateral bundle.
- The ACL also plays a role in assisting the capsular structures, collateral ligaments, joint surface, and meniscal geometry in preventing rotational instability.
- Failure of a primary ACL reconstruction may be due to traumatic re-rupture, stretch-out of the graft, failure to diagnose concomitant injuries (ie, posterolateral corner injury), or technical issues encountered during primary ACL reconstruction (ie, tunnel malposition, fixation failure etc. See Chap. SM-41).

ANATOMY

- The anatomy of the ACL (described in previous chapters) and also that of the secondary stabilizers of the knee are critical in revision surgery. Secondary restraints to anterior translation of the tibia include the medial collateral ligament, the posterior horn of the medial meniscus, and the posterior aspect of the capsule.[6]
- Unrecognized rotatory instability patterns play a significant role in failures of primary ACL reconstruction. Posterolateral instability may involve injury to the popliteus tendon and the popliteofibular and lateral collateral ligaments, and may require repair, advancement, or reconstruction of these structures.[6]
- Primary ACL reconstruction has been described with a number of different grafts, including autograft central patellar tendon; hamstring; and quadricep tendon; as well as a number of allograft tendons, including Achilles, patellar, hamstring, and quadriceps.[10]
  - Attempts have been made at using synthetic structures to reconstruct the ACL but to date have had poor outcomes.
- Fixation techniques are as diverse as the materials used to reconstruct the ACL. In the revision setting it is important to understand the technique and materials used in the initial reconstruction, because it often is necessary to remove fixation devices to obtain optimal results when revising a failed ACL reconstruction.

PATHOGENESIS

- Poor outcomes following ACL reconstruction can be due to a multitude of factors and commonly are grouped into one of four areas: recurrent instability; motion loss; persistent pain; or extensor mechanism dysfunction. This chapter focuses on recurrent instability.
- The incidence of recurrent instability after primary ACL reconstruction is 3% to 10%.[9]
- Graft failure has been reported as the primary cause of recurrent instability. Three different categories of graft failure have been described: failure of graft incorporation; suboptimal sugical technique (eg, tunnel malposition, loss of fixation); and traumatic re-rupture. Although these categories may occur together, a critical step in the successful outcome of treatment for a failed ACL reconstruction is to define the primary cause of failure.

NATURAL HISTORY

- The natural history of the ACL-deficient knee is not well understood.
  - It is commonly thought that patients who continue to experience episodes of instability place the knee at risk of further damage to the articular cartilage and menisci.
  - While it may be possible for some patients to avoid activities that result in instability, others may continue to participate in sports, and still others may experience episodes of instability with activities of daily living.

PATIENT HISTORY AND PHYSICAL FINDINGS

- A detailed history of the primary injury and reconstruction, postoperative course, ability to return to activity, and current symptoms is helpful to determine the optimal treatment.
  - It also is helpful to know the time from the initial injury to the index reconstruction.
  - An explanation of the postoperative therapy program and progress should be obtained, and any traumatic episodes after surgery should be noted.
- A copy of the operative report from the previous repair should be obtained from the primary surgeon to note graft type, tunnel placement, fixation methods and materials, and condition of the articular surfaces and menisci at the time of that procedure.
- An antalgic gait may suggest persistent pain after surgery, or a recent second traumatic event.
  - A varus thrust during gait is highly suggestive of incompetence of the lateral or posterolateral structures and requires further evaluation with long-film standing anteroposterior radiographs for mechanical alignment.
  - Buckling of the knee, especially in the initial phase of gait, may suggest quadriceps weakness, and may give the patient the subjective sensation of knee instability.
- Sensory status and palpation of pulses must be noted in all cases. Any decreases may suggest an initial dislocation of the knee and require appropriate workup to rule out a vascular injury.
- Common examinations to determine instability patterns of the knee include:
  - Anterior drawer test. When compared to the contralateral knee, increased anterior laxity may indicate an ACL-deficient knee.
  - Posterior drawer test. When compared to the contralateral knee, increased posterior laxity may be indicative of a posterior cruciate ligament (PCL)-deficient knee.

- Lachman's test. Sensitive test for ACL deficiency, especially when the contralateral knee has intact native ACL.
- Varus/valgus stress testing. Opening in 30 degrees of flexion is consistent with injury to collateral ligaments alone. If opening in both 0 and 30 degrees, injury to collateral ligaments and other structures, such as the cruciate ligaments or capsule, is suggested.
- Pivot shift. Highly sensitive test for the ACL-deficient knee. It often is difficult for the patient to relax in the setting of a painful knee, however.
- Posterolateral drawer test. Increased posterolateral translation compared with the intact, contralateral knee may suggest posterolateral rotatory instability.
- Dial test. Difference of more than 10 degrees at 30 degrees flexion is consistent with injury to the posterolateral corner (PLC). Difference of more than 10 degrees at 90 degrees flexion is consistent with injury to both PLC and PCL.
  - The varus recurvatum test reveals varus angulation, hyperextension, and external rotation of the tibia. It suggests posterolateral rotatory instability of the knee.
- Testing for concurrent intra-articular injuries should be performed to detect possible meniscal, articular cartilage, or patellofemoral pathology.
- Large effusions are common in the setting of a ruptured native ACL. In the revision setting, rupture of the graft may not lead to a large hemarthrosis, because of decreased vascularity of the graft material compared to the native ACL. Effusions in the setting of a failed ACL reconstruction may be small or even nonexistent.

IMAGING AND OTHER DIAGNOSTIC STUDIES

- Routine radiographs, including weight-bearing anteroposterior and lateral views as well as patellar views, should be performed. In the revision setting, these images allow for critical assesment of previous tunnel placement and assesment for possible bone loss at previous tunnels, which may require further evaluation and treatment.
  - Metallic fixation devices make previous tunnel placement easy to identify, but bioabsorbable screws and other types of fixation also can be evaluated for tunnel placement on these images (**FIG 1**).
  - These images also allow evaluation for possible evidence of osteoarthritis.
- If concern regarding a significant amount of bone loss is present after initial radiographic evaluation, CT imaging allows more precise evaluation of possible tunnel enlargement. MRI also may allow evaluation of tunnel size, along with further evaluation of possible intra-articular pathology.
  - Metallic fixation devices may create significant artifacts on both of these imaging techniques, at times limiting their usefulness.

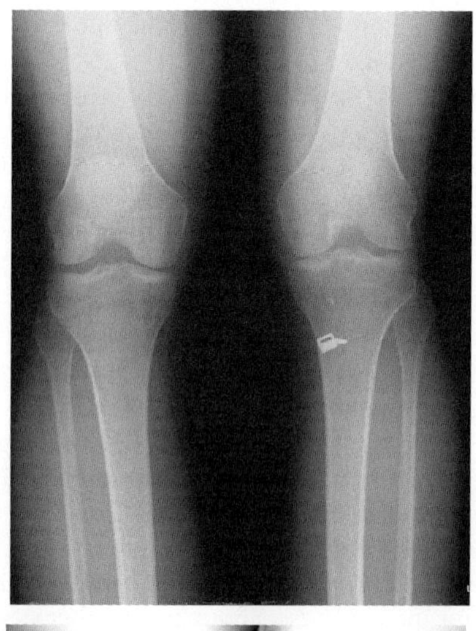

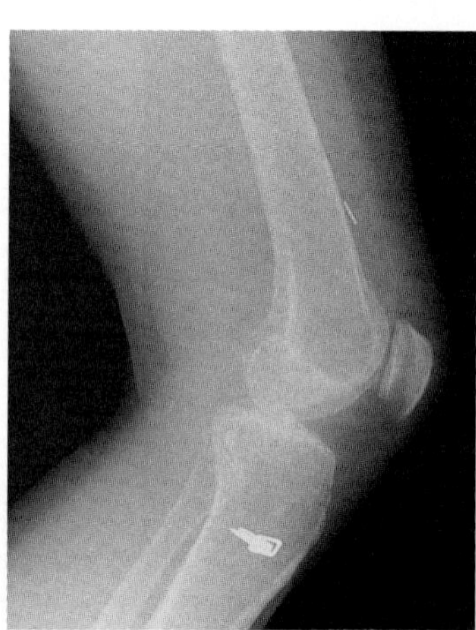

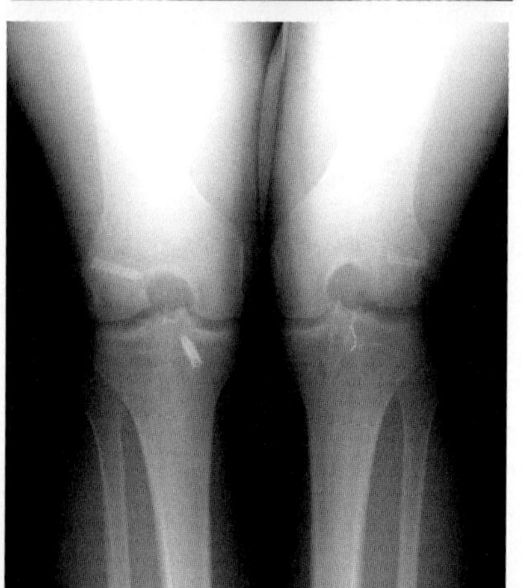

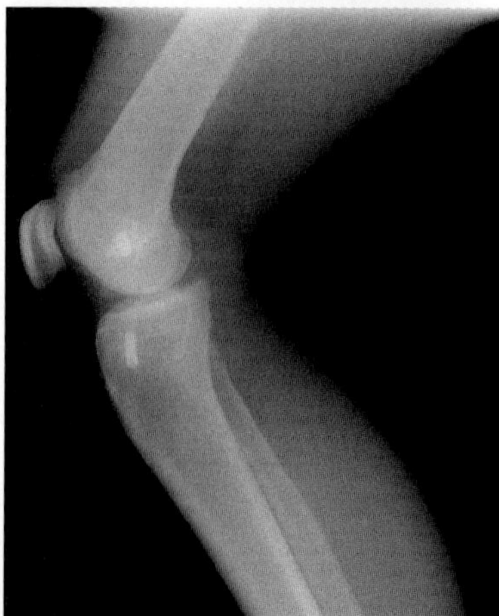

FIG 1 • **A,B.** Anterior cruciate ligament (ACL) reconstruction performed with an EndoButton (Smith & Nephew, Andover, MA) on the femur and staple fixation of the graft on the tibia. **C,D.** Anterior placement of the femoral tunnel in this primary ACL reconstruction performed with a two-incision technique.

- For varus alignment, or chronic posterolateral rotatory instability, radiographs that allow full evaluation of mechanical alignment may be necessary. These will help the surgeon to determine whether there is a significant varus alignment of the knee.
  - In ACL-deficient knees with varus bony alignment, any reconstruction may be doomed to failure if the alignment is not first addressed with an osteotomy procedure.
- Bone scan and serologic tests, including complete blood count, erythrocyte sedimentation rate, C-reactive protein, and bacterial cultures of knee aspirates, should be performed in any setting suggestive of infection, including those cases with significant osteolysis of previous tunnels.

DIFFERENTIAL DIAGNOSIS

- Meniscal injury
- Osteochondral injury
- Subjective weakness or anterior knee pain secondary to quadriceps weakness
- Patella subluxation or dislocation
- Multiligamentous injury (eg, PCL, PLC, medial collateral ligament, lateral collateral ligament)

NONOPERATIVE MANAGEMENT

- Patients with painful ACL-deficient knees after attempted reconstruction must understand that reconstruction of the ACL will not address their pain symptoms and that nonoperative management might be a better approach to address their complaints.
- The basis of any nonoperative treatment for an ACL-deficient knee is to avoid those activities that put the knee at risk, such as cutting sports.
- Strengthening the dynamic stabilizers of the knee, such as the hamstrings (an antagonist to anterior translation of the tibia) may increase stability of the knee for routine activities.
- Bracing

SURGICAL MANAGEMENT

- The primary indication for revision ACL surgery is a patient whose chief complaint is symptomatic instability with his or her activities.
  - ACL reconstruction does not address the pain symptoms of an ACL-deficient knee, and other intra-articular pathology should be investigated as the cause of the subjective pain complaints.
  - ACL reconstruction may decrease the progression of intra-articular pathology, but will not, in itself, treat other lesions that may be present.

Preoperative Planning

- A common cause of failure related to surgical technique is anterior placement of a femoral tunnel, which often is detected on the lateral radiograph (**FIG 1D**).[6,10] This may lead to tightening of the graft with knee flexion resulting in graft stretch-out or failure.
- A preoperative plan should include evaluation of the knee based on history, examination, and imaging for possible other intra-articular pathology, such as meniscal tears or cartilage lesions. The surgeon should be prepared to address these comorbidities at the time of revision surgery.
  - Even if the surgeon does not expect to discover such findings, the possibility of their existence, and their treatment options, must be covered in all preoperative discussions with the patient.
- In the setting of possible posterolateral rotational instability, varus malalignment, or significant bone loss requiring bone grafting, the patient must be aware of the possible need for staged procedures, and the necessary postoperative course should this become the case.
- The possiblity of hardware removal requires knowledge of any previous implants used, and extraction tools, such as a commercially available ACL revision tray. These should be available in the operating room at the time of surgery.
- Once anesthesia has been induced, a thorough examination of the knee as compared to the contralateral extremity is critical. Concerns regarding posterolateral or varus and valgus instability will not be answered during arthroscopic evaluation and are best assessed prior to prepping and draping.

Positioning

- Our preferred positioning for ACL reconstructive surgery is with the patient in the supine position using a lateral post.
- The lateral post should be placed proximal enough to allow for the surgeon's hand to drill the tibial tunnel without hitting the table when the patient's knee is flexed over the edge of the table (**FIG 2**).

Approach

- A standard superolateral outflow and anteromedial and anterolateral portals are used for diagnostic arthroscopy.
  - If the previous incisions were adequately positioned, they may be used, but the placement of portal incisions should not be compromised for the sole purpose of reusing the previous incisions.
- A complete diagnostic arthroscopic evaluation of the knee should be performed.
- Treatment of other comorbid conditions should be performed before the ACL reconstruction is done. These include repair or débridement of meniscal tears, removal of loose bodies, débridement with possible microfracture of osteochondral lesions, and hardware removal, if necessary.

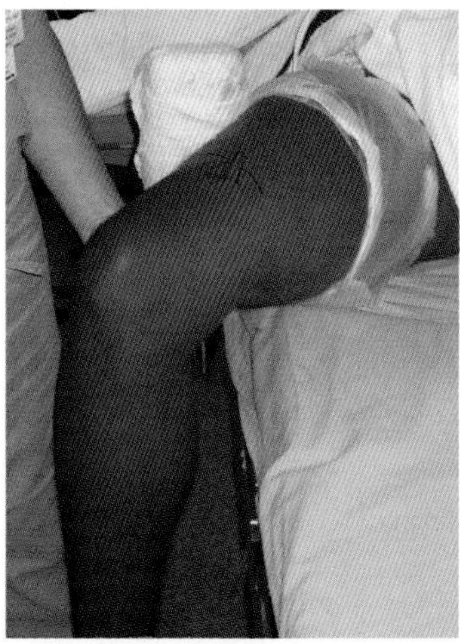

FIG 2 • The lateral post is placed high against the lateral femur to allow adequate room on the medial aspect of the tibia to drill a tibial tunnel without interference from the operative table.

ARTHROSCOPY AND NOTCHPLASTY

- The ACL-deficient knee is diagnosed at the time of examination under anesthesia.
- After completion of the arthroscopic inspection of the knee and treatment of any other intra-articular pathology, the tourniquet is inflated.
- The knee is flexed 90 degrees over a bump under the distal thigh, with the popliteal space free, allowing the neurovascular structures to fall posterior to the posterior capsule of the knee and thus remain out of harm's way.
- The previous graft is removed with a 5.5-mm shaver down to the footprint of the native ACL.
  - The shaver also is used to remove any fat pad obstructing the view, periosteum off the lateral wall of the notch, and any scar tissue present in the notch.
- In revision ACL reconstruction, the notch often is overgrown and narrow, likely as a result of the previous ACL reconstruction (TECH FIG 1A).
  - A notchplasty is completed with use of a 5.5-mm burr, starting at the anterior opening of the notch if necessary.
  - The location of the previous femoral tunnel is noted.
  - Notchplasty is carried back to the posterior wall as needed. A small, curved curette may be used to inspect the back of the notch. A thin white strip of periosteum usually identifies the posterior wall (TECH FIG 1B). Careful attention to localizing the posterior wall is critical, especially because the sides and roof of the notch often are irregular owing to the previous surgery.
- Anterior placement of the femoral tunnel is the primary cause of recurrent laxity for ACL reconstructions, so in many cases there is enough room to place a second femoral tunnel in the appropriate position without interference or compromise from the previous tunnel. If this is the case, the previous interference screw can be left in place or removed (TECH FIG 1C,D).
  - A curved curette is used to remove a small area of bone to localize the desired position of the new femoral tunnel.
- A more difficult scenario is the situation where the femoral tunnel was well placed. In this case, it can be difficult to create a new tunnel that does not overlap with the old tunnel.
  - We have found that transtibially placed femoral tunnels often can be revised by drilling the revision tunnel through the anteromedial portal. In this way, the tunnels diverge, with only the intra-articular outlets overlapping (TECH FIG 1E).
  - Likewise, if a previously well-placed femoral tunnel was placed via the anteromedial portal, it often can be revised by drilling transtibially.

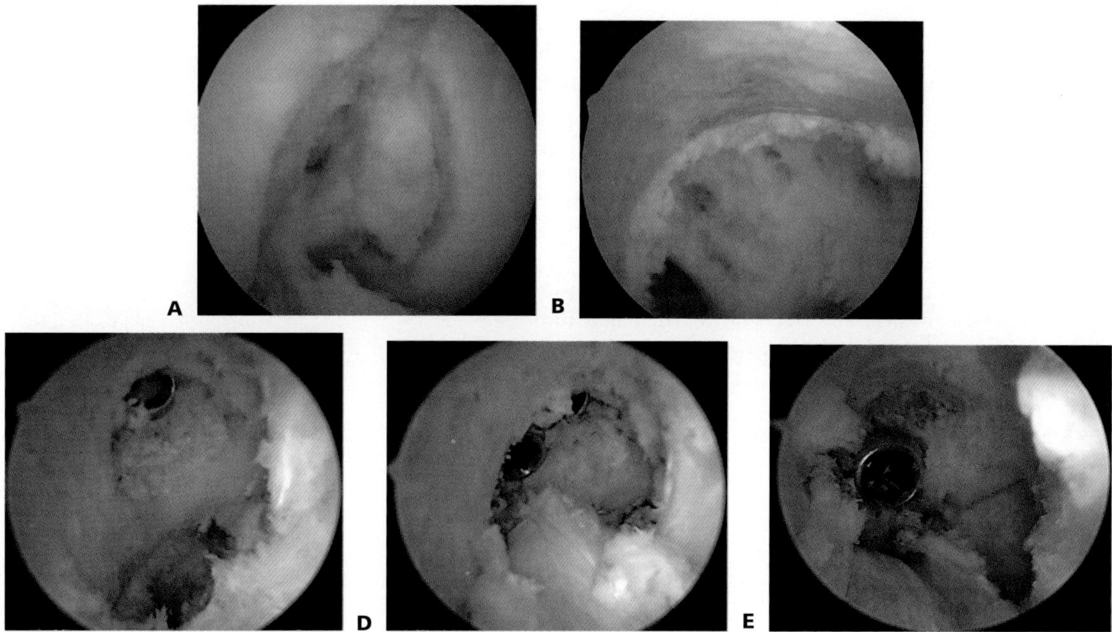

TECH FIG 1 • **A.** Significant overgrowth of the notch noted at the time of revision anterior cruciate ligament (ACL) reconstruction. **B.** A thin layer of periosteum is easily visualized at the posterior wall of the notch. **C.** Note the anterior placement of the femoral tunnel interference screw used during the primary ACL reconstruction. The femoral tunnel for the revision can be placed at the appropriate location without removing the interference screw used in the primary procedure. **D.** The new femoral tunnel and interference screw are placed in the appropriate location without compromise from the screw used in the index procedure. **E.** View of femoral notch after placement of femoral tunnel and interference screw via anteromedial portal. This allows divergence of the old and new femoral tunnels.

GRAFT PREPARATION

- We usually wait to prepare the graft until the tunnels are drilled. This way the bone plugs on the graft can be oversized, in the unlikely event that the new tunnel and old tunnel substantially overlap and create a bony defect that is considerably larger than the standard tunnel size.
- The graft of choice can be used.
  - We do not reharvest previously harvested tendons.
  - Graft options include both autogenous and allogenic grafts.
  - We commonly use bone–patellar tendon–bone allograft.
- Both bone plugs are cut to a length of 25 mm, with a height of 10 mm and width of 10 mm using a micro oscillating saw.
- A small rongeur is used to contour the bone plugs to fit through a 10-mm tunnel.
- A 2-mm drill is used to drill one hole between the proximal two thirds and the distal one third of the bone plug from the patella.
  - Two similar holes are drilled in the tibial bone plug at one- and two-thirds the length of the plug, at a 90-degree angle to each other.
  - No. 5 Ethibond (Ethicon, Inc.) sutures, loaded on Keith needles, are then passed through each hole.
- The graft is then passed through a 10-mm sizer. The graft should slide easily while still having contact with the sides of the sizer.
- The length of the tendon part of the graft is then measured from bone plug to bone plug.
- The graft is wrapped in saline-soaked gauze and protected on the back table.

TUNNEL PLACEMENT

- Neither tibial nor femoral tunnel placement should be compromised based on the location of the previous tunnels.
- The tibial tunnel guidewire is placed the same as for a primary ACL reconstruction, using a commercially available tibial guide.
  - We set the tibial guide at $n + 7$, with n being the length of the graft between the two bone plugs ($n + 7$ rule).[8]
  - The tip of the guide is placed in the posteromedial aspect of the native ACL footprint. The difficulty is that the native ACL footprint is no longer visible. Therefore, we place the guidewire so that it penetrates the joint 6 to 7 mm anterior to the PCL and in a line that intersects the posterior aspect of the anterior horn insertion of the lateral meniscus (TECH FIG 2A).
- The guide is placed in the joint through the anteromedial portal, and a 1.5-cm skin incision is placed just medial to the tibial tubercle, in line with the anteromedial portal for placement of the guidewire.
- If a metallic tibial interference screw was used in the previous reconstruction, it usually is in a location that necessitates its removal.
  - At this point the leg is brought back onto the table, and the interference screw is localized.
  - All overgrown soft tissue and bone is carefully removed, and then the appropriate driver (based on the operative note from the previous procedure) is placed into the head of the screw and it is removed.
- Next, the guide is rechecked, with the sliding bullet placed down to bone. The measurement on the bullet should be just longer than the tendinous portion of the graft ($n + 2$ rule).[11]

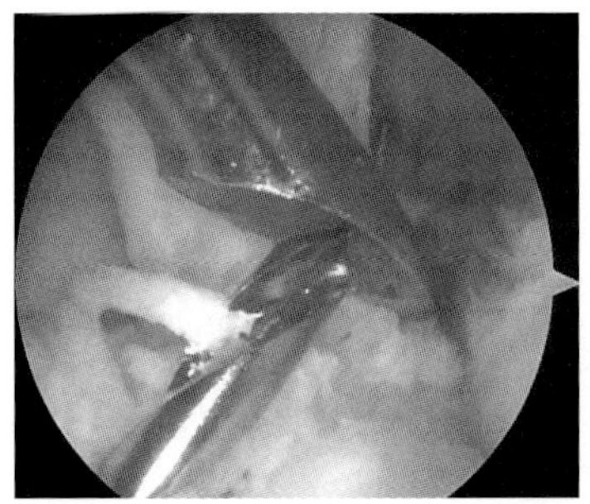
A

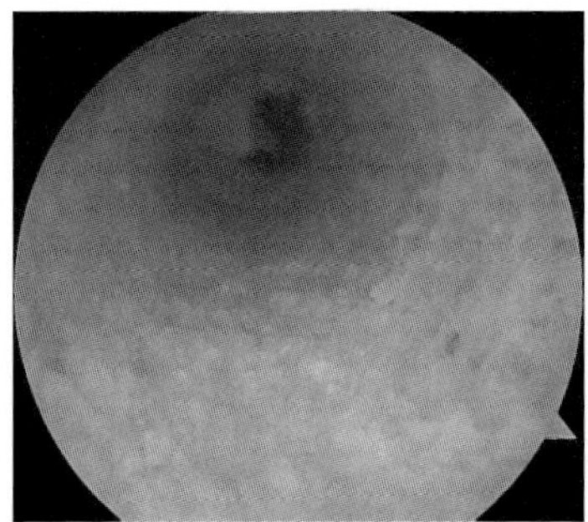
B

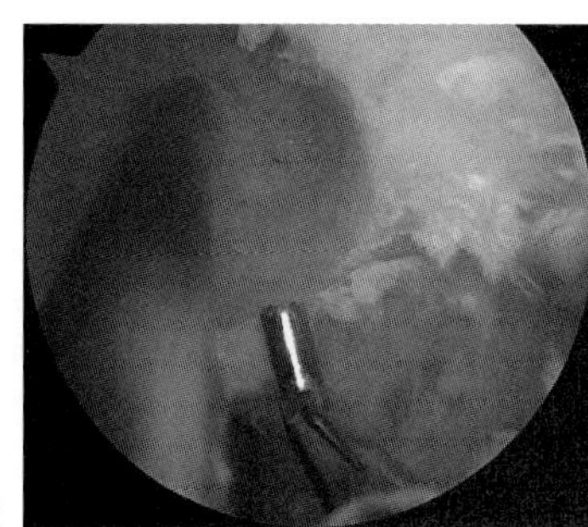
C

TECH FIG 2 • **A.** Placement of the tibial tunnel guidewire just anterior to the native posterior cruciate ligament (PCL). **B.** Appearance of the revision tibial tunnel using the arthroscope to inspect for compromise from the index procedure. **C.** After reaming the femoral tunnel to a depth of 10 mm, the tunnel is inspected to ensure the posterior wall is intact.

- The guidewire is then advanced, and, if correctly placed, the tibial tunnel is made with a 10-mm drill.
- The tunnel is inspected with the arthroscope for wall compromise from the previous tunnel (TECH FIG 2B). This can be performed by placing the arthroscope up the tibial tunnel.
  - If there is concern for fixation strength with the interference screw, the tibial bone plug can be reinforced by tying the suture previously placed through the bone plug over a post just distal to the tibial tunnel.
- Attention is then directed to the femoral notch.
  - A point is marked with a curette in the femoral notch 6 mm (for a 10-mm graft) anterior to the posterior wall in the 1:00 to 1:30 position (left knee) or the 10:30 to 11:00 position (right knee).
  - A Beath pin is advanced across the joint to the previously marked site on the femur. This usually can be done transtibially.
    - In some cases, it is not possible to get the pin to the desired location. In such a case, the knee is flexed to 120 degrees and the Beath pin is passed through the anteromedial portal.
    - As previously mentioned, this technique also can be used when the previous femoral tunnel was placed in an acceptable position transtibially.
    - This allows for divergence of the new tunnel with respect to the old without compromising the entry point into the femoral notch.
- A 10-mm acorn reamer is then advanced by hand through the joint, using care not to damage the PCL.
  - The reamer is advanced to a depth of 10 mm.
  - It is then brought back into the notch so that the back wall can be inspected (TECH FIG 2C).
- At this time, the tunnel also is inspected to ensure that the previous femoral tunnel does not compromise the new tunnel.
  - If there is compromise, one of the other techniques mentioned in the following sections is performed.
  - If the back wall is intact, the reamer is advanced to a depth of 30 mm.

GRAFT PASSAGE AND TENSIONING

- Once appropriate tunnels have been drilled, the single suture from the bone plug from one end of the graft is passed through the Beath pin and then advanced into place.
- The bone plug is advanced into the femoral tunnel under careful visualization to ensure the graft does not rotate and the bone plug is in the anterior aspect of the tunnel.
- The knee is flexed to 120 degrees, and the interference screw is placed while gentle tension is maintained on the graft.
  - Again, careful visualization is used to ensure the graft is not cut by the threads of the advancing screw.
  - The screw is advanced so that it is recessed 1 to 2 mm from the tunnel opening (TECH FIG 3).
- After checking for appropriate isometry of the graft by palpating the tibial bone plug through an arc of motion, the graft is manually tensioned.
  - While maintaining tension, the knee is flexed to about 10 to 20 degrees, and the tibial interference screw is placed.

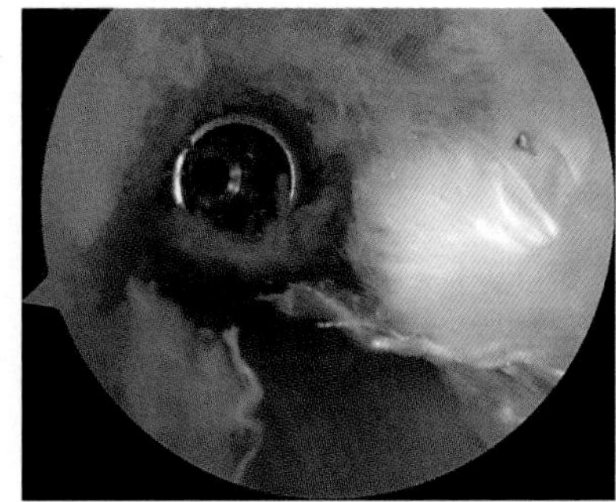

TECH FIG 3 • The femoral interference screw is seated approximately 1 to 2 mm beyond the opening into the notch.

- A final range-of-motion check is performed, and a gentle Lachman test is performed to ensure that stability has been restored.

TWO-INCISION TECHNIQUE

- In cases in which the previous femoral tunnel was placed in the location that would have been preferred for the current one, or osteolysis around the previous tunnel makes placement of the new tunnel difficult, the two-incision technique may be used to create the femoral tunnel.
  - This technique uses the same tunnel aperture, but at a different angle.
  - This allows for fixation of the femoral bone plug at the lateral cortex of the distal femur, a location typically not affected by previous ACL reconstruction.
  - In cases in which the primary ACL reconstruction was performed with a two-incision technique, our standard endoscopic technique usually works without difficulty for placement of the femoral tunnel.
- After drilling the tibial tunnel, and assessment that the femoral tunnel location necessitates two-incision technique, a commercially available, rear-entry, drill guide is used.
- A lateral incision is performed over the distal metaphyseal region.

- The tip of the guide is placed at the posterior aspect of the lateral wall of the notch in the 1:30 position (left knee) or 10:30 position (right knee).
  - The sliding bullet is advanced to bone, and the guidewire is advanced.
- While protecting the PCL with a large curette, the femoral tunnel is reamed with a 10-mm reamer.
- After graft passage using suture material in the bone plugs of the graft, an interference screw is placed at the lateral cortex and advanced until it is adjacent with the bone plug (TECH FIG 4).
- The remainder of the procedure is performed as previously described.

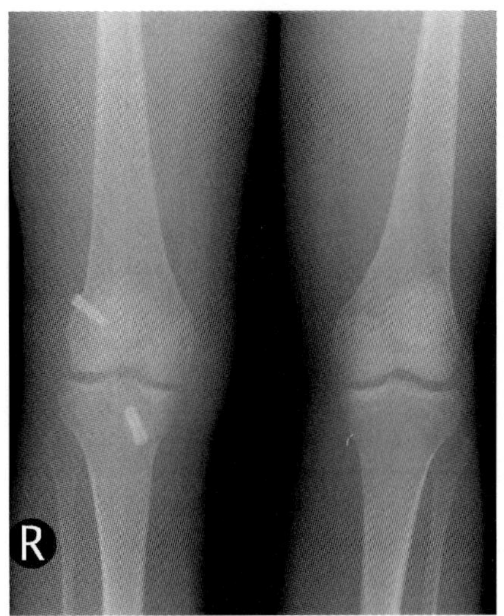

TECH FIG 4 • The femoral interference screw is placed into the femoral tunnel through the lateral cortex.

BONE GRAFTING OF TIBIAL TUNNELS

- If significant bone loss has occurred around the previous tibial tunnel, bone grafting may be necessary, followed by staged revision ACL reconstruction. This is common with synthetic grafts, which can cause an immune reaction to the graft material, and also has been proposed to occur more frequently with hamstring grafts owing to the theoretical "windshield wiper" effect of the graft with fixation at the distal end of the tunnel.[3,13]
- After removal of the fixation devices, the previous tunnels are fully débrided of soft tissue using a shaver, curette, and rasp.
  - If sclerotic bone is encountered, a 2-mm drill can be used to drill the wall of the tunnel.
  - The old tunnels and regions of bony deficiency can be filled with autograft bone (taken in dowels from the iliac crest[13]), or allograft dowels (commonly available from tissue banks[3]).
    - Allograft dowels, when used, should be about 1 mm larger than the diameter of the tunnel and placed using a press-fit technique.
- Reconstruction must be staged to allow time for incorporation of the bone graft.
  - Incorporation of the bone graft can be monitored on CT imaging; it usually takes 4 to 6 months.[13]

PEARLS AND PITFALLS

Indications	■ It is critical to determine whether the patient's chief complaint is instability or pain. ■ For patients 25 years of age and younger, a good reason is needed not to perform revision reconstruction of an ACL-deficient knee. ■ For patients 45 years of age and older, a good reason is needed to consider revision reconstruction in an ACL-deficient knee. ■ Subjective and objective findings of instability should be present to support consideration of revision surgery. Some patients with objective instability are able to participate at a high level of competition in cutting sports without symptomatic instability.
Interference screws	■ In our experience, metallic screws allow easy identification of tunnel placement. We currently do not use "bioabsorbable" screws because we have found that they commonly do not absorb and can be difficult to drill across and difficult to remove during revision surgery.
Synthetic grafts	■ Careful débridement of all synthetic material must be performed to prevent further immune reaction around the new graft.

POSTOPERATIVE CARE

- In the operating room the knee is placed in a hinged knee brace locked in extension, and the patient is permitted to bear weight as tolerated with the brace.
- At all other times, the brace can be removed and immediate postoperative range of motion is begun.
  - Once adequate quadriceps control has been regained, the hinged knee brace is discontinued.

- A cold therapy device, compression stockings, and elevation are used to control edema.
- The first postoperative appointment is on day 2. A wound check is performed, and Steri-strips (3M, St. Paul, MN) are changed as needed.
- The initial physical therapy appointment is scheduled for 3 to 5 days postoperatively and focuses on immediate ROM.
  - The patient is educated regarding use of the knee brace, ROM therapy, and operative findings.
- At the second postoperative visit, on day 8 to 10, sutures are removed, an ROM examination is done, and ROM exercises are explained, especially with focus on extension. In addition, the knee extension brace is discontinued at this time.
- The postoperative rehabilitation schedule is as follows:
  - Months 1–3: focus on ROM and quadriceps strengthening
  - Months 3–4: progress to eccentric quadriceps strengthening and running
  - Months 4–7: continue strengthening
  - Months 7–8: begin agility drills
  - Months 8–9: begin sport-specific drills.
- No contact sports are permitted until 9 to 12 months postoperatively.

OUTCOMES

- The critical factor in successful revision ACL reconstruction is to determine why the initial ACL reconstruction failed before planning the revision surgery. The ultimate clinical outcome likely is based on a combination of factors, including laxity, chondral injury, and meniscal status.
- Grossman et al,[5] in a study that focused on failure of revision ACL reconstruction based on patholaxity, found fairly similar outcomes for subjective and objective measures when compared with primary ACL reconstruction studies.
  - However, only 68% of these patients were able to return to the level of activity and sport they had before the initial injury, significantly lower than the commonly reported 75% to 85% return to pre-injury level sports with primary ACL reconstruction.
- A prospective study by Noyes and Barber-Westin[9,10] looking at revision ACL reconstructions using autogenous bone-patellar tendon–bone grafts resulted in an improvement in subjective scores in 88% of patients, with 62% of these patients able to return to athletics without symptoms.
  - The authors did report an overall graft failure rate of 24%, a threefold increase compared to a previous study by the same authors looking at primary ACL reconstruction.
- In both of the studies by Noyes and Barber-Westin, the condition of the articular cartilage had a significant effect on the subjective scores.
  - In their later study, Noyes and Barber-Westin[10] reported that 93% of patients had compounding problems such as articular cartilage damage, meniscal pathology, loss of secondary ligament restraints, and varus malalignment.
  - While reconstruction of the ACL may provide stability to the knee, these compounding problems play a significant role in patient satisfaction and in patients' ability to return to their level of activity before the primary surgery.

COMPLICATIONS

- Loss of motion
- Graft failure
- Anterior knee pain secondary to damage to the patellofemoral cartilage or quadriceps weakness
- Unrealistic expectations in those patients with articular cartilage damage regarding their ability to return to strenuous sports
- Complex regional pain syndrome

REFERENCES

1. Anderson K, Williams RJ, Wickiewicz TL, et al. Revision ACL surgery: how I do it. In: Insall JN, Scott WN, eds. Surgery of the Knee. Philadelphia: Churchill Livingstone, 2001:813–840.
2. Bach BR Jr, Warren RF, Wickiewicz TL. The pivot shift phenomenon: results and a description of a modified clinical test for anterior cruciate ligament insufficiency. Am J Sports Med 1988;16:571–576.
3. Battaglia TC, Miller MD. Management of bony deficiency in revision anterior cruciate ligament reconstruction using allograft bone dowels: surgical technique. Arthroscopy 2005;21:767.
4. Fox JA, Pierc M, Bochuk J, et al. Revision anterior cruciate ligament reconstruction with nonirradiated fresh-frozen patellar tendon allograft. Arthroscopy 2004;20:784–794.
5. Grossman MG, ElAttrache NS, Shields CL, et al. Revision anterior cruciate ligament reconstruction: three- to nine-year follow-up. Arthroscopy 2005;21:243–247.
6. Harner CD, Giffin JR, Dunteman RC, et al. Evaluation and treatment of recurrent instability after anterior cruciate ligament reconstruction. J Bone Joint Surg Am 2000;82A:1652–1664.
7. Hughston JC, Norwood LA Jr. The posterolateral drawer test and external rotational recurvatum test for posterolateral rotatory instability of the knee. Clin Orthop Rel Res 1980;147:82–87.
8. Miller MD, Hinkin DT. The N+7 rule for tibial tunnel placement during endoscopic ACL reconstruction. Arthroscopy 1996;12:124–126.
9. Noyes FR, Barber-Westin SD. A comparison of results in acute and chronic anterior cruciate ligament ruptures of arthroscopically assisted autogenous patellar tendon reconstruction. Am J Sports Med 1997;25:460–471.
10. Noyes FR, Barber-Westin SD. Revision anterior cruciate surgery with use of bone-patellar tendon-bone autogenous grafts. J Bone Joint Surg Am 2001;83A:1131–1143.
11. Olszewski AD, Miller MD, Ritchie JR. Ideal tibial tunnel length for endoscopic anterior cruciate ligament injuries. Arthroscopy 1998;14:9–14.
12. Spindler KP, Warren TA, Callison JC, et al. Clinical outcome at a minimum of five years after reconstruction of the anterior cruciate ligament. J Bone Joint Surg Am 2005;87A:1673–1679.
13. Thomas NP, Kankate R, Wandless F, et al. Revision anterior cruciate ligament reconstruction using a 2-stage technique with bone grafting of the tibial tunnel. Am J Sports Med 2005;33:1701–1709.
14. Torg JS, Conrad W, Kalen V. Clinical diagnosis of anterior ligament instability in athletes. Am J Sports Med 1976;4:84–93.
15. Wilson TC, Kantaras A, Atay A, et al. Tunnel enlargement after anterior cruciate ligament surgery. Am J Sports Med 2004;32:543–549.

Chapter 44 Posterior Cruciate Ligament Repair

Craig S. Mauro, Anthony M. Buoncristiani, and Christopher D. Harner

DEFINITION

- The posterior cruciate ligament (PCL) serves as the primary restraint to posterior translation of the tibia relative to the femur.
- PCL injuries are uncommon, may be partial or complete, and rarely occur in isolation.
- Our understanding of the PCL with respect to its natural history, surgical indications and technique, and postoperative rehabilitation is improving rapidly.

ANATOMY

- The PCL has a broad femoral origin in a semicircular pattern on the medial femoral condyle.
  - It inserts on the posterior aspect of the tibia, in a depression between the medial and lateral tibial plateaus, 1.0 to 1.5 cm below the joint line.
  - Its width, on average, is 13 mm, which is variable along its course; the average length is 38 mm.
- Anatomic studies have delineated separate characteristics of the anterolateral (AL) and posteromedial (PM) bundles within the PCL.
  - The AL bundle origin is more anterior on the intercondylar surface of the medial femoral condyle, and the insertion is more lateral on the tibia, relative to the PM bundle.
  - The larger AL bundle has increased tension in flexion, whereas the PM bundle becomes more taut in extension.
- The meniscofemoral ligaments, which arise from the posterior horn of the lateral mensicus and insert on the posterolateral aspect of the medial femoral condyle, also contribute to the overall strength of the PCL.

PATHOGENESIS

- Acutely, there usually is a history of a direct blow to the anterior lower leg. Common mechanisms include high-energy trauma and athletic injuries.
  - In motor vehicle trauma, the "dashboard injury" occurs when the proximal tibia strikes the dashboard, causing a posteriorly directed force to the proximal tibia.
  - Athletic injuries usually involve a direct blow to the anterior tibia or a fall onto a flexed knee with the foot in plantar flexion.
- Hyperextension injuries, which often are combined with varus or valgus forces, often result in combined ligamentous injuries.

NATURAL HISTORY

- There is little conclusive clinical information regarding the natural history of patients with PCL tears treated nonoperatively.
  - Most studies suggest that patients with isolated grade I–II PCL injuries usually have good subjective results, but few achieve good functional results.[11,13,14]
- A high incidence of degeneration, primarily involving the medial femoral condyle and patellofemoral joint, has been noted in patients treated nonoperatively. This finding is especially prevalent in those patients with grade III injuries or combined ligamentous injuries.
- Consequently, pain rather than instability may be the patient's primary symptom following a PCL injury treated nonoperatively.

PATIENT HISTORY AND PHYSICAL FINDINGS

- The initial history should focus on the mechanism of injury, its severity, and associated injuries.
- With acute injuries, the patient often does not report feeling a "pop" or "tear," as often is described with ACL injuries.
- The history also should focus on assessing the chronicity of the injury and the instability and pain experienced by the patient.
- A complete knee examination, including inspection, palpation, range of motion (ROM) testing, neurovascular examination, and special tests, should be performed.
  - Posterior drawer test: the most accurate clinical test for PCL injury
  - Posterior sag (Godfrey) test: A positive result is an abnormal posterior sag of the tibia relative to the femur from the force of gravity. This result suggests PCL insufficiency if it is abnormal compared to the contralateral side.
  - Quadriceps active test: useful in patients with combined instability. A posteriorly subluxed tibia that reduces anteriorly is a positive result.
  - Reverse pivot shift test: A palpable reduction of the tibia occuring at 20 to 30 degrees indicates a positive result. The contralateral knee must be examined, because a positive test may be a normal finding in some patients.
  - Dial test: A positive test is indicated by asymmetry in external rotation. Asymmetry of more than 10 degrees at 30 degrees rotation indicates an isolated posterolateral corner (PLC) injury, while asymmetry at 30 and 90 degrees suggests a combined PCL and PLC injury.
  - Posterolateral external rotation test: Increased external rotation of the tibia is a positive result. Increased posterior translation and external rotation at 90 degrees indicate a PLC or PCL injury, while subluxation at 30 degrees is consistent with an isolated PLC injury.
- It is important to assess the neurovascular status of the injured limb, especially if there is a history of a knee dislocation.

IMAGING AND OTHER DIAGNOSTIC STUDIES

- Radiographs of the knee should be performed following an acute injury to assess for a fracture. An avulsion of the tibial insertion of the PCL may be identified on a lateral radiograph (**FIG 1A**).

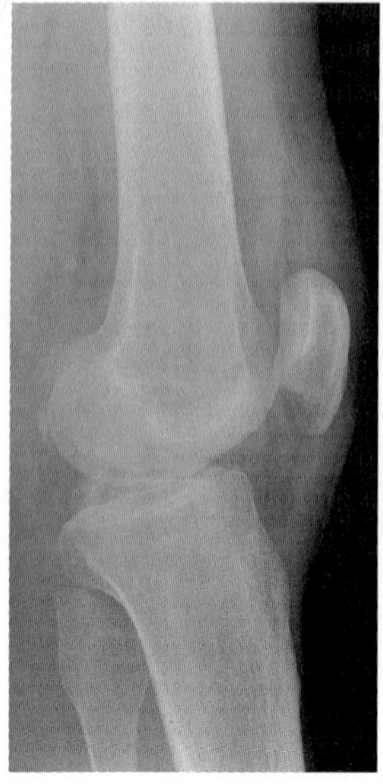
A

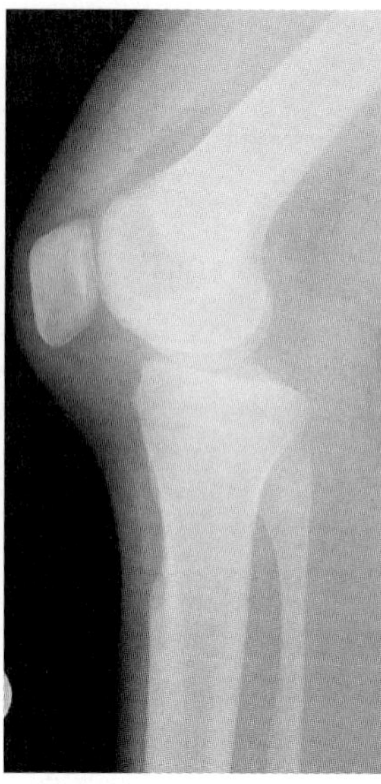
B

FIG 1 • **A.** Avulsion fracture of the tibial insertion of the posterior cruciate ligament (PCL). **B.** Posterior subluxation of the tibia in a case of chonic PCL deficiency.

- In the chronic setting, radiographs may identify posterior tibial subluxation (**FIG 1B**) or medial and patellofemoral compartmental arthrosis.
- Stress radiographs may be used to confirm and quantify dynamic posterior tibial subluxation.[8]
- Long-cassette films should be obtained if coronal malalignment is suspected.

- MRI is important to confirm a PCL injury, determine its location and completeness, and assess for concomitant injury, including meniscal and PLC pathology.

DIFFERENTIAL DIAGNOSIS

- Combined ligament injury
- PLC injury
- ACL tear
- Tibial plateau fracture
- Articular cartilage injury
- Medial or lateral collateral ligament tear
- Meniscal tear
- Patellar or quadriceps tendon rupture
- Patellofemoral dislocation

NONOPERATIVE MANAGEMENT

- Most experts advocate nonoperative management of isolated, partial PCL injuries (grades I and II).
  - In these cases, we recommend immobilization in full extension with protected weight bearing for 2 weeks. The goal is to protect the healing PCL/PLC.
- ROM exercises are advanced as tolerated, and strengthening is focused on the quadriceps muscles.
  - Closed chain exercises (foot on the ground) are recommended.
  - Applying an axial load across the knee causes anterior translation of the tibia because of the sagittal slope.[4] This important biomechanical principle allows early ROM exercises and protects PCL/PLC healing.
- The patient usually can return to athletic activities after isolated grade I and II PCL injuries in 4 to 6 weeks. It is important to protect the knee from injury during this time to prevent progression to a grade III injury.
  - Functional bracing is of little benefit after return to sports activities.
- Isolated grade III injuries are more controversial, and nonoperative management may be appropriate in certain patients.
  - We recommend immobilization in full extension for 2 weeks to prevent posterior tibial subluxation. Weight bearing is protected during these 2 weeks, then slowly advanced.
  - Quadriceps strengthening such as quadriceps sets and straight leg raises is encouraged; hamstring loading is prohibited until later in the rehabilitation course.
  - After 1 month, ROM, full weight-bearing, and progression to functional activities are instituted.
  - Return to sports usually is delayed for 2 to 4 months in patients with grade III injuries.

SURGICAL MANAGEMENT

- Surgical indications include those patients with displaced bony avulsions, acute grade III injuries with concomitant ligamentous injuries, and chronic grade II–III injuries with symptoms of instability or pain.
  - With any PCL injury, it is imperative to assess the PLC to rule out injury, because surgery is indicated for combined injuries.
- In higher-level athletes, surgical treatment may be considered for acute isolated grade III PCL injuries.
- The timing of PCL reconstruction depends on the severity of the injury and the associated, concomitant ligamentous injuries.
  - Displaced bony avulsions and knees with multiligamentous injuries should be addressed within the first 3 weeks to provide the best opportunity for anatomic repair.[5]
- A number of graft options are available for PCL reconstruction.
  - Autologous tissue options include bone–patellar tendon–bone, hamstring tendons, and quadriceps tendons.
  - Allograft options include tibialis anterior tendon, Achilles tendon, bone–patellar tendon–bone, and quadriceps tendon.
  - Advantages of allograft tissue include decreased surgical time and no harvest site morbidity. Disadvantages include the possibility of disease transmission. The operating surgeon should discuss these issues with the patient preoperatively.
- Currently, allograft tibialis anterior tendon is our graft of choice for single- and double-bundle PCL reconstructions (**FIG 2**).

Preoperative Planning

- In the office setting, the surgeon should have a variety of options available and explain that the final surgical plan will depend on the examination under anesthesia (EUA) and the diagnostic arthroscopy.

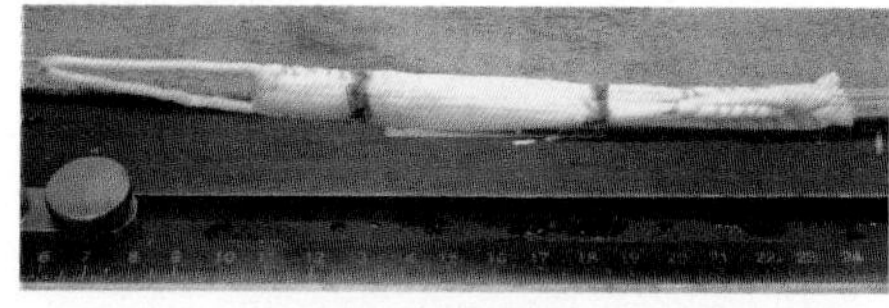

FIG 2 • Double-stranded tibialis anterior allograft sutured through an EndoLoop (Ethicon, Inc).

- In the preoperative holding area, sciatic and femoral nerve block catheters may be placed by the anesthesiology staff.
  - No anesthetic is introduced, however, until neurologic assessment has been completed.
- After anesthesia induction in the operating room, an EUA is performed on both the nonoperative and the operative knees.
  - A detailed examination is performed to determine the direction and degree of laxity.
  - Data from the contralateral knee may be particularly helpful with combined injuries.
- Fluoroscopy may be used after the EUA to assess posterior tibial displacement.

Positioning

- The patient is positioned supine on the operating room table.
- We do not use a tourniquet.
- Depending on the anticipated length of the planned procedure, a Foley catheter may be used.
- A padded bump is taped to the operating room table to hold the knee flexed to 90 degrees. A side post is placed on the operative side just distal to the greater trochanter to support the proximal leg with the knee in flexion (**FIG 3A**). Padded cushions are placed under the nonoperative leg.
- For the inlay technique, a gel pad bump is placed under the contralateral hip to facilitate later exposure to the posteromedial knee of the operative extremity in the figure 4 position.
- After prepping and draping the operative site, a hole is cut in the stockinette for access to the dorsalis pedis pulse throughout the case (**FIG 3B**).

Approach

- Several techniques have been described for PCL reconstruction. We have developed the following treatment algorithm:
  - For acute injuries, we employ the single-bundle technique.
  - If some component of the native PCL remains, we spare this tissue and use the augmentation technique.
    - This technique can be time-consuming and difficult, but preservation of PCL tissue may provide enhanced posterior stability of the knee and may promote graft healing.
  - We most commonly perform the double-bundle technique in the chronic setting, when any remaining structures are significantly incompetent.
  - Some authors advocate the tibial inlay technique for all settings. We typically do not use this technique, but have included a description of an open double-bundle technique here as part of a comprehensive overview. All arthroscopic tibial inlay techniques also have recently been described.[6,9]
  - In cases of displaced tibial avulsion, we use the technique described in the Techniques box.

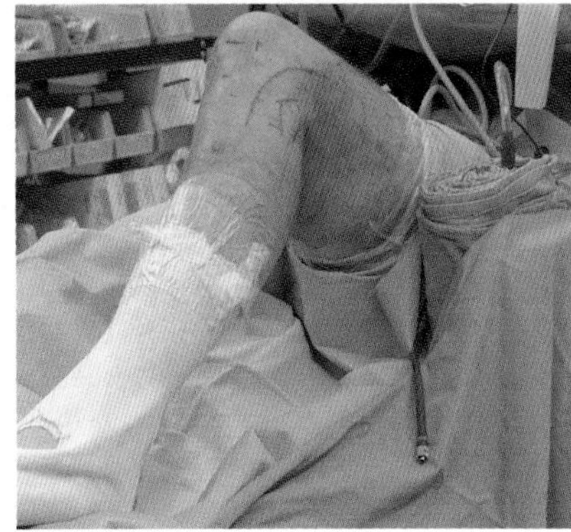

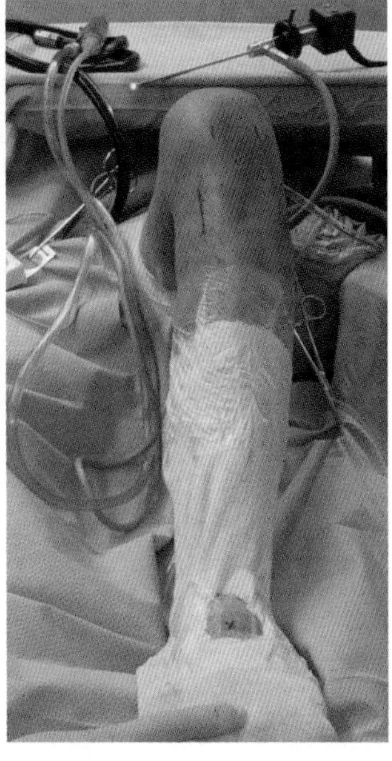

FIG 3 • **A.** Operative field setup, demonstrating the bump holding the knee flexed to 90 degrees and a side post supporting the proximal leg with the knee in flexion. **B.** Stockinette with hole cut out to palpate the dorsalis pedis pulse.

SINGLE-BUNDLE TECHNIQUE

Diagnostic Arthroscopy

- A bump is placed between the post and the leg to stabilize the knee in a flexed position while the foot rests on the pre-positioned sandbag.
  - The knee is flexed to 90 degrees, and the vertical arthroscopy portals are delineated.
- The anterolateral portal is placed just lateral to the lateral border of the patellar tendon and adjacent to the inferior pole of the patella.
- The anteromedial portal is positioned 1 cm medial to the medial border of the superior aspect of the patellar tendon.
- Diagnostic arthroscopy is conducted to determine the extent of injury and evaluate for other cartilage or meniscal derangements.
  - The notch is examined for any remaining intact PCL fibers. If augmentation is to be performed, care should be taken to preserve these fibers (see Single-Bundle Augmentation Technique).

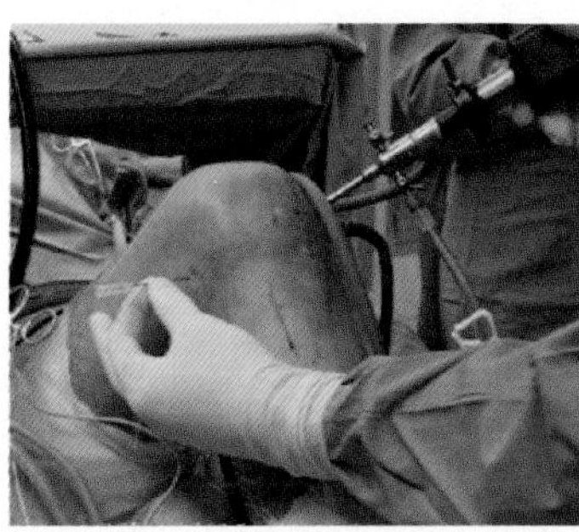

TECH FIG 1 • The posteromedial portal is established under direct visualization using a spinal needle.

- Using an arthroscopic electrocautery device and shaver, overlying synovium and ruptured PCL fibers are débrided, and the superior interval between the ACL and PCL is defined.
- An accessory posteromedial portal is created just proximal to the joint line and posterior to the MCL.
  - A 70-degree arthroscope is placed between the PCL remnants and the medial femoral condyle to assess the posterior horn of the medial meniscus and to localize the posteromedial portal with a spinal needle (TECH FIG 1).
  - A switching stick can be placed into the posteromedial portal to facilitate exchange of the arthroscope. The 30-degree arthroscope is used when viewing via the posteromedial portal.
  - A transseptal portal also may be created for better visualization of and access to the tibial PCL insertion.[1,10]

Preparation and Exposure of the Tibia

- Correct preparation and exposure of the tibia is essential for drilling the tunnel safely in the appropriate position.
- First the 70-degree arthroscope is placed into the anterolateral portal, and a commercially available PCL curette is introduced through the anteromedial portal.
  - A lateral fluoroscopic image can be obtained to confirm its position.
- The 30-degree arthroscope is then introduced through the posteromedial portal. The soft tissue on the posterior aspect of the tibia is carefully elevated centrally and slightly laterally.
- A shaver can be placed through the anterolateral portal to débride some of the surrounding synovium.
- The 70-degree arthroscope is returned to the anterolateral portal and the shaver placed in the posteromedial portal to complete the exposure.

Creating the Tibial Tunnel

- A commercially available PCL tibial drill guide set to 55 degrees is advanced through the anteromedial portal and placed just distal and lateral to the PCL insertion site, 1.5 cm distal to the articular edge of the posterior plateau along the sloped face of the posterior tibial fossa (TECH FIG 2A).
  - The position is checked fluoroscopically using a lateral view and arthroscopically via the posteromedial portal.
- An incision and dissection through periosteum to bone is made on the anteromedial aspect of the tibia in line with the guide.
- The PCL guide is set, and its position is confirmed with fluoroscopy and arthroscopy (TECH FIG 2B).
- A guidewire is drilled to but not through the posterior cortex.
  - Fluoroscopy is used to confirm the path of the guidewire (TECH FIG 2C,D).
- With the 30-degree arthroscope in the posteromedial portal, the PCL curette is introduced through the anteromedial portal and is used to protect the posterior knee

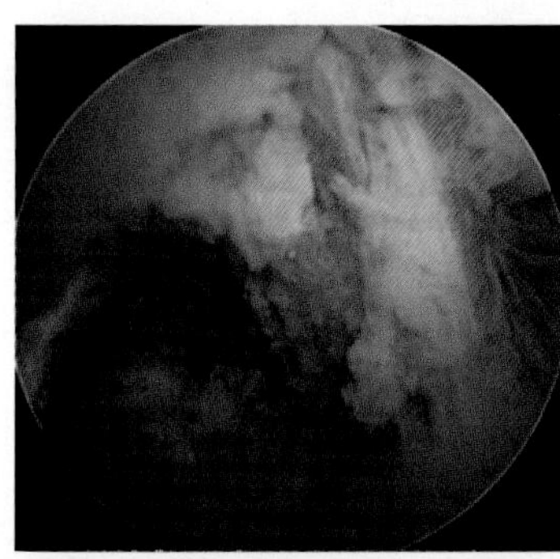

A

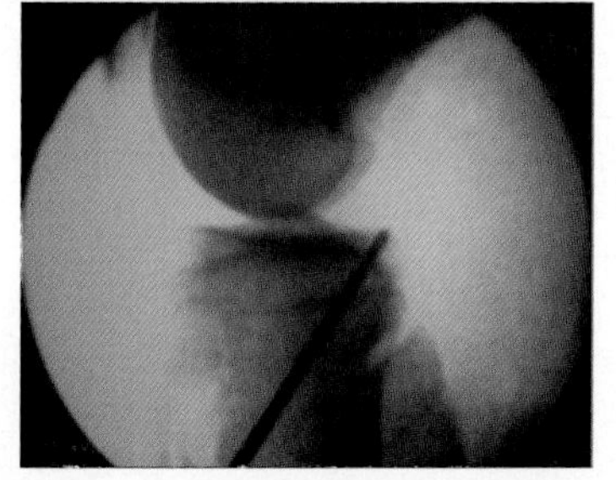

D

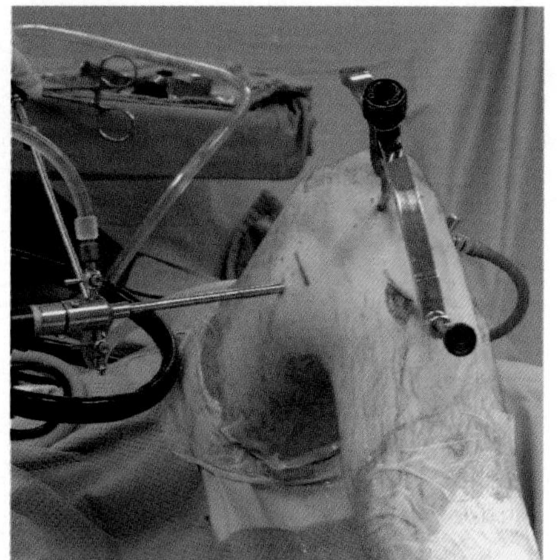

B

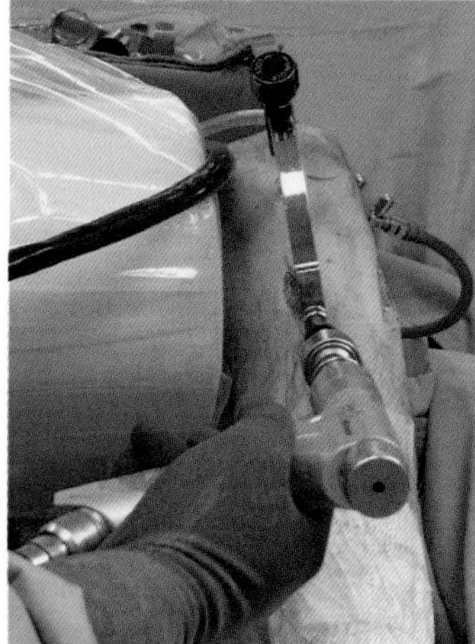

C

TECH FIG 2 • **A.** Posterior cruciate ligament (PCL) drill guide positioned to facilitate guide pin exit at the PCL insertion. **B.** Once the PCL drill guide is set, it is confirmed arthroscopically and fluoroscopically. **C.** The tibial guidewire is drilled under fluoroscopic guidance. **D.** The tibial guidewire position is confimed with fluoroscopy.

structures as the guidewire is carefully advanced through the posterior cortex under arthroscopic visualization.
  - A parallel pin guide can be used to make small pin placement corrections if necessary.
- A cannulated compaction reamer is used to drill the tibial tunnel.
  - The tibial cortex is cautiously perforated by hand reaming under arthroscopic visualization.
  - The tunnel is irrigated, and increasing serial dilators are used under arthroscopic visualization up to the graft size.

Creating the Femoral Tunnel

- An angled awl, via the anterolateral portal, is used to create a starting hole at the 1:00 (right knee) or 11:00 (left knee) position.
  - The anteroposterior position depends on the size of the graft, but the hole should be positioned so the tunnel edge is located at the junction with the articular cartilage (TECH FIG 3).
  - A guidewire is impacted into the starting hole via the anterolateral portal.
  - An appropriately sized cannulated acorn reamer is carefully passed over the guidewire, taking into consideration the close proximity of the patellar articular surface.
- The tunnel is drilled to a depth of approximately 30 mm, taking care to avoid penetrating the outer cortex of the medial femoral condyle.
  - Increasing serial dilators are passed to match the size of the graft.
- A smaller EndoButton drill (Smith & Nephew, Andover, MA) is used to perforate the outer cortex of the medial femoral condyle, and a guidewire is inserted through the anterolateral portal into the femoral tunnel.
- An incision is made parallel to Langer's lines over the anteromedial aspect of the distal medial femoral condyle, at the estimated exit of the guidewire from the bone.
  - The vastus medialis obliquus fascia and muscle is split in line with their fibers, and the muscle and periosteum are elevated off the anteromedial distal femur.
  - The drill hole is exposed and guidewire is removed.

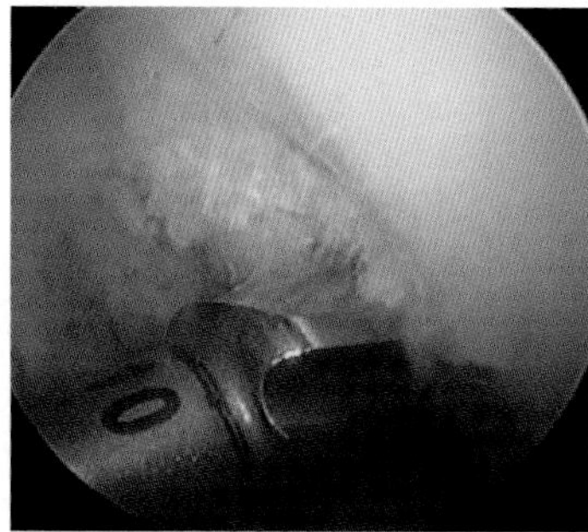

TECH FIG 3 • The femoral tunnel is positioned so the tunnel edge is located at the junction with the articular cartilage.

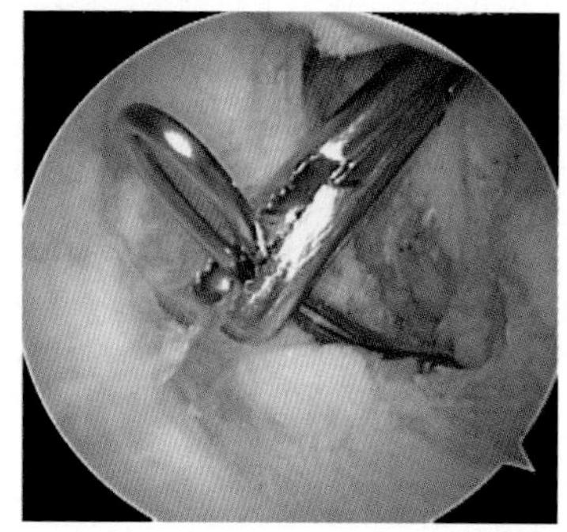

TECH FIG 4 • A long 18-gauge bent wire loop, used to pass the sutures through the tibial tunnel in an anterograde fashion, is retrieved through the anterolateral portal.

Graft Passage

- Passage of the graft may require enlarging the anterolateral portal.
- The 30-degree arthroscope is placed in the posteromedial portal, and a long 18-gauge bent wire loop is passed with the loop bent upward from anterior and distal to posterior and proximal through the tibial tunnel.
  - A tonsil is introduced through the anterolateral portal and through the notch to retrieve the bent wire loop (TECH FIG 4).
  - Leading sutures from the free ends (tibial side) of the graft are placed through the wire loop.
  - The wire and sutures are pulled back through the tibial tunnel in an anterograde fashion.
- A small scooped malleable retractor is introduced through the anterolateral portal and placed just posterior to the femoral tunnel to retract the fat pad and provide an unobstructed path for a Beath pin.
  - A Beath pin is then passed through the anterolateral portal and through the femoral tunnel.
  - The lead suture limbs from the EndoLoop (Ethicon, Inc.) side of the graft are threaded through the eye of the Beath pin.
  - The pin, with the suture limbs, is pulled proximally.
- Traction on the suture limbs pulls the graft into the femoral tunnel to the marked line, while traction of the tibial suture limbs pulls the graft into the femoral tunnel.
  - The position of the graft is confirmed arthroscopically.

Graft Fixation

- Graft fixation is achieved by placing the EndoLoop along the medial femur with a tonsil to estimate its most proximal extent.
- A 3.2-mm drill bit is used to make a unicortical hole at the most proximal extent of the EndoLoop.
  - After the hole is measured and tapped, a 6.5-mm cancellous screw and washer are placed through the EndoLoop into the femur.
  - The screw is tightened as the graft is pulled tight distally.
- The fixation is palpated to ensure the EndoLoop limbs are tight distal to the screw and washer.

- An anterior tibial force is applied to reduce the tibia before and during final tibial fixation.
  - A cortical 4.5-mm screw and washer are placed from anteromedial to posterolateral within the proximal tibia.
  - The graft is fixed at 90 degrees flexion.
  - Before the screw advances to the second cortex, the suture limbs from the tibial side of the graft are tied with tension over the post. The screw is then tightened.
- The arthroscope is inserted to confirm adequate position, tension, and fixation of the graft.

Wound Closure

- The incisions are irrigated, and the fascia in the anterolateral femoral incision is closed with size 0 Vicryl suture.
- The subcutaneous layer is approximated with interrupted, inverted 3-0 Vicryl suture, and the skin is closed with a running 4-0 absorbable suture.
- The portals are closed with 3-0 nylon suture.
- The dorsalis pedis and posterior tibialis pulses are assessed by palpation and a Doppler ultrasound examination if necessary.
- The incisions are covered with adaptic gauze and sterile gauze, then wrapped in cast padding and bias wrap.

SINGLE-BUNDLE AUGMENTATION

- For single-bundle augmentation, much of the technique is identical to the single-bundle technique already described.
  - Often, the AL bundle is ruptured and the PM bundle remains intact. Consequently, for the purposes of this chapter, AL bundle augmentation will be described.
- The diagnostic arthroscopy is performed.
- If the AL bundle is found to be intact, special care is taken to preserve this bundle while the overlying synovium and ruptured PCL fibers are débrided (TECH FIG 5A).
- When preparing the posterior aspect of the tibia, preservation of the PCL origin is essential.
- Tibial tunnel preparation is performed similarly to the single-bundle technique.
  - The exit point for the guide pin along the sloped face of the posterior tibial fossa is just distal and lateral to the intact PCL insertion site (TECH FIG 5B).
- When preparing the medial femoral condyle for tunnel drilling, care again is taken to preserve the intact PCL bundle.
  - The starting hole is placed at the 1:00 (right knee) or 11:00 (left knee) position.
  - The hole should be positioned in the anteroposterior plane so the tunnel edge is located at the junction with the articular cartilage.
  - This location depends on the size of the graft and the distance from the intact PM bundle.
- The graft is passed around the intact bundle, which is the final augmentation consideration.
- Fixation and closure are then performed.

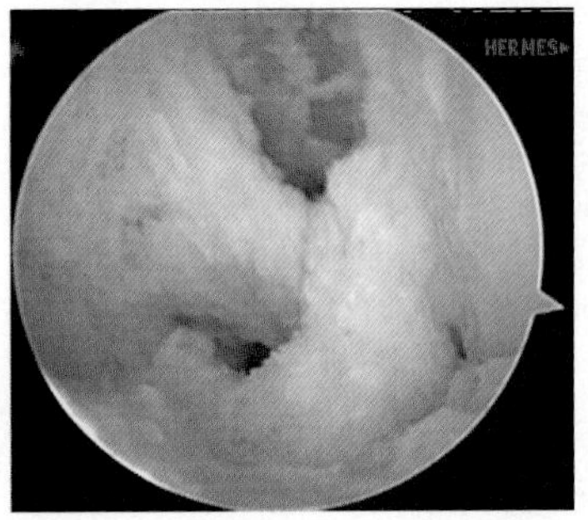

A

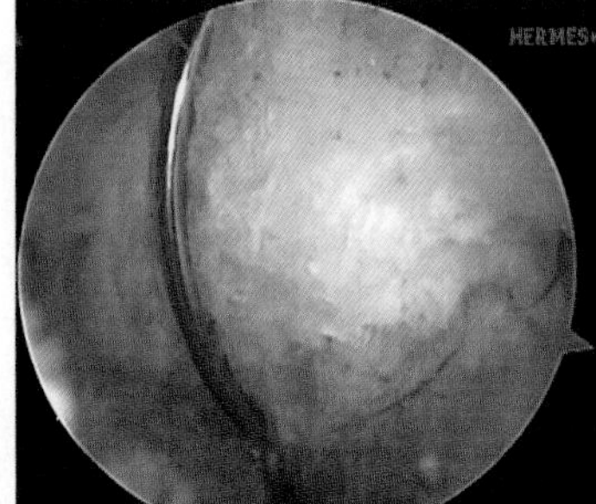

B

TECH FIG 5 • **A.** An intact AL bundle is preserved and the overlying synovium and ruptured PCL fibers are débrided. **B.** The exit point for the tibial tunnel along the sloped face of the posterior tibial fossa is just distal and lateral to the intact PCL insertion, as demonstrated by a long 18-gauge bent wire loop.

DOUBLE-BUNDLE RECONSTRUCTION

- For double-bundle PCL reconstruction, the initial aspects of the technique are identical to those of single-bundle reconstruction, including portal placement, arthroscopy, and preparation for drilling.

Tibial Tunnel Creation

- Throughout this process, care must be taken to avoid tunnel convergence and ensure an adequate bony bridge between the two tibial tunnels.
- First, the guide pin for the AL tunnel is positioned using the same technique as with single-bundle reconstruction.
  - It exits the tibia just distal and lateral to the PCL insertion site, 1.5 cm distal to the articular edge of the posterior plateau.
- The PCL guide is reintroduced into the joint.
- The same steps and precautions are repeated for placement of the PM tibial guidewire.
  - The PM tibial guidewire enters the tibia on the anteromedial aspect of the tibia, slightly more proximal and medial than the AL guidewire.
  - Conversely, the PM guidewire can be introduced through the anterolateral tibia, crossing the AL guidewire on the coronal view, but remaining proximal to the AL guidewire throughout its course on the sagittal view. It exits the tibia in the footprint more medial and slightly proximal to the AL tibial guidewire (TECH FIG 6A).
  - It is important to ensure adequate separation between the two guide pins to accommodate both tunnels with a bony bridge separation.

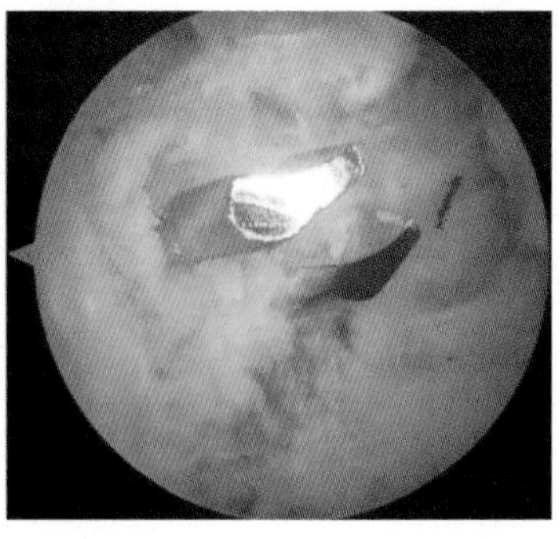
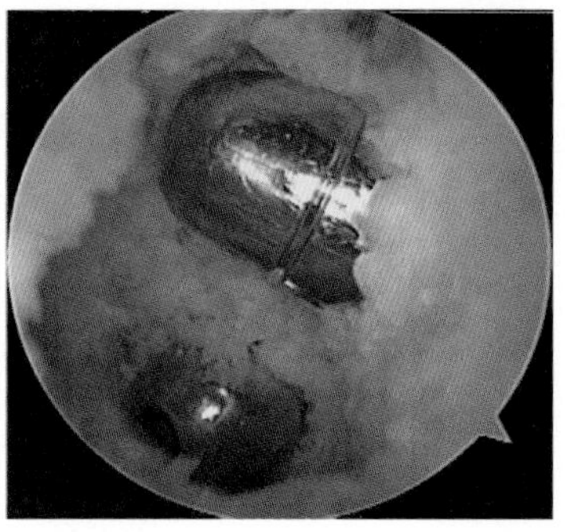

TECH FIG 6 • **A.** Both the AL and PM guidewires are positioned in the proximal posterior tibia. The PM guidewire, and subsequently the tunnel, exits the tibia in the footprint more medial and slightly proximal to the AL tibial guidewire. **B.** Dilators demonstrate the position of the AL and PM tunnels in the proximal posterior tibia.

- Once the guidewire positions are satisfactory, a cannulated compaction reamer is used to first drill the AL tibial tunnel.
  - The drill is advanced under fluoroscopic guidance.
  - The posterior tibial cortex is cautiously perforated by hand reaming under arthroscopic visualization.
  - The tunnel is irrigated, and increasing serial dilators are used under arthroscopic visualization.
- The steps are repeated for drilling the PM tibial tunnel with a 7-mm cannulated compaction reamer (TECH FIG 6B).

Femoral Tunnel Creation

- An angled awl is used to create the starting holes.
- For the AL bundle, the starting hole is placed at the 1:00 (right knee) or 11:00 (left knee) position.
  - The hole should be positioned in the anteroposterior plane so the tunnel edge is located at the junction with the articular cartilage.
  - The guidewire is passed via the anterolateral portal and impacted into the starting hole.
  - The appropriately sized cannulated acorn reamer is passed over the guidewire.
  - The reamer should be passed carefully, given the close proximity of the patellar articular surface.
  - The tunnel is drilled to a depth of about 30 mm, with care taken to avoid penetration of the outer cortex of the medial femoral condyle.
  - Increasing serial dilators are passed to match the size of the graft.
  - A smaller EndoButton drill (Smith & Nephew, Andover, MA) is used to perforate the outer cortex of the medial femoral condyle.
- This inside-out femoral tunnel preparation technique is then repeated for the PM tunnel.
  - The angled awl is used to create the starting hole at the 3:00 (right knee) or 9:00 (left knee) position.
  - The PM tunnel is placed parallel or slightly posterior to the AL tunnel.
  - The guide pin is then placed via the anterolateral portal and impacted into the starting hole.
  - A 7-mm acorn reamer is passed over the guidewire and drilled to a depth of approximately 30 mm (TECH FIG 7).
  - The medial femoral condylar cortex is perforated with the EndoButton drill.

Graft Placement and Fixation

- The AL graft is passed first, using the same technique as with single-bundle reconstruction.
- This process is then repeated for the PM graft (TECH FIG 8).
  - It is helpful to keep tension on the AL graft suture ends when passing the PM graft to ensure that the AL graft does not get pulled into the joint.
- Graft fixation is performed first on the femoral side.
  - The AL bundle is secured as previously described.
  - This process is repeated for the PM bundle, ensuring that adequate separation exists between the two screws and washers to prevent overlap.
- An anterior tibial force is applied to reduce the tibia before and during final tibial fixation.
  - Two 4.5-mm cortical screws and washers are placed from anteromedial to posterolateral within the proximal tibia, just distal to the respective tunnels.
  - As with the single-bundle technique, before the screw advances to the second cortex, the suture limbs from the tibial side of the graft are tied with tension over the post, and then the screw is tightened.
  - The AL graft is secured first at 90 degrees flexion, and the PM bundle then is secured at 15 degrees of flexion.
  - The arthroscope is inserted to confirm adequate position, tension, and fixation of the grafts.

TECH FIG 7 • The femoral tunnels, with the AL tunnel at the 11:00 position and the PM tunnel at the 9:00 position.

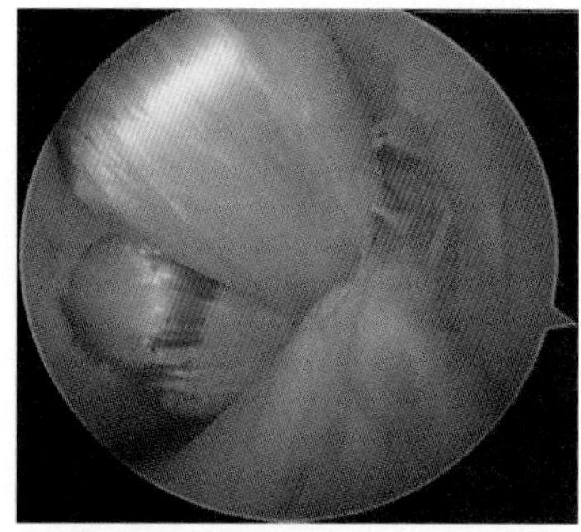

TECH FIG 8 • The double-bundle reconstruction with the grafts in place.

Tibial Inlay

- For the double-bundle tibial inlay PCL reconstruction, the initial aspects of the technique are similar to those for single-bundle reconstruction, including portal placement, arthroscopy, and débridement.
- A whole, nonirradiated, frozen patellar tendon allograft is prepared with two bundles attached to a common tibial bone block and distinct femoral bone blocks.
  - The tibial bone block is fashioned from the tibial side of the graft and should measure 20 mm long, 13 mm wide, and 12 mm thick.
    - A single 4.5-mm gliding hole is placed in the center of the block for later fixation.
  - The tendon bundles stemming from the tibial bone block should measure 11 mm (AL bundle) and 9 mm (PM bundle).
  - The femoral bone plugs from the patellar side of the graft are shaped to 20 mm in length and 11 mm (AL bundle) and 9 mm (PM bundle) in diameter.
    - The femoral bone plugs are each drilled with two separate 2.0-mm holes, through which Fiberwire (Arthrex, Naples, FL) passing sutures are placed (**TECH FIG 9A**).
- The leg is brought into a figure 4 position, with the knee flexed to 90 degrees and the bump repositioned under the lateral ankle.
  - A 6-cm incision is made over the posterior border of the tibia from the crease of the popliteal fossa and curving distally along the posteromedial border of the tibia (**TECH FIG 9B**).
- The dissection is continued through the subcutaneous fat to the sartorius fascia and the fascia overlying the medial head of the gastrocnemius.
  - The fascia is incised along the palpable posteromedial tibial border.
  - The semimembranosus and pes anserinus tendons are retracted anteriorly and proximally.
  - The medial head of the gastrocnemius is elevated from the tibial cortex and retracted posteriorly.
  - The medial border of the gastrocnemius is followed distally along the posterior tibia, and the proximal border of the popliteus muscle is identified. The popliteus muscle is elevated subperiosteally off the posteromedial surface of the tibia and mobilized laterally and distally (**TECH FIG 9C**).
- Attention is then turned to drilling an 11-mm AL and a 9-mm PM femoral tunnel, performed as described for the double-bundle technique.
- The leg is returned to the figure 4 position, and the tibial trough is prepared by creating a vertical arthrotomy between the palpable prominences of the medial and lateral tibial plateaus at the native PCL tibial insertion.
- The remaining PCL is identified and débrided, and a ¼-inch curved osteotome is used to create a trough measuring 13 mm wide, 12 mm deep, and 20 mm long (**TECH FIG 9D**).
  - A 3.2-mm transtibial drill hole is placed in the trough that corresponds to the 4.5-mm gliding hole in the tibial bone block.

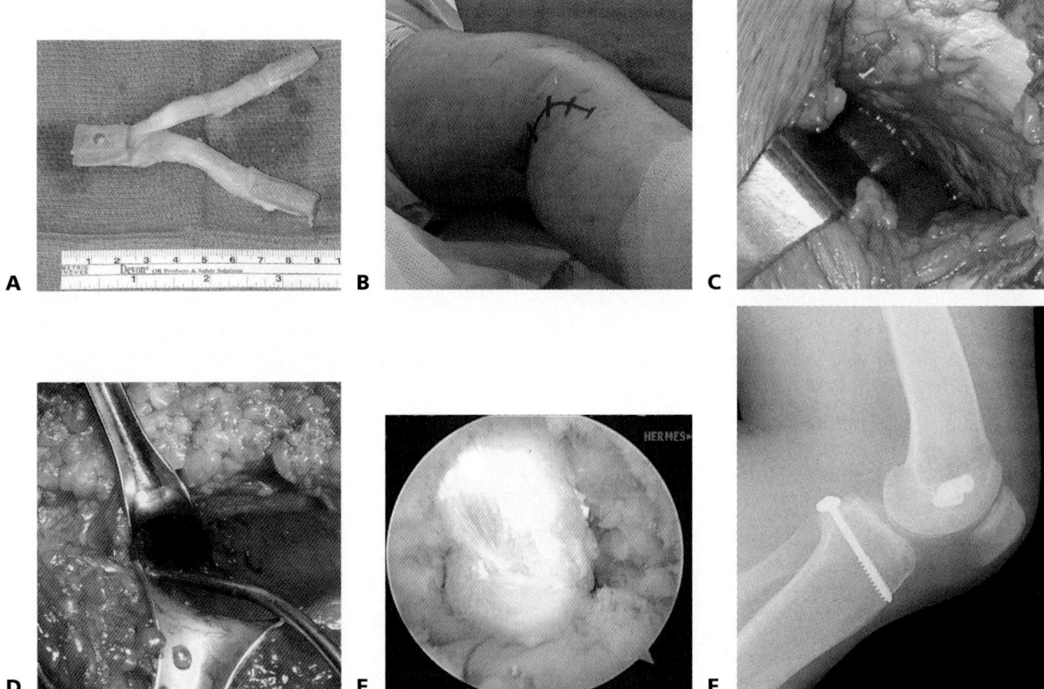

TECH FIG 9 • A. The tibial inlay graft. **B.** The approach for the tibial inlay begins with a 6-cm incision over the posterior border of the tibia from the crease of the popliteal fossa, which curves distally along the posteromedial border of the tibia. **C.** The posterior aspect of the tibia after the popliteus muscle has been elevated subperiosteally off the posteromedial surface of the tibia and mobilized laterally and distally. **D.** The posterior aspect of the tibia after the inlay trough has been created. **E.** The double-bundle tibial inlay graft after being positioned in the tunnels. **F.** Lateral radiograph demonstrating the tibial inlay fixation with a 4.5-mm fully threaded cortical screw on the tibial side, and interference screws on the femoral side.

- The graft is passed through the joint via an enlarged anteromedial portal into the tibial trough.
  - A 4.5-mm fully-threaded cortical screw is used to lag the bone block into the trough.
  - Fluoroscopy is used to verify the position of the graft.
- A 4-cm incision is made along the posterior border of the vastus medialis at the center of the medial femoral condyle, and the femoral tunnels are identified.
  - The AL and PM bundle grafts are then passed through their respective femoral tunnels using a suture passer.
  - Several cycles of flexion and extension are performed to pretension the graft.
- The bundles are secured with metal interference screws placed outside-to-in (**TECH FIG 9E,F**).
  - The AL graft is secured first at 90 degrees flexion, and the PM bundle then is secured at 15 degrees of flexion.
  - A gentle anterior drawer is applied during screw insertion to recreate the natural tibial step-off.
  - Any remaining bone plug protruding from the femoral tunnels is removed with a rongeur, and sutures are tied together over the tunnel bone bridge.

Tibial Avulsion

- The PCL tibial avulsion is approached similarly to tibial inlay reconstruction.
- The patient is positioned supine, as in the tibial inlay technique, to facilitate arthroscopic examination.
- The skin incision and the dissection are performed as described for the tibial inlay technique.
- A vertical arthrotomy is made, and the avulsed fragment of the tibia with the attached PCL is identified.
- The bone fragment and PCL are reduced and secured with a 4.0-mm cortical or a 6.5-mm cancellous screw and spiked washer, depending on the size of the fragment.
- The reduction is confirmed with fluoroscopy or a radiograph (**TECH FIG 10**).

A 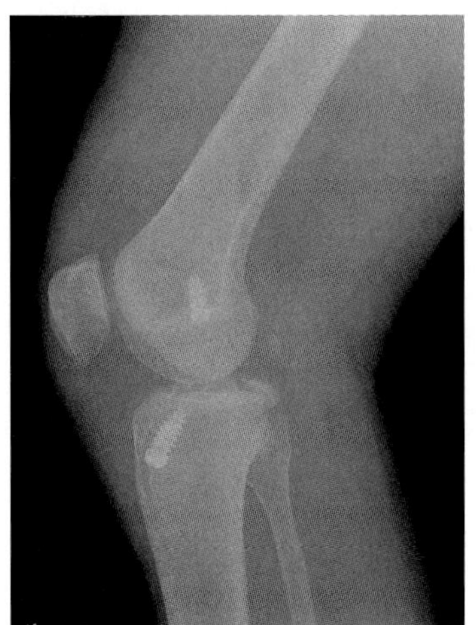

B 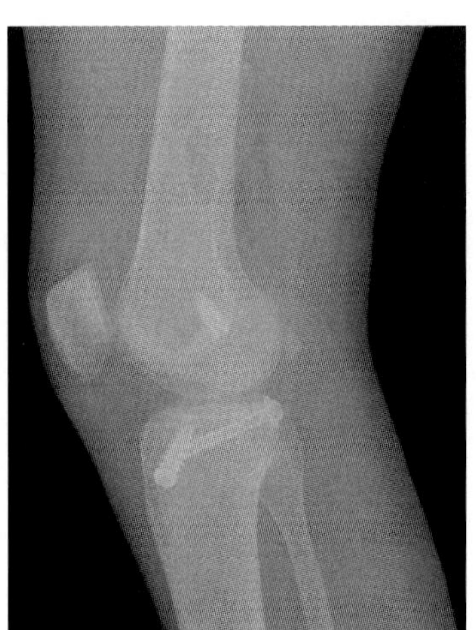

C 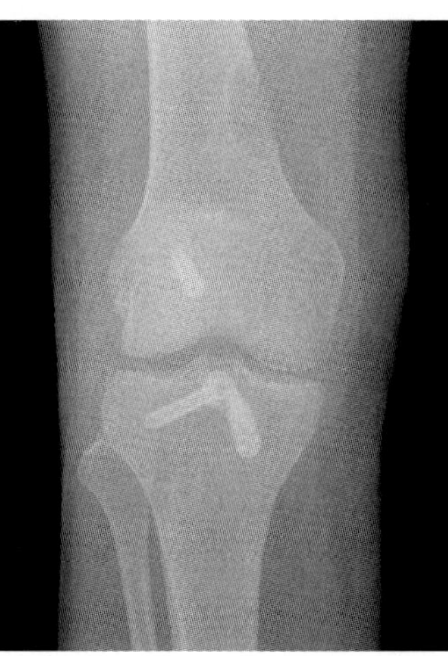

TECH FIG 10 • **A.** PCL tibial avulsion in a patient with a previous ACL reconstruction. **B,C.** Lateral and PA radiographs after fixation of the tibial avulsion.

PEARLS AND PITFALLS

Indications	■ Assess for concomitant PLC injury on the EUA and following PCL reconstruction, because deficiency of these structures may lead to PCL graft failure. ■ Employ the appropriate technique based on the chronicity of the injury and remaining native PCL.
Arthroscopy	■ Exposure of the posterior tibia may be tedious but is essential for appropriate, safe tunnel placement. ■ When working in the posterior knee joint, be certain the shaver or electrocautery device always faces anteriorly, away from the popliteal vessels. ■ Fluid extravasation and lower extremity compartments must be monitored throughout the procedure.
Tunnel placement	■ A parallel pin guide can be used to make small corrections in tunnel placement. ■ Perforate the posterior tibial cortex by hand with the guide pins or reamers in a controlled fashion under direct arthroscopic visualization to avoid neurovascular injury. ■ If the patella causes resistance to the acorn reamer when drilling the femoral tunnels, use a smaller reamer to make a starting hole, then hand-dilate the tunnel to the appropriate size with larger reamers.
Graft management	■ An arthroscopic switching rod, placed via the posteromedial portal between the graft and the posterior tibial cortex, can facilitate graft passage by decreasing friction. ■ Avoid penetrating soft tissue with the Beath pin while passing through the anterolateral portal to prevent the graft from getting caught in the soft tissue.
Fixation	■ An anterior tibial force should be applied during fixation to prevent posterior subluxation.
Rehabilitation	■ Closed-chain exercises that apply an axial load across the knee protect the PCL reconstruction owing to the sagittal slope of the tibial plateau.

POSTOPERATIVE CARE

- A hinged knee brace is applied and locked in extension. The patient is awakened and taken to the recovery room, where pain and neurovascular status are reevaluated.
- Patients may be kept overnight for pain management and to monitor their neurovascular status.
- Patients are given instructions for exercises (quadriceps sets, straight-leg raises, and calf pumps) and crutch use.
- All dressing changes are performed while an anterior tibial force is applied.
- Patients are instructed to maintain touch-down weight bearing for 1 week.
- Partial weight bearing is initiated after the first postoperative visit.
- The brace is unlocked after 4 to 6 weeks, and usually is discontinued after 8 weeks.
- Symmetric full hyperextension is achieved, and passive prone knee flexion, quadriceps sets, and patellar mobilization exercises are performed with the assistance of a physical therapist for the first month.
- Mini-squats are performed from 0 to 60 degrees after the first week and from 0 to 90 degrees after the third week.
- Once full, pain-free ROM is achieved, strengthening is addressed.
- The goals for achievement of flexion are 90 degrees at 4 weeks and 120 degrees at 8 weeks.

OUTCOMES

- Choice of graft (autograft vs allograft) has not been shown to affect overall outcome.[3]
- Acute single-bundle reconstructions have been demonstrated to have significantly better outcomes than chronic reconstructions.[12]
- The clinical outcomes after single-bundle and tibial inlay reconstructions have produced a satisfactory return of function and improvement in symptoms.[3,12]
- Neither transtibial or tibial inlay has been shown to be superior with regard to overall outcome.[7]
- No studies have specifically addressed the long-term clinical outcomes of double-bundle reconstructions and PCL augmentation reconstructions.

COMPLICATIONS

- Failure to carefully position the extremity with adequate padding may result in neuropraxia.
- Loss of motion (usually decreased flexion) can result from errors in graft positioning or excessive tensioning during graft fixation. Inadequate rehabilitation also may lead to loss of motion.
- Residual laxity also can occur as a result of graft positioning or failure to address concomitant ligamentous injury.
- Injury to the popliteal vessels is rare, but may be a very serious complication. Care must be taken to prevent overpenetration of the posterior tibial cortex.
- The thigh and calf should be routinely palpated to ensure no compartment syndrome develops from fluid extravasation into the soft tissues.

REFERENCES

1. Ahn JH, Ha CW. Posterior trans-septal portal for arthroscopic surgery of the knee joint. Arthroscopy 2000;16:774–779.
2. Ahn JH, Yoo JC, Wang JH. Posterior cruciate ligament reconstruction: double-loop hamstring tendon autograft versus Achilles tendon allograft: clinical results of a minimum 2-year follow-up. Arthroscopy 2005;21:965–969.
3. Cooper DE, Stewart D. Posterior cruciate ligament reconstruction using single-bundle patella tendon graft with tibial inlay fixation: 2- to 10-year follow-up. Am J Sports Med 2004;32:346–360.
4. Giffin JR, Vogrin TM, Zantop T, et al. Effects of increasing tibial slope on the biomechanics of the knee. Am J Sports Med 2004;32:376–382.
5. Harner CD, Waltrip RL, Bennett CH, et al. Surgical management of knee dislocations. J Bone Joint Surg Am 2004;86A:262–273.
6. Kim SJ, Park IS. Arthroscopic reconstruction of the posterior cruciate ligament using tibial-inlay and double-bundle technique. Arthroscopy 2005;21:1271.
7. MacGillivray JD, Stein BE, Park M, et al. Comparison of tibial inlay versus transtibial techniques for isolated posterior cruciate ligament reconstruction: minimum 2-year follow-up. Arthroscopy 2006;22:320–328.
8. Margheritini F, Mancini L, Mauro CS, et al. Stress radiography for quantifying posterior cruciate ligament deficiency. Arthroscopy 2003;19:706–711.
9. Mariani PP, Margheritini F. Full arthroscopic inlay reconstruction of posterior cruciate ligament. Knee Surg Sports Traumatol Arthrosc 2006;14:1038–1044. Epub 2006 Sep 8 2006.
10. Mauro CS, Margheritini F, Mariani PP. The arthroscopic transeptal approach for pathology of the posterior joint space. Tech Knee Surg 2005;4:120–125.
11. Parolie JM, Bergfeld JA. Long-term results of nonoperative treatment of isolated posterior cruciate ligament injuries in the athlete. Am J Sports Med 1986;14:35–38.
12. Sekiya JK, West RV, Ong BC, et al. Clinical outcomes after isolated arthroscopic single-bundle posterior cruciate ligament reconstruction. Arthroscopy 2005;21:1042–1050.
13. Shelbourne KD, Davis TJ, Patel DV. The natural history of acute, isolated, nonoperatively treated posterior cruciate ligament injuries. A prospective study. Am J Sports Med 1999;27:276–283.
14. Toritsuka Y, Horibe S, Hiro-Oka A, et al. Conservative treatment for rugby football players with an acute isolated posterior cruciate ligament injury. Knee Surg Sports Traumatol Arthrosc 2004;12:110–114.

Chapter 45 Repair of Acute and Chronic Knee Medial Collateral Ligament Injuries

Christian Lattermann and Darren L. Johnson

DEFINITION

- A medial collateral ligament (MCL) injury usually is the result of a valgus stress on the knee.
  - Forced external rotation injuries with a valgus component also have been described as a mechanism that can disrupt the MCL.
- While the direct valgus force is more likely to injure the superficial MCL, external rotation and valgus stress often causes additional injuries to the deep MCL, the anterior cruciate ligament (ACL), the posteromedial corner, or the posterior oblique ligament.
- The most common combined injury is an ACL and MCL injury, followed by meniscus injuries.

ANATOMY

- The medial side of the knee can be divided into three layers: superficial (I); intermediate (II); and deep (III).
  - Layer I: the crural fascia extending from the quadriceps fascia into the tibial periosteum
  - Layer II: the superficial medial collateral ligament (SMCL) and the medial patellofemoral ligament (MPFL)
  - Layer III: the deep MCL (ie, the meniscotibial and meniscofemoral ligaments) and the posteromedial corner (ie, semimembranosus and posterior oblique ligament [POL])
- The superficial MCL originates from the medial femoral epicondyle. It inserts approximately 4 to 6 cm distal to the medial joint line and can be divided into an anterior and a posterior portion. The anterior portion tightens in flexion; the posterior portion tightens in extension.
- The deep MCL tightens in knee flexion and is lax in full knee extension.
- The posteromedial corner provides rotational stability to the medial side of the knee. Injuries to these structures cause anteromedial rotatory instability.
- The semimembranosus has five main attachments to the posterior capsule of the knee:
  - Pars reflexa, attaching directly to the proximal medial tibia
  - Direct arm, attaching to the posteromedial tibia
  - Insertion to the proximal medial capsule
  - Attachment to the POL
  - Attachment to the popliteus aponeurosis

PATHOGENESIS

- The typical mechanism for an MCL injury is a valgus stress acting on the knee joint with the foot planted. This mechanism often leads to a disruption of the deep and superficial MCL.
- If an external rotational component is added, a disruption of additional restraints such as the ACL and the posteromedial corner is likely. In particular, an injury to the POL indicates a significant capsular injury that leads to a higher grade of medial and rotatory instability.[3]
- MCL injuries can be partial or complete. A complete MCL injury involves disruption of the superficial and deep MCL and usually results initially in inability to ambulate.
- MCL injuries can be on either the femoral or tibial side. It is important for the treatment algorithm to differentiate whether the tear involves the femoral origin of the MCL or the tibial insertion.

NATURAL HISTORY

- Acute isolated MCL injuries usually are treated nonoperatively with protective weight bearing and bracing for 2 to 6 weeks.
  - In particular, partial tears of the MCL (grade I or II) heal well with conservative treatment.
  - Complete MCL injuries (grade III injuries) initially can be treated conservatively if they are femoral-based ligament ruptures.[3]
  - A complete tibial-sided MCL avulsion with POL extension is less likely to tighten up with nonoperative management and may require repair or reconstruction.
- Grade 3 MCL injuries in combination with other ligament injuries of the knee may require acute surgical repair in case of a complete tibial avulsion with POL extension.[5]

PATIENT HISTORY AND PHYSICAL FINDINGS

- A description of the mechanism of injury (eg, valgus mechanism, valgus rotation mechanism) must be elicited.
- The examination includes inspection for peripheral hematoma along the medial side of the knee, palpation of hamstrings, joint line (meniscal injury) and the femoral origin and tibial insertion of the MCL stability testing.
- Valgus stress at 0 and 30 degrees: grade 1 (0- to 4-mm opening) and 2 (5- to 9-mm opening) injuries usually can be treated nonoperatively; grade 3 (10- to 15-mm opening) injuries are associated with other ligament tears (ie, ACL, POL) in over 75% of cases.
- Slocum's modified anterior drawer test: disruption of the deep MCL allows the meniscus to move freely and allows the medial tibial plateau to rotate anteriorly, leading to an increased prominence of the medial tibial condyle.
- Anterior drawer test in external rotation: disruption of the MCL alone should not lead to an increased anteromedial translation. An increased anteromedial translation indicates an anteromedial rotatory instability that involves an injury of the posteromedial capsule (eg, POL, semimembranosus attachments, as well as deep MCL).
- A thorough examination of the knee should always include the following assessments:
  - Meniscus: tenderness directly at the joint line is a sensitive sign for a meniscus injury. The McMurray test or a flexion–rotation–compression maneuver may accentuate medial

joint line pain, suggesting a medial meniscus tear. (This test may not be helpful in an acute setting.)

- ACL: An immediate (within 24 hours) intra-articular effusion after the injury indicates a high likelihood of ACL injury. Positive Lachman test (acute) and pivot shift test (chronic) indicate an associated ACL tear. In the acute or subacute setting, these tests may be difficult to perform. Instrumented laxity testing (KT-1000) may be helpful in these situations. An increased valgus laxity in full extension almost always indicates something more than an MCL injury.
- PCL: A positive posterior drawer test indicates a PCL injury. The endpoint is important to assess the grade of the PCL injury.
- Patella: The apprehension sign and localized tenderness on the lateral or medial aspect of the patella or the lateral trochlea indicates a possible patella dislocation, which can go hand-in-hand with an intra-articular effusion. Tenderness at the medial femoral epicondyle also can be caused by an avulsion of the MPFL.

IMAGING AND OTHER DIAGNOSTIC STUDIES

- Plain radiographs help to assess the bony integrity of the knee joint. They may show indirect signs of ligament injury (eg, Segond fracture), but they usually are not helpful for the diagnosis of an acute MCL injury.
- In the case of chronic MCL instability, a Pellegrini-Stieda lesion (bony spur originating at the femoral origin of the MCL, usually visualized on the flexion weight-bearing posteroanterior radiograph) may be present (**FIG 1A**).
- MRI with or without contrast is helpful to identify medial collateral ligament damage.
  - Edema or MCL disruption can be visualized.
  - The location and extent of the disruption (femoral vs tibial) can be determined.
  - The amount of bone bruising can be assessed, and associated pathology (eg, meniscal tears, ACL tears, posteromedial corner injuries) can be visualized.
- Arthroscopic examination is a formidable tool to assess the true nature of the MCL injury.
  - An ipsilateral "drive-through" sign (ie, opening of the medial compartment of more than 10 mm, allowing for complete insertion of the arthroscope into the medial compartment [**FIG 1B**]) should arouse suspicion for a significant MCL injury that may require repair or reconstruction.
  - The location of the acute or chronic injury —femoral or tibial—also can be evaluated. Separate inuries of the POL also can be visualized (**FIG 1C**).

DIFFERENTIAL DIAGNOSIS

- Medial meniscus tear
- ACL tear
- Posteromedial corner injury
- Patella dislocation
- Pes-anserine bursitis

NONOPERATIVE MANAGEMENT

Grade 1 and 2 Medial Collateral Ligament Sprains

- Rest, ice compression, elevation (RICE) for 24 hours or until swelling is controlled
- Once swelling is controlled, partial weight bearing, range-of-motion (ROM) exercises, and electrical stimulation can be started. A simple hinged brace is applied.
- Full weight bearing can be allowed once ROM over 90 degrees of flexion as well as motor control of the thigh musculature has beeen demonstrated.[2,4]
- Once full ROM and 80% strength of the opposite side have been achieved, closed kinetic chain exercises, jogging, and treadmill exercise may begin.
- In athletes, a return to sport-specific training is safe once 80% of the maximum running speed is achieved.[2,4]
- Return to play depends on the grade of the sprain:
  - Grade 1: 10 to 14 days
  - Grade 2: 3 to 4 weeks

Grade 3 Medial Collateral Ligament Sprains

- MCL sprains without associated ACL or meniscus tear account for less than 20% of all grade 3 sprains.
- The knee is re-evaluated frequently (every 7 to 10 days) to assess whether the MCL "tightens up." Tibial-sided complete avulsions of the MCL may not heal and require acute surgical repair if they do not tighten up within the first 4 weeks.
- It is important to check for combined ACL/MCL tears. Grade 3 MCL tears with POL extension in combination with

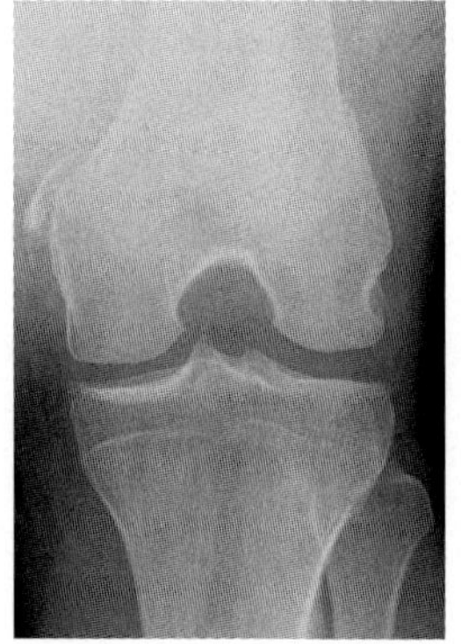
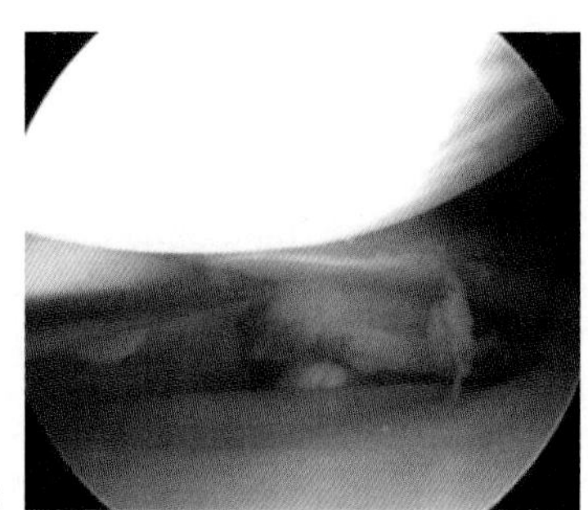
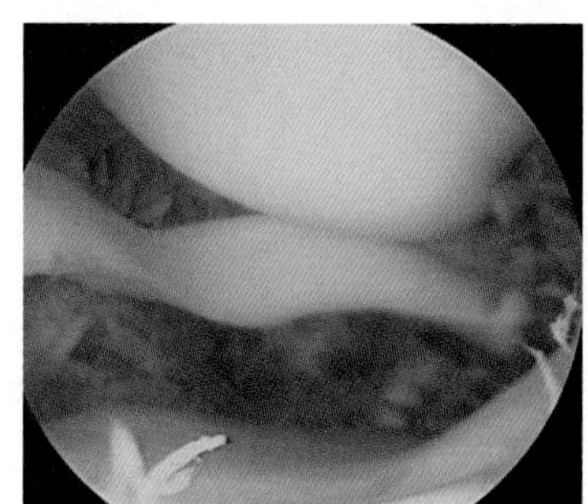

FIG 1 • **A.** Pellegrini-Stieda lesion indicating chronic medial collateral ligament (MCL) insufficiency. **B.** Arthroscopic ipsilateral medial drive-through sign. The joint space opens more than 10 mm and permits complete passage of the arthroscope into the back of the medial compartment. **C.** The arthroscopic examination permits direct evaluation of the injured structure, including the posterior oblique ligament (POL) and tibial- or femoral-sided deep MCL The meniscus tends to follow the noninjured structure. A proximal meniscal lift-off suggests a tibial-sided tear, whereas a distal lift-off suggests a femoral-sided tear.

an acute ACL tear often require surgical repair or even augmentation because of the rotational laxity that results from the POL injury.

- RICE is maintained until the swelling is controlled.
  - 0 to 4 weeks: restoration of ROM, quadriceps/hamstring strengths, normal gait pattern, full weight bearing with hinged knee brace
  - 4 to 6 weeks: full ROM, full quadriceps/hamstring strengths, closed kinetic chain exercises, stair-stepper exercise, proprioceptive exercises
  - 6 to 10 weeks: full squatting, jogging, light agility drills, slow return to competition, brace discontinued for non-contact sports

SURGICAL MANAGEMENT

Preoperative Planning

- All radiographs and MRIs are reviewed before surgery.
- Associated injuries must be addressed at the same time and often determine the sequence of the surgery (PCL before ACL before MCL)
- In case of a chronic MCL injury and associated ACL or PCL tears, the appropriate allograft tissue must be available.
- Examination under anesthesia must include a full ligamentous examination (ie, Lachman test, pivot shift test, varus/valgus stress test, dial test, anteromedial drawer test).

Positioning

- The patient is positioned in the supine position.
- We prefer to use an arthroscopic leg holder. This enables the surgeon to sit during the MCL reconstruction and balance the patient's foot on his or her knee to adjust the flexion angle.
- The procedure also can be performed on a regular operating table with the patient in the supine position with a bolster positioned under the knee.

Approach

- We use the 6- to 8-cm mid-medial approach over the posterior aspect of the superficial MCL.

TECHNIQUES

INCISION AND DISSECTION FOR MID-MEDIAL APPROACH

- The incision should be centered over the joint line and can be extended proximally or distally, as necessary.
- In case of a proximal extension, the incision should be slightly curved posteriorly over the medial femoral epicondyle.
- Retraction of the skin exposes the sartorius fascia, which must be split in a longitudinal or T fashion. Underneath the sartorius fascia (layer I), the superficial MCL is exposed.
- The posterior border of the superficial MCL and the anterior border of the POL are identified, and a vertical incision is made along this interval, exposing the deep MCL.
- This incision can be carried down through the capsule to expose the meniscal attachments. An avulsion of the POL from the posterior capsule may be identified in select cases.
- A plane can be developed between the superficial and the deep MCL.
  - This plane allows for a separate repair of the deep MCL against the POL to tension the POL.
  - It also exposes the medial tibial plateau and allows for easy placement of a suture anchor for a repair of the deep MCL at the level of the joint line, which is critical.

ACUTE REPAIR OF TIBIAL-SIDED ISOLATED GRADE 3 MCL TEARS

- Tibial avulsion is documented arthroscopically by a positive "drive-through" sign (>10 mm of medial opening).
  - The medial meniscus lifts off from the tibial plateau during this maneuver, revealing the tibial-sided tear of the deep MCL.
- A limited direct medial approach is performed through a 5- to 6-cm incision along the posterior aspect of the MCL.
- The sartorius fascia is divided, which usually exposes acute avulsion of the deep MCL from the tibia. The superficial MCL also usually is torn but can be sharply divided from the deep MCL.
- Three or four double-loaded suture anchors are then placed along the medial border of the tibial plateau about 5 mm below the joint line.
  - The meniscotibial ligament can be secured to the suture anchors, allowing for an excellent repair of the deep MCL along with the coronary ligament and medial meniscus.
  - The sutures can be left long after the initial knots are tied and also can be used to tie down the superficial MCL (TECH FIG 1).

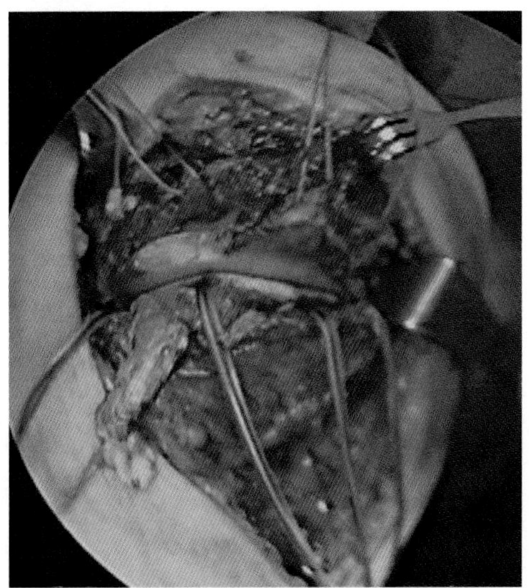

TECH FIG 1 • Acute suture anchor repair of the deep MCL with imbrication of the capsule. The suture anchors are placed just distal to the joint surface and allow for reefing of the torn deep MCL to the proximal tibia.

TECHNIQUES

AUTOGRAFT RECONSTRUCTION OF ISOLATED CHRONIC MCL TEARS

- Reconstruction of the superficial MCL requires stabilization of the central pivot of the knee. Any associated ACL or PCL injury must be addressed simultaneously with or before the MCL reconstruction.
- The reconstruction includes repair and tightening of the deep MCL/POL complex, which should be tightened at 0 degrees. The superficial MCL reconstruction should be tightened at 30 degrees of flexion.
- The deep MCL and POL can be identified through the midmedial incision and can be retightened using suture anchors, as with the primary repair of the MCL (**TECH FIG 2A,B**).
- Chronic MCL injuries should be augmented with a superficial MCL reconstruction.
- Autograft MCL reconstruction can be done using a Bosworth reconstruction.
  - In the Bosworth reconstruction, a semitendinosus tendon is harvested using the open or closed tendon stripper. The femoral origin of the MCL is identified. A K-wire is inserted into the insertion site, and isometry is tested to avoid a flexion contracture after the superficial MCL repair.
  - Once the isometric site is identified, the semitendinosus can be routed around a screw and washer femorally and can be attached distally using a staple or bone tunnels. This allows for reconstruction of the posterior and anterior bundles of the superficial MCL (**TECH FIG 2C,D**).

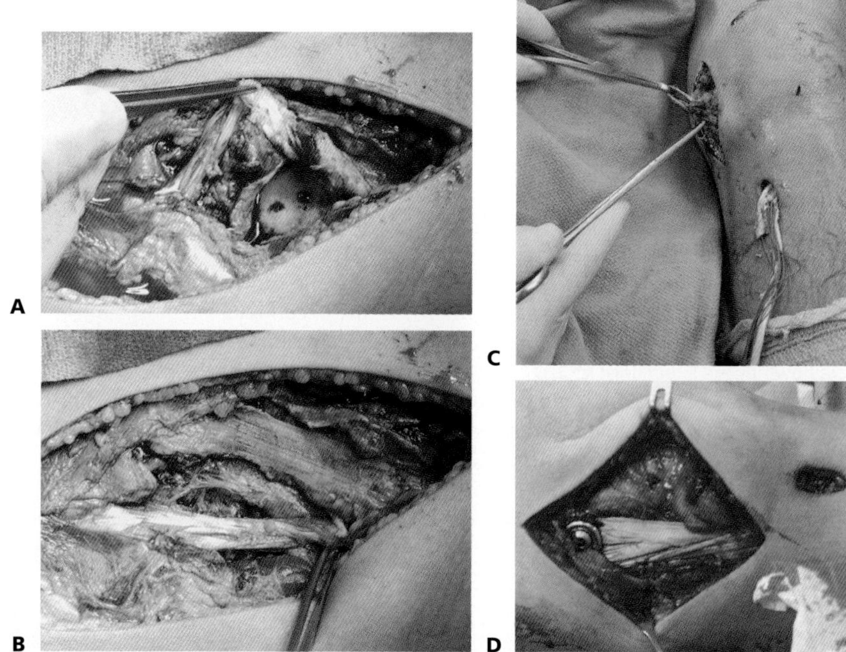

TECH FIG 2 • **A.** Medial incision allowing access to freshly avulsed MCL. **B.** The sartorius fascia is split, and the superficial MCL attachment is recovered. **C,D.** Reconstruction of the MCL over a femoral screw and washer using a semitendinosus allo- or autograft. **C.** Routing of the semitendinosus tendon and the skin incisions. **D.** The final tensioned construct and the screw and washer at the origin of the MCL on the medial femoral epicondyle. (Courtesy of Mark D. Miller, MD.)

ALLOGRAFT RECONSTRUCTION OF ISOLATED CHRONIC MCL TEARS

- Borden et al[1] have described an allograft reconstruction of the MCL.
- A double anterior tibialis tendon or a split Achilles or patella tendon can be used for this technique.
- The surgical approach is the same as that described for autograft reconstruction.
- The origin of the MCL on the medial epicondyle must be identified. The femoral fixation is positioned at the anatomic insertion of the MCL.
- Fixation can be achieved in various ways—bone tunnel using a soft tissue screw fixation, bone block using an interference screw fixation, bone trough, or screw and washer fixation.

- The distal tibial fixation has to reconstruct the anterior and posterior aspect of the native MCL (TECH FIG 3).
- The allograft can be anchored anteriorly and posteriorly along the anatomic attachment sites using an interference screw (as depicted), a screw and washer, or a staple.

Distal Fixation in Chronic Injuries

- In chronic MCL injuries, it often is the distal end of the MCL that has failed to heal.
- Using the standard medial approach, the distal end of the MCL often can be identified (TECH FIG 4A).
  - This attachment can be used in the reconstruction if the length is adequate; if not, it can be sutured to the reconstruction.
- The allograft is then fixed femorally (as described earlier) and routed along the course of the superficial MCL (TECH FIG 4B).
- The posterior and anterior portions of the superficial MCL can then be individually attached to the tibia.

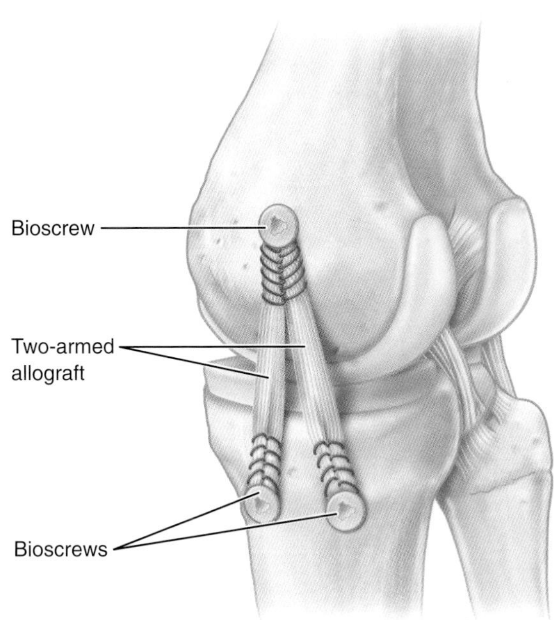

TECH FIG 3 • Double-bundle MCL allograft reconstruction technique using bioabsorbable screw fixation. (Courtesy of Mark D. Miller, MD.)

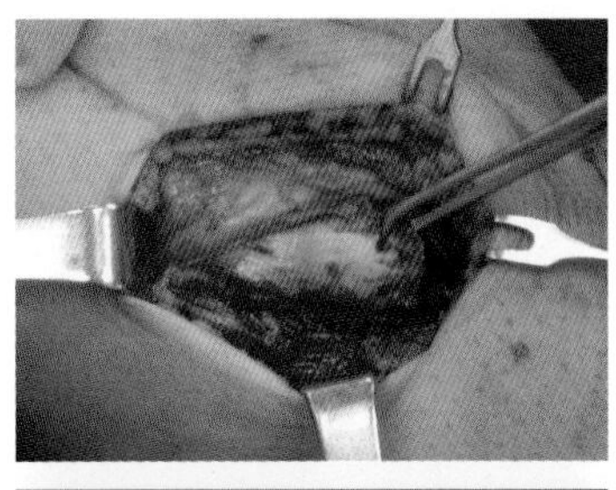

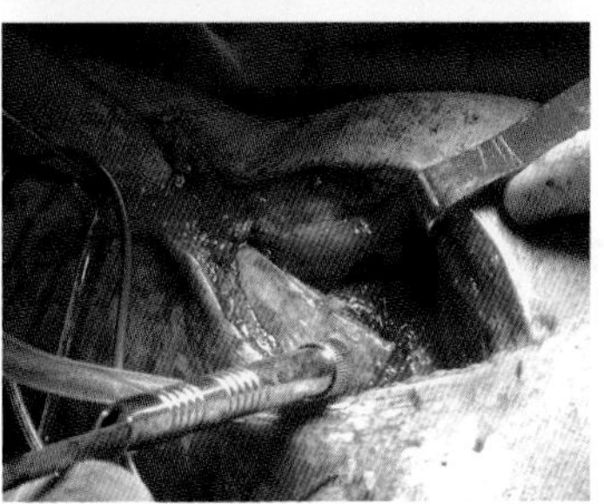

TECH FIG 4 • **A.** Medial incision. The chronically disrupted MCL stump can be visualized through the sartorius fascia. **B.** An Achilles tendon allograft has been sized to fit in a bone trough at the epicondylar origin of the MCL (depth gauge shown in preparation for screw fixation of the bone block). The allograft has been routed along the course of the MCL and fans out to provide the posterior and anterior portion of the MCL. (Courtesy of Mark D. Miller, MD.)

PEARLS AND PITFALLS

Grade 3 MCL tear	■ Obtain MRI and check for tibial-sided avulsions, which may require surgical repair. ■ Be sure to follow patients closely if conservative management is chosen. The MCL should tighten up after 4 to 6 weeks. If it fails to tighten in valgus stress, reconstruction may be necessary. ■ Diagnose associated injuries with clinical examination and MRI. ■ When doing multiple ligament surgery, make sure that the ACL and PCL tunnels have been drilled before positioning of the MCL tunnels.

POSTOPERATIVE CARE

- The postoperative course is as follows:
  - 0 to 3 weeks: touch-down weight bearing, hinged brace locked in 30 to 90 degrees of flexion, hamstring/quadriceps strengthening in brace
  - 3 to 6 weeks: progress to full weight bearing, ROM free in brace, quadriceps/hamstring strengthening, closed kinetic chain exercises. The repair must be protected.
  - 6 to 12 weeks: the brace is discontinued. Light jogging and stair-stepper exercise are begun.
  - 12 to 18 weeks: progressive return to sports with sport-specific drills and return to play once 90% of quadriceps and hamstring strength and 75% of maximum running speed have been regained.

OUTCOMES

- Grade 1 and 2 MCL sprains should be treated nonoperatively. The average time to return to athletic activities is between 19 and 23 days, on average, for grade 1 and 2 injuries, respectively.[2]

- Grade 3 MCL sprains can be treated nonoperatively with good success if several pitfalls are avoided:
  - Conservative treatment of an isolated Grade 3 MCL injury allows most athletes to return to play after an average of 34 days.[2]
  - Tibial-side avulsions of the deep and superficial MCL with POL extension tend to progress toward chronic MCL laxity. Either early surgical treatment or repetitive clinical examination to assess the gradual return of valgus stability over the course of 4 weeks is advisable. If valgus laxity is still present after 4 weeks, surgical treatment is advised.
  - Concomitant ACL injuries are common and often will result in residual chronic MCL laxity if treated nonoperatively.

COMPLICATIONS

- Failure to diagnose associated ligament, meniscal, and articular cartilage injuries
- Deep venous thrombosis
- Infection

REFERENCES

1. Borden PS, Kantaras AT, Caborn DN. Medial collateral ligament reconstruction with allograft using a double-bundle technique. Arthroscopy 2002;18(4):E19.
2. Giannotti BF, Rudy T, Graziano J. The non-surgical management of isolated medial collateral ligament injuries of the knee. Sports Med Arthr 2006;14:74–77.
3. Indelicato PA. Isolated medial collateral ligament injuries in the knee. J Am Acad Orthop Surg 1995;3:9–14.
4. Reider B, Sathy MR, Talkington J, et al. Treatment of isolated medial collateral ligament injuries in athletes with early functional rehabilitation: a five-year follow-up study. Am J Sports Med 1994;22:470–477.
5. Wilson TC, Satterfield WH, Johnson DL. Medial collateral ligament "tibial" injuries: indication for acute repair. Orthopedics 2004;27:389–393.

Chapter 46 Management of Posterolateral Corner Injuries

Richard J. Thomas and Mark D. Miller

DEFINITION

- The posterolateral corner (PLC) of the knee is a complex area, both anatomically and functionally, that has the potential to cause great disability when injured.
- Injuries to the structures of the PLC are uncommon, accounting for only 2% of all acute ligamentous knee injuries.[6]
- Because of the high incidence of combined ligament injuries associated with PLC injuries,[2] other ligament injuries in the knee always should be suspected when treating the PLC.
- Conversely, cruciate ligament reconstructions have a tendency to fail if PLC injuries are left untreated,[8,17] so one must always have a high index of suspicion for PLC injuries when treating other injuries in the knee.
- The significance of a PLC knee injury can be great.
  - Chronic instability due to the untreated PLC injury can be debilitating.
- The complex biomechanical relationships among the structures of the PLC are important in resisting varus and external rotation forces.
- Insufficiency in the posterolateral structures of the knee can lead to a varus-thrust gait and the sensation of instability, especially when the knee is in extension during the toe-off phase of walking.[2]
  - The convexity of the lateral tibial plateau and lateral femoral condyle may contribute to this instability.[17]
  - This instability may hinder stair-climbing or cutting activities, and patients may complain of lateral knee pain.
- Chronic PLC insufficiency also may lead to tricompartmental degenerative joint disease.[2]
- An increase in patellofemoral joint contact pressure has been found to occur with PLC and posterior cruciate ligament (PCL) sectioning in cadaveric studies.[26]

ANATOMY

- Before treating a patient with a PLC injury, one must be familiar with the complex anatomy of the area.
- The PLC is made up of both dynamic and static stabilizers.[5]
- Seebacher et al[25] organized the posterolateral structures into three layers (**FIG 1A**).
  - The *superficial layer* is made up of the iliotibial tract anteriorly and the biceps femoris posteriorly.
    - The common peroneal nerve lies deep and posterior to the biceps femoris in this layer at the level of the distal femur.
    - The iliotibial (IT) tract or band, which inserts on Gerdy's tubercle on the tibia, is tight and moves posteriorly in knee flexion. It actually places an external rotation force on the tibia during knee flexion. During knee extension, the IT band moves anteriorly and becomes less taut. Because of its relaxed state in knee extension, this structure rarely is injured in PLC injuries, so it is a good reference point for the location of other structures in surgery.
    - The biceps femoris inserts on the fibular head, but also has attachments to the IT band, Gerdy's tubercle, the lateral collateral ligament (LCL), and the posterolateral capsule.[2,6] It adds dynamic stability to the PLC.
  - The *middle layer* of the PLC consists of the quadriceps retinaculum anteriorly, the patellofemoral ligaments posteriorly, and the patellomeniscal ligament.[25]
    - These structures add accessory static stability to the PLC.
  - The *deep layer,* which is the most important (**FIG 1B**), consists of the lateral part of the joint capsule and the coronary ligament, which inserts on the lateral meniscus; the popliteus tendon and the popliteofibular ligament; the arcuate ligament; the LCL; and the fabellofibular ligament.[25]
    - The popliteus originates on the posterior tibia, passes through the hiatus of the coronary ligament, and inserts on the lateral femoral condyle.[2] It also has attachments to the lateral meniscus.
    - The popliteofibular ligament exists as a direct static attachment of the popliteus tendon from the posterior fibular head to the lateral femoral epicondyle.
    - The arcuate ligament is a Y-shaped ligament that reinforces the posterolateral capsule of the knee and runs from the fibular styloid to the lateral femoral condyle. In radiographs, the arcuate fracture shows an avulsion of this ligament off of the fibular styloid.[14]
    - The LCL originates on the lateral epicondyle of the femur and inserts on the fibular head. This ligament is the primary static restraint to varus stress from 0 to 30 degrees of knee flexion.[6,7,17] The LCL becomes progressively more lax in greater degrees of flexion, however. Aponeurotic layers of the biceps femoris provide tension to the LCL to assist in dynamic resistance to varus stress.[7,17] The LCL also provides resistance to external rotation stress.[2]
- Much anatomic variation has been noted in the structures of the deep layer, especially the arcuate and fabellofibular ligaments.[25]
- Hughston et al[9] described the importance of an arcuate ligament complex consisting of the LCL, arcuate ligament, popliteus, and the lateral head of the gastrocnemius. This complex acts as a "sling" of static and dynamic restraint to rotation of the lateral tibiofemoral articulation.

PATHOGENESIS

- PLC knee injuries most commonly are caused by sports injuries (40%), motor vehicle accidents, and falls.[2,5]
- Any mechanism that can cause a knee dislocation theoretically can cause an injury to the PLC.
- The most common mechanism for an isolated PLC injury is hyperextension of the knee with a varus moment. This mechanism can be caused by blunt posterolaterally forced trauma to the medial proximal tibia, such as a helmet to the knee in football.

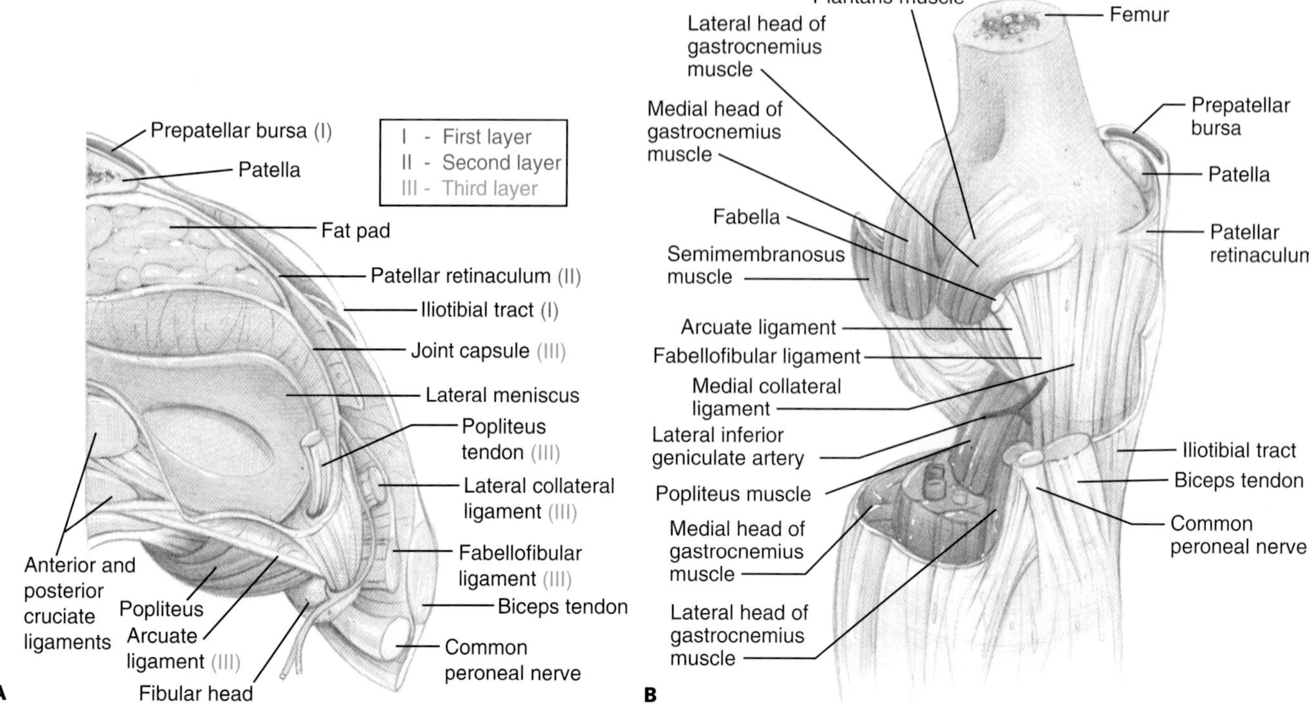

FIG 1 • **A.** The posterolateral corner is made up of three layers. **B.** The deep layer of the posterolateral corner consists of the joint capsule and the coronary ligament, the popliteofibular ligament, the arcuate ligament, the lateral collateral ligament, and the fabellofibular ligament.

- Other mechanisms of injury include hyperextension alone, hyperextension with an external rotation force, a severe varus force alone, or a severe external rotation torque to the tibia.
- As mentioned earlier, an isolated PLC knee injury is rare.[6]
- A flexed knee with tibial external rotation and posterior translation can cause a PCL/PLC combined injury.

NATURAL HISTORY

- Posterolateral knee injuries rarely occur as isolated ligament disruptions.
- They most often are associated with injury to the PCL, the ACL, or both. Therefore, the true natural history of these injuries is unknown.
- If left untreated, they will contribute to failure of other ligament reconstruction.
- Repair, and often supplementation with exogenous grafts, is recommended in all cases of combined PLC injury.

HISTORY AND PHYSICAL FINDINGS

- Methods for examining the PLC include the following:
  - Dial test. More than 10 degrees difference between limbs is consistent with ligamentous PLC injury.[28] Increased rotation at 30 degrees but not at 90 degrees indicates isolated PLC injury. Increased rotation at both 30 degrees and 90 degrees indicates PLC and PCL injuries.
  - Posterolateral external rotation test.[5] Increased posterior translation and external rotation at 90 degrees are suspicious for PLC or PCL injury. Subluxation at 30 degrees is consistent with isolated PLC injury.
  - Posterior drawer test (PCL testing). More than 10 mm translation is highly suggestive of multiligamentous knee injury.
  - Varus stress test (LCL testing). An isolated tear of the LCL causes maximal varus angulation at 30 degrees.
  - Quadriceps active test. Forward translation of the tibia after attempted knee extension is positive for PCL insufficiency (reduction of posterior tibial sag).
  - Gait. The patient may walk with a slightly flexed knee to avoid pain and instability with hyperextension of the knee.[5] Varus thrust also may be present.
  - Reverse pivot-shift test. Palpable shift of the lateral tibial plateau is positive, but not specific for PLC injury. This test is difficult to perform on the awake patient.
  - External rotation recurvatum test.[2] Hyperextension and increased varus of the knee and external rotation of the tibia are positive for PLC injury.
  - Range of motion (ROM). The normal range is 0 to 135 degrees of motion. Loss of extension may be due to a displaced meniscus tear. Loss of flexion may be due to effusion.
  - Effusion. A large effusion suggests other intra-articular pathology, such as an ACL or PCL tear or a peripheral meniscus tear. Effusion may be diminished if the capsule is torn.
  - Neurovascular examination (serial). The incidence of popliteal artery injury is increased in knee dislocations. An arteriogram should be obtained if the vascular examination is different from that in the contralateral leg. The incidence of peroneal nerve injury is increased by 10% to 33% with PLC injuries.[1,6,16]
- It is important to obtain a good history from the patient with an acute PLC injury.

- Pain and swelling of the posterolateral knee are common.
  - A rapid knee effusion suggests the possibility of intra-articular pathology, such as a cruciate ligament injury or peripheral meniscus tear.
  - It also is important to obtain history about the presence or absence of a true tibiofemoral dislocation, because there is an association between PLC injuries and knee dislocations.
  - Neurologic changes also must be investigated because of the increased incidence of peroneal nerve injuries in the patient with an injured PLC.[1,6,16]
- Patients with chronic posterolateral instability commonly present with the sensation of instability with the knee in extension and lateral or posterolateral aching pain in the knee.
- PLC injuries can be graded as 1, 2, or 3.[5]
  - Grade 1 injuries involve minimal tearing of the ligaments and are not associated with abnormal joint motion.
  - Grade 2 injuries have partial tearing, but still have no abnormal joint motion.
  - Grade 3 injuries have complete tearing of the ligaments and abnormal joint motion.
- Hughston et al[28] graded PLC injuries based on ligamentous instability. Cases of mild, moderate, and severe instability are graded as 1+, 2+, and 3+, respectively.
- Because PLC knee injuries have such a high association with combined ligament injuries, a careful examination for other knee pathology is necessary.
  - PCL injury can be recognized by a positive posterior drawer test, tibial sag or recurvatum, and hemarthrosis.
  - A positive Lachman test is the most sensitive test for an ACL tear. The examiner should not be fooled by a false endpoint caused by a tight effusion or a displaced meniscal tear. A positive pivot shift also is a sensitive test for an ACL tear, although it is difficult to perform on an acute patient because of discomfort.
  - Meniscal tears can also be associated with PLC injuries. Joint line tenderness is the most sensitive test for meniscal tears. A lateral meniscus tear may give lateral-sided knee pain, which could be confused with a posterolateral knee injury. Mechanical symptoms also raise concern for meniscal tears. Loss of full extension of the knee hints at the possibility of a locked bucket handle meniscus tear.
  - Although it is rare to have LCL and medial collateral ligament (MCL) tears in the same injury, one must examine all ligaments of the knee in a traumatic injury. The MCL is tested by valgus stress at 0 and 30 degrees of knee flexion. Medial knee tenderness and ecchymosis also are present in an MCL injury.

IMAGING AND DIAGNOSTIC STUDIES

- The initial diagnostic imaging examination should begin with standard anteroposterior (AP) and lateral radiographs of the knee.
  - Laprade and Wentorf[17] recommend obtaining full-length standing AP radiographs to evaluate for varus malalignment in chronic patients.
  - Plain radiographs may show increased joint space laterally or a frank knee dislocation.[2,5]
  - Plain radiographs also can be obtained to evaluate associated fractures, such as an arcuate avulsion fracture of the fibular head, a Gerdy's tubercle avulsion, and a Segond fracture, which is an avulsion of the lateral capsule off of the tibia.[5]
  - Segond fractures typically are thought to be associated with ACL injuries, but they also can be associated with posterolateral ligament injuries.
  - Patellofemoral or tricompartmental arthritis may be associated with chronic instability. Typically, the lateral compartment is more involved than the medial compartment.[2]
  - An effusion in the suprapatellar pouch also can be visualized on plain radiographs and hints at the presence of an intra-articular pathology, such as an ACL or PCL tear.
  - Varus stress films may be used to evaluate the integrity of the LCL as well.
- MRI also is helpful in evaluating a PLC injury.
  - Laprade et al[14] recommend obtaining not only the standard coronal, sagittal, and axial cuts of the knee but also coronal oblique 2-mm thin cuts to include the entire fibular head and styloid, to better evaluate the popliteus tendon and the LCL.
  - Laprade and Wentorf[17] also recommend using a magnet with a signal of at least 1.5 T.
  - MRI is useful in evaluating the soft tissues of the knee and for evaluating the bone for contusions or edema.
  - A bony contusion of the anteromedial femoral condyle is concerning for a PLC injury.[24]
- Arthroscopy can be useful in diagnosing posterolateral ligament pathology.[17]
  - An avulsion of the popliteus off of the femur can be visualized directly, as can injuries to the coronary ligament of the posterior horn of the lateral meniscus (**FIG 2A**).
- The "drive-through" sign is another arthroscopic finding in the patient with a PLC injury.[13] This is defined as more than 1 cm of the lateral joint line opening to varus stress during arthroscopic evaluation of a posterolaterally insufficient knee (**FIG 2B**).

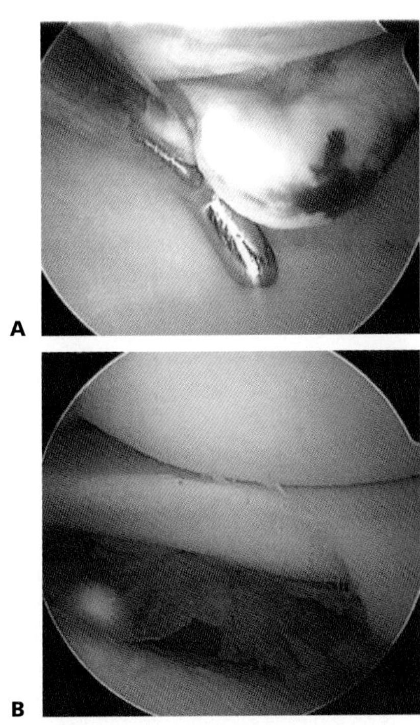

FIG 2 • Lateral compartment. Arthroscopic views demonstrating popliteal tendon injury (**A**) and excessive opening, or "drive-through" sign (**B**).

DIFFERENTIAL DIAGNOSIS

- Lateral meniscus tear
- Other ligamentous injury (eg, PCL, ACL)
- Tibial plateau fracture
- Supracondylar femur fracture
- Contusion
- Degenerative joint disease with varus malalignment

NONOPERATIVE MANAGEMENT

- Grade 1 and most grade 2 posterolateral ligament injuries of the knee usually are treated successfully without surgery.[2] These patients typically do well without significant lingering symptoms or instability.
- For grade 1 and 2 injuries, patients are immobilized for 2 to 4 weeks in either an immobilizer or cast.
- Quadriceps sets and straight leg raises are allowed in the immobilizer only.[17]
- Weight bearing also is restricted during this period.[17]
- After 3 or 4 weeks in an immobilizer, protected ROM exercises are initiated in a hinged knee brace.
- The patient is allowed to bear weight as tolerated, and closed-chain quadriceps strengthening is begun.
- Hamstring strengthening is avoided for 6 to 10 weeks after the injury.[17]
- Because of altered gait mechanics, formal gait instruction also should be initiated once the patient begins weight bearing.
- Although patients with grade 1 or 2 injuries typically do well with nonoperative treatment, residual laxity and instability may require surgical intervention.

SURGICAL MANAGEMENT

- Grade 3 PLC injuries tend to do poorly with nonoperative management.[11]
  - Indications for operative treatment of PLC injuries consist of 5 to 10 mm of opening to varus stress at 30 degrees of knee flexion and a positive dial test or posterolateral external rotation test.[2] These findings are consistent with a grade 3 PLC injury.
- Ideally, PLC injuries should be treated between 10 days and 3 weeks after injury.[2,4,12,23]
  - Before 10 days, the knee usually is significantly swollen and still is in the acute inflammatory stage of the injury.
  - It also is possible to regain some quadriceps tone and ROM if surgery is postponed more than 10 days. Theoretically, the risk of arthrofibrosis would, therefore, be diminished.[23]
  - Waiting more than 3 weeks to operate results in increased scarring and difficulty in repairing the posterolateral structures primarily.[23]
  - Identifying and protecting the peroneal nerve becomes more difficult with increased scarring.[17]
  - Results of chronic repair are inferior to those of acute repair.[2]

Preoperative Planning

- In treating posterolateral ligament injuries, one must decide whether to repair the torn structures primarily, augment the repair, do an advancement, or perform a reconstruction of the posterolateral corner using allograft or autograft.
- Much of the preoperative planning is contingent on whether the PLC injury is isolated or combined with other ligamentous injuries.
- Preoperative radiographs are important to evaluate for fractures or other bony abnormalities.
  - Hip-to-ankle films may be helpful in chronic cases to evaluate for varus malalignment.
  - If malalignment is present, a valgus opening wedge osteotomy of the medial tibia should be considered, because unrecognized varus malalignment may lead to failure of a PLC reconstruction.[2]
- MRI helps evaluate for other associated ligamentous or meniscal injuries and should be used in preoperative planning if possible.
- If cruciate ligamentous injuries exist, they should be reconstructed prior to or concurrently with the PLC repair and reconstruction; otherwise, there is an increased risk that the PLC reconstruction will fail.[2]

Positioning

- Positioning for posterolateral surgery is contingent on the presence of other ligamentous injuries.
- Placing the patient in a lazy lateral position with a beanbag allows the surgeon to rotate the hip and leg externally for arthroscopic and cruciate ligament work as well as to internally rotate the leg into the lateral decubitus position for the lateral knee work.
- We have found a foot holder to be helpful for arthroscopic work.
- A well-padded tourniquet is placed high on the patient's thigh to avoid interference with the operative field.

Approach

- Arthroscopic visualization of the lateral compartment may demonstrate injuries or excessive opening (the "drive-through" sign).
- After arthroscopy and additional procedures, as indicated, the surgical approach is carried out as described in Techniques.

TECHNIQUES

EXPOSURE

- A lateral hockey-stick, straight, or curvilinear incision can be used in the approach to the posterolateral structures.[5] The incision typically measures 12 to 18 cm, begins just superior to the lateral epicondyle, and runs along the posterior border of the IT band (**TECH FIG 1**). The incision typically ends midway between the fibular head and Gerdy's tubercle.[23]
- The peroneal nerve first is identified proximally as it runs posterior to the biceps femoris tendon.[23] The nerve is traced distally around the fibular head and is protected throughout the case.
- Blunt dissection is taken down between the IT band and the biceps femoris.
- At this point, the structures of the PLC are identified and evaluated for pathology.

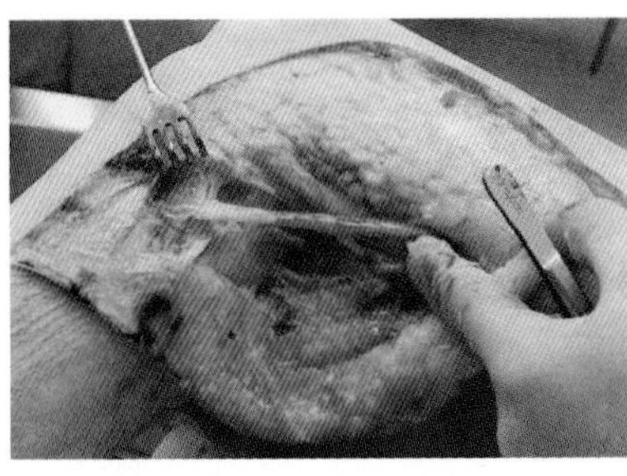

TECH FIG 1 • Exposure begins with an incision along the posterior border of the iliotibial band.

- Terry and Laprade[27] described three fascial incisions for exposure of the PLC:
  - The first incision bisects the IT band.
  - The second incision is made between the posterior border of the IT band and the short head of the biceps femoris.
  - The third incision is made along the posterior border of the long head of the biceps.
- A capsular incision can be made along the anterior border of the LCL.

DIRECT PRIMARY REPAIR

- For best results, primary repair should be done within 2 to 3 weeks of injury.[17]
- The structures should be repaired with the knee in 60 degrees of flexion and neutral tibial rotation.[23]
- A tibial avulsion of the popliteus can be repaired directly to the posterolateral tibia using suture anchors, sutures, or a cancellous screw with soft tissue washer (TECH FIG 2).
- A femoral avulsion of the popliteus typically occurs with an avulsion of the LCL.
  - Both of these structures can be sutured back to the lateral femoral condyle using transosseous drill holes.
- Laprade and Wentorf[17] described the use of a recess procedure for treatment of a femoral avulsion of the popliteus or LCL.
- In this procedure, a whipstitch is placed in the proximal popliteus, a small bone tunnel is made at the original femoral insertion of the popliteus, a stylette pin is used to pass the sutures from the whipstitch to the medial side of the knee, and the popliteus is pulled into the tunnel with the sutures.
  - The sutures are then tied over a button medially.
- A popliteofibular ligament avulsion off the fibula can be treated with tenodesis of the popliteus tendon to the posterior fibular head using suture anchors.[2]
  - The tenodesis can be reinforced with the fabellofibular ligament.
  - An avulsion of the LCL and arcuate ligament off of the fibular head can be reattached with transosseous sutures into the fibular head.[2]

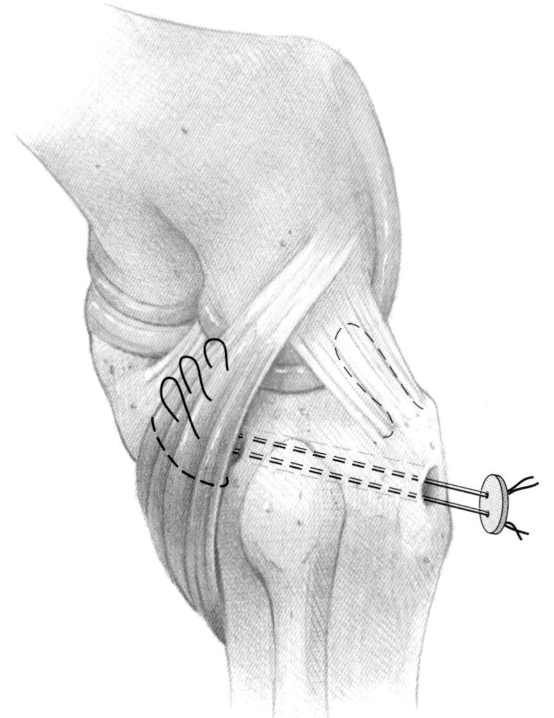

TECH FIG 2 • Direct primary repair of the popliteus tendon using a transosseous suture and button.

AUGMENTATION

- If the repair of the structures of the PLC is tenuous or the tissue is poor, the surgeon should consider augmentation of the repair.
- The tibial attachment of the popliteus can be augmented with a strip of IT band left attached distally to Gerdy's tubercle (TECH FIG 3A).
  - The strip is passed through a drill hole in the proximal tibia from anterior to posterior and sutured to the popliteus.[2]
- The popliteofibular ligament can be augmented using a central slip of the biceps femoris.[29]
  - The biceps distal attachment is left intact, and the slip is sutured to the posterior fibula, passed under the remaining biceps posteriorly, and attached to the lateral femur with suture anchors or screw and soft tissue washer (TECH FIG 3B).

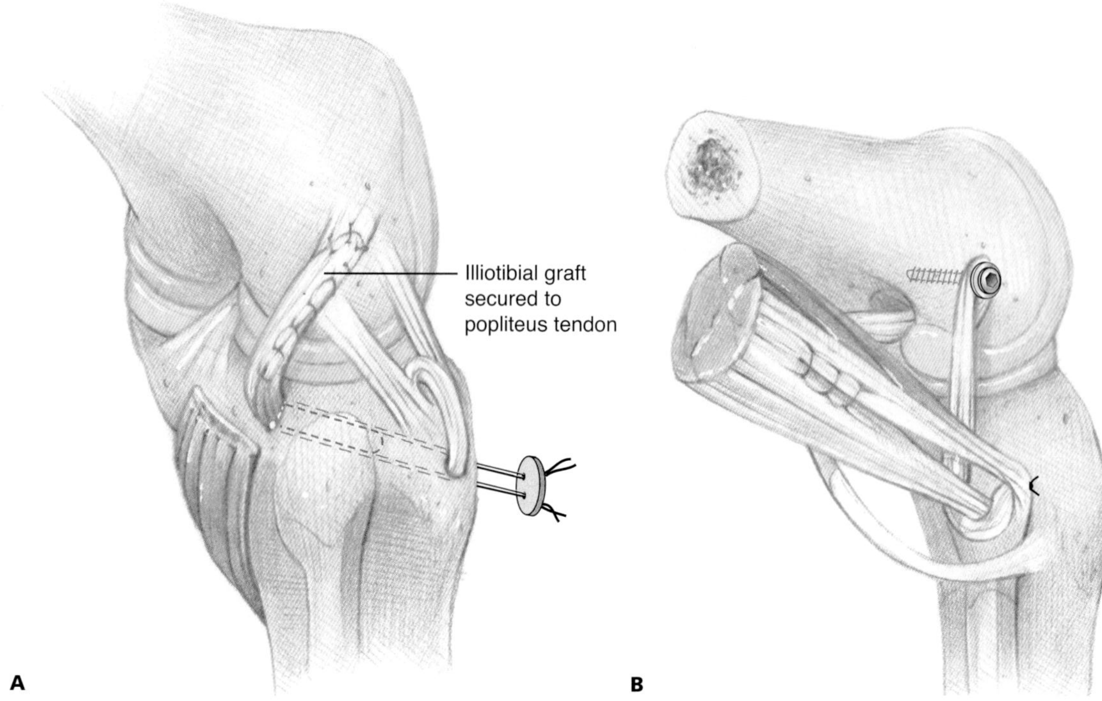

TECH FIG 3 • **A.** Augmentation with the iliotibial (IT) band. **B.** Augmentation with a central slip of biceps femoris passed posteriorly around the remaining biceps and inserted into the distal lateral femur using a soft tissue washer.

ADVANCEMENT

- In the patient in whom the posterolateral structures are insufficient for primary repair or in chronic cases, an arcuate complex advancement can be performed.[10]
- The LCL must be of normal integrity, and the popliteofibular ligament must be intact.
- The LCL, popliteus, lateral gastrocnemius, arcuate ligament, and posterolateral capsule are advanced en bloc in line with the LCL, tensioned with the knee at 30 degrees of flexion and neutral tibial rotation, and inserted into a trough in the distal lateral femur (TECH FIG 4).
- The disadvantage of this procedure is that the advancement does not restore isometry, thus leading to stretching of the reconstruction over time.[20]

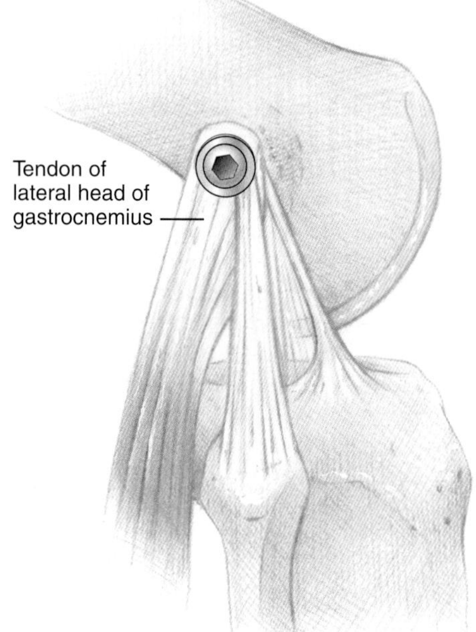

TECH FIG 4 • Proximal arcuate complex advancement. The lateral collateral ligament (LCL), popliteus, lateral head of the gastrocnemius, arcuate ligament, and posterolateral capsule are advanced and inserted en bloc to the distal lateral femur.

RECONSTRUCTION

- Reconstruction of the posterolateral corner is used in acute injuries when the tissue is poor or irreparable and in chronic cases in which the tissues are scarred and attenuated.
- The lateral collateral ligament, the popliteofibular ligament, and the popliteus are the three most important structures to be reconstructed in the PLC.[20]
- Reconstruction of the lateral collateral ligament using local tissue, allograft, and autograft has been described.

BICEPS TENODESIS TECHNIQUE

- Clancy et al[3] reconstructed the lateral collateral ligament using a biceps tenodesis technique (TECH FIG 5).
- In this technique, the entire biceps is transferred to the lateral femoral condyle 1 cm anterior to the LCL origin.
- The distal biceps is left attached to the fibular head.
- Disadvantages of this technique are that it does not reconstruct the popliteus or popliteofibular ligament, and it sacrifices the dynamic stabilizing effect of the biceps femoris.[20]

Collateral Ligament Reconstruction

- Isolated LCL reconstruction also can be performed using Achilles tendon allograft, patellar tendon auto- or allograft, or a central tubularized slip of the biceps tendon (TECH FIG 6).
  - Fluoroscopy can be used to ensure proper placement of the proximal end of the graft to the lateral femoral epicondyle.[2,27]
  - Plication of the remaining posterolateral structures can be performed.

Two-Graft Technique

- Laprade et al[15] have described an anatomic posterolateral knee reconstruction (TECH FIG 7) using a two-graft technique (ie, Achilles tendon allograft split in half).
- The first graft is used to reconstruct the popliteus.
  - The bone plug is secured in the anatomic location of the popliteus insertion on the femur, and the graft is passed from posterior to anterior through an anatomically placed tibial tunnel.
- The second graft is used to reconstruct both the LCL and the popliteofibular ligament.
  - The bone plug is secured in the femoral tunnel at the anatomic location of the LCL origin.

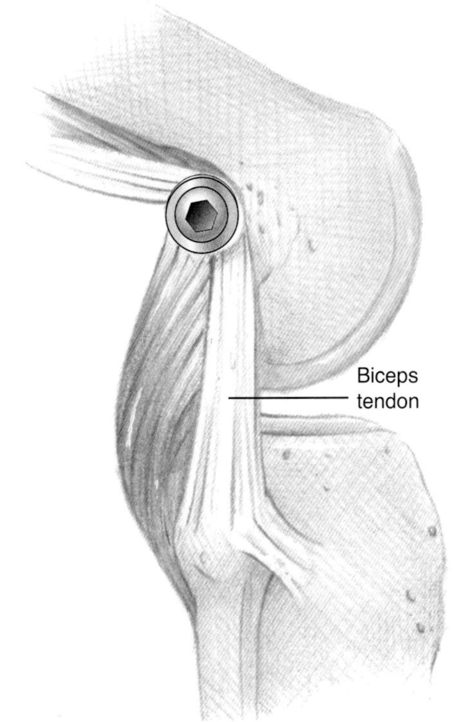

TECH FIG 5 • LCL reconstruction using the biceps tenodesis. The biceps femoris is transferred 1 cm anterior to the LCL origin while leaving the distal insertion on the fibular head intact.

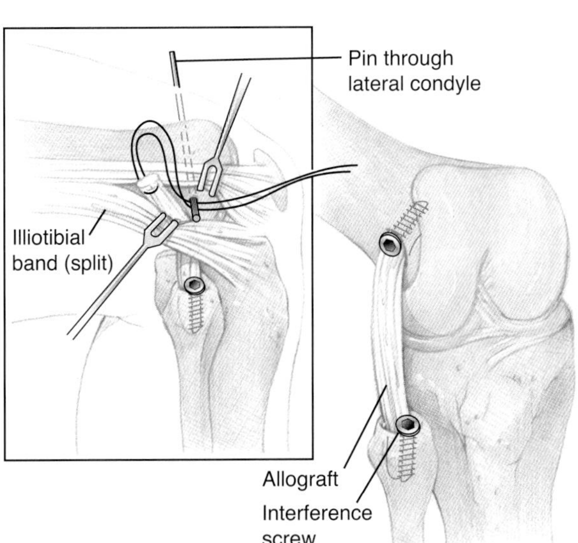

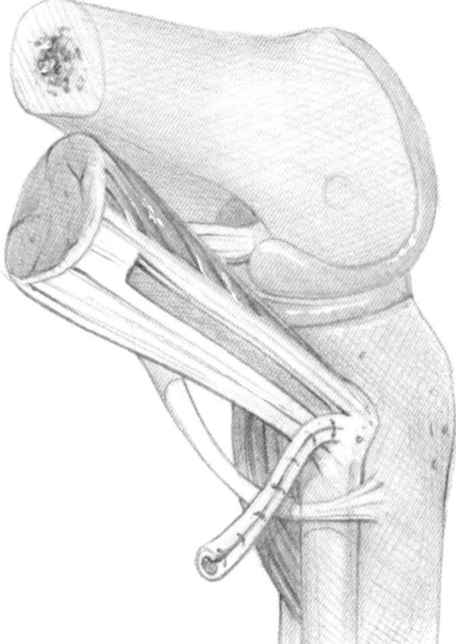

TECH FIG 6 • **A.** LCL reconstruction with tendon allo- or autograft. **B.** LCL reconstruction using a central tubularized slip of the biceps tendon. The distal insertion of the slip on the fibular head is left intact while the proximal portion is inserted on the lateral femoral epicondyle.

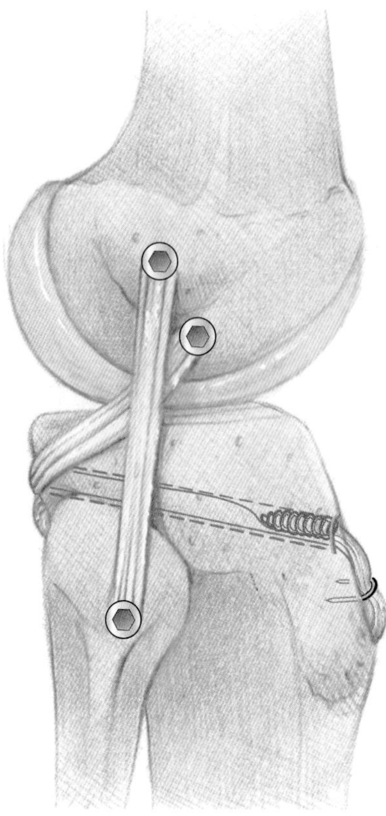

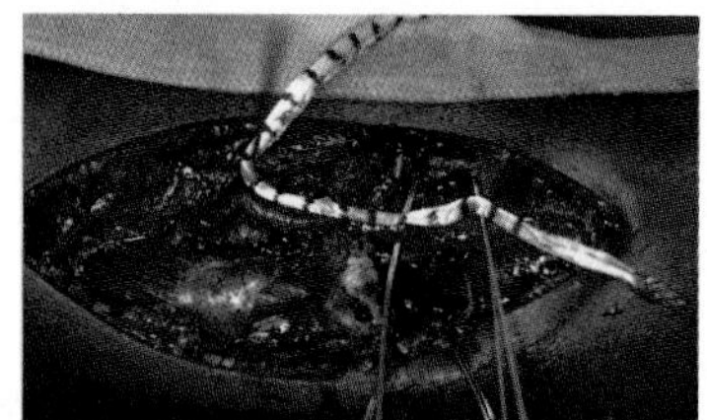

TECH FIG 7 • Two-graft technique for posterolateral corner reconstruction. **A.** The graft labeled *PLT* is inserted to the femur in the anatomic insertion site of the popliteus and then passed from posterior to anterior in the tibia. The graft labeled *FCL* is inserted to the lateral epicondyle and is passed from lateral to posteromedial in the fibula and then into the same tibial tunnel used by the PLT graft. Both the FCL graft and the PLT graft are secured to the tibia using either an interference screw or suture button. **B.** A hamstring graft can be used for this reconstruction. We tubularize our grafts using a whip stitch and ensure that no extraneous soft tissue remains on the graft that could hinder graft passage.

- The graft is then passed through a tunnel from lateral to posteromedial and then pulled through the same tibial tunnel from posterior to anterior.
- Interference screws are used to secure the grafts in their tunnels, and soft tissue staples are used for secondary fixation.

Split Patellar Tendon Technique

- Veltri and Warren[29] have described a technique of reconstructing the PLC using a split patellar tendon allograft or autograft (**TECH FIG 8**).
- The patellar bone plug is fixed in a tunnel in the lateral femoral condyle using a suture button on the medial femoral cortex.
- The graft is then split. The anterior limb is brought from posterior to anterior through a tunnel in the fibular head reproducing the popliteofibular ligament. The posterior limb is brought through a tibial tunnel from posterior to anterior. Both limbs are secured with suture buttons.
- A central slip of biceps can be used to reconstruct the LCL, as described earlier.

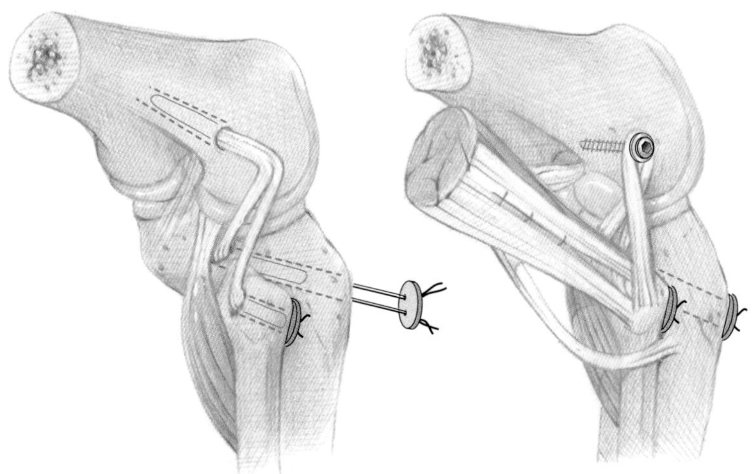

TECH FIG 8 • Reconstruction with a split patella tendon graft.

Popliteus Bypass Technique

- Muller[21] described a popliteus bypass technique (TECH FIG 9) in which a free graft is passed through a tibial tunnel from anterior to the posterolateral proximal tibia and secured to the anterior aspect of the lateral femoral condyle.
- This technique does not reproduce either the LCL or the popliteofibular ligament.

Figure 8 Technique

- Semitendinosus and gracilis autograft have been used to reconstruct the popliteofibular ligament and LCL concurrently.
- Larson[18] described a figure 8 technique in which he used hamstring autograft passed through a fibular tunnel, crossed in a figure 8 pattern, and wrapped around a screw and soft tissue washer at an isometric point on the lateral femoral condyle (TECH FIG 10).

Lateral Collateral Ligament Reconstruction Using Bone–Patellar Tendon–Bone Allograft

- Lattimer et al[19] described using a bone–patellar tendon–bone allograft fixed distally to the fibular head with an interference screw and proximally to the lateral femoral condyle 5 mm anterior to the femoral origin of the LCL.
- The graft is tensioned with a valgus forced placed on the 30-degree flexed knee.
- The large cross-sectional area of the graft theoretically restores LCL and arcuate and popliteofibular ligament function.
- This reconstruction neglects the popliteus, however.

Authors' Preferred Technique

- We have found at our institution that a combination of the Larson and Muller techniques is the most effective approach to reconstructing the LCL, popliteofibular ligament, and popliteus.

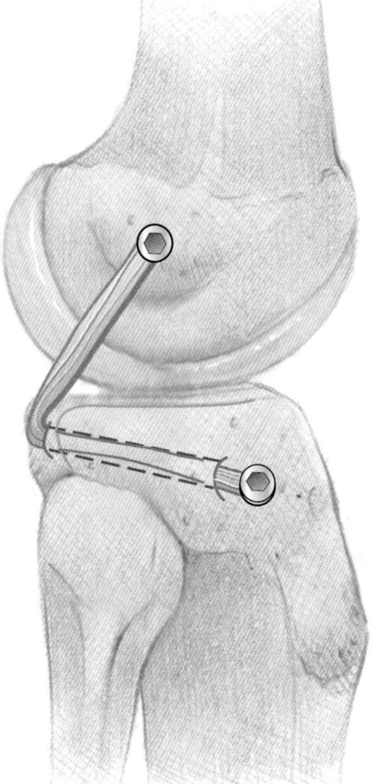

TECH FIG 9 • Popliteus bypass reconstruction technique. A hamstring graft is passed from anterior to posterolateral in the tibia. The graft is then passed from the posterolateral tibia to the anterior aspect of the lateral femoral condyle. The graft may be secured with suture buttons, soft tissue screws, or staples.

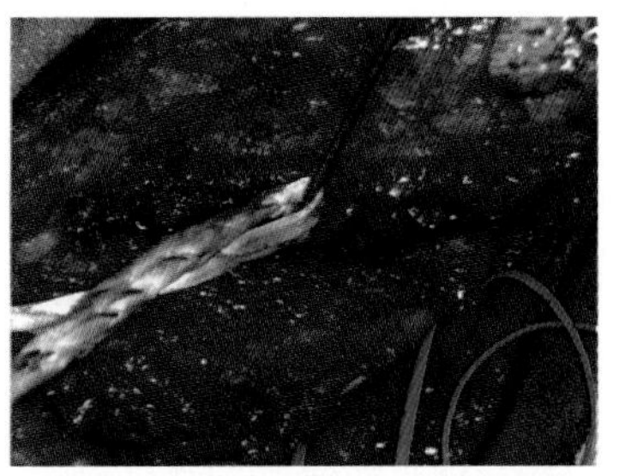

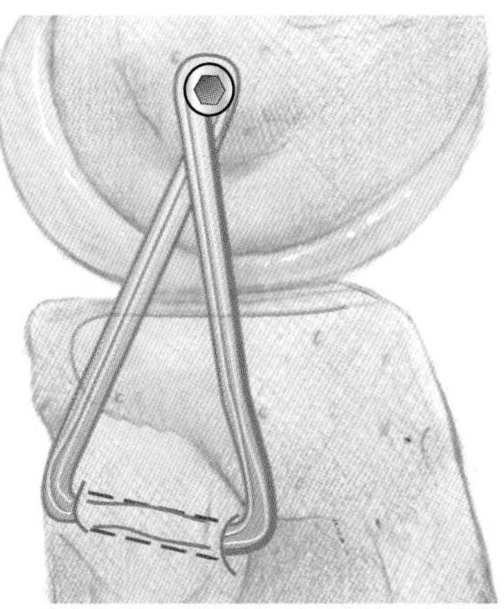

TECH FIG 10 • Figure 8 reconstruction technique. **A.** A guide pin is placed in the lateral femoral condyle and is checked by fluoroscopy to ensure proper placement. The hamstring is then wrapped around the guide pin in a figure 8 fashion and secured with a cannulated soft tissue screw and washer. The pin is then removed. **B.** The graft is passed through the fibular head and secured by sewing the graft to itself or using a soft tissue staple. This step is done after proper tensioning of the graft has been achieved.

PEARLS AND PITFALLS

- Monitor for fluid extravasation and increased compartment pressures during the arthroscopic portion of the procedure, because the capsule usually is disrupted in PLC injuries.
- Do not miss PLC injury when treating cruciate ligament injuries, to avoid failed cruciate ligament reconstruction.
- Reconstruct the cruciate ligaments before or concurrently with PLC reconstruction.
- Repair structures of the PLC beginning from deep to superficial.
- Varus malalignment may lead to failed PLC reconstruction; therefore, valgus osteotomy may be needed in chronic PLC insufficiency.
- Determine safe ROM of the knee before leaving the operating room, to guide postoperative rehabilitation.

POSTOPERATIVE CARE

- A hinged knee brace locked in extension should be used, and protected weight bearing should be followed for 3 weeks following a reconstruction and 6 weeks following a direct primary repair.[2,17]
  - Weight bearing theoretically places tension on the repair because of the normal mechanical axis of the leg.
- Straight leg raises may be allowed in the knee brace initially.
- Active knee extension and closed chain kinetic quadriceps strengthening may be initiated at 4 to 8 weeks postoperatively.
- Gentle leg presses, proprioceptive training, and squats may be initiated at 3 months.
- Hamstring exercises should be strictly avoided until 12 to 16 weeks postoperatively.[2,17]
- A fairly intensive rehabilitation protocol should be followed for 9 to 12 months.
  - The goal of rehabilitation is to achieve symmetrical quadriceps strength, knee stability, and full knee ROM.

OUTCOMES

- Hughston and Jacobsen[10] reported good functional results at 4 years in 12 of 19 patients treated with arcuate complex advancement combined with distal primary repair.
- DeLee et al[6] also reported that 8 of 11 patients treated with advancement surgery had good results, with no arthritis or revisions at 7.5 years.
- Noyes and Barber-Westin[22] reported on 42 months of follow-up in 21 patients treated with Achilles tendon allograft reconstruction of the LCL with plication or advancement of attenuated posterolateral structures.
  - Failure occurred in 2 patients, and good to excellent functional results were reported in 16 (76%) patients.
- Lattimer et al[19] reported on 10 patients treated with bone–patellar tendon–bone reconstruction of the LCL as well as cruciate ligament reconstruction at 28 months of follow-up.
  - All 10 patients had a reduction in their sensation of instability.
  - The patients all had less than 5 mm of lateral opening to varus stress and less than 5 degrees of external rotation.
  - Nine of the 10 patients returned to within one level of their preinjury level of activity.
- The long-term incidence of degenerative arthritis following PLC injuries treated with surgery remains unknown.
  - No long-term prospective studies exist that evaluate the different ways to ligamentously reconstruct the knee with a PLC injury. Because this injury is uncommon, large study populations are difficult to obtain.
  - Consequently, it is difficult to determine the clinically best method of treating this injury.

COMPLICATIONS

- Because of the extensive trauma usually incurred by the PLC-injured knee, arthrofibrosis is one of the most common complications associated with this injury.
- Residual knee instability also can occur, especially in grade 3 PLC injuries treated nonoperatively.
  - These two conflicting complications make postoperative management as important as the surgical treatment itself for a good result.
- Neurovascular complications are more often associated with the initial trauma rather than the surgical management. Delayed surgical treatment increases the incidence of iatrogenic peroneal nerve injury, however.
- The incidence of wound complications can be decreased by delaying surgery until the skin has recovered from the acute phase of the injury, which usually is 10 days or more after the initial injury.
  - Bulky compressive dressings and elevation of the leg also may help decrease swelling before surgery.
  - Skin incisions should be planned to avoid skin bridges less than 7 cm wide.
- The incidence of degenerative joint disease is increased in patients with PLC injuries due to abnormal joint motion.[2,17]
- The goal of surgical intervention is to reconstruct knee motion and stability to be as normal as possible.
- The lateral compartment and patellofemoral compartments are most commonly affected by PLC injuries.
- Because of long surgical times and use of graft material, infection is a possible complication of PLC surgery.
  - Infection is a devastating complication, because to clear the infecting organism, it is often necessary to débride the grafts that were used to reconstruct the knee.

REFERENCES

1. Baker CL Jr, Norwood LA, Hughston JC. Acute posterolateral rotatory instability of the knee. J Bone Joint Surg Am 1983;65A:614–618.
2. Chen FS, Rokito AS, Pitman MI. Acute and chronic posterolateral rotatory instability of the knee. J Am Acad Orthop Surg 2000;8:97–110.
3. Clancy WG Jr, Meister K, Craythorne CB. Posterolateral corner collateral ligament reconstruction. In: Jackson DW, ed. Reconstructive Knee Surgery. New York: Raven Press, 1995:143–159.
4. Cooper DE, Warren RF, Warner JJP. The posterior cruciate ligament and posterolateral structures of the knee: anatomy, function, and patterns of injury. Instr Course Lect 1991;40:249–270.
5. Covey DC. Injuries of the posterolateral corner of the knee. J Bone Joint Surg Am 2001;83A:106–118.

6. DeLee JC, Riley MB, Rockwood CA Jr. Acute posterolateral rotatory instability of the knee. Am J Sports Med 1983;11:199–207.
7. Gollehan, DL, Torzilli PA, Warren RF. The role of the posterolateral and cruciate ligaments in the stability of the human knee: a biomechanical study. J Bone Joint Surg Am 1987;69A:233–242.
8. Harner CD, Vogrin TM, Hoher J, et al. Biomechanical analysis of a posterior cruciate ligament reconstruction: deficiency of the posterolateral structures as a cause of graft failure. Am J Sports Med 2000; 28:32–39.
9. Hughston JC, Andrews JR, et al. Classification of knee ligament injuries. Part II. The lateral compartment. J Bone Joint Surg Am 1976; 58A:173–179.
10. Hughston JC, Jacobson KE. Chronic posterolateral instability of the knee. J Bone Joint Surg Am 1985;67A:351–359.
11. Kannus P. Nonoperative treatment of grade II and III sprains of the lateral ligament compartment of the knee. Am J Sports Med 1989;17: 83–88.
12. Krukhaug Y, Moister A, Rodt A, Strand T. Lateral ligament injuries of the knee. Knee Surg Sports Traumatol Arthrosc 1998;6:21–25.
13. Laprade RF. Arthroscopic evaluation of the lateral compartment of knees with grade 3 posterolateral complex knee injuries. Am J Sports Med 1997;25:596–602.
14. Laprade RF, Bollom TS, Gilbert TJ, et al. The MRI appearance of individual structures of the posterolateral knee: a prospective study of normal and surgically verified grade 3 injuries. Am J Sports Med 2000;28:191–199.
15. Laprade RF, Johansen S, Wentorf FA, et al. An analysis of an anatomical posterolateral knee reconstruction: an in vitro biomechanical study and development of a surgical technique. Am J Sports Med 2004;32:1405–1414.
16. Laprade RF, Terry GC. Injuries to the posterolateral aspect of the knee: association of injuries with clinical instability. Am J Sports Med 1997;25:433–438.
17. Laprade RF, Wentorf F. Diagnosis and treatment of posterolateral knee injuries. Clin Orthop Rel Res 2002;402:110–121.
18. Larson RV. Isometry of the lateral collateral and popliteofibular ligaments and techniques for reconstruction using a free semitendinosus tendon graft. Oper Tech Sports Med 2001;9:84–90.
19. Lattimer HA, Tibone JE, El Attrache NS, et al. Reconstruction of the lateral collateral ligament of the knee with patellar tendon allograft: report of a new technique in combined ligament injuries. Am J Sports Med 1998;26:656–662.
20. Lee MC, Park YK, Lee SH, et al. Posterolateral reconstruction using split Achilles tendon allograft. Arthroscopy 2003;19:1043–1049.
21. Muller W. Die Rotationsinsabilitat am Kniegelenk. Hefte Unfallhk. 1990;125:51–68.
22. Noyes FR, Barber-Westin SD. Surgical reconstruction of severe chronic posterolateral complex injuries of the knee using allograft tissues. Am J Sports Med 1995;23:2–12.
23. Rihn JA, Cha PS, Groff YJ, et al. The acutely dislocated knee: evaluation and management. J Am Acad Orthop Surg 2004;12:334–346.
24. Ross G, Chapman AW, Newberg AR, et al. Magnetic resonance imaging for the evaluation of acute posterolateral complex injuries of the knee. Am J Sports Med 1997;25:444–448.
25. Seebacher JR, Inglis AE, Marshall JL, et al. The structure of the posterolateral aspect of the knee. J Bone Joint Surg Am 1982;64A:536–541.
26. Skyhar MJ, Warren RF, Ortiz GJ, et al. The effects of sectioning of the posterior cruciate ligament and the posterolateral complex on the articular contact pressures within the knee. J Bone Joint Surg Am 1993;75A:694–699.
27. Terry GC, Laprade RF. The posterolateral aspect of the knee: anatomy and surgical approach. Am J Sports Med 1996;24:732–739.
28. Veltri DM, Warren RF. Isolated and combined posterior cruciate ligament injuries. J Am Acad Orthop Surg 1993;1:67–75.
29. Veltri DM, Warren RF. Operative treatment of posterolateral instability of the knee. Clin Sports Med 1994;13:615–627.

Chapter 47 Management of the Multiple Ligament–Injured Knee

Ralph W. Passarelli, Bradley B. Veazey, Daniel C. Wascher, Andrew J. Veitch, and Robert C. Schenck

DEFINITION

- Multiligament knee injuries result from both high-energy (eg, motor vehicle collisions) and low-energy (eg, athletic injuries, falls) events. Dislocation of the tibiofemoral joint is common, with or without spontaneous reduction.

ANATOMY

- Put very simply, knee dislocations can be viewed as injuries to one or both cruciate ligaments (ie, anterior cruciate ligament [ACL] or posterior cruciate ligament [PCL]), with variable involvement of the collateral ligaments (ie, the medial collateral ligament [MCL] and the fibular collateral ligament [FCL]) with important musculotendinous stabilizers—the biceps femoris and popliteus posterolaterally, and the pes anserine complex medially, all of which must be considered in restoring knee function. Palpable bony landmarks about the knee are crucial to aid in orientation for examination and when planning subsequent surgical approaches.
- The lateral femoral epicondyle and the fibular head are critical to identify the placement of lateral incisions, as are anatomic structures such as the FCL and peroneal nerve. Medially, the femoral epicondyle, tibial tubercle, pes insertion site, and posteromedial tibial edge are crucial landmarks for medial surgical exposures for inlay and MCL reconstruction.
- The intrinsic structure of the vascular system of the knee consists of an anastomotic ring of five geniculates: the superomedial, superolateral, inferomedial, inferolateral, and middle geniculates, as well as muscular and articular branches.
  - The extrinsic system plays a crucial role when parallel medial or lateral incisions are made about the knee in the sagittal plane.
  - Proper planning should allow 7 to 10 cm between superficial parallel incisions to greatly lessen the risk of skin bridge loss, but it has been our experience that such incisions should be avoided if possible. This network alone cannot support vascularity distal to the knee with popliteal vessel occlusion.
- The surgical anatomy of the knee usually is described in layers, going from the superficial structures to the deep structures.
  - *Layer I* is commonly described as consisting of Marshall's layer (arciform) anteriorly, the sartorius medially, and the iliotibial band and biceps femoris fascia laterally.
  - *Layer II* includes the FCL, patellar tendon, and superficial MCL.
  - *Layer III* includes the posterior oblique, arcuate ligament, and deep portion of the MCL. Layer III is thin anteriorly and has distinct, structurally important thickenings posteromedially (posterior oblique ligament) and posterolaterally (arcuate ligament). A Segond fracture is caused by avulsion of the thickened middle third of the lateral knee capsule in this layer.
  - Posterolateral reconstructions are complex because of this anatomy and variability and require restoration of both the FCL and popliteofibular (PFL) ligaments.
- The surgeon should understand the important anatomic relationships of the posterior structures of the knee, especially in regard to the popliteal neurovascular bundle.
  - The medial and lateral heads of the gastrocnemius are the borders of the popliteal fossa distally, the pes anserinus tendons medially, and the biceps femoris tendon laterally. The popliteus, posterior joint capsule, oblique popliteal ligament, and posterior femoral cortex form the floor of the fossa. Through this fossa run the plantaris muscle and the neurovascular structures. The popliteal artery enters through the adductor magnus superiorly as it leaves Hunter's canal, courses through the fossa, and exits through the soleal arch. The popliteal vein enters superolateral to the artery and continues superficial to the artery, but is located deep to the tibial and common peroneal nerves, leaving the fossa medial to the popliteal artery.
  - The vascular structures are located directly behind the posterior horns of the medial and lateral menisci. The vascular structures are protected during posteromedial and posterolateral approaches if the surgeon remains anterior to the medial and lateral heads of the gastrocnemius during dissection and careful retraction; of course, further dissection towards the midline can injure the bundle with either approach.
- With the advent of posterior procedures to the tibial side of the PCL, it is critical to understand the posterior neurovascular anatomy. The posteromedial approach also is useful to gain access to the tibial insertion of the PCL.
  - Deep dissection along the posterior tibial surface and femoral condyles provides additional safety for this approach. Use of a tourniquet during dissection provides improved visualization of the surgical planes.
  - Unlike the vascular surgeon, who uses a posteromedial approach for the neurovascular (popliteal) bundle, the orthopedic surgeon dissecting posteromedially should avoid the neurovascular bundle. Staying anterior to the medial gastrocnemius and hugging the posterior aspect of the knee joint protects the bundle in the orthopedic approach.
  - It is important to stop the dissection at the PCL, because further dissection laterally with this approach eventually will reach and potentially injure the bundle.

NATURAL HISTORY

- Before the development of modern surgical techniques for management of multiligament injuries, scores of patients were left with stiff, unstable, or even amputated limbs. Today, even with aggressive evaluation and treatment, patients ultimately may have residual instability with a lower level of activity, decreased range of motion (ROM), and even amputation. The use of allografts in multiligament-injured knees is a recent advance, although occasionally it is complicated by deep infection.

PATIENT HISTORY AND PHYSICAL FINDINGS

- During the initial evaluation of a patient with a suspected multiligament knee injury, the clinician should be cognizant of the potential for concomitant injuries. High- or low-energy knee trauma can have potentially life- or limb-threatening injuries, which must be identified acutely.
  - Once any life-threatening injuries have been treated, careful examination of the injured limb focuses both above and below the knee to evaluate for fracture as well as continuity of the extensor mechanism.
- A careful injury history should be obtained if possible, including pre-hospital neurovascular status of the limb, time of injury, and mechanism. Patients often relate a history of hyperextension of the knee in sporting events or a flexed knee that struck the dashboard during a motor vehicle accident.
  - Any evidence of current dislocation of the tibiofemoral joint should be addressed emergently, with attempted reduction under sedation, splinting, careful neurovascular examination pre- and post-reduction, and high-quality radiographic evaluation following reduction.
    - The radiographic evaluation should include an anteroposterior and lateral radiographs of the knee with the limb in a long-leg splint to demonstrate that a successful reduction has been achieved.
- Any asymmetry in the vascular examination from the uninjured extremity, even pre-hospital, necessitates further evaluation, with the specifics often dictated by vascular surgery protocols and regional preference.[24]
  - Many clinicians routinely obtain angiograms regardless of the vascular examination findings with multiligament injured knees.[2] Nonetheless, the current trend toward using sequential clinical examinations in the *reduced* dislocation with normal pulses is becoming more popular and is considered safe.
  - Use of Doppler or other noninvasive vascular laboratory studies in conjunction with an ankle brachial index is very useful, because these studies can provide objective information (rather than the subjective findings of pulses), and also avoids the invasiveness of angiography.
  - The surgeon must be aggressive in the management of any abnormal vascular findings, with immediate vascular consultation and immediate surgical exploration of ischemia in the reduced knee dislocation. Ischemia in the dislocated knee requires reduction and pulse or vascularity reevaluation. Continued ischemia for more than 6 to 8 hours results in amputation rates of up to 80%.[10]
- Medial puckering of the soft tissues of the knee usually suggests a posterolateral dislocation with buttonholing of the medial femoral condyle through the joint capsule, MCL incarceration into the joint, and irreducibility with closed methods of reduction.[7,28]

IMAGING AND OTHER DIAGNOSTIC STUDIES

- An integral part of evaluation of the multiligamentously injured knee is plain radiographs before and after reduction to confirm congruity of the joint, evaluate for associated fractures, and detect ligament avulsion injuries that may aid in timing of the treatment plan.
- MRI is an excellent adjunct to delineation of the extent of injury and pattern of ligament injury and musculotendinous and osteoarticular injuries. These studies are combined with a careful examination of the ligamentous structures with and without anesthesia, which are compared to the uninjured extremity.
- MRI cannot replace a careful clinical examination under anesthesia, which can determine ligament function and the need for ligament reconstruction.

CLASSIFICATION

- Multiple classification systems have been used to describe dislocations of the knee.
  - Historically, the most commonly used system has been based on a positional description of the relationship of the femur on the tibia when the knee is dislocated.[9] However, this system is not without problems.
    - First, most knee dislocations present spontaneously reduced, making classification based on position at the time of injury difficult, if not impossible.
    - Second, this system does not provide information regarding the energy of the injury, the ligaments injured, or associated neurovascular injuries, all of which play a part in the overall treatment plan.
- Classifying dislocations based on the anatomic injury pattern (ie, ligaments torn and associated neurovascular injuries) allows for adequate physician communication (especially for future reconstructions) and preoperative planning.[3] The anatomic classification is shown in Table 1.

DIFFERENTIAL DIAGNOSIS

- Knee dislocations can be difficult to assess in the presence of gross knee swelling or with the presentation of multi-trauma.
- Accurate detection of associated neurovascular injuries is critical.
- Identification of the ligaments injured is based on the initial examination, imaging studies, and examination under anesthesia.

NONOPERATIVE MANAGEMENT

- Many patients today are treated with surgical management of some type; however, depending on their injury pattern,

Table 1 Anatomic Classification of Knee Dislocations

Class	Description
KD I	Single cruciate torn and knee dislocated, ACL/collateral ligament usually torn, PCL intact *or* PCL/collateral ligament torn, ACL intact
KD II	Both cruciates torn, collaterals intact
KD III	Both cruciates torn, one collateral torn Subset KD III M (M = ACL, PCL, MCL torn) *or* KD III L (L = ACL, PCL, LCL torn)
KD IV	All four ligaments torn
KD V	Periarticular fracture–dislocation

C and N may be added to include arterial (C) and nerve (N) injury.
KD, knee dislocation; L, lateral; M, medial.

there are still subsets that are treated nonoperatively. These include patients with severe comorbidities that increase the risks of surgery or those with open dislocations or greatly damaged soft tissue envelopes, where the focus is on restoring the envelope and treating infection.

Cast Immobilization

- Although cast immobilization technique was used for many years to treat multiligament injuries to the knee before modern reconstructive procedures were available, closed treatment as definitive management rarely is indicated.
- Immobilization in extension for 6 weeks, as described by Taylor,[26] can result in a stable knee, but in our experience should be used only in circumstances where the preferred technique of ligamentous reconstruction is not applicable or feasible.

External Fixation

- External fixation may be used to span the knee joint with fixation in the tibia and femur, and is useful in patients who have poor rehabilitation potential. It also may be used as a temporary stabilizing measure in open knee dislocations, severe soft tissue injuries, and vascular reconstructions while awaiting optimal conditions for operative ligamentous reconstructions.
- Advantages include adequate maintenance of reduction, access to soft tissue wounds, and protection of maturing reverse saphenous vein grafts.
- However, the potentials for loss of knee motion and exuberant scar formation (arthrofibrosis) exist, and these often require later manipulation under anesthesia and lysis of adhesions.

Hinged Knee Brace

- The patient is placed in a hinged knee brace, and supervised ROM exercises are initiated in the first few weeks following the injury.
- This treatment method is ineffective in creating a stable knee but is an extremely important step in the process to a successful multiligamentous reconstruction.
- Gaining extension, a more normal gait pattern, full flexion, and decreased swelling (resolution of inflammation) add to an easier postoperative course, with avoidance of postoperative stiffness and heterotopic ossification with multiligamentous reconstruction. In our experience, early multiligamentous reconstruction has tremendous risks for stiffness and a poor result.
- The work of Shelbourne[21] and others with ACL/MCL injuries with preoperative rehabilitation is even more applicable to multiligament knee injuries. Obtaining preoperative ROM before PCL, ACL, and collateral ligament reconstruction is extremely useful in obtaining a stable, pain-free knee after dislocation.

SURGICAL MANAGEMENT

Indications

- Operative reconstruction is recommended to most patients with multiligament knee injuries. In some cases, an external fixator is used temporarily followed by surgical reconstruction; in most cases, early braced knee motion is instituted with delay of reconstruction of ligament injuries undertaken only once motion is restored and inflammation is resolved.
  - Ligamentous repair (ie, suture repair) is less and less commonly used, because the results are variable, and the use of early postoperative ROM, in our experience, results in failure of the suture repair.
- Crucial to the immediate care of these injuries is a meticulous neurovascular examination. Any vascular deficit necessitates emergent vascular surgery consultation and consideration for an open popliteal artery exploration and reverse saphenous vein graft reconstruction.
  - Patients with open injuries, popliteal artery reconstructions, severe soft tissue injuries, or complex injury patterns (concomitant fractures) should be considered for external fixation for 2 to 4 weeks to allow healing of the soft tissue envelope and maturation of the arterial repair or reconstruction. Once conditions have been optimized and wounds are healed without infection, reconstruction can be performed.
- The optimal timing for surgical intervention is not clearly defined, although many investigators recommend waiting for several weeks after the injury before performing surgical repair or reconstruction of these multiligamentous injuries. The operating surgeon must have a good working knowledge of ligamentous reconstructions and should proceed according to his or her level of experience and preference.
  - In our experiences, it is best to wait for preoperative motion, gait, and swelling to improve. Over 15 years of experience with knee dislocations has led to the following guidelines:
    - Delayed reconstruction is better than immediate surgery.
    - Preoperative rehabilitation is useful to regain motion, and resolution of swelling and inflammation is critical to surgical success.
    - Reconstruction is done with allo- and autografts, avoiding surgical repairs.
    - Both cruciates and involved collateral(s) are reconstructed simultaneously.

Approach

Graft Choice

- Many graft choices are available for ACL reconstruction in the multiligament-injured knee. We prefer a bone–patellar tendon–bone (BTB) allograft.
- While a BTB autograft is the gold standard in an isolated ACL reconstruction, the comorbidities of ipsilateral graft harvest in combined ACL-PCL injuries can result in stiffness, especially in simultaneous cruciate reconstruction.
- The ipsilateral hamstring autograft should not be considered in a type III knee dislocation (KDIIIM) injury, because the hamstrings provide a secondary restraint to valgus load and may be required for MCL reconstruction.
- Allografts are ideal for the multiligamentous knee injury.

Posterior Cruciate Ligament Reconstruction

- A number of approaches to modern PCL reconstruction are available, including (1) transtibial and femoral tunnels (with or without dual femoral socket) and (2) tibial inlay using a single or dual femoral tunnel in which tibial fixation is achieved by securing a bone plug into a trough positioned at the anatomic insertion of the PCL.
  - The inlay technique places the bone–tendon junction of the graft at the joint line of the proximal tibia and may avoid the risk of the "killer curve" graft impingement seen experimentally with the transtibial tunnel technique.
- One of the senior authors prefers a dual femoral socket (ie, double-bundle femoral) and tibial inlay PCL reconstruction through a posteromedial approach.

- The Achilles tendon allograft is ideal for such a reconstruction. The calcaneal bone plug is fashioned for the tibial inlay, and the tendon portion is split into 6- and 8-mm graft bundles for posteromedial and anterolateral PCL bundle reconstruction, respectively. Cannulated, fully threaded 4.0-mm screws are used for the tibial inlay fixation, and soft tissue interference and biodegradable screw fixation (7- and 9-mm) are used in double-bundle femoral fixation.

- PCL reconstructions often have failed to reestablish normal posterior translation at long-term follow-up.
  - Authors have proposed that two major factors are responsible for late loosening and resultant residual posterior tibial translation following this surgical method.
    - The first factor is the acute angle the graft must make to round the posterior lip of the tibia when exiting the transtibial tunnel. This has been described as the "killer turn" or "killer curve," which may cause graft abrasion and subsequent failure.[11] A biomechanical study reported an increased failure rate of transtibial over tibial inlay technique (32% transtibial, 0% inlay) following cyclic testing. Significant differences also were reported in graft thinning and elongation between the two techniques, favoring the inlay technique. The inlay grafts demonstrated 13% thinning and 5.9 mm of graft elongation over 2000 cycles, compared with 41% thinning and 9.8 mm of graft elongation with the transtibial technique.[13]
    - The second factor involves the distinct anatomic bundles of the PCL, which function at different degrees of knee flexion.[4] Reconstructing the specific PCL bundles may produce more normal function than the single femoral tunnel technique (anterolateral PCL bundle).
  - Clinically, long-term cadaveric studies are needed to fully verify these biomechanical differences. Clinical studies to this point have shown no difference in outcome between transtibial and inlay techniques.[11]
  - The double-bundle technique allows reconstruction of both the anterolateral and posteromedial bundles of the PCL.
- Although tibial inlay techniques may appear cumbersome, advances have been made that reduce the technical difficulties encountered during this procedure.
- We believe the posteromedial approach to PCL reconstruction described here simplifies this technique by maintaining the patient in the supine position during ACL and PCL reconstruction, avoiding the prone position altogether, preserving the origin of the medial head of the gastrocnemius, and simplifying graft passage.

BONE–PATELLAR TENDON GRAFT FOR BONE–ANTERIOR CRUCIATE LIGAMENT RECONSTRUCTION

- The patient is positioned supine with a lateral post or leg holder in place.
- Standard arthroscopy portals are used, and a systematic examination of the knee is performed.
- Tibial and femoral tunnels 10 to 11 mm in diameter are drilled using standard methods.
- The allograft BTB bone plugs for the ACL are fashioned to match the tunnel diameter, and the femoral plug is fashioned to a length of 25 mm.
- A small drill is used to place a hole in the femoral bone plug of the graft and a no. 2 braided composite suture (Fiberwire, Arthrex, Naples, FL) is passed through the hole for graft passage.
- Two holes are drilled in the tibial bone plug and a no. 2 suture is passed to aid in graft passage, and even potential post or staple fixation in case of graft length mismatch.
- A critical step in planning the depth of the femoral tunnel is factoring in the length of the allograft.
  - The femoral tunnel should be drilled to a length of 30 to 35 mm.
  - Most patients require an intra-articular graft length of 25 mm.
  - Sixty millimeters (35 mm for the femoral tunnel plus 25 mm for the intra-articular portion) should be subtracted from the length of the entire graft to yield the ideal tibial tunnel length.
  - This method ensures that optimal fixation of the bone plug in the tibial tunnel will be possible.
- A guide pin is placed endoscopically through the tibial tunnel into the femoral ACL origin and drilled out the anterolateral cortex of the femur and through the skin.
  - A no. 2 braided composite suture from the femoral bone plug is placed through the eyelet of the guide pin.
  - The guide pin and suture are pulled up into the femoral ACL socket, passing into the femoral tunnel.
- Fixation on the femoral side is performed using an interference screw through the inferomedial portal with a protective sleeve.
- Fixation and tensioning of the tibial side of the ACL graft are delayed until after PCL reconstruction.
- At this point, the PCL dual femoral socket sites are selected and drilled (discussed later in this section).
- Sutures are placed in the PCL femoral tunnels to allow graft passage.
- Once the PCL graft is securely fixed, then, and only then, is the ACL allograft tensioned in full extension and secured to the tibial tunnel using a metal interference screw.
- If graft tunnel mismatch occurs and the ACL tibial bone plug is not completely within the tibial tunnel, tibial interference fixation can be performed with an oversized soft tissue biodegradable interference screw, or staple–post fixation can be performed externally on the tibial surface.
- In our experience, simultaneous bicruciate reconstruction, although complex, can be simplified by the following steps, performed in this order:
  - ACL femoral and tibial tunnel preparation; dual femoral PCL tunnel preparation; ACL graft passage with fixation of the femoral side only; tibial inlay via the posteromedial approach; PCL graft passage and fixation; ACL tibial fixation; and, lastly, collateral reconstruction as indicated.
  - Such steps allow for the most time-efficient process for simultaneous cruciate reconstruction.

DOUBLE-BUNDLE POSTERIOR CRUCIATE LIGAMENT RECONSTRUCTION

Positioning and Preparation

- The patient is positioned supine on the operating table with the use of a lateral post. A careful examination under anesthesia is performed to confirm the ligament injury and diagnosis.
- Standard inferomedial and inferolateral arthroscopy portals are used.
- A 30-degree arthroscope is inserted and diagnostic arthroscopy performed to confirm the PCL tear.
- The PCL remnant is removed and the anatomic origin identified.

Double-Bundle Tunnel Preparation

- A long drill-tip guidewire is placed through the inferolateral portal with the knee positioned at 90 degrees, viewing the pin placement from an inferomedial portal. This allows sequential femoral bundle pin placement and reaming for the anterolateral bundle of the PCL (8-mm tunnel) followed by posteromedial tunnel creation (6 mm).
- The guidewire is inserted in the anatomic site of the anterolateral bundle (usually high in the notch, near the articular surface), drilled into the condyle and exiting out of the skin overlying the distal medial thigh.
- The slotted end of the guidewire is used to pass a suture into the tunnel, with the loop remaining in the tunnel.
- At our institution, both tunnels are reamed endoscopically through the medial cortex to allow for adequate graft tensioning.
- At this point, both femoral sockets have been reamed, passing sutures are in place (exiting the inferomedial portal), and the posteromedial approach is performed.

Posteromedial Approach and Tibial Inlay Site Preparation

- All arthroscopic instruments are removed from the knee, and the leg is placed in the figure 4 position.
- The primary surgeon is positioned on the contralateral side of the operating table with the assistant on the ipsilateral side of the injured knee.
- The leg is exsanguinated, and the tourniquet is inflated with the knee hyperflexed.
- A posteromedial approach to the knee is utilized, with a 6- to 10-cm incision centered over the posterior joint line. The incision should follow the posterior cortex of the proximal tibia and the medial femoral epicondyle.
- The sartorius fascia is exposed and incised in line with the skin incision. The gracilis and semitendinosus tendons are retracted posteriorly and distally. The fascia between the medial head of the gastrocnemius muscle and the posterior border of the semimembranosus muscle is divided in line with the incision. The semimembranosus muscle is then dissected off of its tibial insertion and tagged with a nonabsorbable suture for later repair.
- The remainder of the exposure is performed by blunt dissection following the posterior border of the joint line and remaining anterior to the medial head of the gastrocnemius muscle at all times to protect the popliteal neurovascular structures.
- The popliteus muscle is elevated, and a blunt Hohmann retractor is placed just lateral to the PCL insertion onto the tibia. This provides excellent visualization of the posterior tibia to create the trough.
  - The remnant of the PCL, the posterolateral edge of the medial femoral condyle, the joint surface, and the lateral meniscus are palpable anatomic landmarks that are used to position the trough in the center of the posterior tibia.
- A burr is used to cut a trough 10 mm wide × 10 mm deep × 25 mm long extending from the joint line and centered over the midline, posterior tibia.
  - The trough should correspond to the size and shape of the allograft bone block.
  - The trough should not be placed too distally, because such placement could possibly create the killer curve effect on the graft.
- A posterior capsulotomy is made at the mid-joint line, and a curved Kelly clamp or similar arthroscopic instrument is used to perform the posterior capsulotomy, through the notch medial to the ACL graft and through the inferolateral portal.
- The dual socket passing sutures are transferred out the back of the knee into the posteromedial exposure.
- We routinely use dry arthroscopy to ensure that the sutures are on the correct side of the ACL as well as to aid in grasping the sutures when reaching from the posterior approach.
- At this time, the tourniquet is released and hemostasis is evaluated. Release of the tourniquet often is indicated at this stage, especially if it was inflated prior to making the posteromedial approach, during notchplasty, ACL tunnel fixation, graft passage, and PCL dual socket formation.

Graft Preparation

- As noted earlier, our preferred graft for PCL reconstruction is an Achilles tendon allograft.
- This graft allows for either a single- or double-bundle femoral technique, depending on surgeon preference and experience.
- The graft can easily be fashioned into a double-bundle graft.
- The ends are prepared by placing a traction stitch with a no. 2 Fiberwire suture to facilitate graft tubulization and eventual passage.
- The calcaneal bone plug is fashioned to maintain the double-bundle tendons and can vary in size (often, it is 15 mm wide × 15 mm deep × 35 mm long). Hence, graft preparation must be performed before tibial trough creation.

Tibial Graft Passage and Fixation

- The tibial inlay graft is positioned into the tibial trough with care taken to ensure that the bone–tendon junction is positioned at the joint line.
- The tibial side of the graft is fixed first to ensure that the bone–tendon junction is positioned at the joint line to avoid graft abrasion.

- The inlay is secured with two 4.0-mm cannulated screws over a guidewire, positioned 1 cm apart.
- The screws are placed from posterior to anterior and parallel to the joint line.
  - It is critical to aim the screws anterolaterally in the tibia to avoid inadvertent fixation of the ACL graft.

Femoral Graft Fixation

- Once the inlay is secured, the double-bundle graft ends are sequentially passed.
- In our experience, the posteromedial bundle is passed first and fixed prior to the anterolateral bundle.
  - If both grafts are passed simultaneously, visualization for the posteromedial bundle is obstructed by the anterolateral bundle.
- As noted, we routinely use a 6 mm graft size for the posteromedial bundle with placement of a 7-mm × 30-mm soft tissue biodegradeable interference screw.
- The knee is positioned at 20 degrees of flexion during tensioning, and the screw is placed endoscopically with viewing from the inferomedial portal.
- Next the anterolateral bundle is passed (8-mm graft) and fixed with a 9-mm × 30-mm soft tissue interference screw.
- The knee is ranged through 20 cycles before the anterolateral bundle is fixed, with the knee positioned at 70 degrees of flexion.
- Lastly, the tibial side of the ACL allograft reconstruction is identified and ranged. The ACL graft is fixed with the knee in full extension.

Collateral Reconstruction

- At this point, the ACL and PCL reconstructions are complete, and the associated collateral reconstruction is performed.
- Although it is tempting to delay the collateral reconstruction, it is the senior author's opinion that the bicruciate reconstruction is at risk for failure or loosening by staging the collateral reconstruction.
- We try to limit the number of other procedures scheduled the day of a bicruciate reconstruction to minimize the pressure from those other cases that may tempt the surgeon to delay the collateral reconstruction (TECH FIG 1).

A
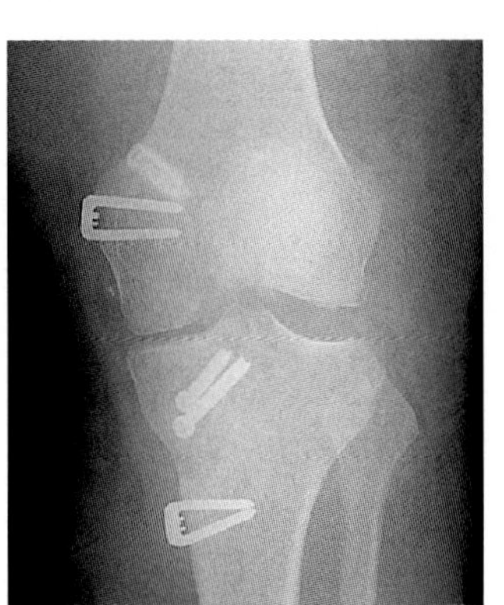

B
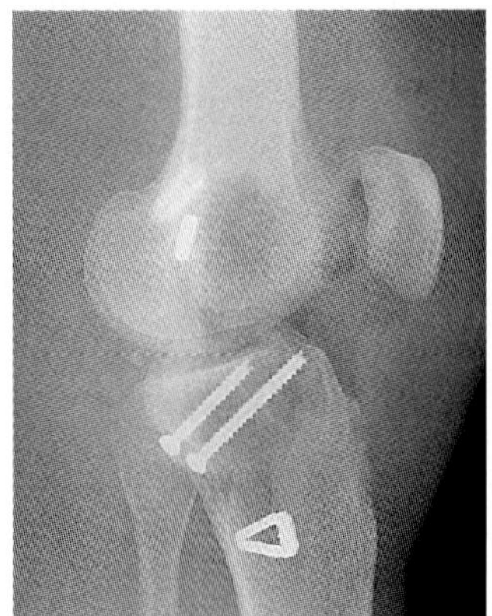

TECH FIG 1 • AP and lateral views of a left knee that has undergone a posterior cruciate ligament (PCL) revision reconstruction (notice retained titanium interference in the medial femoral condyle [MFC]) using tibial inlay technique for the tibial side of the graft and dual femoral tunnel reconstruction with soft tissue interference screws on the femoral side. Staples visible medially are from a simultaneous MCL reconstruction with anterior tibialis allograft.

SINGLE-LOOP POSTEROMEDIAL COMPLEX RECONSTRUCTION

- An incision is made from the medial femoral epicondyle to the posterior aspect of the insertion of the pes anserinus tendon on the tibia. The sartorius fascia is incised in line with the semitendinosus tendon from distal to proximal, and graft harvest is performed, leaving the tibial attachment in place.
- The proximal end of the semitendinosus is cleared of remaining muscle, and a Krackow suture is placed in its free end.
- A subretinacular tunnel is made from distal to proximal, and the graft is passed using this approach.
- Using a high-speed burr, a U-shaped trough is made around the isometric point of the medial epicondyle.
- The graft is laid into this trough and stapled into place.
- The graft is passed back through the fascial tunnel, and the knee is cycled through a ROM.
- The graft is then stapled to the tibia at the insertion of the MCL.
- After wound closure, the limb is placed in a sterile bulky dressing with medial and lateral plaster slabs for 7 to 10 days.
- We monitor these patients carefully and progress them slowly through ROM.

MODIFIED TWO-TAILED RECONSTRUCTION OF THE POSTEROLATERAL CORNER

- The key components of the deep posterolateral corner are the popliteus, the PFL, and the FCL. The modified two-tailed reconstruction[16] addresses each of these components.
- The patient is positioned supine on the operating table, with the injured extremity draped free. The leg is carefully positioned on the operative table, with the foot resting in the seated surgeon's lap.

- The knee is flexed to 90 degrees to relax the peroneal nerve, and a skin incision is made beginning at the lateral epicondyle of the femur toward the fibular head.
- The iliotibial band is incised in line with the fibers from Gerdy's tubercle, extending proximally to the supracondylar process of the femur.
- At this point, the peroneal nerve is identified as it courses from the biceps femoris through the perineural fat to the fibular neck.
  - In our experience, the nerve is identified most easily at the level of the joint line, where it can be palpated. However, depending on the specific injury and the presence of inflammation, the nerve may be identified along the fibular neck or even as it crosses the lateral gastrocnemius head.
  - It is critical to identify the nerve first before any ligamentous exploration or reconstruction is performed.
- Neurolysis is performed distally through the length of the incision. The nerve is protected with a small vessel loop.
- Once the nerve is exposed and protected, the FCL and the posterolateral structures are identified through blunt dissection. The surgeon should not dissect posterior to the lateral gastrocnemius muscle, because this places the popliteal neurovascular structures at risk.
- Once the exposure is complete, a 5-mm tunnel is drilled from anterior to posterior on the lateral tibia, exiting where the popliteus tendon traverses the back of the tibia.
- A retractor is placed posteriorly during the drilling to protect the neurovascular structures.
- The tibial tunnel is tapped with a 7-mm tap to allow fixation with a bioabsorbable interference screw.
- A tibialis tendon allograft is fashioned to approximately 5 mm and passed into the tunnel from posterior to anterior.
  - The allograft tendon must be at least 24 cm long to allow reconstruction of all three components.
- The graft is secured in the tibial tunnel with a 7-mm bioabsorbable interference screw from anterior to posterior.
- A second 5-mm tunnel is made in the fibular head from anterolateral to posteromedial, but is not tapped.
- The isometric point on the lateral femoral condyle is located by finding the intersection of the FCL and the popliteus tendon.
- Using a 3.2-mm drill bit, a hole is made in the lateral femoral condyle at the isometric point from lateral to medial to allow placement of a 4.5-mm bicortical screw.
  - If a concomitant ACL reconstruction is performed, this hole must be drilled from posterior to anterior to avoid interfering with the femoral tunnel of the ACL graft.
- An osteotome is used to decorticate the bone around the screw to allow healing of the allograft to bone. A spiked soft tissue washer is used with the screw.
- The graft is then passed from the posterior aspect of the tibia to the anterior portion of the screw and then posteriorly around to the fibular tunnel.
  - The popliteofibular portion of the graft should lie deep to the popliteus portion of the graft.
- The graft is then passed from posterior to anterior through the fibular tunnel and back to the screw and washer.
- The graft is tensioned with the foot internally rotated and the knee flexed 40 to 60 degrees.
- The screw and washer are then secured to the lateral femoral condyle and graft.
- This completes the reconstruction of all three posterolateral components described earlier. If there is an injury to the PLC, early repair should be considered.

MULTILIGAMENT RECONSTRUCTIONS

Knee Dislocation Type I: Anterior Cruciate and Collateral Ligaments Torn

- The integrity of the ACL determines the timing of reconstruction for a type I knee dislocation.
  - ACL reconstruction is best delayed until ROM is restored, for two reasons:
    - Collateral ligament healing usually occurs nonoperatively.
    - Postoperative stiffness often is avoided.
  - We prefer to regain complete ROM and delay reconstruction for this type of injury. Patients usually regain knee motion within 6 weeks of the injury.
- Graft choice is based on surgeon experience and patient preference and usually involves an ipsilateral bone–tendon–bone autograft.
- Collateral ligament injury associated with only one torn cruciate ligament usually can be treated nonoperatively.

Knee Dislocation Type II: Anterior and Posterior Cruciate Ligaments Torn

- The integrity of the collateral ligaments allows for early ROM and a delayed reconstruction of the cruciate ligaments.
- We prefer allografts for cruciate reconstructions performed simultaneously, but the decision is based on surgeon experience, patient preference, and risk tolerance.
- Our graft of choice for bicruciate injuries is BTB allograft for the ACL and an Achilles tendon allograft for the PCL (dual-bundle femoral with inlay tibial bone plug).
- The patient is positioned supine with the injured extremity draped free. A post is used to assist with arthroscopy.
- Diagnostic arthroscopy is performed through standard portals, and associated injuries are treated as required.
- The remnants of the cruciate ligaments are débrided, and a notchplasty is performed to allow for adequate visualization of ACL femoral tunnel placement and graft passage.
  - The detailed technique for ACL and PCL reconstructions is described earlier in this chapter.
- The ACL tibial and femoral tunnels are prepared first, and the guide pin advanced into the femoral tunnel to be used later for graft passage. The femoral tunnel may be drilled under dry visualization.
- The PCL femoral tunnel(s), either double-socket (preferred) or single, are prepared next under dry visualization. The guide pin is advanced into the femoral tunnel and the attached suture brought through the inferomedial portal for later graft passage.

- The ACL BTB allograft is passed from the tibial tunnel to the femoral tunnel and secured endoscopically to the femur with the knee hyperflexed. The tibial side of the graft is not fixed until after the PCL fixation is complete.
- Arthroscopic instrumentation is removed from the knee and the extremity positioned in the figure 4 position.
- The posteromedial approach is used to gain access to the tibial attachment of the PCL.
- The tibial trough is fashioned as previously described.
- A Kelly clamp or selected arthroscopic instrument is passed from the posterior capsulotomy through the notch medial to the ACL graft to grasp sutures entering the PCL femoral tunnels.
- The sutures are passed to the back of the knee through the capsulotomy.
- The tibial bone plug of the PCL graft is placed in the trough and secured to the tibia using two 4.0-mm cannulated screws. Care must be taken to avoid placement of screws in the ACL tibial tunnel.
- The PCL graft is tensioned through the femoral side, and the knee is put through its ROM 20 times.
- The PCL femoral side is fixed endoscopically sequentially with the knee positioned at 20 degrees (posteromedial bundle) of knee flexion and then at 70 degrees (anterolateral bundle).
- Fixing the PCL graft before final ACL tensioning avoids posterior subluxation of the tibia on the femur.
- The ACL graft is fixed to the tibial side with the knee in extension.
- Again, the ACL must be tensioned after the PCL fixation. Performing ACL tension and fixation before PCL reconstruction could create posterior subluxation of the tibia on the femur.

Knee Dislocation Type IIIM: Tears of the ACL, PCL, and MCL

- The steps for addressing a combined bicruciate injury with a collateral injury are similar to those described for the bicruciate reconstruction through double-bundle passage into the dual femoral sockets.
- During the posteromedial approach, the MCL is exposed as described earlier.
- After double-bundle passage into the dual femoral sockets, the MCL loop graft is tensioned and secured to the femur and the tibia.
- The tibial side of the ACL graft is then tensioned in extension and secured to the tibia.

Knee Dislocation Type IIIL: Torn Anterior and Posterior Cruciate Ligaments and Lateral Complex

- As for the Type IIIM reconstruction, the reconstruction of a Type IIIL injury proceeds through double-bundle passage into the dual femoral sockets.
- After the PCL is tensioned, the lateral approach to the knee is performed, and the FCL and posterolateral corner reconstructed using the technique described earlier.
- The ACL graft is then tensioned in extension and secured to the tibia.

Knee Dislocation Type IV: Torn ACL, PCL, MCL, and Lateral Complex

- This pattern most often is associated with a high-energy injury and represents a complex reconstruction.
- Careful attention to knee position during tensioning of the grafts is required to achieve a stable and concentric reconstruction in which the tibiofemoral joint is not subluxed.
- The initial reconstruction follows bicruciate ligament reconstruction through double-bundle passage into the dual femoral sockets, including exposure of the MCL.
- A lateral approach is used to expose the posterolateral corner, as described earlier.
- The MCL and PLC are prepared.
- The MCL graft is tensioned and fixed.
- The posterolateral graft is tensioned and fixed.
- The ACL graft is tensioned in extension and fixed to the tibia.

PEARLS AND PITFALLS

Neurovascular status	■ Carefully evaluate pulses and the neurologic examination. Use noninvasive studies to objectively document the findings of a normal vascular examination. Aggressively (emergently) evaluate asymmetry or ischemia on vascular examination with vascular consultation and intraoperative arteriography/exploration.
Planning	■ Determine the impact of ligamentous reconstructions on the patient as a whole. Delay reconstructions for multi-trauma, and consider external fixation for such patients to assist in transfers and mobilization. ■ Obtain preoperative ROM with normalized gait prior to reconstruction. This will maximize the final result. The PCL often will heal to a grade I or II, thereby making it possible to perform only an ACL/collateral reconstruction. ■ Use allografts over autografts, depending on patient preference and religious beliefs
Diagnosis	■ Clearly diagnose the ligaments involved. Examination under anesthesia combined with MRI can give an accurate picture of the needed reconstructions. Remember, MRI may overdiagnose ligamentous injuries, which will be found on EUA not to need reconstruction.
Surgery	■ Use reconstructions over repairs. If using repairs, delay postoperative ROM. ■ Perform bicruciate and collateral reconstructions at the same sitting (simultaneously), if possible.

Simultaneous bicruciate reconstruction	■ Drill the ACL femoral and tibial tunnels first. ■ Drill the dual socket PCL femoral tunnels second. ■ Pass the ACL graft and fix on the femoral side. ■ Perform a posteromedial approach for the tibial inlay. ■ Pass sutures from the PCL femoral tunnels through the posterior capsulotomy under dry arthroscopy. ■ Fix the tibial inlay. ■ Pass the posteromedial graft and fix at 20 degree of flexion after 20 cycles of motion under dry arthroscopy. ■ Pass the anterolateral graft and fix at 70 degrees of knee flexion after 20 cycles under dry arthroscopy. ■ Fix tibial side of ACL reconstruction/perform collateral reconstruction.

POSTOPERATIVE MANAGEMENT

- A thorough understanding of the reconstruction and tailoring the treatment plan to each individual patient are crucial to all rehabilitation protocols.
  - Patients who undergo early repair or reconstruction of multiligament knee injuries should begin supervised knee motion exercises within the first 3 days after surgery to decrease the risk of arthrofibrosis.
  - A hinged knee brace is used after bicruciate reconstructions, with non–weight bearing of the extremity recommended for 3 to 4 weeks.
  - Weight bearing is progressed to full, usually at 6 weeks, with a brace and crutches.
  - With medial or lateral procedures consideration is given for a slower return to full weight bearing owing to poor quadriceps tone and potential unfavorable mechanics.
- Early postoperative therapy focuses on control of edema and pain to facilitate return of quadriceps function.
  - Following PCL reconstruction, early return of full extension is paramount.
  - Supervised passive extension exercises are performed with a simultaneous, anteriorly directed force on the proximal tibia twice daily.[23]
  - The knee is kept in a postoperative brace from 0 to 90 degrees for the first 6 weeks.
  - Closed kinetic chain active exercises are allowed in this arc of motion.
  - The goal is to regain full ROM by 3 months.
  - If 90 degrees of flexion is not achieved by 6 to 12 weeks, manipulation under anesthesia (MUA) is strongly recommended.[2,15]
  - Straight-line jogging usually is begun at 5 to 6 months, depending on quadriceps function.
  - Patients may return to full activity in 9 to 12 months.

OUTCOMES

- The trend in recent years of increased surgical management of ligamentous injuries, coupled with earlier motion and a more aggressive approach to the management of stiffness (eg, MUA, arthroscopic lysis of adhesions), has yielded more favorable results than those previously reported regarding function, pain, and the incidence of debilitating instability.
- Studies using Lysholm scores for outcomes favor surgical treatment of these injuries over nonoperative treatment, with an average increase of 20 points reported with operative intervention.[12,18,20,23,25,31]
  - Generally speaking, 93% of patients are able to return to some type of occupation, but may not be able to work at a highly demanding job. In seven studies, approximately 70% of patients returned to their previous occupation.[12,14,17,19,20,25,27]
  - With surgical intervention, many patients ultimately have knees that function well for activities of daily living, and some are able to participate in recreational sports, but only 40% are able to return to their previous level of activity.[17,20,22]

COMPLICATIONS

- One of the most devastating problems encountered in multiligament knee injuries is failure to identify and appropriately manage vascular injuries in the acute phase.
- Another common problem is failure to recognize the full extent of the ligamentous injury, including capsular disruption at the time of surgical management.
- There also is potential for nerve injury, with peroneal nerve involvement more common than tibial nerve injury.
  - Complete nerve dysfunction carries a much worse prognosis than a partial injury, especially regarding the tibial nerve. Fewer than half of these patients have complete functional recovery of the nerve.[5,6,8]
- The necessity of creating multiple femoral and tibial tunnels brings with it the potential risk of tibial plateau fracture, medial femoral condyle avascular necrosis, and subchondral fracture.
  - The potential also exists for intraoperative neurovascular injury, especially with lateral side reconstructions (peroneal nerve) and PCL reconstructions (popliteal neurovascular bundle).
  - Postoperatively, the risks include infection (especially with open injuries), wound healing problems with multiple incisions, and arthrofibrosis (with or without heterotopic ossification).
  - On average, 38% of multiligament knee injuries require at least one surgical intervention to regain motion.[14,15,17,19,22,25,27,30]
  - There also is concern for posttraumatic arthritis (especially of the patellofemoral joint), potential loss of graft or repair fixation, and deep venous thrombosis with pulmonary embolus.

REFERENCES

1. Berg EE. Posterior cruciate ligament tibial inlay reconstruction. Arthroscopy 1995;11:69–76.
2. Chhabra A, Cha PS, Rihn JA, et al. Surgical management of knee dislocations: surgical technique. J Bone Joint Surg Am 2005;87A(Suppl 1):1–21.
3. Eastlack RK, Schenck RC, Guarducci C. The dislocated knee: classification, treatment, and outcome. US Army Med Dept J 1997;11:2–9.

4. Fanelli GC, Gianotti BF, Edson CJ. The posterior cruciate ligament arthroscopic evaluation and treatment. Arthroscopy 1994;10: 673–688.
5. Ferrari JD. Associated injuries. In: Schenck RCJ ed. Multiple ligamentous injuries of the knee in the athlete. AAOS Monograph 2002;22:31–41.
6. Goitz RJ, Tomaino MM. Management of peroneal nerve injuries associated with knee dislocations. Am J Orthop 2003;32:14–16.
7. Good L, Johnson RJ. The dislocated knee. J Am Acad Orthop Surg 1995;3:284–292.
8. Hegyes MS, Richardson MW, Miller MD. Knee dislocation: complications of nonoperative and operative management. Clin Sports Med 2000;19:519–543.
9. Hoover NW. Injuries of the popliteal artery associated with fractures and dislocations. Surg Clin North Am 1961;41:1099–1116.
10. Howard JM, DeBakey ME. The cost of delayed medical care. Mil Med 1956;118:343–357.
11. MacGillivray JD, Stein BE, Park M, et al. Arthroscopy 2006; 22:320–328.
12. Mariani PP, Santoriello P, Iannone S, et al. Comparison of surgical treatments for knee dislocations. Am J Knee Surg 1999;12:214–221.
13. Markolf KL, Zemanovic JR, McAllister DR. Cyclic loading of posterior cruciate ligament replacements fixed with tibial tunnel and tibial inlay methods. J Bone Joint Surg Am 2002;84A:518–524.
14. Martinek V, Steinbacher G, Friedrich NF, et al. Operative treatment of combined anterior and posterior cruciate ligament injuries in complex knee trauma. Am J Knee Surg 2000;13:74–82.
15. Montgomery T, Savioe F, White J, et al. Orthopedic management of knee dislocations: comparison of surgical reconstruction and immobilization. Am J Knee Surg 1999;8:97–103.
16. Noyes FR, Barber-Westin SD. Surgical reconstruction of severe posterolateral complex injuries of the knee using allograft tissues. Am J Sports Med 1993;23:2–12.
17. Noyes FR, Barber-Westin SD. Reconstruction of the anterior and posterior cruciate ligaments after knee dislocation: use of early protected post-operative motion to decrease arthrofibrosis. Am J Sports Med 1997;25:769–778.
18. Richter M, Bosch U, Wippermann B, et al. Comparison of surgical repair of the cruciate ligament versus nonsurgical treatment in patients with traumatic knee dislocations. Am J Sports Med 2002;30: 718–727.
19. Schenck RC. Knee dislocations. Instr Course Lect 1994;43:27–136.
20. Shapiro MS, Freedman EL. Allograft reconstruction of the anterior and posterior cruciate ligaments after traumatic knee dislocation. Am J Sports Med 1995;23:580–587.
21. Shelbourne KD, Carr DR. Instr Course Lect 2003;52:413–418.
22. Sisto DJ, Warren RF. Complete knee dislocation: a follow-up study of operative treatment. Clin Orthop Rel Res 1985;198:94–101.
23. Stannard JP, Riley RS, Sheils TM, et al. Anatomic reconstruction of the posterior cruciate ligament after multiligament knee injuries: a combination of the tibial-inlay and two-femoral-tunnel techniques. Am J Sports Med 2003;31:196–202.
24. Stannard JP, Shiels TM, Lopez-Benn RR, et al. Vascular injuries in knee dislocations: the role of physical examination in determining the need for arteriography. J Bone Joint Surg Am 2004;86A: 910–915.
25. Stannard JP, Wilson TC, Shiels TM, et al. Heterotopic ossification associated with knee dislocation. Arthroscopy 1995;18:835–839.
26. Taylor AR, Arden GP, Rainey HA. Traumatic dislocations of the knee: a report of forty-three cases with special reference to conservative treatment. J Bone Joint Surg Br 1972;54B:96–102.
27. Walker DN, Hardison R, Schenck RC. A baker's dozen of knee dislocations. Am J Sports Med 1994;7:117–124.
28. Wand JS. A physical sign denoting irreducibility of a dislocated knee. J Bone Joint Surg Br 1989;71B:862.
29. Wascher DC. Bicruciate injuries. In: Schenck RCJ ed. Multiple ligamentous injuries of the knee in the athlete. AAOS Monograph 2002;22:91–99.
30. Wascher DC, Dvirnak PC, DeCoster TA. Knee dislocation: initial assessment and implications for treatment. J Orthop Trauma 1997;11: 525–529.
31. Yeh WL, Tu YK, Su JY, et al. Knee dislocation: treatment of high-velocity knee dislocation. J Trauma 1999;46:693–701.

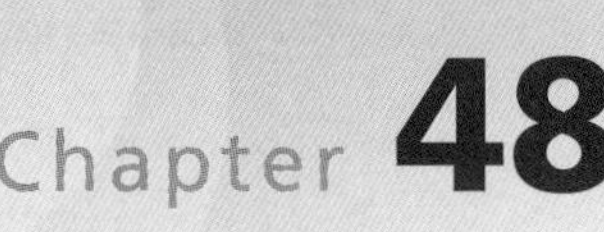

Chapter 48 Repair of Acute and Chronic Patella Tendon Tears

Thomas M. DeBerardino and Brett D. Owens

DEFINITION

- Complete tears of the patella tendon are best classified into acute versus chronic.
- Partial tears often can be managed nonoperatively. The functional integrity of the extensor mechanism is the key to determining the need for surgical repair.
- This chapter focuses on the surgical treatment of complete tendon disruption.

ANATOMY

- The patella tendon is approximately 30 mm wide × 50 mm long, with a thickness of 5 to 7 mm.[1]
- The origin on the inferior pole of the patella is juxtaposed to the articular cartilage on the deep side and becomes confluent with the periosteum of the patella anteriorly.[2]
- The tibial insertion is narrower and invests the entirety of the tibial tubercle.
- The overlying peritenon is thought to be the cellular source for healing of tendon injuries.

PATHOGENESIS

- Tendon rupture usually is the result of underlying tendinosis.[6]
- There is some evidence of genetic predisposition to tendon rupture.
- Certain conditions predispose individuals to tendon rupture, including renal dialysis, chronic corticosteroid use, fluoroquinolone antibiotics, and corticosteroid use.

NATURAL HISTORY

- The natural history of an untreated patella tendon is complete extensor mechanism dysfunction.
- Untreated acute ruptures result in chronic lesions that are more difficult to manage surgically. These often require reconstructive procedures and have inferior functional results.

PATIENT HISTORY AND PHYSICAL FINDINGS

- Patients with acute tendon tears may report an audible "pop" or the sensation of their knee giving way.
- Patients with chronic injuries may report ambulatory difficulty and pain. These injuries often are treated with bracing before definitive evaluation.
- The loss of active knee extension is the key physical examination finding when evaluating for patella tendon rupture.
- Loss of tension in the patella tendon with the knee at 90 degrees of flexion and patella alta are indirect signs of rupture.

IMAGING AND OTHER DIAGNOSTIC STUDIES

- Plain radiographs may reveal patella alta, avulsion fractures, Osgood-Schlatter lesions, or other concomitant knee injuries.
- MRI scans may be helpful in determining the exact location of the rupture and evaluating concomitant intraarticular knee lesions.

DIFFERENTIAL DIAGNOSIS

- Quadriceps tendon rupture
- Patella fracture
- Tibial tubercle avulsion fracture

NONOPERATIVE MANAGEMENT

- Nonoperative management should be considered only for patients who are not surgical candidates because of medical comorbidities.

SURGICAL MANAGEMENT

- Although not considered to be a surgical emergency, prompt surgical management of acute patella tendon ruptures is recommended.

Preoperative Planning

- Repairs of chronic injuries often require allograft tissue availability and careful surgical planning.
- Significant patella alta may require proximal release in conjunction with the repair.

Positioning

- Supine postioning is recommended.
- Use of a tourniquet may preclude proper repair tensioning in chronic injuries.
- Prepping and draping of both lower extremities allows use of contralateral limb as a template for patella positioning.

Approach

- An anterior approach is used, regardless of the repair technique.
- A midline longitudinal incision is made over the patella tendon.
- The peritenon is incised longitudinally and dissected away from the underlying tendon.

ACUTE REPAIR

Midsubstance

- Grossly pathologic tendon tissue is aggressively débrided.
- The full length of the patella tendon is exposed.
- Two Krackow locking stitches are placed in each tendon stump with no. 2 or no. 5 Fiberwire (Arthrex, Inc., Naples FL; TECH FIG 1).
- Any required retinacular repair stitches are placed with absorbable suture before the tendon repair.
- The four proximal core sutures are tied to the four distal core sutures with the knee in full extension.
- Integrity of the repair is evaluated by checking the maximal flexion possible prior to gap formation.
- The peritenon is closed with absorbable suture.

Proximal Avulsion

- Grossly pathologic tendon or bone is removed.
- Exposure of the inferior pole of the patella is performed.
- If the transosseous drill hole technique is preferred, superficial exposure of the superior pole of the patella is required.
  - A smaller exposure is required for suture anchor technique.
- Three suture anchors are placed in the inferior pole of the patella, equally spaced along the anatomic tendon footprint.
  - We prefer the 5.0 Bio-Corkscrew FT Suture Anchor (Arthrex, Inc., Naples, FL) loaded with no. 2 Fiberwire (Arthrex, Inc., Naples, FL).
- The suture is pulled through the anchor eyelet to produce long and short suture arms.
  - The long suture arm is passed down and back up the tendon stump in a locking Krackow fashion (TECH FIG 2).
- The tendon is manually reduced to the inferior pole of the patella, and the slack is taken out by the short arm of suture pulled through the eyelet.
- Each suture pair is tied securely to complete the repair.
- Repair integrity is evaluated by checking the maximal flexion possible before gap formation.
- The peritenon is closed with absorbable suture.

Distal Avulsion

- Grossly pathologic tendon or bone is removed.
- The tibial tubercle is exposed.
- Two suture anchors are placed in the tibial tubercle.
  - We prefer the 5.0 Biocorkscrew FT Anchor loaded with no. 2 Fiberwire (Arthrex, Inc., Naples, FL).
- The suture is pulled through the anchor eyelet to produce long and short suture arms. The long suture arm is passed up and back down the tendon stump in a locking Krackow fashion (TECH FIG 3).
- The tendon is manually reduced to the tibial tubercle, and the slack is taken out by the short arm of suture pulled through the eyelet.
- Each suture pair is tied securely to complete the repair.
- Repair integrity is evaluated by checking maximal flexion possible before gap formation.
- The peritenon is closed with absorbable suture.

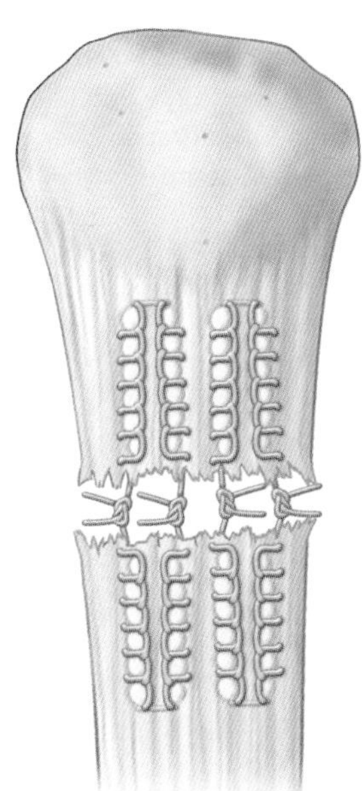

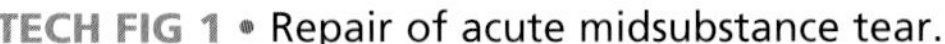

TECH FIG 1 • Repair of acute midsubstance tear.

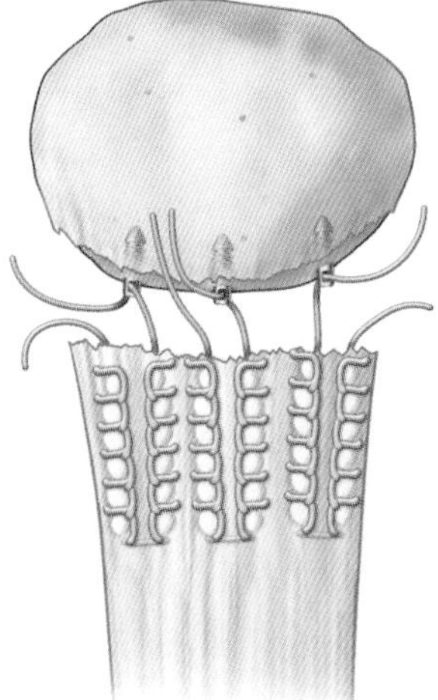

TECH FIG 2 • Repair of acute proximal avulsion.

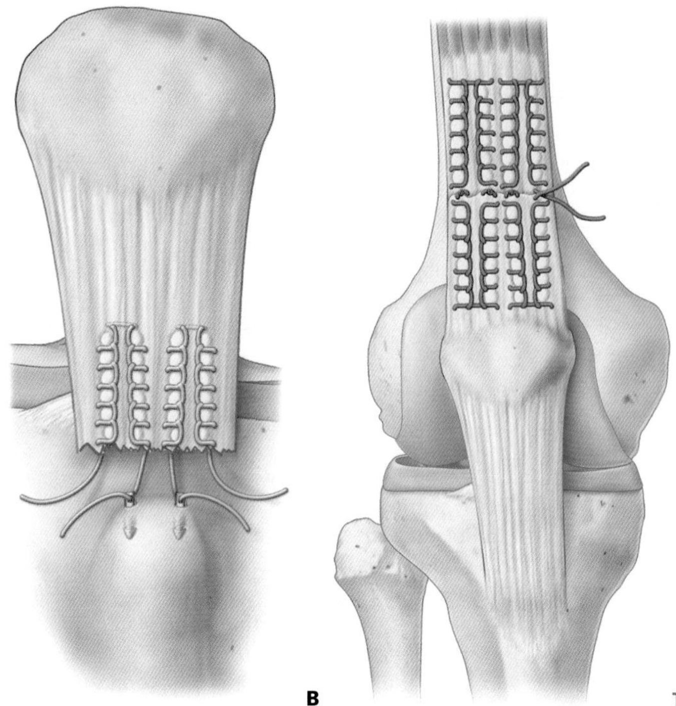

TECH FIG 3 • Repair of acute distal avulsion.

RECONSTRUCTION OF CHRONIC TEARS

- Reconstruction of a chronic tear begins with aggressive débridement of dysplastic tissue.
- Remaining tendon tissue is assessed for possible repair.
- The tibial tubercle is exposed.
- The Achilles allograft is prepared with 15-mm × 25-mm bone block.
- A rectangular box is cut out of the tubercle with an oscillating microsurgical saw and osteotomes to receive the bone block.
- The block is secured to the tubercle with 2-mm × 3.5-mm cortical screws (TECH FIG 4A).
- Suture anchors are placed into the distal pole of the patella and onto the anterior cortex of the patella to secure allograft tendon to the patella (TECH FIG 4B).
- The allograft tendon is draped over the quadriceps tendon and muscle fascia and secured with nonabsorbable suture.

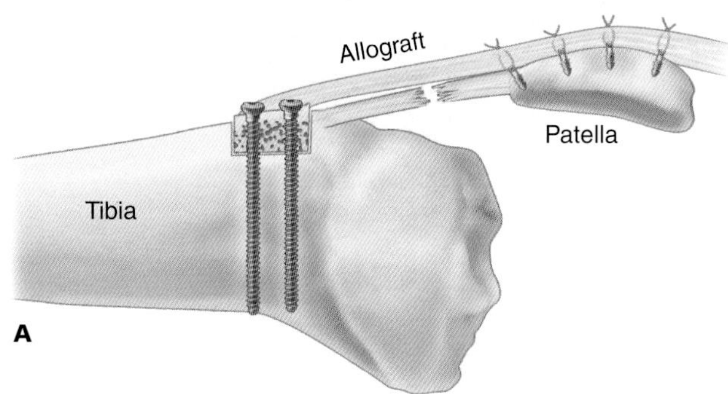

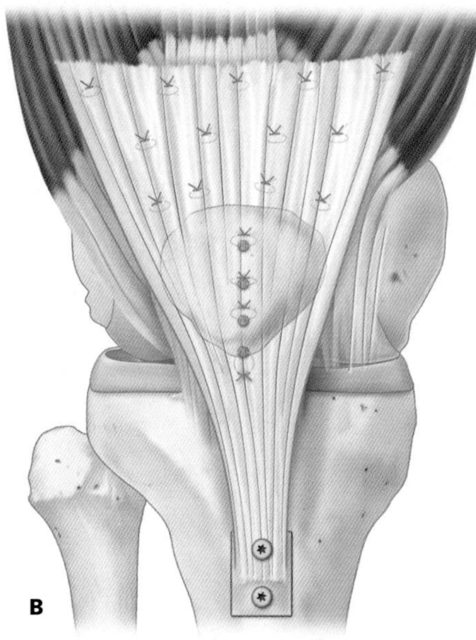

TECH FIG 4 • Chronic reconstruction with Achilles tendon allograft. The bone block is inlayed into the tibial tubercle and fixed with screws or staples. The soft tissue end of the graft is sutured into the patella with suture anchors and into the quadriceps with heavy nonabsorbable sutures. **A.** Lateral view. **B.** AP view.

AUGMENTATION PROCEDURES

- After the repair has been completed, it is assessed for any need for augmentation.
- The following materials can be used for augmentation. They are placed in a box-stitch fashion through drill holes in the patella and tubercle (**TECH FIG 5A**):
  - Mersilene tape
  - No. 5 Fiberwire
  - No. 5 Ethibond
  - Steel wire
  - Cerclage cables
  - Tibialis tendon allograft
- A semitendinosus autograft also may be harvested proximally (while leaving its distal insertion intact) and passed through a drill hole in the patella and either through a drill hole in the tubercle or potted into the proximal tibia if the length is insufficient (**TECH FIG 5B**).

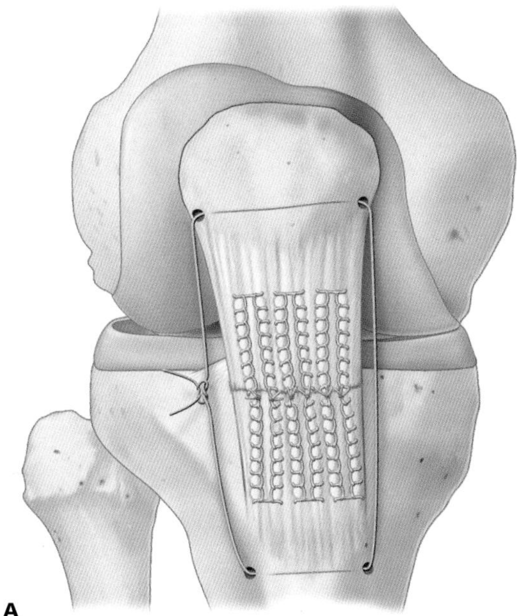

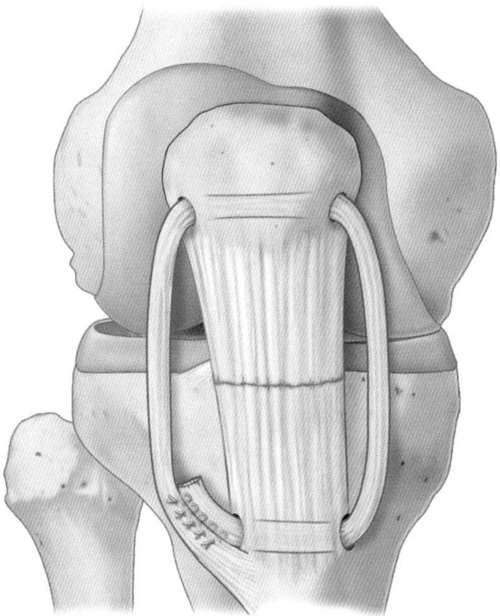

TECH FIG 5 • Augmentation of the repair can be with a box-stitched suture (**A**) or a soft tissue graft (**B**).

PEARLS AND PITFALLS

Preoperative planning	■ Failure to recognize significant patella alta may lead to abnormal knee kinematics and weakness of extension.
Surgical technique	■ Reattachment of the patella tendon into its anatomic footprint on the patella is essential for re-establishing normal patellofemoral kinematics.
Intraoperative assessment	■ Maximum allowed knee flexion angle without repair gap formation is determined immediately after repair.

POSTOPERATIVE CARE

- Weight bearing is allowed with the knee braced in extension.
- Early flexion allowances are determined intraoperatively by the quality of the tendon tissue and repair.
- Active-assisted range of motion is advanced as tolerated with the goal of 90 degrees of flexion by 4 to 6 weeks and full motion by 10 to 12 weeks after repair.
- Strengthening is initiated immediately with isometric quadriceps contractions and progressed to straight-leg raises at 6 weeks.
- Return to unrestricted activities is delayed until 6 months.

OUTCOMES

- Marder and Timmerman[9] reported excellent results in 12 of 14 patients treated with acute repair without augmentation.
- Larson and Simonian[7] reported excellent results (mean Lysholm score, 97.5) in four cases of acute repair augmented with autologous semitendinosus graft placed in a looped fashion.
- Lindy et al[8] reported excellent results in 24 patients repaired acutely and augmented with Mersilene tape placed in a looped configuration.
- Fujikawa[5] reported good results with a patella tendon repair augmented with a synthetic figure-8 weave performed on six

patella tendon ruptures. They noted that the augmentation device allowed for early mobilization and good functional outcome.

- Two recent biomechanical studies show that an augmented repair is stronger than an unaugmented repair[11] and that suture anchor repair is at least as strong as repair through drill holes.[3]
- Two cases of successful treatment of chronic patella tendon ruptures with Achilles allograft reconstruction have been reported.[4,10]

COMPLICATIONS

- Rerupture is the most worrisome complication.
- Infection is uncommon but devastating.
- Residual quadriceps weakness and extensor lag are more common with repairs of chronic injuries.

REFERENCES

1. Andrikoula S, Tokis A, Vasiliadis HS, et al. The extensor mechanism of the knee joint: an anatomical study. Knee Surg Sports Traumatol Arthrosc 2006;14:214–220.
2. Basso O, Johnson DP, Amis AA. The anatomy of the patellar tendon. Knee Surg Sports Traumatol Arthrosc 2001;9:2–5.
3. Bushnell BD, Byram IR, Weinhold PS, et al. The use of suture anchors in repair of the ruptured patellar tendon. Am J Sports Med 2006;34:1492–1499.
4. Falconiero RP, Pallis MP. Chronic rupture of a patellar tendon: a technique for reconstruction with Achilles allograft. Arthroscopy 1996;12:623–626.
5. Fujikawa K, Ohtani T, Matsumoto H, et al. Reconstruction of the extensor apparatus of the knee with the Leeds-Keio ligament. J Bone Joint Surg Br 1994;76B:200–203.
6. Kannus P, Jozsa L. Histopathological changes preceding spontaneous rupture of a tendon. A controlled study of 891 patients. J Bone Joint Surg Am 1991;73A:1507–1525.
7. Larson RV, Simonian PT. Semitendinosus augmentation of acute patellar tendon repair with immediate mobilization. Am J Sports Med 1995;23:82–86.
8. Lindy PB, Boynton MD, Fadale PD. Repair of patellar tendon disruptions without hardware. J Orthop Trauma 1995;9:238–243.
9. Marder RA, Timmerman LA. Primary repair of patellar tendon rupture without augmentation. Am J Sports Med 1999;27:304–307.
10. McNally PD, Marcelli EA. Achilles allograft reconstruction of a chronic patellar tendon rupture. Arthroscopy 1998;14:340–344.
11. Ravalin RV, Mazzocca AD, Grady-Benson JC, et al. Biomechanical comparison of patellar tendon repairs in a cadaver model. Am J Sports Med 2002;30:469–473.

Chapter 49

Repair of Acute and Chronic Quadriceps Tendon Ruptures

Krishna Mallik

DEFINITION

- Quadriceps tendon ruptures result in disruption of the fibers of this tendon, thereby disrupting the extensor mechanism of the knee.
- Injury is prevalent in patients more than 40 years old and is more common in men.
- Ruptures usually occur transversely through the tendon at a pathologic area approximately 2 cm proximal to the superior pole of the patella, and then progress obliquely into the medial and lateral retinacula based on the amount and duration of force.
- Ruptures can occur at the bone–tendon interface (older patients), or at the midtendinous or musculotendinous area (younger patients).[9]
- Unilateral ruptures are more common; bilateral ruptures may occur because of a predisposition from an underlying systemic condition.
- Acute repair of the tendon provides a higher rate of return of function.

ANATOMY

- The quadriceps tendon consists of the coalescence of the rectus femoris, vastus medialis, vastus lateralis, and vastus intermedius, about 3 to 5 cm proximal to the patella, and inserts into the superior pole of the patella.
- The quadriceps tendon averages 8 mm in thickness and 35 mm in width.[11]
- Normal quadriceps tendon layers include three layers:
  - Superficial layer, which originates from the posterior fascia of the rectus femoris
  - Deep layer, which originates from the anterior fascia of the vastus intermedius
  - Middle layer, which originates from the deep fascia separating the vastus medialis and lateralis from the vastus intermedius.[11]
- The tendon recieves its blood supply from multiple contributions: branches of the lateral cicumflex femoral artery, the descending geniculate artery, and the medial and lateral superior geniculate arteries.[8]
- The distribution of the blood supply in the tendon is asymmetric[8]:
  - The superficial tendon vascular supply is complete from the musculotendinous junction to the patella.
  - The deep portion of the tendon has an oval avascular area.

PATHOGENESIS

- Quadriceps tendon rupture typically occurs through a site of pathologic degeneration in the tendon caused by repetitive microtrauma.[4,5]
- Rupture is the result of eccentric contraction of the extensor mechanism against a sudden load of body weight with the foot planted and the knee flexed.[7]
- Rupture can be due to trauma, use of corticosteroids, and systemic diseases (eg, gout, pseudogout, systemic lupus erythematosus, renal failure, hyperparathyroidism, diabetes mellitus).[2]
- Fluoroquinolone antibiotics (eg, ciprofloxacin) also have contributed to tendon weakness.
- Bilateral ruptures typically are the result of systemic medical conditions.

NATURAL HISTORY

- Unrepaired quadriceps tendon rupture can lead to chronic extensor lag and weakness.
- Long-term rupture may lead to quadriceps fibrosis as well as patella baja.

PATIENT HISTORY AND PHYSICAL FINDINGS

- Immediate pain, occasional swelling, subcutaneous hematoma
- Occasionally hears or feels a "pop"
- Inability to bear weight
- Pre-existing pain and symptoms related to quadriceps tendon (tendinitis) prior to injury
- Effusion can be indicative of hemarthrosis.
- Loss of extension (straight leg raise) indicates lack of continuity of the extensor mechanism (*note:* ability to extend may be due to intact retinacula).
- Suprapatella gap (ie, soft tissue defect proximal to the superior pole of the patella) is indicated by loss of continuity of the extensor mechanism at the quadriceps tendon attachment.
- Patella baja (ie, patella of the injured knee more inferior than the contralateral knee) is indicated by loss of proximal extensor mechanism.

IMAGING AND OTHER DIAGNOSTIC STUDIES

- Plain radiographs (especially lateral view) may demonstrate bony avulsion fractures at the superior patella or soft tissue calcific depositions in chronic tendinosis.
  - Tooth sign[6]: on Merchant's view, vertical ridging of osteophytes at the quadriceps tendon attachment site
- Ultrasound, while operator dependent and not as specific, may demonstrate a discrete break in the tendon with abnormal overlying soft tissue.
- Arthrography is invasive; however, it is positive with extravasation of contrast dye from the suprapatellar pouch and along the tendon sheath of the tendon.[1]
- MRI remains the gold standard in diagnosing partial and complete quadriceps tendon ruptures, in addition to associated soft tissue injuries.
  - Notable findings include focal tendon discontinuity, increased signal in the tendon, wavy patella tendon, as well as possible pre-existing pathology.

DIFFERENTIAL DIAGNOSIS

- Patella tendon rupture
- Quadriceps tendon rupture
- Patella femoral contusion
- Cartilage contusion
- Neural injury

NONOPERATIVE MANAGEMENT

- Patients with partial quadriceps tear may be treated nonoperatively.
- For the first 6 weeks, the knee is immobilized in extension to assist with tendon healing and maintenance of tendon length.
  - This can be done with a long-leg brace locked in extension or with a long-leg cylinder cast.
  - Patients should be non–weight bearing with crutches.
  - In the first 6 weeks, the patient may begin isometric straight leg raises.
- In the next phase, regaining flexion is emphasized and the brace is unlocked to allow restoration of normal gait.
  - The patient is advanced to full weight bearing.
- In the last phase, strengthening is emphasized.
- Patients can return to activity once full range of motion and strength are restored, usually in 4 months.

SURGICAL MANAGEMENT

- All complete tendon ruptures should be repaired acutely to restore extensor function.
- Any partial rupture that has progressed to a complete rupture should also be repaired as soon as diagnosed.

PREOPERATIVE PLANNING

- Review all imaging studies.
- Confirm any associated injuries that will require surgical attention.

POSITIONING

- The patient should be placed supine on the operating table with all bony prominences padded.
- A bump under the ipsilateral hip can prevent external rotation of the operative leg.
- If an examination under anesthesia is necessary, care must be taken not to convert a partial tear to a complete rupture.

Approach

- A midline patella incision, centering over the bone–tendon interface, provides access to the tendon repair as well as evaluation and repair of the medial and lateral retinaculae (**FIG 1**).

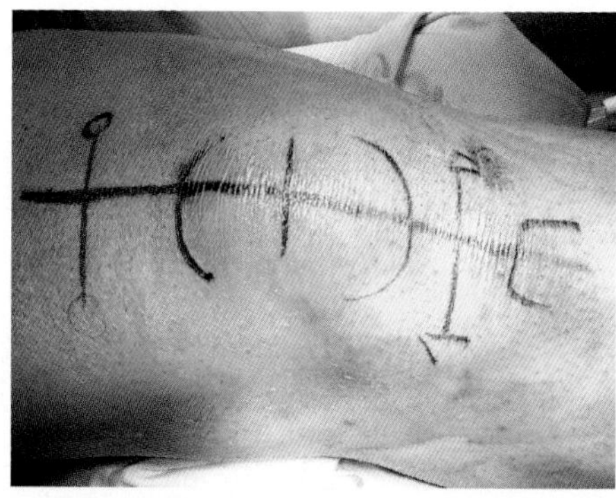

FIG 1 • Planning for a midline longitudinal incision of the knee.

ACUTE TENDON REPAIR AT THE TENDON–BONE INTERFACE

Tendon Preparation

- A straight 10-cm midline incision is made, centered over the bone–tendon interface.
- The superficial layers are retracted to examine the deep tissue layers (**TECH FIG 1A**).
- Hematoma is irrigated.
- The medial and lateral retinaculae are evaluated (**TECH FIG 1B**).
- The tendon edge of necrotic and degenerative tissue is débrided to normal-appearing healthy tendon tissue (**TECH FIG 1C,D**).
- Ability to reapproximate tendon ends without undue tension (**TECH FIG 1E,F**) is confirmed.

Suturing

- Using no. 2 or no. 5 nonabsorbable suture, beginning near the lateral free edge of the tendon, a continuous running-type stitch (eg, Krackow stitch, Mason-Allen stitch) is placed, exiting back at the free end of the tendon (**TECH FIG 2A**).
- This is repeated for the medial aspect of the tendon.
- When completed, there should be four equal strands of sutures exiting the free tendon edge (**TECH FIG 2B,C**).
- A trough is made at the superior pole of the patella to assist with tendon reattachment. The trough should not be placed too anteriorly, to avoid patellar tilt.
- Three longitudinal drill holes, 1 to 1.5 cm apart, are placed, exiting out of the inferior pole of the patella.
- Using a suture passer, beginning at the inferior pole of the patella, each of the four strands of suture is brought longitudinally through the patella (**TECH FIG 2D,E**).
- Holding the sutures provisionally, knee flexion is evaluated with patellar tracking and rotation.
- The tendon is reduced to the superior pole of the patella, and the sutures are tied with the knee in full extension (**TECH FIG 2F**).
- Knots are buried behind the patellar tendon at the inferior pole.
- To complete the repair, no. 0 nonabsorbable sutures are used in interrupted fashion to repair the medial and lateral retinacula (**TECH FIG 2G**).
- Patellar positioning, tracking, and tensioning of the repaired tendon are evaluated.
- The position of knee flexion at which tension begins on the repair should be noted, because this will determine the amount of maximum knee flexion allowed in postoperative rehabilitation.

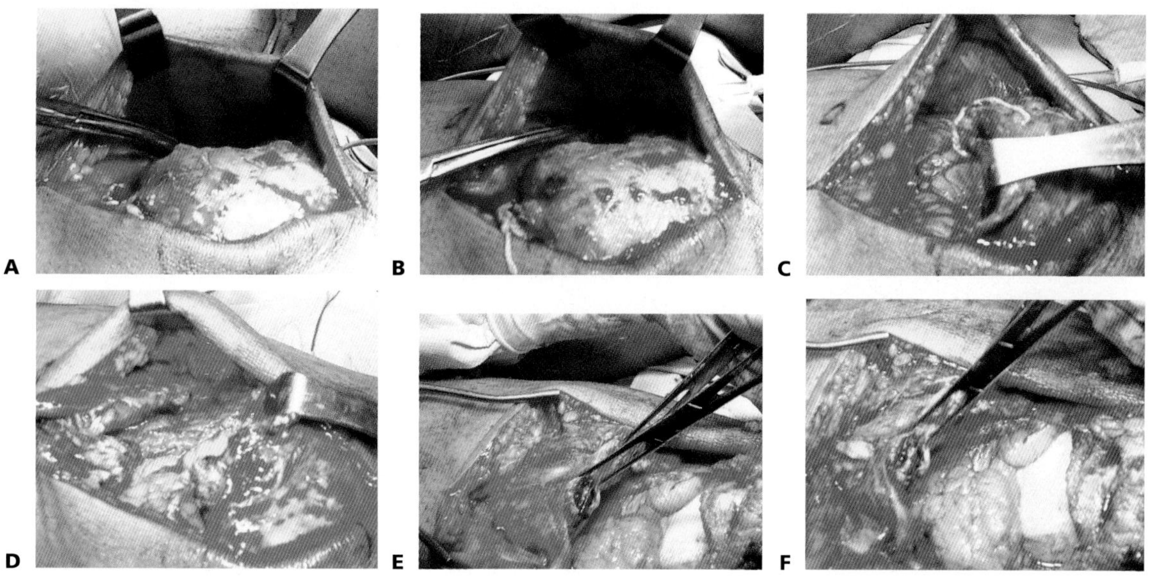

TECH FIG 1 • Evaluating the deep tissue layers (**A**) and the medial and lateral retinacula (**B**). **C.** Patella retracted inferiorly, demonstrating tear. **D.** Alice clamps on quadriceps tendon demonstrating mobility of soft tissue. **E.** Reapproximating the quadriceps tendon to the patella. **F.** Confirmation that there is no excess tension on reapproximation for tendon repair.

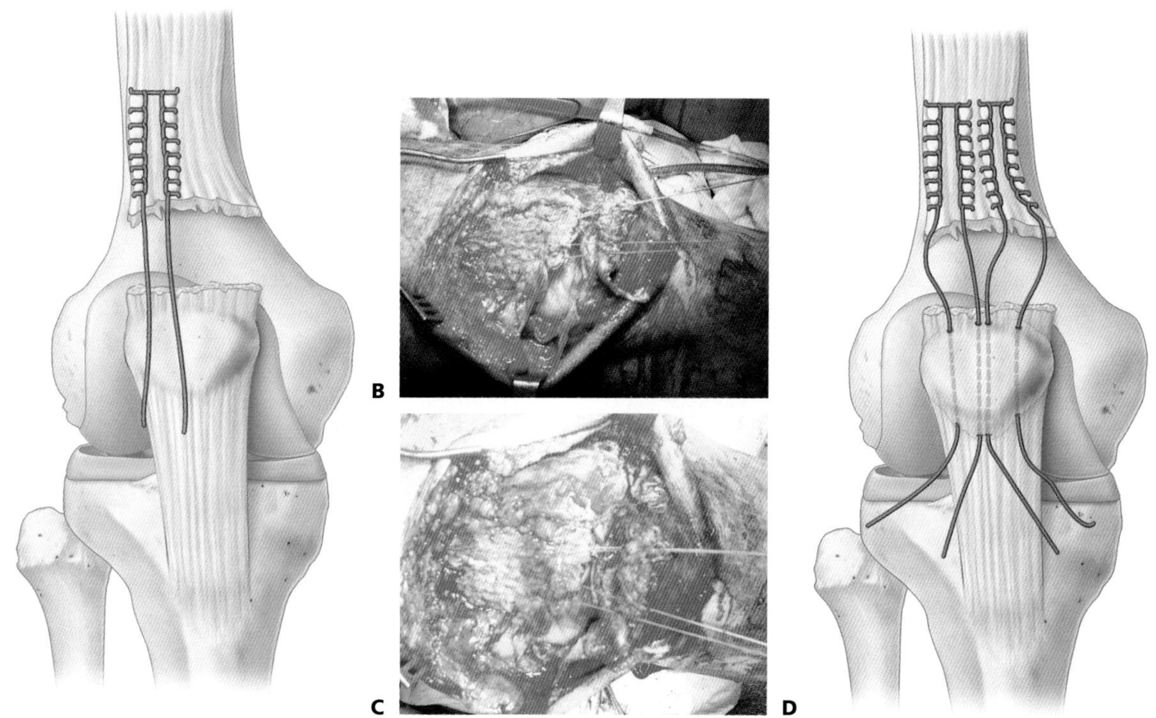

TECH FIG 2 • **A.** Placement of a continuous running stitch, beginning laterally and exiting back at the free edge of the tendon. **B.** Four sutures exiting the free edge of the quadriceps tendon. **C.** Close-up of the four exiting sutures. **D.** Four sutures from the free edge of the quadriceps tendon brought inferiorly through three longitudinal drill holes in the patella. *(continued)*

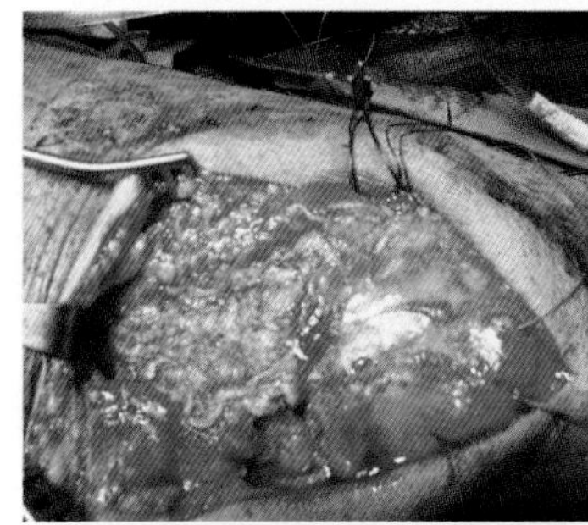

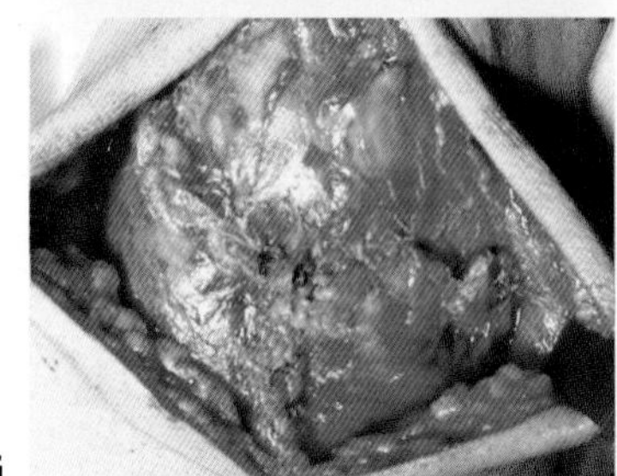

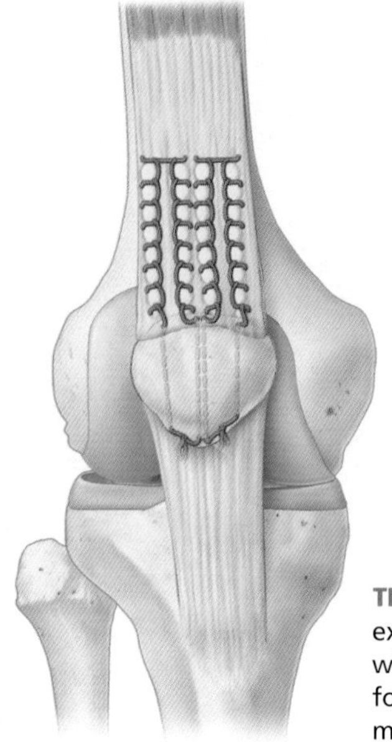

TECH FIG 2 • *(continued)* **E.** The center two sutures exit through a central drill hole. **F.** Sutures are secured with their continuous loop mate—first the lateral set, followed by the medial set. **G.** Repair of lateral and medial retinacula.

ACUTE TENDON REPAIR AT MUSCULOTENDINOUS AND MIDTENDINOUS AREAS

- A straight 10-cm midline incision is made centered over the bone–tendon interface.
- Hematoma is irrigated.
- The tendon edge of necrotic and degenerative tissue is débrided down to normal-appearing healthy tendon tissue.
- Ability to reapproximate tendon ends without undue tension (see Tech Fig 1E,F) is confirmed.
- No. 2 or no. 5 nonabsorbable sutures are used for a continuous running stitch to reapproximate both proximal and distal free lateral edges of the tendon (TECH FIG 3A).
  - Procedure is repeated for the proximal and distal medial edges of the tendon.
- Tendon edges are reapproximated by provisionally tensioning sutures together and evaluating knee flexion with patellar tracking and rotation.
- The sutures are tied together with the knee in full extension, making sure not to overtension or overlap the reattachment (TECH FIG 3B).
- No. 0 nonabsorbable suture is used, if necessary, to reinforce repair with interrupted figure 8 stitches.
- To complete the repair, no. 0 nonabsorbable suture is used in interrupted fashion to repair the medial and lateral retinacula.
- Patellar positioning, tracking, and tensioning of the repaired tendon are evaluated.
- The position of knee flexion at which tension on the repair begins should be noted, because this will determine the amount of maximum knee flexion allowed in postoperative rehabilitation.

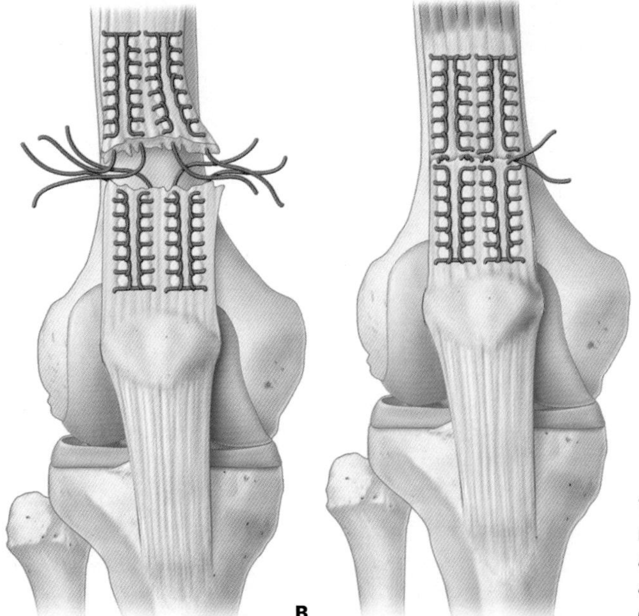

TECH FIG 3 • **A.** Placement of two sets of continuous running stitches laterally and medially in both the proximal and distal stumps. **B.** Alignment of four exiting proximal and distal sutures that makes it possible to secure them to each other as tension is applied on the untied suture sets.

CHRONIC TENDON REPAIR

- Chronic ruptures have scar tissue present in addition to shortening.
- A longitudinal midline incision is used.
- The tendon is mobilized by releasing adhesions to the surrounding soft tissues, skin, and underlying femur.
- The tendon edges are débrided down to healthy tissue, and scar tissue is removed from the tendon gap.
- If the tendon can be reapproximated, it is repaired similarly to an acute repair.
- If the tendon cannot be apposed without undue tension, a reinforcement (Scuderi technique) or lengthening (Codivilla technique) procedure is indicated.

Scuderi Technique

- The tendon edges are débrided to healthy tissue, and scar tissue is removed from the tendon gap (TECH FIG 4A).
- The quadriceps edges are reapproximated and repaired together with interrupted no. 0 nonabsorbable sutures (TECH FIG 4B).
- An inverted V is incised through the full thickness of the proximal quadriceps tendon, with the base of the V ending approximately 1 cm proximal to the rupture (TECH FIG 4C).
- The apex of the V is folded distally and sutured in place (TECH FIG 4D).
- This technique also can be used for acute repairs.[10]

Codivilla Technique

- The tendon edges are débrided to healthy tissue, and scar tissue is removed from the tendon gap (TECH FIG 5A).
- The quadriceps edges are apposed and repaired together with interrupted no. 0 nonabsorbable sutures (TECH FIG 5B).
- An inverted V is incised through the full thickness of the proximal quadriceps tendon, with the base of the V ending approximately 1 cm proximal to the rupture (TECH FIG 5C).
- The apex of the V is folded distally and sutured in place (TECH FIG 5D).
- The proximal length of the V is closed longitudinally with interrupted no. 0 nonabsorbable sutures.
- If further augmentation is required, autograft or allograft of fascia lata, semitendinosus and gracilis tendons, or Mersilene tape can be used.

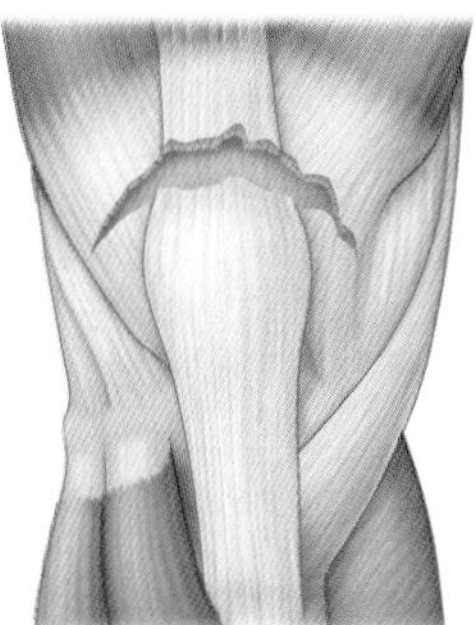
A
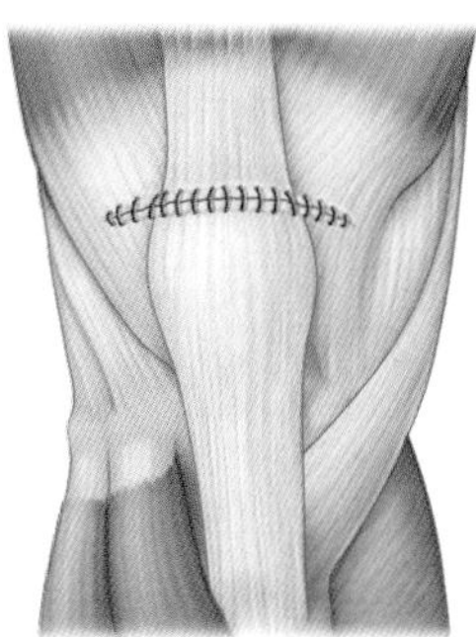
B
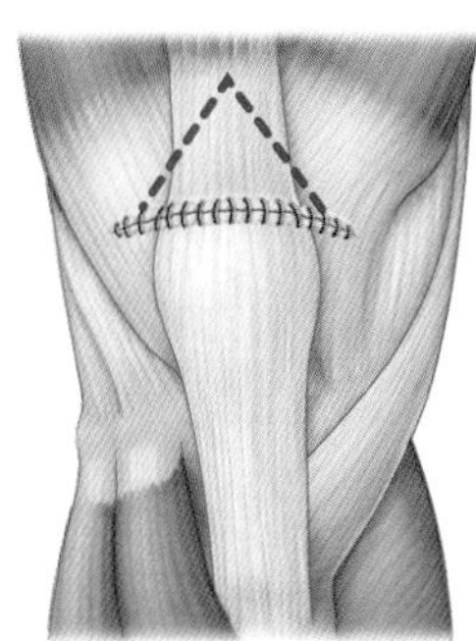
C
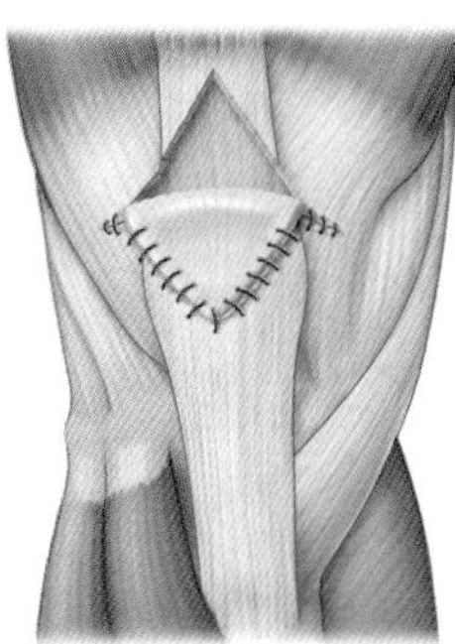
D

TECH FIG 4 • **A.** Proximal tendon edge following débridement of scar tissue. **B.** Apposition and repair of quadriceps tendon to distal quadriceps stump. **C.** Incision of inverted V through full thickness of proximal quadriceps tendon. **D.** Apex of V folded distally and secure in place.

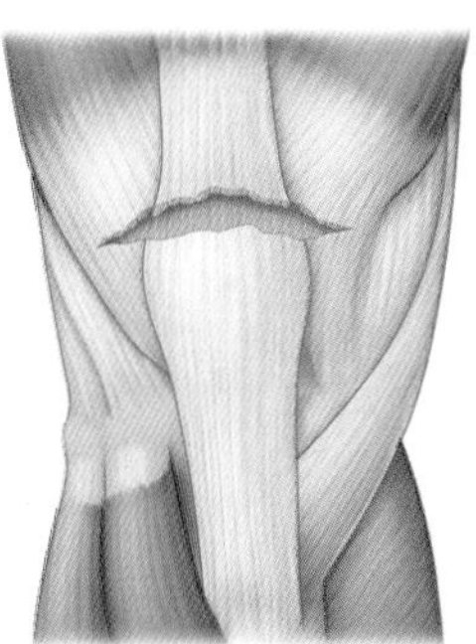
A
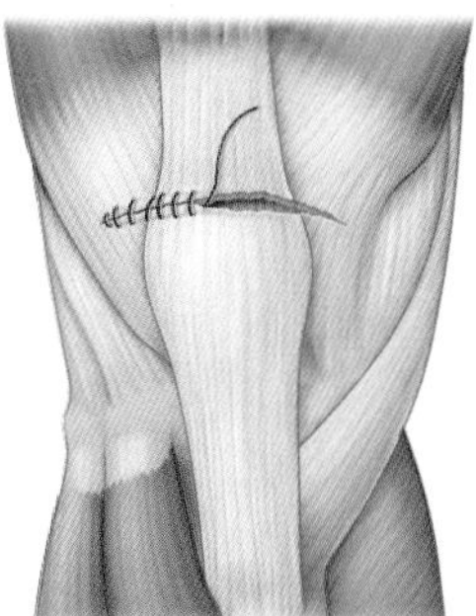
B
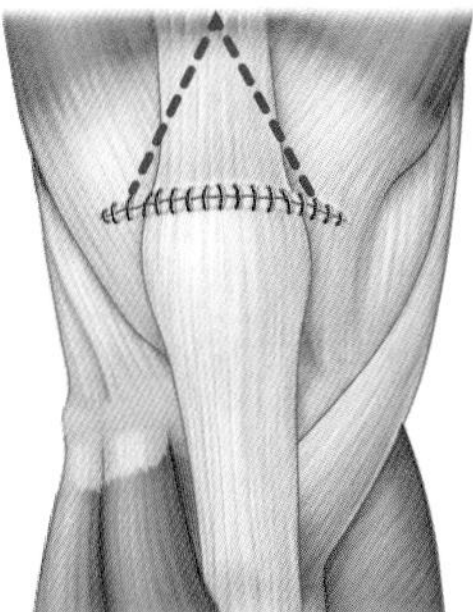
C
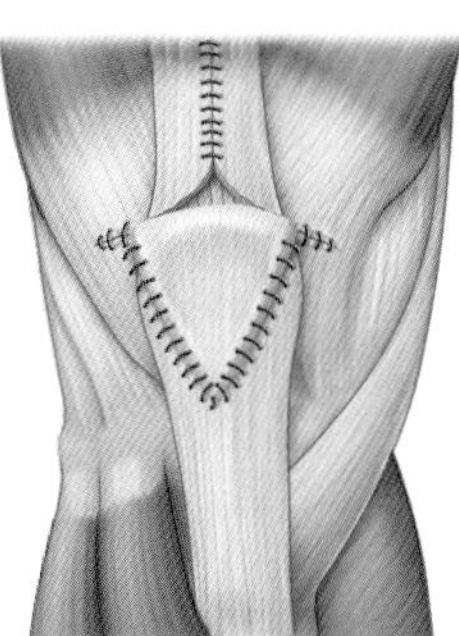
D

TECH FIG 5 • **A.** Following débridement of tendon to healthy tissue, excess tension is placed on the tendon for reapproximation. **B.** Reapproximate the quadriceps edges and secure with sutures. **C.** Incision of inverted V through full thickness of quadriceps tendon for the purpose of lengthening the tendon as it is reapproximated. **D.** Apex of V folded distally and secured, as proximal tendon is closed to each other to allow for lengthening and repair of tendon without excess tension.

PEARLS AND PITFALLS

Proper diagnosis	▪ Complete history and physical examination ▪ Review of radiographs and MRI
Medial or lateral patellar tilt	▪ Anatomic and balanced repair of medial and lateral retinacula
Excessive patellofemoral contact stress	▪ Avoid excessive shortening of the extensor mechanism.
Patella baja	▪ Avoid overtightening of the tendon repair.
Superior patellar tilt	▪ Avoid anterior reattachment of tendon to the superior pole of the patella.

POSTOPERATIVE CARE

- A long-leg hinged brace with the knee locked in full extension is used for 6 weeks (a long-leg cast may be used for unreliable patients).
- The patient is instructed to observe toe-touch weight bearing for the first 1 to 2 weeks, followed by weight bearing as tolerated with crutches during the remainder of the 6-week period.
- Compliant patients can begin range-of-motion (ROM) exercises within the parameters of the hinged brace, which usually is set from 0 to 90 degrees.
  - This flexion amount is the value attained interoperatively following complete repair to determine when tension begins stressing the repair.
- At 6 weeks, the long-leg hinged brace is unlocked gradually to full flexion.
- Once 90 degrees of knee flexion is achieved and quadriceps strength is sufficient, use of the brace can be discontinued.
- The patient may advance bearing weight without crutches as function returns.
- Therapy is continued to achieve full ROM and quadriceps strength.

OUTCOMES

- Following acute quadriceps tendon repair and rehabilitation, most patients achieve normal gait, regain full quadriceps strength, and regain satisfactory flexion (some knee flexion may be lost owing to tendon shortening during débridement of necrotic tissue for repair).[2,9]
- Chronic repairs are associated with persistent quadriceps weakness and extensor lag.
- Older patients often have pre-existing patellafemoral chondromalacia and degeneration, often causing exacerbation of anterior knee pain.[5]
- Recurrence of tendon rupture is rare.
- Nearly half of all patients are unable to return to their preinjury activity level.[2]

COMPLICATIONS

- Loss of full knee flexion
- Residual weakness of quadriceps
- Infection
- Wound complications
- Patella tilt
- Excessive patellofemoral contact stress
- Patella baja
- Residual extensor lag

REFERENCES

1. Aprin H, Broukhim B. Early diagnosis of acute rupture of the quadriceps tendon by arthrography. Clin Orthop 1985;5:185–190.
2. Gregory K, Chen D, Lock T, et al. Outcomes following repair of quadriceps tendon ruptures. J Orthop Trauma 1998;12:273–279.
3. Insall J, Salvati E. Patella position in the normal knee joint. Radiology 1971;101:101–104.
4. Kannus P, Jozsa L. Histopathological changes preceding spontaneous rupture of a tendon. J Bone Joint Surg 1991;73:1507–1525.
5. Kelly DW, Carter VS, Jobe FW, et al. Patellar and quadriceps tendon ruptures—jumper's knee. Am J Sports Med 1984;12:375–380.
6. Kuivila TE, Brems JJ. Diagnosis of acute rupture of the quadriceps tendon by magnetic resonance imaging. Clin Orthop 1991;262:236–241.
7. McLaughlin HL, Francis KC. Operative repair of injuries to the quadriceps extensor mechanism. Am J Surg 1956;91:651–653.
8. Petersen W, Stein V, Tillmann B. Blood supply of the quadriceps tendon (BlutgefaBversorgung der Quadrizepssehne). Unfallchirurg 1999; 102:543–547.
9. Rasul AT, Fischer DA. Primary repair of quadriceps tendon ruptures. Clin Orthop Rel Res 1993;289:205–207.
10. Scuderi C, Schrey EL. Ruptures of the quadriceps tendon. Arch Surg 1950;61:42–54.
11. Zeiss J, Saddemi SR, Ebraheim NA. MR Imaging of the quadriceps tendon: normal layered configuration and its importance in cases of tendon rupture. Am J Roentgenol 1992;159:1031–1034.

Chapter 50 Knee Loss of Motion

Gregory C. Fanelli, Justin D. Harris, Daniel J. Tomaszewski, and John A. Scanelli III

DEFINITION

- *Loss of motion* is a generic term that can refer to a loss of flexion, extension, or both. It does not specifically imply a particular etiology.
- *Flexion contracture* implies a loss of extension secondary to contracture or relative shortening of the posterior soft tissues (capsular or muscular).
- *Arthrofibrosis* describes knee loss of motion (ie, flexion, extension, or both) caused by diffuse adhesions or fibrosis within a joint.
- *Ankylosis* describes immobility of a joint, usually secondary to fibrous, cartilaginous, or bony overgrowth.
- Knee loss of motion is a common and serious complication of knee ligament injury or reconstruction. Surgeon understanding of the pathogenesis, preventive measures, and surgical management of this condition is vital for optimum patient care.

ANATOMY

- The knee has been described as a ginglymus (simple hinge-type) articulation.
  - In actuality, knee motion is complex and requires at least six degrees of freedom (ie, translation in the anteroposterior, mediolateral, and tibial axial planes with rotational moments corresponding to abduction-adduction, flexion-extension, and internal-external rotation).
- The knee joint consists of three independent articulations: the patellofemoral, medial tibiofemoral, and lateral tibiofemoral articulations.
- Constraint of the knee joint is complex and dynamic. It depends on the position of the knee, the direction and nature of a given load, and the integrity of its bony and soft tissue restraints.
- The knee joint is the largest in the body. Its capsular attachments extend from the suprapatellar pouch proximally to posteromedially and from the posterolateral recesses distally.
  - Fibrosis can occur anywhere within these confines and ultimately may lead to loss of motion.
- Normal knee motion varies from person to person.
  - Most people achieve some degree of recurvatum in full extension, with men averaging 5 degrees and women averaging 6 degrees of hyperextension.
  - Normal knee flexion ranges from 140 degrees in men to 143 degrees in women.
- Slight losses of flexion are much better tolerated than slight losses of extension.[2,20] Full extension is required to allow quadriceps relaxation during the stance phase of gait. Small deficits in terminal flexion may go unnoticed by all but the elite athlete.

PATHOGENESIS

- Loss of motion after a knee injury can vary, depending on patient predisposition, the extent and nature of the injury, the timing and technique of surgery, and postoperative management (Table 1).
- Motion loss in an injured or reconstructed knee can be associated with any of a wide variety of conditions.
- A complete understanding of the terminology associated with knee loss of motion is essential to diagnose and communicate the patient's condition appropriately (Table 2).[12]
- Each area has its own pathoanatomy and relevant physical findings.

NATURAL HISTORY

- Loss of knee motion, particularly extension, can have a tremendous effect on clinical outcomes and overall patient satisfaction.
- Pressures across the patellofemoral joint during stance increase from 0 to 30% of body weight when comparing full extension to a 15-degree flexed position.[20]
- These altered mechanics can lead to pain, apprehension regarding motion, and, ultimately, worsening stiffness. Aggressive intercession via a carefully directed physical therapy protocol or appropriate surgical intervention is essential.

PHYSICAL FINDINGS

- Knee motion after ligament reconstruction must be monitored vigilantly.
- Motion should be compared with the contralateral extremity.
  - Any loss of motion in the flexion or extension plane should be considered abnormal.

Table 1 Pathogenesis of Knee Loss of Motion

Patient factors	Underlying arthritis or neuromuscular imbalance can affect final motion.
Injury pattern	Knee dislocations and multiple ligament injured knees typically do worse in regard to incidence and extent of motion loss. This may result from the greater extent of injury, surgery, or both.
Timing of surgery	Acute ligament repair has been identified by some as a risk factor for restricted motion postoperatively.[7,14,23] Surgery in patients with a robust post-injury inflammatory response and subsequent loss of motion should be delayed, if possible, until normal motion can be achieved.
Technical factors	Improper graft positioning and tensioning will prevent normal knee kinematics and has resulted in motion loss.[6] Performing concomitant extra-articular procedures has resulted in poorer postoperative motion.[7]
Postoperative factors	Prolonged immobilization, poor rehabilitation, infection, and reflex sympathetic dystrophy all can contribute to motion loss after surgery.

Table 2 Terms Associated with Knee Loss of Motion

Term	Definition
Arthrofibrosis	Diffuse fibrosis or adhesions
ACL nodule	Described as a "cyclops lesion," this is a dense fibrous scar that can form after bone–patellar tendon–bone autograft for ACL reconstruction. It typically is located anterolateral to the tibial tunnel and can lead to impingement on the intercondylar notch, preventing full extension.
Infrapatellar contracture syndrome	Pathologic fibrous hyperplasia of the anterior fat pad leads to adherence of the patellar tendon to the tibia. This leads, in turn, to limited patellar excursion and can be a cause of patella infera.
Soft tissue calcifications	Calcification and contracture of the capsuloligamentous structures about the knee are a less common, but well-described, cause of motion limitation.
Muscle contracture	Prolonged immobilization, in either flexion or extension, may lead to deficits in motion due to muscle contracture.

- A complete examination of the knee is essential and can help determine the etiology.
- Inspection
  - Swelling or erythema may indicate infection, reflex sympathetic dystrophy, or reinjury.
- Palpation
  - Effusion may indicate infection or reinjury.
  - Allodynia may indicate reflex sympathetic dystrophy.
  - Crepitus may indicate fibrosis, soft tissue calcification, or an anterior cruciate ligament (ACL) nodule.
  - A "clunk" may indicate an ACL nodule.
- Range of motion (ROM)
  - Extension loss may indicate posterior capsular contracture, infrapatellar contracture syndrome, medial collateral ligament (MCL) calcification, hamstring contracture, notch impingement, ACL nodule, or graft malposition or tension.
  - Loss of flexion may indicate quadriceps contracture, infrapatellar contracture syndrome, graft malposition or tension, patellar entrapment, or suprapatellar adhesions.
  - Loss of flexion and extension may indicate arthrofibrosis, infection, soft tissue calcification, infrapatellar contracture syndrome, or graft malposition or tension.

IMAGING AND DIAGNOSTIC STUDIES

- Plain radiographs—including anteroposterior, lateral, sunrise, and tunnel views—are the essential first step in imaging.
  - Hardware failure, osteochondral defects, MCL calcifications, patellar height, patellofemoral alignment, and tunnel placement can be assessed with these images.
- MRI can be obtained to more clearly evaluate the soft tissues.
  - The extent and nature of adhesions, graft position, graft failure, and the presence of an ACL nodule can be clarified by MRI.

DIFFERENTIAL DIAGNOSIS

- Arthrofibrosis
- ACL nodule
- Graft malposition
- Infection
- Infrapatellar contracture syndrome
- Muscle contracture
- Reflex sympathetic dystrophy

NONOPERATIVE MANAGEMENT

- Rest, ice and anti-inflammatory medications should be the first-line intervention for any knee with an acute process as found on physical examination: ie, an inflamed, warm, swollen knee with motion loss.
- Controlled, guided physical therapy is an excellent tool to help regain motion.
  - Quadriceps strengthening, active ROM exercises, use of continuous passive motion machines, hanging weights, and extension bracing or casting may all have a role. Each intervention depends on the clinical picture and pathogenesis.
- Our rehabilitation protocol for a multiple ligament knee reconstruction typically involves four phases (Table 3).
- Manipulation under anesthesia has been used by some to improve postoperative motion.[4]
  - Manipulation should be done with caution, because the procedure itself can cause an inflammatory reaction and lead to further fibrosis.

SURGICAL MANAGEMENT

- Failure to progress with nonoperative treatment is a general indication for operative management.
- Identification of the primary cause of the knee stiffness is essential to maximize outcomes.
- Indications for surgical intervention include:
  - Loss of flexion of 10 degrees or more
  - Extension deficits of 10 degrees or more
  - Failure to improve despite 2 months of intense therapy
- The primary goal of operative treatment is restoration of normal knee motion without causing iatrogenic damage to the joint.
- In both acute and chronic knee stiffness, resolution of the inflammatory phase of the condition is mandatory before proceeding with surgical intervention.
- Epidural or regional anesthesia can be used to assist with postoperative pain control to allow more intensive physical therapy in the immediate postoperative period.
- Millett et al[10,13] have outlined a systematic nine-step evaluation of potential causes for knee loss of motion, all of which must be addressed whether surgical intervention is performed in an open fashion or arthroscopically.

Open Surgical Treatment

- In severe cases of loss of motion of the knee, open releases may be indicated.
- Indications for open débridement and soft tissue release typically include patients with severe arthrofibrosis or patients who have failed previously attempted arthroscopic releases.
- Our general approach is to restore flexion by releasing capsular contractures, by lysing intra-articular fibrosis, and by mobilizing the extensor mechanism.

Table 3 Rehabilitation of Knee Loss of Motion

Goals	Program
Phase I: 0 to 6 weeks	
Maximum protection of grafts during early healing phase	Full-leg hinged knee brace locked in extension for 3 weeks; may begin passive ROM exercises in neutral weeks 4 through 6 and beyond
Maintain patellar mobility	Patellar mobilization exercises
Maintain quadriceps tone	Straight leg raises in brace
Control pain and swelling	Cryotherapy
Maintain full passive extension	Non–weight bearing with crutches
Phase II: 6 to 12 weeks	
Increase flexion ROM	Begin full flexion in brace
Initiate weight bearing	Partial weight bearing, slowly progress to full weight bearing by postoperative week 10
Quadriceps strengthening	Stationary bike, patella mobilization, prone hangs
Proprioceptive training	Closed chain strengthening after full weight bearing
Phase III: 3 to 6 months	
Increase knee flexion to within 10 degrees of uninvolved side by end of 6th month	Aggressive ROM exercises
Improve strength and proprioception	
Incorporate functional drills	Advance proprioceptive training
Phase IV: 6 to 12 months	Agility drills/sport-specific practice sessions without contact at 6th month
Return to sport if minimal pain and swelling, functional strength within 10% of uninvolved side, successful participation in practice drills	
Multidirectional functional brace recommended for sports up to 18 months	

- Extension is restored by addressing notch pathology, posterior capsular contractures, and anterior fibrosis.

Positioning

- The patient is placed supine on the operating table.
- A pneumatic tourniquet is placed high on the thigh over a cotton wrap. It is not routinely inflated.

Preoperative Planning

- Examination under anesthesia is performed.
- Flexion, extension, and patellar mobility should all be assessed preoperatively.
- With the patient fully anesthetized, the hip should be flexed to 90 degrees.
- Gravity should then be allowed to flex the knee. This reveals the true flexion limit.
- With the hip extended, the heel should be supported; the extension limit is then measured.
- Patellar mobility should then be documented with regard to superior–inferior glide, mediolateral glide, and patellar tilt.
- Comparison to the normal, uninvolved knee is extremely useful.

ARTHROSCOPIC EVALUATION

- The affected limb is then prepped and draped in standard fashion.
- A side post is utilized under the drapes along the lateral thigh.
- All surgical landmarks and proposed incisions are then drawn on the skin with a surgical marker.
- A surgical timeout is then performed, confirming the patient, the procedure, and the operative limb.
- Perioperative antibiotics are administered within 30 minutes of the surgical incision.
- In severely fibrotic knees, capsular distention using 120 to 180 mL of saline may be necessary to gain safe access to the knee joint without causing iatrogenic damage to the articular cartilage.
- A standard superolateral inflow portal is then created, followed by an inferolateral viewing portal, and, lastly, by an inferomedial working portal.
  - Portals are interchanged as necessary, and additional arthroscopic surgical portals are established when necessary (TECH FIG 1).

Suprapatellar Pouch

- In a normal knee, a view of the suprapatellar pouch should reveal the vastus intermedius rising off of the femoral shaft.
- The suprapatellar pouch should extend 3 to 4 cm proximal to the superior pole of the patella.

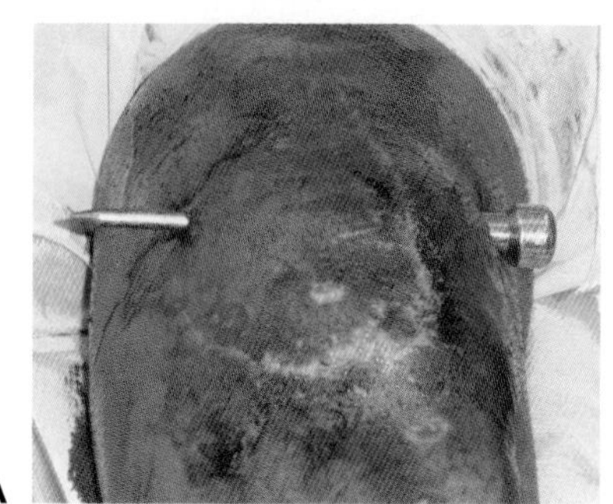

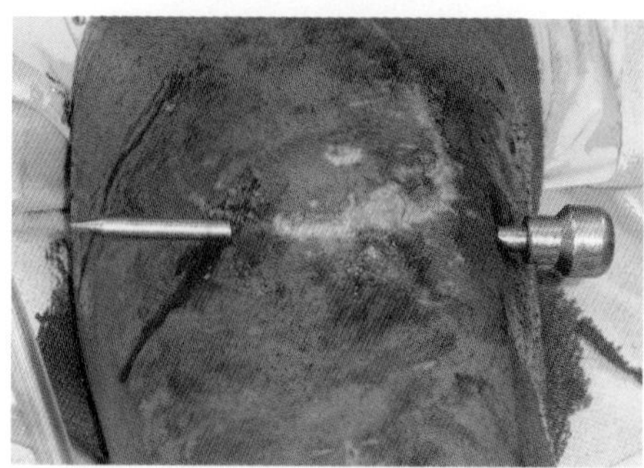

TECH FIG 1 • Establishment of the arthroscopic superior medial and lateral patellar portals (**A**) and the inferior medial and lateral patellar portals (**B**).

- Scarring in the suprapatellar pouch is the most common cause of loss of flexion and, in certain cases, may preclude safe passage of instruments between the femur and patella (TECH FIG 2).
  - Lateral or medial retinacular release, or both, may be necessary before suprapatellar pouch débridement can be done.
- Dense fibrous tissue may make it difficult to visualize normal articular cartilage.
- Using a combination of electrocautery, motorized shavers, arthroscopic knives, or heavy scissors, the suprapatellar pouch is reconstituted by performing aggressive releases.
- Care must be employed to avoid damage to the overlying quadriceps tendon or surrounding articular cartilage.

Medial and Lateral Gutters

- Adhesions in the gutters also are common causes of flexion loss.
- Dense bands of fibrous tissue course between the femoral condyles and the medial and lateral retinaculi.
- The surgeon should then clear all abnormal tissue, moving proximally to distally from the femur to the retinaculum.
- The gutters should be débrided to the level of the tibial plateau, both medially and laterally.
- Ninety degrees of knee flexion should be attainable at this point of the procedure.
- Failure to reach 90 degrees of knee flexion at this point mandates further débridement of the suprapatellar pouch or medial–lateral gutters.

Anterior Interval

- Débridement of the infrapatellar fat pad and pretibial recess is then performed (TECH FIG 3).
- Care must be undertaken to avoid the intermeniscal ligament.
- The release should proceed 1 cm distal to the level of the meniscus along the anterior tibial cortex.
- Hemostasis is essential in the pretibial recess to avoid recurrent scarring of the infrapatellar fat pad.
- Visualization in the anterior interval often can be difficult. A small, medial parapatellar tendon arthrotomy often is used to initiate débridement in the anteroinferior aspect of the knee.

Lateral and Medial Retinaculum

- Using electrocautery, selective lateral and medial retinacular releases are performed.
- This improves patellar mobility and increases the effective joint space in the knee.
- Adequate release is achieved when the patella can be everted at least 45 degrees.

Intercondylar Notch

- Scarring over the anterior aspect of the ACL, "cyclops" lesions, or graft impingement within the notch can all be addressed.
- A notchplasty is performed if there is evidence of graft impingement as the knee nears maximal extension.
- Cyclops lesions should be débrided and excised.
- In severe cases, malpositioned cruciate grafts may require débridement or release to achieve full extension.

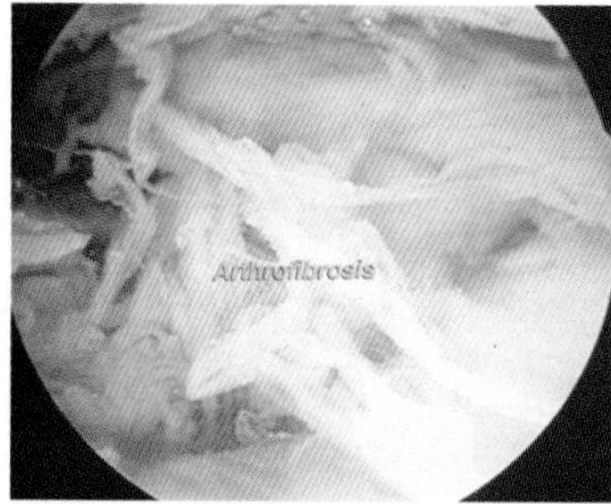

TECH FIG 2 • Arthroscopic view of arthrofibrosis in the suprapatellar pouch.

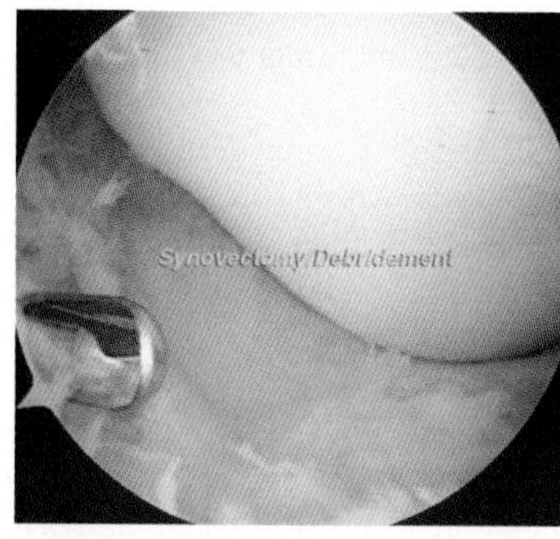

TECH FIG 3 • Arthroscopic débridement of the infrapatellar fat pad, and the pretibial recess.

Menisci

- Normal menisci have significant anteroposterior excursion with knee motion.
- In cases of knee stiffness, the menisci can become scarred in a posterior position during knee flexion, which will limit full extension.
- A probe can be used to assess for meniscal mobility.
- If anterior meniscal excursion is poor, a gutter should be created along the periphery of the meniscus from the midbody, working anteriorly until normal mobility is restored.
- This should help achieve full extension, but a posterior capsular release may be necessary in severe cases.

Posterior Capsule

- If full extension cannot be achieved after release of all the tissues just discussed, open posterior capsular release may be indicated.
- Posteromedial and posterolateral approaches commonly are used.
- The posteromedial approach uses an interval between the superficial MCL anteriorly and the pes anserine tendons posteriorly, revealing the underlying medial head of the gastrocnemius and the posterior oblique ligament.
- The posterior oblique ligament is then released from its femoral attachment, and extension is reassessed.
- If extension is still limited, a posterolateral release is necessary.
- The lateral approach courses over the anterior aspect of the biceps tendon distally to the fibular head.
- The short head of the biceps is reflected posteriorly, revealing the lateral head of the gastrocnemius, which often is intimately attached to the lateral capsule.
- The capsule is then incised anterior to the gastrocnemius tendon, releasing the posterolateral capsule.
- Care is taken to avoid the lateral collateral ligament, the popliteus tendon, and the popliteofibular ligament.

OPEN SURGICAL TREATMENT

Open Anterior Release

- Positioning and examination under anesthesia are performed just as described in the arthroscopic section.
- An anterior extensile approach to the knee is used. Previous vertical incisions can be used, or arthroscopic portal incisions may be extended (TECH FIG 4A).
- The subcutaneous tissues are dissected sharply, and full-thickness flaps are raised medially over the extensor mechanism.
- A medial parapatellar arthrotomy is then employed to gain access to the joint.
  - Care must be taken to protect the medial meniscus and the intermeniscal ligament (TECH FIG 4B).
- A medial release is performed by subperiosteally dissecting the soft tissues off of the medial proximal tibia.
  - The release is extended posteriorly, and the deep MCL and semimembranosus are elevated to assist in mobilizing the tibia. The insertion of the superficial MCL must be protected.
- Débridement of the medial and lateral gutters is then performed using a combination of finger dissection along with sharp excision of dense adhesions and fibrosis (TECH FIG 4C,D).

A 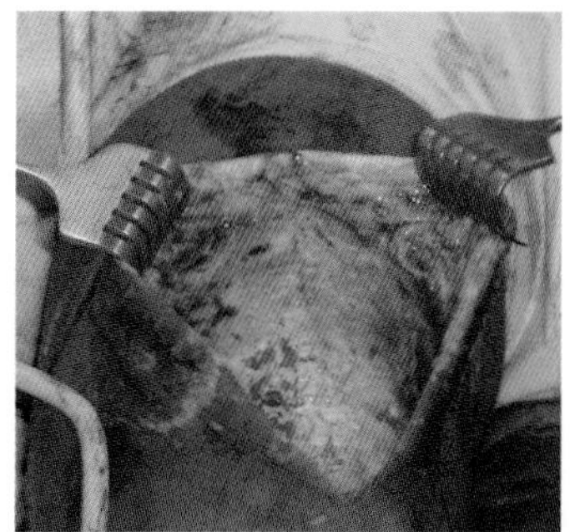

B 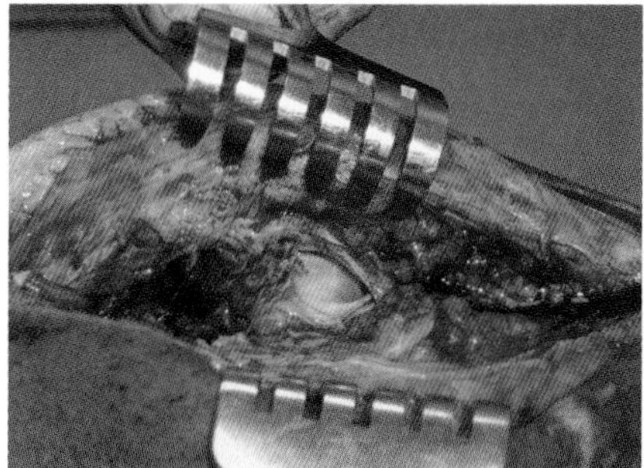

C 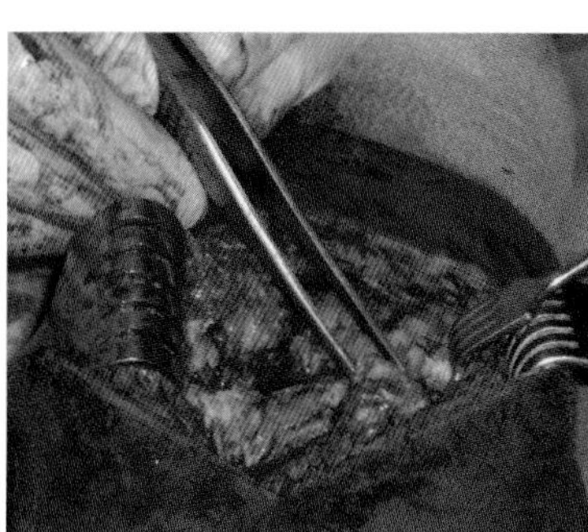

D 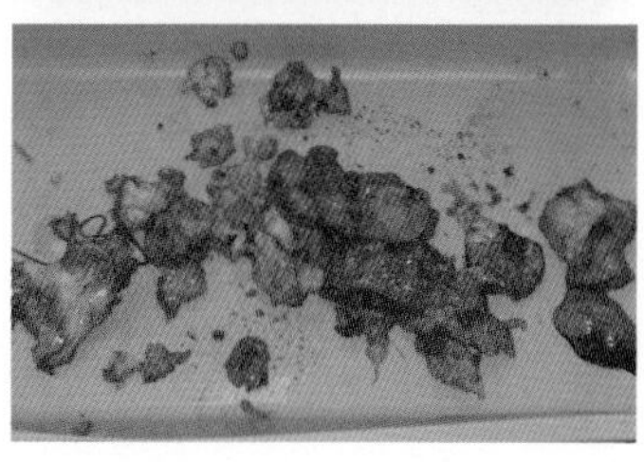

TECH FIG 4 • **A.** Anterior extensile exposure of the knee is used in the open surgical treatment of arthrofibrosis. **B.** Medial parapatellar arthrotomy is used to gain access to the knee joint. Note the severity of the intra-articular fibrous adhesions. **C.** Débridement of the medial and lateral gutters using a combination of sharp and blunt dissection. **D.** A large quantity of pathologic fibrous tissue was excised during the débridement.

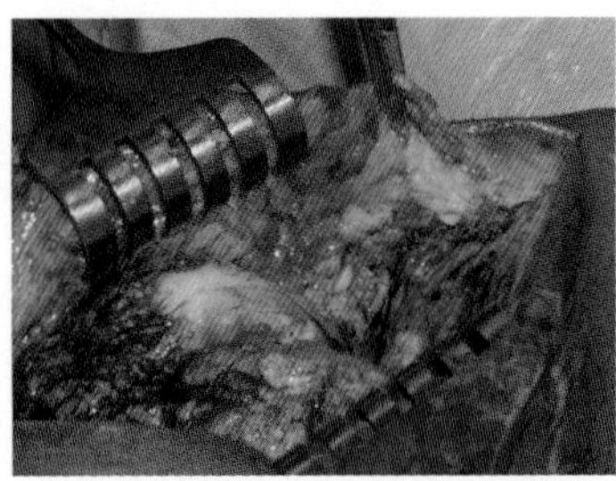

TECH FIG 5 • Establishment of the pretibial recess. The patellar tendon is adherent to the proximal tibia, proximal to its normal insertion site. Establishment of the normal pretibial recess is essential to motion restoration.

Extensor Mechanism Release

- The patellar tendon is dissected free from encasing fibrosis on all sides.
- The infrapatellar fat pad is excised in its entirety. The insertion of the patellar tendon on the tibial tubercle must be protected (TECH FIG 5).
- Adhesions between the quadriceps tendon and the distal femur must be released prior to patellar mobilization.
- An inside-out lateral release is then employed, and the patella is then everted or translated laterally to assist with notch visualization.
- Patellar tracking is then assessed throughout the entire ROM.

Notch Débridement

- If full extension is still unattainable at this point of the procedure, graft impingement and malposition must be addressed.
- Residual cyclops lesions are débrided.
- It may be necessary to excise anteriorly positioned ACL grafts, with removal of involved hardware (TECH FIG 6A).
- Posterior capsular contractures can be released by peeling the capsule off the posterior aspect of the femoral condyles.
- The PCL is then evaluated for impingement and is released if found to be a block to extension.
- Finally, a posterior capsular release from the proximal tibia may be needed if full extension has not yet been achieved (TECH FIG 6B,C).

Closure

- Meticulous hemostasis is achieved using electrocautery following deflation of the tourniquet.
- A medium Hemovac drain is placed intra-articularly to reduce postoperative hematoma formation and is left in place for 1 to 2 days.
- The medial parapatellar arthrotomy is closed with absorbable suture if it can be performed without significant tension on the extensor mechanism.
- The subcutaneous tissues and skin are then closed in standard fashion, and compressive dressings are applied.
- The knee is placed in a hinged knee brace and locked if necessary.

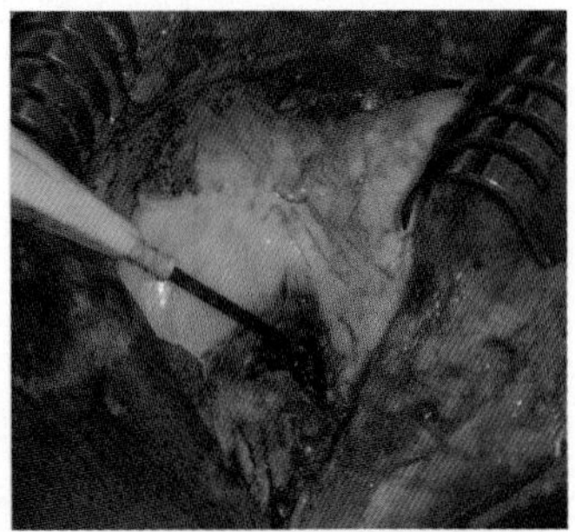

A

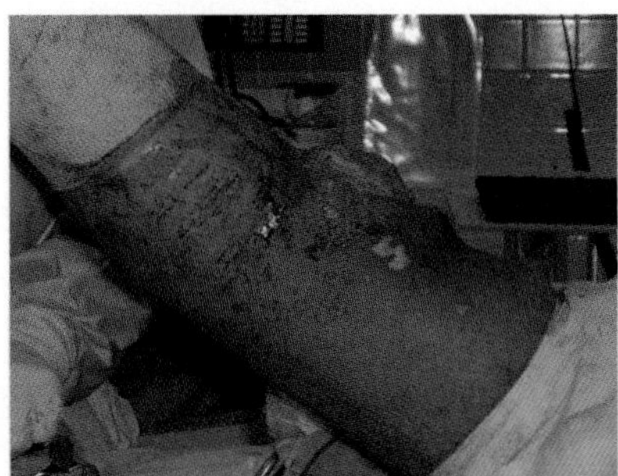

B

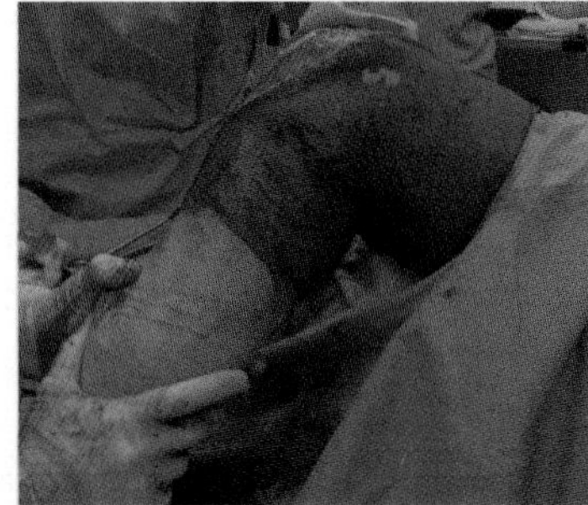

C

TECH FIG 6 • **A.** Intercondylar notch débridement is performed to address the issue of graft impingement and malpositioned grafts. **B,C.** Intraoperative range of motion achieved after open surgical débridement for severe post-traumatic arthrofibrosis. Preoperative range of motion was 10 to 30 degrees of knee flexion.

POSTOPERATIVE CARE

- If epidural anesthesia or regional blocks were used during the operative procedure, patients may benefit by continuing their use in the postoperative period. Additionally, intra-articular injections of bupivacaine combined with morphine given in the operating room can assist with postoperative pain control.
  - Adequate pain relief is essential for the patient to tolerate the immediate postoperative rehabilitation.
- Continuous passive motion (CPM) is used in the immediate postoperative period to assist with knee ROM.
  - When patients are not using the CPM machine, they are placed in a hinged knee brace locked in extension.
  - Home CPM usually is needed for 2 to 3 weeks.
- Outpatient physical therapy also is implemented early in the postoperative period.
  - Gentle ROM exercises are encouraged initially, so as not to exacerbate the inflammatory process that originally created

the knee loss of motion. Additionally, articular cartilage may be prone to injury by forced motion or excessive activity.

- Prone hangs, knee sags, patellar mobilization, and active quadriceps contraction are emphasized to maintain full extension.
- More aggressive strengthening exercises are begun as the patient continues to progress and improve.

- Multiple modalities are implemented to minimize postoperative swelling and pain.
  - A cryotherapy device is applied in the recovery room and used in both the inpatient and outpatient settings.
  - Nonsteroidal anti-inflammatory medications (NSAIDs) or short courses of oral corticosteroids can be given to reduce inflammation.
  - Compressive dressings are used.
  - Knee aspiration may be necessary for effusions that are large enough to cause pain, inhibit quadriceps activity, or limit ROM.
- In severe cases, it may be necessary to restrict weight bearing postoperatively to protect compromised articular cartilage.
  - Initiation of weight-bearing activities is at the surgeon's discretion.
  - Extension bracing often can be discontinued once patients have full return of quadriceps function.

OUTCOMES

Nonsurgical Results

- Few studies have been written regarding nonoperative management of knee loss of motion.
- Noyes and associates[11] reported on 18 patients who did not regain full motion following ACL reconstruction despite implementation of an early active and passive motion protocol.
  - Six knees were treated with serial extension casts, nine had early gentle manipulation under anesthesia, and three required arthroscopic lysis of adhesions.
  - Thirteen of the 15 patients treated nonsurgically regained full ROM of the knee.
- In a separate study, Noyes et al[15] prospectively evaluated 443 knees and reported that 23 developed arthrofibrosis following ACL reconstruction.
  - Twenty knees (87%) were treated successfully using manipulation under anesthesia, extension casting, and continuous epidural anesthesia.
  - The authors stated that nonsurgical management often can be successful if initiated early.
  - Loss of knee motion that is present more than 3 months following ligament reconstruction surgery is less likely to respond to nonsurgical means.
- Dodds et al[4] evaluated the results of knee manipulations performed for loss of motion in 42 knees that previously had undergone intra-articular ACL reconstruction.
  - The average time from reconstruction to manipulation was 7 months.
  - Ten knees had concomitant arthroscopic débridement.
  - Average flexion increased from 95 to 136 degrees, and extension improved from 11 to 3 degrees.
  - No complications were reported.

Arthroscopic Results

- Most studies in the literature pertaining to knee loss of motion contain a mixed group of patients with varying degrees of severity, chronicity, and etiology. Results should be interpreted based on the specific variant of motion loss.
- ACL nodule
  - The term "cyclops syndrome" was coined by Jackson and Schaefer[9] after reviewing 13 patients with loss of knee extension after ACL reconstruction.
    - All patients were treated with arthroscopic débridement and manipulation. Patients gained an additional 10 degrees of extension and 27 degrees of flexion immediately postoperatively.
    - Motion continued to improve with longer follow-up.
    - Six of the patients required more than one procedure to achieve these results.
  - Marzo et al[11] reported on 21 patients with restricted knee extension following ACL reconstruction.
    - All patients had a cyclops lesion at surgery and were treated with arthroscopic débridement, with 10 patients requiring an additional notchplasty for graft impingement.
    - All patients had good results, with an average extension gain of 8 degrees leaving them with an average final extension deficit of 3 degrees.
  - Fisher and Shelbourne[5] reported on 42 patients who required arthroscopic débridement for symptomatic extension loss following ACL reconstruction.
  - Both pain relief and ROM improved postoperatively.
  - No complications were reported.
- Diffuse arthrofibrosis
  - Multiple studies have documented successful treatment of diffuse intra-articular arthrofibrosis with arthroscopic débridement and release.[1,3,17,24–26]
  - Shelbourne and Johnson[22] reported on nine consecutive patients with symptomatic knee loss of motion following ACL surgery.
    - Eight of the nine patients underwent ACL reconstruction within 2 weeks of the initial injury and were immobilized in flexion postoperatively.
    - The patients underwent arthroscopic débridement of adhesions in the superior patellar pouch, medial and lateral gutters, and in the anterior interval. Notchplasties also were performed followed by manipulations to regain flexion. Extension casting and physical therapy were used postoperatively.
    - At an average of 31 months follow-up, patients had gained 23 degrees of extension and 18 degrees of flexion. Eight of the nine patients returned to sports.
  - Hasan and associates[8] reviewed 17 knees with symptomatic extension deficits following ACL reconstruction.
    - All knees were treated with arthroscopic débridement of intra-articular adhesions with excision of cyclops lesions and revision notchplasties.
    - Postoperative ROM yielded 7- and 8-degree improvements in extension and flexion, respectively.
  - Harner and colleagues[7] reviewed 21 of 27 patients who developed motion deficits following ACL reconstruction.
    - Fourteen of the patients were successfully treated arthroscopically, although three of those required a second procedure.
    - Six of the knees underwent formal open débridement for more severe intra- and extra-articular adhesions.
    - Sixty-seven percent of the patients had a good or excellent result at final follow-up.

Open Results

- Open débridement and lysis of adhesions are indicated in cases of severe knee loss of motion, infrapatellar contracture syndrome, and failed arthroscopic intervention.

Infrapatellar Contracture Syndrome

- Paulos et al[18] described infrapatellar contracture syndrome (IPCS) as an exaggerated pathologic fibrous hyperplasia of the anterior soft tissues of the knee.
  - Patients with this condition presented with loss of knee flexion and extension, patellar entrapment, and patella infera. The authors recommended open débridement in cases with extra-articular involvement.
  - Aggressive rehabilitation was done postoperatively.
  - Patients gained an average of 12 degrees of extension and 35 degrees of flexion at final follow-up.
  - Eighty percent of patients had signs and symptoms of patellofemoral arthrosis, however, with 16% of patients demonstrating patella baja.
- A long-term follow-up study of IPCS reported on 75 patients who had undergone previous surgical intervention.
  - Depending on the severity of patellar involvement, arthroscopic and open releases were performed.[19] In cases of patella infera, DeLee tibial tubercle osteotomies were performed.
  - Significant gains in ROM were achieved, but numerous patients required revision lysis of adhesions and manipulations.
  - The authors concluded that the longer the knee was without acceptable motion, the more likely the patient was to have a poor final outcome.
- Richmond and Al Assal[21] reported on arthroscopic treatment of IPCS. Their results revealed a total increase in knee ROM of 45 degrees in 12 patients with that condition.
- Severe and revision cases
  - Millett et al[13] retrospectively reviewed eight patients who had undergone an open débridement and soft tissue release for severe knee loss of motion.
    - All patients had failed previous arthroscopic intervention. The average arc of motion preoperatively was 62.5 degrees.
    - At final follow-up, the average motion had increased to 124 degrees.
    - Patient satisfaction scores were high, but there was a significant incidence of patellofemoral arthritis.
    - The authors concluded that an aggressive open release is a reasonable option for stiff knees that are recalcitrant to less invasive procedures.
  - A recent study detailed a mini-invasive extra-articular quadricepsplasty followed by an intra-articular arthroscopic lysis of adhesions for severe cases of knee arthrofibrosis.[27]
    - Twenty-two patients were treated with the aforementioned technique, in which a five-stage quadricepsplasty is performed to regain knee flexion. Knee arthroscopy was then performed to remove any intra-articular adhesions and to address pathology within the notch and the anterior interval.
    - At 44 months of follow-up, the average maximum degree of flexion had increased from 27 to 115 degrees.
    - Complications were rare: one superficial wound infection and one persistent 15-degree extension lag were reported.

COMPLICATIONS

- The primary complication of surgical intervention for knee loss of motion is recurrence of knee stiffness.
  - Rates of reoperation following arthroscopic débridement range from 6% to 43%.[5,24,25]
- Failure of surgical treatment is directly proportional to the severity of the preoperative stiffness.
- The more invasive the procedure necessary to regain full knee motion, the higher is the risk of potential complications.
- Other complications related to arthroscopic or open débridement and release include the following:
  - Skin tearing or necrosis
  - Wound dehiscence
  - Postoperative infection
  - Septic arthritis
  - Neurovascular injury
  - Extensor mechanism disruption
  - Hemarthrosis
  - Patellofemoral pain syndrome

REFERENCES

1. Achalandabaso J, Albillos J. Stiffness of the knee—mixed arthroscopic and subcutaneous technique: results of 67 cases. Arthroscopy 1993;9:685–690.
2. Benum P. Operative mobilization of stiff knees after surgical treatment of knee injuries and posttraumatic conditions. Acta Orthop Scand 1982;53:625–631.
3. Cosgarea AJ, DeHaven KE, Lovelock JE. The surgical treatment of arthrofibrosis of the knee. Am J Sports Med 1994;22:184–191.
4. Dodds JA, Keene JS, Graf BK, et al. Results of knee manipulations after anterior cruciate ligament reconstructions. Am J Sports Med 1991;19:283–287.
5. Fisher SE, Shelbourne KD. Arthroscopic treatment of symptomatic extension block complicating anterior cruciate ligament reconstruction. Am J Sports Med 1993;2:558–564.
6. Fu FH, Bennett CH, Lattermann C, et al. Current trends in anterior cruciate ligament reconstruction. Part II. Operative procedures and clinical correlations. Am J Sports Med 1999;28:124–130.
7. Harner CD, Irrgang JJ, Paul J, et al. Loss of motion after anterior cruciate ligament reconstruction. Am J Sports Med 1992;20:499–506.
8. Hasan SS, Saleem A, Bach BR Jr, et al. Results of arthroscopic treatment of symptomatic loss of extension following anterior cruciate ligament reconstruction. Am J Knee Surg 2000;13:201–210.
9. Jackson DW, Schaefer RK. Cyclops syndrome: loss of extension following intra-articular anterior cruciate ligament reconstruction. Arthroscopy 1990;6:171–178.
10. Kim DH, Gill TJ, Millett PJ. Arthroscopic treatment of the arthrofibrotic knee. Arthroscopy 2004;20:187–194.
11. Marzo JM, Bowen MK, Warren RF, et al. Intraarticular fibrous nodule as a cause of loss of extension following anterior cruciate ligament reconstruction. Arthroscopy 1992;8:10–18.
12. Millett PJ, Wickiewicz TL, Warren RF. Motion loss after ligament injuries to the knee. Part I: Causes. Am J Sports Med 2001;29:664–675.
13. Millett PJ, Williams RJ III, Wickiewicz TL. Open debridement and soft tissue release as a salvage procedure for the severely arthrofibrotic knee. Am J Sports Med 1999;27:552–561.
14. Mohtadi NGH, Webster-Bogaert S, Fowler PJ. Limitation of motion following anterior cruciate ligament reconstruction: a case-control study. Am J Sports Med 1991;19:620–625.
15. Noyes FR, Berrios-Torres S, Barber-Westin SD, et al. Prevention of permanent arthrofibrosis after anterior cruciate ligament reconstruction alone or combined with associated procedures: a prospective study in 443 knees. Knee Surg Sports Traumatol Arthrosc 2000;8:196–206.
16. Noyes FR, Mangine RE, Barber SD. The early treatment of motion complications after reconstruction of the anterior cruciate ligament. Clin Orthop Rel Res 1992;277:217–228.

17. Parisien JS. The role of arthroscopy in the treatment of postoperative fibroarthrosis of the knee joint. Clin Orthop Rel Res 1988;229: 185–192.
18. Paulos LE, Rosenberg TD, Drawbert J, et al. Infrapatellar contracture syndrome. An unrecognized cause of knee stiffness with patella entrapment and patella infera. Am J Sports Med 1987;15:331–341.
19. Paulos LE, Wnorowski DC, Greenwald AE. Infrapatellar contracture syndrome: diagnosis, treatment, and long-term followup. Am J Sports Med 1994;22:440–449.
20. Perry J, Antonelli D, Ford W. Analysis of knee-joint forces during flexed-knee stance. J Bone Joint Surg Am 1975;57A:961–967.
21. Richmond JC, Al Assal M. Arthroscopic management of arthrofibrosis of the knee including infrapatellar contracture syndrome. Arthroscopy 1991;7:144–147.
22. Shelbourne KD, Johnson GE. The outpatient surgical management of arthrofibrosis after anterior cruciate ligament surgery. Am J Sports Med 1994;22:192–197.
23. Shelbourne KD, Wilckens JH, Mollabashy A, et al. Arthrofibrosis in acute anterior cruciate ligament reconstruction. The effect of timing of reconstruction and rehabilitation. Am J Sports Med 1991;19:332–336.
24. Sprague NF. Motion-limiting arthrofibrosis of the knee: the role of arthroscopic management. Clin Sports Med 1987;6:537–549.
25. Sprague NF, O'Connor RL, Fox JM. Arthroscopic treatment of postoperative knee fibroarthrosis. Clin Orthop Rel Res 1982;166:165–172.
26. Vaquero J, Vidal C, Medina E, et al. Arthroscopic lysis in knee arthrofibrosis. Arthroscopy 1993;9:691–694.
27. Wang JH, Zhao JZ, He YH. A new treatment strategy for severe arthrofibrosis of the knee. J Bone Joint Surg Am 2006;88A:1245–1250.

Chapter 51

Arthroscopic Lateral Release of the Knee

Carl H. Wierks and Andrew J. Cosgarea

DEFINITION

- Patellofemoral pain is a common symptom in active adolescents and adults.
- The diagnosis of patellofemoral pain is nonspecific. It may be caused by trauma, instability, or overuse. It also may be caused by lateral compression of the patella on the femur.
- The patella is guided through its normal course in the trochlea of the femur by the static soft tissue as well as the dynamic muscular stabilizers.[11]
- The lateral retinaculum and patellofemoral ligament make up the lateral static soft tissue stabilizers and can lead to painful compression between the patella and femur if excessively tight.
- This scenario has been described as *excessive lateral pressure syndrome (ELPS)*,[7] *patellar compression syndrome*,[11] and *patellofemoral stress syndrome*.[14]
- This chapter describes the surgical treatment of ELPS.

ANATOMY

- The patella acts as a fulcrum and provides a smooth surface on which the extensor mechanism can function.[5]
- The thickest articular cartilage in the body is located in the patellofemoral joint.
- Forces across the patellofemoral joint are about three times body weight during ascending and descending stairs and can reach up to 20 times body weight during activities such as jumping.[3]
- As the knee flexes from a fully extended position, the patella is drawn into the trochlear groove at approximately 20 degrees.
- In extension, the medial patellofemoral ligament is the primary restraint to excessive lateral translation.
- In early flexion, the lateral trochlear ridge is the primary restraint.
- A tight lateral retinaculum and patellofemoral ligament are responsible for constricting the patella in ELPS.

PATHOGENESIS

- An abnormally tight lateral retinaculum can cause pressure and subsequent pain and degeneration of articular cartilage on the lateral aspect of the patella as it encounters the femoral condyle.
- Some conditions, such as a weak vastus medialis obliquus, malalignment (abnormal Q angle), internal tibial torsion, and femoral anteversion predispose to lateral tracking.
- Other conditions, such as direct trauma (eg, dashboard injury) and dislocation, can result in degeneration of the lateral patellofemoral articular cartilage.

NATURAL HISTORY

- No good long-term natural history studies of ELPS have been reported to date.
- It is well known, however, that disruption of articular cartilage results in progressive degenerative changes.

PATIENT HISTORY AND PHYSICAL FINDINGS

- Patients typically report insidious onset of anterior knee pain that is activity-related, although some may have experienced trauma in the past.
- Pain typically is exacerbated by prolonged sitting and stair climbing.
- Symptoms and clinical findings of instability do not play a part in ELPS.
- A thorough physical examination should include the following:
  - Examination for effusion. Effusion may indicate traumatic or degenerative disruption of the articular surface.
  - Observation of patellar tracking (J-sign)
  - Patellar tilt test. If the lateral facet cannot be tilted to neutral, the lateral retinaculum is abnormally tight.
  - Patellar glide test. A lateral glide of up to two quadrants is normal. More than this may indicate excessive lateral translation. Comparison should be made to the normal extremity.
  - Patellar apprehension test. Apprehension suggests an unstable patella.
  - Examination for quadriceps tightness, which often is associated with patellofemoral pain.
  - Patellar grind test. Pain may indicate patellofemoral athritis but also may be found in normal articular surfaces.
  - Inspection for bony knee malalignment (Q angle)

IMAGING AND OTHER DIAGNOSTIC STUDIES

- Radiographs of the knee should include anteroposterior, tunnel, Merchant (sunrise), and 30-degree lateral views. If arthritis is suspected, a posteroanterior flexed 45-degree view should be obtained.
- Lateral subluxation can be measured on the Merchant radiograph. If the line through the patellar apex is lateral to a line bisecting the trochlear sulcus angle, then the patella is subluxed laterally (**FIG 1A**).
- A CT scan is the best way to evaluate patellar tilt radiographically. Using an axial image, a line is drawn parallel to the posterior femoral condyles and is compared to a line along the lateral patellar facet. If these lines converge laterally, then the patella has excessive lateral tilt (**FIG 1B**).
- An MRI may be beneficial in evaluating the integrity of articular cartilage and also may show concominant meniscal and ligamentous pathology (**FIG 1C**).

DIFFERENTIAL DIAGNOSIS

- Patellofemoral pain (without excessive lateral pressure syndrome)
- Patellar instability
- Lateral meniscal tear
- Patellar fracture

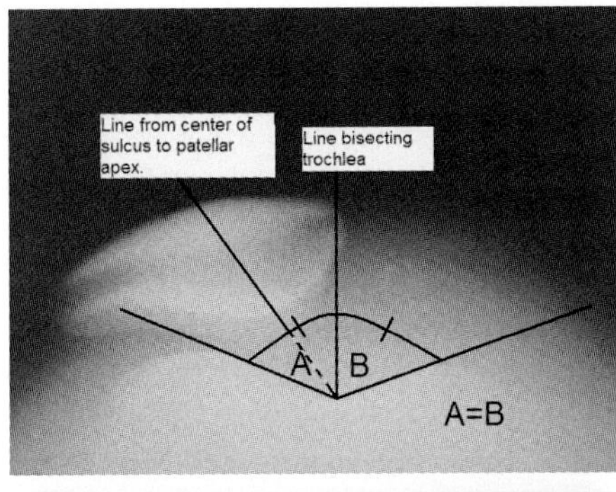

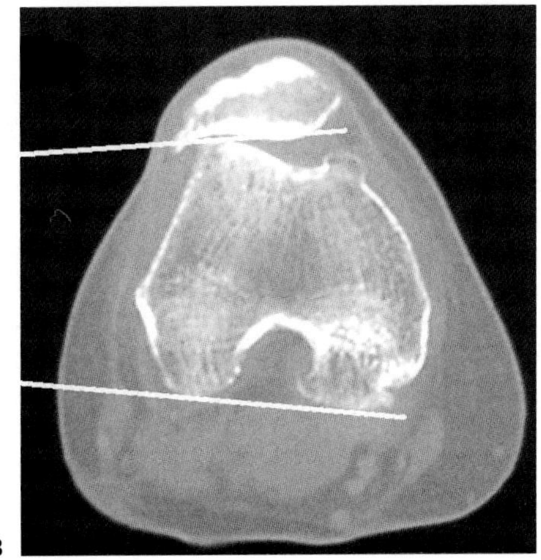

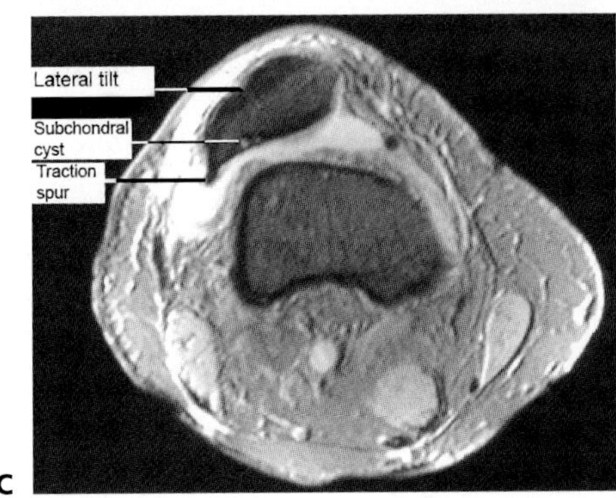

FIG 1 • **A.** Merchant radiograph of right knee showing measurement of lateral patellar subluxation. **B.** Axial CT image of a right knee demonstrating how to measure patellar tilt. **C.** Axial MRI scan of the right knee of a patient with excessive lateral pressure syndrome.

- Iliotibial band syndrome
- Prepatellar bursitis
- Neuroma
- Osteochondritis dissecans of the patella or trochlea

NONOPERATIVE MANAGEMENT

- The mainstay of treatment is nonoperative, with most patients benefiting from quadriceps stretching and selective strengthening exercises.
- Oral analgesics and bracing also can be beneficial.
- Corticosteroid injection or viscosupplementation may be helpful in patients with concomitant arthritis.

SURGICAL MANAGEMENT

- The indication for lateral retinacular release is failure of an adequate trial of rehabilitation in a patient with symptomatic patellofemoral pain, excessive lateral retinacular tightness, and lateral tilt.[8]
- Lateral release usually is not a successful treatment for lateral patellar instability and, in some cases, can result in iatrogenic medial patellar instabilty.
- Successful lateral retinacular release can be performed using either arthroscopic or open techniques.

Preoperative Planning

- Range of motion, patellar tilt and subluxation, and ligamentous stability should be examined while the patient is under anesthesthia.
- Particular attention should be paid to patellar tracking as the knee is taken through a range of motion (ROM).
- The operative knee should be compared to the contralateral side.

Positioning

- The patient is placed in the supine position with the operative leg supported according to the surgeon's preference for standard knee arthoscopy (**FIG 2**).
- A nonsterile tourniquet is placed around the thigh.

Approach

- A superolateral inflow portal is established just lateral to the vastus lateralis obliquus.
- Standard inferomedial and inferolateral portals are used.

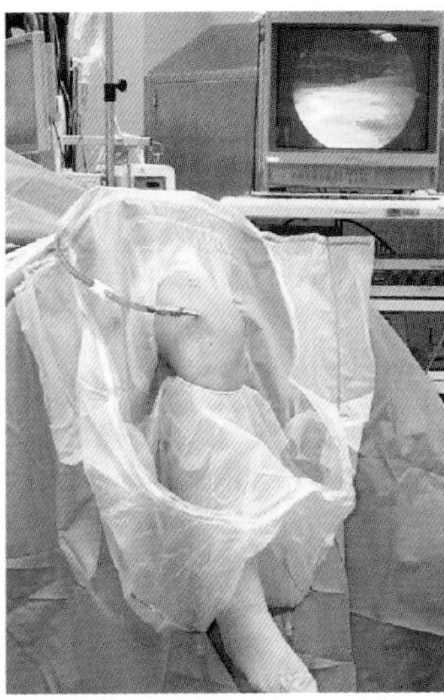

FIG 2 • Patient positioning for standard knee arthroscopy using a leg holder and superolateral portal.

TECHNIQUES

ARTHROSCOPIC LATERAL RELEASE

- Diagnostic arthroscopy is performed with the 30-degree arthroscope placed in the anterolateral portal.
- The entire knee is examined to rule out concomitant intra-articular pathology.
- The posteromedial and posterolateral compartments are visualized using the Gillquist technique.
- Meniscal tears, articular cartilage lesions, and loose bodies are identified and addressed sugically when indicated.
- Patellofemoral tracking is visualized as the knee is put through its ROM.
- Once the diagnostic arthroscopy is completed, an Esmarch bandage is used to exsanguinate the leg, and the tourniquet is inflated.
- The camera is placed in the inferomedial portal and a hooked coagulation device in the inferolateral portal.
- Under direct arthroscopic visualization, the release is started just distal to the inflow cannula (TECH FIG 1A).
- First the synovium is cut, exposing the underlying retinaculum.
- The retinaculum, which has a distinct firm feel, is then cut using multiple passes with the electrocaudery device (TECH FIG 1B).
- The release should extend down to the level of the inferolateral portal.
- Great care should be taken to not cut the vastus lateralis muscle or tendon.
- If the superior lateral geniculate vessels are seen, they should be aggressively coagulated.
- Patellar tilt is assesed after release. The surgeon should be able to tilt the patella 30 to 45 degrees with the knee fully extended.
- Excessive lateral release may result in medial instability.
- After the release is completed, the tourniquet is gradually deflated to assess for excessive bleeding.
- The portal sites are closed, and a sterile compression dressing and cryotherapy device are applied.
- Use of a drain may be considered on a case-by-case basis.

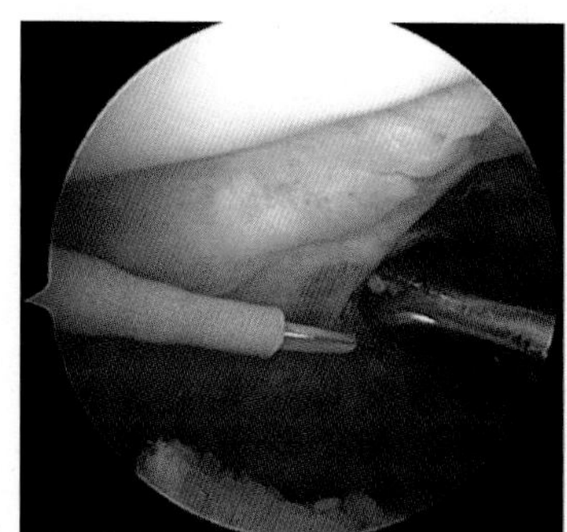
A

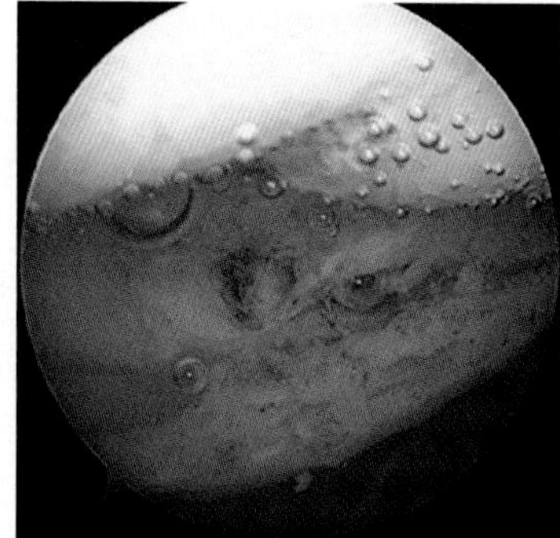
B

TECH FIG 1 • **A.** The proximal starting point for lateral retinacular release is just distal to the superolateral inflow cannula. **B.** Arthroscopic view demonstrating successful release of the capsule and tight lateral retinaculum.

PEARLS AND PITFALLS

Indications	■ The indication for isolated lateral release is retropatellar pain from the lateral patellofemoral joint secondary to soft tissue tightness. Lateral retinacular release should not be performed as an isolated procedure if patellar instability is the primary problem.[8,17]
Instability	■ It is important to not transect the vastus lateralis obliquus muscle and tendon during release, because that can predispose to medial instability.
Hemostasis	■ The superior lateral geniculate vessels are at risk during lateral release. Deflating the tourniquet before closing can help identify excessive bleeding. Use of a cryotherapy device and a compression dressing will also decrease the risk of hemarthrosis.
Landmarks guiding length of release	■ The superolateral inflow cannula is an excellent guide for the most proximal starting point of the release. The release should extend distally to the inferolateral portal.

POSTOPERATIVE CARE

- A compression dressing and a cryotherapy device are used to decrease risk of hemarthrosis.
- Patients are allowed to progress to weight bearing as tolerated and discard crutches when they are ambulating safely.
- Patients are initially seen 1 week after surgery to assess knee motion and quadriceps function and to remove sutures.
- Some patients benefit from formal physical therapy for ROM and quadriceps strengthening to facilitate ruturn to normal function.

OUTCOMES

- Arthroscopic isolated lateral retinacular release has a success rate ranging from 70% to 93%.[12,13,15]

- One prospective, randomized study[13] found that 93% of patients returned to presymptomatic activity level.
- The same study found quadriceps strength deficits in 40% of patients, but in almost all cases the strength was within 10% of the normal leg.[13]
- Arthroscopic and open techniques have similar success rates.[5,11–13,15]
- Success rates of lateral release are lower when performed for instability alone[4,6,9] or when advanced patellofemoral arthritis is present.[1,17]

COMPLICATIONS

- Hemarthrosis is the most common complication, followed by infection.[10]
- Medial instability from overaggressive release can be especially difficult to manage. The diagnosis of medial instability can be difficult to make. Patients may report a sensation of lateral instability if the patella sits in a medially subluxed position during early flexion, then snaps laterally during continued flexion. This is important because if the clinician incorrectly treats the presumed lateral instability with a medial stabilization procedure, the symptoms could worsen.[16]
- Other potential complications include quadriceps tendon rupture, patella baja, thermal injury, and arthrofibrosis.[10]

REFERENCES

1. Aderinto J, Cobb AG. Lateral release for patellofemoral arthritis. Arthroscopy 2002;18:399–403.
2. Aglietti P, Insall JN, Cerulli G. Patellar pain and incongruence. I: Measurements of incongruence. Clin Orthop Rel Res 1983;176: 217–224.
3. Aglietti P, Menchetti PPM. Biomechanics of the patellofemoral joint. In: Scuderi GR, ed. The Patella. New York: Springer-Verlag, 1995:25–48.
4. Betz RR, Magill JT III, Lonergan RP. The percutaneous lateral retinacular release. Am J Sports Med 1987;15:477–482.
5. Ceder LC, Larson RL. Z-plasty lateral retinacular release for the treamtent of patellar compression syndrome. Clin Orthop Rel Res 1979;144:110–113.
6. Christensen F, Soballe K, Snerum L. Treatment of chondromalacia patellae by lateral retinacular release of the patella. Clin Orthop Rel Res 1988;234:145–147.
7. Ficat P. The syndrome of lateral hyperpressure of the patella. Acta Orthop Belg 1978;44:65–76.
8. Fithian DC, Paxton EW, Post WR, et al. Lateral retinacular release: a survey of the International Patellofemoral Study Group. Arthroscopy 2004;20:463–468.
9. Kolowich PA, Paulos LE, Rosenberg TD, et al. Lateral release of the patella: indications and contraindications. Am J Sports Med 1990; 18:359.
10. Kunkle KL, Malek MM. Complications and pitfalls in lateral retinacular release. In: Malek MM, ed. Knee Surgery: Complications, Pitfalls and Salvage. New York: Springer-Verlag, 2001:161–170.
11. Larson RL, Cabaud HE, Slocum DB, et al. The patellar compression syndrome: surgical treatment by lateral retinacular release. Clin Orthop Rel Res 1978;134:158–167.
12. McGinty JB, McCarthy JC. Endoscopoic lateral retinacular release. A preliminary report. Clin Orthop Rel Res 1981;158:120–125.
13. O'Neill DB. Open lateral reinacular lengthening compared with arthroscopic release. J Bone Joint Surg Am 1997;79A:1759–1769.
14. O'Neill DB, Micheli LJ, Warner JP. Patellofemoral stress. A prospective analysis of exercise treatment in adolescents and adults. Am J Sports Med 1992;20:151–156.
15. Panni AS, Tartarone M, Patricola A, et al. Long-term results of lateral retinacular release. Arthroscopy 2005;21:526–531.
16. Post WR. Anterior knee pain: diagnosis and treatment. J Am Acad Orthop Surg 2005;13:534–543.
17. Shea KP, Fulkerson JP. Preoperative computed tomography scanning and arthroscopy in predicting outcome after lateral retinacular release. Arthroscopy 1992;8:327–334.

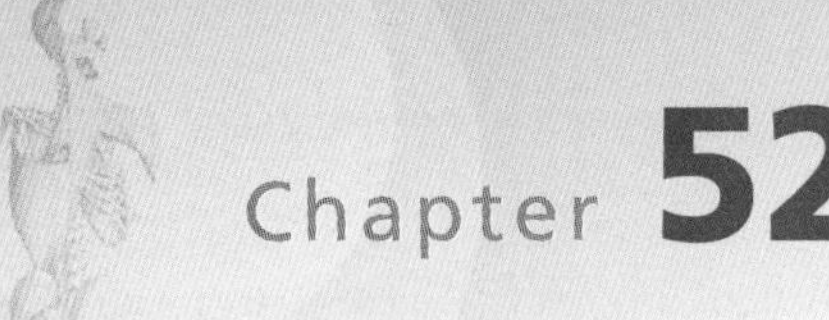

Chapter 52 Proximal Realignment of the Medial Patellofemoral Ligament

Donald C. Fithian, Samuel S. Park, and Erik Stark

DEFINITION

- In most cases, patellar dislocation results in injury to the medial retinacular ligaments, including the medial patellofemoral ligament (MPFL), leading to increased lateral patellar mobility.
- The MPFL is the primary ligamentous restraint against lateral patellar displacement.
- Competency of the MPFL is both necessary and sufficient to restore lateral patellar mobility to a normal range[9]; consequently, surgical treatment should aim for restoration of a functional MPFL.

ANATOMY

- The main stabilizer of the patella in normal knees is the bony congruence between the patella and trochlear groove.
  - When the trochlear groove is dysplastic, as it is in many patients with patellar instability, the medial retinacular ligaments (ie, the MPFL) take on a greater role.
  - Even in the presence of a normal trochlea, MPFL deficiency can result in symptomatic lateral patellofemoral instability.
- The patellotibial and patellomeniscal ligament complex play a secondary role in restraining lateral patellar displacement, whereas the medial patellofemoral retinaculum contributes little to patellofemoral stability.
- The MPFL is an extra-articular ligament that lies in layer 2, between the medial retinaculum superficially and the joint capsule on its deep surface. The vastus medialis obliquus (VMO) tendon lies superficially anteriorly and inserts onto the anterior third of the MPFL.
- In a recent cadaveric study, the MPFL was moderately or well developed in 17 of 20 (85%) specimens, and poorly developed in 3 of 20 (15%).[19]
- The MPFL is about 58 mm long, with a width and thickness of 12 mm and 0.44 mm, respectively, at its midpoint.[19]
- The MPFL fans out anteriorly, inserting on the proximal two thirds of the patella.
- The femoral attachment of the MPFL is posterosuperior to the medial femoral epicondyle and just distal to the adductor tubercle when the knee is fully extended. The center of the anterior edge of the femoral attachment is located 9.5 mm proximal and 5.0 mm posterior to the center of the medial femoral epicondyle (**FIG 1**).[19]

PATHOGENESIS

- Patellar dislocations usually occur when the foot is planted, the knee is partially flexed, and the body pivots abruptly, resulting in internal rotation of the femur. Patients may or may not have sustained a direct blow.
- Patients may report that something "popped out" medially, as the uncovered medial femoral condyle becomes prominent.
- The knee usually gives way secondary to pain inhibition of the quadriceps and disruption of the mechanical advantage of the extensor mechanism, and the patient falls down.
- If the knee remains flexed, the patella may remain dislocated over the lateral femoral condyle.
- The history of injury may be unclear, especially if the patella rapidly and spontaneously reduced.
- In one cohort of 189 patients, 61% of first-time dislocations occurred during sports activity.[2]

NATURAL HISTORY

- Fithian et al[8] reported a 17% incidence of redislocation in a cohort of first-time dislocators followed over 2 to 5 years.
- On the other hand, patients presenting with recurrent patellar instability are much more likely to continue experiencing additional dislocations than patients who present with their first dislocation.
  - The risk of a repeat dislocation in patients presenting with a history of prior patellar dislocation is about 50% over a 2- to 5-year period.[8]
- The strongest risk factor for recurrent patellar instability is a history of prior patellar subluxation or dislocation.[8]
  - Other risk factors include female gender and younger age (less than 18 years old).[8,13]
  - In one study, girls with open tibial apophyses had the worst prognosis for instability.[13]
- It is unclear whether patellar dislocation leads to premature arthritis.
  - Crosby and Insall[3] reported that degenerative changes were uncommon after patellar dislocation.
  - In a more recent study, however, the incidence of degenerative changes was significantly higher at 6- to 26-year follow-up in first-time dislocators treated nonoperatively.[11]

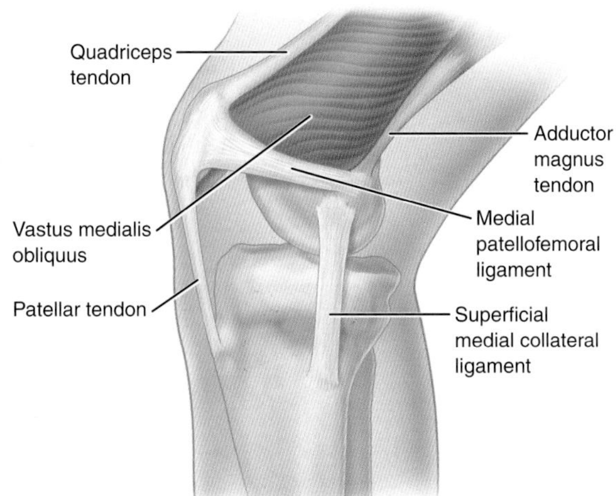

FIG 1 • Schematic diagram of the medial knee. The medial patellofemoral ligament (MPFL) arises between the adductor tubercle and medial epicondyle, then runs forward just deep to the distal vastus medialis obliquus (VMO) to attach to the superior two thirds of the medial patellar margin.

PATIENT HISTORY AND PHYSICAL FINDINGS

- The patient should be asked about mechanical complaints of locking or catching, because osteochondral loose bodies off the medial patellar facet or lateral trochlea (kissing lesion), impaction fracture of the lateral femoral condyle, or avulsion fragments off the medial patella may result from a patellar dislocation.
- Physical examination should include:
  - Lateral-medial patellar translation. Increased laxity is signified by more than two quadrants of translation; 10 mm or more of lateral translation; or the absence of an endpoint.
  - Apprehension sign. Inability to fully translate the patella laterally because of patient guarding may lead to a false-negative result.
  - J-sign. The patella abruptly translates laterally as the knee is fully extended, moving in an upside-down "J" pattern.
  - Check-rein sign. A positive test (no endpoint) signifies MPFL laxity (analogous to a Lachman test).
  - Patellar facet palpation. Tenderness may indicate an osteochondral or avulsion injury.
  - Medial retinacular palpation. Tenderness may indicate retinacular injury. A palpable defect may be felt in the retinaculum or even the VMO.
  - Effusion. A tense effusion or hemarthrosis (on aspiration) after an acute dislocation raises suspicion for an osteochondral fracture. MRI or arthroscopy should be considered.
- The examination also should evaluate associated injuries and rule out differential diagnoses:
  - Anterior cruciate ligament (ACL) injury results from a similar noncontact pivoting mechanism and also leads to an acute effusion. The Lachman test is highly sensitive for an ACL disruption. Pivot shift also may be attempted, but may be difficult to perform on an acutely injured knee. To rule out ACL injury definitively, ligament arthrometry or stress radiography is recommended for all patients presenting with knee injury.
  - If posterior cruciate ligament (PCL) injury is suspected, the patient is checked for normal tibial stepoff with the knee flexed to 90 degrees. A posterior drawer and quadriceps active test also may be done.
  - Medial collateral ligament (MCL) and lateral collateral ligament (LCL) injuries result in joint space opening with valgus or varus stresses, respectively. These tests are performed in both full extension and 30 degrees of flexion. Comparison stress radiographs can be useful to control for individual variation.
  - A posterolateral corner (PLC) injury results in 10 degrees or more of external rotation asymmetry (dial test) and a positive posterolateral drawer test.
  - Medial patellar instability can occur following prior lateral retinacular release. Medial patellar instability can be distinguished from lateral instability by the DeLee sign. The patient is placed in the lateral decubitus position with the injured side up. With medial patellar instability, gravity subluxates the patella medially. As the knee is flexed, the patella reduces in the trochlea with pain. The DeLee sign is positive if the application of a laterally directed force on the patella (which reduces the patella from its subluxated position) eliminates the pain caused by flexion of the knee.
  - Meniscal tears are indicated by joint line tenderness and also possibly by positive McMurray and Appley's grind tests.
  - Diagnosis of extensor mechanism disruption should be obvious based on an inability to straight-leg raise and actively extend the knee.
  - Patellofemoral osteoarthritis may be obvious on plain radiographs, but early stages require MR arthrography or arthroscopy for diagnosis.

IMAGING AND OTHER DIAGNOSTIC STUDIES

- Recommended plain radiographs include a standing anteroposterior view, a true lateral view with the knee flexed 30 degrees, and a standard axial patellar view at 30 or 45 degrees flexion.
- On the lateral radiograph, patellar height is measured according to the method of Caton and Deschamps (ie, the ratio between the distance from the lower edge of the patellar articular surface to the upper edge of the tibial plateau and the length of the patellar articular surface).[2]
  - A ratio of 1.2 or greater indicates patella alta, which predisposes to patellar instability due to late engagement of the patella in the trochlea as the knee flexes.
  - If present, a tibial tubercle osteotomy and distalization may be considered.
- Trochlear morphology can be assessed on the true lateral radiograph (the posterior borders of both femoral condyles are strictly superimposed).
  - Trochlear dysplasia is evident when the floor of the trochlea crosses the anterior border of both femoral condyles (crossing sign)[4] (**FIG 2A**).
  - Alternatively, the positive trochlear prominence (ie, the sagittal distance between the trochlear groove and the anterior femoral cortex) on the lateral view has been shown to correlate well with trochlear dysplasia[4,5] (**FIG 2B**). A trochlear groove prominence of 3 mm indicates trochlear dysplasia (**FIG 2C**).
- The axial patellar view may demonstrate lateral patellar subluxation or even frank dislocation. It may demonstrate medial patellar avulsion fractures, although these may be missed on plain radiographs.
- Stress radiography has been advocated to demonstrate abnormal patellar mobility.
  - With the knee flexed to 30 degrees, an axial patellar view is taken with a laterally directed force applied to the medial side of the patella.
  - Measurements are made on both the symptomatic and asymptomatic knees.
  - A side-to-side increase of 3.7 mm of lateral translation on the symptomatic side compared to the asymptomatic side is considered abnormal.[24]
- MRI identifies osteochondral injuries on the patella and femur, as well as loose bodies, that may be missed on plain radiographs.
  - A tense effusion should be aspirated.
  - Presence of gross hemarthrosis on joint aspiration is an indication for MRI to assess for osteochondral fracture and loose body.
- The TT–TG offset is the transverse distance between the anterior tibial tuberosity (TT) and the center of the trochlear groove (TG).[4]
  - It can be measured on axial CT or MRI (**FIG 2D**).
  - Lateral offsets of 20 mm or more should be corrected with medialization of the tibial tubercle.

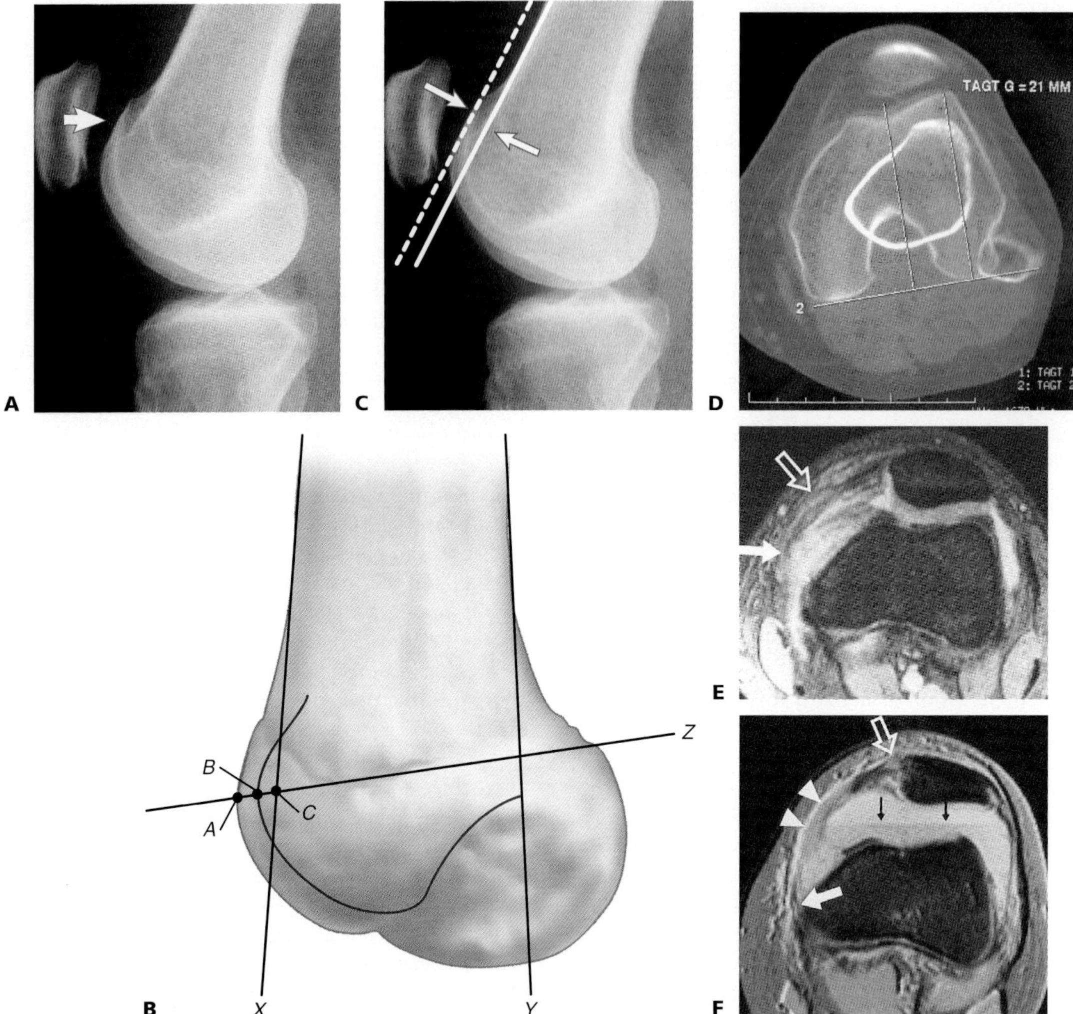

FIG 2 • **A.** On a true lateral radiograph, trochlear dysplasia is evident when the floor of the trochlea crosses the anterior borders of both femoral condyles (ie, the "crossing" sign). **B.** Measurement of the trochlear prominence on the lateral view according to Dejour et al. *X* and *Y* are lines tangential to the anterior and posterior cortices of the distal femoral metaphysis, respectively. Line *Z* crosses the most prominent point of the line of the trochlear groove (point *B*) and the upper aspect of the posterior border of the condyles. Line *Z* crosses the anterior aspect of the lateral condyle (point *A*) and line *X* (point *C*). The distance *BC* (in mm) is the trochlear prominence. **C.** Lateral radiograph demonstrating a knee with positive trochlear prominence. Note that the floor of the trochlea lies anterior to the line tangential to the anterior cortex of the distal femur. **D.** Measurement of the tibial tuberosity–trochlear groove (TT-TG) offset, the transverse distance between the apex of the anterior tibial tuberosity and the center of the trochlear groove. Measurements are made on superimposed axial CT or MRI images. **E,F.** MPFL injury appearance on MRI. **E.** Transverse gradient-echo image of the knee obtained at the level of the insertion of the adductor magnus tendon 3 weeks after lateral patellar dislocation demonstrates a complete tear of the femoral origin of the MPFL, with MPFL fibers retracted anteriorly (*solid arrow*). Partial injury, with surrounding edema, to the midsubstance of the patellar retinaculum (*open arrow*) also is seen. **F.** Transverse gradient-echo image of the knee in a different patient 2 days after lateral patellar dislocation showing partial injury to the femoral origin of the MPFL. The MPFL fibers (*solid white arrow*) are wavy and show longitudinal split, and there is extensive surrounding edema. A complete tear (*open arrow*) is seen in the patellar insertion of the medial patellar retinaculum. A large joint effusion with layering (*black arrows*) is present, consistent with hemarthrosis. Note also the inferior fibers of the VMO (*arrowheads*).

- MRI also is useful in identifying the location and degree of medial soft tissue injury preoperatively.
  - MPFL injuries occur commonly in the form of tears near the femoral attachment or avulsions off the femur, but also may occur as midsubstance tears or avulsions off the patella (**FIG 2E,F**). Injuries to multiple sites in the medial ligamentous stabilizers may occur.[5]

DIFFERENTIAL DIAGNOSIS

- Ligament/capsular injury (ACL, PCL, MCL, LCL, PLC)
- Osteochondral injury
- Medial patellar dislocation
- Extensor mechanism disruption
- Meniscal tear

- Patellofemoral osteoarthritis
- Contusion

NONOPERATIVE MANAGEMENT

- Nonoperative treatment usually is indicated for acute, first-time dislocators without associated osteochondral fracture and loose bodies.
  - Randomized prospective studies comparing operative and nonoperative treatment of initial patellar dislocation found no benefit from immediate medial retinacular repair.[1,13,14]
- Although there is evidence suggesting that immobilization following patellar dislocation may lower the risk of redislocation, patients often do not accept prolonged cast or splint immobilization. As a result, nonoperative management relies on brace protection during early progressive moblization and functional rehabilitation.
  - After an acute dislocation, patients initially are placed in knee immobilizers for comfort and weight bearing as tolerated.
  - As soon as comfort allows, passive ROM exercises and resisted closed-chain exercises in a patella-stabilizing brace are begun.
  - Patients are allowed to return to stressful activities, including sports, on resolution of the effusion, attainment of a full ROM, and return to at least 80% of their quadriceps strength compared to the noninjured limb.
  - Patients are encouraged to continue wearing the patella-stabilizing brace during participation in pivoting activities and sports.

SURGICAL MANAGEMENT

- An associated osteochondral fracture and loose body occurs in 3% to 4% of first-time dislocators and is an indication for acute surgical treatment.
  - In this case, primary MPFL repair should be performed after fixation of the osteochondral fracture. Preoperative MRI can help in localizing the site of MPFL injury.
- Surgical management usually is indicated for any patient with at least two documented patellar dislocations and a physical examination demonstrating excessive lateral patellar laxity.
  - For these recurrent dislocators, MPFL reconstruction should be done.

Preoperative Planning

- Appropriate imaging studies should be reviewed.
- Plain radiographs should be reviewed for the presence of trochlear dysplasia (ie, crossing sign and trochlear prominence of 3 mm or more), avulsion fractures, and loose bodies.
  - If signs of trochlear dysplasia are present, an axial CT or MRI scan should be obtained to measure the TT-TG offset. Offset of 20 mm or more should be treated with medialization of the tibial tubercle.
  - If patella alta is present (ie, Caton-Deschamps ratio of 1.2 or greater), then distalization of the tibial tubercle should be considered.
- MRI scans should be reviewed for the presence of avulsion fractures, osteochondral fractures, and loose bodies.
  - If MPFL repair is to be performed, MRI should be reviewed to identify all locations of MPFL disruption. Failure to identify and treat each location of MPFL disruption may jeopardize the repair.
- Examination under anesthesia should confirm excessive lateral patellar mobility.
  - The patella should displace more than 10 mm laterally from the centered position with the knee flexed 30 degrees, and there should be a soft endpoint or no endpoint with the knee extended.

Positioning

- The patient is positioned supine.
- If an osteochondral fracture and loose body amenable to reduction and fixation are present, surgery may proceed with an open approach (see Primary MPFL Repair at the Patellar Insertion, in the Techniques section).
- If a diagnostic arthroscopy is performed before MPFL reconstruction, then the limb is placed in an adjustable leg holder to adjust knee flexion during the procedure.

Approach

- The surgical approach depends on whether a primary MPFL repair or reconstruction is to be performed.
- During MPFL repair, the surgical approach is determined by the location of MPFL and retinacular injury. MPFL injury may be seen as a proximal or distal avulsion, or as a tear near the femoral origin, the midsubstance, or the patellar insertion. Multiple sites of injury may coexist.

DIAGNOSTIC ARTHROSCOPY

- Standard anterolateral and anteromedial portals are used.
- A superolateral portal is used to facilitate viewing of the patellar articular surface and passive patellar tracking and mobility.
- Articular cartilage lesions are addressed.
  - Specifically, the patellofemoral compartment is assessed for the severity of articular cartilage injury and the presence of degenerative changes.
  - Unstable cartilage flaps are débrided.
- Loose bodies are removed.

PRIMARY MPFL REPAIR AT THE PATELLAR INSERTION

- A midline skin incision is made extending from the superior pole of the patella to the midaspect of the patellar tendon.
- After dissection through the subcutaneous tissue, the superficial medial patellar retinaculum (layer 1) is identified. It is incised and reflected medially, exposing the underlying MPFL.
- The MPFL is inspected both visually and digitally along its entire length to identify all sites of injury.
  - The deep synovial layer (layer 3) can be dissected off the deep surface of the ligament to aid in inspection.
- The knee is then flexed to 30 degrees with the patella manually reduced in the trochlear groove.

- Avulsions are repaired with suture anchors.
- Tears of the substance of the MPFL are repaired with with no. 2 Fiberwire (Arthrex, Naples, FL) in a modified Kessler fashion (TECH FIG 1).[10]
- After the repair, proper tensioning is assessed.
  - The knee is taken through a full passive ROM to evaluate patellar tracking, looking for abrupt or gradual deflection of the patella that might indicate either excessive or insufficient medial tightening.
  - With the knee extended, a laterally directed force should reproduce a firm endpoint ("check rein" sign).
  - Patellar mobility is assessed by applying medial and lateral forces of about 5 pounds with the knee flexed to 30 degrees. This should produce 5 to 10 mm of medial and lateral translation, respectively. If lateral displacement is less than 5 mm or more than 10 mm, then the medial repair is retensioned.
- The wound is closed in layers.

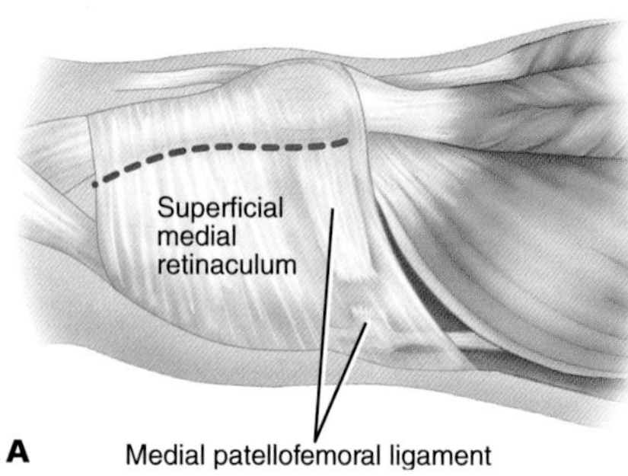

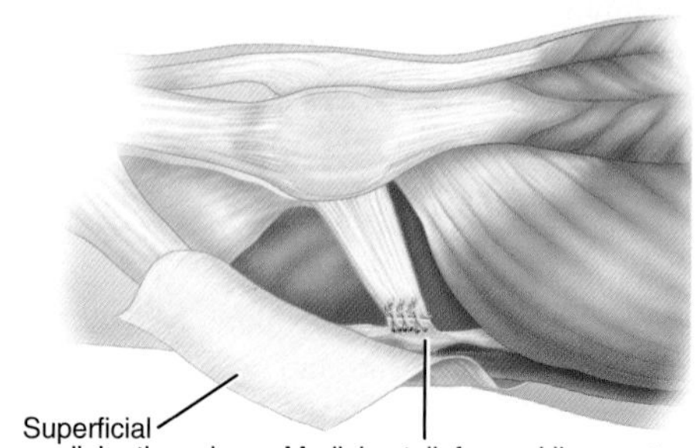

TECH FIG 1 • **A.** Disruption of the medial patellofemoral ligament (MPFL) near its femoral origin. **B.** For repair at this site, the superficial medial patellar retinaculum (layer 1) is reflected medially, exposing the torn MPFL. With the knee flexed 30 degrees, midsubstance MPFL tears are repaired primarily while avulsions are repaired using suture anchors.

AUGMENTED MEDIAL PATELLOFEMORAL LIGAMENT REPAIR AT ITS FEMORAL ORIGIN

- The femoral origin of the MPFL may be accessed through an extensile midline skin incision.
  - Alternatively, the origin may be approached through a separate posterior incision centered between the medial epicondyle and the adductor tubercle.
- The dissection is carried down through the subcutaneous tissue, and the injured medial retinacular tissue is identified.
- MPFL avulsions off the femur are repaired with suture anchors placed at a point 9 mm proximal and 5 mm posterior to the medial epicondyle, just distal to the adductor tubercle.
- To augment the repair, a 10-mm × 60-mm strip of medial retinacular tissue (layer 1) is dissected off the femur, leaving the patellar attachment intact (TECH FIG 2).[20]
- This medial retinaculum strip may be placed over the repaired MPFL and anchored into the adductor tubercle using a cancellous screw and either a spiked washer or suture anchor.

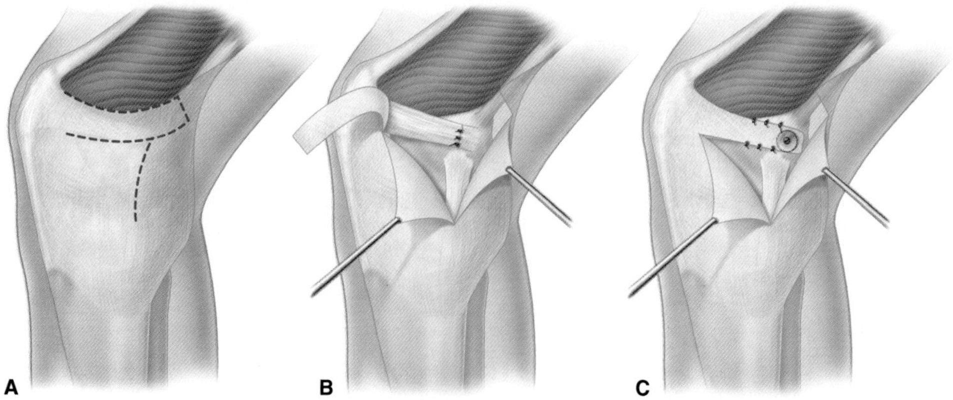

TECH FIG 2 • Schematic diagram of augmented MPFL repair at its femoral origin. **A.** Preparation of patellar-based medial retinaculum slip (10 mm × 60 mm). **B.** Avulsed MPFL repaired to femoral origin. **C.** Slip of medial retinaculum laid over MPFL and anchored to adductor tubercle with spiked washer and screw. (Redrawn from Nomura E, Inoue M, Osada N. Augmented repair of avulsion-tear type medial patellofemoral ligament injury in acute patellar dislocation. Knee Surg Sports Traumatol Arthrosc 2005;13:346–351.)

MEDIAL PATELLOFEMORAL LIGAMENT RECONSTRUCTION

Semitendinosus Tendon Graft Harvest and Preparation

- The sartorial fascia is exposed through a 2- to 3-cm skin incision made 2 cm medial and distal to the medial border of the tibial tubercle (TECH FIG 3).
- The sartorial fascia is incised in line with the palpable gracilis tendon.
  - Avoid making this incision too deep, to avoid injury to the underlying superficial MCL.
- Identify and isolate both the gracilis (proximal) and semitendinosus (distal) tendons from their deep aspect, ie, from within the bursal layer.
- Apply tension to the semitendinosus while freeing it from the crural fascia at the posteromedial corner with tissue scissors.
- Place stay sutures of no. 0 or 1 absorbable on a tapered needle, and then divide the tendon from the tibial insertion.
- Once all tendinous slips have been freed, harvest the semitendinosus tendon using a closed (preferred) or open tendon stripper.
- Baseball stitches are placed on both free ends for later graft passage throught the two patellar tunnels. The remaining free ends are discarded after graft fixation.
- The graft is prepared on the back table by first sizing the graft to 240 mm, then folding it in half, leaving a doubled graft of 120 mm. The excess is removed.
- A pullout suture of no. 5 polyester is placed through the loop to be used for pulling the doubled graft into the blind femoral tunnel.
- A baseball stitch 25 mm in length is placed in the looped end of the graft.

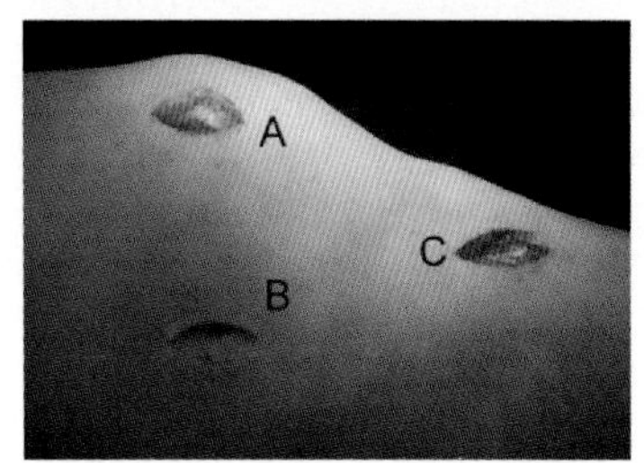

TECH FIG 3 • Incisions used for MPFL reconstruction at the left knee. **A.** Over the medial patella. **B.** Over the femoral origin of the MPFL, which lies between the adductor tubercle and the medial epicondyle. **C.** Over the pes anserinus, which is used to harvest the semitendinosus graft.

Patellar Tunnel Placement

- A longitudinal incision the length of the patella is made at the junction of the medial and middle thirds of the patella (in line with the medial border of the patellar tendon at the distal patellar pole).
- The medial 8 to 10 mm of the patella is exposed by subperiosteal dissection with a no. 15 scalpel.
- The dissection extends medially and dorsally around the patella through layers 1 (longitudinal retinaculum) and 2 (native MPFL), stopping after the transverse fibers of the native MPFL have been cut. The capsule (layer 3) is left intact (TECH FIG 4A).
- A 4.5-mm drill hole is placed on the medial side of the upper pole of the patella adjacent to the articular margin (TECH FIG 4B).
  - A corresponding drill hole is placed on the anterior surface of the patella approximately 8 mm from the

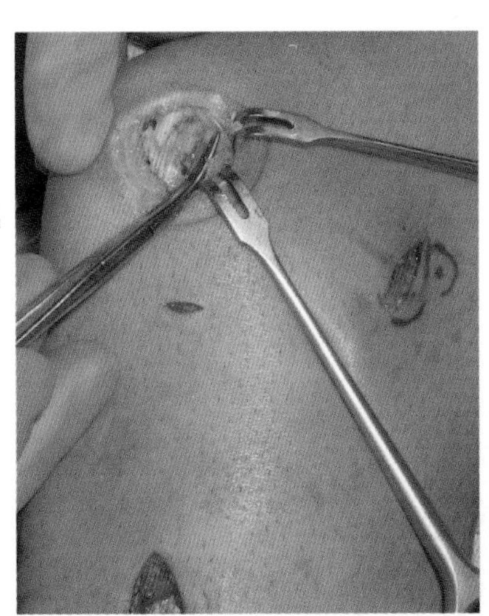

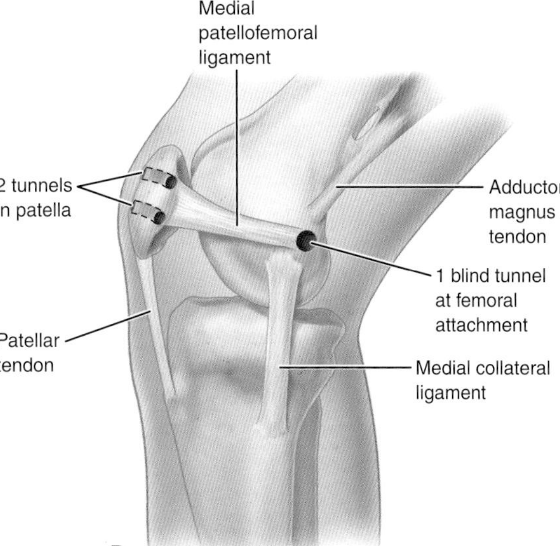

TECH FIG 4 • **A.** Exposure of the medial patella of the right knee. The medial 8 to 10 mm of the patella is exposed by subperiosteal dissection. The native MPFL is dissected off the medial border of the patella, leaving the capsule (layer 3) intact. **B.** Schematic diagram of the medial knee demonstrating the locations of the two patellar tunnels and the blind femoral tunnel, reproducing the anatomic femoral origin and patellar insertion of the native MPFL.

  - medial border (this point corresponds to the lateral edge of the original retinacular dissection).
  - The two drill holes are connected with a curved curette.
- A second 4.5-mm drill hole is placed on the medial side of the patella at a point two thirds down the length of the patella.
  - Again, a corresponding drill hole is placed on the anterior surface of the patella about 8 mm from the medial border, and the two holes are connected with a curved curette.
- If the semitendinosus graft is more than 4.5 mm in diameter, the drill holes are enlarged slightly to facilitate graft passage.
- It is important to avoid placing the distal patellar tunnel distal to the native insertion of the MPFL to avoid constraining the distal pole of the patella.

Femoral Tunnel Placement and Checking Isometry

- A skin incision is made just anterior to the palpable ridge connecting the medial femoral epicondyle and the adductor tubercle (see Tech Figs 3 and 4).
  - The knee is flexed slightly to facilitate palpation of this landmark (flexion moves the hamstrings posteriorly away from the medial epicondyle).
  - If the patient is obese and the landmarks are difficult to palpate, a small skin incision is made and palpation is done through the wound to identifty the ridge.
- The graft may be placed between layers 1 and 2 or between layers 2 and 3 (joint capsule) (ie, it may lie superficial or deep to the native MPFL).
  - Placing the graft between layers 2 and 3 is preferred, because blind dissection superficial to the native MPFL may disrupt the insertion of the VMO into the anterior portion of the MPFL; in addition, by placing the graft deep to the native MPFL, the latter may be repaired to the graft during wound closure.
  - The graft should not be placed deep to the capsule, because it should remain extra-articular to avoid graft abrasion and facilitate complete healing.
- Using a long, curved clamp, the selected interval is developed (again, preferably between layers 2 and 3) from the patellar incision anteriorly to the medial femoral epicondyle posteriorly.
- With the tip of the clamp overlying the ridge between the medial epicondyle and adductor tubercle, layers 1 and 2 are incised using a no.15 blade.
- The tip of a Beath pin is placed at a point 9 mm proximal and 5 mm posterior to the medial epicondyle; the pin is then passed toward the lateral side of the femur.
- A loop of no. 5 braided polyethylene suture is passed through the Beath pin, through the dissected retinacular tunnel, then through one of the patellar tunnels.
- The knee is taken through the ROM to evaluate isometry.
  - If lengthening occurs in flexion, a second Beath pin is placed more distally toward the medial epicondyle. The first pin is left in place to facilitate repositioning while drilling the second Beath pin. The loop of no. 5 suture is passed through the second Beath pin, and the knee is put through ROM again. If isometry is acceptable, then the first Beath pin is removed.
  - If lengthing occurs in extension, a second Beath pin is placed more proximally toward the adductor tubercle. Again, the first pin is left in place to facilitate repositioning while drilling the second Beath pin. The loop of no. 5 suture is passed through the second Beath pin and the knee put through ROM again. If isometry is acceptable, then the first Beath pin is removed.
- Once the femoral pin site is accepted, a blind tunnel is reamed into the femur the size of the doubled graft. For a semitendinosus graft, this usually is 6 to 7 mm in diameter.
- The femur is reamed to a depth of at least 20 mm, with a preferred depth of 25 mm.

Graft Passage and Fixation

- No. 5 suture is passed through the Beath pin on the looped end of the graft, and the pin then is advanced out the lateral femoral cortex to pass the graft into the femoral tunnel.
- Fixation to the femur may be achieved reliably with a 20-mm absorbable interference screw.
- The looped isometry suture, if left in place in the retinacular tunnel, may be used to pass the free ends of the graft through the retinacular interval created previously (TECH FIG 5A,B).
- The free graft arms are passed individually through their respective patellar tunnels using double 22-gauge stainless steel wire or a curved suture passer.
- The graft arms enter the medial border of the patella and exit anteriorly (TECH FIG 5C).
- The free graft arms are then doubled back and sutured on themselves just medial to the patella using two figure 8 mattress sutures of no. 2 nonabsorbable suture on a tapered needle.

A 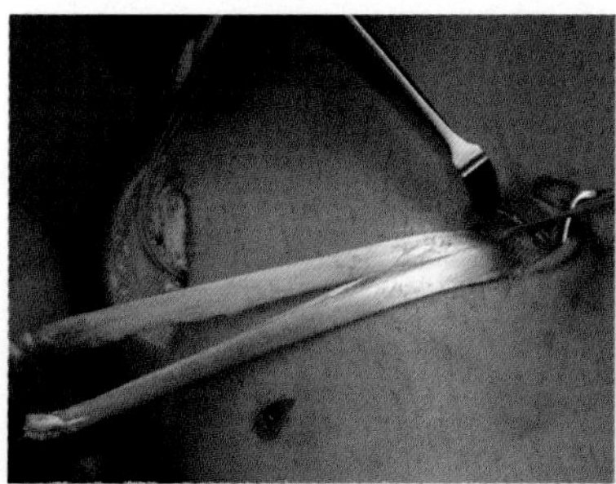

B 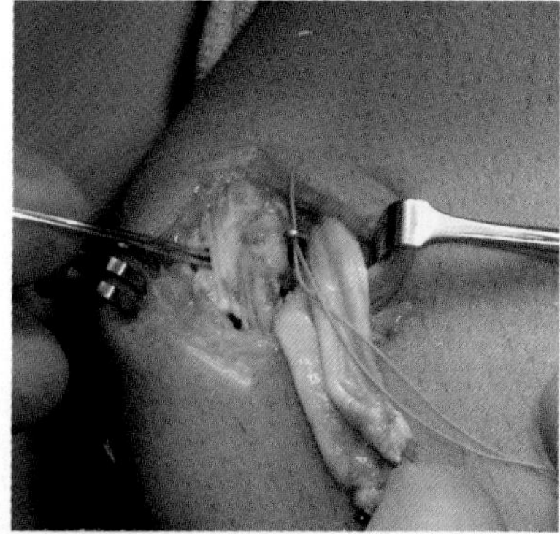

TECH FIG 5 • **A.** The synthetic isometry suture is in place. After correct placement of the femoral attachment site is confirmed using the isometry suture, the semitendinosus graft has been fixed to the femur using an interference screw. **B.** The isometry suture is used to shuttle the graft anteriorly out the medial patellar incision. The graft will then be fixed to the two patellar tunnels. *(continued)*

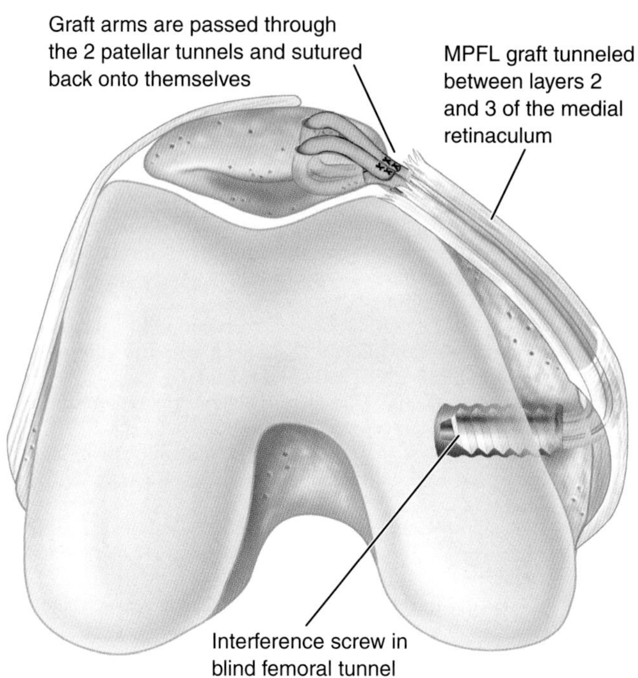
Graft arms are passed through the 2 patellar tunnels and sutured back onto themselves
MPFL graft tunneled between layers 2 and 3 of the medial retinaculum
Interference screw in blind femoral tunnel
C

TECH FIG 5 • *(continued)* **C.** Schematic diagram demonstrating fixation of the graft posteriorly into a blind femoral tunnel, and anteriorly to two patellar tunnels. At the patella, each limb of the graft enters into respective medial drill hole, exits the anterior drill hole, then is sutured back to itself medial to the patella.

- Patellar mobility is checked after the first suture is placed. There should be a good endpoint, or checkrein, with the knee in full extension and at 30 degrees of flexion, full knee ROM, and 7 to 9 mm of lateral patellar displacement from the centered position at 30 degrees of flexion.
- Excess graft is sharply removed.
- The native MPFL is sutured to the graft, and then the retinaculum is closed over the graft.
- The wounds are closed in standard fashion.

PEARLS AND PITFALLS

Indications	■ Perform examination under anesthesia to confirm excessive lateral patellar mobility. ■ Perform arthroscopy to stage articular cartilage lesions and rule out preexisting arthritis, a contraindication to MPFL reconstruction.
Femoral tunnel placement	■ This is one of the most critical steps in the operation. ■ Adjust the tunnel placement to ensure appropriate graft behavior during flexion and extension, recreating isometry.
MPFL graft tensioning	■ Center the patella in the patellar groove and ensure that the MPFL graft is lax throughout a range of motion, becoming tight only when the patella is displaced laterally from its centered position. ■ The patella should enter the trochlea from the lateral side as the knee is flexed.
Overtightened graft resulting in excessive medial constraint	■ If the patella enters the trochlea from the medial side as the knee is flexed or if there is less than 5 mm of lateral patellar glide with gentle manual force at 30 degrees of knee flexion, then the graft is overtensioned. The sutures should be removed and the graft retensioned.
Breakage of patellar bone bridge	■ May occur during preparation of the two patellar tunnels or during passage of an oversized graft through a tight patellar tunnel. ■ If this occurs, then drill a second exit hole more laterally on the anterior patellar surface or drill the tunnel transversely across the patella, exiting at the lateral patellar margin. ■ The graft can be secured by tying the sutures over a button or suturing the end of the graft to the soft tissues on the lateral patellar border.

POSTOPERATIVE CARE

- Weight bearing as tolerated is allowed immediately postoperatively in a drop-lock or knee extension brace.
  - Bracing may be continued for up to 6 weeks during ambulation to prevent falls until quadriceps control is restored.
- After the soft tissue procedure, passive ROM exercises and resisted closed-chain exercises are begun as soon as possible to restore ROM and quadriceps control.
- If a tibial tubercle osteotomy is performed, passive ROM using heel slides is begun postoperatively. No active extension is allowed for 6 postoperative weeks. At that time, full active ROM is begun, followed by closed-chain resistance exercises at 3 postoperative months.
- Patients are allowed to return to stressful activities, including sports, when they attain full ROM and have regained at least 80% of their quadriceps strength compared to the noninjured limb.
- If at least 90 degrees of flexion is not achieved by 6 postoperative weeks, then the intensity of the therapy program must be increased; manipulation under anesthesia (MUA) may be needed between 9 and 12 postoperative weeks if stiffness does not resolve with therapy alone.

OUTCOMES

- In a series of 92 knees treated with MPFL reconstruction, Fithian et al[7] reported only 7 failures or reoperations (7.6%) and only one case of frank patellar redislocation (1.1%). Most of the reoperations were for stiffness and were treated successfully with MUA.
- Schottle et al[22] reported 86% good and excellent results at 47 months after MPFL reconstruction using semitendinosus autograft. In their series of 15 MPFL reconstructions, there was one case of bilateral recurrent instability.
- Steiner et al,[23] in a series of 34 patients treated with MPFL reconstruction using a variety of graft sources, reported 91.1% good and excellent results at 66 months and no recurrent dislocations.
- In series by both Schottle et al[22] and Steiner et al,[23] the presence of trochlear dysplasia did not affect the outcome of MPFL reconstruction.
- Nomura and Inoue[18] reported on 12 knees after hybrid MPFL reconstruction using semitendinosus graft at a minimum of 3 years follow-up. There were 83% good and excellent results, and no cases of recurrent patellar subluxation or dislocation.

COMPLICATIONS

- Stiffness
- Redislocation
- Excessive medial patellar constraint resulting in a painful, overconstrained patella[6,12,16,17]
- Patellar fracture

REFERENCES

1. Andrade A, Thomas N. Randomized comparison of operative vs. nonoperative treatment following first time patellar dislocation. Presented at the European Society for Sports, Knee and Arthroscopy, Rome, 2002.
2. Caton J, Deschamps G, Chambat P, et al. Patella infera. Apropos of 128 cases. Rev Chir Orthop Reparatrice Appar Mot 1982;68: 317–325.
3. Crosby EB, Insall J. Recurrent dislocation of the patella: relation of treatment of osteoarthritis. J Bone Joint Surg Am 1976;58A:9–13.
4. Dejour H, Walch G, Nove-Josserand L, et al. Factors of patellar instability: an anatomic radiographic study. Knee Surg Sports Traumatol Arthrosc 1994;2:19–26.
5. Elias DA, White LM, Fithian DC. Acute lateral patellar dislocation at MR imaging: injury patterns of medial patellar soft-tissue restraints and osteochondral injuries of the inferomedial patella. Radiology 2002;225:736–743.
6. Elias JJ, Cosgarea AJ. Technical errors during medial patellofemoral ligament reconstruction could overload medial patellofemoral cartilage. Am J Sports Med 2006;34:1478–1485.
7. Fithian DC, Gupta N. Patellar instability: principals of soft tissue repair and reconstruction. Tech Knee Surg 2006;5:19–26.
8. Fithian DC, Paxton WE, Stone ML, et al. Epidemiology and natural history of acute patellar dislocation. Am J Sports Med 2004;32: 1114–1121.
9. Hautamaa PV, Fithian DC, Kaufman KR, et al. Medial soft tissue restraints in lateral patellar instability and repair. Clin Orthop Rel Res 1998;349:174–182.
10. Kessler I. The grasping technique for tendon repair. Hand 1973;5: 253–255.
11. Maenpaa H, Lehto MU. Patellofemoral osteoarthritis after patellar dislocation. Clin Orthop Rel Res 1997;339:156–162.
12. Muneta T, Sekiya I, Tsuchiya M, et al. A technique for reconstruction of the medial patellofemoral ligament. Clin Orthop Rel Res 1999; 359:151–155.
13. Nikku R, Nietosvaara Y, Aalto K, et al. Operative treatment of primary patellar dislocation does not improve medium-term outcome: a 7-year follow-up report and risk analysis of 127 randomized patients. Acta Orthop 2005;76:699–704.
14. Nikku R, Nietosvaara Y, Kallio PE, et al. Operative versus closed treatment of primary dislocation of the patella: similar 2-year results in 125 randomized patients. Acta Orthop Scand 1997;68:419–423.
15. Nomura E, Horiuchi Y, Inoue M. Correlation of MR imaging findings and open exploration of medial patellofemoral ligament injuries in acute patellar dislocations. Knee 2002;9:139–143.
16. Nomura E, Horiuchi Y, Kihara M. Medial patellofemoral ligament restraint in lateral patellar translation and reconstruction. Knee 2000;7:121–127.
17. Nomura E, Horiuchi Y, Kihara M. A mid-term follow-up of medial patellofemoral ligament reconstruction using an artificial ligament for recurrent patellar dislocation. Knee 2000;7:211–215.
18. Nomura E, Inoue M. Hybrid medial patellofemoral ligament reconstruction using the semitendinosus tendon for recurrent patellar dislocation: minimum 3 years' follow-up. Arthroscopy 2006;22: 787–793.
19. Nomura E, Inoue M, Osada N. Anatomical analysis of the medial patellofemoral ligament of the knee, especially at the femoral attachment. Knee Surg Sports Traumatol Arthrosc 2005;13:510–515.
20. Nomura E, Inoue M, Osada N. Augmented repair of avulsion-tear type medial patellofemoral ligament injury in acute patellar dislocation. Knee Surg Sports Traumatol Arthrosc 2005;13:346–351.
21. Remy F, Chantelot C, Fontaine C, et al. Inter- and intraobserver reproducibility in radiographic diagnosis and classification of femoral trochlear dysplasia. Surg Radiol Anat 1998;20:285–289.
22. Schottle PB, Fucentese SF, Romero J. Clinical and radiological outcome of medial patellofemoral ligament reconstruciton with a semitendinosus autograft for patella instability. Knee Surg Sports Traumatol Arthrosc 2005;13:516–521.
23. Steiner TM, Torga-Spak R, Teitge RA. Medial patellofemoral ligament reconstruction in patients with lateral patellar instability and trochlear dysplasia. Am J Sports Med 2006;34:1254–1261.
24. Teitge RA, Faerber WW, Des Madryl P, et al. Stress radiographs of the patellofemoral joint. J Bone Joint Surg Am 1996;78A:193–203.

Chapter 53 Tibial Tubercle Transfer

John P. Fulkerson

DEFINITION

- Tibial tubercle transfer is a versatile surgical alternative in the treatment of difficult and resistant patellofemoral disorders ranging from patellofemoral instability to patellofemoral arthritis.
- Patients with combined instability and arthritis often benefit from tibial tubercle transfer.
- Tibial tubercle transfer may be best regarded as "compensatory." In other words, if a multiplicity of structure and alignment factors leads to patellar instability or arthritis, carefully planned repositioning of the tibial tubercle can compensate for other deficiencies, providing permanent relief of pain and instability.

ANATOMY

- The patella articulates within the femoral trochlea in such a way that the distal aspect of the patella enters the trochlea from a slightly lateralized position upon initiation of knee flexion. Normally the patella enters the trochlea promptly within the first 10 degrees of flexion, first making contact with the distal aspect of the patella.
- As the knee flexes further, load is transferred more proximally on the patella such that in full flexion, contact is on the proximal aspect of the patella. The intervening flexion transfers load more gradually along the patella, moving proximally with each degree of flexion load.[11]
- As the patella enters the trochlea with further knee flexion, the trochlea becomes deeper, so that containment of the patella is improved. Therefore, in most people, the point of greatest instability is early flexion of the knee, when the trochlea is at its shallowest and containment of the patella is most limited.
- The position of the tibial tuberosity relative to the femoral trochlea further complicates the process of patella entry into the trochlea.[4]
  - This relationship has been referred to as the tibial tuberosity to trochlea groove (TT-TG) index, measured in millimeters using superimposed tomographic images of the position of the central trochlea and the tibial tubercle (**FIG 1**).
- The patella is contained within a soft tissue investing layer of tendon and retinacular structure.
  - The lateral retinaculum extends to the iliotibial band but also proximally to the lateral femur and to the tibia (the patellofemoral and patellotibial components, respectively, of the lateral retinaculum).
  - On the medial side is the medial patellofemoral ligament (MPFL), which extends from the proximal half of the patella to the adductor tubercle region.[1]
  - The patellar tendon is located distally, with the quadriceps tendon proximally connecting the patella to the quadriceps muscle. The quadriceps tendon is a massive tendon, including a major vastus lateralis tendon component on the proximal lateral aspect of the patella.
  - The superolateral corner of the patella is supported dynamically by the vastus lateralis obliquus, which interdigitates with the lateral intermuscular septum.[14]

PATHOGENESIS

- The pathogenesis of problems around the patellofemoral joint relates to dysplasia of anterior knee anatomy, malalignment, and trauma.
- Most patients with significant dysplasia have a congenital underlying imbalance of the extensor mechanism, which leads to improper morphologic development.

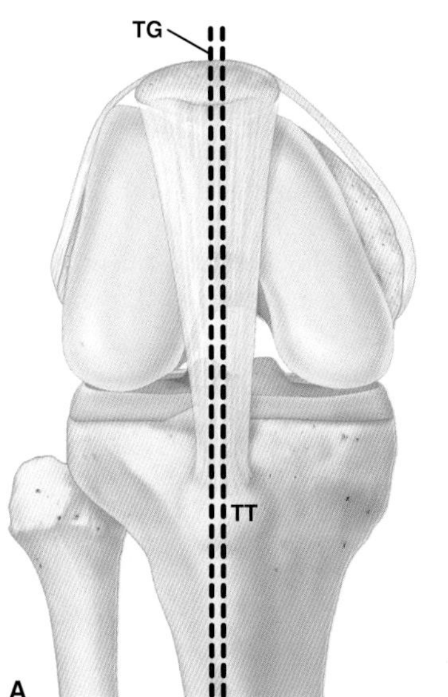

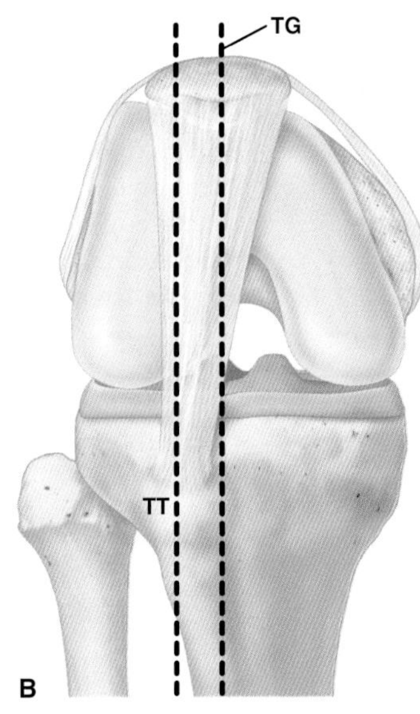

FIG 1 • The relation of the tibial tubercle (TT) to the central trochlear groove (TG)—the TT-TG relationship—pertains to patella instability. **A.** Normal TT-TG relationship, in which the tibial tubercle and trochlear groove are lined up. **B.** Lateralized tibial tubercle.

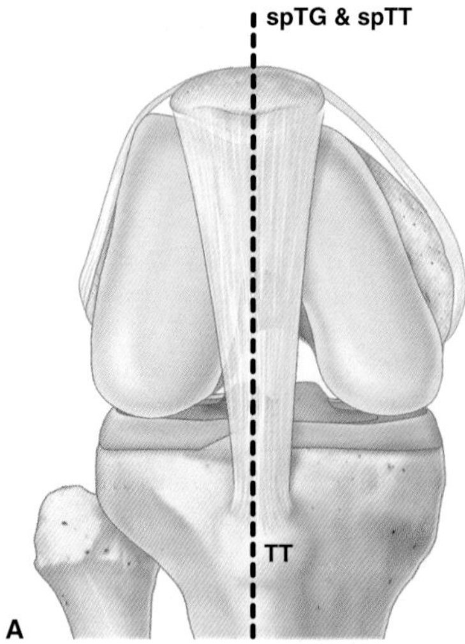

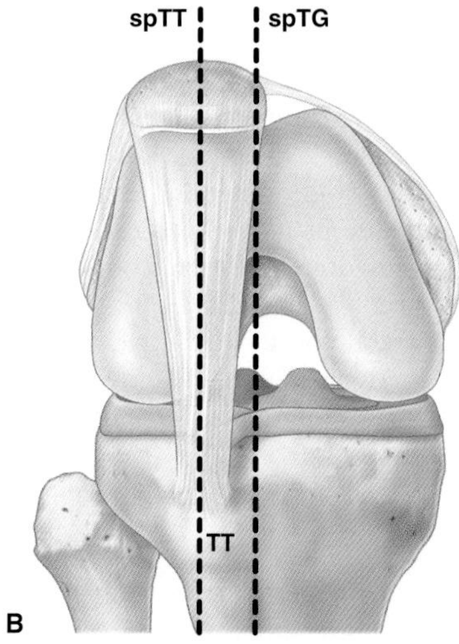

FIG 2 • **A.** Normal trochlear groove. **B.** With prolonged lateral patella tracking, the lateral trochlea becomes flattened, further aggravating lateral patella instability and stretching the medial patella support structure (including the medial patellofemoral ligament). *, center of trochlea; *spTG,* sagittal plane of trochlear groove; *spTT,* sagittal plane of tibial tubercle; *TT,* tibial tubercle.

- A chronically lateralized extensor mechanism is likely to cause abnormally high lateral pressure on the femoral trochlea, thereby leading to developmental flattening of the lateral trochlea and also flattening of the patella (**FIG 2**). Although it is not always the case, this pattern of development most likely explains the poor development of the lateral trochlea and persistent instability in patients with abnormal extensor mechanism alignment. Such patients stretch the medial patella support structure over time, leading to subluxation and tilt of the patella in many cases.
  - This stretching can lead to chronic instability, chronic overload of the lateral patellofemoral joint, dislocation (which often causes *medial* patella articular damage), breakdown of the lateral patellofemoral joint, and pain related to overload of the joint and peripatellar retinacula.[13]
- Some patients have anterior knee pain as the result of blunt trauma, usually with the knee flexed.
- An impact to the flexed knee and resulting trauma to the patellofemoral joint usually leads to proximal patella injury. This is important, because anteriorization of the tibial tubercle shifts contact on the patella proximally and can, therefore, exacerbate a lesion on the proximal patella related to blunt injury.
- Because movement of the tibial tubercle was not involved in the injury in many patients who have had blunt trauma, the problem usually is not one of abnormal extensor mechanism alignment requiring correction.

NATURAL HISTORY

- The natural history of patellofemoral pain, instability, or arthrosis often relates to the imbalance noted earlier. With chronic lateral tracking of the patella in the trochlea, overload occurs with increased point loading on the patella and trochlea, particularly the patella.
- Eventually this can lead to breakdown of articular cartilage and what Ficat[7] has called *excessive lateral pressure syndrome* (**FIG 3**).
  - Schutzer [21]demonstrated a high incidence of patellofemoral tilt and subluxation in patients with patellofemoral pain, compared with controls.
- With dislocation of the patella, the medial patellofemoral ligament is torn and, even after healing, elongated. This further exacerbates any tendency toward lateral displacement of the patella out of the trochlea.
- With blunt trauma, pain is related to impact and subchondral bone injury, generally on the proximal patella. This pain, then, originates from injured subchondral bone, because there are no nerves in cartilage.

PATIENT HISTORY AND PHYSICAL FINDINGS

- With the patient who may be a candidate for tibial tubercle transfer, it is important to establish that this definitive surgery truly is indicated because of a structural alignment imbalance or articular overload condition leading to instability or pain.
  - The physical examination should emphasize a very critical look at patella tracking within the femoral trochlea, the condition of the medial patellofemoral ligament, evidence of articular breakdown of the patellofemoral joint, evidence of retinacular or soft tissue pain, and a search for other possible causes of pain such as medial or lateral compartment disease or referred pain from the hip or back.
- Careful palpation of the retinacular structure around the patella will indicate whether there is soft tissue or retinacular overload contributing to pain.[18]
  - In some cases, simple release of the painful retinacular structure may be all that is needed.
- When examining the medial patellofemoral ligament, holding the patella laterally in extension is recommended, then slowly

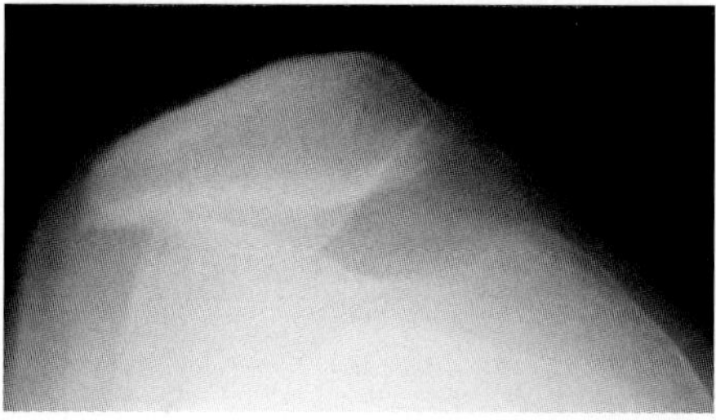

FIG 3 • Excessive lateral pressure leads to lateral patella chondropathy and breakdown. (Courtesy of David Dejour.)

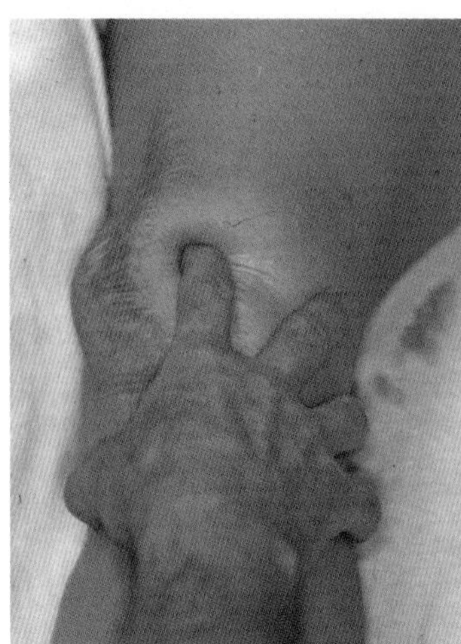

FIG 4 • Test for medial patella subluxation. The patella is held medial and knee is flexed abruptly. If patella relocation reproduces the patient's symptom, pathologic medial subluxation probably is present.

flexing the knee to see whether the medial patellofemoral ligament delivers the patella into the central trochlea by 20 to 30 degrees of knee flexion. A distinct pressure, pushing the examining finger back as the patella enters the trochlea, should be encountered using this technique.

- If the patella remains lateralized with the examining finger holding it lateral as the knee is flexed to 20 to 30 degrees of flexion, the medial patellofemoral ligament is incompetent.[10]

- Similarly, in a patient who has had previous extensor mechanism surgery, the examiner should hold the patella medially in extension and flex the knee abruptly to 30 to 40 degrees of flexion (**FIG 4**).
  - If the patella enters the trochlea very suddenly and reproduces the patient's symptom, he or she actually may have a medial instability problem (ie, medial subluxation) that requires repair or reconstruction of the lateral support structure or even lateralization of the tibial tubercle if it previously was over-medialized.
- The patella is held in the central trochlea, and the knee is flexed with compression of the patella to see if this elicits crepitus or pain. The degree of flexion at which this crepitus or pain occurs is important in localizing the location of the lesion, bearing in mind that the articulation surface of the patella moves proximally as the knee is flexed. This compression of the patella in the trochlea should be repeated as the patient extends the knee actively against resistance of the other examining hand from full flexion up to full extension, taking note of where pain or crepitus occurs with active extension against resistance.
- Every patient should be examined prone so that the hip can be rotated internally and externally to see if there is a source of pain within the hip. With the patient prone, the pelvis is flat, and, therefore, flexion of the knee may be completed to compare with the contralateral side to establish whether the quadriceps and extensor mechanism are overly tight. The patient should be taught at this time how to stretch the extensor mechanism.
- Nonoperative treatment should be exhausted before considering surgical intervention.

IMAGING AND OTHER DIAGNOSTIC STUDIES

- In diagnosis of the anterior knee, a standardized office radiograph with the knee flexed 45 degrees and standardized axial radiograph of the patellofemoral joint with the knee flexed exactly to 30 degrees is very important.[15]
  - By 45 degrees of knee flexion, the patella normally is centralized in the femoral trochlea. This is a good screening test in the office to determine whether there is significant imbalance of the extensor mechanism.
  - Radiographs taken in more than 45 degrees knee flexion are not particularly useful in most patients.
  - Our practice has not found 30-60-90–degree radiographs useful.
  - Many patients present for evaluation with axial radiographs taken only at 90 degrees of flexion. This probably is easier for radiology technicians, because they can simply hang the patient's legs over the side of an examining table and take the axial radiograph in this fashion. It is very important to standardize flexion to 45 degrees, using a support frame as needed.
- The other important office radiograph is the true lateral view[16] (**FIG 5**), which is taken with the knee at 30 degrees of flexion and standing. The posterior femoral condyle should be overlapped.
  - This view is technically demanding, but most radiology technicians with reasonable experience can palpate the posterior condyles, and with one or sometimes two tries, obtain a good lateral view with overlap (or near-complete overlap) of the posterior condyles.
  - This study shows the femoral trochlea completely, so that the central sulcus can be identified as well as both medial and lateral aspects of the trochlea from proximal to distal.
- Other imaging studies include CT, MRI, and radionuclide scan. Relatively few patients require these studies.
  - If CT is done, it is best performed at 0, 15, 30, and 45 degrees of knee flexion, obtaining mid-patella transverse images to see how the patella enters the trochlea. This should be done with reproduction of normal standing alignment on the tomographic table.
  - MRI is less useful in many patients but can be helpful in evaluating articular cartilage and soft tissue structure, as well as gaining insight into subchondral bone reaction.

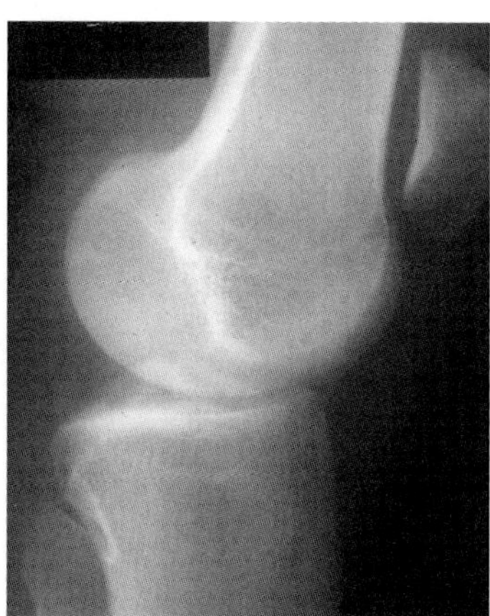

FIG 5 • The true lateral radiograph defines the osseous structure of the trochlea most accurately.

- Radionuclide scanning is not often used but can be extremely helpful in determining subchondral bone reaction to overload.[5] It may be most applicable in patients with trauma to the anterior knee, unexplained anterior knee pain, or chronic patella overload, and in cases involving workers' compensation litigation where objective findings beyond the normal studies needed to determine appropriate treatment are particularly important.
- In some cases, a single photon emission computed tomographic (SPECT) scan also can be helpful in accurately locating a source of subchondral bone overload. SPECT may play a role, selectively, in patients who require a patella unloading or resurfacing procedure.

NONOPERATIVE MANAGEMENT

- Before tibial tubercle transfer is considered, all patients must exhaust nonoperative management, including complete lower extremity core stability therapy, patellofemoral taping and bracing (I prefer the Tru-Pull brace that I helped design, DJ ORTHO, Vista, CA), and modification of activity.
- Viscosupplementation may be helpful in some patients with patellofemoral arthritis but has not been very helpful in most cases?

SURGICAL MANAGEMENT

- In patients with more severe extensor mechanism malalignment, instability, pain, and eventual articular cartilage breakdown are fairly common. When specific factors such as disruption of the MPFL cause instability, reconstruction of the deficient structure should be considered first.
  - In many patients with patella instability, restoration of medial support, either by imbrication (open or arthroscopic) or reconstruction of the medial patellofemoral ligament and release of tight lateral retinaculum, may be the procedure of choice. In general, this is the first line of surgical treatment after failed nonoperative measures in a patient with patella instability related to deficiency of medial support structure.
- In patients with more severe dysplasia, a high TT-TG index (see Fig 1B), and degenerative change in the patella or trochlea, tibial tubercle transfer offers an opportunity to improve balance permanently and provide long-term relief of instability.
- Tibial tubercle transfer in the treatment of patella instability is best used when the TT-TG index is high (>20 in most cases), the Q angle is high (usually >20 degrees) or the lateral trochlea is dysplastic, such that soft tissue reconstruction alone will either be less likely to succeed or require excessive tension resulting in overload of the medial patellofemoral joint.[20]
  - Anteriorization alone is best reserved for patients with patella arthritis alone without malalignment.
  - The primary concern with MPFL reconstruction in the face of more serious malalignment and patella instability is the need to "pull" the patella in a posteromedial direction to gain stability, thereby adding load to the patella that eventually might lead to patellofemoral joint degeneration. For this reason, the wise surgeon will recognize the inherent benefit of tibial tubercle transfer in selected patients with more severe patella instability to compensate for the malalignment problems leading to the instability in a way that limits or avoids point articular loading on the patella.[6]
  - Tibial tubercle transfer also provides immediate fixation and stability, making early ROM possible, further reducing the risk of stiffness, tightness, and chronic pain in the anterior knee following reconstructive surgery for instability.
- In the treatment of patellofemoral arthritis, tibial tubercle transfer plays an important role in joint preservation.
  - Many patients have patellofemoral arthritis as a result of excessive lateral pressure, as originally described by Ficat.[7] This excessive lateral pressure eventually causes erosion of the lateral patellofemoral joint, sometimes to bone, because of the constant lateralization of the patella related to lateral subluxation and high lateral pressure on the lateral patella facet. Lateral release has been used to reduce some of this pressure and is helpful in the early stages when patella tilt is prominent.
  - Tibial tubercle transfer is a powerful procedure for unloading and rebalancing the extensor mechanism, however, placing the patella into the center trochlea and maintaining it there through a range of motion.
- By adding some anteriorization to a medial tibial tubercle transfer (ie, anteromedial tibial tubercle transfer) the distal articular surface of the patella also may be unloaded.[19] This is important, because many patients with patellofemoral chondrosis or arthrosis have distal patella articular breakdown or pain. Anteriorization of the tibial tubercle unloads the distal articular surface of the patella permanently, and the medialization component of this procedure rebalances the patella in the central trochlea, unloading the lateral facet.
  - Most patients with chronic lateralization of the extensor mechanism develop lateral facet breakdown and distal patella degeneration over time because of the abnormal shear stress and lateral overload. Anteromedial tibial tubercle transfer compensates for this and is, therefore, the procedure of choice for treating articular degeneration and pain emanating from the distal or lateral patella articular surface.
- Anterolateral tibial tubercle transfer[9] may be best regarded as a salvage procedure in patients who have had previous overmedialization of the tibial tubercle. It has been helpful in relieving pain related to chronic medial patellofemoral arthritis resulting from a previous Hauser procedure in which the tibial tubercle was moved posteriorly, medially, and distally to stabilize the extensor mechanism at an earlier time.

TECHNIQUES

MEDIAL TIBIAL TUBERCLE TRANSFER

Incision and Dissection

- Medial tibial tubercle transfer is best approached through a midline incision from the mid patella to a region approximately 5 to 7 cm distal to the tibial tubercle.[3]
- The medial and lateral borders of the patella tendon are identified, the anterior tibialis muscle is reflected posteriorly and retracted, the skin edges are retracted, and a cut is made deep to the tibial tubercle.

Osteotomy

- A flat incision is made posterior to the tibial tubercle, tapered anteriorly at its distal extent such that only about 1 mm of bone is left at the distal tip of the osteotomy and the proximal cut is made about 2 mm above the patellar tendon insertion.
  - This cut should be made perpendicular to the anterior surface of the tibia such that a flat ledge is left to add

additional stability to the transferred tibial tubercle. This proximal cut must be made in such a way that the tibial tubercle may be freely moved medially, ie, so that the medial side of the proximal cut is more proximal than the lateral side of the proximal cut, open medially.
- The thickness of the cut deep to the tibial tubercle will vary depending on the individual patient's need for medialization.
  - In patients with a severe dysplasia requiring more than 1 cm of medialization, a deeper cut will be required.
  - In patients requiring 1 cm of medialization, a proximal tibial tubercle thickness of 1 to 1.5 cm is ample in most cases.
- Care must be taken to taper this osteotomy anteriorly at the distal extent of the cut to allow for easy greenstick fracturing of the tip of the osteotomy to move the tubercle medially.

Completion of the Transfer

- After the osteotomy has been completed with an oscillating saw, the proximal cut usually is made with a ½-inch osteotome.
- The osteotomized fragment is elevated and then displaced medially. If there is an overhang of bone medially, it can be removed with the saw or a rongeur.
- The fragment is then stabilized securely with two cortical lag screws (TECH FIG 1), carefully measuring the depth of the drill hole, overdrilling the proximal fragment, and lagging the fragment down using the posterior cortex to hold the cortical screw.
  - Care must be taken not to allow the cortical screw tip to protrude any more than necessary beyond the posterior cortex.

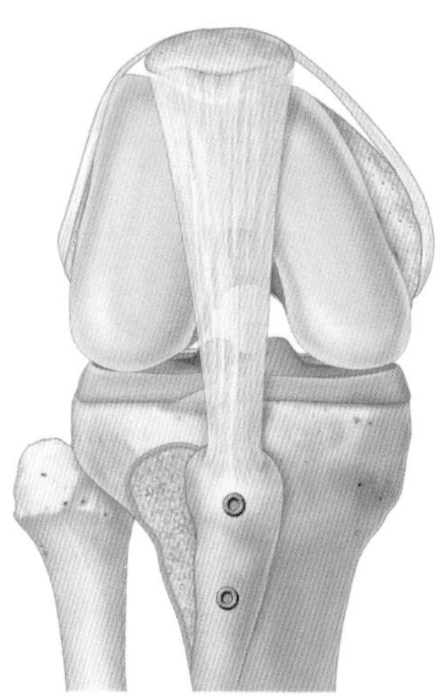

TECH FIG 1 • Correction of abnormal TT-TG relationship by medialization of tibial tubercle.

- The surgeon releases the lateral retinaculum either arthroscopically or by open surgery to achieve the needed balance of the extensor mechanism upon tibial tubercle transfer.
- Some thickening and even mild infrapatellar contracture may be observed in patients who have had longstanding and more severe imbalance of the extensor mechanism. This also should be released at the time of surgery.
- Tracking of the patella within the central trochlea should be confirmed arthroscopically or openly after the tibial tubercle transfer.

ANTEROMEDIAL TIBIAL TUBERCLE TRANSFER

Incision and Dissection

- To unload both the distal and lateral aspects of the patella, an oblique osteotomy must be created deep to the tibial tubercle, and the tibial tubercle transferred in both anterior and medial directions.[8,12]
- To perform anteromedial tibial tubercle transfer, a longitudinal incision close to midline, extending from a region about halfway between the patella and the tibial tubercle to about 7 cm distal to the tibial tubercle usually is sufficient.
- After isolating the patellar tendon, the anterior tibialis muscle is released and reflected posteriorly.
- Because an oblique osteotomy will be made from medial to lateral, a large retractor must be placed to retract the anterior tibialis muscle laterally to view the saw making the osteotomy cut as it exits on the posterolateral aspect of the tibia. The entire lateral side of the tibia must be under direct view[11] (TECH FIG 2).

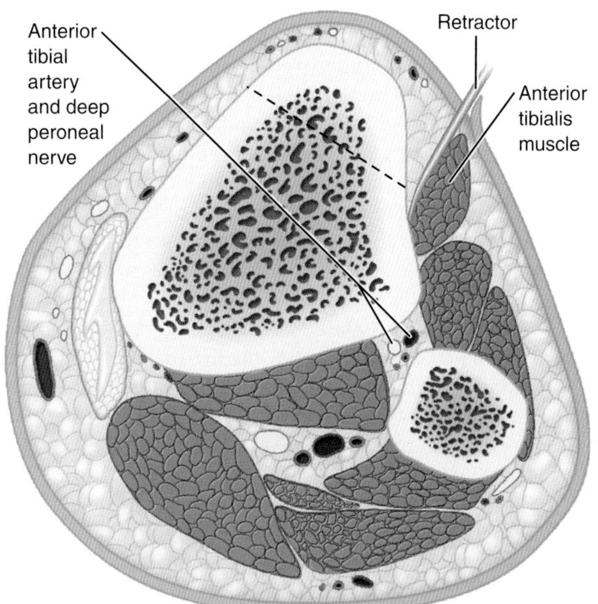

TECH FIG 2 • Retraction of the tibialis anterior gives a full view of the entire lateral proximal tibia.

Osteotomy

- At this point, it usually is best to use a guide, such as the Tracker guide (Mitek, Norwood, MA), to ensure an accurate osteotomy cut. With experience, some surgeons can

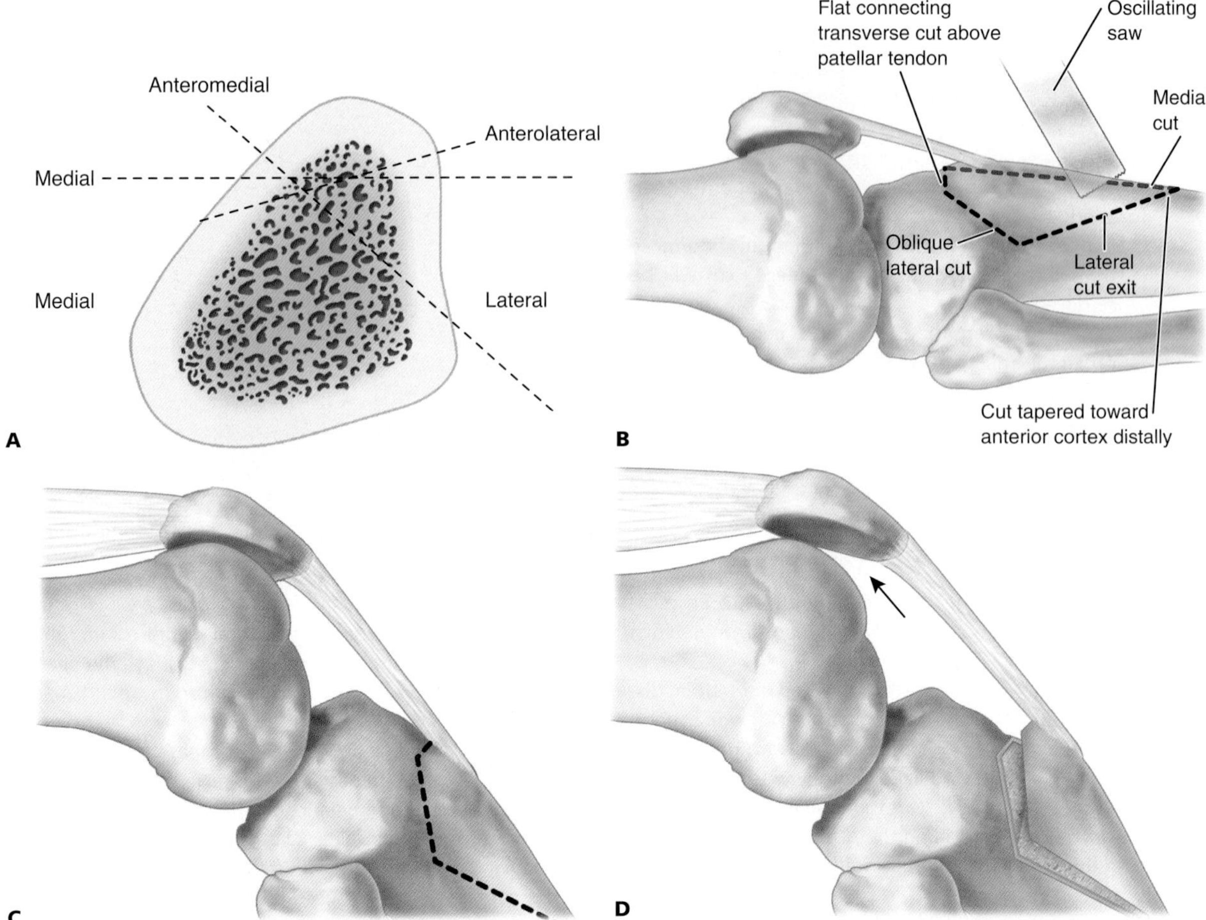

TECH FIG 3 • A. Displacement of the tibial tubercle transfer showing planes for cuts. **B.** For anteromedial tibial tubercle transfer, the cut proceeds obliquely from medial to lateral, tapering toward the anterior crest distally. After transferring the tibial tubercle along the osteotomy (**C**), both anteriorization and medialization of the tibial tubercle are achieved (**D**).

make this cut without a guide, but only a surgeon who is doing this type of surgery on a regular basis will feel comfortable without guide control.

- An external fixator block also may be used to create an appropriate orientation for the osteotomy (**TECH FIG 3A**). A drill bit is left at the top and bottom of the osteotomy.
- The osteotomy usually extends from the level of the tibial tubercle to a level of about 7 to 9 cm distally on the tibia and again must exit at the level of the anterior cortex of the tibia to avoid a large fragment distally.
  - Making a deep cut distally increases the risk of tibia fracture; this should be avoided.
- After the guide is placed at the desired angle to create an oblique osteotomy from medial to lateral, a cut is made from the region immediately adjacent to the patella tendon insertion medially and angled posterolaterally so that the saw blade will exit on the lateral cortex (**TECH FIG 3B**).
  - This strategy avoids injury to the anterior tibial artery and deep peroneal nerve, which are around the posterolateral corner of the tibia posteriorly.
  - The cut should start distally first where it is most visible, and as the oblique cut proceeds proximally, it will become more posterior.
- Once the proximal extent of the cut has reached the level of the mid to posterior portion of the lateral tibia cortex, it should be stopped at the lateral side. An osteotome or saw then is used to make a back cut from the corner of the proximal lateral corner of the osteotomy up to a point proximal to the patellar tendon laterally.
  - This allows for release of the lateral cortex when the osteotomy has been completed, and the osteotomized fragment will be displaced anteromedially.
- The third cut for anteromedial tibial tubercle transfer is directly proximal to the patellar tendon insertion on the tibia, about 2 mm above the patellar tendon insertion.
  - This cut usually is made with a ¼- or ½-inch osteotome under direct vision using an Army-Navy retractor to hold the patellar tendon anteriorly.
  - It is best made from medial to lateral and connects the proximal extent of the medial osteotomy cut to the oblique back cut on the lateral side so that the osteotomy is now free to displace anteromedially.
  - It is moved anteromedially by greenstick fracturing the anterior cortex distally, which should be no more than 1 to 2 mm thick at its distal extent.
  - The osteotomized fragment is moved about 1 cm but may be moved slightly more, as needed, to achieve more anteriorization or medialization.

- The obliquity of this osteotomy will be determined by how much anteriorization and how much medialization the surgeon wants (TECH FIG 3C,D).
  - When there is a greater need for realignment of the extensor mechanism, the cut should be made flatter, so that more medialization can be achieved.
  - When it is more urgent to unload a damaged or painful distal patella, the cut should be made more oblique (steeper), allowing more anteriorization.
  - Thus, this osteotomy is customized for each patient, depending on the specific need.

Completion of the Transfer

- The osteotomized fragment is fixed securely with two cortical lag screws.
  - These screws must be carefully positioned to ensure that they remain within the cortex and that they have good cortical bone purchase on both sides.
  - If the most proximal cut has been made carefully, there will be a ledge of bone on which the osteotomized fragment will rest, which will add stability to the osteotomy beyond what the screws offer.
- Lateral release is accomplished as needed to free the patella. In patients with any retropatellar tendon contracture, this tendon also is released to free up the extensor mechanism.
- After tibial tubercle transfer, hemostasis must be meticulous, and then the subcutaneous tissue and skin are closed. We prefer skin sutures or skin clips rather than subcuticular sutures.

ANTEROLATERAL TIBIAL TUBERCLE TRANSFER

- In the very small number of patients who have had previous overmedialization of the tibial tubercle, an osteotomy cut deep to the previously transferred tibial tubercle may be made in a slightly oblique lateral-to-medial direction, and the tibial tubercle transferred anterolaterally.
- Fixation and rehabilitation are similar to anteromedial tibial tubercle transfer.

PEARLS AND PITFALLS

Avoiding complications	■ Patients should stay on crutches for at least 6 weeks, because fracture is a risk with weight bearing that is too aggressive. ■ Smoking should be stopped before surgery and not resumed for at least 2 months because of its adverse effect on bone healing. ■ Surgery should be accurate and fixation secure. ■ Patients should start ROM very soon after surgery to avoid stiffness. ■ All patients should receive some form of postoperative anticoagulation, and should have prophylactic antibiotics at the time of surgery. ■ Hemostasis should be meticulous, and proper drainage of hematoma implemented as needed.

POSTOPERATIVE CARE

- Following tibial tubercle transfer, immediate ROM is important.
  - If stability is secure, patients are started immediately on ROM exercises.
  - These may start with a single cycle of flexion a day if proximal reconstruction has been done and there is concern about stretching out a proximal repair.
  - In such cases, a short period of immobilization in extension may be appropriate for soft tissue healing, but a single cycle of knee flexion daily after the first 10 to 12 days is important to ensure full ROM later and maximal ROM ultimately.
- Patients are kept on crutches for 6 to 8 weeks and resume weight bearing as tolerated after 6 weeks.
- During the initial 6 weeks, we recommend toe-touch or light weight bearing on the affected side.
- We recommend anticoagulation with aspirin for at least 4 to 6 weeks for most patients.
- Most of our patients go home from same-day surgery and are seen in 1 to 3 days as needed and then for suture removal and radiographs at 10 to 12 days.
- Steri-strips are applied and kept in place for 4 to 6 weeks to minimize wound spread.

COMPLICATIONS

- The primary concerns following tibial tubercle transfer are fracture of the tibia,[22] stiffness, thrombophlebitis, nonunion, infection, and hematoma.
- These complications usually can be avoided with proper care.
- Gross obesity increases the risk of complications.

OUTCOMES

- Buuck[2] reviewed the results of anteromedial tibial tubercle transfer in patients 4 to 12 years following the procedure and demonstrated that good results are maintained over time.
- Our follow-up studies have consistently revealed a satisfactory outcome in 85% to 90% of patients. Pidoriano et al[17]

demonstrated that results are closely related to the location of articular lesions. Patients with lateral and distal patellar lesions are more likely to experience relief than patients with proximal (dashboard) or medial (s/p dislocation) lesions.

REFERENCES

1. Amis AA, Firer P, Mountney J, et al. Anatomy and biomechanics of the medial patellofemoral ligament. Knee 2003;10:215–220.
2. Buuck DA, Fulkerson JP. Anteromedialization of the tibial tubercle: a 4- to 12- year follow-up. Oper Tech Sports Med 2000;8:131–137.
3. Cox JS. Evaluation of the Roux-Elmslie-Trillat procedure for knee extensor realignment. Am J Sports Med 1982;10:303–310.
4. Dejour H, Walch G, Nove-Josserand L, et al. Factors of patellar instability: an anatomic radiographic study. Knee Surg Sports Traumatol Arthrosc 1994;2:19–26.
5. Dye SF, Chew MH. The use of scintigraphy to detect increased osseous metabolic activity about the knee. J Bone Joint Surg Am 1993; 75A:1388–1406.
6. Farr J. Anteromedialization of the tibial tubercle for treatment of patellofemoral malpositioning and concomitant isolated patellofemoral arthrosis. Tech Orthop 1997;12:151–164.
7. Ficat P. The syndrome of lateral hyperpressure of the patella (translated from French). Acta Orthopaedica Belgica 1978;44(1):65–76.
8. Fulkerson JP. Anteromedialization of the tibial tuberosity for patellofemoral malalignment. Clin Orthop Rel Res 1983;177: 176–181.
9. Fulkerson JP. Anterolateralization of the tibial tubercle. Tech Orthop 1997;12:165–169.
10. Fulkerson JP. A clinical test for medial patella tracking. Tech Orthop 1997;12:144.
11. Fulkerson JP. Disorders of the Patellofemoral Joint. Philadelphia: Lippincott Williams & Wilkins, 2005.
12. Fulkerson JP, Becker GJ, Meaney JA, et al. Anteromedial tibial tubercle transfer without bone graft. Am J Sports Med 1990;18:490–497.
13. Fulkerson JP, Tennant R, Jaivin JS, et al. Histologic evidence of retinacular nerve injury associated with patellofemoral malalignment. Clin Orthop Rel Res 1985;197:196–205.
14. Hallisey MJ, Doherty N, Bennett WF, et al. Anatomy of the junction of the vastus lateralis tendon and the patella. J Bone Joint Surg Am 1987;69A:545–549.
15. Merchant AC, Mercer RL, Jacobsen RH, et al. Radiographic analysis of patellofemoral congruence. J Bone Joint Surg Am 1974;56A: 1391–1396.
16. Murray TF, Dupont J-Y, Fulkerson JP. Axial and lateral radiographs in evaluating patellofemoral malalignment. Am J Sports Med 1999; 27:580–584.
17. Pidoriano AJ, Weinstein RN, Buuck DA, et al. Correlation of patellar articular lesions and results from anteromedial tibial tubercle transfer. Am J Sports Med 1997;25:533–537.
18. Post WR. Clinical evaluation of patients with patellofemoral disorders [current concepts]. Arthroscopy 1999;15:841–851.
19. Saleh KJ, Arendt EA, Eldridge J, et al. Operative treatment of patellofemoral arthritis. J Bone Joint Surg Am 2005;87A:659–671.
20. Schepsis AA, DeSimone AA, Leach RE. Anterior tibial tubercle transposition for patellofemoral arthrosis: a long-term study. Am J Knee Surg 1994;7:13–20.
21. Schutzer SF, Ramsby GR, Fulkerson JP. Computed tomographic classification of patellofemoral pain patients. Orthop Clin North Am 1986;17:235–248.
22. Stetson WB, Friedman MJ, Fulkerson JP, et al. Fracture of the proximal tibia with immediate weightbearing after a Fulkerson osteotomy. Am J Sports Med 1997;25:570–574.

Chapter 54 Chronic Exertional Compartment Syndrome

Jocelyn R. Wittstein, L. Scott Levin, and Claude T. Moorman III

DEFINITION

- Compartment syndrome can be either acute or chronic.
- Acute compartment syndrome usually is due to trauma to, or reperfusion of, the extremity. Chronic exertional compartment syndrome (CECS) often is associated with the repetitive loading or microtrauma of endurance activities.
- Both acute and chronic compartment syndromes are due to increased interstitial pressure within a compartment, resulting in decreased perfusion and ischemia of soft tissues.
  - In contrast to the reversible nature of CECS, acute compartment syndromes progress rapidly and require urgent fasciotomy to avoid irreversible soft tissue necrosis in the affected compartment.
- Wilson first described the concept of CECS in 1912, but Mavor[12] was the first to successfully treat a patient with anterior compartment syndrome of the leg using a fasciotomy.
- Clinical manifestations of exercise-induced pain relieved by rest, swelling, numbness, and weakness of the extremity have long been attributed to elevated intracompartmental pressures.[5,17]
- The true incidence of CECS is unknown, but one study reported a prevalence of 14% among individuals with lower leg pain.[16]
- CECS often is bilateral and is equally prevalent among males and females.
- Case reports of CECS of the forearm, thigh, and gluteal regions exist, but are rare.[7,9,10]
  - The leg is the most common site, with the anterior and lateral compartments most frequently affected. This chapter focuses on CECS of the leg.

ANATOMY

- The leg contains four compartments: anterior, lateral, superficial posterior, and deep posterior (**FIG 1**).
- The anterior compartment contains the anterior tibial artery, the deep peroneal nerve, and four muscles (tibialis anterior, extensor digitorum longus, extensor hallucis longus, and peroneus tertius). Its borders are the tibia, fibula, interosseus membrane, anterior intermuscular septum, and deep fascia of the leg.

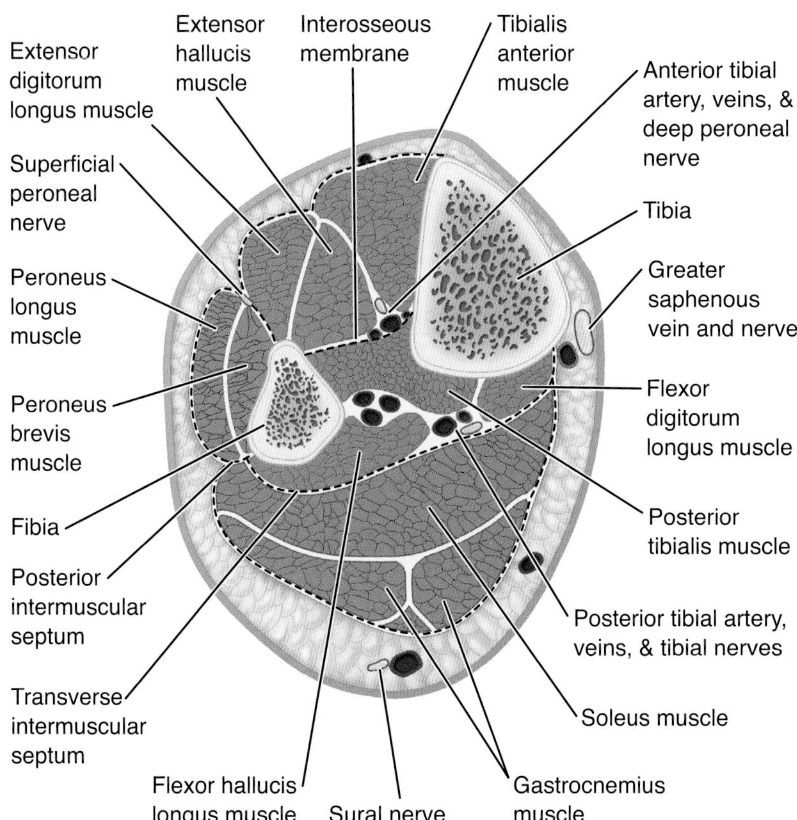

FIG 1 • Cross-sectional anatomy of the leg.

- The lateral compartment contains the superficial peroneal nerve and two muscles (peroneus longus and peroneus brevis).
  - The common peroneal nerve braches into the superficial and deep peroneal nerves within the substance of the peroneus longus after passing along the neck of the fibula.
  - The superficial peroneal nerve continues within the lateral compartment, while the deep peroneal nerve wraps around the fibula deep to the extensor digitorum longus until reaching the anterior surface of the interosseus membrane.
  - The lateral compartment does not contain a large artery; the peroneal muscles receive their blood supply via several branches of the peroneal artery.
  - The lateral compartment is bordered by the anterior intermuscular septum, the fibula, the posterior intermuscular septum, and the deep fascia.
- The superficial posterior compartment contains the sural nerve and three muscles (gastrocnemius, soleus, and plantaris) and is surrounded by the deep fascia of the leg.
- The deep posterior compartment contains the posterior tibial and peroneal arteries, tibial nerve, and four muscles (flexor digitorum longus, flexor hallucis longus, popliteus, and tibialis posterior).
  - It is bordered anteriorly by the tibia, fibula, and interosseus membrane, and posteriorly by the deep transverse fascia.
- A fifth compartment that encloses the tibialis posterior muscle has been described,[3] but its existence is controversial. It has been suggested that the presence of an extensive fibular origin of the flexor digitorum longus muscle may create a subcompartment within the deep posterior compartment that may develop elevated pressures.[8]

PATHOGENESIS

- The etiology of CECS is not entirely understood. It is thought to be due to an abnormal increase in intramuscular pressure during exercise resulting in impaired local perfusion, tissue ischemia, and pain.
  - Contributing factors may include exertion-induced swelling of the muscle fibers, increased perfusion volume, and increased interstitial fluid volume within a constrictive compartment.
  - The elevated intramuscular pressure decreases arteriolar blood flow and diminishes venous return.
  - This, in turn, results in tissue ischemia and accumulation of metabolites.
  - Elevated lactate levels and water content have been documented in muscle biopsies from compartments with elevated pressures following exercise.[16]
- Muscle hypertrophy and increased perfusion volume with exertion do not explain the elevated resting pressure seen in patients with CECS, however. The mechanical damage theory hypothesizes that heavy exertion results in myofibril damage, release of protein-bound ions, increased osmotic pressure in the interstitial space, and, therefore, decreased arteriolar flow in the compartment.
- Additionally, in some cases focal fascial defects may be a contributing factor.
  - Anterolateral fascial hernias are present in 39% to 46% of patients with CECS, as compared to less than 5% of asymptomatic individuals.[6,25]

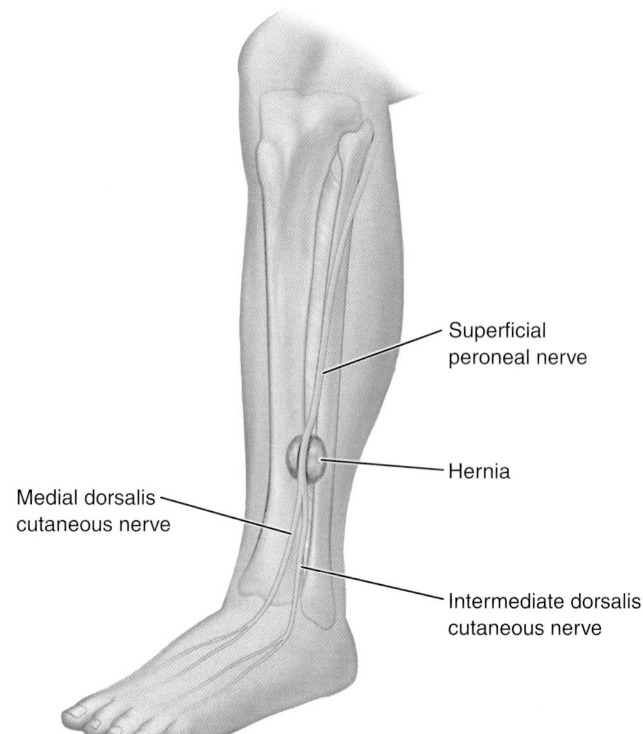

FIG 2 • The superficial peroneal nerve can become entrapped at a fascial defect.

  - These defects typically are located near the anterior intermuscular septum between the anterior and lateral compartments and can entrap the superficial peroneal nerve exiting the junction of the middle and distal thirds of the leg (**FIG 2**).
- None of the existing theories explain all the available data on the etiology of CECS. Most likely, the pathogenesis of the elevated intracompartmental pressures seen in CECS is multifactorial.

NATURAL HISTORY

- CECS of the leg is a common injury in people involved in running and endurance sport activities, such as young athletes and military personnel.
- Pain, as well as occasional numbness and weakness, develops at a predictable interval after initiation of a repetitive, endurance type activity and resolves with rest.
- The symptoms are longstanding and recurrent, because patients tend to self-limit but then subsequently attempt to resume activities.

PATIENT HISTORY AND PHYSICAL FINDINGS

- The following symptoms may be present upon exertion and resolve with rest:
  - A sensation of cramping, burning, aching, or tightness in the region of the affected compartment(s)
  - Numbness or weakness in the extremity
    - A transient footdrop may develop if the deep peroneal nerve is affected.

      - A temporary loss of eversion strength may occur if the superficial peroneal nerve is affected.
- Physical examination of the resting lower extremity often is unremarkable.
- Examination following exercise may reveal:
  - Increased tightness of the involved compartments
  - If a fascial defect is present, a focal area of tenderness and swelling may develop as the underlying muscle bulges through the defect.
    - A positive Tinel's sign over the defect if the superficial peroneal nerve is compressed
- When the history and physical examination findings are consistent with CECS, the diagnosis should be confirmed with pre- and postexercise compartment pressure measurements.
  - Most clinicians follow the diagnostic criteria of Pedowitz et al,[15] in which a resting pressure greater than or equal to 15 mm Hg or a 1-minute postexercise measurement greater than or equal to 30 mm Hg or a 5-minute postexercise measurement greater than or equal to 20 mm Hg is considered abnormal and diagnostic of CECS.
  - The exercise performed at the time of testing must be intense enough to reproduce the patient's symptoms; otherwise, the postexercise pressure measurements may be falsely low.
  - Several methods for measuring compartment pressures have been described in the literature.
    - These include the slit catheter, wick catheter, needle manometery, digital pressure monitor, microcapillary infusion, and solid-state transducer intracompartmental catheter methods.[1,2,13,14,19,25]
    - The Stryker inracompartmental pressure monitor (Kalamazoo, MI) is a handheld digital monitor that can be used to check multiple compartments. It can be used with a side port needle or with an indwelling slit catheter to obtain serial measurements in a single compartment.
    - A new handheld digital device recently developed by Synthes (Paoli, PA) also allows placement of indwelling catheters and may be useful for obtaining serial measurements.
- Near-infrared spectroscopy has been used to determine tissue oxygen saturation.[26] This may be a noninvasive, painless alternative to intracompartmental pressures in the diagnosis of CECS, but is not currently standardized or readily available.
- The vibration test consists of placing a vibrating tuning fork over bone at the area of suspected stress; an elicitation of pain is consistent with a stress fracture.
- Pain when performing resisted ankle dorsiflexion and inversion is consistent with tibialis posterior tendinitis or posteromedial periostitis.

IMAGING AND OTHER DIAGNOSTIC STUDIES

- When pressure measurements are not consistent with CECS, further diagnostic studies may be necessary to explore the differential diagnosis.
- Plain radiographs may demonstrate a periosteal reaction in patients with tibial stress fractures or posteromedial tibial periostitis.
- Bone scan will show increased uptake, and MRI may show edema or a black line at the site of a stress fracture.
- Tingling, numbness, or a positive Tinel's sign at a specific location may warrant an EMG and nerve conduction study to evaluate for peripheral nerve entrapment.

DIFFERENTIAL DIAGNOSIS

- Tibial stress fractures
- Posteromedial tibial periostitis
- Tenosynovitis of posterior tibialis or ankle dorsiflexors
- Peripheral nerve entrapment
- Radiculopathy secondary to lumbar pathology
- Complex regional pain syndrome
- Peripheral vascular disease
- Popliteal artery entrapment syndrome
- Deep venous thrombosis

NONOPERATIVE MANAGEMENT

- Nonoperative management usually requires activity limitation.
- Symptoms usually return with resumption of prior activity level. Surgery, therefore is indicated in patients who cannot tolerate activity restriction.

SURGICAL MANAGEMENT

- Surgical treatment involves fasciotomy of the affected compartments, sometimes with partial fasciectomy.
- Patients who are unable to maintain their desired activity level owing to symptoms of CECS are appropriate operative candidates.

Preoperative Planning

- It is critical to identify which compartments are affected.
  - All symptomatic compartments should be addressed at the time of surgery. It is common for a failed index procedure to be due to a failure to release an affected compartment.
- The appropriate approach should be selected based on the compartments that need to be released.

Positioning

- The patient is placed in the supine position for each technique.

Approach

- A single- or dual-incision technique can be used to release the lateral and anterior compartments.
- The perifibular approach can be used to access all four compartments.
- A second posteromedial approach offers easier access to the superficial and deep posterior compartments.
- Endoscopically assisted fasciotomies allow access to the entire length of the compartment, allow visualization of fascial hernias, and may minimize surgical complications such as postsurgical fibrosis and injury to the superficial peroneal nerve.
  - The safety and effectiveness of endoscopically assisted compartment release has been demonstrated in cadavers.[11]
  - A technique using balloon dissectors and carbon dioxide insufflation is described in the Technique section.[27]

SINGLE-INCISION LATERAL APPROACH FOR ANTERIOR AND LATERAL COMPARTMENT FASCIOTOMY

- The patient is placed in the supine position on the operating table.
- A 5-cm vertical incision is made halfway between the fibular shaft and the tibial crest at the midportion of the leg. The incision should lie over the anterolateral intermuscular septum (TECH FIG 1A).
  - If a focal fascial defect is present, the incision should be adjusted so that the defect can be incorporated.
- A small transverse incision is made just through the fascia, and the septum and the superficial peroneal nerve, which lie near the septum in the lateral compartment and exit the fascia near the distal aspect of the incision, are identified (TECH FIG 1B).
- Longitudinal releases of the anterior and lateral compartments are performed using long Metzenbaum scissors in a proximal and distal direction from the transverse incision in the fascia that crosses over the anterolateral intermuscular septum (TECH FIG 1C).
- A partial fasciectomy may be performed, particularly in cases of recurrence following a prior fasciotomy.
- The fascia is left open.
- The subcutaneous tissue is approximated using 2-0 absorbable suture material.
- The skin is closed with a running subcuticular 4-0 nonabsorbable suture material and Steri-strips.

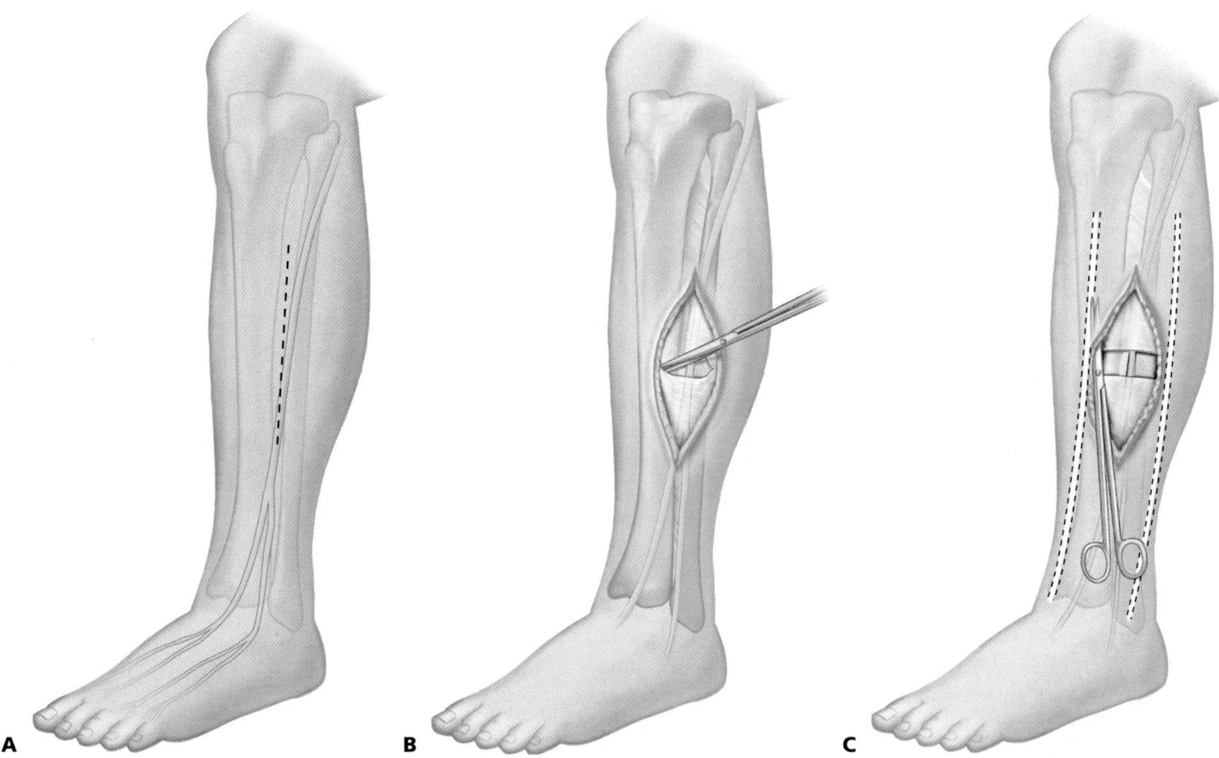

TECH FIG 1 • Single-incision lateral approach. **A.** A 5-cm vertical incision is made halfway between the fibular shaft and the tibial crest over the anterolateral intermuscular septum. **B.** A small transverse incision is made just through the fascia, and the superficial peroneal nerve is identified. **C.** Longitudinal releases of the anterior and lateral compartments are performed using long Metzenbaum scissors.

DUAL INCISION LATERAL APPROACH FOR ANTERIOR AND LATERAL COMPARTMENT FASCIOTOMY

- The patient is placed in a supine position.
- The leg is divided into thirds, and two 3-cm incisions are placed at the junction of the thirds over the anterolateral intermuscular septum (TECH FIG 2A,B).
- The superficial peroneal nerve is identified as it exits the fascia near the distal incision (TECH FIG 2C).
- Fasciotomies of the anterior and lateral compartments are performed on each side of the intermuscular septum (TECH FIG 2D).
- The incisions in the fascia are connected using Metzenbaum scissors to divide the fascia from the proximal incision toward the knee (TECH FIG 2E), then from

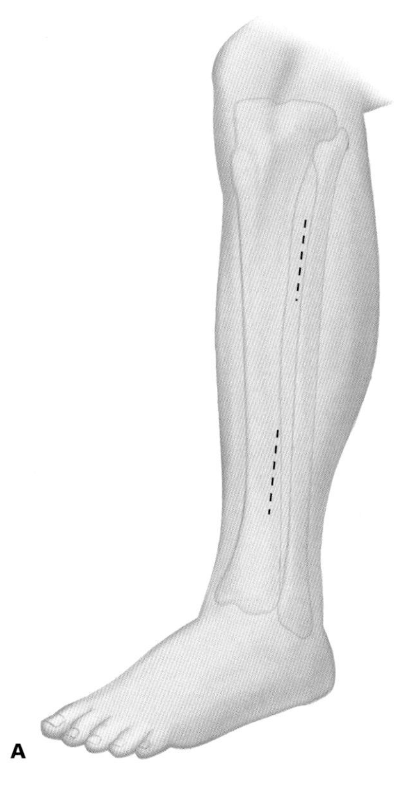

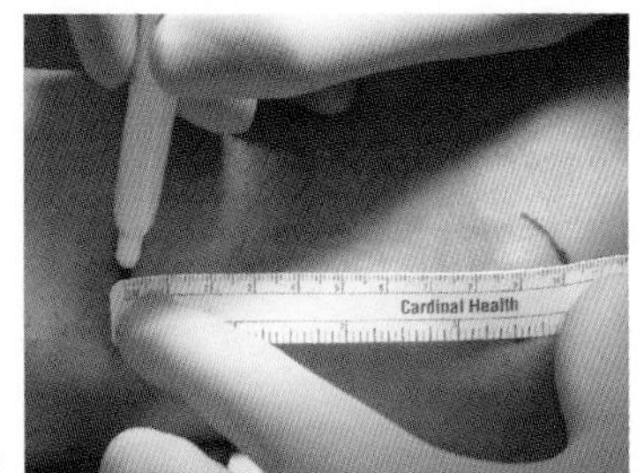

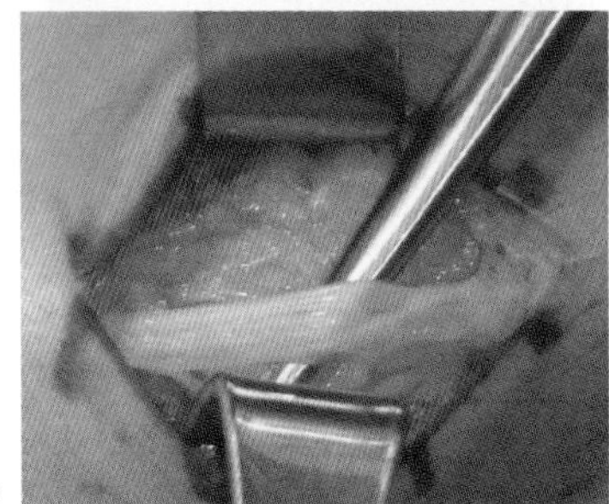

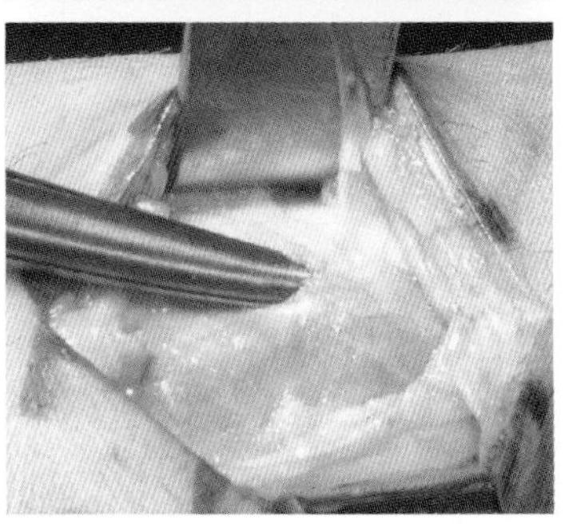

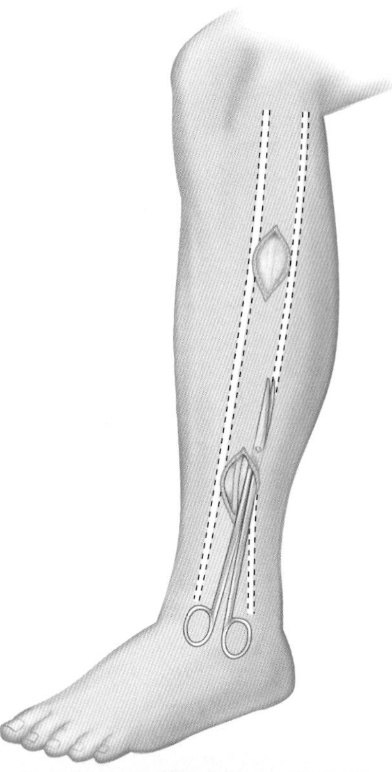

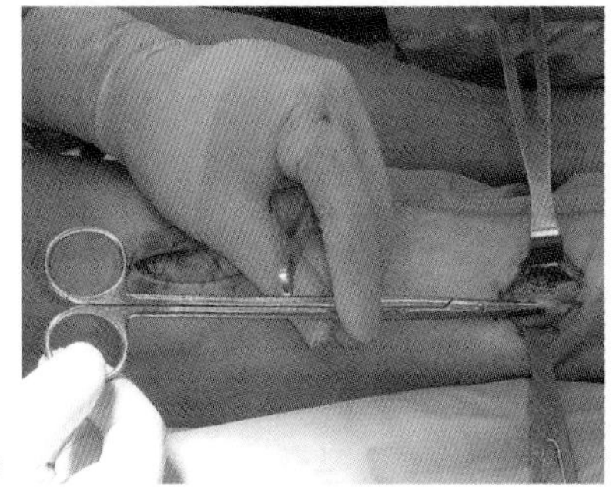

TECH FIG 2 • Dual-incision approach. **A.** The leg is visually split into thirds, and two 3-cm incisions are placed at the junction of the thirds over the anterolateral intermuscular septum. **B.** The superficial peroneal nerve is located 10 to 12 cm proximal to the tip of the lateral malleolus. The inferior incision is centered over this area. **C.** Dissection of the superficial peroneal nerve. **D.** A fascial defect often is present in this area, and compartment releases should be centered over these areas if possible. **E.** The incisions in the fascia are connected using Metzenbaum scissors to divide the fascia. **F.** Long scissors are used and are opened only slightly at the tips. (**B–D,F:** Courtesy of Mark D. Miller, MD.)

the proximal incision toward the distal incision, and finally from the distal incision toward the ankle (TECH FIG 2F).
  - Distally, the fasciotomy should extend to 4 to 6 cm proximal to the ankle.
  - At the distal aspect of the anterior compartment, the release should be directed more toward the midline to minimize risk of injuring cutaneous sensory nerves at the lateral aspect of the compartment.
  - The distal aspect of the lateral compartment fasciotomy should be directed more laterally.
- The subcutaneous tissue is closed with 2-0 absorbable suture material.
- The skin is closed with running subcuticular 4-0 sutures and Steri-strips.

PERIFIBULAR APPROACH FOR FOUR-COMPARTMENT FASCIOTOMY

- The patient is placed in the supine position.
- A 10-cm incision is made directly over the midportion of the fibula (TECH FIG 3A).
- The skin is retracted anteriorly and the fascia of the anterior and lateral compartments is released longitudinally in a proximal and distal direction (TECH FIG 3B).
- The skin is retracted posteriorly.
- The fascia overlying the lateral head of the gastrocnemius is released.
  - The fascia over the superficial posterior compartment is incised for a distance of about 15 cm.

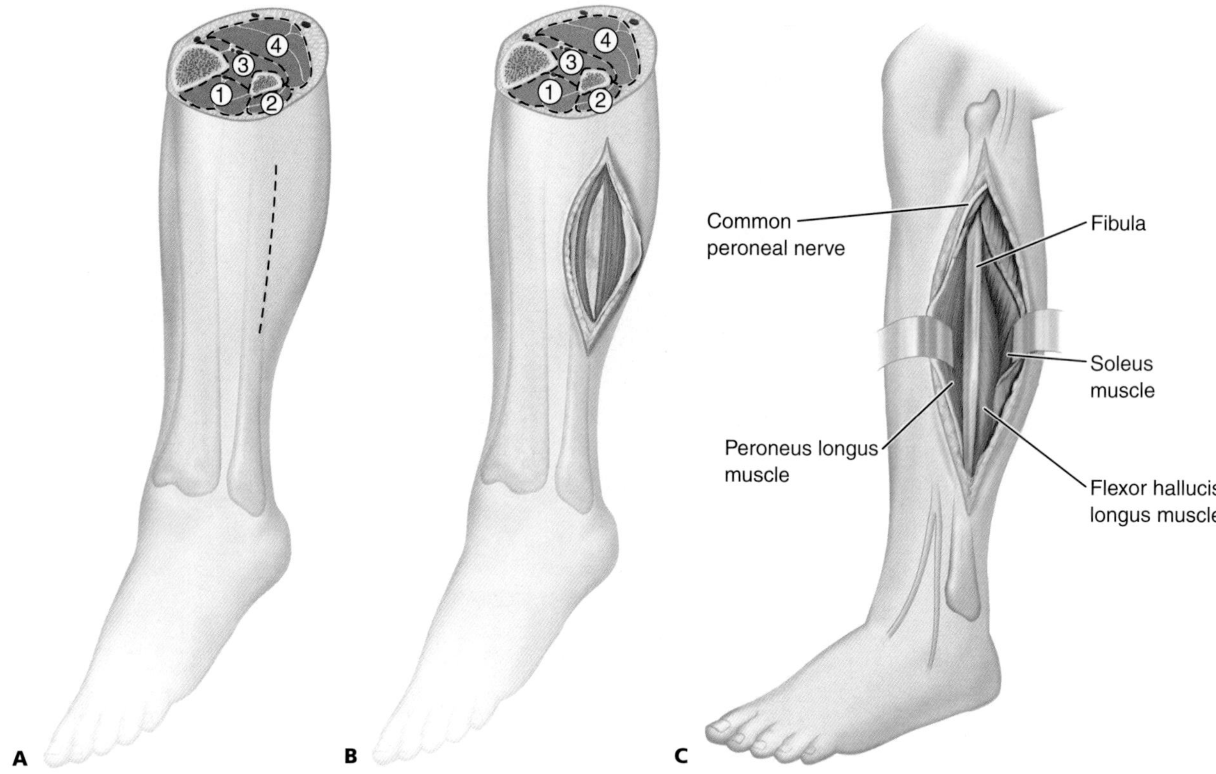

TECH FIG 3 • Perifibular approach. **A.** A 10-cm incision is made directly over the midportion of the fibula. **B.** The skin is retracted anteriorly, and the fascia of the anterior and lateral compartments is released longitudinally. **C.** The anterior and lateral compartments are retracted anteriorly and the superficial posterior compartment posteriorly, and the soleal bridge is released from the fibula.

- The anterior and lateral compartments are retracted anteriorly and the superficial posterior compartment posteriorly. The soleal bridge must be released from the fibula (**TECH FIG 3C**).
- The fascia over the flexor hallucis longus is identified and incised.
- The gastrocsoleus is retracted posteriorly and the flexor hallucis longus laterally to expose the posterior tibial artery, tibial nerve, and peroneal artery overlying the tibialis posterior.
- The fascia is incised around the tibialis posterior and the interval between the muscle and the origins of the flexor hallucis longus is widenend if it is constrictive.
- The subcutaneous tissue is approximated with 2-0 absorbable suture.
- The skin is closed with running subcuticular nonabsorbable 4-0 suture.

POSTEROMEDIAL INCISION FOR FASCIOTOMY OF THE POSTERIOR COMPARTMENTS

- A vertical incision 8 to 10 cm in length is made over the midportion of the leg approximately 1 cm posterior to the posteromedial edge of the tibia (**TECH FIG 4A**).
- The saphenous vein and nerve are identified in the subcutaneous tissue and retracted anteriorly.
- The fascia over the superficial posterior compartment is incised for a distance of about 15 cm (**TECH FIG 4B,C**).
- To fully access the deep posterior compartment, the origin of the soleus from the proximal tibia and fibula must be detached (**TECH FIG 4D**).
- The deep fascia can then be sharply divided with Metzenbaum scissors (**TECH FIG 4E–G**).
  - The fasciotomy should extend distally to 8 to 10 cm above the ankle.
- The opening between the origins of the flexor hallucis longus and the tibialis posterior is enlarged if constrictive.
- The subcutaneous tissue is closed with 2-0 absorbable suture.
- The skin is closed with running subcuticular nonabsorbable 4-0 suture.

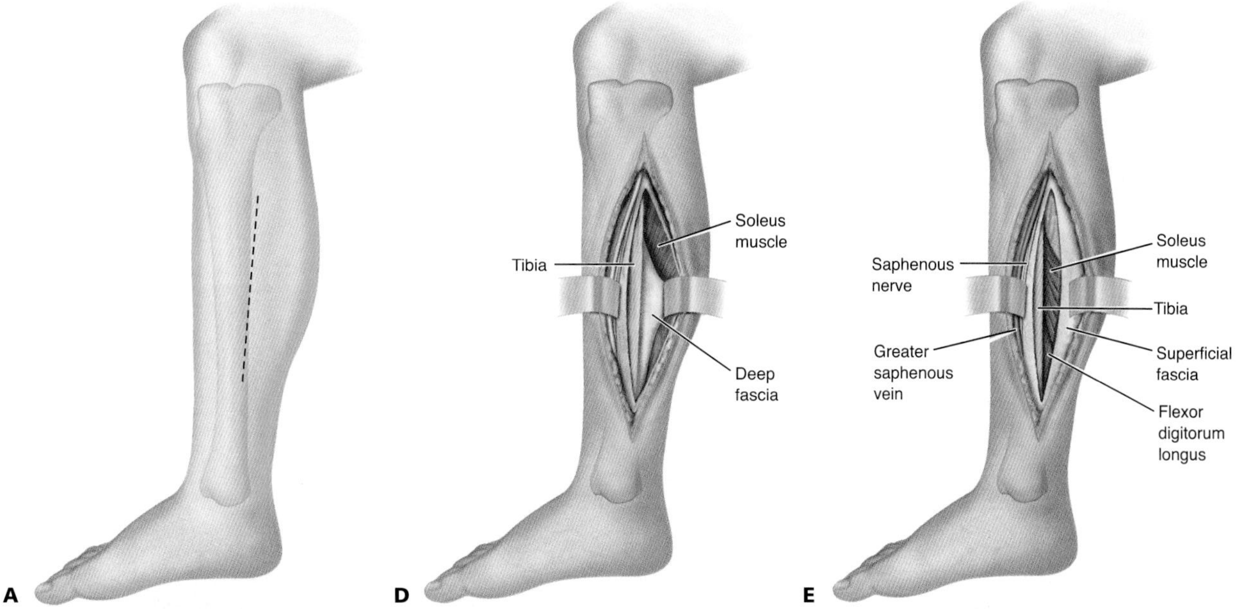

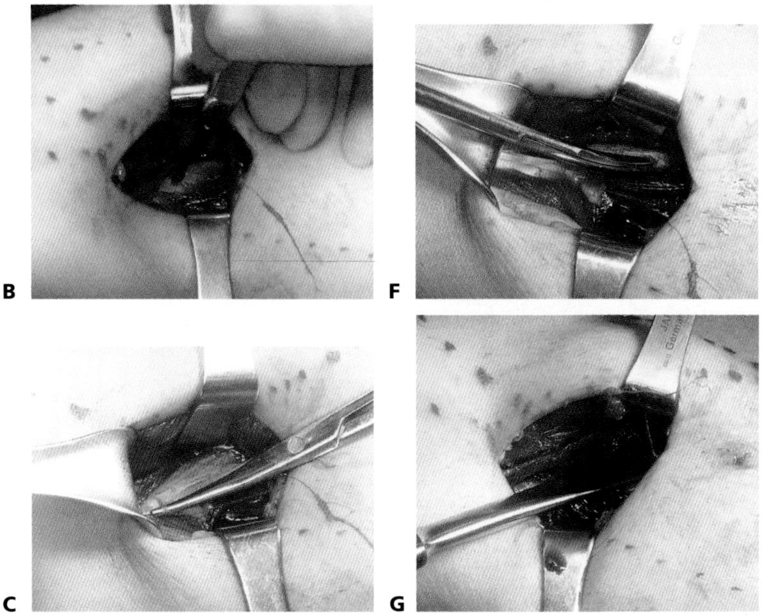

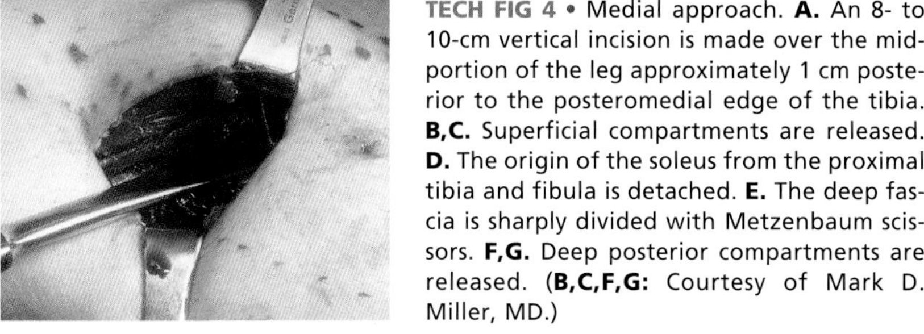

TECH FIG 4 • Medial approach. **A.** An 8- to 10-cm vertical incision is made over the midportion of the leg approximately 1 cm posterior to the posteromedial edge of the tibia. **B,C.** Superficial compartments are released. **D.** The origin of the soleus from the proximal tibia and fibula is detached. **E.** The deep fascia is sharply divided with Metzenbaum scissors. **F,G.** Deep posterior compartments are released. (**B,C,F,G:** Courtesy of Mark D. Miller, MD.)

ENDOSCOPICALLY ASSISTED COMPARTMENT RELEASE

- The patient is placed in a supine position.
- Balloon dissectors can be used to create an optical cavity at the fascial cleft, which is the potential space between the superficial fascia (the deepest layer of the skin and subcutaneous tissue) and the deep fascia (the fascia overlying a muscle compartment; TECH FIG 5).
  - To insert the balloon dissector, a 2-cm transverse incision is made either at the anterolateral aspect of the knee between the fibular head and Gerdy's tubercle or at the posteromedial aspect of the knee at the level of the tibial crest.
  - Dissection is carried down through the subcutaneous fat and superficial fascia until the deep fascia overlying the muscle is visualized.
- The balloon dissector with a sheath around it is inserted between the superficial and deep fascial layers under direct observation and manual palpation to the level of the ankle.
- The sheath is removed and the balloon is inflated to create a cavity within the fascial cleft.
- The balloon is then deflated and removed.
- A one-way cone-shaped cannula is inserted in the skin at the site of balloon insertion.
- The optical cavity between the superficial and deep fascial layers can be maintained subsequently with 15 mm Hg of carbon dioxide insufflation to allow adequate visualization of the fascia to be released and to allow adequate space to perform soft tissue dissection with the endoscopic equipment.

- Alternatively, the cavity is not insufflated, but is maintained with towel clips externally.
- Next, the fascia is released with endoscopic scissors down to the level of the ankle under direct vision.
- If necessary, a distal instrument portal with a pneumatic lock can be placed, but the fasciotomies usually are carried out proximal to distal through the initial portal.
- After the release, the cannula is removed and the cavity is deflated.
- The wound is closed in a two-layer fashion with 2-0 Vicryl for the deep layer and a running subcuticular stitch for the skin over a medium Hemovac drain.

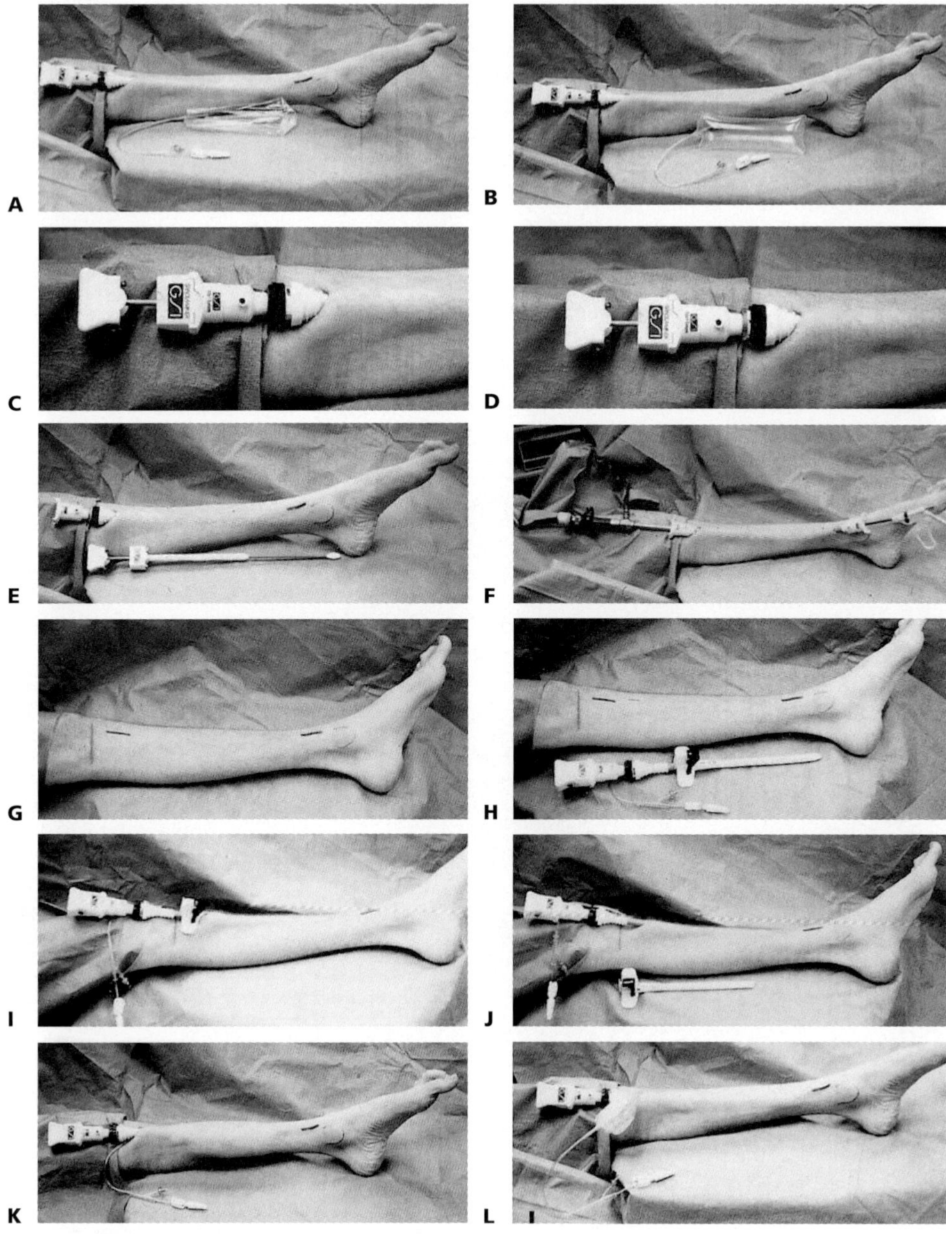

TECH FIG 5 • Sequential demonstration of balloon placement in the lower extremity. **A.** Portal incisions for balloon insertion. **B.** Balloon parallel to the leg in disassembled position. **C.** Entry of balloon. **D.** Sheath removed. **E.** Balloon inflated. **F.** Balloon deflated. **G.** Balloon removed. **H.** Balloon inflated to confirm complete removal of dissector balloon. **I.** Portal advancement. **J.** Portal placed into skin by turning clockwise. **K.** Guide rod withdrawn. **L.** Endoscope inserted proximally. (Reprinted with permission from Zobrist R, Aponte R, Levin LS. Endoscopic access to the extremities: the principle of fascial clefts. J Orthop Trauma 2002;16:264–271.)

PEARLS AND PITFALLS

Superficial peroneal nerve injury	■ Identify the nerve as it exits the fascia at the junction of the distal and middle thirds of the leg; direct the anterior fasciotomy medially and the lateral fasciotomy posteriorly at the distal extent.
Saphenous vein and nerve injury	■ Identify the structures in the subcutaneous tissue at the medial aspect of the leg. Avoid excessive traction on the saphenous nerve, which results in a traction paresthesia.
Incomplete fascial release	■ Muscle herniates at the bottom of the "V" of the fasciotomy, resulting in pain. Extend lateral and anterior fasciotomies to 4 to 6 cm above the ankle and posterior fasciotomies to 8 to 10 cm above the ankle.

POSTOPERATIVE CARE

- Active range of motion at the ankle and knee should begin immediately.
- Crutches can be used as needed in the initial postoperative period, but patients are encouraged to bear weight as tolerated and perform light activities.
- Elevation of the legs while at rest may help to decrease pain and swelling.
- Full activity usually can be resumed 4 to 6 weeks after surgery.

OUTCOMES

- Various techniques of compartment release have reports of success rates ranging from 81% to 100%.[4,6,18,20,22,24]
  - These techniques include open fasciotomies, one- or two-incision minimally invasive subcutaneous fasciotomies, and fasciotomies with partial fasciectomies.
- Adequate long-term follow-up is lacking in the literature.
  - Slimmon et al reported on long-term follow-up of patients treated with fasciotomy with partial fasciectomy and noted a good or excellent outcome in 60% at a mean follow-up of 51 months. Thirteen of 62 had reduced activity levels due to recurrence of symptoms or development of a different lower extremity compartment syndrome.[23]
- Fasciotomy appears to be less effective in alleviating pain in the deep posterior compartment than in other compartments.
  - Some authors have postulated that failure of the fasciotomy may be due to an incomplete fasciotomy or not identifying and releasing the fascia around the tibialis posterior.[3,18,20]

COMPLICATIONS

- Recurrence rates of 3% to 17% have been reported after fasciotomy.[4,18,20,22]
  - Recurrence may be due to a number of factors, including inadequate fascial releases, failure to decompress a compartment that was believed to be asymptomatic, nerve compression by an unrecognized fascial hernia, and the development of prolific scar tissue.[21]
- Other reported complications of fasciotomies with some degree of subcutaneous or blind dissection include arterial injury, hematoma or seroma formation, superficial wound infections, peripheral cutaneous nerve injuries, and deep venous thromboses.[4,6,23]
  - The superficial peroneal nerve is particularly vulnerable as it exits the fascia over the lateral aspect of the leg at the junction of the middle and distal thirds.

REFERENCES

1. Awbrey BJ, Sienkiewicz PS, Mankin HJ. Chronic exercise-induced compartment pressure elevation measured with a miniaturized fluid-pressure monitor. A laboratory and clinical study. Am J Sports Med 1988;16:610–615.
2. Brace RA, Guyton AC, Taylor AE. Reevaluation of the needle method for measuring interstitial fluid pressure. Am J Physiol 1976; 229:603–607.
3. Davey JR, Rorabeck CH, Fowler PJ. The tibialis posterior muscle compartment. An unrecognized cause of exertional compartment syndrome. Am J Sports Med 1984;12:391–397.
4. Detmer DE, Sharpe K, Sufit RL, et al. Chronic compartment syndrome: Diagnosis, management, and outcomes. Am J Sports Med 1985;13:162–170.
5. French EB, Price WH. Anterior tibial pain. BMJ 1962;2:1290–1296.
6. Fronek J, Mubarak SJ, Hargens AR, et al. Management of chronic exertional compartment syndrome of the lower extremity. Clin Orthop Relat Res 1987;220:217–227.
7. Hallock GG. An endoscopic technique for decompressive fasciotomy. Ann Plast Surg 1999;43:668–670.
8. Hislop M, Tierney P, Murray P, et al. Chronic exertional compartment syndrome: the controversial "fifth" compartment of the leg. Am J Sports Med 2003;31:770–776.
9. Kuklo TR, Tis JE, Moores LK, et al. Fatal rhabdomyolysis with bilateral gluteal, thigh, and leg compartment syndrome after the Army Physical Fitness Test. A case report. Am J Sports Med 2000;28: 112–116.
10. Kutz JE, Singer R, Linday M. Chronic exertional compartment syndrome of the forearm: a case report. J Hand Surg Am 1985;10: 302–304.
11. Leversedge FJ, Casey PJ, Seiler JG, et al. Endoscopically assisted fasciotomy: description of technique and in vitro assessment of lower-leg compartment decompression. Am J Sports Med 2002;30: 272–278.
12. Mavor GE. The anterior tibial syndrome. J Bone Joint Surg Br 1956; 38B:513–517.
13. McDermott AG, Marble AE, Yabsley RH, Phillips MB. Monitoring dynamic anterior compartment pressures during exercise: a new technique using the STIC catheter. Am J Sports Med 1982;10:83–89.
14. Murabak SJ, Hargens AR, Owen CA, et al. The wick catheter technique for measurement of intramuscular pressure: a new research and clinical tool. J Bone Joint Surg Am 1976;58A:1016–1020.
15. Pedowitz RA, Hargens AR, Mubarak SJ, et al. Modified criteria for the objective diagnosis of chronic compartment syndrome of the leg. Am J Sports Med 1990;18:35–40.
16. Qvarfordt P, Christenson JT, Eklof B, et al. Intramuscular pressure, muscle blood flow, and skeletal muscle metabolism in chronic anterior tibial compartment syndrome. Clin Orthop Relat Res 1983;179: 284–290.
17. Reneman RS. The anterior and the lateral compartment syndrome of the leg due to intensive use of muscles. Clin Orthop Rel Res 1975;113:69–80.
18. Rorabeck CH, Bourne RB, Fowler PJ. The surgical treatment of exertional compartment syndrome in athletes. J Bone Joint Surg Am 1983;65A:1245–1251.

19. Rorabeck CH, Castle GS, Hardie R, et al. Compartment pressure measurements: an experimental investigation using the slit catheter. J Trauma 1981;21:446–449.
20. Rorabeck CH, Fowler PJ, Nott L. The results of fasciotomy in the management of chronic exertional compartment syndrome. Am J Sports Med 1988;16:224–227.
21. Schepsis AA, Fitzgerald M, Nicoletta R. Revision surgery for exertional compartment syndrome of the lower leg. Am J Sports Med 2005;33:1040–1047.
22. Schepsis AA, Martini D, Corbett M. Surgical management of exertional compartment syndrome of the lower leg: long term follow up. Am J Sports Med 1993;21:811–817.
23. Slimmon D, Bennell K, Brunker P, et al. Long-term outcome of fasciotomy with partial fasciectomy for chronic exertional compartment syndrome of the lower leg. Am J Sports Med 2002;30:581–588.
24. Styf JR, Korner LM. Chronic exertional compartment syndrome of the leg: results of treatment by fasciotomy. J Bone Joint Surg Am 1986;68A:1338–1347.
25. Styf JR, Korner LM. Microcapillary infusion technique for measurement of intramuscular pressure during exercise. Clin Orthop Rel Res 1986;207:253–262.
26. Van den Brand JGH, Verleisdonk EJMM, van der Werken C. Near infrared spectroscopy in the diagnosis of chronic exertional compartment syndrome. Am J Sports Med 2004;32:452–456.
27. Zobrist R, Aponte R, Levin LS. Endoscopic access to the extremities: the principle of fascial clefts. J Orthop Trauma 2002;16: 264–271.

Chapter 55 Common Peroneal and Lateral Femoral Cutaneous Nerve Injuries

Ivica Ducic and Jeffrey M. Jacobson

BACKGROUND

- Care of peripheral nerve problems requires knowledge and understanding of nerve pathology, anatomic nerve variations, patterns of nerve damage and entrapment that follow trauma and common operative procedures, and specialized surgical techniques for manipulation of the damaged peripheral nerve.
- Unlike other surgical disciplines, a large proportion of peripheral nerve surgery attempts to correct neuropathy in the postoperative patient and, therefore, is reoperative in nature.
- Lateral femoral cutaneous nerve (LFCN) neuropathy can be encountered in the orthopedic patient after injuries or procedures in proximity to the anterior superior iliac spine (ASIS), the inguinal region, or the anterior thigh.
  - The symptoms are limited to pain or paresthesias in the distribution shown in **FIGURE 1**, because this nerve carries only sensory signals.
- Surgical procedures and trauma to the lateral knee both represent potential for common peroneal nerve (CPN) injury.
  - The nerve can become entrapped in postoperative scar tissue, stretched with knee or ankle dislocations, or inadvertently directly damaged, resulting in neuropathy.

ANATOMY

Lateral Femoral Cutaneous Nerve

- The LFCN arises from the lumbar plexus through contributions from the dorsal divisions of the L2 and L3 spinal roots. In most people, the nerve courses medial to the ASIS and traverses the groin crease under the inguinal ligament as it descends to innervate the thigh.
- The nerve is prone to iatrogenic injury when its anatomy is aberrant; the surgeon should be aware that the LFCN can run through the inguinal ligament and against the ASIS or over the most medial portion of ASIS rather than in its usual course.
- The surface anatomy and the most common site of impingement can be seen in **FIGURE 2**.

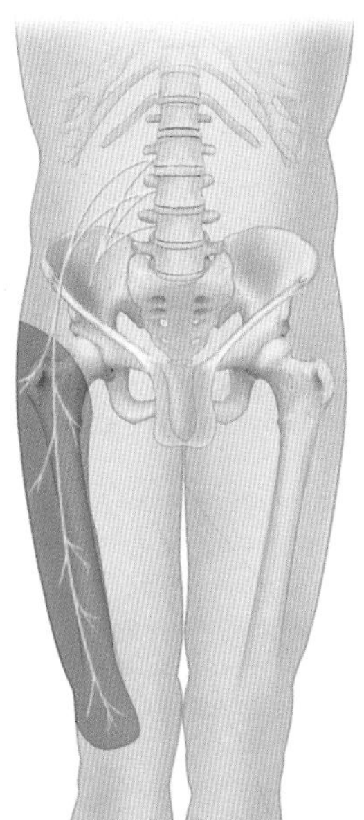
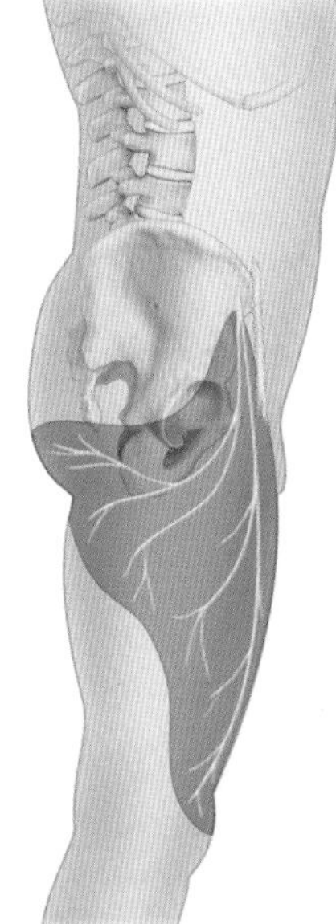

FIG 1 • Sensory innervation of the lateral femoral cutaneous nerve

Common Peroneal Nerve

- The CPN is a branch of the sciatic nerve, formed from contributions from the sacral plexus from L4 to S2.
- Pathology of the CPN classically is seen as it wraps around the neck of the fibula, deep to the peroneus longus muscle just before it splits into its deep and superficial branches (**FIG 3**).
- The CPN innervates the muscles for foot dorsiflexion and eversion and provides sensory innervation to the anterolateral lower leg and the majority of the dorsum of foot and toes.

General Nerve Anatomy

- The peripheral nerve has a significant intrinsic blood supply that permits the surgeon to lift the nerve from its anatomic bed, open the epineurium, and operate between the fascicles.[1]
- The endoneurial and perineurial microvessels maintain excellent vascularity to the peripheral nerve. Segmental blood vessels enter the peripheral nerve through the mesoneurium. In addition, an extensive number of longitudinal vessels in the epineurium, perineurium, and endoneurium supply the nerve.[2]
- Maki et al[3] have demonstrated that the "safe" length a nerve can be elevated from its bed (its segmental vascular supply) is a distance of about 60 times the diameter of the nerve. Therefore, the surgeon should consider primarily the need to move the nerve into an area that is free from forces that might externally compress it and, thus, cause symptomatic neuropathy but also should acknowledge internal

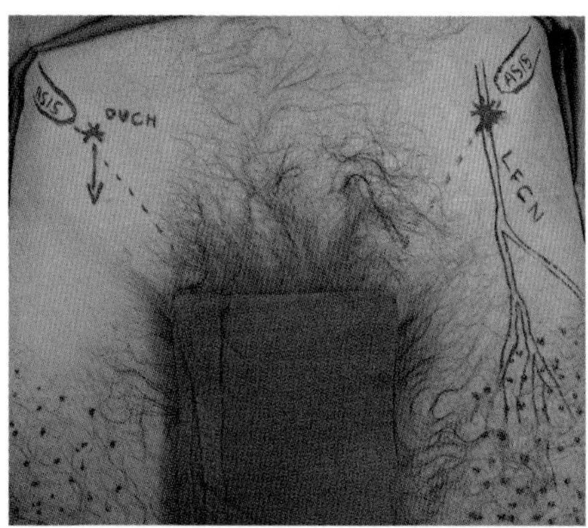

FIG 2 • Surface anatomy of the lateral femoral cutaneous nerve. Note the approximate site of compression at the level of the inguinal ligament

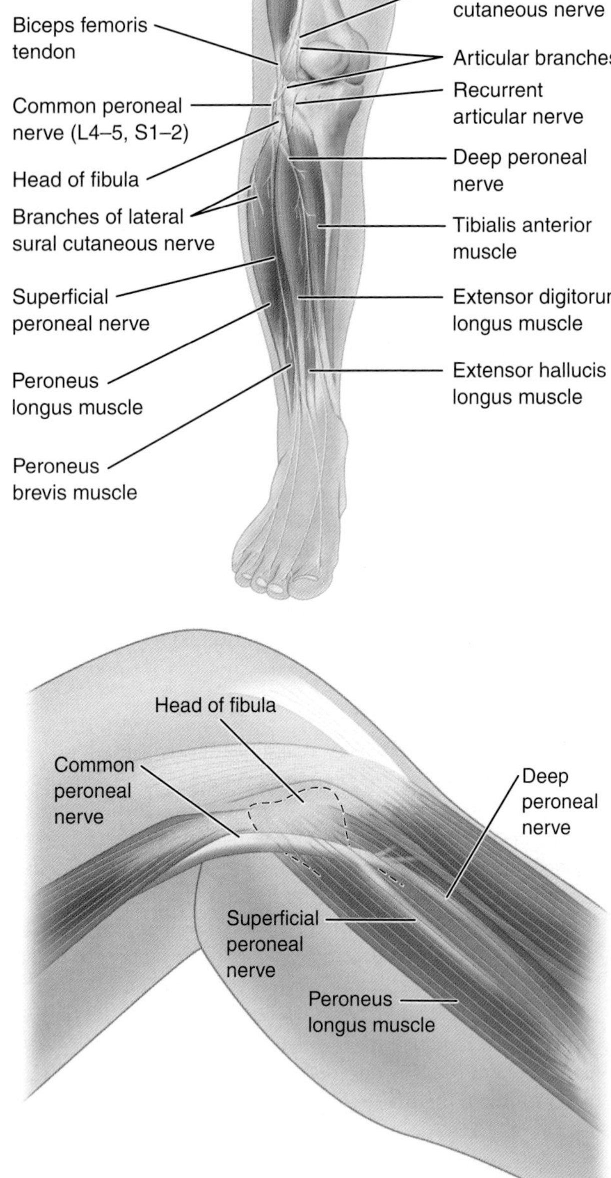

FIG 3 • Anatomy of the common peroneal nerve. Note the proximity of the nerve to the fibula as it wraps anteriorly on the lower leg.

vascular properties of the nerve when effective mobilization is considered.

- Extreme caution should be exercised in repeat neurolysis of a peripheral nerve, because of repeated nerve devascularization.

PATHOGENESIS

- Peripheral nerve pathology is due to any process that interferes with neuronal conduction outside of the central nervous system.
  - Those processes amenable to surgical intervention include nerve damage due to physical compression related to various metabolic conditions and surgeries around or adjacent to a nerve.
- Peripheral nerve surgery encompasses repair of two common pathophysiologic entities:
  - Accidental nerve transection or direct crush injury leads to nerve dysfunction and possible painful neuroma formation.
  - Scar formation from any surgery or trauma can engulf a peripheral nerve and compress it; symptomatic relief can then be accomplished through surgical decompression of the peripheral nerve.
- Peripheral nerve injury becomes symptomatic either when a critical function is lost or when paresthesia and pain replace normal sensory signaling.
- Partial or complete nerve transection causes loss of sensory or motor function because of loss of nerve continuity or disruption of the nerve's blood supply. The nerve's regenerative capacity then either re-establishes neuronal continuity or forms a disorganized scar within a mature end-bulb neuroma.
- Similarly, compression on a peripheral nerve causes ischemia and neuroma formation.[1]
  - A neuroma contains bundled, disorganized nerve endings within a collagenous mass, and is an anatomic source of the localized pain and paresthesia following peripheral nerve damage.

PATIENT HISTORY AND PHYSICAL FINDINGS

- History and physical examination, particularly a thorough neurologic examination, often suggest the diagnosis by demonstrating a dermatomal distribution of pain or paresthesia. Further imaging and electrodiagnostic testing may be necessary, mainly to evaluate other causes for the symptoms.[2,4]
  - Central nervous system disease, particularly spinal root impingement, shares many of the same symptoms and must be excluded.
- Diagnostic workup must evaluate and exclude other etiologies for postoperative pain, particularly infection, loosened hardware, mechanical misalignment, spinal involvement, and neoplasm.
  - The timing of the sensory or motor symptoms needs to be considered when taking the history and performing the physical examination, because that can aid in understanding the cause of neuropathy.
- When encountering potential neuropathies in the knee or lower leg, the clinician must consider that, although the common peroneal nerve is the major peripheral nerve affected following knee surgery, neuromas of sensory nerves supplying the knee and its surroundings may develop when they are severed or encased in scar tissue.
  - These smaller peripheral nerves can be the source of chronic postoperative knee pain and can be mistaken for CPN neuropathy or mask the CPN involvement.
  - Therefore, the examining physician should be aware of the different possible causes of pain in this anatomic area and should be able to distinguish deep and superficial paresthesias and pains in the knee area.
  - The most commonly affected sensory nerves involved in deep knee pain are the lateral retinacular nerve, the medial retinacular nerves, and the articular branch of the common peroneal nerve, whereas superficial knee pain is caused mainly by involvement of the infrapatellar branch of the saphenous nerve and the medial and anterior cutaneous nerves of the thigh.

- If any of these smaller nerves is suspected as the cause of a patient's symptoms, referral to a peripheral nerve surgeon is suggested.

IMAGING AND DIAGNOSTIC STUDIES

- Current imaging techniques—including CT, MRI, and radiolabeled bone scans—have limited, if any, value confirming the diagnosis of a malfunctioning nerve.
- Electrodiagnostic studies also can have a false-negative rate as high as 33%, whereas nerve blocks, because of anatomic variations, can give a false-negative result.
- For these reasons, it cannot be overstated that a diagnostic workup must be interpreted cautiously.

NONOPERATIVE MANAGEMENT

- Medical management of paresthesias and pain from injured peripheral nerves centers on symptom management:
  - Activity and lifestyle modification
  - Narcotic and nonnarcotic analgesics
  - Centrally acting agents such as gabapentin and pregabalin
  - Nerve blocks
  - Physical and occupational therapy
- Although medical management offers temporary relief in most patients, it can be complicated by increasing dosage requirements and narcotic dependence, as an acute insult develops into a chronic pain syndrome.[5]
- Among the first steps to focus on are eliminating possible causes of neuropathy and optimizing the patient's medical condition if comorbidities are present.
- Nonoperative management is considered a failure when patients with neuropathy do not achieve a reasonable recovery by approximately 12 weeks.
  - At that point, additional evaluation by a peripheral nerve surgeon or electrodiagnostic workup is appropriate to determine whether surgical intervention or continued observation is indicated.

TECHNIQUES

LATERAL FEMORAL CUTANEOUS NERVE

- The patient is placed in the supine position, and an incision of about 6 cm is made anterior to the anterior superior iliac spine, extending toward the thigh.
- Careful dissection is then carried to deep fascia and toward the inguinal ligament (TECH FIG 1A).
- The use of loupe magnification as well as proper microsurgical instruments and bipolar electrocautery is essential when identifying the LFCN because of the variability in its anatomy (TECH FIG 1B).
  - The LFCN could be encountered at any point in the dissection of the inguinal ligament and must not be damaged.
- Once identified, the nerve is first decompressed distally approximately 4 to 6 cm and then proximally at the inguinal ligament and internal oblique and transversalis deep muscle fascia, where most compression typically occurs (TECH FIG 1C).
- After this release, retroperitoneal decompression is performed by retraction of the muscle and excision of the deep fascia sitting on the top of the nerve (TECH FIG 1D,E).
  - Great caution must be exercised dissecting in this area because of the proximity of the deep circumflex iliac artery that crosses the nerve in the retroperitoneum.

A
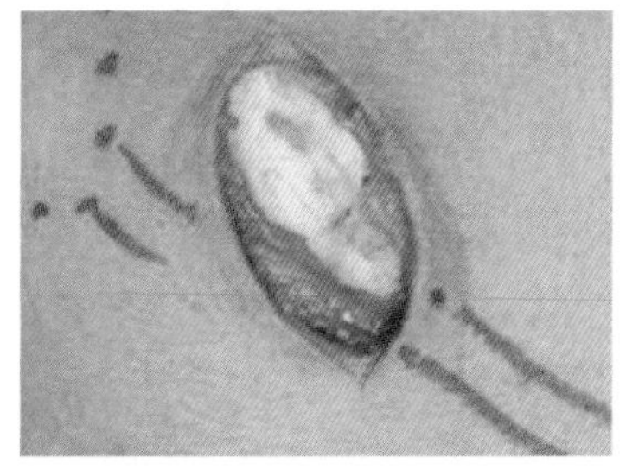
B
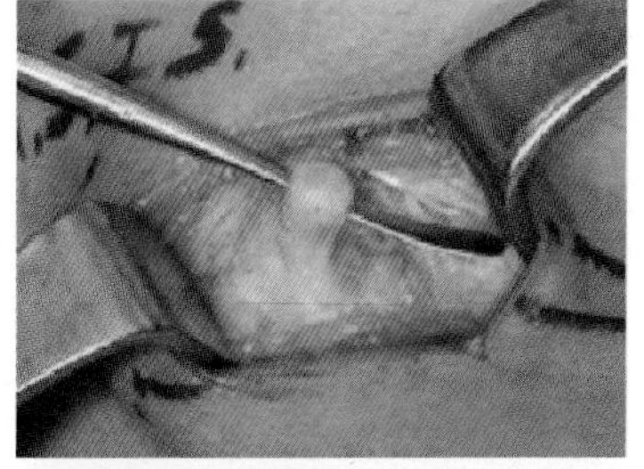
C
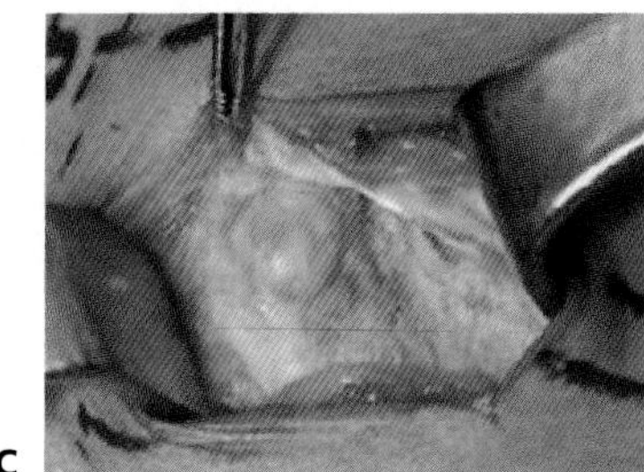
D
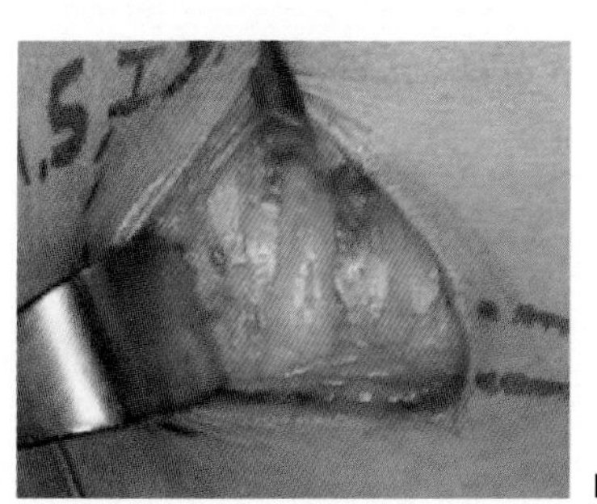
E
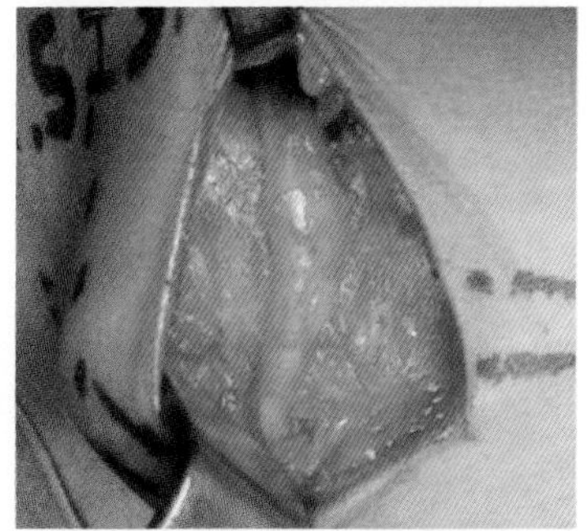

TECH FIG 1 • **A.** Exposure for dissection of the lateral femoral cutaneous nerve (LFCN). **B.** Identification of LFCN. **C.** Internal oblique muscle elevated off LFCN at compression site. **D,E.** LFCN proximally and distally decompressed. Note the cuff of internal oblique that has been removed around the LFCN proximally

TECHNIQUES

COMMON PERONEAL NERVE

- With the patient in a supine position, a thigh tourniquet is placed—as long as the patient does not have previous vascular bypasses in this area—and an incision is made 1 to 2 fingerbreadths below the fibular head (TECH FIG 2A).
- Dissection is carried to the deep fascia under loupe magnification, because proper identification of the nerve is critical (TECH FIG 2B).
  - The nerve can easily be mistaken for yellow fat, particularly if it runs abnormally superficially or was displaced with trauma.
- Proximal decompression is performed first by release of the gastrocnemius fascia and its attachment to hamstring and iliotibial fascial tissues (TECH FIG 2C).
- Distal dissection is performed by incising the peroneus longus fascia and retracting this muscle laterally.
  - A fascial band that causes both a kink in the nerve as well as compression against the fibula can then be visualized and addressed (TECH FIG 2D).
- Closure is then performed in anatomic layers, sparing the deep fascia, which is not closed, to avoid recreating the nerve compression.
- Great caution should be exercised in patients with a history of previous knee trauma or dislocation, because the anatomy of the nerve may be aberrant, which could lead to iatrogenic nerve injury during surgical approach and manipulation.

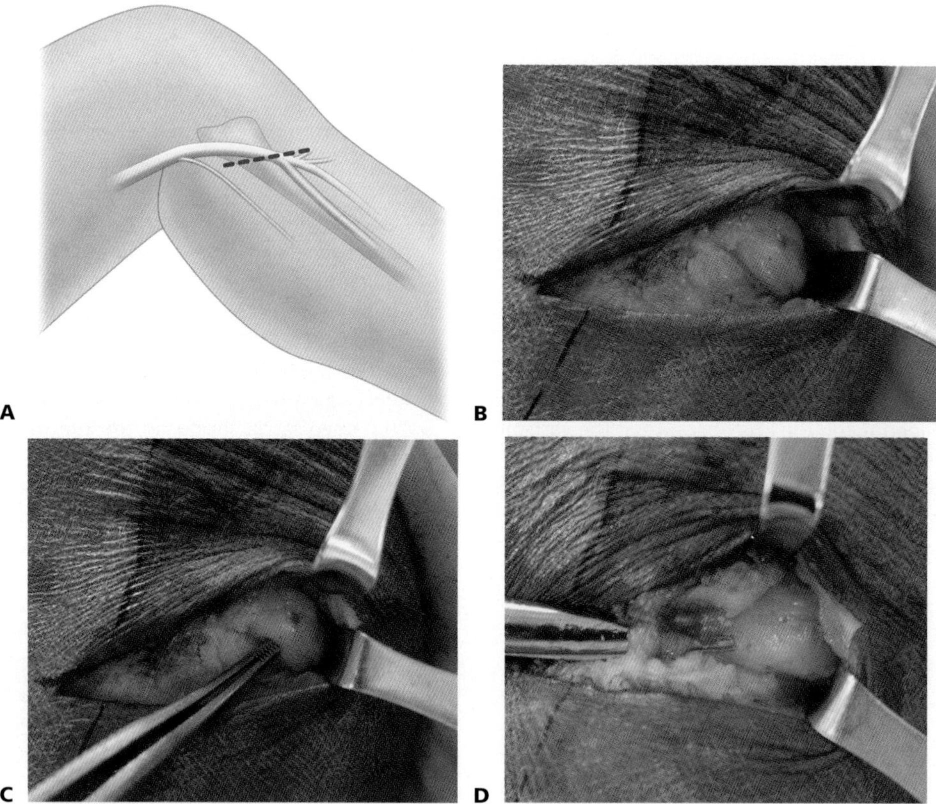

TECH FIG 2 • **A.** Schematic for skin incision to access the common peroneal nerve. **B.** Exposure of CPN through surgical incision. **C.** Identification of CPN. **D.** Identification of compressive band of peroneus longus muscle fascia over CPN.

PEARLS AND PITFALLS

Indications	▪ Complete history and physical examination, with particular focus on the neurologic examination ▪ Document any nerve function compromise: loss of function, paresthesias, positive Tinel's sign, or tenderness over nerves. ▪ Obtain electrodiagnostic confirmation of diagnosis if possible.
Lateral femoral cutaneous nerve	▪ Careful dissection with appropriate magnification and instruments ▪ Consider anatomic variations of the nerve in relation to the ASIS and the inguinal ligament. ▪ Careful retroperitoneal decompression because of the proximity of the deep circumflex iliac artery
Common peroneal nerve	▪ Careful initial dissection, because nerve can easily be mistaken for fat ▪ Recognize that the nerve can be more superficial than expected: with a history of trauma, it tends to be more anterior and superior. ▪ Careful dissection with appropriate magnification and instruments
Postoperative management	▪ If a nerve decompression was performed, early mobilization should be encouraged. ▪ If nerve reconstruction was performed, limited ambulation or immobilization is advised.

POSTOPERATIVE CARE

- Wound healing concepts should be applied to the peripheral nerve.
- During the first week after surgery, the nerve will lie in an environment that is predominantly inflammatory. Collagen is not deposited into the wound until the second week, and cross-linking of the collagen does not occur until after the third week.
- If the nerve is kept immobile during the second and third postoperative weeks, it will become adherent to the surrounding tissues.
  - Conversely, for the nerve to be loose and able to slide through its surrounding tissues, it is necessary to allow the nerve to move with respect to its bed following the first week of splinting.
- The fact that a nerve will not adhere to a bed of cut muscle and fibrous tissue if it is allowed to glide early in the postoperative period was demonstrated for the ulnar nerve at the elbow in a baboon model.[7]
  - Therefore, in operation on the peripheral nerve, it is essential that the postoperative regimen include some movement of the joints during the first week and splinting be reserved mainly for cases involving nerve grafting.

REFERENCES

1. Lundborg G, Rydevik B. Effects of stretching the tibial nerve of the rabbit: a preliminary study of the intraneural circulation and the barrier function of the perineurium. J Bone Joint Surg Br 1973;55B:390–401.
2. Mackinnon SE, Dellon AL. Physical examination. In: Surgery of the Peripheral Nerve. New York: Thieme, 1988.
3. Maki Y, Firrell JC, Breidenbach WC. Blood flow in mobilized nerves: results in a rabbit sciatic nerve model. Plast Reconstr Surg 1997;100:627–633.
4. Dellon AL. Physical examination in nerve compression. In: Gelberman R, ed. Operative Management of Peripheral Nerve Injury. Philadelphia: JB Lippincott, 1991.
5. Vernadakis AJ, Koch H, Mackinnon SE. Management of neuromas. Clin Plast Surg 2003;30:247–268.
6. Ducic I, Taylor NS, Dellon AL. Decompression of the lateral femoral cutaneous nerve in the treatment of meralgia paresthetica. J Reconstr Microsurg 2006;22:113–117.
7. Dellon AL, Mackinnon SE, Hudson AR, et al. Effect of submuscular versus intramuscular placement of ulnar nerve: experimental model in the primate. J Hand Surg Br 1986;11B:117–119.

Exam Table for Sports Medicine

Examination	Technique	Illustration	Grading & Significance
The Shoulder			
Range of motion (ROM)	The examiner observes active and passive ROM for forward elevation (20 to 30 degrees in sagittal plane), external rotation and internal rotation (both at side and 90 degrees of abduction).	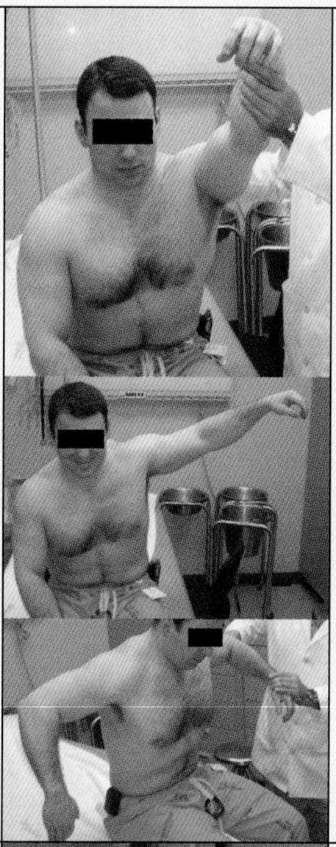	Average normal ROM: forward flexion 180 degrees, abduction 180 degrees, adduction 50 degrees, internal rotation at the side 80 degrees, external rotation at the side 90 degrees. Loss of ROM may indicate adhesive capsulitis, rotator cuff pathology (tendinitis or rotator cuff tear), degenerative changes. ROM is compared to contralateral side. Patients with impingement may have limited internal rotation from posterior capsular tightness. Active motion is typically more painful than passive motion, especially in descending phase of elevation.
Jobes sign ("empty can" test)	Arm is placed in 90 degrees of elevation in the scapular plane with the hand in the thumbs-down position. Manual resistance is provided by the examiner to elevation and weakness or pain is recorded.	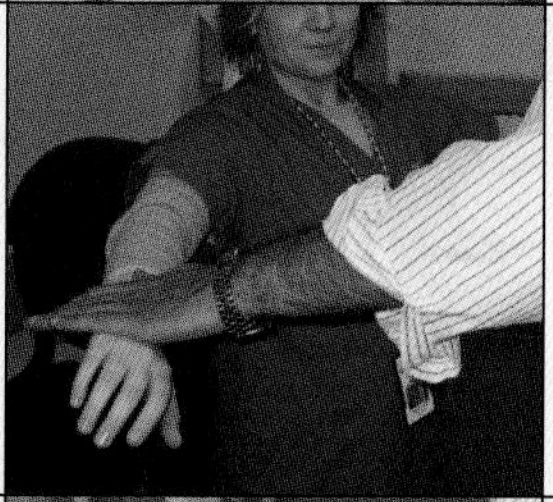	Weakness or pain represents dysfunction of the supraspinatus tendon.
Resisted external rotation in adduction	Arm is placed in full adduction, elbows are bent at 90 degrees, and the shoulder is internally rotated 20 to 30 degrees. Manual resistance is provided by the examiner to external rotation, and weakness is recorded.	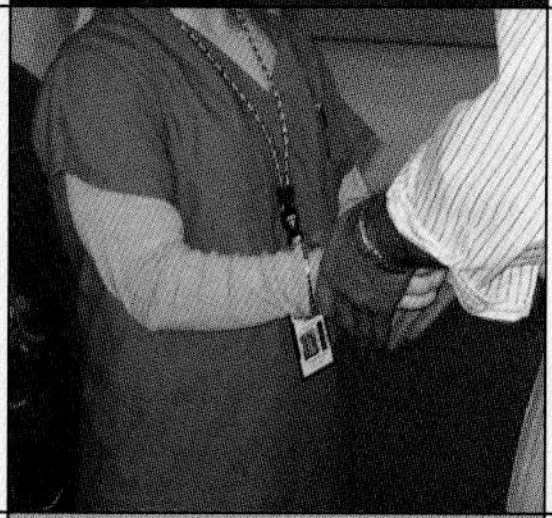	Weakness represents dysfunction or tearing of the infraspinatus tendon.
Apprehension test	With the patient supine, the arm is passively abducted to 90 degrees and externally rotated. The examiner can then push the proximal humerus posteriorly (relocation).	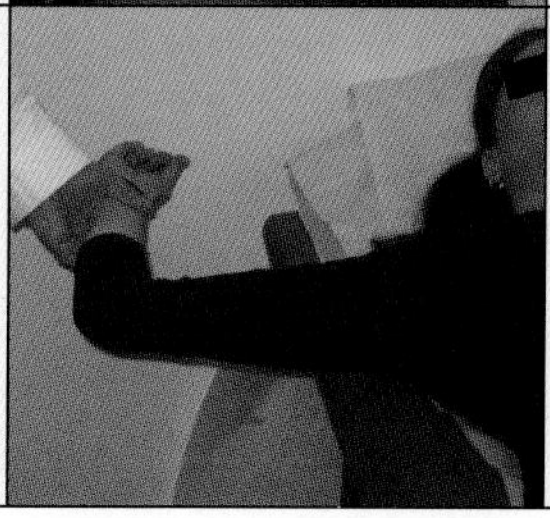	Patients with anterior instability will have apprehension in this position. This will resolve with posterior force on the proximal humerus.

(continued)

Examination	Technique	Illustration	Grading & Significance
Kim test	With the patient seated, the arm is placed in 90 degrees of abduction and the elbow and hand are supported by the examiner. An axial and upward elevating force of 45 degrees is applied to the distal arm while an inferior and posterior force is applied to the proximal arm.	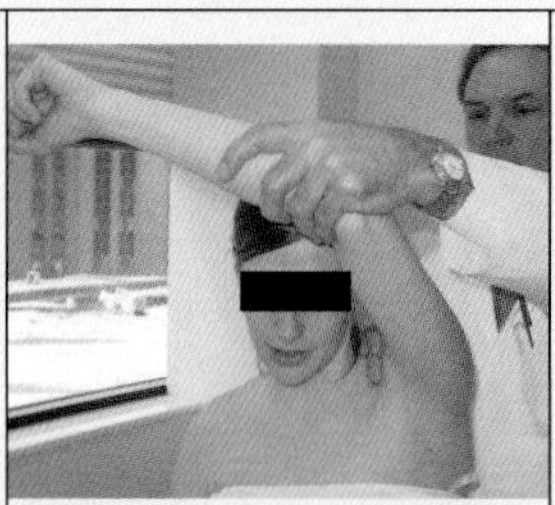	A sudden onset of posterior shoulder pain is considered a positive test result. A positive Kim test is suggestive of a posterior inferior labral tear or subluxation.
Neer impingement sign	Passive elevation of the arm while stabilizing the scapula	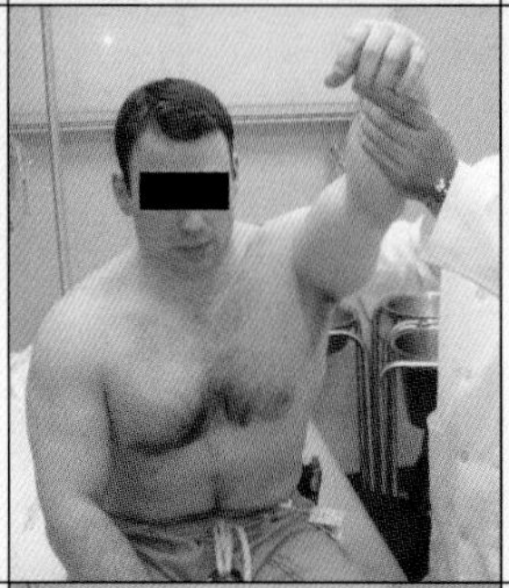	Presence or absence of pain or facial grimace. This maneuver compresses the critical area of the supraspinatus tendon against the anterior inferior acromion, reproducing impingement pain. The pain will resolve following subacromial lidocaine injection.
Hawkins sign	The examiner forward flexes the shoulder to 90 degrees and then passively internally rotates the shoulder.	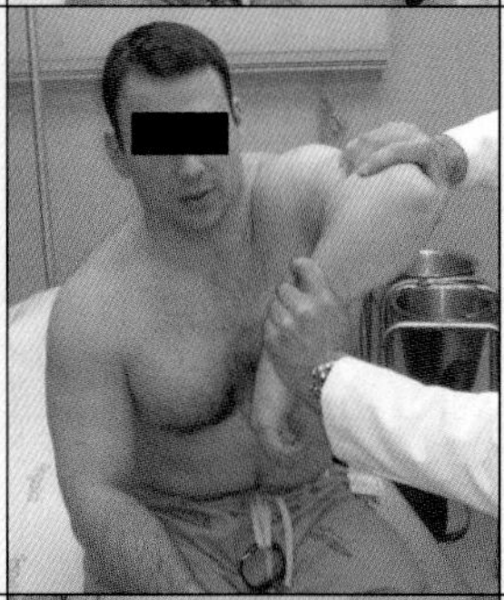	Presence or absence of pain. This maneuver compresses the supraspinatus tendon against the coracoacromial ligament, reproducing the pain of impingement. High sensitivity but low specificity.
Painful abduction arc	The patient is asked to abduct the arm in the coronal plane.	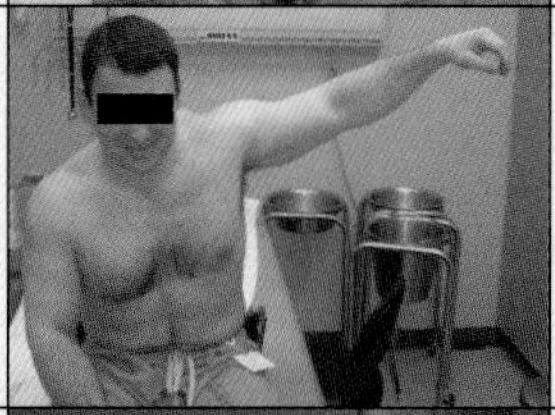	Abduction is compared to the contralateral side. Pain from 60 to 120 degrees (maximally at 90) suggests impingement. Patients may externally rotate at 90 degrees to clear the greater tuberosity from the acromion and increase motion.
Yergason test	Resistance of attempted forearm supination with the elbow flexed to 90 degrees and the forearm in a pronated position	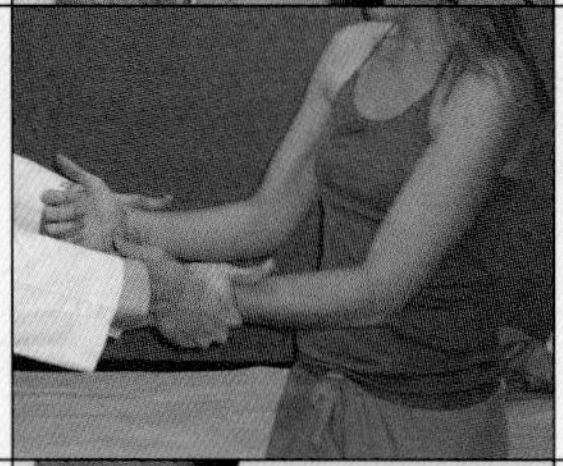	Positive or negative. A positive test is defined as one in which the patient experiences shoulder pain in the bicipital groove with this maneuver. Suggestive of biceps tendonopathy in appropriate clinical context.
Lift-off test	Arm is brought into maximal passive internal rotation behind the back with the hand off the spine by the examiner; the examiner releases the hand in this position.	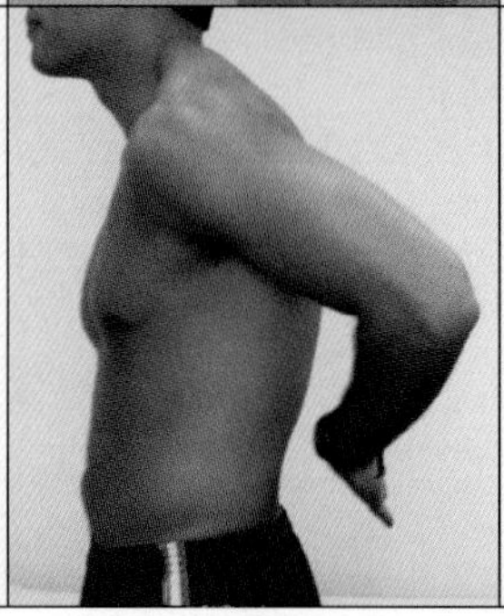	Ability to maintain active maximal internal rotation with hand off the lumbar spine without extending the elbow. Inability indicates impaired subscapularis function.

Examination	Technique	Illustration	Grading & Significance
Belly-press test	Hand is placed on abdomen; patient presses abdomen with flat hand and attempts to keep arm in maximum internal rotation and the elbow anterior to the mid-sagittal plane of the trunk.		Ability to maintain maximum internal rotation without the elbow dropping posterior to the midsagittal plane of the trunk. Inability indicates impaired subscapularis function.
Napoleon test (modified belly press)	The patient presses his or her hand against the belly at the umbilicus. The wrist should be straight and the elbow in front of the body. This creates the classic pose seen in pictures of Napoleon.		Negative test: the patient is able to "strike the pose." Intermediate test: wrist flexed 30 to 60 degrees. Positive test: wrist flexed 90 degrees and elbow posteriorly positioned. Negative test: less than 50% of the subscapularis tendon is torn. Intermediate test: more than 50% of the subscapularis tendon is torn. Positive test: the entire subscapularis tendon is torn. With a significant subscapularis tendon tear the patient flexes the wrist, the elbow drops backward, and the posterior deltoid acts to pull the hand against the belly.
Bear hug test	The patient places the hand of the affected extremity on the opposite shoulder. The elbow is elevated in a forward position and the wrist and fingers are straight and collinear. The physician attempts to pull the hand off the patient's shoulder while the patient resists.		Negative test: the physician is unable to pull the patient's hand off the shoulder. Positive test: the physician is able to pull the patient's hand off the shoulder. The bear hug test is the most sensitive test for an upper subscapularis injury (eg, a partial tear involving the superior aspect of the subscapularis tendon).
External rotation lag sign	Arm is positioned in full adduction with the elbow at 90 degrees of flexion and the shoulder in maximal external rotation by the examiner. Inability of the patient to maintain shoulder in an externally rotated position is recorded.	45°	Inability to maintain the shoulder in a fully externally rotated position indicates is positive for significant dysfunction or tearing of the infraspinatus muscle.
Hornblower sign	Arm is positioned in 90 degrees of abduction with the elbow flexed to 90 degrees and the shoulder in neutral rotation. External rotation of the shoulder to a position of full abduction–external rotation is performed and weakness or inability to achieve full external rotation is noted.	Examiner resistance Patient force	Ability to fully externally rotate in an abducted position indicates good teres minor function. Weakness or inability to achieve full external rotation in abducted position indicates teres minor dysfunction or tearing.

(continued)

Examination	Technique	Illustration	Grading & Significance
ROM	The examiner observes active and passive ROM (flexion–extension of the elbow, rotation of the forearm) and compares it to the uninjured side. Palpable and auditory crepitus should be noted.	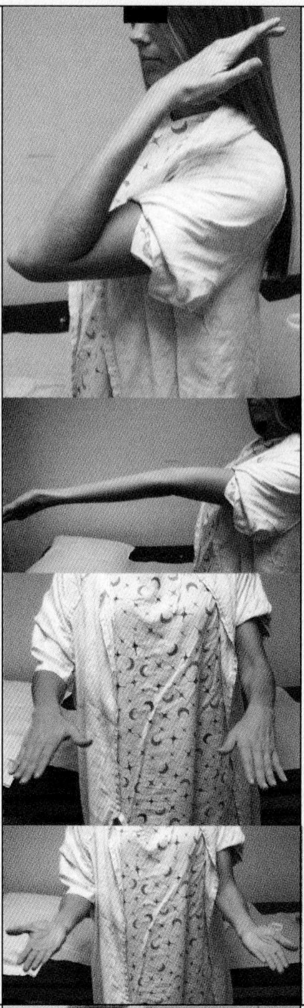	Normal ROM is 0 to 150 degrees flexion–extension, 80 degrees pronation–supination; functional ROM is 30 to 130 degrees flexion–extension, 50 degrees pronation–supination. Locking of the elbow could represent loose bodies. Stiffness may indicate intrinsic capsular contracture.
Effusion	The examiner palpates the posterolateral gutter of the elbow and ballotes the soft tissue.	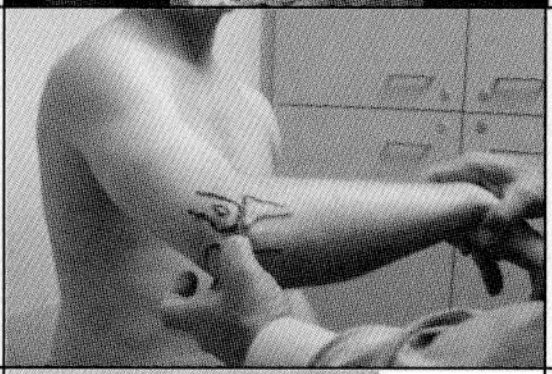	Most clinicians simply grade as none, mild, moderate, large. Normally, fluid is not present. Effusion indicates intra-articular irritation and may be consistent with a loose or unstable osteochondritis dissecans lesion or loose body.
Capitellum tenderness	Examiner's thumb pushes against the posterior capitellum while taking the elbow through a range of motion of flexion to extension.	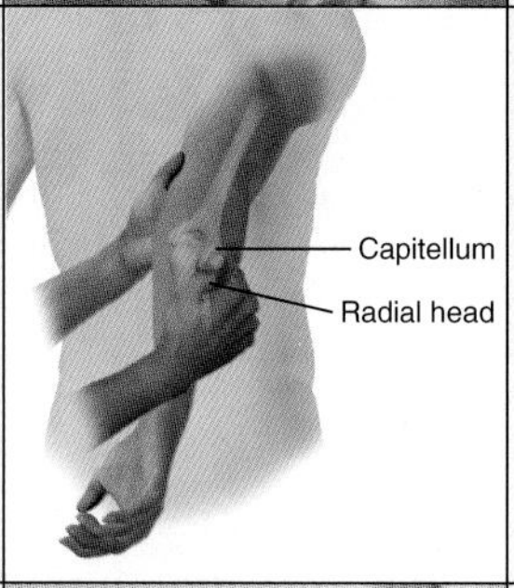 Capitellum Radial head	Most clinicians just grade this as none, mild, moderate, or significant pain. Tenderness may be present with osteochondritis dissecans.
Active radiocapitellar compression test	Forearm pronation and supination with the elbow in full extension is performed.	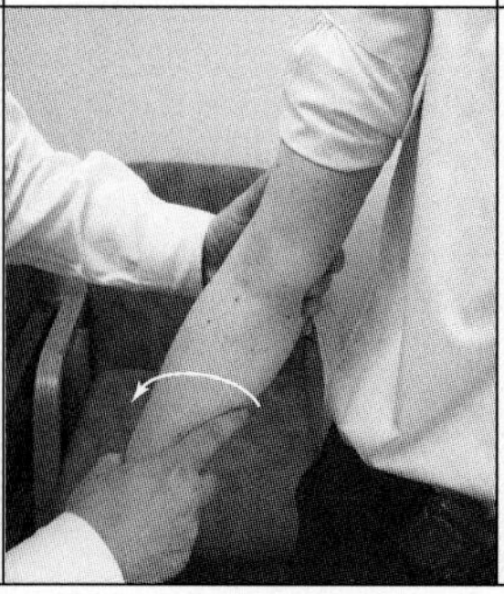	Most clinicians just grade this as none, mild, moderate, or significant pain. This test loads the radiocapitellar joint in pronation. Pain on pronation that is reduced in supination may be present in osteochondritis dissecans.

Examination	Technique	Illustration	Grading & Significance
Milking maneuver	With forearm fully supinated, elbow is placed in greater than 90 degrees of flexion. The examiner pulls on the patient's thumb.	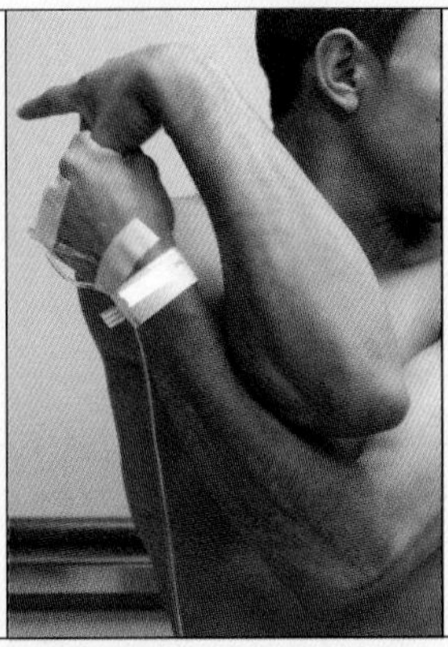	Maneuver eliciting pain, apprehension, or instability is indicative of ulnar collateral ligament (UCL) insufficiency. Posterior bundle of anterior band of UCL.
The Knee			
ROM	The examiner observes passive and active ROM—flexion–extension; pronation–supination.	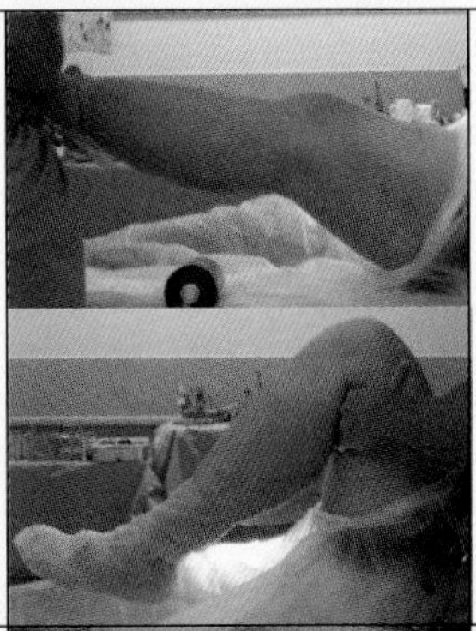	Normal ROM is 0 to 145 degrees and 60 degrees of pronation and supination. Loss of extension (flexion contracture) is frequently present. Loss of pronation is less common. May be due to capsular irritation, loose bodies, or displaced chondral flap.
Lachman test	With the knee flexed 30 degrees, the examiner stabilizes the thigh with the hand that is closest to the head and uses the other hand to passively displace the proximal tibia anteriorly.	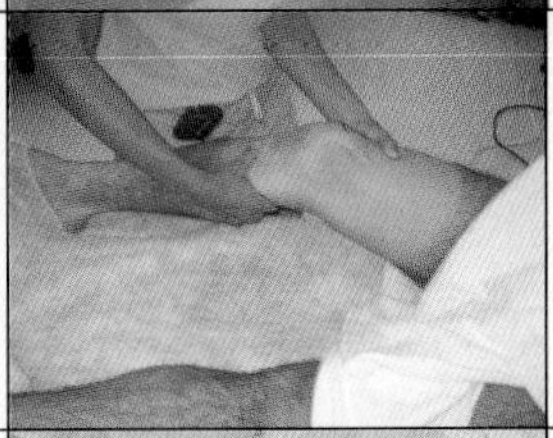	Anterior displacement more than the normal side indicates an anterior crucial ligament injury.
Posterior drawer test	With knee in 70 to 90 degrees of flexion, a posterior-directed force is applied to the proximal tibia.	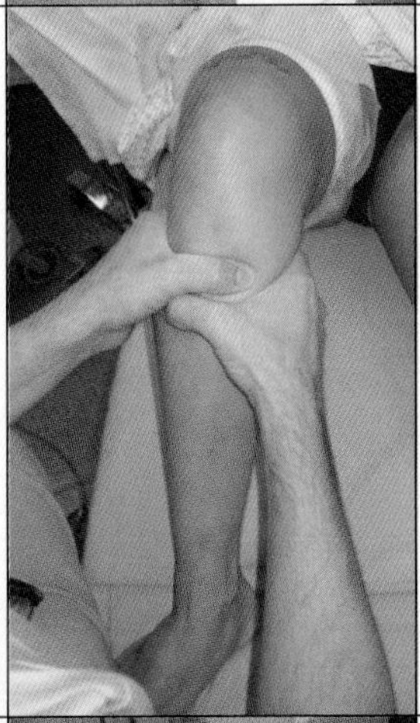	0 = no abnormal translation; 1 = 1 to 5 mm; 2 = 6 to 10 mm (but medial tibial plateau [MTP] not beyond medial femoral condyle [MFC]); 3 = >10 mm, or translation of MTP beyond MFC. When compared to contralateral knee, may be indicative of posterior cruciate ligament-deficient knee.
Varus and valgus laxity	A valgus and varus force is applied to the knee in both 30 degrees of flexion and full extension.	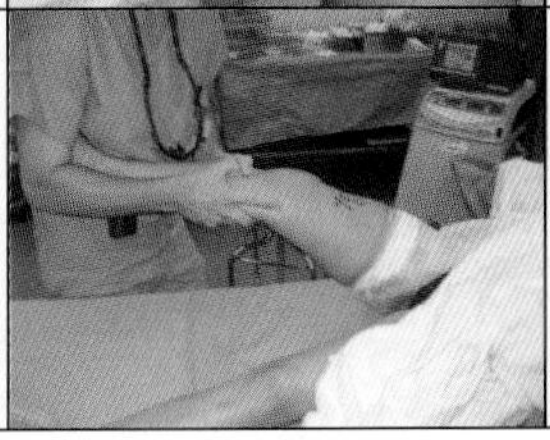	Classically, displacement of <5 mm is considered a grade I injury, 5 to 10 mm a grade II injury, and >10 mm a grade III injury. Opening in full extension implies a combined injury to the collateral ligament and at least one cruciate ligament.

(continued)

Examination	Technique	Illustration	Grading & Significance
Dial test	With the patient in prone position, the tibia is externally rotated at 30 and 90 degrees. The foot-to-thigh angle is compared between the two legs.	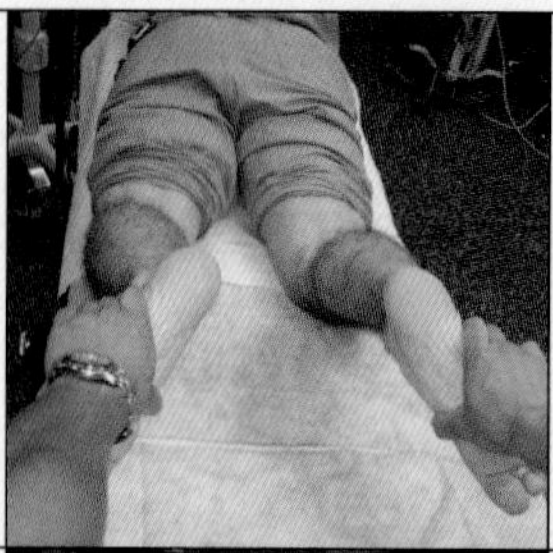	Difference of more than 10 degrees at 30 degrees is consistent with injury to posterolateral corner (PLC). Difference of more than 10 degrees at 90 degrees is consistent with injury to PLC and posterior cruciate ligament.
Varus recurvatum test	With the patient supine, the examiner lifts both feet by the big toes and watches for varus angulation, hyperextension, and external rotation of the tibia.	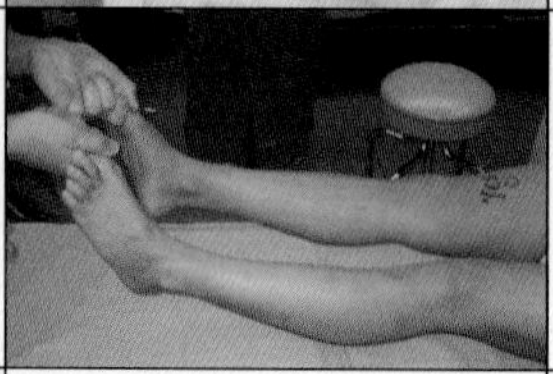	Suggestive of posterolateral rotatory instability of the knee.
McMurry test	With the patient supine and the knee acutely and forcibly flexed, the examiner can check the medial meniscus by palpating the posteromedial margin of the joint with one hand while grasping the foot with the other hand. Keeping the knee completely flexed, the leg is externally rotated as far as possible and then the knee is slowly extended. As the femur passes over a tear in the meniscus, a click may be heard or felt. The lateral meniscus is checked by palpating the posterolateral margin of the joint, internally rotating the leg as far as possible, and slowly extending the knee while listening and feeling for a click. With the knee maximally flexed, it is extended to 90 degrees while applying internal rotation and valgus force to the foot and ankle. Repeat with external rotation and varus force.	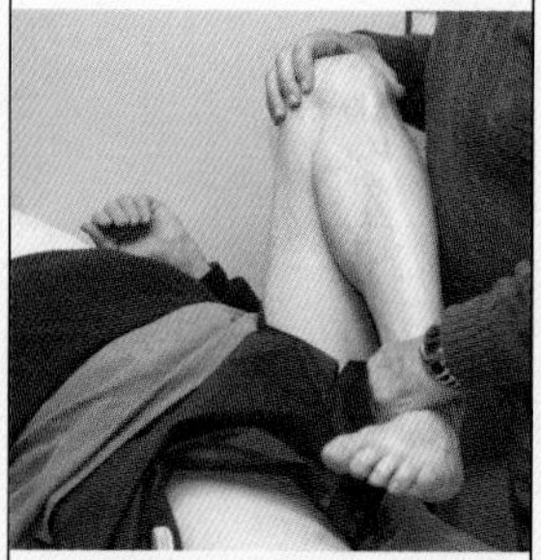	A click produced by the McMurray test usually is caused by a posterior peripheral tear of the meniscus and occurs between complete flexion of the knee and 90 degrees. Popping, which occurs with greater degrees of extension when definitely localized to the joint line, suggests a tear of the middle and anterior portions of the meniscus. Thus, the position of the knee when the click occurs may help locate the lesion. A positive McMurray click localized to the joint line is additional evidence that the meniscus is torn; a negative McMurray test does not rule out a tear. A palpable or audible pop in combination with pain is considered positive. Results are variable, but a positive McMurray test is indicative of a meniscus lesion and not a chondral lesion.
Apley grind test	With the patient prone, the knee is flexed to 90 degrees and the anterior thigh is fixed against the examining table. The foot and leg are then pulled upward to distract the joint and rotated to place rotational strain on the ligaments. Next, with the knee in the same position, the foot and leg are pressed downward and rotated as the joint is slowly flexed and extended.	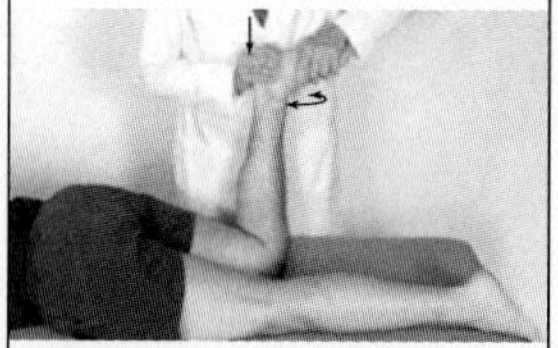	When the ligaments have been torn, pulling the leg upward and rotating it usually are painful. When the foot and leg are pressed downward and rotated, popping and pain localized to the joint line usually indicate a torn meniscus.

Examination	Technique	Illustration	Grading & Significance
The Hip			
ROM	The hip is flexed to its maximum extent and the examiner records the degrees of flexion. The hip is then flexed to 90 degrees and passively internally and externally rotated.	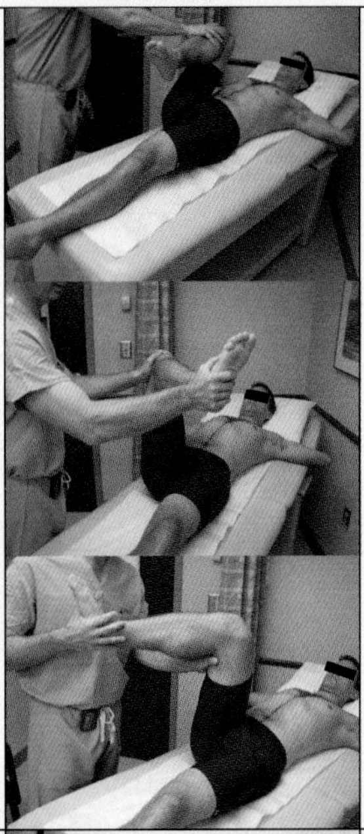	Loss of motion is often associated with arthritis.
Abduction external rotation test	The hip is passively forced into maximal abduction with external rotation.	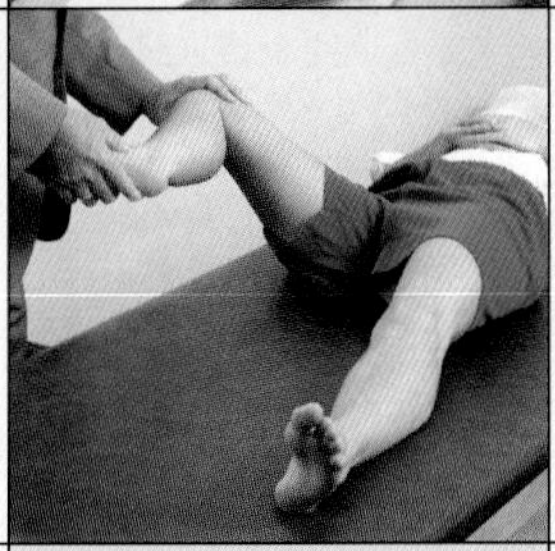	May create symptoms associated with posterior joint pathology by compression, or anterior pathology by anterior translation of the femoral head.
C sign	Patient cups hand above greater trochanter, gripping fingers into groin.	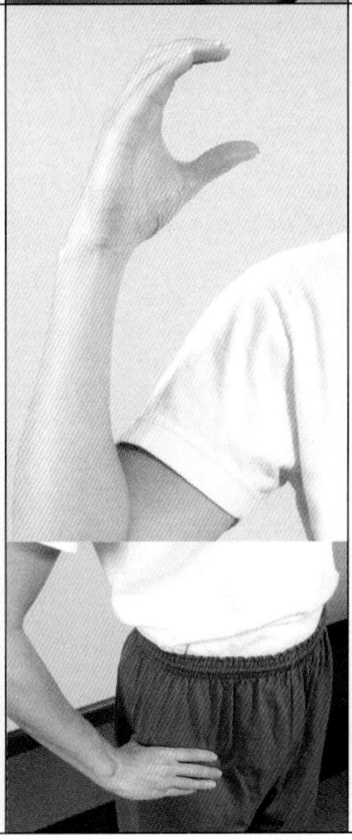	Common observation with patients describing interior hip pain.

(continued)

Examination	Technique	Illustration	Grading & Significance
Log roll test	With the patient supine, the affected leg is simply rolled back and forth.	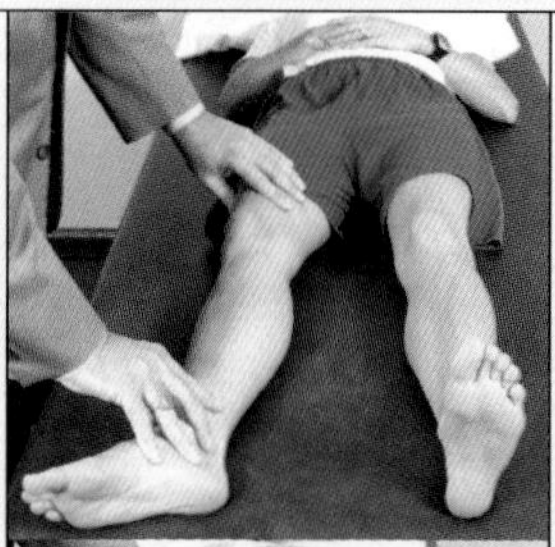 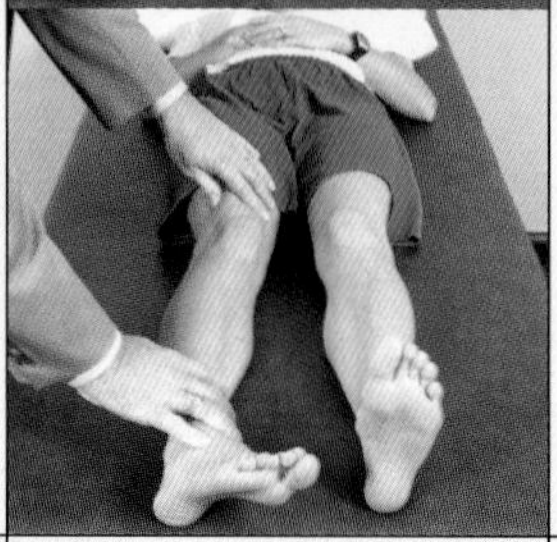	Most specific test for hip joint pathology since femoral head is being rotated in relation to the acetabulum and capsule without stressing any of the extra-articular structures.
Patrick test (Faber test)	Patient is supine on examination table and placed such that one half of the buttock is off the table while the ipsilateral leg is placed in a figure 4 position on the other (extended) knee. The pelvis is stabilized with one of the examiner's hands and a downward force is applied to the flexed knee with the examiner's other hand.	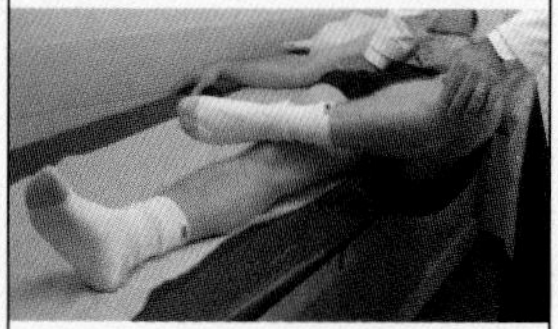	Pain may be felt with the downward stress on the flexed knee. Pain in the posterior pelvis may be considered positive for the pain coming from the sacroiliac (SI) joint. Indicative of SI abnormalities or iliopsoas spasm.
Ober test	Patient is placed in lateral decubitus position, with the down hip and knee flexed for stability. The examiner flexes the other hip to 90 degrees and then abducts the hip fully and extends the hip past neutral with the knee in 90 degrees of flexion. The hip and knee are allowed to adduct while the hip is held in neutral rotation.	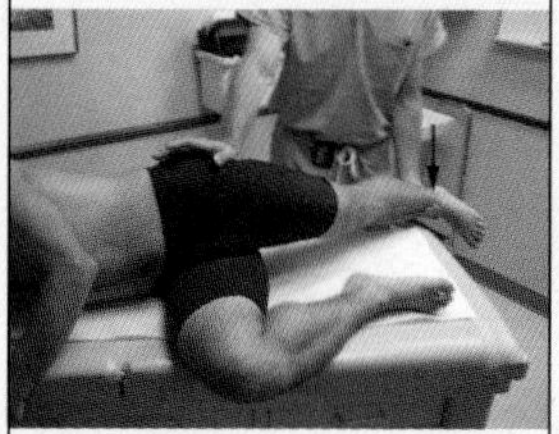	The test is positive when the upper knee remains in the abducted position after the hip is passively extended and abducted and then adducted with the knee flexed. Used to evaluate iliotibial band tightness. If, when the hip and knee are allowed to adduct while the hip is held in neutral rotation, the knee adducts past midline, the hip abductors are not tight; if the knee does not reach to midline, then the hip abductors are tight.
Impingement test	The hip is passively forced into maximal flexion, adduction, and internal rotation.	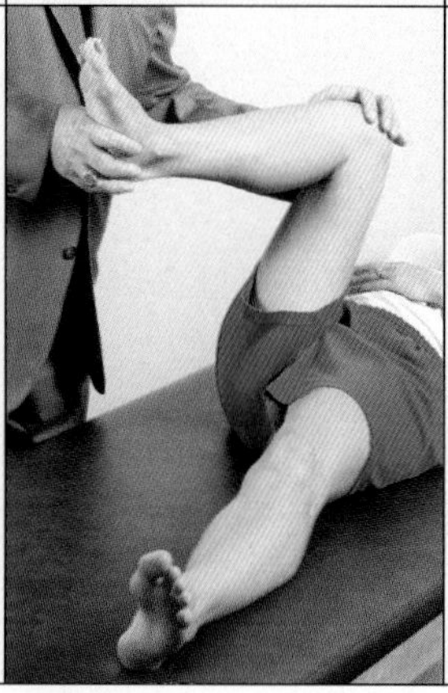	A more sensitive test for detecting hip joint irritability. This is associated with impingement findings but is positive with most sources of hip pathology.

Examination	Technique	Illustration	Grading & Significance
Anterior compression of the iliopsoas tendon	Firm digital pressure over the anterior hip capsule may block the snapping.	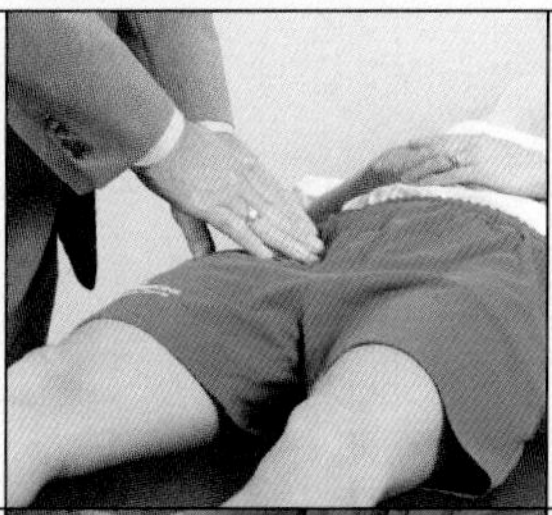	Applying pressure to block the snapping of the tendon substantiates the diagnosis. However, often this maneuver is uncomfortable and not well tolerated by the patient.
Squeeze test	Supine subject actively attempts adduction by squeezing legs against resistance provided by examiner.	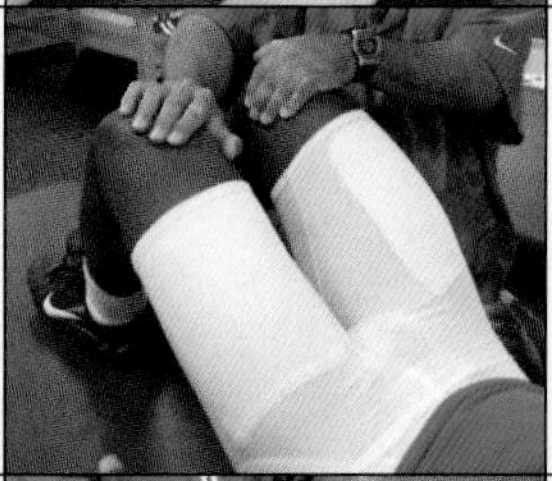	The presence or absence of pain is noted. Strength is graded as mild (minimal loss of strength); moderate (clear loss of strength); or severe (complete loss of strength). Pain with or without a strength deficit implies adductor-related groin pain.
Hamstring strength	Patient lies prone. Patient attempts knee flexion against resistance.	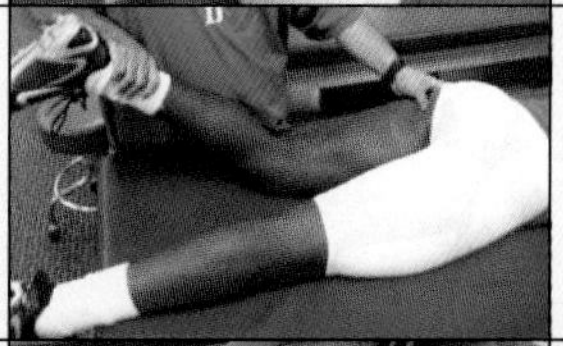	Mild: minimal loss of strength; moderate: clear loss of strength; severe: complete loss of strength. Severe injury implies proximal avulsion.
Passive hamstring stretch	Patient performs a hurdler's stretch.	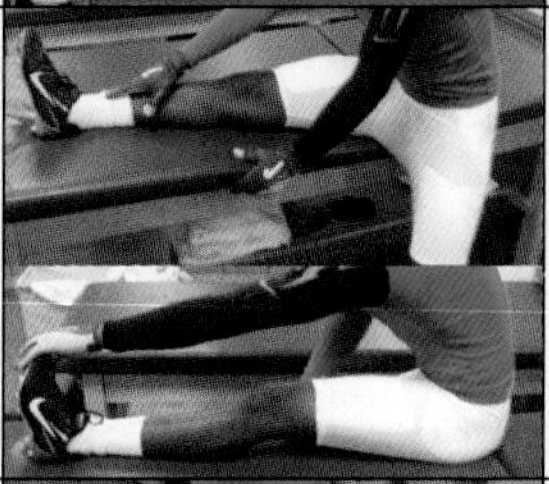	Apparent hamstring flexibility is compared to the uninjured side. An obvious increase in apparent hamstring flexibility of injured extremity implies proximal avulsion.
Passive adductors stretch	The subject lies supine. The examiner either abducts the leg or places the leg in a figure 4 position.	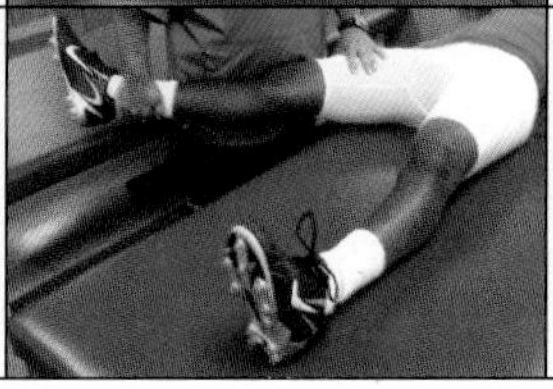	The presence or absence of pain is noted. Pain localized to the adductor implies adductor-related groin pain.

INDEX

Page numbers followed by *f* and *t* indicated figures and tables, respectively.

B

C

T